Laboratory Tests and Diagnostic Procedures

Sixth Edition

EDITED AND AUTHORED BY

Cynthia C. Chernecky, PhD, RN, CNS, AOCN, FAAN
Professor
Department of Physiological and Technological Nursing
College of Nursing
Georgia Regents University Augusta
Augusta, Georgia

Barbara J. Berger, MSN, RN, CNS
Director of Clinical Management
SummaCare, Inc.
Akron, Ohio

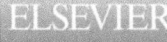

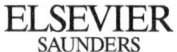

3251 Riverport Lane
St. Louis, Missouri 63043

Notices

Knowledge and best practice in this field are constantly changing. As new research and experience broaden our understanding, changes in research methods, professional practices, or medical treatment may become necessary.

Practitioners and researchers must always rely on their own experience and knowledge in evaluating and using any information, methods, compounds, or experiments described herein. In using such information or methods they should be mindful of their own safety and the safety of others, including parties for whom they have a professional responsibility.

With respect to any drug or pharmaceutical products identified, readers are advised to check the most current information provided (i) on procedures featured or (ii) by the manufacturer of each product to be administered, to verify the recommended dose or formula, the method and duration of administration, and contraindications. It is the responsibility of practitioners, relying on their own experience and knowledge of their patients, to make diagnoses, to determine dosages and the best treatment for each individual patient, and to take all appropriate safety precautions.

To the fullest extent of the law, neither the Publisher nor the authors, contributors, or editors, assume any liability for any injury and/or damage to persons or property as a matter of products liability, negligence or otherwise, or from any use or operation of any methods, products, instructions, or ideas contained in the material herein.

Library of Congress Cataloging-in-Publication Data

Laboratory tests and diagnostic procedures / edited by Cynthia C. Chernecky, Barbara J. Berger. – 6th ed.
   p. ; cm.
Includes bibliographical references and index.
ISBN 978-1-4557-0694-5 (pbk. : alk. paper)
I. Chernecky, Cynthia C.   II. Berger, Barbara J.
[DNLM: 1. Clinical Laboratory Techniques–Handbooks. QY 39]
616.07'5–dc23

                                                                          2012041501

Content Strategist: Tamara Myers   *Project Manager:* Bridget Healy
Publishing Services Manager: Deborah Vogel   *Design Direction:* Maggie Reid

Printed in the United States of America

Last digit is the print number: 9   8   7   6   5

REVIEWERS

Reviewers

JoAnn Acierno, MSN, RN
Carol A. Biscardi, PA-C, PhD
Teresa Brenan Turi, MSN, RN, CNM
Yvette P. Conley, PhD
Joseph R. Hawkins
Sheryl Hutchinson, PhD, MSN, RN, ANP-C
Stephen D. Krau, PhD, RN, CNE, CT
Dr. Geralyn Lopez-de-Victoria

Carla R. Lynch, MS, RN
Dana Sue Parker, DNP, RN, APN
Mary Lou Robinson, PhD, RN
Jennifer Sweat, BSN Student, (Georgia Health Sciences University)
Bonnie L. Welniak, RN
Alan H. Wu, PhD, DABCC

The Editors Acknowledge the Contributors to the Third, Fourth, and Fifth Editions

Christine Alichnie, PhD, RN
John T. Benjamin, MD
Barbara J. Berger, MSN, RN, CNS
Amy Bieda, MSN, RN, CNP
Martha J. Bradshaw, PhD, RN
Wendy Gram Brick, MD
Russell E. Burgess, MD
Patricia A. Catalano, MSN, RN, CCRN
Cynthia C. Chernecky, PhD, RN, CNS, AOCN, FAAN
Robyn DeGennaro, RN, CCRN
Michelle Ficca, PhD, RN
Michael E. Fincher, MD
Mark S. Green, MS, PA-C
Annette Gunderman, PhD, RN
Sharon Haymaker, PhD, RN
Steve S. Lee, BSN, RN

Ronald W. Lewis, MD
Kathryn S. McLeod, MD
Shelli McLeod, BSN, RN-C, CCE
Kenneth P. Miller, PhD, RN, CFNP, FAAN
Marguerite J. Murphy, RN, DNP
David Nicolaou, MD, MS, FACEP
Carl E. Rosenberg, MD, MBA
William H. Salazar, MD
Robert R. Schade, MD
Kevin Navin Sheth, MD
Judith Banks Stallings, BS, PA-C
Benjamin H. Taylor, Jr., MPAS, PA-C
Saundra L. Turner, EdD, RN-CS, FNP
Rachel Vaneck, MSN, RN, CNP
Eric Walsh, MD
Kristy Woods, MD
Timothy L. Wren, RN, DNP

PREFACE

We are pleased to announce the arrival of the sixth edition of *Laboratory Tests and Diagnostic Procedures*. The text is completely alphabetical, fully cross-referenced, and indexed. There is no need to know which body system is tested or whether the test uses blood or urine or is diagnostic to locate the test. The best advantage, we believe, is that all the information is complete and contained within one cover. There is no need to waste time referring to multiple texts or flipping between sections to obtain test-specific information. Valuable features include designation of the most common tests used for diseases, conditions, or symptoms (Part One), norms throughout all age-groups, drug and herbal and natural-remedy effects on test results, inclusion of medicolegal implications, panic levels and symptoms and emergency treatment for panic levels, dialysis implications for timing of blood draws or treating high levels, client and family teaching, risks of and contraindications for procedures, and whether informed consent is required or recommended. The content is concise enough for novices and complete enough for seasoned practitioners. It has significant value for both students and practitioners of allied health, medicine, and nursing and is the kind of reference to use throughout one's career. It is appropriate for the many specialties within the professions, and it includes information from across the life span.

The text is organized into two parts. Part One is designed to help the practitioner confirm a suspected diagnosis or condition. The most common tests or procedures used for the suspected diagnosis are indicated. Items with a • symbol next to them are significant tests for the listed condition. Part Two lists the tests and diagnostic procedures in alphabetical order with normal values; panic-level symptoms and treatment, including whether the substance is dialyzable; usage or conditions in which the values may be abnormal; and a concise description of the test and its significance. This edition also includes expanded information on genetic tests, consent requirements, risks and contraindications, client and family teaching, and the details of the test and client care, as well as integration of the most current scientific literature. Other features include the use of shading in Part Two for ease of use, reduction of blood sample volumes to the minimum amount required (to help avoid iatrogenic anemia), information on whether blood samples can be drawn during hemodialysis, expansion of age-specific norms, and improved quality-assurance information on factors that interfere with results. Finally, a comprehensive, international, up-to-date bibliography of specific resources is included to direct practitioners to additional information.

Other features of this edition include the newest tests in many fields. Cross-referencing of the test and procedure names includes associated acronyms to expedite the location of each test or procedure. The index now includes a synthesis of diseases, tests, and procedures for the entire book in one place. The format of this text is the product of years of clinical practice and expertise. It has been written by practitioners for practitioners. The invaluable contributions of a large number of clinical experts and their contacts who freely shared the most up-to-date information about the tests, procedures, and medical conditions are a most valued feature.

The purpose of this text is to provide complete information to guide practitioners or students in the clinical care of patients. Applicability of information in a text of this type is relative. Although we have used reliable and current sources in the compilation of the book, variations in laboratory techniques and client conditions must be considered for interpretation. The normal and panic levels listed are not meant to be used as rigid separations of normal and abnormal but rather as guidelines for consideration within the context of individual client conditions and laboratory specifications.

We have provided information regarding procedures that may require separate consent forms, or those beyond the general institutional consent form. Certainly there is much variation among institutions regarding whether a consent form is necessary. At the minimum, oral consent is generally documented. We have provided what is general practice according to the literature and the experience of our expert contributors across the country. However, we caution that institutional protocols vary and should, of course, be consulted and followed. Regardless of whether formal consent is obtained, it is the responsibility of all health care professionals to educate clients undergoing any test or procedure. Teaching about the test or procedure must be tailored to the client's and the client's family's condition, language, comprehension, anxiety level, clinical goals, and other specific needs.

Most drugs in this text are listed by their generic names. This includes specific tests to determine drug levels in either blood or urine and includes within these tests names of drugs that may interfere with the test results. Generic names have been used to save valuable printed space and to avoid confusion attributable to multiple trade names. We must stress that, in judging possible drug interferences, the clinical evaluation of the client should remain primary in the process of interpreting test values. Clearly it is impractical to discontinue all medications to get a "pure value." If, however, a drug is known to cause severe interferences with the test results, it is clearly stated, and the drug should be discontinued when possible.

With concern about the transmission of bloodborne pathogens and in view of the content of this text, it is imperative to address the safe handling of specimens. In 1994 (revised 1996), the Centers for Disease Control and Prevention (CDC) published "Standard Precautions," which include guidelines for isolation precautions in hospitals, designed to prevent the transmission of the hepatitis B virus and the human immunodeficiency virus (HIV). A condensed and current version of these recommendations is provided. Most institutions currently follow these guidelines in some version, and we recommend referral to individual institutional protocol. In addition the CDC in 2007 developed the "2007 Guideline for Isolation Precautions: Preventing Transmission of Infectious Agents in Healthcare Settings" and in 2011 developed a "Guide to Infection Prevention for Outpatient Settings: Minimum Expectations for Safe Care" that speaks to hand hygiene, personal protective equipment, injection safety, environmental cleaning, medical equipment and respiratory hygiene/cough etiquette.

Years of research and writing went into the completion of this text. It could not have been done without our many dedicated professional contributors, without the assistance and support of our editor Tamara Myers, and without the support of our families, friends, and professional colleagues. We know that we have acquired much knowledge through the process of writing and editing this book. We believe that the book is a valuable tool for all health care professionals.

Cynthia C. Chernecky
Barbara J. Berger

ACKNOWLEDGMENTS

It is with humble thanks that I dedicate this book to all those who have helped in its creation, support, and update and in particular to those who use it in their practice and education. Particular thanks to Jennifer Sweat, BSN student at GHSU, who helped with research and editing. This book has been a labor of love and continues to be used on both the national and international levels. I fully believe that an excellent clinical book on labs and diagnostics is what the clinical caregiver needs to give excellent care to persons who are ill and to all persons who have a right to disease prevention. There are others who, though they did not write, were supportive in ways that we can all understand—these are people who have integrity, caring souls, faith, and a sense of humor: my mother Olga, late father Edward Chernecky, godmother Helen Prohorik, godsons Jonathon Tarutis and Vincent Hunter, goddaughters Ekaterina McNeill and Dawn Priscilla Payne, brother Dr. Richard Chernecky, nieces Ellie Burton and Annie Chernecky, nephew Michael Chernecky, great nephew William "Liam" Burton, Cliff Burton, Budnik family; cousins Paula Smart, Karyn Tarutis, Philip Prohorik, Ed Sztuka, Eileen Sztuka, Tyler Sztuka, and Benjamin Sztuka; friends Olga, Don and Peter McNeill, Yelena and Igor Senko, Elaine Calugar, Phyllis Skiba, David and Janice Douglass, Frankie Ekroyd, Andrea Burton, Molly Loney; colleagues Dr. Joyceen Boyle, Dr. Jean Brown, Dr. Linda Burnes-Bolton, Dr. Mary Cooley, Dr. Leda Danao, Kitty Garrett, Beverly George-Gay, Dr. Rich Haas, Becki Hodges, Dr. Ann Kolanowski, Dr. Elisabeth Monti-Siebert, Dr. Ruth McCorkle, Dr. Linda Sarna, Dr. Geri Padilla, Dr. Autumn Schumacher, Dr. Shirley Quarles, Denise Macklin, Dr. Marlene Rosenkoetter, Dr. Georgia Narsavage, Dr. Beverly Roberts, Dr. May Wykle, Rebecca Rule, Paula T. Rieger, Dr. Rob Lafferty; and those who keep me focused in life itself: Mother Thecla (Abbess), and Mother Helena and Mother Luybov of Saints Mary and Martha Ortho-dox Monastery in South Carolina, Priest Gregory and Presbytera Raisa Koo, Priest Antonio and Matushka Elizabeth Perdomo, and Heirmonk Fr. Cyprian DuRant. It never fails to surprise me when I meet an Orthodox member of His Holy, Catholic, and Apostolic Church who has found true joy in that he or she has found the truth in the faith that we trace back to the time of Christ himself. I know from my life that the truth is worth the search.

To the universities that have shared their knowledge with me, I thank the University of Connecticut, Yale University, University of Pittsburgh, Clemson University, Case Western Reserve University, University of Wisconsin Oshkosh, and the University of California at Los Angeles.

As we continue in further editions of this book, I do not know what else to say about my coeditor, coauthor, friend, and colleague Barb Berger. We work well together, know how to laugh, know how to work hard, and have a commitment to care with an eye for quality research to make each and every edition packed with quality information and timely updates. This book is a massive project, and I could not have accomplished it without trust, equality, respect, and admiration, which is what Barb and I have for one another and why we make such a great team. Barb, you are a distinguished professional and a great role model, which adds not just to this book but to the discipline and profession of nursing.

To all nurses, physicians, attorneys, and other health care professionals who give true meaning to this book by using it, we respect your comments and suggestions—after all we are all striving for the same goals in our respective services.

Cynthia (Cinda) Cecilia Chernecky

My thanks and gratitude for their meticulous attention to detail and sharing of their expertise go to current and past contributors and reviewers of this text. I am appreciative of our oh-so-meticulous experts at Elsevier, Tamara Myers and Bridget Healy, who made the process from manuscript-to-production go smoothly and stay on schedule. Thanks go to my husband,

Stephan Berger, who shares my pride in this work and does more than his fair share keeping the home front running so that I can spend time working on the manuscript. My mother, Alice Adams, once again supported and encouraged my work on this sixth edition. Finally, massive thanks to Cinda Chernecky, my **awesome** and excellent coeditor and friend, who never fails to amaze me with her depth and breadth of knowledge, pitch-in attitude and unending optimism!

Barbara J. Berger

HOW TO USE THIS BOOK

This book contains two major sections: Part One is a selected alphabetical listing of diseases, conditions, and symptoms that will aid in the diagnosis and monitoring of illnesses. Part Two presents information on laboratory and diagnostic tests in alphabetical order, using a consistent, time-saving format.

PART ONE: DISEASES, CONDITIONS, AND SYMPTOMS

The purpose of this section is to assist practitioners in diagnosing and monitoring the progress of illness or wellness.

Part One is a selected alphabetical listing of diseases, conditions, and symptoms. Under each topic is a list of laboratory and diagnostic tests, also in alphabetical order. It is not expected that all the tests listed would necessarily be required or be abnormal for any one disease, condition, or symptom. Rather, any of the listed tests or a combination of tests would likely be performed to aid, confirm, monitor, or rule out that diagnosis or condition. Where appropriate, the tests and/or procedures considered diagnostic or significant in determining a diagnosis are highlighted with a bullet.

PART TWO: LABORATORY TESTS AND DIAGNOSTIC PROCEDURES

The purpose of this section is to provide a comprehensive, concise, ready reference of practitioner "need-to-know" information about laboratory tests and diagnostic procedures. Features of this section, in format order, include:

- **Alphabetical list of laboratory tests and diagnostic procedures:** This saves you time in looking up any test. You will also find combined laboratory profiles listed such as CBC, CMP, and Chemistry Profile.
- **Norms** are listed for all known age-groups and for all known units (i.e., national and international units). Also included are therapeutic peak and trough norms, toxic and panic levels, as well as associated signs, symptoms, and emergency treatment for overdose when applicable. Tests with toxic and/or panic levels include symptoms and treatment. Treatments listed are generally accepted treatments. The listing of these does not imply that some or all of them should be used. Selection of treatments must be based on the client's history and condition, as well as the history of the episode.
- **Usage:** states the typical conditions or monitoring for which the diagnostic test or procedure is commonly used (i.e., cardiac catheterization).
- **Increased**, **Decreased** or **Positive**, **Negative** are categories to describe conditions that cause abnormal laboratory test results. Also listed, in alphabetical order, are medications and herbal and natural remedies that interfere with the laboratory results.
- **Description:** A concise description of the test or procedure is provided, including interpretation of results and significance for various conditions.
- **Professional Considerations** include seven types of information:
  1. **Consent, Risks**, and **Contraindications:** Indicate whether a separate special consent form IS or IS NOT required. Where tests or procedures carry significant risks, the risks that should be explained to the client are included in a highlighted alert box. Contraindications are in a list of generally accepted conditions (in a highlighted alert box labeled Risks) in which the test or procedure should not be performed and Relative Contraindications in which the test or procedure should be modified, where applicable.
  2. **Preparation:** Includes supplies needed, assessment for allergies, unusual scheduling requirements, procedural preparation requirements, such as establishing intravenous access, equipment/medications needed to treat anaphylaxis, and medicolegal handling.
  3. **Procedure:** Gives step-by-step description of specimen collection or procedural steps, including safety "time out" for correct site or procedure verification, client positioning

and participation, and monitoring required during the procedure. NOTE: For blood samples, mini-volumes (1 to 3 mL) are listed for tests in which special manual tests may be run on smaller volumes for clients in whom blood preservation is essential. For pediatric clients, microtainers may be used, but volumes should equate to those specified in the text (e.g., two 1-mL sized microtainers would be needed for a 2-mL specimen). For clients not at risk for iatrogenic anemia as a result of frequent blood sampling, the quickest turnaround times are achieved with higher volumes, which enable automated testing.

4. **Postprocedure Care:** Provides aftercare instructions regarding specimen handling, site dressing, activity restriction, vital signs, and postsedation monitoring.
5. **Client and Family Teaching:** Includes instructions the client or family should be informed about, including precare, procedural care, aftercare, and monitoring, as well as disease-specific information, time frame for test results, and follow-up recommendations.
6. **Factors That Affect Results:** Gives quality assurance information about items that will interfere with the accuracy of results, such as improper collection techniques, improper specimen handling, drugs and herbals that cause false-positive or false-negative results, and cross-reactivity of other diseases or conditions.
7. **Other Data:** Provides selected information from current research that may not yet be generalizable but could be helpful in decision-making for individuals or groups of clients; recommendations for confirmatory testing if the results are positive; direction to other tests related to the same diagnosis or condition and known association between tests; and national guideline information and recommendations, when available.

CONTENTS

PART ONE

DISEASES, CONDITIONS, AND SYMPTOMS

Abdominal Aortic Aneurysm
(see Aneurysm, Abdominal aortic; Aneurysm, Cerebral; or Aneurysm, Thoracic aortic)

Abortion, Spontaneous
Alpha-fetoprotein, Blood
Amniotic fluid, Alpha$_1$-fetoprotein, Specimen
Amniotic fluid, Chromosome analysis, Specimen
Amniotic fluid, Erythroblastosis fetalis, Specimen
Chorionic villi sampling, Diagnostic
Complete blood count, Blood
Endometrium, Anaerobic, Culture
Estriol, Serum or 24-hour urine
Glucose tolerance test, Blood
• Histopathology, Specimen
• Human chorionic gonadotropin, Beta-subunit, Serum
• Pregnancy test, Routine, Serum and qualitative urine
Progesterone, Serum
Type and crossmatch, Blood

Abscess
Actinomyces, Culture
• Biopsy, Site-specific, Specimen (Anaerobic culture, fungus culture)
• Body fluid (Abscess), Anaerobic, Culture
Bronchial aspirate, Routine, Culture
Histopathology, Specimen
Magnetic resonance imaging, Diagnostic
Skin, *Mycobacterium*, Culture
Sputum, Routine, Culture
Wound, Culture
Wound, Fungus, Culture
Wound, *Mycobacterium*, Culture

Achlorhydria
• Gastric analysis, Specimen
Gastrin, Serum
• Histopathology, Specimen
Intrinsic factor antibody, Blood
Pepsinogen I antibody, Blood
pH, Urine
Urinalysis, Urine
Vitamin B$_{12}$, Serum

Acidosis
(see Metabolic acidosis or Respiratory acidosis)

Acne Vulgaris
Biopsy, Site-specific, Specimen (Anaerobic culture)
Follicle-stimulating hormone, Serum
• Histopathology, Specimen

Luteinizing hormone, Blood
Testosterone, Blood

Acquired Immune Deficiency Syndrome
• Acquired immune deficiency syndrome evaluation battery, Diagnostic
Beta$_2$-microglobulin, Blood and 24-hour urine
Biopsy, Site-specific, Specimen
Bronchoscopy, Diagnostic
Cerebrospinal fluid, Routine, Culture and cytology
Chest radiography, Diagnostic
Cryptococcal antibody titer, Serum
Cryptococcal antigen titer, Cerebrospinal fluid, Specimen
Cryptococcal antigen titer, Serum
Cryptosporidium diagnostic procedures, Stool
Cytomegalovirus antibody, Serum
Diffusing capacity for carbon monoxide, Diagnostic
Hepatitis B surface antigen, Blood
Lymphocyte subset enumeration, Blood
Mantoux skin test, Diagnostic
Oral mucosal transudate, Specimen
OraQuick Rapid HIV tests, Specimen
Pneumocystis immunofluorescent assay, Serum
Pulmonary function tests, Diagnostic
Single-photon emission computed tomography, Brain, Diagnostic
Skin, Mycobacteria, Culture
• T- and B-lymphocyte subset assay, Blood
Throat culture for *Candida albicans*, Culture
Toxoplasmosis serology, Serum

Acromegaly
(see also Hyperpituitarism)
Alkaline phosphatase, Isoenzymes, Serum
Alkaline phosphatase, Serum
Calcium, Total, Serum
Calcium, Urine
Computed tomography of the body (Chest, head), Diagnostic
Glucose, Blood
• Glucose tolerance test, Blood in combination with growth hormone and growth hormone–releasing hormone, Blood
Hydroxyproline, Total, 24-hour urine
• Insulin-like growth factor-I, Blood
Magnetic resonance imaging, Diagnostic
Phosphorus, Serum
Single-photon emission computed tomography, Diagnostic

Actinomycosis
Acid-fast stain, *Nocardia* species, Culture
• *Actinomyces*, Culture
• Biopsy, Site-specific, Specimen (Anaerobic culture, fungus culture, routine culture)
Body fluid (Abscess), Anaerobic, Culture
Bronchial aspirate, Routine, Culture
Bronchial washing, Specimen
Brushing cytology, Specimen
Cervical-vaginal cytology, Specimen
Chest radiography, Diagnostic
Complete blood count, Blood
Computed tomography of the body, Diagnostic
Endometrium, Anaerobic, Culture
Foreign body, Routine, Culture
Histopathology, Specimen
Sedimentation rate, Erythrocyte, Blood
Sputum fungus, Specimen
Ultrasonography, Diagnostic (Various sites)
Wound culture

Acute Myocardial Infarction
(see Myocardial infarction)

Acute Respiratory Distress Syndrome
• Blood gases, Arterial, Blood
• Chest radiography, Diagnostic
Complete blood count, Blood
CO-oximeter profile, Blood
C-reactive protein, Plasma or serum
Culture, Blood
Electrolytes, Plasma or serum
KeyPath MRSA/MSSA Blood culture test, Blood
Oximetry, Diagnostic
Prothrombin time and international normalized ratio, Plasma
• Pulmonary artery catheterization, Diagnostic
Sputum culture and sensitivity, Specimen
Urea nitrogen, Plasma or serum

Addison's Disease
• ACTH stimulation test, Diagnostic
Alkaline phosphatase, Isoenzymes, Serum
Alkaline phosphatase, Serum
Calcium, Total, Serum
Calcium, Urine
Computed tomography of the body (Abdomen), Diagnostic
• Cortisol, Plasma or serum
Flat-plate radiography of abdomen, Diagnostic
Glucose, Blood
Growth hormone and growth hormone–releasing hormone, Blood

Hydroxyproline, Total, 24-hour urine
Insulin-like growth factor-I, Blood
Magnesium, Serum
Metyrapone test, Serum
Phosphorus, Serum

Adenovirus Infection
• Adenovirus antibody titer, Serum
Ocular cytology, Specimen
• Viral culture, Specimen

Adrenalectomy
• Cortisol, Serum
Magnesium, Serum

Adult Respiratory Distress Syndrome
(see Acute respiratory distress syndrome)

Agranulocytosis
Blood culture, Blood
• Bone marrow aspiration analysis, Specimen
• Complete blood count, Blood
Culture, Skin, Specimen
Culture, Urine
• Differential leukocyte count, Peripheral blood

Ahaptoglobinemia
• Haptoglobin, Serum

AIDS
(see Acquired immune deficiency syndrome)

Albright Syndrome
Alkaline phosphatase, Serum
Blood gases, Arterial, Blood
Bone radiography, Diagnostic
Comprehensive metabolic panel, Blood
Dexamethasone suppression test, Diagnostic
Estradiol, Serum
Follicle-stimulating hormone, Serum
Growth hormone and growth hormone–releasing hormone, Blood
Human chorionic gonadotropin, Beta-subunit, Serum
• Hydroxyproline, Total, 24-hour urine
Luteinizing hormone, Blood
Testosterone, Blood
Thyroid function tests, Blood

Alcoholism
Alanine aminotransferase, Serum
Albumin, Serum, Urine, and 24-hour urine
• Alcohol, Blood
Alkaline phosphatase, Isoenzymes, Serum
Alkaline phosphatase, Serum
Ammonia, Blood
Amylase, Serum and urine

Anion gap, Blood
Aspartate aminotransferase, Serum
Bilirubin, Direct, Serum
Bilirubin, Total, Serum
Blood gases, Arterial, Blood
Blood indices (MCV), Blood
Chemistry profile, Blood
Complete blood count, Blood
Differential leukocyte count, Peripheral
   blood
Electrolytes, Plasma or serum
Folic acid, Serum
Gamma-glutamyltranspeptidase, Blood
Glucose, Blood
Heavy metals, Blood and 24-hour urine
Hepatitis C antibody, Serum
Hepatitis serologies
Histopathology, Specimen
Ketones, Semiquantitative, Urine
Ketone bodies, Blood
Lactate dehydrogenase, Blood
Lactate dehydrogenase, Isoenzymes, Blood
Lactic acid, Blood
Lipid profile, Blood
• Liver battery, Serum
Magnesium, Serum
5′-Nucleotidase, Blood
Occult blood, Stool, Diagnostic
Osmolality, Calculated test, Blood
Osmolality, Serum
Phosphorus, Serum
Platelet count, Blood
Prothrombin time and international
   normalized ratio, Plasma
Red blood cell morphology, Blood
Sedimentation rate, Erythrocyte, Blood
• Toxicology, Volatiles group by GLC, Blood
   or urine
Transferrin, Carbohydrate-deficient, Serum
Transthyretin (Prealbumin), Serum
Triglycerides, Blood
Uric acid, Serum
• Vitamin B_{12}, Serum
Zinc, Blood

Alkalosis
(see Metabolic alkalosis or Respiratory
alkalosis)

Allergic Reaction
(see Hypersensitivity reaction)

Alzheimer's Disease
Apolipoprotein E4 genotyping, Plasma
• Beta-amyloid protein 40/42, CSF
Blood gases, Arterial, Blood
Bromides, Serum

Cerebral computed tomography, Diagnostic
Cerebrospinal fluid, Oligoclonal bands,
   Specimen
Cerebrospinal fluid, Protein, Specimen
Cerebrospinal fluid, Routine analysis,
   Specimen
Cerebrospinal fluid immunoglobulin G,
   Immunoglobulin G ratios and
   immunoglobulin G index,
   Immunoglobulin G synthesis rate,
   Specimen
Ceruloplasmin, Serum
Comprehensive metabolic panel, Blood
Copper, Serum
Copper, Urine
Electroencephalography, Diagnostic
Heavy metals, Blood and 24-hour urine
HIV antibodies (see Acquired immune
   deficiency syndrome evaluation battery,
   Diagnostic)
Magnetic resonance spectroscopy,
   Diagnostic
Positron emission tomography, Diagnostic
Protein electrophoresis, Cerebrospinal
   fluid, Specimen
• Single-photon emission computed
   tomography, Brain, Diagnostic
• Tau test, Cerebrospinal fluid
Toxicology drug screen, Blood or urine
   (Urine)
Transthyretin (Prealbumin), Serum

Amaurosis Fugax
Cerebral angiogram (Carotid arteries),
   Diagnostic
Computed tomography of the body,
   Diagnostic
Creatinine, Serum
Doppler ultrasonic flow studies (Carotid
   arteries), Diagnostic
Echocardiogram, Diagnostic
Electrolytes, Plasma or serum
Glucose, Fasting, Blood
Lipid profile, Blood
Magnetic resonance angiography,
   Diagnostic
Urea nitrogen, Plasma or serum
• Viscosity, Serum

Amenorrhea
Adrenocorticotropic hormone, Serum
Chromosome analysis, Blood
Cortisol, Plasma or serum
Cortisol, Urine
Dehydroepiandrosterone sulfate, Serum
Estradiol, Serum

Estrogens, Nonpregnant, 24-hour urine
• Estrogens, Serum and 24-hour urine
• Follicle-stimulating hormone, Serum
Histopathology, Specimen
Hormonal evaluation, Cytologic, Specimen
17-Hydroxycorticosteroids, 24-hour urine
Luteinizing hormone, Blood
Pap smear, Diagnostic
Pregnancy test, Routine, Serum and
  qualitative, Urine
Prolactin, Serum
Testosterone, Free, Bioavailable and total,
  Blood
• Thyroid-stimulating hormone, Blood
Thyroid test, Free thyroxine index, Serum

Amikacin
(see Aminoglycoside toxicity)

Aminoglycoside Toxicity
(see Amikacin and Gentamicin)
Amikacin sulfate, Blood
Beta$_2$-microglobulin, Blood and 24-hour
  urine
Bicarbonate, Blood
Blood gases, Arterial, Blood
Blood urea nitrogen/creatinine ratio, Blood
Blood volume, Blood
• Creatinine, Serum
Creatinine, Urine (Spot)
Creatinine clearance, Serum, Urine
Digoxin level
Electrolytes, Urine
Gentamicin, Blood
Kidney ultrasonography, Diagnostic
Osmolality, Calculated test, Blood
Osmolality, Serum
Osmolality, Urine
Renal indices (Fractional excretion of
  sodium), Diagnostic
Sodium, Plasma, Serum or urine
Specific gravity, Urine
Tobramycin, Serum
Urinalysis, Urine

Amputation
*(see Surgery, Preoperative; Surgery,
Postoperative)*

Amyloidosis
Apolipoprotein A-I, Plasma
Biopsy, Site-specific, Specimen
Bone marrow aspiration analysis, Specimen
Chemistry profile, Blood
Chest radiography, Diagnostic
Computed tomography of the body
  (HRCT), Diagnostic

Concentration test, Urine
• Creatinine, Serum
Creatinine clearance, Serum, Urine
Cytologic study of gastrointestinal tract,
  Diagnostic
D-Xylose absorption test, Diagnostic,
  Serum or urine
Echocardiography, Diagnostic
Globulin, Serum
• Histopathology, Specimen
Immunoelectrophoresis, Serum and urine
Leukocyte cytochemistry, Specimen
Liver battery, Serum
Liver biopsy, Diagnostic
Liver ^{131}I scan, Diagnostic
• Protein electrophoresis, Serum
Protein electrophoresis, Urine
Protein, Quantitative, Urine
Protein, Semiquantitative, Urine
Sedimentation rate, Erythrocyte, Blood
Skin, Mycobacteria, Culture
Thyroid function tests, Blood
• Transthyretin, Serum or vitreous fluid
  (Familial Amyloidosis)
Urea nitrogen, Plasma or serum
Urinalysis, Urine

Amyotrophic Lateral Sclerosis
Barium swallow, Diagnostic
Biopsy, Site-specific (Muscle), Specimen
Creatine kinase, Serum
Creatinine clearance, Serum, Urine
• Electromyography and nerve conduction
  (electromyelogram) studies, Diagnostic
• Magnetic resonance neurography,
  Diagnostic

Anaphylaxis
(see Shock)

Anemias
*(see Aplastic, Dyserythropoietic, Folic acid,
G6PD deficiency, Galactokinase deficiency,
Heinz body, Hemolytic, Iron [hypochromic]
deficiency, Megaloblastic, Pernicious, or
Sickle cell anemias)*

Anesthesia
*(see Surgery, Preoperative; Surgery,
Postoperative)*

Aneurysm
*(see Aneurysm, Abdominal aortic; Aneurysm,
Cerebral; Aneurysm, Thoracic aortic)*

Aneurysm, Abdominal Aortic
• Abdominal aorta ultrasonography,
  Diagnostic
Cardiac catheterization, Diagnostic

Chest radiography, Diagnostic
• Computed tomography of the body (Abdomen), (Spiral), Diagnostic
• Flat-plate radiography of abdomen, Diagnostic
Fluorescent treponemal antibody–absorbed double-stain test, Serum
Lipid profile, Blood
• Magnetic resonance angiography, Diagnostic
• Magnetic resonance imaging, Diagnostic
Rapid plasma reagin test, Blood
Venereal Disease Research Laboratory test, Serum

Aneurysm, Cerebral
Activated partial thromboplastin time and partial thromboplastin time, Plasma
• Cerebral angiography, Diagnostic
• Cerebral computed tomography, Diagnostic
Cerebrospinal fluid, Protein, Specimen
Computed tomography of the body (HRCT), Diagnostic
Doppler ultrasonographic flow studies, Diagnostic (Transcranial)
Lumbar puncture, Diagnostic
• Magnetic resonance angiography, Diagnostic
• Magnetic resonance imaging (Brain), Diagnostic
Prothrombin time and international normalized ratio, Plasma

Aneurysm, Thoracic Aortic
• Chest radiography, Diagnostic
• Computed tomography of the body (Abdomen, chest), (Spiral), Diagnostic
Fluorescent treponemal antibody–absorbed double-stain test, Serum
Lipid profile, Blood
• Magnetic resonance angiography, Diagnostic
• Pulmonary angiography, Diagnostic
Rapid plasma reagin test, Blood
• Transesophageal ultrasonography, Diagnostic
Venereal Disease Research Laboratory test, Serum

Angina Pectoris
Anticardiolipin antibody, Serum
Antimyocardial antibody, Serum
Aspartate aminotransferase, Serum
Cardiac calcium scoring, Diagnostic
Cardiac catheterization, Diagnostic
Chest radiography, Diagnostic

Complete blood count, Blood (Hemoglobin)
Computed tomography of the body (EBCT), Diagnostic
• Coronary intravascular ultrasonography, Diagnostic
C-reactive protein (High sensitivity), Serum
Creatine kinase, Serum (Isoenzymes)
D-Dimer test, Blood
Echocardiography, Diagnostic
• Electrocardiography, Diagnostic
Ergonovine provocation test, Diagnostic
Glucose, Blood
Heart scan, Diagnostic
Holter monitor, Diagnostic
Homocysteine, Plasma or urine
Lactate dehydrogenase, Isoenzymes, Blood
• Lipid profile, Blood
Positive emission tomography, Diagnostic
• Stress exercise test, Diagnostic
• Stress test, Pharmacologic, Diagnostic
Troponin I, Plasma and troponin T, Serum

Ankylosing Spondylitis
Antinuclear antibody, Serum
Bone scan, Diagnostic
Computed tomography of the body, Diagnostic
• C-reactive protein, Plasma or serum
Human leukocyte antigen B27, Blood
• Immunoglobulin G, Serum
Immunoglobulin M, Serum (Rheumatoid factor)
Magnetic resonance imaging (Sacroiliac spine), Diagnostic
Protein electrophoresis, Serum
• Radiography (Bone), Diagnostic
Rheumatoid factor, Blood
• Sedimentation rate, Erythrocyte, Blood

Anorexia Nervosa
Bone densitometry, Diagnostic
Complete blood count, Blood
Comprehensive metabolic panel, Blood
Differential leukocyte count, Peripheral blood
Electrocardiography, Diagnostic
Electrolytes, Plasma or serum
• Estradiol, Serum
17-Hydroxycorticosteroids, 24-hour urine
Low-density lipoprotein cholesterol, Blood
• Luteinizing hormone, Blood
Phenolphthalein test, Diagnostic
Potassium, Plasma or serum

Protein-bound iodine, Blood
Sedimentation rate, Erythrocyte, Blood
Thyroid test, Free thyroxine index, Serum
Thyroid test, Thyroxine, Blood
• Thyroid test, Triiodothyronine, Blood
• Transthyretin (Prealbumin), Serum

Anoxia

Apnea test, Diagnostic
Bicarbonate, Blood
• Blood gases, Arterial, Blood
Blood gases, Capillary, Blood
Blood gases, Venous, Blood
Carbon dioxide, Partial pressure, Blood
Carbon dioxide, Total content, Blood
Chest radiography, Diagnostic
Diffusing capacity for carbon monoxide,
   Diagnostic
Doppler ultrasonographic flow studies
   (Transcranial), Diagnostic
Electroencephalography, Diagnostic
Lactic acid, Blood
Magnetic resonance angiography,
   Diagnostic
Magnetic resonance imaging, Diagnostic
• Oxygen saturation, Blood
Single-photon emission computed
   tomography, Brain, Diagnostic
Ultrasonography, Brain, Diagnostic

Anthrax

Biopsy, Site-specific, Specimen
• Blood culture, Blood
• Chest radiography, Diagnostic
Complete blood count, Blood
Computed tomography of the body
   (Chest), Diagnostic
Culture, (Body fluid), Routine, Specimen
• Culture, Skin, Specimen
Differential leukocyte count, Peripheral
   blood
Gram stain, Diagnostic
Hypersensitivity pneumonitis serology,
   Blood

Antigens
(see Immunoglobulin A)

Anxiety

Blood gases, Arterial, Blood
Catecholamines, Urine
Complete blood count, Blood
Creatinine, Urine
Electrocardiography, Diagnostic
Epinephrine, Blood
Glucose, Blood
Holter monitor, Diagnostic

Metanephrine, Total, 24-hour urine, and
   free, Plasma
• Norepinephrine, Serum
Thyroid function tests, Blood
Toxicology drug screen, Blood or urine
   (Urine)
Toxicology drug screen, Urine
Vanillylmandelic acid, Urine

Aortic Aneurysm
(see Aneurysm, Abdominal aortic)

Aortic Valvular Stenosis

Blood gases, Arterial, Blood
Cardiac catheterization, Diagnostic
Chest radiography, Diagnostic
Digital subtraction angiography and
   transvenous-digital subtraction,
   Diagnostic
• Echocardiography, Diagnostic
Electrocardiography, Diagnostic
• Magnetic resonance angiography,
   Diagnostic
Transesophageal ultrasonography,
   Diagnostic

Aortitis

• Abdominal aortic ultrasonography,
   Diagnostic
• Complete blood count, Blood
Lipid profile, Blood
Rapid plasma reagin test, Blood
Venereal Disease Research Laboratory test,
   Serum

Aplastic Anemia

• Bone marrow aspiration analysis,
   Diagnostic
• Complete blood count, Blood
Differential leukocyte count, Peripheral
   blood
Hepatitis B core antibody, Blood
Hepatitis C antibody, Serum
Mixed leukocyte culture, Specimen
Red blood cell morphology, Blood
Reticulocyte count, Blood

Appendicitis

Blood culture, Blood
Body fluid (Abscess), Anaerobic, Culture
• Complete blood count, Blood
Compression ultrasonography, Diagnostic
Computed tomography of the body
   (Abdomen), Diagnostic
• Differential leukocyte count, Peripheral
   blood
Histopathology (Postoperatively),
   Specimen

Infectious mononucleosis screening test, Blood

Occult blood, Stool

Pregnancy test, Routine, Serum, and Qualitative, Urine

Urinalysis, Urine

ARDS
(see Acute respiratory distress syndrome)

Arrhythmias
(see Dysrhythmias)

Arterial Ischemic Leg Ulcer
(see Peripheral vascular disease)

Arterial Occlusion
(see Occlusion, Acute arterial)

Arterial Thrombosis
(see Thrombosis)

Arteriosclerosis
Activated partial thromboplastin time and partial thromboplastin time, Plasma

Anticardiolipin antibody, Serum

C-reactive protein, Blood

Cholesterol, Blood

Computed tomography of the body (EBCT, MDCT), Diagnostic

• Coronary intravascular ultrasonography, Diagnostic

• Doppler ultrasonographic flow studies, Diagnostic

Electrocardiography, Diagnostic

High-density lipoprotein cholesterol, Blood

Homocysteine, Plasma or urine

• Lipid profile, Blood

Low-density lipoprotein cholesterol, Blood

Mean platelet volume, Blood

Prothrombin time and international normalized ratio, Plasma

Single-photon emission computed tomography, Myocardial perfusion, Diagnostic

Stress exercise test, Diagnostic

Stress plasma reagin, Pharmacologic, Diagnostic

Triglycerides, Blood

Arteriosclerotic Heart Disease
(see Arteriosclerosis)

Arteritis
• Biopsy, Site-specific (Temporal artery), Specimen

• Complete blood count, Blood

C-reactive protein, Serum

Liver battery, serum

• Sedimentation rate, Erythrocyte, Blood

Arthritis
(see Osteoarthritis, Rheumatoid arthritis)

Asbestosis
(see Industry-related diseases)

Ascites
• Albumin, Serum, Urine and 24-hour urine

Amylase, Serum and urine (Serum)

Body fluid analysis, Cell count, Specimen

• Body fluid cytology, Specimen

Flat-plate radiography of the abdomen (Kidneys, ureters, bladder), Diagnostic

Lactate dehydrogenase (isoenzymes), Blood

Lipase, Serum

Liver battery, Serum

Paracentesis, Diagnostic

• Ultrasonography, Abdomen, Diagnostic

ASHD/Arteriosclerotic Heart Disease
(see Arteriosclerosis)

Aspiration Pneumonia
(see Pneumonia)

Aspirin Poisoning
(see Poisonings)

Asterixis
(see Liver failure)

Asthma
• Allergen-specific IgE antibody, Serum

Bicarbonate, Blood

Blood gases, Arterial, Blood

Carbon dioxide, Partial pressure, Blood

Carbon dioxide, Total content, Blood

• Chest radiography, Diagnostic

Complete blood count, Blood

Differential leukocyte count, Peripheral blood

Diffusing capacity for carbon monoxide, Diagnostic

Eosinophil count, Blood

Eosinophil peroxidase, Serum

Esophageal manometry

Hypersensitivity pneumonitis serology, Blood

Immunoglobulin E, Serum

Low-density lipoprotein cholesterol, Blood

Methacholine challenge test, Diagnostic

Ova and parasites, Stool

Oximetry, Diagnostic

• Pulmonary function tests, Diagnostic

Skin test for hypersensitivity, Diagnostic

Sputum cytology, Specimen

Theophylline, Blood

Ataxia
Alcohol, Blood
Antistreptolysin-O titer, Serum
Benzodiazepines, Plasma and urine
• Cerebral Computed Tomography,
   Diagnostic
Echocardiography, Diagnostic
Electrocardiography, Diagnostic
FMR1 testing for fragile X associated
   disorders, Blood (males over age 50)
Heavy metals, Blood and 24-hour urine
Lead, Blood and urine
Magnesium, Serum
Nerve conduction studies, Diagnostic
• Oculoplethysmography, Diagnostic
Oculopneumoplethysmography,
   Diagnostic
Phenothiazines, Blood
Phenytoin, Serum
SCA gene test, Diagnostic
Streptozyme, Blood
Venereal Disease Research Laboratory test,
   Cerebrospinal fluid, Specimen

Atelectasis
• Blood gases, Arterial, Blood
• Chest radiography, Diagnostic
Complete blood count, Blood

Atherosclerosis
(see Arteriosclerosis)

Athlete's Foot
• Culture, Skin, Specimen

Atransferrinemia
Transferrin, Serum

Atrial Septal Defect
• Blood gases, Arterial, Blood
Cardiac catheterization, Diagnostic
Chest radiography, Diagnostic
• Echocardiography, Diagnostic
Electrocardiography, Diagnostic
Heart scan, Diagnostic
• Magnetic resonance imaging, Diagnostic
Pulmonary artery catheterization,
   Diagnostic
• Ventriculography, Diagnostic

Australian Antigen
(see Hepatitis)

Autoimmune Diseases
*(see Amyloidosis, Ankylosing spondylitis,
Goodpasture's syndrome, Raynaud's
phenomenon, Rheumatic fever, Rheumatoid
arthritis, Scleroderma, Sjögren's syndrome,
Systemic lupus erythematosus, or Vasculitis)*

Azotemia
Blood urea nitrogen/creatinine ratio, Blood
Calcium, Total, Serum
Chemistry profile, Blood
• Creatinine, Serum
Creatinine, Urine (Spot)
Creatinine clearance, Serum, Urine
• Electrolytes, Plasma or serum
Electrolytes, Urine
Flat-plate radiography of the abdomen
   (Kidneys, ureters, bladder), Diagnostic
Kidney ultrasonography (Kidneys, ureters,
   bladder), (Doppler) Diagnostic
Occult blood, Stool
Osmolality, Calculated test, Blood
Osmolality, Serum
Osmolality, Urine
Phosphorus, Serum
Phosphorus, Urine
Protein, Semiquantitative, Urine
• Urea nitrogen, Plasma or serum
Uric acid, Serum
Urinalysis, Urine

Bacteremia
(see Sepsis)

Bacterial Endocarditis
(see Endocarditis)

Barrett's Esophagus
Biopsy, Site-specific, Specimen
• Endoscopy, Diagnostic

Bartonella Infection
(see Cat-scratch disease)

Bell's Palsy
Electromyography and nerve conduction
   studies, Diagnostic

Benign Prostatic Hyperplasia
Acid phosphatase, Serum
Alkaline phosphatase, Serum
Bicarbonate, Blood
Body fluid (Urine), Routine, Culture
Chemistry profile, Blood
Complete blood count, Blood
Cytologic study of urine, Diagnostic
Electrolytes, Plasma or serum
Kidney ultrasonography, Diagnostic
Occult blood, Urine
Prostate-specific antigen, Blood
Renal function tests, Diagnostic
• Urinalysis, Urine
Urinary bladder ultrasonography,
   Diagnostic
Uroflowmetry, Diagnostic

Berger's Disease
Biopsy, Site-specific (Renal), Specimen
Creatinine, Serum
Creatinine clearance, 12- or 24-hour urine
• Immunoglobulin A, Serum
Intravenous pyelography, Diagnostic
• Urinalysis, Urine

Beriberi
Chest radiography, Diagnostic
Electrocardiography, Diagnostic
Electromyography and nerve conduction
    studies, Diagnostic
• Vitamin B_1, Serum or urine

Bernard-Soulier Syndrome
• Platelet adhesion test, Diagnostic
• Platelet aggregation, Blood
Platelet aggregation, Hypercoagulable state,
    Blood
Platelet count, Blood
von Willebrand factor assay, Blood

Beta-Glucuronidase Syndrome
• Mucopolysaccharides, Qualitative, Urine

Biliary Calculi
• Bile, Urine
Urobilinogen, Urine

Bilirubinuria
Bile, Urine
Gallbladder and biliary system
    ultrasonography, Diagnostic

Black Lung Disease
(see Silicosis)

Bladder Cancer
Cytologic study of breast cyst, Effusions,
    Gastrointestinal tract, Nipple discharge,
    Respiratory tract, or Urine, Diagnostic
    (Urine)
Cystoscopy, Diagnostic
Fluorescence in situ hybridization Test,
    Urine
Tissue polypeptide antigen (TPA), Plasma
    or serum

Blepharitis
Culture (Eye margin), Routine, Specimen

Botulism
Body fluid (Abscess), Anaerobic, Culture
• Botulism, Diagnostic procedures, Stool
Clostridium difficile toxin assay, Stool
Complete blood count, Blood
• Culture, Stool, Specimen
Electromyography and nerve conduction
    studies, Diagnostic

Bowel Obstruction
(see Obstruction)

Bradycardia
• Complete blood count, Blood
Creatine kinase, Blood (Isoenzymes)
Digoxin, Serum
Disopyramide phosphate, Serum
Echocardiography, Diagnostic
• Electrocardiography, Diagnostic
• Electrolytes, Plasma or serum
Electrophysiologic study, Diagnostic
Holter monitor, Diagnostic
Propranolol, Blood
Quinidine, Serum
Thyroid profile, Blood
Toxicology drug screen, Blood or urine
Troponin I, Plasma and troponin T,
    Serum

Brain Abscess
(see Abscess)

Brain Cancer
(see Brain tumors)

Brain Death
Apnea test, Diagnostic
Autopsy, Diagnostic
Brain scan, Cerebral flow and pathology,
    Diagnostic
• Brainstem auditory evoked potential,
    Diagnostic
Carbon dioxide, Partial pressure, Blood
Cerebral angiography, Diagnostic
Doppler ultrasonographic flow studies
    (Transcranial), Diagnostic
• Electroencephalography, Diagnostic
Magnetic resonance angiography,
    Diagnostic
Magnetic resonance imaging, Diagnostic

Brain Tumors
• Brain biopsy, Diagnostic
Carcinoembryonic antigen, Serum
Cerebral angiography, Diagnostic
• Cerebral computed tomography,
    Diagnostic
Cerebrospinal fluid, Protein, Specimen
Cerebrospinal fluid, Routine analysis,
    Specimen
Electroencephalography, Diagnostic
Doppler ultrasonographic flow studies,
    Diagnostic
Dual modality imaging, Diagnostic
Histopathology, Specimen
Homovanillic acid, 24-hour urine
Lumbar puncture, Diagnostic

Magnetic resonance angiography,
  Diagnostic
• Magnetic resonance imaging (Diffusion-
  weighted), Diagnostic
Magnetic resonance spectroscopy,
  Diagnostic
Metanephrines, Total, 24-hour urine and
  free, Plasma
Neuron-specific enolase, Serum
Octreotide scan, Diagnostic
Positron emission tomography, Diagnostic
Telomerase enzyme marker, Blood
Vanillylmandelic acid, Urine
Vascular endothelial growth factor,
  Specimen

Breast Cancer
Alanine aminotransferase, Serum
Alkaline phosphatase, Serum
Alpha-fetoprotein, Blood
• Biopsy, Site-specific (Breast, lymph
  nodes), Specimen
Bone scan, Diagnostic
BRCA (Breast cancer tumor suppressor
  genes) 1 and 2, Serum
• Breast ultrasonography, Diagnostic
CA 15-3, Serum
CA 50, Blood
CA 125, Blood
CA 549, Blood
Calcitonin, Plasma or serum
Calcium, Total, Serum
Carcinoembryonic antigen, Serum
Chest radiography, Diagnostic
Circulating tumor cell test, Blood
Complete blood count, Blood
DNA ploidy, Specimen
Dual modality imaging, Diagnostic
Estradiol receptor and progesterone
  receptor in breast cancer, Diagnostic
• Estrogen receptor assay, Tissue specimen
Follicle-stimulating hormone, Serum
• HER-2/*neu* oncogene, Specimen
Liver battery, Serum
• Magnetic resonance imaging, Diagnostic
Magnetic resonance spectroscopy,
  Diagnostic
• Mammography, Diagnostic
Mitogen-activated protein kinase, Specimen
Mucinlike carcinoma–associated antigen,
  Blood
Needle aspiration cytology (Breast cysts
  and abscesses), Diagnostic
Positron emission tomography, Diagnostic
• Progesterone receptor assay, Specimen

Prolactin, Serum
Scintimammography, Diagnostic
Sentinel lymph node biopsy, Diagnostic
• Stereotactic breast biopsy, Specimen
Telomerase enzyme marker, Blood
Tissue polypeptide antigen, Plasma or serum

Bronchitis, Acute or Chronic
Bicarbonate, Blood
Blood gases, Arterial, Blood
Blood gases, Venous, Blood
Bronchial aspirate, Fungus, Culture
Bronchial aspirate, Routine (Anaerobic),
  Culture
Bronchoscopy, Diagnostic
Carbon dioxide, Partial pressure, Blood
Carbon dioxide, Total content, Blood
• Chest radiography, Diagnostic
Chloride, Sweat, Specimen
Complete blood count, Blood
Low-density lipoprotein cholesterol, Blood
• Pulmonary function tests, Diagnostic
Sputum, Routine, Culture
Theophylline, Blood

Brucellosis
Bone marrow aspiration analysis, Specimen
• Brucellosis agglutinins, Blood
• Brucellosis skin test, Diagnostic
Culture, Site-specific, Specimen
Differential leukocyte count, Peripheral
  blood
Liver battery, Serum

Buerger's Disease
(*see Thromboangiitis obliterans*)

Bulimia Nervosa
Complete blood count, Blood
Comprehensive metabolic panel, Blood
Electrocardiography, Diagnostic
• Electrolytes, Plasma or serum
Electrolytes, Urine
Follicle-stimulating hormone, Serum
Ghrelin, Plasma
Glucose, Fasting, Blood
Luteinizing hormone, Blood
• Phenolphthalein test, Diagnostic
Protein, Total, Serum
Sedimentation rate, Erythrocyte, Blood
Thyroid function tests, Blood

Bulimarexia
(*see Anorexia nervosa or Bulimia nervosa*)

Burns
Activated partial thromboplastin time and
  partial thromboplastin time, Plasma
Albumin, Serum, Urine and 24-hour urine

Albumin/globulin ratio, Serum
Blood culture, Blood
Blood gases, Arterial, Blood
Blood urea nitrogen/creatinine ratio, Blood
Carbon monoxide, Blood
Chest radiography, Diagnostic
Complete blood count, Blood
Creatine kinase, Serum
Culture, Routine, Specimen
D-Dimer test, Blood
Electrocardiography, Diagnostic
• Electrolytes, Plasma or serum
Electrolytes, Urine
Fibrinogen, Plasma
Glucose, Blood
Hemoglobin, Plasma and qualitative, Urine
Myoglobin, Qualitative, Urine
Occult blood, Urine
Osmolality, Calculated test, Blood
Osmolality, Serum
• Protein, Total, Serum
Prothrombin time and international
   normalized ratio, Plasma
Pseudocholinesterase, Plasma
Type and crossmatch, Blood
Urea nitrogen, Plasma or serum

Bursitis
Body fluid analysis, Cell count, Specimen
Needle aspiration, Diagnostic
Radiography, Diagnostic

CABG
(see Coronary artery bypass graft)

Cachexia
(see Kwashiorkor or Marasmus)

Calculi
(see Renal calculi or Biliary calculi)

Canavan Disease
• Ashkenazi Jewish genetic carrier screening
   profile

Cancer
*(see Brain tumors, Breast cancer, Cervical
cancer, Colorectal cancer, Endocrine tumors,
Esophageal cancer, Ganglioneuroblastoma,
Gastric cancer, Glucagonoma, Head and
neck cancer, Hepatomas, Insulinomas,
Leukemia, Liver cancer, Lung cancer,
Lymphoma, Melanoma, Metastasis, Multiple
myeloma, Neuroblastoma, Ovarian cancer,
Pancreatic cancer, Pheochromocytoma,
Prostate cancer, Renal cell cancer, Sarcoma,
Testicular cancer, Thyroid cancer, Uterine
cancer, Vaginal cancer, or Wilms' tumor)*

Candidiasis
(see Thrush, Vaginitis)

Cannabis Drug Abuse
(see Drug abuse)

Carbohydrate-Deficient Glycoprotein Syndrome
• Transferrin, Carbohydrate-deficient,
   Serum

Carbon Monoxide Poisoning
Bicarbonate, Blood
• Blood gases, Arterial, Blood (Oxygen
   saturation)
• Carbon monoxide, Blood
Carboxyhemoglobin, Blood
Cardiac enzymes/isoenzymes, Blood
CO-oximeter profile, Blood
Creatine kinase, Serum
Diffusing capacity for carbon monoxide,
   Diagnostic
Electrocardiography, Diagnostic
Electrolytes, Plasma or serum
Methemoglobin, Blood
Myoglobin, Qualitative, Urine
Oximetry, Diagnostic
Toxicology drug screen, Blood or Urine

Carcinoma
(see Cancer)

Cardiogenic Shock
(see Shock)

Cardiomyopathy
Alanine aminotransferase, Serum
Aspartate aminotransferase, Serum
Biopsy, Site-specific (Right ventricular
   endomyocardium), Specimen (in
   children)
Cardiac catheterization, Diagnostic
Cardiac enzymes/isoenzymes, Blood
Cardiac output, Diagnostic
Chemistry profile, Blood
• Chest radiography, Diagnostic
Complete blood count, Blood
Computed tomography of the body
   (Abdomen), Diagnostic
Coronary intravascular ultrasonography,
   Diagnostic
Creatine kinase, Serum
Doppler ultrasonic flow studies
   (Transthoracic), Diagnostic
• Echocardiography, Diagnostic
Electrocardiography, Diagnostic
Electron microscopy (for Cardiomyopathy),
   Diagnostic

Histopathology, Specimen
Hydroxybutyrate dehydrogenase, Blood
Lactate dehydrogenase, Blood
Lactate dehydrogenase, Isoenzymes, Blood
Magnetic resonance imaging, Diagnostic
Natriuretic peptides, Plasma
Stress/exercise test, Diagnostic
Stress test, Pharmacologic, Diagnostic
Thyroid-stimulating hormone, Sensitive
  assay, Blood
Transesophageal ultrasonography,
  Diagnostic
Viral culture, Specimen

Carpal Tunnel Syndrome
Electromyography and nerve conduction
  studies, Diagnostic
• Magnetic resonance neurography,
  Diagnostic

Cat-Scratch Disease
• Biopsy, Site-specific (Lymph node),
  Specimen
Bone scan, Diagnostic
Complete blood count, Blood
Computed tomography of the body
  (Abdomen), Diagnostic
• Culture, Routine, Specimen
Differential leukocyte count, Peripheral
  blood
Liver battery, Serum
Lupus test, Blood
• *Rochalimaea henselae*, Antibody, Serum
Sedimentation rate, Erythrocyte, Blood
Skin test for hypersensitivity, Diagnostic

Cataracts
Galactokinase, Blood
Visual acuity test, Diagnostic

Celiac Sprue
Barium enema, Diagnostic
Barium swallow, Diagnostic
Biopsy, Site-specific (Small bowel/jejunum),
  Specimen
Carotene, Serum
Chemistry profile, Blood
Complete blood count, Blood
• D-Xylose absorption test, Diagnostic,
  Serum
• Endomysial antibody, Serum
• Fecal fat, Quantitative, 72-hour stool
Prothrombin time and INR, Blood
Raji cell immune complex assay, Blood
Red blood cell morphology, Blood
Red blood cell size distribution width, Blood
Sigmoidoscopy, Diagnostic

Cerebral Aneurysm
(see Aneurysm, Cerebral)

Cerebral Arteriovenous Malformations
• Magnetic resonance angiography,
  Diagnostic

Cerebral Infarction
(see Cerebrovascular accident)

Cerebral Infections
(see Encephalitis or Meningitis)

Cerebral Palsy
Ammonia, Blood and urine (Blood)
Brain ultrasonography, Diagnostic
Cerebral computed tomography, Diagnostic
Chloride, Serum
Chromosome analysis, Blood
Electroencephalography, Diagnostic
Electromyography and nerve conduction
  studies, Diagnostic
Magnetic resonance imaging (Brain, spinal
  cord), Diagnostic
• Potassium, Plasma or serum
• Sodium, Plasma, Serum or urine
Thyroid function test, Blood

Cerebrovascular Accident
Activated partial thromboplastin time and
  partial thromboplastin time, Plasma
Basic metabolic panel, Blood
Brain scan, Cerebral flow and pathology,
  Diagnostic
• Cerebral computed tomography,
  Diagnostic
Cerebrospinal fluid, Lactic acid, Specimen
Cerebrospinal fluid, Routine analysis,
  Specimen
Chest radiography, Diagnostic
Complete blood count, Blood
Computed tomography of the body
  (Spiral), Diagnostic
Creatine kinase, Serum
Differential leukocyte count, Peripheral
  blood
Doppler ultrasonographic flow studies
  (Carotid), Diagnostic
Electrocardiography, Diagnostic
Electrolytes, Plasma or serum
Homocysteine, Plasma or urine
Magnetic resonance angiography,
  Diagnostic
• Magnetic resonance imaging (of Brain)
  (Diffusion-weighted), Diagnostic
Magnetic resonance spectroscopy,
  Diagnostic
Oximetry, Diagnostic

Platelet count, Blood
Prothrombin time and international
  normalized ratio, Plasma
Transesophageal ultrasonography,
  Diagnostic

Cervical Cancer
• Cervical-vaginal cytology, Specimen
Colposcopy, Diagnostic
Conization of cervix, Diagnostic
Dual modality imaging, Diagnostic
Human papillomavirus in situ
  hybridization, Specimen
• Pap smear, Diagnostic
Pap smear, Ultrafast, Diagnostic
Squamous cell carcinoma antigen,
  Serum
Telomerase enzyme marker, Blood
Thymidylate synthase, Specimen
Urinary chorionic gonadotropin peptide,
  Urine

Cervical Spondylosis
Computed tomography of body (Spine),
  Diagnostic
• Magnetic resonance imaging, Diagnostic
Radiography (Cervical disks of spine),
  Diagnostic

Cervicitis
• Cervical-vaginal cytology, Specimen
Chlamydia culture and group titer,
  Specimen (Culture)
Chlamydia screening, Specimen
Genital, *Neisseria gonorrhoeae*, Culture
Herpesvirus antigen, Direct fluorescent
  antibody, Specimen
• Histopathology, Specimen
Human papillomavirus in situ
  hybridization, Specimen
Rapid plasma reagin test, Blood
Trichomonas preparation, Specimen
Urinary chorionic gonadotropin peptide,
  Urine
Urine culture and nucleic acid
  amplification tests for *Neisseria*
  gonorrhoeae, Urine
Venereal Disease Research Laboratory test,
  Serum

Chancroid
Culture, Routine, Specimen
• Genital, Bacillus *Haemophilus ducreyi*,
  Culture
Herpesvirus antigen, Direct fluorescent
  antibody, Specimen
Tzanck smear, Specimen

Venereal Disease Research Laboratory test,
  Serum
Viral culture, Specimen (for Herpes
  simplex)

Chest Pain
*(see Angina pectoris, Myocardial infarction,
Pleurisy, or Pneumonia)*

Chickenpox
Chest radiography, Diagnostic
Complete blood count, Blood
Differential leukocyte count, Peripheral
  blood
• Tzanck smear, Specimen
• Varicella-zoster virus serology, Serum
Viral culture, Specimen

Chlamydia
Cervical culture
Cervical-vaginal cytology, Specimen
Chlamydia culture and group titer,
  Specimen (Culture)
• *Chlamydia* screening, Specimen
Leukocyte esterase (see Urinalysis), Urine
Ocular cytology, Specimen

Cholecystitis
Alanine aminotransferase, Serum
Alkaline phosphatase, Serum
Amylase, Serum
Aspartate aminotransferase, Serum
• Bilirubin, Serum
Computed tomography of the body
  (Abdomen), Diagnostic
Differential leukocyte count, Peripheral
  blood
Endoscopic retrograde
  cholangiopancreatography, Diagnostic
• Gallbladder and biliary system
  ultrasonography, Diagnostic
Gamma-glutamyltranspeptidase, Blood
Glucose, Serum (Random)
Hepatobiliary scan, Diagnostic
Histopathology, Specimen
Ornithine carbamoyltransferase, Blood

Cholelithiasis
Alanine aminotransferase, Serum
Amylase, Serum
Bile, Urine
Bile fluid examination, Diagnostic
• Bilirubin, Serum
Chemistry profile, Blood
Chorionic villi sampling, Diagnostic
Endoscopic retrograde
  cholangiopancreatography, Diagnostic
Endoscopic ultrasonography, Diagnostic

Flat-plate radiography of the abdomen,
Diagnostic
• Gallbladder and biliary system
ultrasonography, Diagnostic
Histopathology, Specimen
Leucine aminopeptidase, Blood
Lipase, Serum
• Magnetic resonance
cholangiopancreatography, Diagnostic
T-tube cholangiography (Postoperative),
Diagnostic

Christmas Disease
(see Factor IX deficiency)

Chronic Fatigue Syndrome
Alanine aminotransferase, Serum
Albumin, Serum, Urine and 24-hour, Urine
(Serum)
Alkaline phosphatase, Serum
Calcium, Total, Serum
Complete blood count, Blood
Creatinine, Serum
Differential leukocyte count, Peripheral
blood
• Dexamethasone suppression test,
Diagnostic
Electrolytes, Plasma or serum
Glucose, Blood
Heterophile agglutinins, Blood
Phosphorus, Serum
Protein, Total, Serum
Sedimentation rate, Erythrocyte, Blood
Thyroid-stimulating hormone, Sensitive
assay, Blood
Urea nitrogen, Plasma or serum
Urinalysis, Urine

Chronic Obstructive Pulmonary Diseases
(see Bronchitis or Emphysema)

Cirrhosis
Alanine aminotransferase, Serum
• Albumin, Serum, Urine and 24-hour
urine
Albumin/globulin ratio, Serum
Aldosterone, Serum and urine
Alkaline phosphatase, Heat stable, Serum
Alkaline phosphatase, Isoenzymes, Serum
Alkaline phosphatase, Serum
Alpha$_1$-antitrypsin, Serum
Alpha-fetoprotein, Serum
• Ammonia, Blood
Antimitochondrial antibody, Blood
Antinuclear antibody, Serum
Anti–smooth muscle antibody, Serum

Antithrombin III test, Diagnostic
Aspartate aminotransferase, Serum
• Bilirubin, Direct, Serum
Ceruloplasmin, Serum
Chemistry profile, Blood
Cold agglutinin titer, Serum
Complete blood count, Blood
• Computed tomography of the body
(Abdomen, chest), Diagnostic
Copper, Serum or urine (Serum)
Cryoglobulin, Qualitative, Serum
Des-gamma-carboxy prothrombin, Serum
Electrolytes, Plasma or serum
Endoscopic retrograde
cholangiopancreatography, Diagnostic
Ferritin, Serum
Gamma-glutamyltranspeptidase, Blood
Hepatitis B surface antibody, Blood
Hepatitis B surface antigen, Blood
Hepatitis C antibody, Serum
Histopathology, Specimen
Immunoglobulin M, Serum
Iron, Serum
Iron and total iron-binding capacity/
transferrin, Serum
Lactate dehydrogenase, Blood
Lactate dehydrogenase, Isoenzymes, Blood
Leucine aminopeptidase, Blood
• Liver battery, Serum
Liver biopsy, Diagnostic
Liver ultrasonography, Diagnostic
Mucinlike carcinoma–associated antigen,
Blood
5′-Nucleotidase, Blood
Ornithine carbamoyltransferase, Blood
Protein electrophoresis, Serum
• Prothrombin time and international
normalized ratio, Plasma
Red blood cell morphology, Blood
Renal function tests, Diagnostic
Sodium, Serum
Urobilinogen, Urine
Zinc, Blood

Coarctation of the Aorta
Blood gases, Arterial, Blood
Cardiac catheterization, Diagnostic
• Chest radiography, Diagnostic
Echocardiography, Diagnostic
• Electrocardiography, Diagnostic

Coccidioidomycosis
Acquired immune deficiency syndrome
evaluation battery, Diagnostic
Biopsy, Site-specific (Lung, duodenum,
skin, skeleton), Specimen

Blood culture, Blood
Body fluid (Abscess), Anaerobic, Culture
Bone scan, Diagnostic
• Chest radiography, Diagnostic
• *Coccidioides* serology, Blood or CSF
• *Coccidioides* skin test, Diagnostic
Complete blood count, Blood
• Culture (Sputum, urine), Routine,
  Specimen
Eosinophil count, Blood
Sedimentation rate, Erythrocyte, Blood
Stool culture, Routine, Stool

Coccidiosis
(see Coccidioidomycosis)

Cold, Common
(see also Rhinitis)
Complete blood count, Blood
Viral culture, Specimen

Colitis
(see Ulcerative colitis)

Collagen Diseases
(see Arthritis, Autoimmune diseases, Rheumatoid arthritis, Scleroderma, Sjögren's syndrome, or Systemic lupus erythematosus)

Colorectal Cancer
Barium enema, Diagnostic
Brushing cytology, Specimen
CA 19-9, Blood
CA 50, Blood
CA 72-4, Blood
Calcium, Ionized, Blood
Calcium, Total, Serum
Carcinoembryonic antigen, Serum
Chest radiography, Diagnostic
• Colonoscopy, Diagnostic
Colorectal cancer allelotyping for
  chromosomes 17p and 18q, Specimen and
  blood
ColoSure test, Stool™
Complete blood count, Blood
Computed tomography of the body
  (Abdomen, pelvis), Diagnostic
Dual modality imaging, Diagnostic
Endoscopic ultrasonography, Diagnostic
Ferritin, Serum
• Histopathology, Specimen
• Immunochemical fecal occult blood
  testing, Stool
Iron and total iron-binding capacity/
  transferrin, Serum
K-ras, Blood or specimen
Liver battery, Serum
Microsatellite instability test, Specimen

Mitogen-activated protein kinase, Specimen
Occult blood, Stool
Sedimentation rate, Erythrocyte, Blood
  Telomerase enzyme marker, Blood
Thymidylate synthase, Specimen
Transferrin, Serum
Vascular endothelial growth factor,
  Specimen

Condyloma Latum
• Condyloma latum, Vulvar or anal culture
  for cytology, Specimen

Congenital Heart Disease
Denver Developmental Screening test II
Magnetic resonance angiography,
  Diagnostic
• Magnetic resonance imaging, Diagnostic
Mean platelet volume, Blood
Oximetry, Pulse, Diagnostic

Congestive Heart Failure
Alanine aminotransferase, serum
Albumin, Serum, Urine and 24-hour urine
Aspartate aminotransferase, Serum
Biopsy, Site-specific, Specimen
  (Endomyocardial) (limited situations)
Body fluid analysis, Cell count, Specimen
Cardiac enzymes/isoenzymes, Blood
• Chemistry profile, Blood
• Chest radiography, Diagnostic
Complete blood count, Blood
Comprehensive metabolic panel, Blood
Creatine kinase, Serum (Isoenzymes)
Diffusing capacity for carbon monoxide,
  Diagnostic
Digoxin, Serum
Disopyramide phosphate, Serum
• Echocardiography, Diagnostic
• Electrocardiography, Diagnostic
Electrolytes, Plasma or serum
Electrolytes, Urine
Gamma-glutamyltranspeptidase, Blood
Heart scan, Diagnostic
Lactate dehydrogenase, Isoenzymes, Blood
Lidocaine, Serum
Liver battery, Serum
• Natriuretic peptides (Atrial, B-Type),
  Plasma
Osmolality, Calculated test, Blood
Osmolality, Serum
Osmolality, Urine
Positron emission tomography, Diagnostic
Procainamide, Serum
Propranolol, Blood
Protein, Quantitative, Urine
Sedimentation rate, Erythrocyte, Blood

Sodium, Plasma or serum
Thyroid profile, Blood (TSH)
Transesophageal ultrasonography,
  Diagnostic
Troponin I, Plasma and troponin T, Serum
Urea nitrogen, Plasma or serum
Ventriculography, Diagnostic

Conjunctivitis
Chlamydia culture and group titer,
  Specimen (Culture)
• *Chlamydia* screening, Specimen
• Conjunctivae, Routine, Culture
Culture, Routine, Specimen
Ocular cytology, Specimen
Sjögren's antibodies, Blood

Constrictive Pericarditis
(see Pericarditis)

Convulsions
(see Seizures)

COPD
(see Bronchitis or Emphysema)

Coronary Artery Bypass Graft (CABG)
Activated coagulation time, Automated,
  Blood
Blood gases, Arterial, Blood
Cardiac catheterization, Diagnostic
Cardiac output, Diagnostic
Coronary intravascular ultrasonography,
  Diagnostic

Coronary Artery Disease
(see Arteriosclerosis)

Cough
Acid-fast bacteria, Culture and stain
  (Sputum)
• Chest radiography, Diagnostic
Complete blood count, Blood
Sputum, Gram stain, Diagnostic
Sputum culture and sensitivity, Specimen

Cretinism
(see Hypothyroidism)

Crohn's Disease
Albumin, Serum
Anti–neutrophil cytoplasmic antibody
  screen, Serum
Barium enema, Diagnostic
Biopsy, Site-specific, Specimen
Chemistry profile, Blood
Clostridium difficile toxin assay, Stool
• Colonoscopy, Diagnostic
Complete blood count, Blood
Computed tomography of the body
  (Abdomen), Diagnostic

C-reactive protein, Plasma or serum
• Cytologic study of gastrointestinal tract,
  Diagnostic
Electrolytes, Plasma or serum
Esophagogastroduodenoscopy, Diagnostic
Fecal fat, Quantitative, 72-hour stool
Flat-plate radiography of the abdomen,
  Diagnostic
Histopathology, Specimen
Muramidase, Serum
Occult blood, Stool
Oxalate, 24-hour urine
Parasite screen, Stool
Raji cell immune complex assay, Blood
Sedimentation rate, Erythrocyte, Blood
Sigmoidoscopy, Diagnostic
Small bowel series, Diagnostic
Upper gastrointestinal series, Diagnostic
Urea nitrogen, Plasma or serum
Vitamin B_{12}, Serum
Yersinia enterocolitica antibody, Blood

Cushing's Syndrome and Cushing's Disease
Adrenocorticotropic hormone, Serum
Aldosterone, Serum
Androstenedione, Serum
Calcitonin, Plasma or serum
Calcium, Urine
Chemistry profile, Blood
Chloride, Urine
Complete blood count, Blood
Computed tomography of the body
  (Adrenal glands), Diagnostic
• Cortisol, Plasma or serum (Late night)
• Cortisol, Urine
Creatinine, Serum
Creatinine, Urine
• Dexamethasone suppression test,
  Diagnostic
Differential leukocyte count, Peripheral
  blood
Electrolytes, Plasma or serum
Glucose, Blood
Glucose tolerance test, Blood
Histopathology, Specimen
17-Hydroxycorticosteroids, 24-hour urine
Low-density lipoprotein cholesterol,
  Blood
• Magnetic resonance imaging, Diagnostic
Metyrapone test, Plasma
Renin activity, Plasma
Sodium, Plasma or serum
Testosterone, Free, Bioavailable and total,
  Blood

Cutaneous Lupus Erythematosus
Biopsy, Site-specific (Skin), Specimen
Chemistry profile, Serum
Complete blood count, Blood
Lupus panel, Blood
Sedimentation rate, Erythrocyte, Blood
Urinalysis, Urine

CVA
(see Cerebrovascular accident)

Cyanosis
Bicarbonate, Blood
Blood gases, Capillary, Blood
• Blood gases, Venous, Blood
Carbon dioxide, Partial pressure, Blood
Carbon dioxide, Total content, Blood
Carboxyhemoglobin, Blood
Glucose, Blood
Heavy-metal drug screen, Blood and
    24-hour urine
5-Hydroxyindoleacetic acid, Quantitative,
    24-hour urine
Methemoglobin, Blood
Serotonin, Serum or blood

Cystectomy
*(see Surgery, Preoperative; Surgery,
Postoperative)*

Cystic Fibrosis
Albumin, Serum
Ashkenazi Jewish genetic carrier screening
    profile
Chest radiography, Diagnostic
• Chloride, Sweat, Specimen
Cystic fibrosis CFTR mutations, Specimen
D-Xylose absorption test, Diagnostic,
    Serum or urine
Electrolytes, Plasma or serum
Fat, Semiquantitative, Stool
Immunoglobulin E, Serum
Immunoglobulin G, Serum
Liver battery, Serum
Pulmonary function tests, Diagnostic
Semen analysis, Specimen
Sputum, Routine, Culture
Trypsin, Plasma or serum
Trypsin, Stool
Vitamin E_1, Serum

Cystitis
Body fluid (Urine), Routine, Culture
Cystoscopy, Diagnostic
Gram stain (Urine), Diagnostic
Histopathology, Specimen
Nitrite, Bacteria drug screen, Urine
Occult blood, Urine

Urinalysis, Fractional, Urine
• Urinalysis, Urine
Urine, Fungus, Culture
• Urine cytology, Urine

Cytomegalic Inclusion Disease
(see Cytomegalovirus)

Cytomegalovirus
Acquired immune deficiency syndrome
    evaluation battery, Diagnostic
Anti-RNP test, Diagnostic
Biopsy, Site-specific (Gastrointestinal tract,
    lungs, liver, skin), Specimen
Blood indices, Blood
Body fluid (Bronchoalveolar lavage, CSF,
    saliva, urine), Routine, Culture
Brushing cytology, Specimen
Chemistry profile, Blood
Chest radiography, Diagnostic
Complete blood count, Blood
Culture, routine, Specimen (Sputum)
Cytomegalic inclusion disease, Cytology,
    Urine
• Cytomegalovirus antibody, Serum
Differential leukocyte count, Peripheral
    blood
Endoscopy, Diagnostic
Heterophile agglutinins, Blood
Histopathology, Specimen
Infectious mononucleosis screening test,
    Blood
Magnetic resonance imaging (Brain),
    Diagnostic
Red blood cell, Blood
Sputum cytology, Specimen
Toxoplasmosis, Rubella, Cytomegalovirus,
    Herpesvirus serology, Blood
Urine cytology, Urine
• Viral culture, Specimen

Deafness
(see Hearing disorders)

Decubiti
Biopsy, Site-specific, Specimen (Anaerobic
    culture, routine culture)
Blood culture, Blood
Culture, Routine, Specimen

Deep Vein Thrombosis
Activated partial thromboplastin time and
    partial thromboplastin time, Plasma
Antiphospholipid antibodies, Serum
Antithrombin III test, Diagnostic
Arteriography, Diagnostic
Color duplex ultrasonography, Diagnostic
Compression ultrasound, Diagnostic

Computed tomography of the body
(Spiral), Diagnostic
D-Dimer test, Blood
• Doppler ultrasonographic flow studies,
Diagnostic
Factor V, (Leiden mutation), Blood
Fibrinogen, Plasma
Hemoglobin, Blood
^{125}I-Labeled fibrinogen leg scan, Diagnostic
Lung scan, Perfusion and ventilation,
Diagnostic
Magnetic resonance angiography,
Diagnostic
Magnetic resonance imaging, Diagnostic
Plasminogen assay, Blood
Platelet count, Blood
Protein C, Blood
Protein S, Total and free, Blood
Prothrombin time and international
normalized ratio, Plasma
Pulse volume recorder testing of peripheral
vasculature (Impedance
plethysmography), Diagnostic
Soluble fibrin monomer complex, Serum
Urinalysis, Urine
• Venography, Diagnostic

Degenerative Arthritis
(see Cervical spondylosis)

**Degenerative Disorders of
Nervous System**
(see Alzheimer's disease)

Degenerative Joint Disease
(see Osteoarthritis)

Dehydration
(see Hypovolemia)

Delirium Tremens
• Alcohol, Blood
Electrolytes, Plasma or serum

Dementia
Brain scan, Cerebral flow and pathology,
Diagnostic
Cerebral computed tomography,
Diagnostic
Cerebrospinal fluid, Routine analysis,
Specimen
• Chemistry profile, Blood
Chest radiography, Diagnostic
• Complete blood count, Blood
Drug levels
Electroencephalography, Diagnostic
Electrolytes, Plasma or serum
Folic acid, Serum

HIV antibodies (see Acquired immune
deficiency syndrome evaluation battery,
Diagnostic)
Lipid profile, Blood
Liver battery, Serum
Magnetic resonance imaging, Diagnostic
• Magnetic resonance spectroscopy,
Diagnostic
Rapid plasma reagin test, Blood
Sedimentation rate, Erythrocyte, Blood
• Thyroid profile, Blood
Transcranial Doppler ultrasonography,
Diagnostic
Venereal Disease Research Laboratory test,
Cerebrospinal fluid, Specimen
Venereal Disease Research Laboratory test,
Serum
Vitamin B_1, Serum or urine
Vitamin B_{12}, Serum

Demyelinization
(see Multiple sclerosis)

Dengue Fever
Differential leukocyte count, Peripheral
blood
• Immune complex assay, Blood

Depressant Drug Abuse
*(see Drug abuse: Barbiturates, Meprobamate,
and Methaqualone)*

Depression
Chemistry profile, Blood
Chromosome analysis, Blood
Complete blood count, Blood
Cortisol, Plasma or serum
• Dexamethasone suppression test,
Diagnostic
Electrocardiography, Diagnostic
Electroencephalography, Diagnostic
Liver battery, Serum
Selective serotonin reuptake inhibitors,
Blood
Serotonin, Serum or blood
Thyroid function testing, Blood
Urinalysis, Urine

Dermatitis
Allergen-specific IgE, Serum
Antinuclear antibody, Serum
Biopsy (Punch biopsy of the skin),
Site-specific, Specimen
Chromium, Serum
Complete blood count, Blood
Differential leukocyte count, Peripheral
blood
Eosinophil count, Blood

Heavy-metal screen, 24-hour urine
• Histopathology, Specimen
Immunoglobulin E, Serum
Porphyrins, Quantitative, Blood
Skin, Fungus, Culture

Diabetes, Gestational
• Glucose tolerance test, Blood

Diabetes Insipidus
Antidiuretic hormone, Serum
Chloride, Sweat, Specimen
• Concentration test, Urine
Creatinine, Serum
Cyclic adenosine monophosphate, Urine
Electrolytes, Plasma or serum
Glucose, Blood
Intravenous pyelography, Diagnostic
Magnetic resonance imaging, Diagnostic
• Osmolality, Calculated test, Blood
Osmolality, Serum
Osmolality, Urine
• Sodium, Plasma or serum
• Sodium, Urine
Specific gravity, Urine
Urea nitrogen, Plasma or Serum

Diabetes Mellitus
Anion gap, Blood
Body fluid (Urine), Routine, Culture
Chemistry profile, Blood
Complete blood count, Blood
C-peptide, Serum
C-reactive protein, Plasma or serum
Creatinine, Serum
Creatinine clearance, Serum, Urine
Differential leukocyte count, Peripheral
  blood
Electrocardiography, Diagnostic
Electrolytes, Plasma or serum
Electrolytes, Urine
Endomysial antibody, Serum
Ferritin, Serum
Fructosamine, Serum
Glucagon, Plasma
• Glucose, Blood
Glucose, Qualitative, Semiquantitative,
  Urine
Glucose, Quantitative, 24-hour urine
Glucose, 2-hour postprandial, Serum
Glucose-monitoring machines, Diagnostic
Glucose tolerance test, Blood (for screening
  for gestational diabetes mellitus)
• Glycosylated hemoglobin, Blood (Hb A_{1c})
Insulin and insulin antibodies, Blood
Ketone, Semiquantitative, Urine
Ketone bodies, Blood

Lactic acid, Blood
Lipid profile, Blood
Magnesium, Serum
Magnetic resonance spectroscopy,
  Diagnostic
Osmolality, Urine
Potassium, Plasma or serum
Protein electrophoresis, Serum
Red blood cell, Blood
Triglycerides, Blood
Urea nitrogen, Plasma or serum
Urinalysis, Urine
Urine, Fungus, Culture

Diabetic Glomerulosclerosis
Albumin, Serum, Urine and 24-hour urine
  (Urine)
Creatinine, Serum
Creatinine clearance, Serum, Urine
Electrolytes, Plasma or serum
Glycosylated hemoglobin, Blood
Kidney biopsy, Specimen
Kidney ultrasonography, Diagnostic
• Protein, Quantitative, Urine
Urea nitrogen, Plasma or serum
Urinalysis, Urine

Diabetic Ketoacidosis
• Anion gap, Blood
• Beta-hydroxybutyrate, Blood
• Blood gases (pH), Arterial, Blood
• Chemistry profile, Blood
Chest radiography, Diagnostic
• Complete blood count, Blood
Culture (Urine), Routine, Specimen
Electrolytes, Plasma or serum
• Glucose, Serum
Osmolality, Serum
Phosphate, Serum
Potassium, Plasma or serum
Urea nitrogen, Plasma or serum

Dialysis, Hemo-
Activated coagulation time, Automated,
  Blood
Activated partial thromboplastin time and
  partial thromboplastin time, Plasma
Complete blood count, Blood
Creatinine, Serum
Electrolytes, Plasma or serum
Lee-White clotting time, Blood
Parathyroid hormone, Blood
Urea nitrogen, Plasma or serum

Dialysis, Peritoneal
Complete blood count, Blood
Creatinine, Serum

Electrolytes, Plasma or serum
Urea nitrogen, Plasma or serum

Diarrhea
Albumin, Serum
Carotene, Serum
C-difficile amplified probe, Stool
Chemistry profile, Blood
Clostridial toxin, Serum
Clostridium difficile toxin assay, Stool
Colonoscopy, Diagnostic
Cortisol, Plasma or serum
Cryptosporidium diagnostic procedures, Stool
D-Xylose absorption test, Diagnostic, Serum or urine
• Electrolytes, Plasma or serum
Entamoeba histolytica serologic test, Blood
Fat, Semiquantitative, Stool
Fecal fat, Quantitative, 72-hour stool
Fecal leukocytes, Stool, Diagnostic
Gastrin, Serum
Glucagon, Plasma
Glucose, 2-hour postprandial, Serum
Histopathology, Specimen
Homovanillic acid, 24-hour urine
5-Hydroxyindoleacetic acid, Quantitative, 24-hour urine
Magnesium, Serum
Mycoplasma titer, Blood
Occult blood, Stool
Osmolality, Calculated test, Blood
Osmolality, Serum
Osmolality, Urine
Ova and parasites, Stool
pH, Stool
Phenolphthalein test, Diagnostic
Reducing substances, Stool
Rotavirus antigen, Stool
Serotonin, Serum or blood
Specific gravity, Urine
• Stool culture, Routine, Stool
Thyroid profile, Blood
Vasoactive intestinal polypeptide, Blood
Yersinia enterocolitica antibody, Blood

DIC
(see Disseminated intravascular coagulation)

Diphtheria
Gram stain, Diagnostic
• Schick test for diphtheria, Diagnostic
Throat culture for *Corynebacterium diphtheriae*, Culture

Disaccharide Deficiencies
• D-Xylose absorption test, Diagnostic, Serum or urine
pH, Stool
• Reducing substances, Stool
Rotavirus antigen, Stool

Discoid Lupus Erythematosus
(see Systemic lupus erythematosus)

Disseminated Intravascular Coagulation
Activated coagulation time, Automated, Blood
• Activated partial thromboplastin time and partial thromboplastin time, Plasma
Antithrombin III test, Diagnostic
C3 proactivator, Serum
Chest radiography, Diagnostic
• Complete blood count, Blood
• D-Dimer test, Blood
Differential leukocyte count, Peripheral blood
• Fibrinogen, Plasma
Fibrinogen breakdown products, Blood
Fibrinopeptide A, Blood
Fibrin split products, Protamine sulfate test, Blood
Haptoglobin, Serum
Intravascular coagulation screen, Blood
Plasminogen assay, Blood
Protein C, Blood
Protein S, Total and free, Blood
• Prothrombin time and international normalized ratio, Plasma
Red blood cell morphology, Blood
• Soluble fibrin monomer complex, Serum
Thrombin time, Serum

Diverticulitis and Diverticulosis
Barium enema, Diagnostic
Blood indices, Blood
• Colonoscopy, Diagnostic
Complete blood count, Blood
Compression ultrasound, Diagnostic
Computed tomography of the body (Abdomen), Diagnostic
Differential leukocyte count, Peripheral blood
Fecal leukocytes, Stool, Diagnostic
Histopathology, Specimen
Occult blood, Stool
Red blood cell, Blood
• Sigmoidoscopy, Diagnostic
Urinalysis, Urine

Down Syndrome

Amniotic fluid, Chromosome analysis, Specimen
Chorionic villi sampling, Specimen
• Chromosome analysis (Chromosome 21), Blood
Urinary chorionic gonadotropin peptide, Urine

Dracunculiasis

Culture, Skin, Specimen
Eosinophil count, Blood
Radiography, Diagnostic

Drowning, Near

Blood culture, Blood
• Blood gases, Arterial, Blood
Cerebral computed tomography, Diagnostic
Chest radiography, Diagnostic
Complete blood count, Blood
Drug screen, Blood
Electrocardiography, Diagnostic
Electroencephalography, Diagnostic
Electrolytes, Plasma or serum
Glucose, Blood
Radiography of the skull, chest, and cervical spine (Cross-table neck radiography), Diagnostic
Toxicology, Drug screen, Blood or urine

Drug Abuse

(Includes Cannabis, Depressants, Ethanol, Hallucinogens, Narcotics, Stimulants)
Acetaminophen, Serum
Alcohol, Blood
Barbiturates, Quantitative, Blood
Blood fungus, Culture
• Blood gases, Arterial, Blood
Cannabinoids, Qualitative, Blood or urine
Carbamazepine, Blood
Chlordiazepoxide, Blood
Clonazepam, Blood
Cocaine, Blood
Cytologic study of gastrointestinal tract, Diagnostic
Diazepam, Serum
Ethchlorvynol, Blood
Ethosuximide, Blood
Fluorescent treponemal antibody–absorbed double-stain test, Serum
Flurazepam, Serum
Gamma-hydroxybutyric acid, Blood or urine
Glutethimide, Blood
Hepatitis B surface antigen, Blood
Lidocaine, Serum

Lithium, Serum
• Liver battery, Serum
Meprobamate, Blood
Methaqualone, Blood
Methyprylon, Serum
Morphine, Urine
Phencyclidine, Qualitative, Urine
Phenobarbital, Plasma or serum
Phenothiazines, Blood
Phenytoin, Serum
Primidone, Serum
Rapid plasma reagin test, Blood
Salicylate, Blood
• Toxicology, Drug screen, Blood or urine
Toxicology, Volatiles group by GLC, Blood or urine
Tricyclic antidepressants, Plasma or serum

Drug Withdrawal

(see Drug abuse)

Dry Eyes

Fluorescein angiography, Diagnostic
Ocular impression cytology, Specimen
• Schirmer's tearing eye test, Diagnostic

Duchenne Muscular Dystrophy

Aldolase, Serum
Aspartate aminotransferase, Serum
Creatine kinase, Serum (Isoenzymes)
• Muscle biopsy, Specimen

Duodenal Ulcer

(see also Helicobacter pylori)
ABO group and Rh type, Blood
Amylase, Serum
Barium swallow, Diagnostic
Complete blood count, Blood
• Esophagogastroduodenoscopy, Diagnostic
Gastrin, Serum
• Helicobacter pylori, Quick office serology, Serum and titer, Blood
Histopathology, Specimen
Pepsinogen I and pepsinogen II, Blood
Upper gastrointestinal series, Diagnostic
Urea breath test, Diagnostic

Dwarfism

(see Hypopituitarism)

Dysentery

Computed tomography of the body (Abdomen), Diagnostic
• Entamoeba histolytica serologic test, Blood
Fecal leukocytes, Stool, Diagnostic
Liver biopsy, Diagnostic
• Ova and parasites, Stool
Parasite drug screen, Stool
Stool culture, Routine, Stool

Dyserythropoietic Anemia
Blood indices, Blood
Bone marrow aspiration analysis,
  Diagnostic
Complete blood count, Blood
Differential leukocyte count, Peripheral
  blood
Ham's test, Diagnostic
Haptoglobin, Serum
Red blood cell, Blood
• Red blood cell morphology, Blood
Sucrose hemolysis test, Diagnostic

Dysfibrinogenemia
Activated partial thromboplastin time and
  partial thromboplastin time, Plasma
• Fibrinogen, Plasma
Fibrin split products, Protamine sulfate
  test, Blood
Prothrombin time and international
  normalized ratio, Plasma
Reptilase time, Serum
• Thrombin time, Serum

Dysmenorrhea
Complete blood count, Blood
Dilation and curettage, Diagnostic
• Estrogens, Serum and 24-hour urine
Gynecologic ultrasonography, Diagnostic
Herpesvirus antigen, Direct fluorescent
  antibody, Specimen
Human chorionic gonadotropin, Serum
Iron, Serum
Laparoscopy, Diagnostic
Total iron-binding capacity, Serum
• Urinalysis, Urine
Urine culture and nucleic acid amplification
  tests for *Neisseria gonorrhoeae*, Urine
Venereal Disease Research Laboratory test,
  Serum

Dyspepsia
Biopsy, Site-specific (Gastric mucosa),
  Specimen
• Esophageal acidity test, Diagnostic
• Esophagogastroduodenoscopy, Diagnostic
Gastric analysis, Specimen
Gastric pH, Specimen
Gastrin, Serum
• *Helicobacter pylori*, Quick office serology,
  Serum and titer, Blood

Dysphagia
• Esophageal manometry, Diagnostic

Dyspnea
Bicarbonate, Blood
• Blood gases, Arterial, Blood

Carbon dioxide, Partial pressure, Blood
Carbon monoxide, Blood
Carboxyhemoglobin, Blood
• Chest radiography, Diagnostic
• Complete blood count, Blood
Diffusing capacity for carbon monoxide,
  Diagnostic
Heavy metals, Blood and 24-hour urine
Methemoglobin, Blood
• Natriuretic peptides, Plasma
pCO_2, Blood

Dysproteinemia
Blood indices, Blood
Bone marrow aspiration analysis,
  Diagnostic
Chemistry profile, Blood
Complete blood count, Blood
Differential leukocyte count, Peripheral
  blood
Globulin, Serum
Immunoelectrophoresis, Serum and urine
Immunoglobulin A, Serum
Immunoglobulin D, Serum
Immunoglobulin E, Serum
Immunoglobulin M, Serum
Platelet aggregation, Blood
Platelet aggregation, Hypercoagulable state,
  Blood
• Protein electrophoresis, Serum
Protein electrophoresis, Urine
Red blood cell, Blood
• Urinalysis, Urine
Viscosity, Serum

Dysrhythmias
Amiodarone, Plasma or serum
Bicarbonate, Blood
Biopsy, Site-specific, Specimen
  (Endomyocardial) (unexplained atrial
  fibrillation or unexplained ventricular
  arrhythmias)
Blood gases, Arterial, Blood
Calcium, Total, Serum
Carbon dioxide, Partial pressure, Blood
Digoxin, Serum
Disopyramide phosphate, Serum
• Electrocardiography, Diagnostic
Electrolytes, Plasma or serum (Plasma)
Electrophysiologic study, Diagnostic
FAMILION® test, Blood (Long QT
  syndrome)
Flecainide, Plasma or serum
Holter monitor, Diagnostic
Lidocaine, Serum
Magnesium, Serum

Natriuretic peptides, Plasma
Potassium, Plasma or serum
Procainamide, Serum
Propranolol, Blood
Quinidine, Serum
Signal-averaged electrocardiography,
 Diagnostic

Dysuria

Body fluid (Urine), Routine, Culture
Chlamydia culture and group titer,
 Specimen (Culture)
Chlamydia screening, Specimen
Cystoscopy, Diagnostic
Nitrite, Bacteria drug screen, Urine
Occult blood, Urine
Trichomonas preparation, Specimen
• Urinalysis, Urine

Eating Disorders

Bone densitometry, Diagnostic
Complete blood count, Blood
Comprehensive metabolic panel, Blood
Electrocardiography, Diagnostic
Estradiol, Serum (Females)
Follicle-stimulating hormone, Serum
 (Females)
Luteinizing hormone, Blood
Pregnancy test, Routine, Serum and
 Qualitative, Urine (If sexually active)
Thyroid function tests, Blood

Ecchymosis (Spontaneous)

• Activated partial thromboplastin time and
 partial thromboplastin time, Plasma
Bleeding time, Duke, Blood
Bleeding time, Ivy, Blood
Des-gamma-carboxy prothrombin, Serum
Factor VIII, Blood
Factor VIII R:Ag, Blood
Fibrinogen, Plasma
Fibrinogen breakdown products, Blood
Platelet aggregation, Blood
Platelet aggregation, Hypercoagulable state,
 Blood
• Platelet count, Blood
• Prothrombin time and international
 normalized ratio, Plasma
Salicylate, Blood

Echinococcosis

Bile fluid examination, Diagnostic
Cerebrospinal fluid, Cytology specimen
Computed tomography of the body
 (Abdomen, liver), Diagnostic
• Echinococcosis serologic test, Blood
Histopathology, Specimen

Eclampsia (Toxemia)

Activated partial thromboplastin time and
 partial thromboplastin time, Plasma
Albumin, 24-hour urine
Complete blood count, Blood
Creatinine, Serum
D-Dimer test, Blood
Electrolytes, Plasma or serum
Glucose, Qualitative and semiquantitative,
 Urine
Hematocrit, Blood
Liver battery, Diagnostic
Low-density lipoprotein cholesterol, Blood
• Protein, Quantitative, Urine
Prothrombin time and international
 normalized ratio, Serum
Sodium, Plasma, Serum
Urea nitrogen, Plasma or serum
Uric acid, Serum

Ectopic Hyperparathyroidism

Bone densitometry, Diagnostic
Calcium, Ionized, Serum
• Calcium, Total, Serum
Calcium, Urine
Chemistry profile, Blood
• Parathyroid hormone, Blood (Intact)
• Phosphorus, Serum
Sputum cytology, Specimen

Ectopic Pregnancy

• Gynecologic ultrasound, Diagnostic
Histopathology, Specimen
Human chorionic gonadotropin, Beta-
 subunit, Serum
Laparoscopy, Diagnostic
• Pregnancy test, Routine, Serum and
 qualitative, Urine
Type and crossmatch, Blood (Screen)

Eczema

Allergen-specific IgE antibody, Serum
Eosinophil count, Blood
• Histopathology, Specimen
Immunoglobulin E, Serum

Edema

Albumin/globulin ratio, Serum
Chemistry profile, Blood
• Electrolytes, Plasma or serum
Magnetic resonance imaging, Diagnostic
Osmolality, Serum
Osmolality, Urine
• Protein, Total, Serum

Effusions, Abdominal

Body fluid, Amylase, Specimen
Body fluid, Anaerobic, Culture

Body fluid, Glucose, Specimen
Body fluid analysis, Cell count, Specimen
• Body fluid cytology, Specimen
Flat-plate radiography of the abdomen,
  Diagnostic
Gram stain (Effusion specimen),
  Diagnostic
• Paracentesis, Diagnostic
Sputum, Routine, Culture
Synovial fluid analysis, Diagnostic

Effusions, Pericardial

Body fluid analysis, Specimen
Body fluid cytology, Specimen
• Chest radiography, Diagnostic
• Echocardiography, Diagnostic
Electrocardiography, Diagnostic
Pericardiocentesis, Diagnostic

Effusions, Pleural

• Blood gases, Arterial, Blood
Body fluid, Anaerobic, Culture
Body fluid, Glucose, Specimen
Body fluid analysis, Cell count, Specimen
Body fluid analysis, Specimen
Body fluid cytology, Specimen
• Chest radiography, Diagnostic
Computed tomography of the body
  (Lung), Diagnostic
Fluoroscopy, Diagnostic
Gram stain (Effusion specimen),
  Diagnostic
Sputum, Routine, Culture
Synovial fluid analysis, Diagnostic
Thoracentesis, Diagnostic

Embolectomy

(see Fat embolism or Pulmonary embolism)

Emphysema

Alpha₁-antitrypsin, Serum
Bicarbonate, Blood
Blood gases, Arterial, Blood
Carbon dioxide, Partial pressure, Blood
Carbon dioxide, Total content, Blood
• Chest radiography, Diagnostic
Complete blood count, Blood
Diffusing capacity for carbon monoxide,
  Diagnostic
Digoxin, Serum
Electrolytes, Plasma or serum (Plasma)
Histopathology, Specimen
Low-density lipoprotein cholesterol, Blood
Natriuretic peptides, Plasma
• Pulmonary function tests, Diagnostic
Sputum cytology, Specimen
Theophylline, Blood

Empyema

Blood gases, Arterial, Blood
Body fluid, Anaerobic, Culture
Body fluid, Fungus, Culture
Body fluid, Mycobacteria, Culture
Body fluid, Routine, Culture
Body fluid analysis (pH), Specimen
• Body fluid cytology, Specimen
Chest radiography, Diagnostic
C-reactive protein, Plasma or serum
• Gram stain (Empyema specimen),
  Diagnostic
Thoracentesis, Diagnostic

Encephalitis

California encephalitis virus titer, Serum
Cerebral computed tomography, Diagnostic
Cerebrospinal fluid, Immunoglobulin G,
  Immunoglobulin G ratios and
  immunoglobulin G index,
  Immunoglobulin G synthesis rate,
  Specimen
• Cerebrospinal fluid, Protein, Specimen
• Cerebrospinal fluid, Routine analysis,
  Specimen
Eastern equine encephalitis virus titer,
  Specimen
Electroencephalography, Diagnostic
Herpesvirus antigen, Direct fluorescent
  antibody, Specimen
Lumbar puncture, Diagnostic
Magnetic resonance imaging (Brain),
  Diagnostic
Rubeola serology, Serum
St. Louis encephalitis virus serology,
  Serum
Toxoplasmosis, Rubella, Cytomegalovirus,
  Herpesvirus serology, Blood
Toxoplasmosis serology, Serum
Venezuelan equine encephalitis virus
  serology, Serum
Viral culture, Specimen
Western equine encephalitis virus serology,
  Serum

Encephalopathy

Ammonia, Serum
Cerebral angiography, Diagnostic
Chemistry profile, Blood
Computed tomography of brain,
  Diagnostic
Electroencephalography, Diagnostic
Electrolytes, Plasma or serum
Doppler ultrasonographic flow studies,
  Diagnostic
• Magnetic resonance imaging, Diagnostic

Magnetic resonance spectroscopy,
  Diagnostic
Urea nitrogen, Plasma or serum

Endocarditis
(see also Subacute bacterial endocarditis)
Anti-DNA, Serum
Antinuclear antibody, Serum
• Blood culture, Blood
Blood culture with antimicrobial removal
  device, Culture
Blood fungus, Culture
Blood indices, Blood
Clq immune complex detection, Serum
C3 complement, Serum
C4 complement, Serum
Chemistry profile, Blood
Chest radiography, Diagnostic
Complement, Total, Serum
Complete blood count, Blood
C-reactive protein, Plasma or serum
Differential leukocyte count, Peripheral
  blood
• Echocardiography, Diagnostic
Electrocardiography, Diagnostic
5-Hydroxyindoleacetic acid, Quantitative,
  24-hour urine
Immune complex assay, Blood
Minimum bactericidal concentration,
  Culture
Red blood cell, Blood
Rheumatoid factor, Blood
Schlichter test (Body fluid), Diagnostic
• Sedimentation rate, Erythrocyte, Blood
Serotonin, Serum or blood
Teichoic acid antibody, Blood
Transesophageal ultrasonography,
  Diagnostic
• Urinalysis, Urine

Endocrine Tumors
*(see also Addison's disease, Cushing's
syndrome, Hashimoto's thyroiditis,
Hyperparathyroidism, Hyperpituitarism,
Hyperthyroidism, Hypothyroidism, and
Insulinoma)*
Computed tomography of the body,
  Diagnostic
Endoscopic ultrasonography, Diagnostic
Immunoperoxidase procedures,
  Diagnostic
• Magnetic resonance imaging, Diagnostic

Endometritis (Endometriosis)
Body fluid (Abscess), Anaerobic, Culture
CA 125, Blood
Endometrium, Anaerobic, Culture

Foreign body, Routine, Culture
Genital, *Candida albicans*, Culture
Genital, *Neisseria gonorrhoeae*, Culture
• Histopathology, Specimen
• Laparoscopy, Diagnostic

Enteric Fever
• Blood culture, Blood
Complete blood count, Blood
Stool culture, Routine, Stool

Epididymitis
Histopathology, Specimen
• Urinalysis, Urine

Epiglottitis
Blood culture, Blood
• Culture (Throat, nose), Routine,
  Specimen
Culture for *Haemophilus* species, Sputum
Radiography of the skull, chest, and
  cervical spine (Cross-table neck
  radiography), Diagnostic

Epilepsy
Body fluid analysis (Cerebrospinal fluid),
  Cell count, Specimen
Brain scan, Cerebral flow and pathology,
  Diagnostic
Carbamazepine, Blood
Cerebral computed tomography,
  Diagnostic
Cerebrospinal fluid, Glucose, Specimen
Cerebrospinal fluid, Routine, Culture and
  cytology
Clonazepam, Blood
Diazepam, Serum
• Electroencephalography, Diagnostic
Ethosuximide, Blood
• Magnetic resonance imaging, Diagnostic
Mephenytoin, Blood
Methsuximide, Serum
Phenobarbital, Plasma or serum
Phenytoin, Serum
Primidone, Serum
Valproic acid, Blood

Epistaxis
• Activated partial thromboplastin time and
  partial thromboplastin time, Plasma
Bleeding time, Duke, Blood
Bleeding time, Ivy, Blood
• Complete blood count, Blood
Hematocrit, Blood
Hemoglobin, Blood
Platelet count, Blood
Red blood cell morphology, Blood
Thrombin time, Serum

Epstein-Barr Virus
Complete blood count, Blood
Differential leukocyte count, Peripheral
  blood
• Epstein-Barr virus, Serology, Blood
Heterophile agglutinins, Blood
• Infectious mononucleosis screening test,
  Blood

Erectile Dysfunction
Electromyography (of the Penis), Diagnostic
Glucose, Blood
• Glycosylated hemoglobin Hb A$_{1c}$, Blood
Lipid profile, Blood
Prolactin, Serum
Pulse volume recording of peripheral
  vasculature, Diagnostic
Testosterone, Free, Bioavailable and total,
  Blood

Erythroblastosis Fetalis
• ABO group and Rh type, Blood
Amniotic fluid, Erythroblastosis fetalis,
  Specimen

Esophageal Atresia with Tracheoseptal Fistula
• Blood gases, Arterial, Blood
• Esophagogastroduodenoscopy, Diagnostic
Flat-plate radiography of abdomen,
  Diagnostic

Esophageal Cancer
Biopsy, Site-specific, Specimen
Brushing cytology, Specimen
CA 19-9, Blood
CA 72-4, Blood
Carcinoembryonic antigen, Blood
Dual modality imaging, Diagnostic
Endoscopic ultrasonography, Diagnostic
Esophageal radiography, Diagnostic
• Esophagogastroduodenoscopy, Diagnostic
• Histopathology, Specimen
Squamous cell carcinoma antigen, Serum
Telomerase enzyme marker, Blood
Thymidylate synthase, Specimen
Washing cytology, Specimen

Esophageal Varices
(see Varices)

Esophagitis
Biopsy, Site-specific, Specimen (Fungus
  culture)
Brushing cytology, Specimen
Endoscopic ultrasonography, Diagnostic
Esophageal radiography, Diagnostic
• Esophagogastroduodenoscopy, Diagnostic

Herpesvirus antigen, Direct fluorescent
  antibody, Specimen
Histopathology, Specimen

Ethylene Glycol Poisoning
• Anion gap, Blood
Bicarbonate, Blood
• Chemistry profile, Blood
• Electrolytes, Plasma or serum
Heavy metals, Blood
Osmolality, Calculated tests, Blood
  (Osmolar gap)
• Toxicology, Volatiles group by GLC, Blood
  or urine
Urea nitrogen, Plasma or serum

ETOH
(see Alcoholism and Drug abuse)

Factor Deficiency
Activated partial thromboplastin
  substitution test, Diagnostic
Activated partial thromboplastin time and
  partial thromboplastin time, Plasma
• Coagulation factor assay, Blood
Factor, Fitzgerald, Plasma
Factor, Fletcher, Plasma
Factor II, Blood
Factor V, Blood
Factor VII, Blood
Factor VIII, Blood
Factor VIII R:Ag, Blood
Factor IX, Blood
Factor X, Blood
Factor XI, Blood
Factor XII, Blood
Factor XIII, Blood
Fibrinogen, Plasma
Prothrombin time and international
  normalized ratio, Serum
Thrombin time, Serum
von Willebrand factor antigen, Blood
von Willebrand factor assay, Blood

Factor V Deficiency
• Coagulation factor assay, Blood
Factor V, Blood

Factor IX Deficiency (Christmas Disease)
Activated partial thromboplastin time and
  partial thromboplastin time, Plasma
Circulating anticoagulant, Blood
• Coagulation factor assay, Blood
Factor XII, Blood
Plasma recalcification time, Plasma
Prothrombin time and international
  normalized ratio, Plasma

Factor XIII Deficiency

Activated partial thromboplastin time
and partial thromboplastin time,
Plasma
• Coagulation factor assay, Blood
Factor VIII, Blood
Factor VIII R:Ag, Blood
Plasma recalcification time, Plasma
Prothrombin time and international
normalized ratio, Plasma
von Willebrand factor antigen, Blood
von Willebrand factor assay, Blood

Failure to Thrive

Blood gases, Arterial, Blood
Body fluid (Urine), Routine, Culture
• Complete blood count, Blood
Creatinine, Serum
Fat, Semiquantitative, Stool
Growth hormone and growth hormone–
releasing hormone, Blood
Ova and parasites, Stool
• Transthyretin (Prealbumin), Serum
Urea nitrogen, Plasma or serum

Familial Dysautonomia

Ashkenazi Jewish genetic carrier screening
profile

Fanconi Syndrome

Alkaline phosphatase, Serum
Anion gap, Blood
Ashkenazi Jewish genetic carrier screening
profile
Blood gases, Venous, Blood
Calcium, Urine
Chemistry profile, Blood
Complete blood count, Blood
Electrolytes, Plasma or serum
Glucose, Semiquantitative, Urine
Ketone, Semiquantitative, Urine
pH, Urine
• Phosphorus, Serum
Phosphorus, Urine
Protein, Quantitative, Urine
Uric acid, Serum

Farmer's Lung

• Chest radiography, Diagnostic
• Hypersensitivity pneumonitis serology,
Blood

Fascioliasis

• Differential leukocyte count, Peripheral
blood
Eosinophil count, Blood
Liver scan, Diagnostic

Fat Embolism

Bicarbonate, Blood
Blood gases, Arterial, Blood
Carbon dioxide, Total content, Blood
Chemistry profile, Blood
Complete blood count, Blood
Electrolytes, Plasma or serum
Lipase, Serum
• Radiography, Diagnostic
• Venography, Diagnostic

Fatigue

*(see also Cancer, Chronic fatigue syndrome,
Depression, Infectious mononucleosis,
Myasthenia gravis, Sleep disorders, and
Systemic lupus erythematosus)*
Alcohol, Blood
• Complete blood count, Blood
Liver battery, Serum
Thyroid profile, Blood

Fatty Liver

(see Liver dysfunction)

Febrile Diseases

(see Fever of undetermined origin)

Fetal Diseases

(see Pregnancy)

Fever of Undetermined Origin

Acid-fast stain, *Nocardia* species, Culture
Anti-DNA, Serum
Antinuclear antibody, Serum
Biopsy, Site-specific, Specimen
(Mycobacteria culture)
• Blood culture, Blood
Blood culture with antimicrobial removal
device, Culture
Body fluid (Urine), Routine, Culture
Bone marrow aspiration analysis, Specimen
Borrelia burgdorferi C6 peptide antibody,
Serum
Chest radiography, Diagnostic
C-reactive protein, Plasma or serum
• Differential leukocyte count, Peripheral
blood
Histopathology, Specimen
Malaria smear, Blood
Salmonella titer, Blood
Sedimentation rate, Erythrocyte, Blood

Fibrinolysis

D-Dimer test, Blood
Euglobulin clot lysis, Blood
Fibrinogen, Plasma
Fibrinogen breakdown products, Blood
Intravascular coagulation screen, Blood
• Plasminogen assay, Blood

Fibrinopenia
Cryofibrinogen, Serum and plasma
• Fibrinogen, Plasma
Intravascular coagulation screen, Blood
Reptilase time, Serum
Thrombin time, Serum

Fibrocystic Breast
Estrogens, Serum and 24-hour urine
Histopathology, Specimen
• Mammography, Diagnostic
Nipple discharge cytology, Specimen
Scintimammography, Diagnostic

Flank Pain
Antegrade pyelography, Diagnostic
Complete blood count, Blood
Comprehensive metabolic panel, Blood
Computed tomography of the body,
  Diagnostic
Flat-plate radiograph of the abdomen,
  Diagnostic
Intravenous pyelography, Diagnostic
• Kidney ultrasound, Diagnostic
Liver ultrasound, Diagnostic
Magnetic resonance urography, Diagnostic
Nephrotomography, Diagnostic
• Urinalysis, Urine

Folic Acid Anemia
(Folate Deficiency Anemia)
Blood indices, Blood
Bone marrow aspiration analysis,
  Diagnostic
Differential leukocyte count, Peripheral
  blood
Folic acid, Red blood cell, Blood
• Folic acid, Serum
Lactate dehydrogenase, Isoenzymes, Blood
Red blood cell, Blood
Red blood cell morphology (Megalocyte),
  Blood
Vitamin B_{12}, Serum

Forbes-Albright Syndrome
• Prolactin, Serum

Fractures
• Bone radiography, Diagnostic
Complete blood count, Blood
Computed tomography of the body,
  Diagnostic

Fungal Infections
Biopsy, Site-specific, Specimen (fungus
  culture)
• Blood, Fungus, Culture
Bronchial aspirate, Fungus, Culture

Cerebrospinal fluid, Fungus, Culture
Fungal antibody screen, Blood
Genital, *Candida albicans*, Culture
• Skin, Fungus, Culture
• Sputum, Fungus, Culture
• Urine, Fungus, Culture
• Wound, Fungus, Culture

FUO
(see Fever of undetermined origin)

G6PD (Glucose-6-Phosphate Dehydrogenase) Deficiency
Blood indices, Blood
Complete blood count, Blood
Differential leukocyte count, Peripheral
  blood
Glucose-6-phosphate dehydrogenase,
  Quantitative, Blood
• Glucose-6-phosphate dehydrogenase
  screen, Blood
Haptoglobin, Serum
Red blood cell, Blood
Reticulocyte count, Blood

G-Cell Hyperplasia
• Gastrin, Serum
• Histopathology, Specimen
Immunoperoxidase procedures, Diagnostic
Pepsinogen I antibody, Blood

Galactokinase Deficiency
• Galactose, Screening test for galactosemia,
  Urine

Galactorrhea
• Nipple discharge cytology, Specimen
Prolactin, Serum

Galactosemia
Galactokinase, Blood
• Galactose, Screening test for galactosemia,
  Urine
Galactose-1-phosphate, Blood
Galactose-1-phosphate uridyl transferase,
  Erythrocyte, Blood
Galactose-1-phosphate uridyl transferase,
  Qualitative, Blood
Glucose, Qualitative and semiquantitative,
  Urine

Ganglioneuroblastoma
Bone marrow aspiration analysis, Specimen
Bone scan, Diagnostic
• Brain biopsy, Diagnostic
Cerebral computed tomography, Diagnostic
Complete blood count, Blood
Histopathology, Specimen
Homovanillic acid, 24-hour urine

5-Hydroxyindoleacetic acid, Quantitative,
    24-hour urine
Magnetic resonance imaging, Brain,
    Diagnostic
• Magnetic resonance neurography,
    Diagnostic
• Magnetic resonance spectroscopy,
    Diagnostic
    Metanephrines, Total, 24-hour urine and
        free, Plasma
Octreotide scan, Diagnostic
Vanillylmandelic acid, Urine

Gangrene
• Biopsy, Site-specific, Specimen (Anaerobic
    culture)
• Blood culture, Blood
• Blood indices, Blood
• Body fluid (Abscess), Anaerobic,
    Culture
• Complete blood count, Blood
• Creatine kinase, Serum
• Differential leukocyte count, Peripheral
    blood
• Electrolytes, Plasma or serum
• Histopathology, Specimen
• Myoglobin, Qualitative, Urine
• Myoglobin, Serum
• Radiography, Diagnostic

Gastric Cancer
Biopsy, Site-specific, Specimen
CA 72-4, Blood
Carcinoembryonic antigen, Serum
Dual modality imaging, Diagnostic
Endoscopic ultrasonography, Diagnostic
• Gastroscopy, Diagnostic
Helicobacter pylori, Quick office serology,
    Serum and titer, Blood
• Histopathology, Specimen
Iron, Serum
Mucinlike carcinoma–associated antigen,
    Blood
Occult blood, Stool
Pepsinogen I and pepsinogen II, Blood
Telomerase enzyme marker, Blood
Thymidylate synthase, Specimen
Upper gastrointestinal series, Diagnostic

Gastric Ulcer
ABO group and Rh type, Blood
Amylase, Serum
Brushing cytology, Specimen
Complete blood count, Blood
Endoscopic ultrasonography, Diagnostic
Gastrin, Serum
• Gastroscopy, Diagnostic

Helicobacter pylori, Quick office serology,
    Serum and titer, Blood
• Histopathology, Specimen
Lipase, Serum
Occult blood, Stool
Pepsinogen I and pepsinogen II, Blood
Washing cytology, Specimen

Gastrinoma
(see Zollinger-Ellison syndrome)

Gastritis
(see also Helicobacter pylori)
Brushing cytology, Specimen
Campylobacter-like organism test, Specimen
Folic acid, Serum
Gastrin, Serum
• Gastroscopy, Diagnostic
Helicobacter pylori, Quick office serology,
    Serum and titer, Blood
• Histopathology, Specimen
Occult blood, Stool
Pepsinogen I and pepsinogen II, Blood
Urea breath test, Diagnostic
Vitamin B_{12}, Serum

Gastroenteritis
Fecal leukocytes, Stool, Diagnostic
Meat fibers, Stool
• Stool culture, Routine, Stool

Gastroesophageal Reflux
• Esophageal acidity test, Diagnostic
• Esophageal manometry, Diagnostic
Esophageal radiography, Diagnostic

Gastrointestinal Bleeding
Blood urea nitrogen/creatinine ratio, Blood
• Complete blood count, Blood
Esophagogastroduodenoscopy, Diagnostic
Occult blood, Stool
• Type and crossmatch, Blood (Screen)

Gaucher Disease
Acid phosphatase, Serum
Ashkenazi Jewish genetic carrier screening
    profile
Bone marrow aspiration analysis,
    Diagnostic
• Complete blood count, Blood
Magnetic resonance imaging, Diagnostic

Genital Herpes
• Herpes cytology, Specimen
• Herpes simplex antibody, Blood
Histopathology, Specimen
Rapid plasma reagin test, Blood
Tzanck smear, Specimen
Viral culture, Specimen

Gentamycin
(see Aminoglycoside toxicity)

German Measles
(see Rubella)

Giardiasis
Fecal leukocytes, Stool, Diagnostic
Histopathology, Specimen
• Ova and parasites, Stool
Washing cytology, Specimen

Glanzmann Disease
• Bleeding time, Ivy, Blood
• Bleeding time, Mielke, Blood
Platelet adhesion test (Venous blood),
  Diagnostic
Platelet aggregation, Blood
Platelet aggregation, Hypercoagulable state,
  Blood

Glaucoma
Amsler grid test, Screen
Slit-lamp vision test, Diagnostic
• Tonometry test for glaucoma, Screen
Visual acuity tests, Diagnostic

Glomerulonephritis
Addis count, 12-hour urine
Albumin/globulin ratio, Serum
Antideoxyribonuclease-B antibody titer,
  Serum
Anti-DNA, Serum
Antihyaluronidase titer, Serum
Antistreptolysin-O titer, Serum
C1q immune complex detection,
  Serum
C3 complement, Serum
C3 proactivator, Serum
C4 complement, Serum
Chemistry profile, Blood
Complement, Total, Serum
Complement components, Serum
Creatinine clearance, Serum, Urine
Glomerular basement membrane antibody,
  Serum
Hepatitis B surface antigen, Blood
Immune complex assay, Blood
Intravenous pyelography, Diagnostic
Kidney biopsy, Specimen
Mean platelet volume, Blood
Occult blood, Urine
• Protein, Urine
Protein electrophoresis, Serum
Specific gravity, Urine
Streptozyme, Blood
Throat culture for group A beta-hemolytic
  streptococci, Culture

Urea nitrogen, Plasma or serum
• Urinalysis, Urine

Glucagonoma
Chemistry profile, Blood
• Glucagon, Plasma
Glucose, Blood
Insulin and insulin antibodies, Blood

Glycogen Storage Disease
Bone marrow aspiration analysis,
  Specimen
• Glucose, Blood
Glucose, 2-hour postprandial, Serum
Glucose tolerance test, Blood
Histopathology, Specimen
• Ketones, Semiquantitative, Urine
Ketone bodies, Blood
Lipid profile, Blood
Pregnancy test, Routine, Serum and
  qualitative, Urine
Uric acid, Serum

Glycogenosis
(see Glycogen storage disease)

Glycosuria
• Glucose, Qualitative and semiquantitative,
  Urine
Glucose, Quantitative, 24-hour urine
Glucose, 2-hour postprandial, Serum
Glycosylated hemoglobin, Blood
Osmolality, Urine

Goiter
(see Hypothyroidism)

Gonococcal Infection of Pharynx
Rapid plasma reagin test, Blood
• Throat culture for *Neisseria gonorrhoeae*,
  Culture

Gonorrhea
Chlamydia culture and group titer,
  Specimen (Culture)
Chlamydia screening, Specimen
Fluorescent treponemal antibody–absorbed
  double-stain test, Serum
Genital, *Neisseria gonorrhoeae*, Culture
Gram stain (Urine), Diagnostic
• *Neisseria gonorrhoeae* smear, Specimen
Rapid plasma reagin test, Blood
Throat culture for *Neisseria gonorrhoeae*,
  Culture
Urine culture and nucleic acid
  amplification tests for *Neisseria
  gonorrhoeae*, Urine
• Venereal Disease Research Laboratory test,
  Serum

Goodpasture's Syndrome
Bronchial washing, Specimen
Brushing cytology, Specimen
Complete blood count, Blood
Creatinine, Serum
Creatinine, Urine
Electrolytes, Plasma or serum
Electrolytes, Urine
Eosinophil count, Blood
Glomerular basement membrane antibody,
  Serum
• Kidney biopsy, Specimen
Occult blood, Urine
Protein, Quantitative, Urine
Protein, Semiquantitative, Urine
Sputum hemosiderin preparation,
  Specimen
• Urinalysis, Urine
Washing cytology, Specimen

Gout
Body fluid, Routine, Culture
Body fluid analysis, Cell count, Specimen
Chemistry profile, Blood
Heavy-metal screen, Blood and 24-hour
  urine
Mucin clot test, Specimen
Phosphorus, Serum
• Synovial fluid analysis, Diagnostic
Uric acid, Serum
Uric acid, Urine

Granulocytic Leukemia
(see Leukemia)

Granulomas
• Liver ^{131}I scan, Diagnostic

Graves' Disease
(see Hyperthyroidism)

Growth Hormone Deficiency
Chromosome analysis, Blood
• Growth hormone and growth hormone–
  releasing hormone, Blood
Insulin-like growth factor-I, Blood
Zinc, Blood

Guillain-Barré Syndrome
• Cerebrospinal fluid, Routine analysis,
  Specimen
Electromyography and nerve conduction
  studies, Diagnostic
Heavy-metal screen, Blood and 24-hour
  urine
Immunoglobulin G synthesis rate,
  Cerebrospinal fluid, Specimen
Magnetic resonance neurography, Diagnostic

Gynecomastia
Alcohol, Blood
Chemistry profile, Blood
• Estradiol, Serum
Follicle-stimulating hormone, Serum
Histopathology, Specimen
• Human chorionic gonadotropin,
  Beta-subunit, Serum
Liver battery, Serum
Prolactin, Serum
• Testosterone, Free, Bioavailable and total,
  Blood

Haemophilus influenzae Infection
Respiratory antigen panel, Specimen
• Sputum for *Haemophilus* species, Culture
Viral culture, Specimen

Hageman Factor
Activated partial thromboplastin time and
  partial thromboplastin time, Plasma
Coagulation factor assay, Blood
• Factor XII, Blood

Hairy Cell Leukemia
Acid phosphatase, Serum
• Bone marrow aspiration analysis,
  Diagnostic
Histopathology, Specimen
Leukocyte cytochemistry (Bone marrow),
  Specimen
• Tartrate-resistant acid phosphatase,
  Blood

Hallucinogens: LSD, Mescaline, MDA, PCP, Psilocybin
(see Drug abuse)

Hand-Schüller-Christian Disease
Bone scan, Diagnostic
• Chest radiography, Diagnostic

Hansen's Disease
(see Leprosy)

Hartnup Disease
• Indican, Urine

Hashimoto's Thyroiditis
Histopathology, Specimen
Needle aspiration cytology (Thyroid),
  Specimen
Thyroid antithyroglobulin antibody, Serum
Thyroid peroxidase antibody, Blood
• Thyroid profile, Blood
• Thyroid-stimulating hormone, Blood

Hay Fever
Allergen-specific IgE, Serum
• Eosinophil count, Blood

Eosinophil peroxidase, Serum
Immunoglobulin E, Serum

Head and Neck Cancer
Barium swallow, Diagnostic
• Biopsy, Site-specific, Specimen
CA 15-3, Serum
CA 50, Blood (Esophagus, squamous)
Carcinoembryonic antigen, Serum
Chest radiography, Diagnostic
• Computed tomography of the body
   (Head and neck), Diagnostic
Dual modality imaging, Diagnostic
Esophageal radiography, Diagnostic
Magnetic resonance imaging, Diagnostic
Sentinel lymph node biopsy, Diagnostic
Telomerase enzyme marker, Blood or urine
   (Blood)
Transesophageal ultrasonography, Diagnostic

Head Injuries
• Cerebral computed tomography,
   Diagnostic
Cerebrospinal fluid, Routine analysis,
   Specimen
Complete blood count, Blood
Doppler ultrasonographic flow studies
   (Transcranial), Diagnostic
Electroencephalography, Diagnostic
• Magnetic resonance imaging, Diagnostic
Radiography of skull, chest, and cervical
   spine, Diagnostic

Headache
Carbon monoxide, Blood
Carboxyhemoglobin, Blood
Cerebrospinal fluid, Routine analysis,
   Specimen
Cold agglutinin screen, Blood
Cold agglutinin titer, Serum
Heavy-metal screen, Blood and 24-hour
   urine (Urine)
Methemoglobin, Blood
Mycoplasma titer, Blood
Rocky Mountain spotted fever serology,
   Blood
Viscosity, Serum

Hearing Disorders
• Audiometry Test, Diagnostic
   (Vestibular-evoked myogenic potential)
Fluorescent treponemal antibody–absorbed
   double-stain test, Serum
Magnetic resonance imaging (functional),
   Diagnostic
• Tuning fork test of Weber, Rinne, and
   Schwabach, Diagnostic

Heart Cancer
Biopsy, Site-specific, Specimen
   (Endomyocardial)

Heart Failure
(see Congestive heart failure)

Heart-Lung Machine
Activated coagulation time, Automated,
   Blood
Activated partial thromboplastin time and
   partial thromboplastin time, Plasma
Blood gases, Arterial, Blood
Complete blood count, Blood
Prothrombin time and international
   normalized ratio, Plasma

Heart Murmur
Echocardiography, Diagnostic
• Electrocardiography, Diagnostic
Transesophageal ultrasonography, Diagnostic

Heart Transplant
(see Transplants)

Heat Stroke
Calcium, Total, Serum
Complete blood count, Blood
• Electrocardiography, Diagnostic
• Electrolytes, Plasma or serum
Prothrombin time and international
   normalized ratio, Plasma
Urea nitrogen, Plasma or serum
Urinalysis, Urine

Heinz Body Anemia
Blood indices, Blood
Complete blood count, Blood
Differential leukocyte count, Peripheral
   blood
Glucose-6-phosphate dehydrogenase,
   Quantitative, Blood
Glucose-6-phosphate dehydrogenase
   screen, Blood
• Heinz body stain, Diagnostic
Hemoglobin, Unstable, Heat-labile test,
   Blood
Hemoglobin, Unstable, Isopropanol
   precipitation test, Blood
Hemoglobin electrophoresis, Blood
Methemoglobin, Blood
Red blood cell, Blood
Red blood cell morphology, Blood
Reticulocyte count, Blood

Helicobacter Pylori
Campylobacter-like organism test, Specimen
Cytologic study of gastrointestinal tract,
   Diagnostic

Gastric acid analysis test, Diagnostic
Gastric analysis, Specimen
Gastroscopy or gastroduodenojejunoscopy,
   Diagnostic
• *Helicobacter pylori,* Quick office serology,
   Serum and titer, Blood
Helicobacter pylori antigen test, Stool
Immunoglobulin G, Serum
Pepsinogen I and pepsinogen II, Blood
Stool culture, Routine, Stool
Urea breath test, Diagnostic

Hematuria

Addis count, 12-hour urine
Antideoxyribonuclease-B antibody titer,
   Serum
Antihyaluronidase titer, Serum
Antistreptolysin-O titer, Serum
Body fluid (Urine), Routine, Culture
Creatinine, Serum
Creatinine, Urine
Electrolytes, Plasma or serum
Electrolytes, Urine
Glomerular basement membrane antibody,
   Serum
Kidney biopsy, Specimen
Kidney stone analysis, Specimen
Myoglobin, Urine
• Occult blood, Urine
Streptozyme, Blood
Urea nitrogen, Plasma or serum
• Urinalysis, Urine
Urine, Fungus, Culture
Urine, Mycobacteria, Culture
Urine cytology, Urine

Hemochromatosis

Ferritin, Serum
Glucose, Blood
Glucose tolerance test, Blood
Histopathology, Specimen
• Iron, Serum
Iron stain, Bone marrow, Specimen
Liver battery, Serum
• Total iron-binding capacity, Serum

Hemoflagellates

(see Trypanosomiasis)

Hemoglobin C Disease

• Complete blood count, Blood
• Hemoglobin electrophoresis, Blood
Red blood cell morphology, Blood

Hemolytic Anemia

• Bilirubin, Total, Serum
Complete blood count, Blood
Ham's test, Blood

• Haptoglobin, Serum
Red blood cell morphology, Blood
• Reticulocyte count, Blood
Sedimentation rate, Erythrocyte, Blood
Urobilinogen, Urine

Hemophilia

Activated coagulation time, Automated,
   Blood
Activated partial thromboplastin time and
   partial thromboplastin time, Plasma
Aspirin tolerance test, Diagnostic
Circulating anticoagulant, Blood
Complete blood count, Blood
• Factor VIII, Blood
Factor VIII R:Ag, Blood
Occult blood, Urine
Plasma recalcification time, Plasma
Platelet aggregation, Hypercoagulable state,
   Blood

Hemoptysis

Activated partial thromboplastin time and
   partial thromboplastin time, Plasma
Bleeding time, Duke, Blood
Bleeding time, Ivy, Blood
Bronchial washing, Specimen
• Bronchoscopy, Diagnostic
Brushing cytology, Specimen
• Chest radiography, Diagnostic
Complete blood count, Blood
Computed tomography of the body
   (Lung), Diagnostic
Prothrombin time and international
   normalized ratio, Plasma
Sputum, Mycobacteria, Culture and smear
Sputum, Routine, Culture
• Sputum cytology, Specimen

Hemorrhage

• Activated partial thromboplastin time and
   partial thromboplastin time, Plasma
Chemistry profile, Blood
• Complete blood count, Blood
D-Dimer Test, Blood
Hematocrit, Blood
Hemoglobin, Blood
Iron, Serum
Kleihauer-Betke stain, Diagnostic
Occult blood, Stool
Platelet count, Stool
• Prothrombin time and international
   normalized ratio, Plasma
Sputum hemosiderin preparation, Specimen
Total iron-binding capacity, Serum
Type and crossmatch, Blood
Urinalysis, Urine

Hemorrhoids

Complete blood count, Blood
• Proctoscopy, Diagnostic

Hepatic Cirrhosis

• Liver biopsy, Diagnostic
Liver ultrasonography, Diagnostic

Hepatic Coma

(see also Hepatitis or Jaundice)
• Albumin, Serum
• Ammonia, Blood
Amylase, Serum
Antinuclear antibody, Serum
• Bilirubin, Total, Serum
Cerebrospinal fluid, Glucose, Specimen
Cerebrospinal fluid, Protein, Specimen
Cerebrospinal fluid, Routine, Culture and
  cytology
Lactic acid, Blood
Urea nitrogen, Plasma or serum

Hepatic Encephalopathy

Acquired immunodeficiency syndrome
  evaluation battery, Diagnostic
Activated partial thromboplastin time
  and partial thromboplastin time,
  Plasma
• Ammonia, Blood
Blood culture, Blood
Blood gases, Arterial, Blood
Calcium, Total, Serum
Cerebral computed tomography,
  Diagnostic
Complete blood count, Blood
Copper, Serum
Creatinine, Serum
Electroencephalogram, Diagnostic
Electrolytes, Plasma or serum
Glucose, Blood
• Liver battery, Serum
Liver biopsy, Diagnostic
Liver scan, Diagnostic
Liver ultrasonography, Diagnostic
Liver-spleen scan, Diagnostic
Lumbar puncture, Diagnostic
Magnetic resonance spectroscopy,
  Diagnostic
Paracentesis, Diagnostic
Prothrombin time and international
  normalized ratio, Plasma
Thyroid function tests, Blood
Toxicology drug screen, Blood or urine
Ultrasonography, Liver, Diagnostic
• Urea nitrogen, Plasma or serum
Urinalysis, Urine

Hepatitis

Acetaminophen, Serum
Alanine aminotransferase, Serum
Albumin, Serum
Albumin/globulin ratio, Serum
Alkaline phosphatase, Isoenzymes,
  Serum
Alkaline phosphatase, Serum
Alpha-antitrypsin, Serum
Alpha-fetoprotein, Serum
Antimitochondrial antibody, Blood
Anti–smooth muscle antibody, Serum
Aspartate aminotransferase, Serum
• Bilirubin, Direct, Serum
Bilirubin, Indirect, Serum
Bilirubin, Urine
C1q immune complex detection, Serum
C3 complement, Serum
C4 complement, Serum
Chemistry profile, Blood
Cytomegalovirus antibody, Serum
Epstein-Barr virus, Serology, Blood
Gamma-glutamyltranspeptidase, Blood
Hepatitis A antibody, IgM and IgG, Blood
Hepatitis B core antibody, Blood
Hepatitis B e antibody, Serum
Hepatitis B e antigen, Blood
Hepatitis B surface antibody, Blood
Hepatitis B surface antigen, Blood
Hepatitis C antibody, Serum
Hepatitis C genotype, Serum
Hepatitis delta antibody, Serum
• Hepatitis serologies
Histopathology, Specimen
Lactate dehydrogenase, Isoenzymes, Blood
• Liver battery, Serum
Liver biopsy, Diagnostic
Liver scan, Diagnostic
Liver ultrasonography, Diagnostic
Lupus test, Blood
5′-Nucleotidase, Blood
Ornithine carbamoyltransferase, Blood
Protein electrophoresis, Serum
Prothrombin time and international
  normalized ratio, Plasma
Salicylate, Blood
Toxoplasmosis serology, Serum
Urobilinogen, Urine

Hepatomas

Liver ^{131}I scan, Diagnostic
• Liver ultrasonography, Diagnostic

Hepatomegaly

Liver biopsy, Diagnostic
Liver ultrasonography, Diagnostic

Hereditary Nonpolyposis Colorectal Cancer
(see Colorectal cancer)

Herpes Simplex
Herpes simplex antibody, Blood
• Herpesvirus antigen, Direct fluorescent antibody, Specimen
• Tzanck smear, Specimen
Viral culture, Specimen

Herpesvirus Infection
Biopsy, Site-specific, Specimen
Bronchial washing, Specimen
Brushing cytology, Specimen
Cervical-vaginal cytology, Specimen
• Herpes cytology, Specimen
Herpes simplex antibody, Blood
Oral cavity cytology, (Scrape) Specimen
Pap smear, Diagnostic
Sputum cytology, Specimen
Toxoplasmosis, Rubella, Cytomegalovirus, Herpesvirus serology, Blood
Tzanck smear, Specimen
Varicella-zoster virus serology, Serum
Viral culture, Specimen

Herpes Zoster (Shingles)
Tzanck smear, Diagnostic
• Varicella-zoster virus serology, Serum
Viral Culture, Specimen

Hiatal Hernia
Barium swallow, Diagnostic
Esophageal manometry, Diagnostic
• Esophageal radiography, Diagnostic
Upper gastrointestinal series, Diagnostic

Hirschsprung's Disease
• Barium enema, Diagnostic
Histopathology, Specimen

Hirsutism (Hypertrichosis)
ACTH stimulation test, Diagnostic
Androstenedione, Serum
Computed tomography of the body (Adrenal glands), Diagnostic
Cortisol, Urine
• Dehydroepiandrosterone sulfate, Serum
Gynecologic ultrasonography, Diagnostic
17-Hydroxycorticosteroids, 24-hour urine
• 17-Hydroxyprogesterone, Blood
Metyrapone, 24-hour urine
Pregnanetriol, Urine
Prolactin, Serum
• Testosterone, Free, Bioavailable and total, Blood

Histoplasmosis
Biopsy, Site-specific, Specimen (Fungus culture)
Blood, Fungus, Culture
Body fluid, Fungus, Culture
Bone marrow aspiration analysis, Diagnostic
Bronchial aspirate, Fungus, Culture
Bronchial aspirate, Routine, Culture
Bronchial washing, Specimen
Brushing cytology, Specimen
Cerebrospinal fluid, Fungus, Culture
Chest radiography, Diagnostic
Complement fixation, Serum
Computed tomography of the body, Diagnostic
Culture (Tissue), Routine, Specimen
Flucytosine, Serum
Fungal antibody screen, Blood
Histopathology, Specimen
• Histoplasmosis serology, Blood
Needle aspiration cytology, (Lung) Specimen
Platelet count, Blood
Pulmonary function tests, Diagnostic
Sputum, Fungus, Culture
Sputum cytology, Specimen

HNPCC
(see Colorectal cancer)

Hodgkin's Disease
Acquired immune deficiency syndrome evaluation battery, Diagnostic
Biopsy, Site-specific, Specimen
Body fluid cytology, Specimen
Bone marrow aspiration analysis, Diagnostic
Chemistry profile, Blood
Chest radiography, Diagnostic
Chromosome analysis, Blood
Complete blood count, Blood
Computed tomography of the body (Abdomen, chest, pelvis), Diagnostic
C-reactive protein, Plasma or serum
Cryoglobulin, Qualitative, Serum
Differential leukocyte count, Peripheral blood
D-Xylose absorption test, Diagnostic, Serum or urine
Globulin, Serum
Heterophile agglutinins, Blood
• Histopathology, Specimen
Immunoelectrophoresis, Serum and urine
Immunoglobulin A, Serum
Immunoglobulin G, Serum

Immunoglobulin M, Serum
Immunoperoxidase procedures (for
  Antigens), Diagnostic
Laparoscopy, Diagnostic
Leukocyte cytochemistry, Specimen
Liver battery, Serum
• Lymph node biopsy, Specimen
Lymphocyte subset enumeration, Blood
Muramidase, Serum and urine
Needle aspiration cytology, (Mass)
  Specimen
Platelet count, Blood
Pneumocystis immunofluorescent assay,
  Serum
Protein electrophoresis, Serum
Protein electrophoresis, Urine
Sedimentation rate, Erythrocyte, Blood
T- and B-lymphocyte subset assay, Blood
Terminal deoxynucleotidyl transferase,
  Bone marrow
Uric acid, Serum

Hormonal Therapy
Estrogen receptor and progesterone
  receptor in breast cancer, Diagnostic
Progesterone receptor assay, Specimen

Human Papillomavirus
Biopsy, Site-specific, Specimen
Chlamydia culture and group titer,
  Specimen (Culture)
Chlamydia screening, Specimen
• Human papillomavirus, Specimen
Rapid plasma reagin test, Blood
Urine culture and nucleic acid
  amplification tests for *Neisseria
  gonorrhoeae*, Urine
Venereal Disease Research Laboratory test,
  Serum

Humoral Immune Deficiency
Globulin, Serum
• Immunoelectrophoresis, Serum and Urine
Immunoglobulin A, Serum
Immunoglobulin G, Serum
Immunoglobulin M, Serum
Protein electrophoresis, Serum
• T- and B-lymphocyte subset assay, Blood

Hunter's Syndrome
• Mucopolysaccharides, Qualitative, Urine

Hurler's Syndrome
Differential leukocyte count, Peripheral
  blood
Fibroblast skin culture
• Mucopolysaccharides, Qualitative, Urine
S mucopolysaccharide turnover, Diagnostic

Hyaline Membrane Disease
• Alpha$_1$-antitrypsin, Serum
• Amniotic fluid analysis, (Pulmonary
  surfactant) Specimen
Bicarbonate, Blood
Blood gases, Arterial, Blood
Blood gases, Capillary, Blood
Carbon dioxide, Partial pressure, Blood
Chest radiography, Diagnostic

Hydatidiform Mole
Chemistry profile, Blood
Chest radiography, Diagnostic
Complete blood count, Blood
Gynecologic ultrasonography,
  Diagnostic
Histopathology, Specimen
• Human chorionic gonadotropin,
  Beta-subunit, Serum
Pregnancy Test, Routine, Serum and
  Qualitative, Urine
Protein, Quantitative, Urine

Hydration
Albumin, Serum
Chemistry profile, Blood
• Complete blood count, Blood
• Electrolytes, Plasma or serum
Electrolytes, Urine
• Osmolality, Serum
Osmolality, Urine
Parathyroid hormone, Blood
Protein, Total, Serum
Sodium, Plasma, Serum or urine
Urinalysis, Urine (Specific gravity)

Hydronephrosis
Body fluid (Urine), Routine, Culture
Complete blood count, Blood
Computed tomography of the body
  (Kidney), Diagnostic
• Creatinine, Serum
Creatinine clearance, Serum, Urine
Electrolytes, Plasma or serum
Electrolytes, Urine
Intravenous pyelography, Diagnostic
• Kidney ultrasonography, Diagnostic
Magnetic resonance imaging, Diagnostic
Prostate-specific antigen, Serum
Urea nitrogen, Plasma or serum
Urinalysis, Urine
Urine cytology, Urine

Hyperaldosteronism
• Aldosterone, Serum and urine
Basic metabolic panel, Blood
Chemistry profile, Blood

Computed tomography of the body
  (Adrenal glands), Diagnostic
Electrolytes, Plasma or serum
Electrolytes, Urine
Histopathology, Specimen
Osmolality, Calculated test, Blood
Osmolality, Serum
Osmolality, Urine
• Potassium, Plasma or serum
Renin activity, Plasma
Sodium, Plasma, Serum or urine

Hyperalimentation

Albumin, Serum
Albumin/globulin ratio, Serum
Blood, Fungus, Culture
Chemistry profile, Blood
Electrolytes, Plasma or serum
Foreign body, Routine, Culture
Glucose, Blood
Lipid profile, Blood

Hyperbaric Oxygenation

Blood gases, Arterial, Blood

Hyperbilirubinemia

Alanine aminotransferase, Serum
Aspartate aminotransferase, Serum
• Bilirubin, Total, Serum

Hypercalcemia

Albumin, Serum
Alkaline phosphatase, Serum
Anion gap, Blood
Blood urea nitrogen/creatinine ratio, Blood
• Calcium, Total, Serum
Calcium, Urine
Cyclic adenosine monophosphate, Serum
  and urine
Magnesium, Serum
Parathyroid hormone, Blood
• Phosphorus, Serum
Phosphorus, Urine
Vitamin D₃, Plasma or serum

Hypercapnia

Bicarbonate, Blood
• Blood gases, Arterial, Blood
Blood gases, Capillary, Blood
Blood gases, Venous, Blood
Carbon dioxide, Blood
Chest radiography, Diagnostic
pH, Blood
Pulmonary function tests, Diagnostic

Hypercholesterolemia

Cholesterol, Blood
Glucose, Blood
High-density lipoprotein cholesterol, Blood

Low-density lipoprotein cholesterol, Blood
• Lipid profile, Blood
Phospholipids, Serum
Thyroid profile, Blood
Triglycerides, Blood
Uric acid, Serum

Hyperglucagon Syndrome (Hyperglucagonemia)

• Glucagon, Plasma

Hyperglycemia

Chemistry profile, Blood
Cortisol, Plasma or serum
Glucagon, Plasma
• Glucose, Blood
Glucose, 2-hour postprandial, Serum
Glucose-monitoring machines, Diagnostic
Glucose tolerance test, Blood
Glycosylated hemoglobin, Blood
Growth hormone and growth hormone–
  releasing hormone, Blood
Insulin and insulin antibodies, Blood
Ketone bodies, Blood
Urinalysis, Urine

Hyperglycemic Hyperosmolar Nonketotic Coma

Blood gases (pH), Arterial, Blood
Chemistry profile, Blood
Complete blood count, Blood
Creatinine, Serum
Creatinine, Urine
Electrolytes, Plasma or serum
Electrolytes, Urine
• Glucose, Blood
• Osmolality, Serum
Osmolality, Urine
Urea nitrogen, Plasma or serum

Hyperinsulinism

C-peptide, Serum
• Insulin and insulin antibodies, Blood

Hyperkalemia

Aldosterone, Serum and urine
Calcium, Total, Serum
Chemistry profile, Blood
• Electrocardiography, Diagnostic
Electrolytes, Plasma or serum
Glucose, Blood
Magnesium, Serum
• Potassium, Plasma or serum
Potassium, Urine

Hyperlipoproteinemia

Cholesterol, Blood
• Lipid profile, Blood
Triglycerides, Blood

Hypermagnesemia
Anion gap, Blood
Calcium, Total, Serum
Electrolytes, Plasma or serum
• Magnesium, Serum
Magnesium, 24-hour urine

Hypernatremia
Cholesterol, Blood
• Electrolytes, Plasma or serum
Electrolytes, Urine
Glucose, Blood
Glucose, Quantitative, 24-hour urine
Osmolality, Serum
• Sodium, Plasma or serum
Triglycerides, Blood

Hyperparathyroidism
Alkaline phosphatase, Serum
Amylase, Serum and urine (Serum)
Bone densitometry, Diagnostic
Bone radiography, Diagnostic
Calcitonin, Plasma or serum
• Calcium, Total, Serum
Calcium, Urine
Chemistry profile, Blood
Cyclic adenosine monophosphate, Serum
  and urine
Histopathology, Specimen
Magnesium, Serum
Osteocalcin, Plasma or serum
• Parathyroid hormone, Blood (Intact)
Phosphorus, Serum

Hyperphosphatemia
Calcium, Total, Serum
Creatinine, Serum
Electrolytes, Plasma or serum
• Phosphorus, Serum

Hyperpituitarism (Acromegaly or Gigantism)
Adrenocorticotropic hormone, Serum
Alkaline phosphatase, Isoenzymes, Serum
Alkaline phosphatase, Serum
Calcium, Total, Serum
Calcium, Urine
Computed tomography of the body (Head
  or whole body), Diagnostic
Follicle-stimulating hormone, Serum
Glucose, Blood
• Glucose tolerance test, Blood in
  combination with growth hormone and
  growth hormone–releasing hormone,
  Blood
Hydroxyproline, Total, 24-hour urine
Insulin-like growth factor-I, Blood

Luteinizing hormone, Blood
Magnetic resonance imaging (Head),
  Diagnostic
Phosphorus, Serum
Prolactin, Serum
Single-photon emission computed
  tomography, Diagnostic
Thyroid function tests, Blood

Hypersensitivity Pneumonitis
Biopsy, Site-specific (Lung), Specimen
• Chest radiography, Diagnostic
Complete blood count, Blood
Computed tomography of the body (High
  resolution), Diagnostic
• Differential leukocyte count, Peripheral
  blood (WBCs)
Hypersensitivity pneumonitis serology,
  Blood
Pulmonary function tests, Diagnostic
Rheumatoid factor, Blood

Hypersensitivity (Allergic) Reaction
Eosinophil peroxidase, Serum
Immunoglobulin E, Serum
Skin test for hypersensitivity, Diagnostic

Hypertension
Aldosterone, Serum or urine
Angiotensin-converting enzyme, Blood
Blood urea nitrogen/creatinine ratio,
  Blood
Catecholamines, Fractionation free, Plasma
Catecholamines, Urine
• Chemistry profile, Blood
Complete blood count, Blood
Creatinine, Serum
Creatinine clearance, Serum, Urine
Echocardiography, Diagnostic
Electrocardiography, Diagnostic
• Electrolytes, Plasma or serum
Electrolytes, Urine
Mean platelet volume, Blood
Metanephrines, Total, 24-hour urine and
  free, Plasma
Potassium, Plasma or serum
Protein, Quantitative, Urine
Renin activity, Plasma
Sodium, Plasma or serum
Urea nitrogen, Plasma or serum
• Uric acid, Serum
• Urinalysis, Urine
Vanillylmandelic acid, Urine

Hyperthermia
Blood culture, Blood
Chest radiography, Diagnostic

Chloride, Serum
Complete blood count, Blood
Creatine kinase, Serum
• Differential leukocyte count, Peripheral
  blood
Lactic acid, Blood
Myoglobin, Urine
Potassium, Plasma or serum
Sodium, Plasma or serum

Hyperthyroidism (Thyrotoxicosis)
Albumin, Serum
Calcium, Total, Serum
Chemistry profile, Blood
Cholesterol, Blood
Endomysial antibody, Serum
Human leukocyte antigen B27, Blood
Hydroxyproline, Total, 24-hour urine
Magnesium, Serum
Mean platelet volume, Blood
Thyroid antithyroglobulin antibody,
  Serum
Thyroid function tests, Blood
Thyroid peroxidase antibody, Blood
Thyroid scan, Diagnostic
• Thyroid-stimulating hormone, Blood
Thyroid-stimulating hormone,
  Immunoglobulins, Blood
Thyroid-stimulating hormone, Sensitive
  assay, Blood
Thyroid test, Free thyroxine index, Serum
Thyroid test, Thyroid hormone binding
  ratio, Blood
• Thyroid test, Thyroxine, Blood
Thyroid test, Thyroxine free, Serum
• Thyroid test, Triiodothyronine, Blood
Triglycerides, Blood

Hyperventilation
(see Respiratory alkalosis)

Hypervolemia
(see Overhydration)

Hypocalcemia
Albumin, Serum, Urine and 24-hour urine
  (Serum)
Calcium, Ionized, Blood
• Calcium, Total, Serum
Calcium, Urine
Creatinine, Serum
Electrocardiography, Diagnostic
Magnesium, Serum
Parathyroid hormone, Blood
• Phosphorus, Serum
Renal function tests, Diagnostic
Vitamin D, Plasma or serum

Hypochromic Anemia
(see Iron deficiency anemia)

Hypoglycemia
Cortisol, Plasma or serum
C-peptide, Serum
Glucagon, Plasma
• Glucose, Blood
Glucose-monitoring machines,
  Diagnostic
Glucose tolerance test, Blood
Insulin and insulin antibodies, Blood
Tolbutamide tolerance test, Diagnostic
Urinalysis, Urine

Hypogonadism
(see also Erectile dysfunction)
• Luteinizing hormone, Blood
Mendelian inheritance in genetic disorders,
  Diagnostic
Prolactin, Serum
• Testosterone, Free, Bioavailable and total,
  Blood
• Thyroid function tests, Blood

Hypokalemia
Aldosterone, Serum and urine (Serum)
Chloride, Urine
Computed tomography of the body
  (Adrenal glands), Diagnostic
Digoxin, Serum
Electrocardiography, Diagnostic
• Electrolytes, Plasma or serum
Electrolytes, Urine
Magnesium, Serum
pH, Blood
• Potassium, Plasma or serum
Potassium, Urine
Renal function tests, Diagnostic
Renin activity, Plasma

Hypomagnesemia
Calcium, Total, Serum
Electrolytes, Plasma or serum
Electrolytes, Urine
• Magnesium, Serum
Magnesium, 24-hour urine
Phosphorus, Serum

Hyponatremia
Chemistry profile, Blood
Cholesterol, Blood
Concentration test, Urine
Cortisol, Plasma or serum
Creatinine, Serum
Creatinine, Urine
• Electrolytes, Plasma or serum
Electrolytes, Urine

Osmolality, Calculated tests, Blood
(Osmolar gap)
Osmolality, Serum
Osmolality, Urine
• Sodium, Plasma, Serum or urine
Triglycerides, Blood
Uric acid, Serum

Hypoparathyroidism
Alkaline phosphatase, Serum
Calcium, Calculated ionized, Serum
Calcium, Ionized, Serum
• Calcium, Total, Serum
Calcium, 24-hour urine
Chemistry profile, Blood
Cyclic adenosine monophosphate, Serum
and urine
• Magnesium, Serum
Parathyroid hormone, Blood
• Phosphorus, Serum
Phosphorus, Urine
Uric acid, Serum
Vitamin D_3, Plasma or serum

Hypophosphatemia
• Calcium, Total, Serum
Chloride, Serum
Magnesium, Serum
• Phosphorus, Serum
Sodium, Plasma, Serum or urine

Hypophysectomy
Complete blood count, Blood
Luteinizing hormone, Blood
Type and crossmatch, Blood
Urinalysis, Urine

Hypopituitarism (Dwarfism)
Adrenocorticotropic hormone, Serum
Chromosome analysis, Blood
Complete blood count, Blood
Cortisol, Plasma or serum
Electrolytes, Plasma or serum
Estrogens, Serum and 24-hour urine
(Serum)
Follicle-stimulating hormone, Serum
• Growth hormone and growth hormone–
releasing hormone, Blood
Insulin-like growth factor-I, Blood
Luteinizing hormone, Blood
Magnetic resonance imaging (Head),
Diagnostic
Prolactin, Serum
Semen analysis, Specimen
Testosterone, Free, Bioavailable and total,
Blood
Thyroid test, Thyroxine free, Blood

Thyroid-stimulating hormone sensitive
assay, Blood
Zinc, Blood

Hypotension
(see also Orthostatic hypotension)
Aldosterone, Serum and urine
Catecholamines, Fractionation free, Plasma
Catecholamines, Urine
Sodium, Plasma or serum

Hypothermia
Acetone, Serum
Activated partial thromboplastin time and
partial thromboplastin time, Plasma
Amylase, Serum
Blood gases, Arterial, Blood
Cerebral computed tomography, Diagnostic
Chest radiography, Diagnostic
Complete blood count, Blood
Creatinine, Serum
Electrocardiography, Diagnostic
Electrolytes, Plasma or serum
Glucose, Blood
Lactic acid, Blood
Lipase, Serum
Liver battery, Serum
Prothrombin time and international
normalized ratio, Blood
• Specific gravity, Urine
Thrombin time, Serum
Toxicology drug screen, Blood or urine
(Blood)
Urea nitrogen, Plasma or serum
Urinalysis, Urine

Hypothyroidism (Cretinism)
(see also Myxedema)
Alkaline phosphatase, Serum
Chemistry profile, Blood
Chloride, Sweat, Specimen
Cholesterol, Blood
Complete blood count, Blood
Creatine kinase, Serum
Lactate dehydrogenase, Blood
Lactate dehydrogenase, Isoenzymes, Blood
Lipid profile, Blood
Red blood cell morphology, Blood
Sodium, Plasma or serum
• Thyroid antithyroglobulin antibody,
Serum
Thyroid function tests, Blood
Thyroid peroxidase antibody, Blood
• Thyroid-stimulating hormone, Sensitive
assay, Blood
Thyroid-stimulating hormone, Filter paper,
Blood

Thyroid test, Free thyroxine index, Serum
Thyroid test, Thyroid hormone binding
  ratio, Blood
• Thyroid test, Thyroxine, Blood
Thyroid test, Thyroxine, Free, Serum
• Thyroid test, Triiodothyronine, Blood

Hypovolemia
Albumin/globulin ratio, Serum
Anion gap, Blood
Blood volume, Blood
Complete blood count, Blood
Creatinine, Serum
Creatinine, Urine
• Electrolytes, Plasma or serum
Electrolytes, Urine
Osmolality, Serum
• Osmolality, Urine
Potassium, Plasma or serum
Protein, Total, Serum
Sodium, Plasma or serum
• Specific gravity, Urine
Type and crossmatch, Blood
Urinalysis, Urine

Hypoxia
Bicarbonate, Blood
• Blood gases, Arterial, Blood
Carbon dioxide, Total content, Blood
Chest radiography, Diagnostic
Diffusing capacity for carbon monoxide,
  Diagnostic
Doppler ultrasonographic flow studies
  (Lower extremities), Diagnostic
• Oxygen saturation, Blood
Ventilation-perfusion lung scan, Diagnostic

Hysterectomy
• Complete blood count, Blood
Dilation and curettage, Diagnostic
Gynecologic ultrasonography, Diagnostic
Hysteroscopy, Diagnostic
Pap smear, Diagnostic
Potassium, Plasma or serum
Prothrombin time and international
  normalized ratio, Plasma
Sodium, Plasma, Serum or urine
• Type and crossmatch, Blood

Idiopathic Thrombocytopenic Purpura
Acquired immune deficiency syndrome
  evaluation battery, Diagnostic (for HIV
  antibody)
• Bleeding time, Duke, Blood
• Bleeding time, Ivy, Blood
Bone marrow aspiration analysis,
  Diagnostic

Complete blood count, Blood
Computed tomography of the body
  (Spleen), Diagnostic
Differential leukocyte count, Peripheral
  blood
Histopathology, Specimen
Mean platelet volume, Blood
Platelet antibody, Blood
• Platelet count, Blood
Red blood cell, Blood

Ileitis
(see Crohn's disease)

Immune Deficiency
Acquired immune deficiency syndrome
  evaluation battery, Diagnostic
Beta$_2$-microglobulin, Blood and 24-hour
  urine
Blood culture, Blood
Bone marrow aspiration analysis, Specimen
C3 complement, Serum
C4 complement, Serum
Chemistry profile, Blood
Chest radiography, Diagnostic
Complement, Total, Serum
Complete blood count, Blood
Computed tomography of the body
  (Head), Diagnostic
Cytomegalic inclusion disease, Cytology,
  Urine
Cytomegalovirus antibody, Serum
• Differential leukocyte count, Peripheral
  blood
Glucose-6-phosphate dehydrogenase, Blood
Hepatitis B core antibody, Blood
Herpes cytology, Specimen
Immunoglobulin A, Serum
Immunoglobulin D, Serum
Immunoglobulin E, Serum
Immunoglobulin G, Serum
Immunoglobulin M, Serum
Lymph node biopsy, (Tissue) Specimen
Lymphocyte subset enumeration, Blood
Magnetic resonance imaging (Head),
  Diagnostic
Mantoux skin test, Diagnostic
Nocardia culture, All sites, Specimen
Oral cavity cytology, Specimen
Oral mucosal transudate, Specimen
OraQuick Rapid HIV tests, Specimen
Pneumocystis immunofluorescent assay,
  Serum
Protein electrophoresis, Serum
Rapid plasma reagin test, Blood
• T- and B-lymphocyte subset assay, Blood

Toxoplasmosis serology, Serum
Vitamin B$_{12}$, Serum

Immunoglobulin A Deficiency
• Immunoglobulin A, Serum
Immunoglobulin A antibodies, Serum

Immunoglobulin A Nephropathy
(see Berger's disease)

Impetigo
Antistreptolysin-O titer, Serum
Complement components, Serum
• Culture, Skin, Specimen (Bullae for group
 A beta-hemolytic streptococci or
 Staphylococcus aureus)
Gram stain, Diagnostic
Sedimentation rate, Erythrocyte, Blood
Urinalysis, Urine

Impotence
Acid phosphatase, Serum
Alkaline phosphatase, Serum
Complete blood count, Blood
Drug screen, Blood
Estrogens, Serum, Urine and 24-hour urine
 (Serum) (Females)
Follicle-stimulating hormone, Serum
 (Females)
• Glucose, Blood
Glucose, 2-hour postprandial, Serum
Luteinizing hormone, Blood (Females)
Polysomnography, Diagnostic
Prolactin, Serum
Prostate-specific antigen, Blood
Pulse volume recording of peripheral
 vasculature, Diagnostic
Testosterone, Free, Bioavailable and total,
 Blood
Thyroid-stimulating hormone, Blood

Indigestion
(see Dyspepsia)

Industry-Related Diseases
Blood gases, Arterial, Blood
Bronchoscopy, Diagnostic
• Chest radiography, Diagnostic
Chloride, Serum
• Complete blood count, Blood
Computed tomography of the body
 (HRCT) (Lungs), Diagnostic
Lupus test, Blood
Potassium, Plasma or serum
Sedimentation rate, Erythrocyte, Blood
Sodium, Plasma, Serum or urine
Sputum cytology, Specimen

Infarction
(see Cerebral, Myocardial, or Renal infarction)

Infection
*(see Acquired immune deficiency syndrome,
Pulmonary infection, Sepsis, or Urinary tract
infection)*

Infectious Mononucleosis
Alkaline phosphatase, Serum
Antinuclear antibody, Serum
Aspartate aminotransferase, Serum
Bilirubin, Total, Serum
Chemistry profile, Blood
Chest radiography, Diagnostic
Complete blood count, Blood
Cytomegalovirus antibody, Serum
Differential leukocyte count, Peripheral
 blood
• Epstein-Barr virus serology, Blood
Heterophile agglutinins, Blood
Lactate dehydrogenase, Blood
Lactate dehydrogenase, Isoenzymes, Blood
Liver battery, Serum
• Monospot screen, Blood
Ornithine carbamoyltransferase, Blood
Smooth muscle antibody, Blood
Streptozyme, Blood
Tartrate-resistant acid phosphatase, Blood
Toxoplasmosis serology, Serum
Uric acid, Serum

Infertility
Biopsy, Site-specific (Endometrium),
 Specimen
Cervical culture (for *Chlamydia*)
Chlamydia culture and group titer, Specimen
Chlamydia screening, Specimen
Chromosome analysis, Blood
Dilation and curettage, Diagnostic
Estradiol, Serum
Estrogens, Serum and 24-hour urine
FMR1 testing for fragile X associated
 disorders, Blood
Follicle-stimulating hormone, Serum
• Gynecologic ultrasonography, Diagnostic
Histopathology, Specimen
Hysterosalpingography, Diagnostic
Hysteroscopy, Diagnostic
• Infertility screen, Specimen
Laparoscopy, Diagnostic
Luteinizing hormone, Blood
Mercury, Blood and urine
Progesterone, Serum
Prolactin, Serum
Rubin's test, Diagnostic

• Semen analysis, Specimen
Sims-Huhner test, Diagnostic
Testosterone, Blood

Inflammation

Complete blood count, Blood
Computed tomography (Site-specific),
 Diagnostic
C-reactive protein, Plasma or serum
• Differential leukocyte count
 (Neutrophils), Peripheral blood
Procalcitonin, Plasma or serum
Sedimentation rate, Erythrocyte, Blood

Influenza

(see also Haemophilus influenzae)
Chest radiography, Diagnostic
Cold agglutinin titer, Serum
Culture (Sputum), Routine, Specimen
Influenza A and B titer, Blood
Respiratory antigen panel, Specimen
• Viral culture, Specimen

Insecticide Poisoning

• Pseudocholinesterase, Plasma

Insomnia

Cortisol, Plasma or serum
Electroencephalography, Diagnostic
17-Hydroxycorticosteroids, 24-hour urine
Oximetry, Diagnostic
Polysomnography, Diagnostic
Tryptophan, Plasma

Insulinoma

Adrenocorticotropic hormone, Serum
C-peptide, Serum
Electrolytes, Plasma or serum
Gastrin, Serum
Glucagon, Plasma
• Glucose, Blood
Histopathology, Specimen
Human chorionic gonadotropin, Beta-
 subunit, Serum
Insulin and insulin antibodies, Blood
Tolbutamide tolerance test, Diagnostic
Vasoactive intestinal polypeptide, Blood

Intermittent Claudication

(see Peripheral vascular disease)

Intervertebral Disk Abnormalities

Computed tomography of the body,
 Diagnostic
Electromyography and nerve conduction
 studies, Diagnostic
• Magnetic resonance imaging, Diagnostic
Radiography of the skull, chest and cervical
 spine, Diagnostic

Intoxication

Alcohol, Blood
Anion gap, Blood
Bromides, Serum
Cannabinoids, Qualitative, Blood or
 urine
Drug screen, Blood
Osmolality, Calculated tests, Blood
 (Osmolar gap)
Osmolality, Serum
pH, Blood
• Toxicology, Drug screen, Blood or
 urine
• Toxicology, Volatiles group by GLC, Blood
 or urine

Intracerebral Hemorrhage

(see Hemorrhage)

Intracranial Pressure, Increased

Antidiuretic hormone, Serum
• Cerebral computed tomography,
 Diagnostic
Cerebrospinal fluid, Routine analysis,
 Specimen
Electrolytes, Plasma or serum (Plasma)
Specific gravity, Urine

Intracranial Tumors

(see Brain tumors)

Intraductal Papilloma (Breast)

(see Breast cancer)

Intussusception

• Barium enema, Diagnostic
Complete blood count, Diagnostic
Computed tomography of the body,
 Diagnostic (with Contrast)
Flat-plate radiograph of abdomen,
 Diagnostic
Occult blood, Stool
Renal function tests, Diagnostic
Stool culture, Routine, Stool
Urinalysis, Urine

Iron Deficiency Anemia (Uncomplicated)

Blood indices, Blood
Complete blood count, Blood
Ferritin, Serum
Hematocrit, Blood
• Iron, Serum
• Iron and total iron-binding capacity/
 transferrin, Serum
Protoporphyrin, Free erythrocyte, Blood
Red blood cell indices, Blood
Reticulocyte count, Blood

Ischemic Heart Disease
(see Angina pectoris)

Islet Cell Tumors
(see Insulinoma)

Jaundice
Amylase, Serum
• Bilirubin, Serum (Total and direct)
Coombs', Direct, Serum
Coombs', Indirect, Serum
Endoscopic retrograde
 cholangiopancreatography, Diagnostic
Galactose, Screening test for galactosemia,
 Urine
Gallbladder and biliary system
 ultrasonography, Diagnostic
Gamma-glutamyltranspeptidase, Blood
Hemoglobin, Blood
Hepatitis A antibody IgM and IgG,
 Blood
Hepatitis B surface antigen, Blood
Hepatitis C genotype, Serum
Histopathology, Specimen
Infectious mononucleosis screening test,
 Blood
Leptospira serodiagnosis, Blood
Leucine aminopeptidase, Blood
Lipase, Serum
• Liver battery, Serum
Liver biopsy, Diagnostic
Liver scan, Diagnostic
Liver ultrasonography, Diagnostic
Magnetic resonance
 cholangiopancreatography, Diagnostic
Malaria smear, Blood
Ornithine carbamoyltransferase, Blood
Phenobarbital, Plasma or serum
Reticulocyte count, Blood
Urobilinogen, Urine

Jock Itch
(see Tinea cruris)

Kaposi's Sarcoma
Acquired immune deficiency syndrome
 evaluation battery, Diagnostic
• Biopsy, *Mycobacterium*, Culture
Cytomegalovirus antibody, Serum
Ocular cytology, Specimen
Oral mucosal transudate, Specimens
T- and B-lymphocyte subset assay,
 Blood

Keratitis
Ocular cytology, Specimen
Viral culture, Specimen

Ketoacidosis
(see Diabetic ketoacidosis)

Kidney
(see Renal)

Kidney Stone
(see Nephrolithiasis)

Kimmelstiel-Wilson Syndrome
Creatinine, Serum
Creatinine clearance, Serum, Urine
Glycosylated hemoglobin, Blood
• Kidney biopsy, Specimen
Protein, Urine
Urea nitrogen, Plasma or serum
Urinalysis, Urine

Klinefelter's Syndrome
Biopsy, Site-specific (Testes), Specimen
Bone densitometry, Diagnostic
Chromosome analysis, Blood
Estradiol, Serum
• Follicle-stimulating hormone, Serum
• Luteinizing hormone, Blood
Metyrapone, 24-hour urine
Oral cavity cytology, Specimen
• Semen analysis, Specimen
Testosterone, Free, Bioavailable and total,
 Blood

Kwashiorkor
• Albumin, Serum
Amylase, Serum
Carotene, Serum
Cholesterol, Blood
Complete blood count, Blood
Lipase, Serum
Phospholipids, Serum
• Protein, Total, Serum
Protein electrophoresis, Serum
Triglycerides, Blood
Trypsin, Plasma or serum

Lactose Intolerance
Biopsy, Site-specific (Small bowel),
 Specimen
• D-Xylose absorption test, Diagnostic,
 Serum or urine
Small bowel series, Diagnostic
Urea breath test, Diagnostic

Lambert-Eaton Myasthenic Syndrome
• Striational antibody, Specimen

Lead Poisoning
Complete blood count, Blood
Coproporphyrin, Urine
Erythrocyte protoporphyrin, Blood

Flat-plate radiography of abdomen, Diagnostic
Heavy-metal screen, Blood and 24-hour urine
• Lead, Blood and urine
Lead mobilization test, 24-hour urine
Radiography of long bones (for Increased density), Diagnostic
Red blood cell, Blood
Thyroid function tests, Blood

Legionnaires' Disease
Alkaline phosphatase, Serum
• Biopsy, Site-specific (Lung), Specimen
Brushing cytology, Specimen
Chest radiography, Diagnostic
Differential leukocyte count, Peripheral blood
Histopathology, Specimen
Lactate dehydrogenase, Blood
• *Legionella* antigen, Urine
• *Legionella pneumophila*, Culture
Legionella pneumophila, Direct FA smear, Specimen (Lung)
Legionnaires' disease antibodies, Blood
Sodium, Plasma, Serum or urine (Serum)
• Sputum cytology, Specimen

Leprosy (Hansen's Disease)
• Acid-fast bacteria, Culture and stain
Biopsy, Site-specific, Specimen
Histopathology, Specimen
Immune complex assay, Blood
Protein, Total, Serum

Leptospirosis
Alanine aminotransferase, Serum
Blood culture, Blood
Cerebrospinal fluid, Routine, Culture and cytology
Chest radiography, Diagnostic
Electrocardiography, Diagnostic
Electrolytes, Plasma or serum
Electrolytes, Urine
• *Leptospira* culture, Urine
• *Leptospira* serodiagnosis, Blood
Liver battery, Serum

Leukemia
Beta$_2$-microglobulin, Blood and 24-hour urine
Blood culture, Blood
Body fluid (Urine), Routine, Culture
• Bone marrow aspiration analysis, Diagnostic
Chest radiography, Diagnostic
Complete blood count, Blood

Compression ultrasonography (Abdomen), Diagnostic
Creatinine, Serum
Cryoglobulin, Qualitative, Serum
• Differential leukocyte count, Peripheral blood
Immunoelectrophoresis, Serum and urine
Lactate dehydrogenase, Blood
T- and B-lymphocyte subset assay, Blood
Tartrate-resistant acid phosphatase, Blood
Terminal deoxynucleotidyl transferase, Blood or bone marrow
Uric acid, Serum
Vitamin B$_{12}$, Serum
Xanthurenic acid, Urine
Zinc, Blood

Leukocytosis
• Bone marrow aspiration analysis, Diagnostic
• Complete blood count, Blood
• Differential leukocyte count, Peripheral blood
Electrolytes, Plasma or serum

Leukopenia
Blood fungus, Culture
Bone marrow aspiration analysis, Diagnostic
Chest radiography, Diagnostic
• Complete blood count, Blood
Culture (Blood, ulcerative lesions, urine), Routine, Specimen
• Differential leukocyte count, Peripheral blood
Foreign body (Catheters or venous access devices), Routine, Culture
Lymph node biopsy, Specimen

Leukorrhea
• Cervical-vaginal cytology, Specimen
Complete blood count, Blood
Urinalysis, Urine

Lice
• Arthropod identification, Specimen

Liver Abscess
Activated partial thromboplastin time and partial thromboplastin time, Plasma
Alanine aminotransferase, Serum
Albumin, Serum
Alkaline phosphatase, Serum
Bilirubin, Direct, Serum
Bilirubin, Total, Serum
Blood culture, Blood
Chest radiography, Diagnostic
Complete blood count, Blood

Compression ultrasound (Abdomen), Diagnostic
Computed tomography of the body (Abdomen), Diagnostic
Entamoeba histolytica serologic test, Blood
Iron and total iron-binding capacity/transferrin, Serum
Leucine aminopeptidase, Blood
Liver battery, Serum
Liver biopsy, Diagnostic
Liver scan, Diagnostic
• Liver ultrasonography, Diagnostic
Needle aspiration, Diagnostic
Prothrombin time and international normalized ratio, Plasma

Liver Cancer
Alanine aminotransferase, Serum
Albumin, Serum, Urine and 24-hour urine (Serum)
Alkaline phosphatase, Serum
Alpha-fetoprotein, Blood
Aspartate aminotransferase, Serum
Bilirubin, Serum
Complete blood count, Blood
Compression ultrasonography (Abdomen), Diagnostic
Computed tomography of the body (Liver), Diagnostic
• Des-gamma-carboxy prothrombin (DCP), Serum
Dual modality imaging, Diagnostic
Leucine aminopeptidase, Blood
Liver battery, Serum
• Liver biopsy, Diagnostic
Liver scan, Diagnostic
Liver ultrasonography, Diagnostic
Magnetic resonance imaging, Diagnostic (Dual contrast)
Needle aspiration, Diagnostic
5'-Nucleotidase, Serum
Ornithine carbamoyltransferase, Blood
Prothrombin time and international normalized ratio, Plasma
Telomerase enzyme marker, Blood

Liver Dysfunction
Alanine aminotransferase, Serum
Alkaline phosphatase, Serum
Antimitochondrial antibody, Serum
Antinuclear antibody, Serum
Bilirubin, Total, Serum
Ceruloplasmin, Serum
Complete blood count, Blood
Gamma-glutamyltranspeptidase, Blood
Hepatitis serologies, Serum

Leucine aminopeptidase, Blood
• Liver battery, Serum
Liver biopsy, Diagnostic
Liver scan, Diagnostic
Liver ultrasonography, Diagnostic
5'-Nucleotidase, Blood
Ornithine carbamoyltransferase, Blood
Prothrombin time and international normalized ratio, Plasma
Striational antibody, Specimen

Liver Failure
Alanine aminotransferase, Serum
Albumin, Serum
Albumin/globulin ratio, Serum
Alkaline phosphatase, Serum
• Ammonia, Blood
Amylase, Serum
Blood culture, Blood
Complete blood count, Blood
• Creatinine, Serum
Creatinine, Urine
Electrolytes, Plasma or serum
Electrolytes, Urine
Globulin, Serum
Hepatitis serologies, Serum
Leucine aminopeptidase, Blood
Lipase, Serum
• Liver battery, Serum
Liver ultrasonography, Diagnostic
5'-Nucleotidase, Blood
Paracentesis, Diagnostic
Protein, Total, Serum
Prothrombin time and international normalized ratio, Plasma
Toxicology, Drug screen, Blood or urine
Urea nitrogen, Plasma or serum

Long QT Syndrome
FAMILION® test, Blood

Lung Cancer
Alpha$_1$-antitrypsin, Serum
• Biopsy, Site-specific (Lung), Specimen
Bone scan, Diagnostic
Brain scan, Cerebral flow and pathology, Diagnostic
Bronchial washing, Specimen
Bronchoscopy, Diagnostic
Brushing cytology, Specimen
CA 15-3, Blood
CA 15-3, Serum
CA 50, Blood
Chest radiography, Diagnostic
Complete blood count, Blood
Computed tomography of the body (Spiral) (Lung), Diagnostic

Dual modality imaging, Diagnostic
Endoscopic ultrasonography (Guided transesophageal fine-needle aspiration)
Mediastinoscopy, Diagnostic
Mucinlike carcinoma–associated antigen, Blood
Neuron-specific enolase, Serum
Pulmonary function tests, Diagnostic
Renal function tests, Diagnostic
Sputum cytology, Specimen
Squamous cell carcinoma antigen, Serum
Striational antibody, Specimen
Telomerase enzyme marker, Blood
Thoracentesis, Diagnostic
Tissue polypeptide antigen, Plasma or serum

Lupoid Hepatitis
• Lupus panel, Blood

Lupus Erythematosus
(see Cutaneous lupus erythematosus and Systemic lupus erythematosus)

Lyme Disease
Borrelia burgdorferi C6 peptide antibody, Serum
Electrocardiography, Diagnostic
Immunoglobulin G, Serum
Immunoglobulin M, Serum
• Lyme disease antibody, Blood
Sedimentation rate, Erythrocyte, Blood

Lymphadenitis
Blood culture, Blood
Lymph node biopsy, Specimen

Lymphangitis
Blood culture, Blood
Culture, Routine, Specimen

Lymphogranuloma Venereum
Biopsy, Site-specific (Lymph node), Specimen
Chlamydia culture and group titer, Specimen
Complement fixation, Serum (for *Chlamydia*)
Complete blood count, Blood
Culture, Skin, Specimen
Erythrocyte sedimentation rate, Blood
• Histopathology, Specimen

Lymphoma
Acquired immune deficiency syndrome evaluation battery, Diagnostic
Biopsy, Site-specific, Specimen (Excisional, Fine needle aspiration)
Bone marrow aspiration analysis, Specimen

Calcium, Total, Serum
Chest radiography, Diagnostic
Complete blood count, Blood
Computed tomography of the body (Abdomen, chest, pelvis), Diagnostic
Cytologic study of gastrointestinal tract, Diagnostic
Differential leukocyte count, Peripheral blood
Electrolytes, Plasma or serum
Gallium scan of bone, Brain, Breast or liver, Diagnostic
Liver battery, Serum
Lumbar puncture, Diagnostic
• Lymph node biopsy, Specimen
Mediastinoscopy, Diagnostic
Needle aspiration (Lymph node), Diagnostic
O-banding (CSF proteins), Serum
Phosphorus, Serum
Platelet count, Blood
Positron emission tomography, Diagnostic
Potassium, Plasma or serum
Tartrate-resistant acid phosphatase, Blood
Terminal deoxynucleotidyl transferase, Blood or bone marrow
Urea nitrogen, Plasma or serum
Uric acid, Serum
Xanthurenic acid, Urine

Lynch Syndrome
(see Colorectal cancer)

Macroglobulinemia
(see Waldenström's macroglobulinemia)

Malabsorption
Calcium, Total, Serum
Carotene, Serum
• D-Xylose absorption test, Diagnostic, Serum or urine
Fat, Semiquantitative, Stool
• Fecal fat, Quantitative, 72-hour stool
Folic acid, Serum
Glucose, 2-hour postprandial, Serum
Glucose tolerance test, Blood
Lipid profile, Blood
Magnesium, Serum
Phosphorus, Serum
Protein, Total, Serum
Pyridoxal 5′-phosphate, Plasma
Sigmoidoscopy, Diagnostic
Sodium, Plasma, Serum or urine
Transferrin, Serum
Trypsin, Plasma or serum

Trypsin, Stool
Vitamin B$_{12}$, Serum
Vitamin C, Plasma or serum

Malaria
Alanine aminotransferase, Serum
Alkaline phosphatase, Serum
Bilirubin, Total, Serum
Blood indices, Blood
Cold agglutinin titer, Serum
Complement, Total, Serum
Complete blood count, Blood
Differential leukocyte count, Peripheral
  blood
Electrolytes, Plasma or serum
Glucose, Blood
Liver battery, Serum
• Malaria smear, Blood
Parasite screen, Blood
Platelet count, Blood
Protein electrophoresis, Serum
Red blood cell morphology, Blood
Rheumatoid factor, Blood

Malignant Hypertension
(see Hypertension)

Malnutrition
(see Kwashiorkor and Marasmus)

Manic-Depressive Psychosis
Complete blood count, Blood
• Cortisol, Plasma or serum
Creatinine, Serum
Electrolytes, Plasma or serum
Glucose, Blood
• Lithium, Serum
Liver battery, Serum
Thyroid function tests, Blood
Urea nitrogen, Plasma or serum
Valproic acid, Blood

Marasmus
Albumin, Serum
Blood urea nitrogen/creatinine ratio,
  Blood
Complete blood count, Blood
• Protein, Total, Serum
Protein electrophoresis, Serum
• Transthyretin (Prealbumin), Serum
Vitamin B$_6$, Plasma

Marfan Syndrome
Bone scan, Diagnostic
• Echocardiography, Diagnostic
Hydroxyproline, Total, 24-hour urine
Magnetic resonance imaging, Diagnostic

Maroteaux-Lamy Syndrome
• Mucopolysaccharides, Qualitative, Urine

McCune-Albright Syndrome
(see Albright syndrome)

Measles
(see Rubella and Rubeola)

Megaloblastic Anemia
Blood indices, Blood
• Bone marrow aspiration analysis,
  Diagnostic
Complete blood count, Blood
Differential leukocyte count, Peripheral
  blood
Folic acid, Red blood cells, Blood
• Folic acid, Serum
Gastric analysis, Specimen
Gastric pH, Specimen
Gastrin, Serum
Homocysteine, Plasma or urine
Intrinsic factor antibody, Blood
Lactate dehydrogenase, Blood
Lactate dehydrogenase, Isoenzymes, Blood
Pepsinogen I antibody, Blood
Platelet count, Blood
Red blood cell morphology, Blood
Reticulocyte count, Blood
Type and crossmatch, Blood (Screen)
Vitamin B$_{12}$, Serum

Melanoma
• Biopsy, Site-specific, Specimen
Bone marrow aspiration analysis, Specimen
Cerebral computed tomography, Diagnostic
Chest radiography, Diagnostic
Complete blood count, Blood
Computed tomography of the body
  (Melanoma site), Diagnostic
Creatinine, Serum
Electrolytes, Plasma or serum
Histopathology, Specimen
Lactate dehydrogenase, Blood
Liver battery, Serum
Melanin, Urine
Positron emission tomography, Diagnostic
Sentinel lymph node biopsy, Diagnostic
  (for tumors 1-4 mm in thickness)
TA90 immune complex assay, Serum
Urea nitrogen, Plasma or serum

Ménière's Disease
Allergen-specific IgE, Serum
Antinuclear antibody, Serum
• Audiometry test, Diagnostic
Cerebrospinal fluid, Protein, Specimen
Electrocardiography, Diagnostic

Electronystagmography test, Diagnostic
Lyme disease antibody, Blood
Magnetic resonance imaging (Head, inner
  ear), Diagnostic
Thyroid profile, Blood
Venereal Disease Research Laboratory test,
  Serum

Meningitis
Blood culture, Blood
Cerebral computed tomography, Diagnostic
• Cerebrospinal fluid, Cytology, Specimen
Cerebrospinal fluid, Fungus, Culture
Cerebrospinal fluid, Heparin binding
  protein, Myelin basic protein, Oligoclonal
  bands, Protein, and Protein
  electrophoresis, Specimen
Cerebrospinal fluid, *Mycobacterium*,
  Culture
Cerebrospinal fluid, Routine analysis,
  Specimen
Complete blood count, Blood
Computed tomography of brain, Diagnostic
Coxsackie A or B virus titer, Blood
C-reactive protein, Plasma or serum
Cryptococcal antibody titer, Serum
Cryptococcal antigen titer, Cerebrospinal
  fluid, Specimen
Cryptococcal antigen titer, Serum
Differential leukocyte count, Peripheral
  blood
Gastric aspirate, Routine, Culture
Herpes cytology, Specimen
Leptospira serodiagnosis, Blood
Lumbar puncture, Diagnostic
Magnetic resonance imaging, Diagnostic
O-banding (CSF proteins), Plasma
Procalcitonin, Plasma or serum
Sodium, Plasma, Serum or urine
Sputum for *Haemophilus* species, Culture
Toxoplasmosis, Rubella, Cytomegalovirus,
  Herpesvirus serology, Blood
Viral culture, Specimen

Menopause
Biopsy, Site-specific (Endometrium),
  Specimen
Bone densitometry, Diagnostic
Bone scan, Diagnostic
Cholesterol, Blood
Estradiol, Serum
Estrogens, Nonpregnant, 24-hour urine
• Estrogens, Serum
Follicle-stimulating hormone, Serum
Hormonal evaluation, Cytologic, Specimen
Luteinizing hormone, Blood

Mammography, Diagnostic
Metyrapone, 24-hour urine
Thyroid-stimulating hormone, Sensitive
  assay, Blood

Menorrhagia (Hypermenorrhea)
Activated partial thromboplastin time and
  partial thromboplastin time, Plasma
• Complete blood count, Blood
Cortisol, Plasma or serum
Estrogens, Serum and 24-hour urine
Prothrombin time and international
  normalized ratio, Plasma

Menstruation
Estrogens, Serum and 24-hour urine
Follicle-stimulating hormone, Serum
Luteinizing hormone, Blood

Metabolic Acidosis
Beta-hydroxybutyrate, Blood
• Blood gases, Arterial, Blood
• Chemistry profile, Blood
Creatinine, Serum
Dinitrophenylhydrazine test, Diagnostic
Electrolytes, Plasma or serum
Glucose, Blood
Osmolality, Calculated tests, Blood
  (Osmolar gap)
Osmolality, Serum
Salicylate, Blood
Toxicology, Drug screen, Blood or urine
Toxicology, Volatiles group by GLC, Blood
  or urine
Urea nitrogen, Plasma or serum
Urinalysis, Urine

Metabolic Alkalosis
• Blood gases, Arterial, Blood
Electrolytes, Plasma or serum
Potassium, Plasma or serum
Urinalysis, Urine

Metabolic Syndrome
C-reactive protein, Blood
Glucose, Blood (fasting)
Insulin and insulin antibodies, Blood
• Lipid profile, Blood
Triglycerides, Blood
Uric acid, Serum

Metal Poisoning
Arsenic, Blood, Hair, Nails or Urine
Cadmium, Serum and 24-hour urine
Chemistry profile, Blood
Chromium, Serum
Chromium, Urine
• Heavy metals, Blood and 24-hour urine
Lead, Blood or urine

Lithium, Serum
Mercury, Blood
Mercury, 24-hour urine
Thallium, Serum or 24-hour urine
Urinalysis, Urine
Zinc, Blood

Metastasis

Acid phosphatase, Serum
Adrenocorticotropic hormone, Serum
Alkaline phosphatase, Heat stable, Serum
Alkaline phosphatase, Isoenzymes, Serum
Alkaline phosphatase, Serum
Alpha-fetoprotein, Blood
Body fluid cytology, Specimen
Bone marrow biopsy, Diagnostic
Bone scan, Diagnostic
Bronchial washing, Specimen
Brushing cytology, Specimen
CA 15-3, Serum (Breast metastasis)
Calcium, Total, Serum
Carcinoembryonic antigen, Serum
Cathepsin D, Specimen
Cerebrospinal fluid, Cytology, Specimen
Cervical-vaginal cytology, Specimen
Chemistry profile, Blood
Circulating tumor cell test, Blood (Breast
  metastasis)
Complete blood count, Blood
Computed tomography of the body
  (Spiral) (Site-specific), Diagnostic
Differential leukocyte count, Peripheral
  blood
Electrolytes, Plasma or serum
Estrogen receptor and progesterone
  receptor in breast cancer, Diagnostic
Gamma-glutamyltranspeptidase, Blood
Gastrin, Serum
Histopathology, Specimen
Human chorionic gonadotropin,
  Beta-subunit, Serum
Magnetic resonance imaging, Diagnostic
Magnetic resonance spectroscopy,
  Diagnostic
Mucinlike carcinoma–associated antigen,
  Blood
Needle aspiration, Diagnostic
5'-Nucleotidase, Blood
Ocular cytology, Specimen
Parathyroid hormone, Blood
Progesterone receptor assay, Specimen
Serotonin, Serum or blood
Sputum cytology, Specimen
Urine cytology, Urine
Washing cytology, Specimen

Metrorrhagia

Biopsy, Site-specific (Endometrium),
  Specimen
Complete blood count, Blood
Cortisol, Plasma or serum
• Estrogens, Serum and 24-hour urine
Gynecologic ultrasonography, Diagnostic
Human chorionic gonadotropin, Beta-
  subunit, Serum
Hysteroscopy, Diagnostic
Liver battery, Serum
Pap smear, Diagnostic
Prolactin, Serum
Prothrombin time and international
  normalized ratio, Blood
Thyroid function tests, Blood

Microcytic Anemia

Blood indices, Blood
Bone marrow aspiration analysis, Specimen
Complete blood count, Blood
Ferritin, Serum
Fetal hemoglobin, Blood
Heavy-metal screen, 24-hour urine
Hemoglobin A2, Blood
Hemoglobin electrophoresis, Blood
Iron, Serum
Iron and total iron-binding capacity/
  transferrin, Serum
Lead, Blood and urine
Protoporphyrin, Free erythrocyte, Blood
• Red blood cell morphology, Blood
Reticulocyte count, Blood
Total iron-binding capacity, Serum

Migraine Headaches

Arteriography, Diagnostic
Cerebral computed tomography, Diagnostic
Computed tomography of the body
  (Cervical spine), Diagnostic
Magnetic resonance imaging, Diagnostic

Mitral Stenosis

Chest radiography, Diagnostic
• Echocardiography, Diagnostic
Electrocardiography, Diagnostic
Transesophageal ultrasonography, Diagnostic
Ventriculography, Diagnostic

Mitral Valve Regurgitation

Chest radiography, Diagnostic
• Echocardiography, Diagnostic
Electrocardiography, Diagnostic
Pulmonary artery catheterization,
  Diagnostic
Transesophageal ultrasonography,
  Diagnostic

Mongoloidism
(*see Down syndrome*)

Moniliasis
(*see Thrush, Vaginitis*)

Monkeypox
• Biopsy, Site-specific (Lesion), Specimen
• Culture, Routine, Specimen (Oropharynx, Tonsillar area)

Mononucleosis
(*see Infectious mononucleosis*)

Morquio's Syndrome
• Mucopolysaccharides, Qualitative, Urine

Multiple Myeloma
Acid phosphatase, Serum
Albumin, Serum
Alkaline phosphatase, Serum
• Bence Jones protein, Urine
• Bone marrow aspiration analysis, Specimen
Bone radiography (Complete skeleton), Diagnostic
Calcium, Total, Serum
Complement components, Serum
Complete blood count, Blood
Creatinine, Serum
Electrolytes, Plasma or serum
Immunoelectrophoresis, Serum and urine
Protein, Total, Serum
Sedimentation rate, Erythrocyte, Blood
T- and B-lymphocyte subset assay, Blood
Urea nitrogen, Plasma or serum
Uric acid, Serum
Urinalysis (for Protein), Urine
Viscosity, Blood

Multiple Sclerosis
Brainstem auditory evoked potential, Diagnostic
Cerebrospinal fluid, Immunoglobulin G, Specimen
Cerebrospinal fluid, Myelin basic protein, Specimen
• Cerebrospinal fluid, Oligoclonal bands, Specimen
Cerebrospinal fluid, Protein, Specimen
Cerebrospinal fluid, Protein electrophoresis, Specimen
Cerebrospinal fluid, Routine analysis, Specimen
Human leukocyte antigen B27, Blood
• Magnetic resonance imaging (Diffusion-weighted), Diagnostic
Magnetic resonance spectroscopy, Diagnostic

O-banding (CSF proteins), Plasma
Somatosensory evoked potential, Diagnostic
Vestibular-evoked myogenic potential

Mumps
• Mumps antibody, Blood
• Viral culture, Specimen

Muscular Dystrophy
(*see also Duchenne muscular dystrophy*)
Aldolase, Serum
Aspartate aminotransferase, Serum
Catecholamines, Fractionation free, Plasma
Creatine, Urine
Creatine kinase, Serum (Isoenzymes)
Creatinine, Serum
Electromyography and nerve conduction studies, Diagnostic
Lactate dehydrogenase, Blood
Metanephrines, Total, 24-hour urine and free plasma
• Muscle biopsy, Specimen
Myoglobin, Serum and qualitative, Urine

Myasthenia Gravis
Acetylcholine receptor antibody, Serum
Cerebrospinal fluid, Immunoglobulin G ratios and immunoglobulin G index, Specimen
Computed tomography of the body (Mediastinum), Diagnostic
• Electromyography and nerve conduction studies, Diagnostic (Electromyography)
Human leukocyte antigen B27, Blood
Magnetic resonance imaging, Diagnostic
Metanephrines, Total, 24-hour urine and free, Plasma
Pulmonary function tests, Diagnostic (Spirometry)
Striational autoantibody, Specimen
Thyroid peroxidase antibody, Blood
Thyroid profile, Blood

Mycoses
Gastric cytology, Specimen
Sputum cytology, Specimen

Myocardial Conduction Defect
Cardiac enzymes/isoenzymes, Blood
Chemistry profile, Blood
Creatine kinase, Serum (Isoenzymes)
Digoxin, Serum
• Electrocardiography, Diagnostic
Electrolytes, Plasma or serum
• Electrophysiologic study, Diagnostic
Lactate dehydrogenase, Blood
Lactate dehydrogenase, Isoenzymes, Blood

Lidocaine, Serum
Procainamide, Serum
Propranolol, Serum
Quinidine, Serum
Signal-averaged electrocardiography,
  Diagnostic
Toxicology, Drug screen, Blood or urine

Myocardial Infarction
Activated coagulation time, Automated,
  Blood
Activated partial thromboplastin time and
  partial thromboplastin time, Plasma
Anticardiolipin antibody, Serum
Antimyocardial antibody, Serum
Aspartate aminotransferase, Serum
Basic metabolic panel, Blood
Cardiac catheterization, Diagnostic
• Cardiac enzymes/isoenzymes, Blood
Cardiac output, Diagnostic
Chemistry profile, Blood
Chest radiography, Diagnostic
Cholesterol, Blood
Complete blood count, Blood
Coronary intravascular ultrasonography,
  Diagnostic
Creatine kinase, Serum (Isoenzymes)
D-Dimer test, Blood
Digoxin, Serum
Disopyramide phosphate, Serum
Echocardiography, Diagnostic
• Electrocardiography, Diagnostic
Glucose, Blood
Heart scan, Diagnostic
Hydroxybutyrate dehydrogenase, Blood
Lactate dehydrogenase, Blood
Lactate dehydrogenase, Isoenzymes, Blood
Lidocaine, Serum
Low-density lipoprotein cholesterol, Blood
Magnesium, Serum
Myoglobin, Qualitative, Urine and serum
Persantine-sestamibi stress test and scan,
  Diagnostic
Positron emission tomography, Diagnostic
Potassium, Plasma or serum
Procainamide, Serum
Propranolol, Blood
Prothrombin time and international
  normalized ratio, Plasma
P-selectin, Plasma
Quinidine, Serum
Signal-averaged electrocardiography,
  Diagnostic
Stress exercise test, Diagnostic
Stress test, Pharmacologic, Diagnostic

Thyroid-stimulating hormone, Sensitive
  assay, Blood
• Troponin I, Plasma and troponin T,
  Serum
Urea nitrogen, Plasma or serum

Myocarditis
Antimyocardial antibody, Serum
Antinuclear antibody, Serum
Antistreptolysin-O titer, Serum
Aspartate aminotransferase, Serum
Blood culture, Blood
Blood indices, Blood
Cardiac catheterization, Diagnostic
Cardiac enzymes/isoenzymes, Blood
Chest radiography, Diagnostic
Complete blood count, Blood
• Coxsackie A or B virus titer, Blood
Creatine kinase, Serum (Isoenzymes)
Culture, Routine (Nasopharyngeal, rectal),
  Specimen
Differential leukocyte count, Peripheral
  blood
• Echocardiography, Diagnostic
• Electrocardiography, Diagnostic
Histopathology, Specimen
HIV testing (see Acquired
  immunodeficiency syndrome evaluation
  battery, Diagnostic)
Magnetic resonance imaging (with
  Contrast, cardiac), Diagnostic
• Muscle biopsy (Myocardium), Specimen
Sedimentation rate, Erythrocyte, Blood
Transesophageal ultrasonography,
  Diagnostic
Troponin I, Plasma and troponin T,
  Serum

Myoclonus
Cerebral computed tomography, Diagnostic
Electroencephalography, Diagnostic
• Magnetic resonance imaging, Diagnostic

Myxedema (Hypothyroidism)
Complete blood count, Blood
Electrolytes, Plasma or serum
Thyroid antithyroglobulin antibody, Serum
• Thyroid function tests, Blood
  Thyroid peroxidase antibody, Blood
Thyroid-stimulating hormone, Sensitive
  assay, Blood
Thyroid test, Free thyroxine index, Serum
Thyroid test, Thyroid hormone binding
  ratio, Blood
Thyroid test, Thyroxine, Blood
Thyroid test, Thyroxine free, Serum

Narcolepsy
(see Sleep disorders)

Narcotics
(see Drug abuse)

Neoplasia
(see Tumors)

Nephritic Syndrome
Abdominal plain film, Diagnostic
Anti-DNA, Serum
Biopsy, Site-specific (Kidney), Specimen
Body fluid (Urine), Routine, Culture
Chemistry profile, Blood
Complete blood count, Blood
• Creatinine, Urine
Culture, Routine, Specimen
Electrocardiography, Diagnostic
Electrolytes, Urine
Kidney ultrasonography, Diagnostic
Urea nitrogen, Plasma or serum
Urinalysis, Urine

Nephrolithiasis
Abdominal plain film, Diagnostic
Body fluid (Urine), Routine, Culture
Calcium, Total, Serum
Calcium, Urine
Chemistry profile, Blood
• Computed tomography of the body
  (Spiral) (Kidneys), Diagnostic
Creatinine, Serum
Creatinine clearance, Urine
Culture (Urine), Routine, Specimen
Cystine, Qualitative, Urine
Electrolytes, Plasma or serum
Electrolytes, Urine
Flat-plate radiograph of the abdomen,
  Diagnostic
Histopathology, Specimen
Intravenous pyelography, Diagnostic
Kidney stone analysis, Specimen
Kidney ultrasonography, Diagnostic
Magnesium, Serum
Magnesium, 24-hour urine
Magnetic resonance urography,
  Diagnostic
Occult blood, Urine
Oxalate, 24-hour Urine
pH, Urine
Phosphorus, Serum
Phosphorus, Urine
Urea nitrogen, Plasma or serum
Uric acid, Serum
Uric acid, Urine
Urinalysis, Urine (24-hour)

Nephrosclerosis
Complete blood count, Blood
Creatinine, Serum
Urea nitrogen, Plasma or serum
• Urinalysis, Urine

Nephrotic Syndrome
Albumin, Serum
Albumin/globulin ratio, Serum
• Biopsy, Site-specific (Kidney), Specimen
Chest radiography, Diagnostic
Cholesterol, Blood
Complete blood count, Blood
Creatinine, Serum
Creatinine clearance, Serum, Urine
Electrolytes, Plasma or serum
Electrolytes, Urine
Glucose, 2-hour postprandial, Serum
Glucose tolerance test, Blood
HIV testing (see Acquired immune
  deficiency syndrome evaluation battery,
  Diagnostic)
Kidney biopsy, Specimen
Kidney ultrasonography, Diagnostic
Phosphorus, Serum
Protein electrophoresis, Serum
Protein electrophoresis, Urine
Protein, Quantitative (24-hour), Urine
Protein, Total, Serum
Sodium, Urine
Transferrin, Serum
Triglycerides, Blood
Urea nitrogen, Plasma or serum
• Urinalysis, Urine

Neuroblastoma
Biopsy, Site-specific, Specimen
Bone marrow aspiration analysis, Specimen
Bone scan, Diagnostic
Chemistry profile, Blood
Complete blood count, Blood
Computed tomography of the body,
  Diagnostic
• Homovanillic acid, 24-hour urine
Lactate dehydrogenase, Blood
Magnetic resonance imaging, Diagnostic
Magnetic resonance spectroscopy, Diagnostic
• Neuron-specific enolase, Serum
Octreotide scan, Diagnostic
Sedimentation rate, Erythrocyte, Blood
• Vanillylmandelic acid, Urine

Neurodegeneration
Cerebrospinal fluid, Myelin basic protein,
  Specimen
Cerebrospinal fluid, Routine analysis,
  Specimen

Electrocardiography, Diagnostic
Electromyography and nerve conduction
studies, Diagnostic
HIV testing (see Acquired immune
deficiency syndrome evaluation battery,
Diagnostic)
Lead, Blood and urine
• Magnetic resonance spectroscopy,
Diagnostic
Nerve biopsy, Diagnostic

Neurofibromatosis
• Biopsy, Site-specific, Specimen
• Biopsy, Site-specific (Skin, nerves),
Specimen
Bone radiography, Diagnostic
Chest radiography, Diagnostic
Cerebral computed tomography,
Diagnostic
Electroencephalography, Diagnostic
Magnetic resonance imaging (Brain, spine),
Diagnostic
Slit-lamp vision test, Diagnostic

Neurogenic Pulmonary Edema
(see Pulmonary edema)

Neuropathy
Antinuclear antibody, Serum
Cerebrospinal fluid, Routine analysis,
Specimen
Electrocardiography, Diagnostic
• Electromyography and nerve conduction
studies, Diagnostic
Electron microscopy (for Nerve tissue),
Diagnostic
• Epidermal nerve fiber density test,
Specimen
Folate, Serum
Glucose, Blood
Glucose, 2-hour postprandial, Serum
Histopathology, Specimen
HIV testing (see Acquired immune
deficiency syndrome evaluation battery,
Diagnostic)
Lead, Blood
Lumbar puncture, Diagnostic
Magnetic resonance neurography,
Diagnostic
Nerve biopsy, diagnostic
Protoporphyrin, Free erythrocyte,
Blood
Sweat gland nerve fiber density test,
Specimen
Vitamin B$_{12}$, Serum
Vitamin E$_1$, Serum

Neurosyphilis
(see Syphilis)

Niemann-Pick Disease
Biopsy, Site-specific (Skin), Specimen
• Sphingomyelinase, Diagnostic

Non-Alcoholic Fatty Liver Disease
(see Liver dysfunction)

Nontropical Sprue
(see Celiac sprue)

Normal Pressure Hydrocephalus
Brain ultrasonography, Diagnostic
• Cerebral computed tomography,
Diagnostic
Cerebrospinal fluid, Routine analysis,
Specimen (Pressure)
• Cisternography, Radionuclide, Diagnostic
• Lumbar puncture, Diagnostic
Magnetic resonance imaging, Diagnostic

Obesity
Bone densitometry, Diagnostic
C-reactive protein, Blood
• Cholesterol, Blood
Electrocardiography, Diagnostic
Electrolytes, Plasma or serum
• Glucose, Blood
Glucose, Qualitative, Semiquantitative,
Urine
Insulin, Blood
Insulin-like growth factor-I, Blood
Lipid profile, Blood
Melanocyte-stimulating hormone, Urine
Protein, Urine
Thyroid test, Thyroxine, Blood
• Thyroid test, Triiodothyronine, Blood
Urea nitrogen, Plasma or serum

Obstruction, Bowel
Alanine aminotransferase, Serum
Alkaline phosphatase, Serum
Amylase, Serum and urine
Aspartate aminotransferase, Serum
Barium enema, Diagnostic
Chloride, Serum
Complete blood count, Blood
Differential leukocyte count, Peripheral
blood
Doppler ultrasonographic flow studies,
Diagnostic
• Flat-plate radiograph of the abdomen,
Diagnostic
Occult blood, Stool
Potassium, Plasma or serum
Sigmoidoscopy, Diagnostic

Sodium, Plasma or serum
Urinalysis, Urine

Obstructive Jaundice
(see Jaundice)

Occlusion, Acute Arterial
Activated partial thromboplastin time and
  partial thromboplastin time, Plasma
• Arteriography, Diagnostic
Blood gases, Arterial, Blood
Complete blood count, Blood
Glucose, Blood
Magnetic resonance angiography,
  Diagnostic
Prothrombin time and international
  normalized ratio, Plasma

Organic Brain Syndrome
Adrenocorticotropic hormone, Serum
Calcium, Total, Serum
Glucose, Blood
• Potassium, Plasma or serum
Red blood cell, Blood
Thyroid-stimulating hormone, Blood

Orthostatic Hypotension
Catecholamines, Fractionation free,
  Plasma
Complete blood count, Serum
Cortisol, Serum
Tilt table test, Diagnostic

Osteoarthritis
Body fluid cytology, Specimen
• Bone radiography (Spine), Diagnostic
Culture (Synovial fluid), Routine
  Specimen
Histopathology, Specimen
Mucin clot test (Synovial fluid), Specimen
• Radiography of long bones, Diagnostic
Synovial fluid analysis, Diagnostic

Osteomalacia
• Alkaline phosphatase, Serum
Bone scan, Diagnostic
• Calcium, Total, Serum
Calcium, Urine
Creatinine, Serum
Cytologic study of urine, Diagnostic
Electrolytes, Plasma or serum
Liver battery, Serum
• Parathyroid hormone, Blood
• Phosphorus, Serum
• Radiography of long bones, Diagnostic
Thyroid function tests, Blood
Urea nitrogen, Plasma or serum
Vitamin D$_3$, Plasma or serum

Osteomyelitis
Blood culture, Blood
• Bone radiography (Affected area),
  Diagnostic
Bone scan, Diagnostic
Complete blood count, Blood
Computed tomography of the body,
  Diagnostic
C-reactive protein, Serum
Culture (Orthopedic wound; Site sinus),
  Routine, Specimen
Differential leukocyte count, Peripheral
  blood
Magnetic resonance imaging, Diagnostic
Needle aspiration (Bone), Diagnostic
• Sedimentation rate, Erythrocyte, Blood

Osteoporosis
Alkaline phosphatase, Serum
• Bone densitometry, Diagnostic
Bone radiography, Diagnostic
Bone scan, Diagnostic
Bone ultrasonometry, Diagnostic
Calcium, Total, Serum
Calcium (24-hour), Urine
Complete blood count, Blood
Cortisol, Plasma or serum
Creatinine, Serum
Electrolytes, Plasma or serum
Estradiol, Serum
Estrogens, Serum
Glucose, Blood
Liver battery, Serum
Osteocalcin, Plasma or serum
Phosphorus, Serum
Prolactin, Serum
Protein electrophoresis, Urine
Tartrate-resistant acid phosphatase, Blood
Thyroid function tests, Blood
Urea nitrogen, Plasma or serum

Otitis Media
Biopsy, Site-specific, Specimen (Anaerobic
  culture)
Bone radiography (Mastoids), Diagnostic
Complete blood count, Blood
Computed tomography of the body,
  Diagnostic
Ear, Routine, Culture
Gamma-globulin, Plasma
Sputum for *Haemophilus* species, Culture

Ovarian Cancer
CA 15-3, Blood
CA 72-4, Blood
• CA 125, Blood
Complete blood count, Blood

Compression ultrasound (Abdomen),
  Diagnostic
Creatinine, Serum
Dual modality imaging, Diagnostic
Electrolytes, Plasma or serum
Flat-plate radiography of abdomen,
  Diagnostic
Gynecologic ultrasonography, Diagnostic
Human epididymis protein 4, Blood
Mucinlike carcinoma–associated antigen,
  Blood
Osteopontin, Serum
OVA1™ ovarian tumor triage test, Serum
Pregnancy test routine, Serum and
  qualitative, Urine
Telomerase enzyme marker, Blood
Urea nitrogen, Plasma or serum
Urinary chorionic gonadotropin peptide,
  Urine
Vascular endothelial growth factor,
  Specimen

Ovarian Function
Androstenedione, Serum
• Estradiol, Serum
Estrogens, Serum and 24-hour urine
• Follicle-stimulating hormone, Serum
Hormonal evaluation, Cytologic, Specimen
17-Hydroxyprogesterone, Blood
• Luteinizing hormone, Blood
Metyrapone, 24-hour urine
Pregnanetriol, Urine
• Progesterone, Serum

Ovarian Hyperstimulation Syndrome
Activated partial thromboplastin time and
  partial thromboplastin time, Plasma
Alanine aminotransferase, Serum
Albumin, Serum
Alkaline phosphatase, Serum
Aspartate aminotransferase, Serum
Bilirubin, Indirect (Unconjugated), Serum
Blood gases, Arterial, Blood
Body fluid analysis, Cell count, Specimen
Body fluid cytology, Specimen
Chest radiography, Diagnostic
Complete blood count, Blood
C-reactive protein, Plasma or serum
Creatinine, Serum
Differential leukocyte count, Peripheral
  blood
Doppler ultrasonographic flow studies,
  Diagnostic
Electrolytes, Plasma or serum
Estradiol, Serum
Estrogens, Serum and 24-hour, Urine

Gamma-glutamyltranspeptidase, Blood
Gram stain (Effusion specimen),
  Diagnostic
• Gynecologic ultrasonography, Diagnostic
Paracentesis, Diagnostic
Pregnancy test (hCG), Routine, Serum
Progesterone, Serum
Urea nitrogen, Plasma or serum
Vascular endothelial growth factor,
  Specimen

Overdose
(see Poisonings)

Overhydration
(see Hydration)

Ovulation
• Progesterone, Serum

Paget's Disease, Bone
Acid phosphatase, Serum
• Alkaline phosphatase, Serum
• Bone radiography, Diagnostic
• Bone scan, Diagnostic
Calcium, Total, Serum
Calcium, Urine
• Hydroxyproline, Total, 24-hour urine
Osteocalcin, Plasma or serum
Phosphorus, Urine

Paget's Disease, Breast
• Biopsy, Site-specific (Breast), Specimen
Breast ultrasonography, Diagnostic
Mammography, Diagnostic
Needle aspiration, Diagnostic
Prolactin, Serum

Pain, Abdominal
• Acute abdominal series, Diagnostic
Albumin, Serum, Urine and 24-hour urine
  (Serum)
Amylase, Serum
• Complete blood count, Blood
Compression ultrasound (Abdomen),
  Diagnostic
Computed tomography of the body
  (Abdomen), Diagnostic
Cytologic study of urine, Diagnostic
Electrolytes, Plasma or serum
• Flat-plate radiograph of the abdomen,
  Diagnostic
Glucose, Blood
Lipase, Serum
Liver battery, Serum
Nitrite, Bacteria screen, Urine
Occult blood, Stool
Ova and parasites, Stool
Potassium, Plasma or serum

Pregnancy test routine, Serum and
  qualitative, Urine
Protein, Total, Serum
Sedimentation rate, Erythrocyte, Blood
Sodium, Plasma or serum
Upper gastrointestinal series, Diagnostic
Urea breath test, Diagnostic
Urinalysis (Leukocyte esterase; Nitrite),
  Urine

Pain, Back

Bone radiography, Diagnostic
Bone scan, Diagnostic
Calcium, Total, Serum
Complete blood count, Blood
Computed tomography of the body
  (Spine), Diagnostic
Magnetic resonance imaging, Diagnostic
Magnetic resonance neurography,
  Diagnostic
Myelography, Diagnostic
Nerve conduction studies, Diagnostic
Phosphorus, Serum
Red blood cell morphology, Blood
Rheumatoid factor, Blood
Sedimentation rate, Erythrocyte, Blood
Urinalysis, Urine

Pain, Chest

*(see Angina pectoris, Myocardial infarction,
Pleurisy, or Pneumonia)*

Pain, Chronic

Complete blood count, Blood
C-reactive protein, Plasma or serum
Magnetic resonance neurography,
  Diagnostic
Platelet count, Blood
Radiography, Diagnostic
Rheumatoid factor, Blood
Sedimentation rate, Erythrocyte, Blood
Serotonin, Serum or blood
Sickle cell test, Blood
Urea nitrogen, Plasma or serum
Urinalysis, Urine

Pain, Muscle and Bone

Aspartate aminotransferase, Serum
Bone radiography, Diagnostic
Bone scan, Diagnostic
Calcium, Total, Serum
Complete blood count, Blood
Creatine kinase, Serum
Magnetic resonance imaging, Diagnostic
Muscle biopsy, Specimen
Phosphorus, Serum
Thyroid test, Thyroxine, Blood

Thyroid test, Triiodothyronine, Blood
Uric acid, Serum

Pain, Vascular

Activated partial thromboplastin time and
  partial thromboplastin time, Plasma
Ankle-brachial index, Diagnostic
Cerebrospinal fluid, Routine analysis,
  Specimen
Complete blood count, Blood
Doppler ultrasonic flow studies, Diagnostic
Electrocardiography, Diagnostic
Glucose, Blood
Homocysteine, Plasma or urine (Plasma)
Lipid profile, Blood
Platelet count, Blood
Prothrombin time and international
  normalized ratio, Plasma
Urinalysis, Urine

Palpitations, Heart

Alcohol, Blood
Blood gases, Arterial, Blood
Cholesterol, Blood
Complete blood count, Blood
Creatine kinase, Serum
Echocardiography, Diagnostic
• Electrocardiography, Diagnostic
Holter monitor, Diagnostic
Stress test, Diagnostic
Thyroid test, Thyroxine, Blood
Thyroid test, Triiodothyronine, Blood

Pancreatic Cancer

Amylase, Serum and urine, and Amylase
  clearance
• CA 19-9, Blood
CA 50, Blood
Chest radiography, Diagnostic
• Computed tomography of body
  (Abdomen; Pelvis), Diagnostic
Dual modality imaging, Diagnostic
Endoscopic retrograde
  cholangiopancreatography, Diagnostic
• Endoscopic ultrasonography, Diagnostic
Glucose, Blood
K-ras, Blood or specimen
Laparoscopy, Diagnostic
Lipase, Serum
• Magnetic resonance
  cholangiopancreatography, Diagnostic
Needle aspiration, Diagnostic
Occult blood, Stool
• Pancreas ultrasonography, Diagnostic
Pancreatic secretory trypsin inhibitor,
  Diagnostic

Telomerase enzyme marker, Blood
Urobilinogen, Urine

Pancreatic Islet Cell Lesion
Arteriogram, Diagnostic
Computed tomography of the body
  (Abdomen), Diagnostic
• Endoscopic ultrasonography, Diagnostic
Gastrin, Serum
Glucagon, Plasma
Insulin and insulin antibodies, Blood
Magnetic resonance imaging, Diagnostic
• Vasoactive intestinal polypeptide, Blood

Pancreatic Trauma
• Amylase, Serum
Complete blood count, Blood
Glucose, Blood
• Lipase, Serum
Peritoneal fluid analysis, Specimen
Type and crossmatch, Blood (Screen)
Urinalysis, Urine

Pancreatitis
Alcohol, Blood
• Amylase, Serum and urine and amylase
  clearance
Blood indices, Blood
Body fluid, Amylase, Specimen
Calcium, Total, Serum
Carotene, Serum
Chemistry profile, Blood
Complete blood count, Blood
Computed tomography of the body
  (Abdomen), Diagnostic
C-reactive protein, Plasma or serum
Differential leukocyte count, Peripheral
  blood
Endoscopic retrograde
  cholangiopancreatography, Diagnostic
Endoscopic ultrasonography, Diagnostic
Flat-plate radiography of the abdomen,
  Diagnostic
Gamma-glutamyltranspeptidase, Blood
Glucose, Blood
Histopathology, Specimen
Leucine aminopeptidase, Blood
• Lipase, Serum
Lipid profile, Blood
Liver battery, Serum
Magnesium, Serum
Magnetic resonance
  cholangiopancreatography, Diagnostic
Methemoglobin, Blood
Pancreas ultrasonography, Diagnostic
Pancreatic secretory trypsin inhibitor,
  Diagnostic

Protein electrophoresis, Serum
Secretin test for pancreatic function,
  Diagnostic
Soluble fibrin monomer complex, Serum
Trypsin, Plasma or serum
Trypsin, Stool
Trypsinogen-2, Urine

Panic Disorder
Cerebral computed tomography, Diagnostic
Echocardiography, Diagnostic
Electrocardiography, Diagnostic
Stress exercise test, Diagnostic
Upper gastrointestinal series, Diagnostic

Paralytic Ileus
Chloride, Serum
Electrolytes, Plasma or serum
• Flat-plate radiograph of abdomen,
  Diagnostic
Sodium, Plasma or serum

Parkinson's Disease
Cerebral computed tomography, Diagnostic
Ceruloplasmin, Serum
Copper, Serum
Copper, Urine
FMR1 testing for fragile X-associated
  disorders, Blood
Haloperidol, Serum
Magnetic resonance spectroscopy (Brain),
  Diagnostic
Phenothiazines, Blood
Positron emission tomography (F-dopa),
  Diagnostic
Reserpine, Serum
• Single-photon emission computed
  tomography, Brain, Diagnostic
Thyroid function tests, Diagnostic

Paroxysmal Hypertension
(see Pheochromocytoma)

Patent Ductus Arteriosus
• Blood gases, Arterial, Blood
Cardiac catheterization, Diagnostic
• Chest radiography, Diagnostic
• Echocardiography, Diagnostic
Electrocardiography, Diagnostic
Transesophageal ultrasonography,
  Diagnostic

Pelvic Inflammatory Disease
Actinomyces, Culture
Biopsy, Site-specific, Specimen (Endocervix;
  Endometrium; Anaerobic culture;
  Mycobacterium culture)
Body fluid, Anaerobic, Culture

Chlamydia culture and group titer,
  Specimen (Culture)
Complete blood count, Blood
Computed tomography of the body
  (Abdomen), Diagnostic
C-reactive protein, Serum
Endometrium, Anaerobic, Culture
Fluorescent treponemal antibody–absorbed
  double-stain test, Serum
Genital, *Candida albicans*, Culture
Genital, *Neisseria gonorrhoeae*, Culture
Gynecologic ultrasonography, Diagnostic
• Histopathology, Specimen
• Laparoscopy, Diagnostic
Magnetic resonance imaging, Diagnostic
Neisseria gonorrhoeae smear, Specimen
Pap smear, Diagnostic
Pregnancy test routine, Serum and
  qualitative, Urine
Sedimentation rate, Erythrocyte, Blood
Venereal Disease Research Laboratory test,
  Serum
Wound culture

Pemphigus
Brushing cytology, Specimen
Complete blood count, Blood
Fibroblast skin culture
• Histopathology, Specimen
Immunofluorescence, Skin biopsy, Specimen
Oral cavity cytology, (Scrape) Specimen
Pemphigus antibodies, Blood
Tzanck smear, Specimen

Peptic Ulcer
ABO group and Rh type, Blood
Amylase, Serum and urine
Biopsy, Site-specific (Gastric tissue),
  Specimen
Brushing cytology, Specimen
Campylobacter-like organism test,
  Specimen
Complete blood count, Blood
Gastric analysis, Specimen
Gastric pH, Specimen
Gastrin, Serum
• Gastroscopy, Diagnostic
• *Helicobacter pylori*, Quick office serology,
  Serum
Helicobacter pylori titer, Blood
Histopathology, Specimen
Lipase, Serum
Occult blood, Stool
Pepsinogen I and pepsinogen II, Blood
Type and crossmatch, Blood
Upper gastrointestinal series, Diagnostic

Urea breath test, Diagnostic
Washing cytology, Specimen

Pericarditis
Anti-DNA, Serum
Antinuclear antibody, Serum
Body fluid, Routine, Culture
Chest radiography, Diagnostic
Complete blood count, Blood
Coxsackie A or B virus titer, Blood
C-reactive protein, Plasma or serum
Creatine kinase (CK-MB), Serum
Creatinine, Serum
• Echocardiography, Diagnostic
Electrocardiography, Diagnostic
Histopathology, Specimen
Magnetic resonance imaging, Diagnostic
Pericardiocentesis, Diagnostic
Rheumatoid factor, Blood
Sedimentation rate, Erythrocyte, Blood
Troponin I, Plasma and troponin T, Serum
Urea nitrogen, Plasma or serum
Viral culture, Specimen

Peripheral Neuropathy
(see also Neuropathy)
• Electromyography and nerve conduction
  studies, Diagnostic (Electromyography)
Glucose, Blood
Glucose, 2-hour postprandial, Serum
Glutethimide, Blood
Heavy metals, Blood and 24-hour urine
Histopathology, Specimen
Magnetic resonance neurography, Diagnostic
Nerve biopsy, Diagnostic

Peripheral Vascular Disease
Ankle-brachial index, Diagnostic
Antiphospholipid antibodies, Serum
• Doppler ultrasonographic flow studies,
  Diagnostic
Electrocardiography, Diagnostic
Glucose, Blood
Lipid profile, Blood
Prothrombin time and international
  normalized ratio, Plasma
Pulse volume recording of peripheral
  vascular disease, Diagnostic

Peritonitis
Abdominal ultrasound, Diagnostic
Amylase, Serum
Blood culture, Blood
Blood gases, Arterial, Blood
Body fluid (Ascitic fluid), Amylase, Specimen
Body fluid (Ascitic fluid), Anaerobic,
  Culture

Body fluid (Ascitic fluid), Mycobacteria, Culture
Body fluid (Ascitic fluid; Urine), Routine, Culture
Body fluid, Fungus, Culture
Body fluid analysis (Ascitic fluid), Cell count, Specimen
• Body fluid cytology (Ascitic fluid), Specimen
Cerebrospinal fluid, Lactic acid, Specimen
Chest radiography, Diagnostic
Complete blood count, Blood
Computed tomography of the body (Abdomen; with Contrast), Diagnostic
C-reactive protein, Plasma or serum
Electrolytes, Plasma or serum
Flat-plate radiograph of the abdomen, Diagnostic
Genital, *Candida albicans*, Culture
Genital, *Neisseria gonorrhoeae*, Culture
Histopathology, Specimen
Lactate dehydrogenase, Blood
Lactic acid, Blood
Liver battery, Serum
Magnetic resonance imaging, Diagnostic
Paracentesis, Diagnostic
Prothrombin time and international normalized ratio, Blood
Sedimentation rate, Erythrocyte, Blood

Pernicious Anemia
Blood indices, Blood
Bone marrow aspiration analysis, Diagnostic
Complete blood count, Blood
Cytologic study of gastrointestinal tract, Diagnostic
Differential leukocyte count, Peripheral blood
Folic acid, Red blood cells, Blood
Folic acid, Serum
• Gastrin, Serum
• Immunoglobulin G, Serum
• Intrinsic factor antibody, Blood
Lactate dehydrogenase, Blood
Lactate dehydrogenase, Isoenzymes, Blood
• Parietal cell antibody, Blood
Pepsinogen I and pepsinogen II, Blood
Pepsinogen I antibody, Blood
Platelet count, Blood
Red blood cell morphology, Blood
Reticulocyte count, Blood
• Vitamin B_{12}, Serum
Vitamin B_{12}, Unsaturated binding capacity, Serum

Pertussis
(*see Whooping cough*)

Pharyngitis
Antideoxyribonuclease-B antibody titer, Serum
Antihyaluronidase titer, Serum
Antistreptolysin-O titer, Serum
• Complete blood count, Blood
• Culture, Routine (Throat, nose), Specimen
Differential leukocyte count, Peripheral blood
Epstein-Barr virus serology, Blood
Infectious mononucleosis screening test, Blood
• Throat culture, Routine, Culture
Throat culture for *Candida albicans*, Culture
Throat culture for *Corynebacterium diphtheriae*, Culture
Throat culture for group A beta-hemolytic streptococci, Culture
Throat culture for *Neisseria gonorrhoeae*, Culture
Viral culture, Specimen

Phenylketonuria (PKU) Disease
• Guthrie test for phenylketonuria, Diagnostic
Phenylalanine, Blood

Pheochromocytoma
Calcitonin, Plasma or serum
• Catecholamines, Fractionation free, Plasma
Computed tomography of the body (Adrenal glands), Diagnostic
Homovanillic acid, 24-hour urine
Magnetic resonance imaging, Diagnostic
• Metanephrines, Total, 24-hour urine and free, Plasma
• MIBG scan, Diagnostic
• Vanillylmandelic acid, Urine

Phlebitis
(*see Thrombophlebitis*)

PID
(*see Pelvic inflammatory disease*)

Pinworm
• Parasite screen, Stool

Pituitary
(*see Addison's disease or Cushing's syndrome*)

PKU Disease
(see Phenylketonuria)

Pleural Effusion
(see Effusions, pleural)

Pleurisy
Biopsy, Site-specific, Specimen
Blood culture, Blood
Blood gases, Arterial, Blood
• Chest radiography, Diagnostic
Complete blood count, Blood
Coxsackie A or B virus titer, Blood
Histopathology, Specimen
Sputum, Routine, Culture

Pneumoconiosis
(see Black lung disease)

Pneumonia
Blood culture, Blood
Blood gases, Arterial, Blood
Bronchoscopy, Diagnostic
• Chest radiography, Diagnostic
• Complete blood count, Blood
Electrolytes, Plasma or serum
• Gram stain (Sputum), Diagnostic
Legionella pneumophila, Direct fluorescent
   antibody smear, Specimen
Mycoplasma enzyme immunoassay, Blood
Mycoplasma titer, Blood
Oximetry, Diagnostic
Procalcitonin, Plasma or serum
Pulmonary function tests, Diagnostic
Respiratory antigen panel, Specimen
Sputum, Routine, Culture
Thoracentesis, Diagnostic
Viral culture, Specimen

Pneumothorax
Blood gases, Arterial, Blood
• Chest radiography, Diagnostic
Complete blood count, Blood
Electrocardiography, Diagnostic
Oximetry, Diagnostic
Sputum cytology, Specimen

Poisonings
(see also Carbon monoxide poisoning,
Ethylene glycol poisoning, Insecticide
poisoning, Lead poisoning, Metal poisoning)
Acetaminophen, Serum
Anion gap, Blood
Bicarbonate, Blood
Blood gases, Arterial, Blood
Carbon monoxide, Blood
Cyanide, Blood
Heavy metals, Blood and 24-hour urine

Lead, Blood and urine
Morphine, Urine
Salicylate, Blood
• Toxicology, Drug screen, Blood or urine

Polio
(see Poliomyelitis)

Poliomyelitis (Polio)
Cerebrospinal fluid, Routine analysis,
   Specimen
Electromyography and nerve conduction
   studies, Diagnostic
Magnetic resonance imaging, Diagnostic
• Poliomyelitis I, II, III titer, Blood
Viral culture, Specimen

Polycystic Ovary Syndrome
Androstenedione, Serum
Dehydroepiandrosterone sulfate, Serum
Estrogens, Serum and 24-hour urine
• Follicle-stimulating hormone, Serum
Follicle-stimulating hormone, Urine
FSH/LH ratio
Glucose, Blood
Gynecologic ultrasonography, Diagnostic
17-Hydroxyprogesterone, Blood
• Luteinizing hormone, Blood
Prolactin, Serum
Testosterone, Free, Bioavailable and total,
   Blood

Polycythemia Vera
Abdominal ultrasound, Diagnostic
Bilirubin, Serum (Total)
Blood gases, Arterial, Blood (Oxygen
   saturation)
Blood volume, Blood
Bone marrow aspiration analysis,
   Diagnostic
Chest radiography, Diagnostic
• Complete blood count, Blood
Creatinine, Serum
^{51}Cr-labeled red blood cell survival, Blood
Erythropoietin, Serum
Leukocyte alkaline phosphatase, Blood
Red blood cell mass, Blood
Red blood cell morphology, Blood
Uric acid, Serum
Vitamin B$_{12}$, Unsaturated binding capacity,
   Serum

Polyuria
• Glucose, Blood
Glucose, 2-hour postprandial, Serum
Osmolality, Serum
Osmolality, Urine
Urinalysis, Urine

Postoperative
(see Surgery)

Posttraumatic Stress Disorder
No specific laboratory or diagnostic tests
indicated.

Preeclampsia
(see Pregnancy-induced hypertension)

Pregnancy
Alcohol, Blood
Amniocentesis and amniotic fluid analysis,
  Diagnostic
Chorionic villi sampling, Diagnostic
D-Dimer test, Blood
Fetal fibronectin, Specimen
Fetal monitoring, External, Diagnostic
Fetal monitoring, Internal, Diagnostic
Fetoscopy, Diagnostic
Foam stability test, Amniotic fluid
Fructosamine, Serum
Glucose tolerance test, Blood
Hematocrit, Blood
Hemoglobin, Blood
Human chorionic gonadotropin,
  Beta-subunit, Serum
Mendelian inheritance in genetic disorders,
  Diagnostic
Obstetric ultrasonography, Diagnostic
P-selectin, Plasma
• Pregnancy test, Routine, Serum and
  qualitative, Urine
Protein, Urine
Thyroid peroxidase antibody, Blood
Thyroid test, Thyroxine free, Serum

Pregnancy-Induced Hypertension
Activated partial thromboplastin time
  and partial thromboplastin time,
  Plasma
• Chemistry profile, Blood
Complete blood count, Blood
Creatinine, Serum
Kidney biopsy, Specimen
• Liver battery, Serum
Magnesium, Serum
Obstetric ultrasound, Diagnostic
• Platelet count, Blood
Pregnancy test, Routine, Serum and
  qualitative, Urine
Pregnanetriol, Urine
• Protein, Urine (24-hour)
Prothrombin time and international
  normalized ratio, Plasma
Sodium, Plasma or serum
Urea nitrogen, Plasma or serum

• Uric acid, Serum
Urinalysis, Urine

Preoperative
(see Surgery)

Primary Essential Hypertension
(see Hypertension)

Prostate Cancer
Acid phosphatase, Serum
Bone scan, Diagnostic
CA 15-3, Blood
Computed tomography of the body,
  Diagnostic
Creatinine, Serum
Cytologic study of urine, Diagnostic
Dual modality imaging, Diagnostic
Mitogen-activated protein kinase, Specimen
• Prostate-specific antigen, including free
  PSA, Blood
Prostate ultrasonography, Diagnostic
Prostatic acid phosphatase, Blood
Telomerase enzyme marker, Blood or urine
Urea nitrogen, Plasma or serum

Prostatitis
Blood culture, Blood
Body fluid, Routine, Culture (Urine)
• Complete blood count, Blood
Urinalysis, Fractional, Urine
Urinalysis, Urine

Pruritus
Culture, Skin, Specimen
Toxicology, Drug screen, Blood

Psittacosis
Blood culture, Blood
Body fluid (Pleural fluid), Routine, Culture
Chest radiography, Diagnostic
Chlamydia culture and group titer,
  Specimen (Group titer)
Cold agglutinin screen, Blood
Complement fixation, Serum
• Complete blood count, Blood
Protein, Quantitative, Urine
Sedimentation rate, Erythrocyte, Blood
Sputum, Routine, Culture

Psoriasis
Culture, Skin, Specimen
• Histopathology, Specimen

Pulmonary Edema
Albumin, 24-hour urine
Blood gases, Arterial, Blood
Blood urea nitrogen/creatinine ratio, Blood
• Chest radiography, Diagnostic
Complete blood count, Blood

Creatine kinase (CK-MB), Serum
Creatinine, Serum
Digoxin, Serum
Echocardiography, Diagnostic
Electrocardiography, Diagnostic
Electrolytes, Plasma or serum
Natriuretic peptides, Plasma
Oximetry, Diagnostic
Pulmonary artery catheterization,
  Diagnostic
Sputum cytology, Specimen
Thyroid function tests, Blood
Urea nitrogen, Plasma or serum

Pulmonary Embolism

Activated partial thromboplastin time and
  partial thromboplastin time, Plasma
Antithrombin III test, Diagnostic
Blood gases, Arterial, Blood
Chemistry profile, Blood
Chest radiography, Diagnostic
Complete blood count, Blood
Computed tomography of the body (Spiral,
  EBCT), Diagnostic
D-Dimer, Blood
Doppler ultrasonographic flow studies,
  Diagnostic
Echocardiography, Diagnostic
Electrocardiography, Diagnostic
• Lung scan, Perfusion and ventilation,
  Diagnostic
Plasminogen assay, Blood
• Pulmonary angiography, Diagnostic
Sedimentation rate, Erythrocyte, Blood
Venography (with Contrast), Diagnostic

Pulmonary Infection

Blood culture, Blood
Blood gases, Arterial, Blood
• Chest radiography, Diagnostic
• Complete blood count, Blood
Respiratory antigen panel, Specimen
Respiratory Syncytial virus, Culture
Sputum, Routine, Culture

Pulmonic Stenosis

Blood gases, Arterial, Blood
Cardiac catheterization, Diagnostic
• Chest radiography, Diagnostic
• Echocardiography, Diagnostic
• Electrocardiography, Diagnostic

Pyelonephritis

Blood culture, Blood
Body fluid (Urine), Routine, Culture
Chemistry profile, Blood
Complete blood count, Blood

Computed tomography of the body
  (Kidneys), Diagnostic
Creatinine, Serum
Creatinine clearance, Urine
Cystourethrography, Voiding, Diagnostic
Cytologic study of urine, Diagnostic
Differential leukocyte count, Peripheral
  blood
Electrolytes, Plasma or serum
Flat-plate radiography of the abdomen,
  Diagnostic
Intravenous pyelography, Diagnostic
Kidney ultrasonography, Diagnostic
Nitrite, Bacteria screen, Urine
Renal angiogram, Diagnostic
Urea nitrogen, Plasma or serum
• Urinalysis, Urine

Pyrexia

• Blood culture, Blood
Body fluid (Urine), Routine, Culture
Creatine kinase, Serum (Isoenzymes)
Culture, Routine, Specimen (Sputum)

Q Fever

Complete blood count, Serum
Differential leukocyte count, Peripheral
  blood
Liver battery, Serum
• Weil-Felix agglutinins, Blood

Rabies

• Animals and rabies Negri bodies, Brain
  tissue, Specimen
Cerebrospinal fluid, Routine analysis,
  Specimen
Fluorescent rabies antibody (Brain tissue),
  Specimen
Immunofluorescence, Skin biopsy,
  Specimen
Magnetic resonance imaging (Brain, Spinal
  cord), Diagnostic

Rape Trauma

• Acid phosphatase, Vaginal swab
• Blood group antigen of semen, Vaginal
  swab
Body fluid, Amylase, Specimen
Cervical culture for *Neisseria gonorrhoeae*,
  Culture
Chlamydia culture and group titer,
  Specimen (Culture)
Chlamydia Screening, Specimen
Gamma-hydroxybutyric acid, Blood or
  urine
• Motile sperm, Wet mount, Diagnostic
Pap smear, Diagnostic

Precipitin test against human sperm and blood, Vaginal swab
• Pregnancy test, Routine, Serum and qualitative, Urine
Sims-Huhner test, Diagnostic
Syphilis, Serum
Trichomonas preparation, Specimen
• Venereal Disease Research Laboratory test, Serum

Rat-Bite Fever
• Biopsy, Site-specific (Bite site), Specimen
Complete blood count, Blood
Differential leukocyte count, Peripheral blood
Fluorescent treponemal antibody–absorbed double-stain test, Serum

Raynaud's Phenomenon
Antinuclear antibody, Serum
Anti-RNP test, Diagnostic
Anti-Sm test, Diagnostic
Cold agglutinin titer, Serum
Complete blood count, Blood
• Cryoglobulin, Qualitative, Serum
Electrolytes, Plasma or serum
Extractable nuclear antigen, Serum
Protein electrophoresis, Serum
• Raynaud's cold stimulation test, Diagnostic
Sedimentation rate, Erythrocyte, Blood
Urinalysis, Urine

Rectal Cancer
(*see Colorectal cancer*)

Renal Calculi
(*see Kidney stone*)

Renal Cell Cancer
Activated partial thromboplastin time and partial thromboplastin time, Plasma
• Biopsy, Site-specific (Kidney), Specimen
Blood indices, Blood
Bone scan, Diagnostic
Calcium, Total, Serum
Chest radiography, Diagnostic
Complete blood count, Blood
Computed tomography of the body (Abdomen, pelvis), Diagnostic
Creatinine, Serum
Dual modality imaging, Diagnostic
Fibrinogen, Plasma
Intravenous pyelography, Diagnostic
Kidney ultrasonography, Diagnostic
Liver battery, Serum
Magnetic resonance imaging (Abdomen, pelvis), Diagnostic

Nephrotomography, Diagnostic
Prothrombin time and international normalized ratio, Blood
Renal angiogram, Diagnostic
Sedimentation rate, Erythrocyte, Blood
Telomerase enzyme marker, Urine
Urea nitrogen, Plasma or serum
Urinalysis, Urine
Vascular endothelial growth factor, Specimen

Renal Failure
Albumin–Serum, Urine and 24-hour urine
$Beta_2$-microglobulin, Blood and 24-hour urine
Bicarbonate, Blood
Body fluid (Urine), Routine, Culture
Chemistry profile, Blood
Chest radiography, Diagnostic
Complete blood count, Blood
• Creatinine, Serum
Creatinine clearance, Serum, Urine
Cystatin C, Serum (Chronic kidney disease)
Cytologic study of urine, Diagnostic
Differential leukocyte count, Peripheral blood
Electrocardiography, Diagnostic
• Electrolytes, Plasma or serum
Electrolytes, Urine
Flat-plate radiography of the abdomen, Diagnostic
Globulin, Serum
Homocysteine, Plasma or urine
Immunoelectrophoresis, Serum and urine
Intravenous pyelography, Diagnostic
Kidney biopsy, Specimen
Kidney ultrasonography, Diagnostic
Liver battery, Serum
Magnesium, Serum
Magnetic resonance angiography, Diagnostic
Magnetic resonance imaging, Diagnostic
Mean platelet volume, Blood
Myoglobin, Qualitative, Urine
Myoglobin, Serum
pH, Blood
Phosphorus, Serum
Potassium, Plasma or serum
Protein, Semiquantitative, Urine
Protein, Urine (Quantitative, 24-hour)
Retrograde pyelography, Diagnostic
Sodium, Plasma, Serum or urine (Serum)
Technetium-pentaacetic acid clearance, Diagnostic

Transferrin, Serum
• Urea nitrogen, Plasma or serum
Uric acid, Serum
Urinalysis, Urine

Renal Hypertension
• Aldosterone, Serum and urine
Arteriography, Diagnostic
Chloride, Serum
Color duplex ultrasonography, Diagnostic
Intravenous pyelography, Diagnostic
Potassium, Plasma or serum
Renal function tests, Diagnostic
Renal indices, Diagnostic
• Renin activity, Plasma
Renocystogram, Diagnostic (Captopril renography)
Sodium, Plasma, Serum or urine

Renal Infarction
Chemistry profile, Blood
Creatine kinase, Serum (Isoenzymes)
• Histopathology, Specimen
Kidney ultrasonography, Diagnostic
Lactate dehydrogenase, Blood
Lactate dehydrogenase, Isoenzymes, Blood
Urinalysis, Urine

Renin Hypertension
(see Renal hypertension)

Respiratory Acidosis
Bicarbonate, Blood
• Blood gases, Arterial, Blood
Chest radiography, Diagnostic
Complete blood count, Blood
Electrolytes, Plasma or serum
Urinalysis, Urine

Respiratory Alkalosis
• Blood gases, Arterial, Blood
Calcium, Total, Serum
Chest radiography, Diagnostic
Lung scan, Perfusion and ventilation, Diagnostic
Potassium, Plasma or serum
Urinalysis, Urine

Respiratory Failure
Alpha$_1$-antitrypsin, Serum
Bicarbonate, Blood
Blood culture, Blood
• Blood gases, Arterial, Blood
Chest radiography, Diagnostic
Complete blood count, Blood
Culture (Sputum), Routine, Specimen
Differential leukocyte count, Peripheral blood
Electrolytes, Plasma or serum

Lung scan, Perfusion and ventilation, Diagnostic
Pulmonary artery catheterization, Diagnostic
Pulmonary function tests, Diagnostic
Sputum, Routine, Culture

Restless Leg Syndrome
(see Sleep disorders)

Rett Syndrome
MECP2 Full gene sequencing, Blood

Reye's Syndrome
Activated partial thromboplastin time and partial thromboplastin time, Plasma
Alanine aminotransferase, Serum
• Ammonia, Blood
Aspartate aminotransferase, Serum
Bilirubin, Direct, Serum
Cerebrospinal fluid, Routine analysis, Specimen
Computed tomography of the body, Diagnostic
Creatinine, Serum
Electroencephalography, Diagnostic
Glucose, Blood
Histopathology, Specimen
• Liver battery, Serum
Liver biopsy, Diagnostic
Lumbar puncture, Diagnostic
Magnetic resonance imaging, Diagnostic
Prothrombin time and international normalized ratio, Plasma
Toxicology, Drug screen, Blood or urine
Urea nitrogen, Plasma or serum

Rhabdomyolysis
Cocaine, Blood
Complete blood count, Blood
Creatine kinase (CH-MM), Serum
Creatinine, Serum
Cytologic study of urine, Diagnostic
Electrocardiography, Diagnostic
Electrolytes, Plasma or serum
Kidney ultrasonography, Diagnostic
Muscle biopsy, Specimen
• Myoglobin, Qualitative, Urine
• Myoglobin, Serum
Toxicology drug screen, Blood or urine
Urea nitrogen, Plasma or serum
Urinalysis, Urine

Rheumatic Fever
Antideoxyribonuclease-B antibody titer, Serum
• Antistreptolysin-O titer, Serum
Chest radiography, Diagnostic

C-reactive protein, Plasma or serum
Culture (Throat), Routine, Specimen
Echocardiography, Diagnostic
Electrocardiography, Diagnostic
Mean platelet volume, Blood
Sedimentation rate, Erythrocyte, Blood
Streptozyme, Blood

Rheumatoid Arthritis
(see also Osteoarthritis)
Alanine aminotransferase, Serum
Albumin, Serum
Anti-DNA, Serum
Antineutrophil cytoplasmic antibody
  screen, Serum
Antinuclear antibody, Serum
Antistreptolysin-O titer, Blood
Aspartate aminotransferase, Serum
Bilirubin, Serum
Body fluid, Routine, Culture
Body fluid analysis (Synovial fluid),
  Specimen
Bone radiography (Hand, foot),
  Diagnostic
C4 complement, Serum
Chemistry profile, Blood
Complement, Total, Serum
Complement components, Serum
Complete blood count, Blood
C-reactive protein, Plasma or serum
Electrolytes, Plasma or serum
Extractable nuclear antigen, Serum
Genital, *Candida albicans*, Culture
Genital, *Neisseria gonorrhoeae*, Culture
Human leukocyte antigen B27, Blood
Immune complex assay, Blood
Lupus test, Blood
Mean platelet volume, Blood
Mucin clot test (Synovial fluid), Specimen
Occult blood, Stool
Protein electrophoresis, Serum
Prothrombin time and international
  normalized ratio, Blood
Raji cell immune complex assay, Blood
• Rheumatoid factor, Blood
Sedimentation rate, Erythrocyte, Blood
Sjögren's antibodies, Blood
Synovial fluid analysis, Diagnostic
Uric acid, Serum
Uric acid, Urine
Urinalysis, Urine

Rhinitis
Allergen-specific IgE, Serum
Computed tomography of the body
  (Sinuses), Diagnostic

Cytologic study of respiratory tract (Nasal
  smear), Diagnostic
Eosinophil count, Blood
Immunoglobulin E, Serum
Pulmonary function tests (Spirometry),
  Diagnostic
Sinus radiography, Diagnostic

Rickets
(see Osteomalacia)

Riley-Day Syndrome
Ashkenazi Jewish genetic carrier screening
  profile

Ringworm (Tinea Capitis)
Chest radiography, Diagnostic
• Culture, Skin (Scalp for *Microsporum
  audouinii*), Specimen
Skin, Fungus, Culture

Rocky Mountain Spotted Fever
Biopsy, Site-specific (Skin), Specimen
Cerebrospinal fluid, Routine analysis,
  Specimen
Complete blood count, Blood
Differential leukocyte count, Peripheral
  blood
Platelet count, Blood
Red blood cell, Blood
• Rocky Mountain spotted fever serology,
  Serum
Sodium, Plasma, Serum or urine (Serum)
Weil-Felix agglutinins, Blood

Rubella (German Measles)
Immunoglobulin M, Serum
• Rubella serology, Serum and specimen
Toxoplasmosis, Rubella, Cytomegalovirus,
  Herpesvirus serology, Blood
Viral culture, Specimen

Rubeola
Differential leukocyte count, Peripheral
  blood
Histopathology, Specimen
Lymph node biopsy, Specimen
• Rubeola serology, Serum

Salmonellosis
Blood culture, Blood
Complete blood count, Blood
Differential leukocyte count, Peripheral
  blood
Febrile agglutinins, Serum
• *Salmonella* titer, Blood
• Stool culture, Routine, Stool

Sanfilippo Syndrome
• Mucopolysaccharides, Qualitative, Urine
S. mucopolysaccharide turnover,
   Diagnostic

Sarcoidosis
Angiotensin-converting enzyme, Blood
Bronchial washing, Specimen
Brushing cytology, Specimen
Calcium, Urine
• Chest radiography, Diagnostic
Complete blood count, Blood
Computed tomography of the body
   (HRCT), Diagnostic
Creatinine, Serum
Diffusing capacity for carbon monoxide,
   Diagnostic
Echocardiography, Diagnostic
Electrocardiography, Diagnostic
Electrolytes, Plasma or serum
• Histopathology, Specimen
Liver battery, Serum
Liver biopsy, Diagnostic
Liver ^{131}I scan, Diagnostic
Mediastinoscopy, Diagnostic
Muramidase, Serum and urine
Nerve biopsy, Diagnostic
Pulmonary function tests, Diagnostic
Sputum cytology, Specimen
Urea nitrogen, Plasma or serum

Sarcoma
Alkaline phosphatase, Serum
• Biopsy, Site-specific (Bone), Specimen
Bone marrow aspiration analysis,
   Specimen
Bone radiography, Diagnostic
Bone scan, Diagnostic
Chemistry profile, Blood
Complete blood count, Blood
Computed tomography of the body
   (Bone), Diagnostic
Lactate dehydrogenase, Blood
Magnetic resonance imaging, Diagnostic
Sedimentation rate, Erythrocyte, Blood

SARS
(see Severe acute respiratory syndrome)

Scabies
• Culture, Skin (Scrapings for ova or mites),
   Specimen

Scarlet Fever
• Antistreptolysin-O titer, Serum
Throat culture for group A beta-hemolytic
   streptococci, Culture

Schistosomiasis
Complete blood count, Blood
Differential leukocyte count, Peripheral
   blood
Eosinophil count, Blood
Liver battery, Serum
Liver biopsy, Diagnostic
Liver-spleen scan, Diagnostic
• Ova and parasite, Stool
• Urinalysis, Urine

Schizophrenia, Chronic
Cerebral computed tomography, Diagnostic
Chest radiography, Diagnostic
Complete blood count, Blood
Creatinine, Serum
Electroencephalogram, Diagnostic
• Fluorescent treponemal antibody–
   absorbed double-stain test, Serum
HIV antibodies (see Acquired immune
   deficiency syndrome evaluation battery,
   Diagnostic)
Iron, Serum
Liver battery, Serum
Magnetic resonance imaging, Diagnostic
Thyroid function tests, Blood
Toxicology drug screen, Blood or urine
Tricyclic antidepressants, Plasma or serum
Urea nitrogen, Plasma or serum
Urinalysis, Urine
Vitamin B$_{12}$, Serum

Sciatica
Bone radiography, Diagnostic
Bone scan, Diagnostic
Complete blood count, Blood
Computed tomography of the body
   (Spine), Diagnostic
Differential leukocyte count, Peripheral
   blood
Electromyography and nerve conduction
   studies (Electromyography), Diagnostic
Magnetic resonance imaging, Diagnostic
Magnetic resonance neurography,
   Diagnostic
Nerve conduction studies, Diagnostic
Sedimentation rate, Erythrocyte, Blood

Scleroderma
Anti-DNA, Serum
Anti-La/SS-B test, Diagnostic
Antinuclear antibody, Serum
Anti-RNP test, Diagnostic
Anti-Sm test, Diagnostic
Biopsy, Site-specific (Skin), Specimen
Bone radiography (Joint), Diagnostic
Complete blood count, Blood

Creatinine, Serum

D-Xylose absorption test, Diagnostic,
  Serum or urine

Echocardiography, Diagnostic

Electrocardiography, Diagnostic

Histopathology, Specimen

Potassium, Plasma or serum

Pulmonary function tests, Diagnostic

Rheumatoid factor, Blood

• Scleroderma antibody, Blood

Sodium, Serum

Urea nitrogen, Plasma or serum

Urinalysis, Urine

Scurvy

• Vitamin C, Plasma or serum

Secondary Hypertension
(see Hypertension)

Seizures

Alcohol, Blood

Blood gases, Arterial, Blood

Body fluid (Urine), Routine, Culture

Brain scan, Cerebral flow and pathology,
  Diagnostic

Brain ultrasonography, Diagnostic

Calcium, Blood

Carbon monoxide, Blood

Carboxyhemoglobin, Blood

Cerebral computed tomography, Diagnostic

Cerebrospinal fluid, Glucose, Specimen

Cerebrospinal fluid, Routine analysis,
  Specimen

Chemistry profile, Blood

Chlordiazepoxide, Blood

Chromium, Serum

Clonazepam, Blood

Cocaine, Blood

Complete blood count, Blood

Creatine kinase, Serum

Diazepam, Serum

• Electroencephalography, Diagnostic

Electrolytes, Plasma or serum

Ethosuximide, Blood

Flurazepam, Serum

Glucose, Blood

Heavy metals, 24-hour urine

Ketones, Semiquantitative, Urine

Ketone bodies, Blood

Lidocaine, Serum

Lumbar puncture, Diagnostic

Magnesium, Serum

Magnetic resonance imaging (Brain),
  Diagnostic

Mephenytoin, Blood

Methsuximide, Serum

Neuron-specific enolase, Serum

Osmolality, Serum

Phenobarbital, Plasma or serum

Phenytoin, Serum

Primidone, Serum

Pseudocholinesterase, Plasma

Sodium, Plasma, Serum or urine

Theophylline, Blood

Thiocyanate, Blood

Thiocyanate, Urine

Toxicology, Drug screen, Blood or urine

Urinalysis, Urine

Valproic acid, Blood

Vitamin B_6, Plasma

Senile Dementia
(see Dementia)

Sepsis

ACTH stimulation test, Diagnostic

Activated partial thromboplastin time and
  partial thromboplastin time, Plasma

• Blood culture, Blood

Body fluid (Abscess), Anaerobic, Culture

• Body fluid (Urine), Routine, Culture

Chest radiography, Diagnostic

Complete blood count, Blood

Creatinine, Serum

Culture (Sputum), Routine, Specimen

Differential leukocyte count, Peripheral
  blood

Electrocardiography, Diagnostic

Electrolytes, Plasma or serum

Foreign body, Routine, Culture

Glucose, Blood

KeyPath MRSA/MSSA Blood culture test,
  Blood

Lactic acid, Blood

Liver battery, Serum

Lumbar puncture, Diagnostic

• Procalcitonin, Plasma or serum

Prothrombin time and international
  normalized ratio, Blood

Urea nitrogen, Plasma or serum

Urinalysis, Urine

Serum Sickness

C1q immune complex detection, Serum

C3 complement, Serum

C4 complement, Serum

Complete blood count, Blood

Differential leukocyte count, Peripheral
  blood

Heterophile agglutinins, Blood

Immune complex assay, Blood

Protein electrophoresis, Serum
Sedimentation rate, Erythrocyte, Blood
Urinalysis, Urine

Severe Acute Respiratory Syndrome
Blood culture, Blood
Blood gases, Arterial, Blood
Bronchoscopy, Diagnostic
Calcium, Blood
• Chest radiography, Diagnostic
Complete blood count, Blood
Computed tomography of the body
  (Chest), Diagnostic
Creatine kinase, Serum
Electrolytes, Plasma or serum
• Gram stain (Sputum), Diagnostic
Influenza A and B titer, Blood
Lactate dehydrogenase, Blood
Legionella pneumophila culture, IgM titer,
  Blood
Liver battery, Serum
Oximetry, Diagnostic
Respiratory antigen panel, Specimen
• Severe acute respiratory syndrome–
  associated coronavirus antibody and
  reverse transcriptase polymerase chain
  reaction tests, Specimen
Urea nitrogen, Plasma or serum
• Viral culture (Nasopharynx, stool),
  Specimen

Sexual Assault
(see Rape trauma)

Sexually Transmitted Disease
*(see Acquired immune deficiency syndrome,
Chancroid, Chlamydia, Gonorrhea, Human
papillomavirus, Lymphogranuloma
venereum, and Syphilis)*

Shingles
(see Herpes zoster)

Shock
(see also Sepsis and Toxic shock syndrome)
Activated partial thromboplastin time and
  partial thromboplastin time, Plasma
Aspartate aminotransferase, Serum
Blood culture, Blood
• Blood gases, Arterial, Blood
Blood urea nitrogen/creatinine ratio, Blood
• Complete blood count, Blood
Creatinine, Serum
Electrolytes, Plasma or serum
Glucose, Blood
Lactic acid, Blood
Osmolality, Serum
Potassium, Plasma or serum

Prothrombin time and international
  normalized ratio, Plasma
Pulmonary artery catheterization,
  Diagnostic
Urinalysis, Urine

SIADHS (SIADH)
*(see Syndrome of inappropriate antidiuretic
hormone secretion)*

Sickle Cell Disease
Antibody identification, Red cell, Blood
Blood culture, Blood
Body fluid (Pus; Urine), Routine, Culture
Bone radiography, Diagnostic
C3 proactivator, Serum
Complete blood count, Blood
D-Dimer test (for Crisis), Blood
Differential leukocyte count, Peripheral
  blood
Doppler ultrasonic flow studies
  (Transcranial), Diagnostic
Ferritin, Serum
Fetal hemoglobin, Blood
Hemoglobin electrophoresis, Blood
Reticulocyte count, Blood
Sedimentation rate, Erythrocyte, Blood
• Sickle cell test, Blood

Silicosis
• Chest radiography, Diagnostic
Pulmonary function tests, Diagnostic

Sinusitis
Biopsy, Site-specific (Nasal canal; Paranasal
  sinuses), Specimen
Body fluid, Anaerobic, Culture (Abscess)
Cerebral computed tomography,
  Diagnostic
Complete blood count, Blood
• Culture, Routine, Specimen (Nose)
Cytologic study of respiratory tract (Nasal
  smear), Diagnostic
Histopathology, Specimen
Immunoglobulin A, Serum
Sedimentation rate, Erythrocyte, Blood
Sinus radiography, Diagnostic

Sjögren's Syndrome
Anti-La/SS-B test, Diagnostic
Antinuclear antibody, Serum
Anti-RNP test, Diagnostic
Biopsy, Site-specific (Minor salivary gland),
  Specimen
Blood indices, Blood
Complete blood count, Blood
Differential leukocyte count, Peripheral
  blood

Extractable nuclear antigen, Serum
Histopathology, Specimen
Immune complex assay, Blood
Protein electrophoresis, Serum
Red blood cell, Blood
Rheumatoid factor, Blood
Schirmer tearing eye test, Diagnostic
• Sjögren's antibodies, Blood

Skin Cancer
Biopsy, Site-specific, Specimen
Sentinel lymph node biopsy, Diagnostic

Sleep Disorders
(see also Insomnia)
Complete blood count, Blood
Oximetry, Diagnostic
Polysomnography, Diagnostic
Thyroid function tests, Blood
Upper gastrointestinal endoscopy,
  Diagnostic

Snake Bite (Detection of Envenoming)
Activated partial thromboplastin time and
  partial thromboplastin time, Plasma
Creatine kinase, Serum
Prothrombin time and international
  normalized ratio, Plasma (INR)

Spider Bites
• Arthropod identification, Specimen
Complete blood count, Blood
Creatine kinase, Serum
Creatinine, Serum
Electrolytes, Plasma or serum
Glucose, Blood
Haptoglobin, Serum
Urea nitrogen, Plasma or serum
Urinalysis (Dipstick), Urine

Spinal Cord Injury
Activated partial thromboplastin time and
  partial thromboplastin time, Plasma
Bone radiography (Spine), Diagnostic
Calcium, Total, Serum
Cerebral computed tomography,
  Diagnostic
Computed tomography of the body
  (Spine), Diagnostic
• Magnetic resonance imaging, Diagnostic
Phosphorus, Serum
Prothrombin time and international
  normalized ratio, Plasma
Radiography of the skull, chest, and
  cervical spine, Diagnostic
Uric acid, Serum
Urinalysis, Urine

Splenomegaly
Alanine aminotransferase, Serum
Aspartate aminotransferase, Serum
Bone marrow aspiration analysis,
  Diagnostic
• Complete blood count, Blood
Computed tomography of the body
  (Abdomen), Diagnostic
Immunoperoxidase procedures (for
  Antigens), Diagnostic
Liver battery, Serum
Platelet count, Blood
Spleen scan, Diagnostic
• Spleen ultrasonography, Diagnostic
Sputum, Mycobacteria, Culture and smear

Status Epilepticus
Cerebral computed tomography, Diagnostic
• Electroencephalography, Diagnostic
Phenobarbital, Plasma or serum
Phenytoin, Serum
Valproic acid, Blood

Steatorrhea
• Fat, Semiquantitative, Stool

Stein-Leventhal Syndrome
(see Polycystic ovary syndrome)

Sterility
(see Infertility)

Stimulant Drug Abuse
(see also Drug abuse)
Amphetamines, Blood
Cocaine, Blood
Methylphenidate, Serum
Phenmetrazine, Blood

Stomatitis
• Complete blood count, Serum
Differential leukocyte count, Peripheral
  blood
Ferritin, Serum
Glucagon, Plasma
Iron, Serum
Potassium hydroxide preparation, Specimen
Sedimentation rate, Erythrocyte, Blood
T- and B-lymphocyte subset assay, Blood
Throat culture for *Candida albicans*,
  Culture
Tzanck smear, Specimen
Vitamin B_{12}, Serum

Stress
(see also Posttraumatic stress disorder)
Adrenocorticotropic hormone, Serum
Aldosterone, Serum
Cortisol, Plasma or serum

Stress Ulcer
(see Peptic ulcer)

Stroke
(see Cerebrovascular accident)

Subacute Bacterial Endocarditis
(see Endocarditis)

Subarachnoid Hemorrhage
• Cerebral angiography, Diagnostic
Cerebral computed tomography,
  Diagnostic
Cerebrospinal fluid, Routine analysis,
  Specimen
Lumbar puncture, Diagnostic
• Magnetic resonance imaging,
  Diagnostic

Sunstroke
(see Heat stroke)

Surgery, Postoperative
Activated partial thromboplastin time and
  partial thromboplastin time, Plasma
Blood gases, Arterial, Blood
Chloride, Serum
• Complete blood count, Blood
D-Dimer test, Blood
Glucose, Blood
Platelet count, Blood
Potassium, Plasma or serum
Prothrombin time and international
  normalized ratio, Plasma
Sodium, Plasma or serum
Urea nitrogen, Plasma or serum
Urinalysis, Urine

Surgery, Preoperative
Activated partial thromboplastin time and
  partial thromboplastin time, Plasma
Blood gases, Arterial, Blood
• Chest radiography, Diagnostic
• Complete blood count, Blood
Creatinine, Serum
Differential leukocyte count, Peripheral
  blood
Electrocardiography, Diagnostic
Electrolytes, Plasma or serum
Glucose, Blood
Pregnancy test, Routine, Serum and
  qualitative, Urine
Prothrombin time and international
  normalized ratio, Blood
Type and crossmatch, Blood
Urea nitrogen, Plasma or serum
Urinalysis, Urine

Syncope
Carotid phonoangiography, Diagnostic
• Doppler ultrasonographic flow studies
  (Carotid), Diagnostic
Echocardiography, Diagnostic
• Electrocardiography, Diagnostic
Holter monitor, Diagnostic
Oculoplethysmography, Diagnostic
Oculopneumoplethysmography, Diagnostic
Stress test, Exercise, Diagnostic
• Tilt table test, Diagnostic

Syndrome of Inappropriate Antidiuretic Hormone Secretion
• Antidiuretic hormone, Serum
Electrolytes, Plasma or serum
Electrolytes, Urine
Natriuretic peptides, Plasma
Osmolality, Serum
Osmolality, Urine
• Sodium, Plasma, Serum or urine (Serum
  and urine)
Specific gravity, Urine
Urea nitrogen, Plasma or serum
Uric acid, Serum

Syphilis
Automated reagin testing, Diagnostic
Cerebrospinal fluid, Routine analysis,
  Specimen
Chest radiography, Diagnostic
• Fluorescent treponemal antibody–
  absorbed double-stain test, Serum
Hemagglutination treponemal test for
  syphilis, Serum
Histopathology, Specimen
• Immunofluorescence, Skin biopsy,
  Specimen
Microhemagglutination–*Treponema
  pallidum* test, Serum
Rapid plasma reagin test, Blood
Venereal Disease Research Laboratory test,
  Cerebrospinal fluid, Specimen
Venereal Disease Research Laboratory test,
  Serum

Systemic Lupus Erythematosus
Activated partial thromboplastin time and
  partial thromboplastin time, Plasma
Anti-DNA, Serum
Anti-La/SS-B test, Diagnostic
Antinuclear antibody, Serum
Antiphospholipid antibody, Serum
Anti-RNP test, Diagnostic
Anti-Sm test, Diagnostic
C3 complement, Serum
C4 complement, Serum

Chest radiography, Diagnostic
Circulating anticoagulant, Blood
Complement components, Blood
Complete blood count, Blood
Comprehensive metabolic panel, Blood
C-reactive protein, Plasma or serum
Electrocardiography, Diagnostic
Electromyogram and nerve conduction
 studies, Diagnostic
Fibrinopeptide A
Fluorescent treponemal antibody–absorbed
 double-stain test, Serum
Immune complex assay, Blood
• Lupus panel, Blood
Lupus test, Blood
Magnetic resonance spectroscopy,
 Diagnostic
Platelet count, Blood
Protein, Total, Serum
Protein electrophoresis, Serum
Raji cell immune complex assay, Blood
Rheumatoid factor, Blood
Sedimentation rate, Erythrocyte, Blood
Urinalysis, Urine
Viscosity, Serum

Tay-Sachs Disease
• Amniocentesis, Diagnostic
Ashenazi Jewish genetic carrier screening
 profile
Chromosome analysis, Blood
Mendelian inheritance in genetic disorders,
 Diagnostic

Tension
(see Headache)

Testicular Cancer
• Alpha-fetoprotein, Blood
• Biopsy, Site-specific (Testes), Specimen
Computed tomography of the body
 (Retroperitoneum), Diagnostic
Dual modality imaging, Diagnostic
• Human chorionic gonadotropin,
 Beta-subunit, Serum
• Lactate dehydrogenase, Blood
Needle aspiration, Diagnostic
Scrotum and testicles ultrasonography,
 Diagnostic
Telomerase enzyme marker, Blood or
 urine

Tetany
Calcium, Total, Serum
Calcium, Urine
• Chemistry profile, Blood
Complete blood count, Blood

Culture (Wound), Routine, Specimen
• Electrolytes, Plasma or serum
Histopathology (Wound), Specimen
Immunoglobulin G (Tetanus antibody),
 Serum
Magnesium, Serum

Tetralogy of Fallot
Blood gases, Arterial, Blood
Cardiac catheterization, Diagnostic
• Chest radiography, Diagnostic
Complete blood count, Blood
Echocardiography, Diagnostic
• Electrocardiography, Diagnostic
Hematocrit, Blood
Hemoglobin, Blood
Iron, Serum
Magnetic resonance imaging, Diagnostic
Oximetry, Diagnostic
Red blood cell, Blood

Thalassemia
Bilirubin, Total, Direct and indirect, Serum
 (Indirect)
Chorionic villi sampling, Specimen
• Complete blood count, Blood
• Ferritin, Serum
Fetal hemoglobin, Blood
• Hemoglobin electrophoresis, Blood
Iron and total iron-binding capacity/
 transferrin, Serum
Urobilinogen, Urine

Thoracic Aortic Aneurysm
(see Aneurysm)

Thromboangiitis Obliterans
Antinuclear antibody, Serum
Antiphospholipid antibodies, Serum
• Arteriography, Diagnostic
Complement components, Serum
Complete blood count, Blood
C-reactive protein, Serum
Creatinine, Serum
Glucose, Blood
Histopathology, Specimen
Liver battery, Serum
Rheumatoid factor, Blood
Sedimentation rate, Erythrocyte, Blood
Urea nitrogen, Plasma or serum
Urinalysis, Urine

Thrombocytopenia
• Bone marrow aspiration analysis,
 Diagnostic
Complete blood count, Blood
Folic acid, Serum
Liver battery, Serum

Mean platelet volume, Blood
Occult blood, Urine
Platelet antibody, Blood
• Platelet count, Blood
Potassium, Plasma or serum
Red blood cell morphology, Blood
Vitamin B₁₂, Serum

Thrombophlebitis
Activated partial thromboplastin time and
partial thromboplastin time, Plasma
Blood culture, Blood
Circulating anticoagulant, Blood
Color duplex ultrasonography, Diagnostic
Complete blood count, Blood
Culture (Wound), Routine, Specimen
D-Dimer test, Blood
Differential leukocyte count, Peripheral
blood
Magnetic resonance imaging, Diagnostic
Plethysmography, Diagnostic
Pregnancy test routine, Serum and
qualitative, Urine (Serum)
Protein C, Blood
Protein S, Total and free, Plasma
• Prothrombin time and international
normalized ratio, Plasma
Venereal Disease Research Laboratory test,
Diagnostic
Venography (with Contrast), Diagnostic

Thrombosis
(see Deep vein thrombosis)

Thrush (Candidiasis, Moniliasis)
Biopsy, Site-specific (Skin), Specimen
Complete blood count, Blood
Gram stain (Vaginal scraping), Diagnostic
Oral cavity cytology, Specimen
Potassium hydroxide preparation,
Specimen
Skin, Fungus, Culture (with Sensitivity)
Throat culture for *Candida albicans*,
Culture
Vaginal culture

Thyroid
*(see Goiter, Hyperthyroidism,
Hypothyroidism)*

Thyroid Cancer
• Biopsy, Site-specific (Thyroid),
Specimen
Calcitonin, Plasma or serum
Dual modality imaging, Diagnostic
Electrolytes, Plasma or serum
Neuron-specific enolase, Serum
Telomerase enzyme marker, Blood

Thyroid function tests (Thyroglobulin),
Blood
Thyroid scan, Diagnostic
Thyroid ultrasonography, Diagnostic

Thyroidectomy
Calcium, Total, Serum
Cholesterol, Blood
Complete blood count, Blood
Phosphorus, Serum
Thyroid function tests (Thyroglobulin),
Blood
Thyroid test, Thyroxine, Blood
Thyroid test, Triiodothyronine, Blood
Type and crossmatch, Blood

Thyrotoxicosis
(see Hyperthyroidism)

TIA
(see Transient ischemic attack)

Tic Douloureux (Trigeminal Neuralgia)
Complete blood count, Blood
Computed tomography of the body,
Diagnostic
Magnetic resonance angiography,
Diagnostic
Phenytoin, Serum
Platelet count, Blood
Tegretol, Serum

Tinea Capitis
(see Ringworm)

Tinea Cruris
Culture, Skin, Specimen
Potassium hydroxide preparation,
Specimen
Skin, Fungus, Culture

Tinnitus
• Audiometry test, Diagnostic
Cerebral angiography, Diagnostic
Cerebral computed tomography,
Diagnostic
Complete blood count, Blood
Glucose tolerance test, Blood
Salicylate, Blood
• Tuning fork test of Weber, Rinne, and
Schwabach, Diagnostic

Tonsillitis
• Complete blood count, Blood
Computed tomography of the body (Neck),
Diagnostic
Differential leukocyte count, Peripheral
blood
Monospot screen, Blood

Radiography of the body (Neck), Diagnostic
Throat culture for group A beta-hemolytic
  streptococci (with Rapid strep test),
  Culture

Toxemia
(see Pregnancy-induced hypertension)

Toxic Shock Syndrome
Activated partial thromboplastin time and
  partial thromboplastin time, Plasma
Alanine aminotransferase, Serum
Alkaline phosphatase, Serum
Aspartate aminotransferase, Serum
• Bilirubin, Total, Serum
Blood culture, Blood
Body fluid, Routine, Culture
• Chemistry profile, Blood
Chest radiography, Diagnostic
Chloride, Serum
• Complete blood count, Blood
Creatine kinase, Serum
Creatinine, Serum
Culture, Routine, Specimen
Electrocardiography, Diagnostic
Electrolytes, Plasma or serum
Genital, Routine (for *Staphylococcus
  aureus*), Culture
Glucose, Blood
Gynecologic ultrasonography, Diagnostic
pH, Blood
Potassium, Plasma or serum
Prothrombin time and international
  normalized ratio, Plasma
Rocky Mountain spotted fever serology,
  Serum
Sodium, Plasma or serum
Throat culture for group A beta-hemolytic
  streptococci (with Rapid strep test),
  Culture
Urea nitrogen, Plasma or serum
Urinalysis, Urine
Vaginal culture (for *Staphylococcus aureus*)

Transfusion Reaction
Antibody identification, Red blood cell,
  Blood
Blood culture, Blood
Coombs', Direct, Serum
Coombs', Direct IgG, Serum
Haptoglobin, Serum
Hemoglobin, Plasma and qualitative, Urine
Hemosiderin, Urine
Immunoglobulin A antibodies, Serum
Occult blood, Urine
• Transfusion reaction work-up, Diagnostic

Transient Ischemic Attack
Activated partial thromboplastin time and
  partial thromboplastin time, Plasma
Antiphospholipid antibodies, Serum
Antithrombin III test, Diagnostic
Arteriography (Bilateral carotids), Diagnostic
• Carotid Doppler, Diagnostic
Cerebral angiography, Diagnostic
• Cerebral computed tomography, Diagnostic
Chest radiography, Diagnostic
Cholesterol, Blood
Circulating anticoagulant, Blood
Color duplex ultrasonography (Carotids),
  Diagnostic
Complete blood count, Blood
Doppler ultrasonic flow studies
  (Transcranial), Diagnostic
Echocardiography, Diagnostic
Electrocardiography, Diagnostic
Factor V (Leiden), Blood
Folic acid, Serum
Glucose, Blood
Holter monitor, Diagnostic
Homocysteine, Plasma or urine (Plasma)
Lipid profile, Blood
Magnetic resonance angiography,
  Diagnostic
Magnetic resonance imaging, Diagnostic
Oculoplethysmography, Diagnostic
Oculopneumoplethysmography, Diagnostic
Ophthalmodynamometry, Diagnostic
Protein C, Blood
Protein S, Total and free, Blood
Protein electrophoresis, Serum
Prothrombin time and international
  normalized ratio, Plasma
Single-photon emission computed
  tomography, Brain, Diagnostic
Transesophageal echocardiography,
  Diagnostic
Triglycerides, Blood
Urinalysis, Urine
Venereal Disease Research Laboratory test,
  Diagnostic
Viscosity, Serum
Vitamin B_{12}, Serum

Transplant (Bone Marrow, Cornea, Heart, Liver, Kidney)
Biopsy, Site-specific, Specimen
Blood culture, Blood
Blood gases, Arterial, Blood
Calcium, Total, Serum
Carbon dioxide, Partial pressure, Blood
Carbon dioxide, Total content, Blood

Chloride, Serum
• Complete blood count, Blood
Computed tomography of the body, Diagnostic
Creatinine, Serum
Diffusing capacity for carbon monoxide, Diagnostic
Hepatitis C genotype, Diagnostic
Human leukocyte antigen typing, Blood
Kidney biopsy, Specimen
Magnetic resonance imaging, Diagnostic
Mixed leukocyte culture, Specimen
Potassium, Plasma or serum
Renocystography, Diagnostic
Sodium, Plasma or serum
• Type and crossmatch, Blood
Urea nitrogen, Plasma or serum

Transplant Rejection

Activated partial thromboplastin time and partial thromboplastin time, Plasma
Alanine aminotransferase, Serum
Aspartate aminotransferase, Serum
Biopsy, Site-specific, Specimen
Blood gases, Arterial, Blood
Bone marrow aspiration analysis, Diagnostic
Complete blood count, Blood
Creatinine, Serum
Differential leukocyte count, Peripheral blood
Muramidase, Serum and urine
Platelet count, Blood
Prothrombin time and international normalized ratio, Plasma
Urea nitrogen, Plasma or serum

Transposition of the Great Arteries

• Blood gases, Arterial, Blood
Cardiac catheterization, Diagnostic
• Chest radiography, Diagnostic
Echocardiography, Diagnostic
Electrocardiography, Diagnostic
Platelet count, Blood
Red blood cell, Blood

Tremor

Calcium, Ionized, Blood
• Cerebral computed tomography, Diagnostic
Electroencephalography, Diagnostic
Electrolytes, Plasma or serum
FMR1 testing for fragile X associated disorders, Blood (Males over age 50)
Glucose, Blood
Magnetic resonance imaging (Brain), Diagnostic
Thyroid function tests, Blood

Treponema Pallidum
(see Syphilis)

Trichinosis

Aldolase, Serum
Eosinophil count, Blood
Muscle biopsy, Specimen
Muscle profile, Specimen
Parasite screen, Blood
• Trichinosis serology, Serum

Trichomonas
(see Vaginitis)

Tricuspid Atresia

• Blood gases, Arterial, Blood
Cardiac catheterization, Diagnostic
Chest radiography, Diagnostic
• Echocardiography, Diagnostic
Electrocardiography, Diagnostic
• Transesophageal ultrasonography, Diagnostic

Trigeminal Neuralgia
(see Tic douloureux)

Trypanosomiasis

African trypanosomiasis, Blood
Malaria smear, Blood
Microfilaria, Peripheral blood
Parasite screen, Blood
• Trypanosomiasis serologic test, Blood

Tubal Pregnancy
(see Ectopic pregnancy)

Tuberculosis, Pulmonary

• Acid-fast bacteria, Culture and stain (Sputum) (including Nucleic acid amplification test)
Body fluid (Sputum), Routine, Culture (for Mycobacteria)
Cerebrospinal fluid, Routine analysis, Specimen
• Chest radiography, Diagnostic
Computed tomography of the body (HRCT) (Spine), Diagnostic
Histopathology (Biopsy), Specimen
Immunoglobulin G, Serum
Liver ^{131}I scan, Diagnostic
• Mantoux skin test, Diagnostic
Muramidase, Serum and urine
RD1-interferon tests for tuberculosis, Blood (for Latent TB)
Urinalysis (for Kidney tuberculosis), Urine

Tularemia

Blood culture, Blood
Brucellosis agglutinins, Blood
Chest radiography, Diagnostic

Complete blood count, Blood
Culture (Tissue), Routine, Specimen
Differential leukocyte count, Peripheral
  blood
Febrile agglutinins, Serum
Liver battery, Serum
• Tularemia agglutinins, Serum
Weil-Felix agglutinins, Blood

Tumors

*(see Brain tumors, Breast cancer, Cervical
cancer, Colorectal cancer, Endocrine tumors,
Esophageal cancer, Ganglioneuroblastoma,
Gastric cancer, Glucagonoma, Head and
neck cancer, Hepatomas, Insulinomas, Liver
cancer, Lung cancer, Melanoma, Metastasis,
Neuroblastoma, Ovarian cancer, Pancreatic
cancer, Pheochromocytoma, Prostate cancer,
Renal cell cancer, Sarcoma, Testicular cancer,
Thyroid cancer, Uterine cancer, and Wilms'
tumor)*

Turner's Syndrome

Amniocentesis and amniotic fluid analysis,
  Specimen
Audiometry test, Diagnostic
Bone radiography (Long bones),
  Diagnostic
• Chromosome analysis, Blood
Echocardiography, Diagnostic
Follicle-stimulating hormone, Serum
Glucose, Blood
Glucose tolerance test, Diagnostic
Kidney ultrasound, Diagnostic
Luteinizing hormone, Blood
Oral cavity cytology, Specimen
Thyroid function tests, Blood

Typhoid Fever

Alanine aminotransferase, Serum
Alkaline phosphatase, Serum
Aspartate aminotransferase, Serum
Blood culture, Blood
Body fluid (Duodenal fluid; Urine),
  Routine, Culture
Bone marrow aspiration analysis, Specimen
Complete blood count, Blood
Febrile agglutinins, Serum
Liver biopsy, Diagnostic
Salmonella titer, Blood
• Stool culture (for *Salmonella*), Routine,
  Stool

Typhus

Alanine aminotransferase, Serum
Albumin, Serum, Urine and 24-hour urine
  (Serum)

Aspartate aminotransferase, Serum
Complement fixation, Serum
Complete blood count, Blood
Creatinine, Serum
Electrolytes, Plasma or serum
Febrile agglutinins, Serum
Immunoglobulin G, Serum
Immunoglobulin M, Serum
• Typhus titer, Blood
Urea nitrogen, Plasma or serum
Weil-Felix agglutinins, Blood

Ulcerative Colitis

Alanine aminotransferase, Serum
Albumin, Serum
Alkaline phosphatase, Serum
Antineutrophil cytoplasmic antibody
  screen, Serum
Aspartate aminotransferase, Serum
Barium enema, Diagnostic
Bilirubin, Total, Direct and indirect, Serum
Biopsy, Site-specific (Colon), Specimen
Calcium, Total, Serum
Clostridium difficile toxin assay, Stool
• Colonoscopy, Diagnostic
Complete blood count, Blood
Creatinine, Serum
Cytologic study of gastrointestinal tract,
  Diagnostic
Electrolytes, Plasma or serum
Flat-plate radiography of the abdomen,
  Diagnostic
Histopathology, Specimen
Lactate dehydrogenase, Blood
• Occult blood, Stool
Ova and parasites, Stool
Phosphorus, Serum
Prothrombin time and international
  normalized ratio, Blood
Sedimentation rate, Erythrocyte, Blood
Sigmoidoscopy, Diagnostic
Stool, Routine, Culture
Urea nitrogen, Plasma or serum
Uric acid, Serum
Yersinia enterocolitica enteritis

Ulcers

(see Decubiti, duodenal or peptic)

Unstable Angina

(see Angina pectoris)

Uremia

Activated coagulation time, Blood
• Anion gap, Blood
Bleeding time, Duke, Ivy, or Mielke, Blood
Creatinine, Serum

Creatinine clearance, Serum, Urine
• Electrolytes, Plasma or serum
Electrolytes, Urine
Liver battery, Serum
Neuron-specific enolase, Serum
• Platelet count, Blood
• Renal function tests, Diagnostic
• Urea nitrogen, Plasma or serum
Urinalysis, Urine

Ureteral Stents

Activated partial thromboplastin time and
  partial thromboplastin time, Plasma
Body fluid, Routine, Culture (Urine)
Complete blood count, Blood
Creatinine, Serum
Prothrombin time and international
  normalized ratio, Plasma
Urea nitrogen, Plasma or serum
Urinalysis, Urine

Ureterosigmoidostomy

Calcium, Total, Serum
Chloride, Serum
• Complete blood count, Blood
Potassium, Plasma or serum
Prothrombin time and international
  normalized ratio, Plasma
Type and crossmatch, Blood
Urinalysis, Urine

Urinary Tract Infection

• Body fluid (Urine), Routine, Culture
Complete blood count, Blood
Differential leukocyte count, Peripheral
  blood
Foreign body (Indwelling catheter),
  Routine, Culture
Leukocyte esterase (see Urinalysis),
  Urine
Nitrite, Bacteria screen, Urine
Urinalysis, Urine

Uterine Cancer

• Biopsy, Site-specific (Endometrium,
  uterus), Specimen
CA-125, Blood
Complete blood count, Blood
Computed tomography of the body
  (Pelvis), Diagnostic
Dilation and curettage, Diagnostic
Dual modality imaging, Diagnostic
Gynecologic ultrasonography, Diagnostic
Pap smear, Diagnostic
Squamous cell carcinoma antigen, Serum
Telomerase enzyme marker, Blood

Vaginal Cancer

Barium enema, Diagnostic
• Biopsy, Site-specific (Vagina), Specimen
Chest radiography, Diagnostic
Colposcopy, Diagnostic
Computed tomography of the body,
  Diagnostic
Dual modality imaging, Diagnostic
Gynecologic ultrasonography, Diagnostic
Intravenous urography, Diagnostic
Magnetic resonance imaging, Diagnostic
Pap smear, Diagnostic
Squamous cell carcinoma antigen, Serum
Telomerase enzyme marker, Blood
Thymidylate synthase, Specimen

Vaginitis

• Cervical-vaginal cytology, Specimen
Chlamydia culture and group titer,
  Specimen (Culture)
Chlamydia screening, Specimen
Complete blood count, Blood
Differential leukocyte count, Peripheral
  blood
Estrogens, Serum, Urine and 24-hour urine
  (Serum)
Follicle-stimulating hormone, Serum
Genital, *Candida albicans*, Culture
Genital, *Neisseria gonorrhoeae*, Culture
Glucose, Blood
Herpes cytology, Specimen
Luteinizing hormone, Blood
Neisseria gonorrhoeae smear, Specimen
Pap smear, Diagnostic
Potassium hydroxide preparation,
  Specimen
Rapid plasma reagin test, Blood
Trichomonas preparation, Specimen
Urinalysis, Urine
Venereal Disease Research Laboratory test,
  Serum

Varicella
(see Chickenpox)

Varices (Esophageal, Leg)

Activated partial thromboplastin time and
  partial thromboplastin time, Plasma
Alanine aminotransferase, Serum
Alkaline phosphatase, Serum
Aspartate aminotransferase, Serum
Calcium, Total, Serum
Complete blood count, Blood
Electrolytes, Plasma or serum
• Endoscopic ultrasound, Diagnostic
  (Esophageal varices)

Esophagogastroduodenoscopy, Diagnostic
 (Esophageal varices)
Occult blood, Stool
Potassium, Plasma or serum
Prothrombin time and international
 normalized ratio, Blood
Type and crossmatch, Blood
Upper gastrointestinal endoscopy,
 Diagnostic
Urea nitrogen, Plasma or serum

Vasculitis

Antineutrophil cytoplasmic antibody
 screen, Serum
Eosinophil count, Blood
• Histopathology, Specimen
Immunofluorescence, Skin biopsy,
 Specimen
Nerve biopsy, Diagnostic
Raji cell immune complex assay, Blood
Rheumatoid factor, Blood
Sedimentation rate, Erythrocyte, Blood

Venous Stasis Ulcer
(see Ulcers)

Venous Thromboembolism
*(see Deep vein thrombosis or Pulmonary
embolism)*

Ventricular Septal Defect
• Blood gases, Arterial, Blood
Cardiac catheterization, Diagnostic
• Chest radiography, Diagnostic
• Echocardiography, Diagnostic
Electrocardiography, Diagnostic

Vertigo
(see also Tinnitus)
Alcohol, Blood
Audiometry test (Vestibular evoked
 myogenic potential), Diagnostic
Blood gases, Arterial, Blood
Carbon dioxide, Blood
Cerebral computed tomography, Diagnostic
Complete blood count, Blood
Lyme disease antibody, Blood
Magnesium, Serum
Magnetic resonance imaging, Diagnostic
Magnetic resonance neurography,
 Diagnostic

Viral Hepatitis
(see Hepatitis)

Virilization
• Androstenedione, Serum
Dehydroepiandrosterone sulfate, Serum
 and 24-hour urine

• Estrogens, Serum and 24-hour urine
17-Hydroxycorticosteroids, 24-hour urine
17-Hydroxyprogesterone, Serum
Metyrapone, 24-hour, Urine
Pregnanetriol, Urine
• Testosterone, Free, Bioavailable and total,
 Blood

Vitamin D Deficiency
• Vitamin D, Plasma or Serum

Vomiting
Alanine aminotransferase, Serum
Amylase, Serum
Aspartate aminotransferase, Serum
Blood gases, Arterial, Blood
• Chloride, Serum
Complete blood count, Blood
Creatinine, Serum
Lipase, Serum
• Potassium, Plasma or serum
Pregnancy test, Routine, Serum and
 qualitative, Urine
Sedimentation rate, Erythrocyte, Blood
• Sodium, Plasma or serum
Urea nitrogen, Plasma or serum
Urinalysis, Urine

von Willebrand Disease
Activated partial thromboplastin time and
 partial thromboplastin time, Plasma
Aspirin tolerance test, Diagnostic
Bleeding time, Ivy, Blood
Factor VIII, Blood
Factor VIII R : Ag, Blood
Platelet aggregation, Blood
Platelet aggregation, Hypercoagulable state,
 Blood
Prothrombin time and international
 normalized ratio, Blood
• von Willebrand factor antigen, Blood
• von Willebrand factor assay, Blood

VTE
*(see Deep vein thrombosis or Pulmonary
embolism)*

Waldenström's Macroglobulinemia
Alanine aminotransferase, Serum
Alkaline phosphatase, Serum
Aspartate aminotransferase, Serum
Bence Jones protein, Urine
Biopsy, Site-specific, Specimen
Bone marrow aspiration analysis,
 Diagnostic
Complete blood count, Blood
Computed tomography of the body
 (Abdomen, pelvis), Diagnostic

Cryoglobulin, Serum
Electrolytes, Plasma or serum
• Immunoelectrophoresis, Serum and urine
Immunofluorescence, Skin biopsy,
  Specimen
Lactate dehydrogenase, Blood
Leukocyte cytochemistry, Specimen
Magnetic resonance imaging (Spine),
  Diagnostic
Needle aspiration (Abdominal fat),
  Diagnostic
Platelet count, Blood
Protein electrophoresis, Serum
Red blood cell, Blood
Red cell indices, Blood
Sedimentation rate, Erythrocyte, Blood
Urea nitrogen, Plasma or serum
Viscosity, Serum

Wegener's Granulomatosis

• Antineutrophil cytoplasmic antibody
  screen, Serum
Biopsy, Site-specific, Specimen
Chest radiography, Diagnostic
Complete blood count, Blood
Computed tomography of the body (Chest,
  sinuses), Diagnostic
Histopathology, Specimen
Platelet count, Blood
Red blood cell morphology, Blood
Urinalysis, Urine

Weil's Syndrome

(see Leptospirosis)

Whipple's Disease

• Biopsy, Site-specific (Pancreas), Specimen
Cytologic study of gastrointestinal tract,
  Diagnostic
D-Xylose absorption test, Diagnostic,
  Serum or urine
Electron microscopy, Diagnostic (for Small
  bowel mucosa, macrophage laden)
Histopathology, Specimen

Whooping Cough

Blood culture, Blood
• *Bordetella pertussis* (Nasopharyngeal
  swab), Culture
Chest radiography, Diagnostic
Complete blood count, Blood
Differential leukocyte count, Peripheral
  blood

Wilms' Tumor

Activated partial thromboplastin time and
  partial thromboplastin time, Plasma
Basic metabolic panel, Blood

Bone scan, Diagnostic
Chest radiography, Diagnostic
• Chromosome analysis (Deletion of 11p),
  Blood
Complete blood count, Blood
Computed tomography of the body
  (Abdomen), Diagnostic
• Histopathology, Specimen
Intravenous pyelography, Diagnostic
Magnetic resonance imaging, Diagnostic
Prothrombin time and international
  normalized ratio, Blood
Ultrasound (Liver, kidney, adrenal, pelvis),
  Diagnostic

Wilson's Disease

Cerebral computed tomography,
  Diagnostic
Ceruloplasmin, Serum
Chromosome analysis, Blood
• Copper, Serum
Copper, Urine
• Liver biopsy, Diagnostic
Mendelian inheritance in genetic disorders,
  Diagnostic

Wounds

Biopsy, Site-specific, Specimen
Body fluid, Anaerobic, Culture
Gram stain (Wound specimen), Diagnostic
Nocardia culture, All sites, Specimen
Wound, Fungus, Culture
Wound, Mycobacteria, Culture
Wound culture

Xerostomia

Antinuclear antibody, Serum
Complete blood count, Blood
Differential leukocyte count, Peripheral
  blood
Extractable nuclear antigen, Serum
Histopathology, Specimen
Immune complex assay, Blood
Protein electrophoresis, Serum
Rheumatoid factor, Blood
Sedimentation rate, Erythrocyte, Blood
Sjögren's antibodies, Blood

Yaws

Bone scan, Diagnostic
• Culture, Skin, Specimen

Yellow Fever

Alanine aminotransferase, Serum
Albumin, Urine
Alkaline phosphatase, Serum
Aspartate aminotransferase, Serum
• Bilirubin, Total, Serum

Bilirubin, Urine
Blood culture, Blood
Cerebral computed tomography,
  Diagnostic
Chest radiography, Diagnostic
Complete blood count, Blood
Differential leukocyte count, Peripheral
  blood
Electrocardiography, Diagnostic
• Electrolytes, Plasma or serum
Fibrin breakdown products, Blood
Fibrinogen, Plasma
Gastric analysis, Specimen
Glucose, Blood
Liver biopsy, Diagnostic
Prothrombin time and international
  normalized ratio, Blood
Pulmonary artery catheterization,
  Diagnostic
Urea nitrogen, Plasma or serum
Urinalysis, Urine
Viral culture (Group B arbovirus),
  Specimen

Zollinger-Ellison Syndrome

Body fluid analysis (Gastric fluid),
  Specimen
Calcium, Serum
Chloride, Serum
Computed tomography of the body,
  Diagnostic
Endoscopic ultrasonography, Diagnostic
Esophagogastroduodenoscopy, Diagnostic
Fat, Semiquantitative, Stool
Gastric analysis, Specimen
• Gastrin, Serum
Magnetic resonance imaging, Diagnostic
Octreotide scan, Diagnostic
• Pepsinogen I and pepsinogen II, Blood
Pepsinogen I antibody, Blood
Potassium, Plasma or serum
• Secretin test for pancreatic function,
  Diagnostic
Sodium, Plasma or serum

Zoster

(see Herpes zoster)

PART TWO

LABORATORY TESTS AND DIAGNOSTIC PROCEDURES

3-D Body Scan

See **Dual Modality Imaging**—Diagnostic.

Aβ₄₂

See **Beta-Amyloid Protein**—CSF.

Abdominal Aorta Ultrasonography (Abdominal Aorta Echogram, Abdominal Aorta Ultrasound)—Diagnostic

Norm. Negative for presence of aneurysm. Normal cross-sectional diameter of adult aorta (maximum internal diameter) varies from 3 cm at the xiphoid to about 1 cm at the bifurcation. Transverse and vertical diameters should be the same. Measurements should be taken at various points down the length of the aorta. Any significant increase in diameter toward the feet (caudally) is abnormal. Ultrasound underestimates the anteroposterior diameter (mean, 2.16 mm) and transverse diameter (mean, 4.29 mm) of the abdominal aorta.

Usage. Localization, measurement, and monitoring of abdominal aortic aneurysm; follow-up evaluation of surgical graft and aortic attachment after surgery for aneurysm; and detection of abdominal aortic atherosclerosis or thrombus. May be indicated in clients with pulsatile abdominal mass, poor circulation of the legs, recent abdominal trauma, and suspected idiopathic aortitis.

Description. Evaluation of the structure, size, and position of the abdominal aorta and branches (celiac trunk and renal, superior mesenteric, and common iliac arteries) by the creation of an oscilloscopic picture from the echoes of high-frequency sound waves passing over the anterior portion of the trunk (acoustic imaging). The time required for the ultrasonic beam to be reflected back to the transducer from differing densities of tissue is converted by a computer to an electrical impulse displayed on an oscilloscopic screen to create a three-dimensional picture of the abdominal aorta and branches. Ultrasonography allows measurement of the luminal diameter of the aorta. A narrowed lumen would indicate atherosclerosis or thrombus, whereas a wider-than-normal lumen with an irregular border may indicate aneurysm. Scattered internal echoes within the aneurysm may indicate an internal clot. A double lumen may indicate a tear in the wall of the abdominal aorta. Surgical grafts from aneurysm repair appear as bright echo reflections.

Professional Considerations

Consent form NOT required.

Preparation

1. This test should be performed before intestinal barium tests or else after the barium is cleared from the system (with allowance of several days for clearance).
2. An enema may be prescribed to be given before the ultrasonogram is taken.
3. The client should wear a gown.
4. Obtain ultrasonic gel or paste.

Procedure

1. Client is positioned supine on a procedure table.
2. The abdomen is covered with conductive gel.
3. A lubricated transducer is passed slowly along the abdomen at 1-cm intervals along the transverse and then longitudinal lines, covering the area between the xiphoid process and the symphysis pubis. If dissection is suspected, real-time techniques can be used more specifically to locate the site.
4. Photographs are taken of the oscilloscopic images.
5. Procedure takes less than 60 minutes.

Postprocedure Care

1. Cleanse skin of ultrasonic gel.

Client and Family Teaching

1. Eat a low-residue diet the day before the ultrasonogram is taken, fast from food

and fluids after midnight before the test, and refrain from smoking.

2. Lie as still as possible during the procedure, which is painless and carries no risks.

3. Results are normally available within 24 hours.

Factors That Affect Results

1. Dehydration interferes with adequate contrast between organs and body fluids.

2. Intestinal barium or gas obscures results by preventing proper transmission and deflection of the high-frequency sound waves.

3. The more abdominal fat present, the greater is the attenuation (reduction in sound-wave amplitude and intensity), which interferes with the clarity of the picture.

4. Aorta may be displaced by scoliosis, a retroperitoneal mass, or the para-aortic lymph nodes; in some clients, these anomalies can mimic an aneurysm.

Other Data

1. There is some evidence that aneurysms smaller than 4 cm in diameter may be safely followed by ongoing monitoring and any aneurysm larger than 4 cm in diameter should be considered for surgery.

2. Ultrasound ranks below CAT scan (or CT scan) in its accuracy; however, it surpasses CT in screening.

Abdominal Plain Film

See Flat-Plate Radiography of Abdomen—Diagnostic.

Abdominal Ultrasound

See Abdominal Aorta Ultrasonography—Diagnostic; Gallbladder and Biliary System Ultrasonography—Diagnostic; Liver Ultrasonography—Diagnostic; Obstetric Ultrasonography—Diagnostic; Pancreas Ultrasonography—Diagnostic; and Spleen Ultrasonography—Diagnostic.

Abeta

See Beta-Amyloid Protein—CSF.

ABG

See Blood Gases, Arterial—Blood.

ABI

See Ankle-Brachial Index—Diagnostic.

ABO Group and Rh Type—Blood

Norm. Specific to each individual.

Usage. Blood transfusion therapy, erythroblastosis fetalis, paternity determinations, pregnancy, and preoperatively.

Description. The ABO blood group is the phenotype of a client's blood resulting from genetic inheritance. The four most common phenotypes are A, B, AB, and O, referring to the type of antigen present on the surface of red blood cells. Rh type refers to whether an Rh antigen is present (Rh positive) or absent (Rh negative) on the surface of a client's red blood cells. Routine testing usually involves only the $Rh_0(D)$ antigen. If an Rh-negative client receives Rh-positive blood, he or she will develop Rh antibodies, and future Rh-positive transfusions may cause a transfusion reaction. In pregnancy, antibodies from an Rh-negative mother may hemolyze fetal erythrocytes in a fetus that has inherited the Rh-positive antigen from the father (erythroblastosis fetalis, or hemolytic disease of the newborn). This test determines the specific ABO phenotype and Rh type by determining which A and B red blood cell antigens are present as well as whether the $Rh_0(D)$ antigen is present.

Professional Considerations
Consent form NOT required.

Preparation
1. Assess client for history of recent blood transfusion reaction, which can result in a positive antibody screen and require further testing. Write affirmative history on blood bank requisition.
2. Tube: Red topped, red/gray topped, or gold topped, 1 or 2 tubes.

Procedure
1. Ask the client to state full name and compare with the client's name band. Label the sample tube and laboratory requisition with the client's name, identification number, date, time, and initials and sign it. Some institutions require additional data.
2. Draw one or two 10-mL blood samples, depending on institutional requirements.

Postprocedure Care
1. Some institutions require application of a blood band to the client's wrist. The blood bank identification numbers should match the identification numbers on any blood bag used for transfusion for the client.

Client and Family Teaching
1. Results are normally available within 24 hours.

Factors That Affect Results
1. Hemolyzed specimen invalidates results.
2. Specimen drawn from extremity into which blood or dextran is infusing invalidates results.
3. Drugs causing a false-positive Rh test include levodopa, methyldopa, and methyldopate hydrochloride.
4. Abnormal plasma proteins, cold autoagglutinins, positive direct antiglobulin test, and in some cases, bacteremia may interfere with results.

Other Data
1. The test must be performed within 48 hours of specimen collection.
2. Amerindians are blood group O. Incompatible platelet products that are transfused can cause acute intravascular hemolysis.
3. ABO incompatibility is a significant prognostic risk factor in allogeneic bone marrow transplant for acute myelogenous leukemia or myelodysplastic syndrome.
4. See also Type-and-crossmatch, Blood.

Abscess
See **Body Fluid**—Anaerobic Culture.

ACA
See **Antiphospholipid Antibodies**—Serum.

Accu-Chek
See **Glucose Monitoring Machines**—Diagnostic.

ACE
See **Angiotensin-Converting Enzyme**—Blood.

Acetaminophen—Serum

Norm. 2 months to 10 years (received >60 mg of APAP/kg/day) = 0-23 mg/mL.

	4 Hours After Last Dose	SI Units
Therapeutic level	10-30 μg/mL	66-199 μmol/L
Toxic level	>150 μg/mL	>990 μmol/L
Panic level (hepatotoxicity)	>200 μg/mL	>1320 μmol/L

APAP, N-acetyl-p-aminophenol.

Overdose Symptoms and Treatment
Symptoms. Occur in four stages.
1. Stage I (ingestion to 24 hours): Gastrointestinal irritation, pallor, lethargy, diaphoresis, metabolic acidosis, and coma (cases of massive ingestion with serum concentration >800 μg/mL have been reported, but coma is usually attributed to a coingestant such as alcohol).
2. Stage II (24 to 48 hours): Increased serum hepatic enzymes, right upper quadrant abdominal pain, possible decreased renal function.
3. Stage III (72 to 96 hours): Increased AST, increased ALT, nausea, vomiting, jaundice, lethargy, confusion, coma, coagulation disorders, possible decreased renal function.
4. Stage IV (4 days to 2 weeks): Clinical symptoms subside; laboratory values return to baseline.

Treatment
NOTE: Treatment choice(s) depend(s) on client's history and condition and episode history.
1. Establish and maintain adequate airway, respiratory, and circulatory function.
2. If client is obtunded or unconscious, appropriate doses of thiamine, dextrose, and naloxone must be considered.
3. Gastric decontamination: In one study, rapid complete bowel lavage with 4 g of polyethylene glycol electrolyte solution was shown to significantly reduce serum acetaminophen levels. In another study, use of activated charcoal prevented acetaminophen absorption when given within 60 minutes of acetaminophen ingestion. An emetic may be used to induce emesis for recent ingestion, but it must be used with extreme caution. Ondansetron can be used to manage vomiting if acetaminophen ingestion occurred within the previous 8 hours.
4. Oral administration of N-acetylcysteine (Mucomyst by Mead Johnson) for suspected toxic doses (>7.5 g). Mucomyst is most likely to be effective when given within 16 hours after acetaminophen ingestion.
5. Laboratory monitoring: Urine toxicology screen, hepatic profile daily for 3-4 days, BUN, Cr, serum electrolytes, serum acetaminophen concentration level 4 hours after ingestion.
6. Coingestion of other substances that delay gastric emptying is an indication for serial measurement to detect late-rising acetaminophen levels.
7. Chronic alcohol intake enhances acetaminophen hepatotoxicity.
8. Hemodialysis WILL but peritoneal dialysis will NOT remove acetaminophen.

Usage. Drug abuse, hepatitis, monitoring for toxicity during acetaminophen therapy, overdose, poisoning, and suicide.

Description. Acetaminophen (also known as paracetamol) is a p-aminophenol derivative that has antipyretic (direct action on hypothalamus) and moderate analgesic actions. It is absorbed by the gastrointestinal tract and metabolized by liver microsomes. Half-life is 1 to 4 hours with peak blood levels reached in 30 minutes to 1 hour. Used for headache, fever, and relief of pain in clients who cannot tolerate aspirin or those with peptic ulcers or bleeding disorders. It is the drug of choice (antipyretic/analgesic) in children 13 years of age and younger because of the possible development of Reye's syndrome associated with aspirin. In adults, ingestion of more than 4 g/day can be hepatotoxic.

Professional Considerations
Consent form NOT required.

Preparation

1. Tube: Red topped, red/gray topped, gold topped, or lavender topped.
2. Do NOT draw during hemodialysis.
3. Document times of ingestion and sample collection on lab requisition.

Procedure

1. Draw a 4-mL blood sample.

Postprocedure Care

1. None.

Client and Family Teaching

1. Results are normally available within 24 hours.
2. If overdose is suspected, prepare client and family for necessary supportive treatment described above.
3. If activated charcoal was given for elevated levels, client should drink 4 to 6 glasses of water each day for 2 days to prevent constipation. Activated charcoal will also cause stools to be black for a few days.

Factors That Affect Results

1. Cardiovascular, hepatic, gastrointestinal, or renal dysfunction can alter drug absorption and elimination.
2. Toxic levels of acetaminophen positively interfere with glucose-monitoring machine results.
3. Draw two samples, 4 hours apart, to determine the half-life of acetaminophen.

Other Data

1. Acetaminophen is present in many medicines: Anacin 3, Datril, Liquiprin, Panadol, Panex, paracetamol, Phenaphen, Tempra, and Tylenol.
2. Acetaminophen used with aspirin and caffeine alleviates migraine headache pain.
3. Premedication with acetaminophen does not significantly lower the incidence of nonhemolytic transfusion reactions.
4. Acetaminophen poisoning has been found in nearly 50% of all acute liver failure in the United States.
5. Prothrombin time prolongation may be noted in clients with hepatic failure and paracetamol poisoning.

Acetone

See **Acetone**—Urine; **Ketone Bodies**—Blood or Toxicology; **Volatiles Group by GLC**—Blood or Urine.

Acetone—Urine

Norm. Keto-Diastix or Multistix: Negative. Quantitative 0.3-2.0 mg/dL.

Usage. Differentiation of diabetic coma and insulin shock, evaluation of glucose control in diabetics, preadmission screening, pregnancy, screening for ketoacidosis, and monitoring for occupational exposure to isopropyl alcohol. Increased in ethanol hangover and in ingestion of denatured alcohol.

Description. Acetone is a by-product of fat and fatty acid metabolism that provides a source of cellular energy for cells when glucose stores are exhausted or when glucose is prevented from entering cells because of lack of insulin. Acetone entering the bloodstream is almost completely metabolized in the liver. When acetone is formed at a faster-than-normal rate or is present in the bloodstream in higher-than-normal levels, it is excreted in the urine.

Professional Considerations
Consent form NOT required.

Preparation

1. Obtain a clean urine container and acetone testing strips or tablets.
2. Client should empty the bladder 30 minutes before specimen collection and then drink a glass of water.
3. For specimens obtained from an indwelling urinary catheter, also obtain a catheter clamp, a sterile 10-mL syringe and needle, and an alcohol wipe.

Procedure

1. Obtain a 20-mL double-voided urine specimen in a clean container.
2. Specimens from catheter: Clamp the catheter tubing for 15 minutes to allow urine to accumulate above the sample port. Cleanse the sample port with an alcohol wipe and allow to dry. Aspirate

20 mL of urine from the sample port, using a sterile syringe and needle. Collect only fresh urine that has accumulated above the sample port. Unclamp the catheter tubing.
3. Dip the Keto-Diastix, Multistix, or other acetone testing material in fresh urine and hold the strip horizontally for 15 seconds.
4. Compare the color of the ketone patch on the strip with the color chart on the container of acetone testing strips.
5. Alternative method using Acetest tablets: Place a drop of urine on an Acetest tablet and wait 30 seconds. Compare the color with the Acetest color chart.

Postprocedure Care
1. None.

Client and Family Teaching
1. Results are immediately available.

Factors That Affect Results
1. Fasting or dieting may cause acetone to appear in the urine.
2. Use of acetone tablets that are darkened or expired invalidates results.
3. Drugs that may cause false-positive results include captopril, levodopa, paraldehyde, and phenazopyridine hydrochloride.
4. Gender and ingestion of alcohol may affect the basal levels of urinary acetone.

Other Data
1. Refrigerate the specimen if the test cannot be performed within 1 hour of collection.
2. In one study, ratings on scales of well-being and acute symptoms correlated significantly with the concentration of acetone in urine after acute airborne acetone exposure.
3. See also Ketone, semiquantitative—Urine.

Acetylcholine Receptor Antibody—Serum

Norm. ≤0.03 nmol/L.

Usage. Diagnosis and clinical monitoring of myasthenia gravis, Lambert-Eaton myasthenic syndrome, small cell lung carcinoma.

Description. In clients with myasthenia gravis, this antibody interferes with the binding of acetylcholine to receptor sites on the muscle membrane, thus preventing muscle contraction. Assays for acetylcholine receptor (AChR) antibodies are positive in 85%-90% of clients with acute myasthenia gravis and are replacing the Tensilon test as a diagnostic aid for this condition. However, this assay is less sensitive for Lambert-Eaton myasthenic syndrome diagnosis.

Professional Considerations
Consent form NOT required.

Preparation
1. Tube: Red topped, red/gray topped, or gold topped.
2. List on the laboratory requisition any recent immunosuppressive drug therapy the client received.

Procedure
1. Draw a 2-mL blood sample.

Postprocedure Care
1. None.

Client and Family Teaching
1. Results may not be available for several days.

Factors That Affect Results
1. False-positive results may be caused by D-penicillamine.
2. Decrease in titer may be caused by intravenous immunoglobulin (IVIg) therapy.
3. Clients with orthostatic hypotension may have a seropositive AChR antibody.

Other Data
1. Undetectable titer occurs in 33.4% of clients who have only ocular myasthenia gravis.
2. See also Tensilon test—Diagnostic.

Acetylsalicylic Acid

See **Salicylate**—Blood.

ACG—Diagnostic
See **Apexcardiography**—Diagnostic.

Acid-Fast Bacteria—Culture and Stain

Norm. Negative.

Usage. Acquired immune deficiency syndrome (AIDS); suspected *Helicobacter pylori*, intestinal parasites, leprosy, mycobacteriosis, or tuberculosis; and differentiation of tuberculosis from carcinoma and bronchiectasis.

Description. *Mycobacterium tuberculosis* is a rod-shaped bacterium that resists decolorizing chemicals after staining, a property termed "acid-fastness." *M. tuberculosis* is transmitted most commonly by the airborne route to the lungs, where it survives well, causes areas of granulomatous inflammation, and, if not dormant, causes cough, fever, and hemoptysis. The acid-fast bacterium *Mycobacterium avium-intracellulare* is a common cause of infection in clients with AIDS. Culture of sputum is necessary to confirm the diagnosis of tuberculosis and for sensitivity studies for drug therapy. The sensitivity of sputum smears for tuberculosis, however, is only 50%. The CDC recommends that every client with suspected tuberculosis also have nucleic acid amplification testing performed on at least one respiratory specimen. Nucleic acid amplification testing provides earlier confirmation (24-48 hours) of tuberculosis than does culture.

Professional Considerations
Consent form NOT required.

Preparation
1. Obtain three small, sterile containers.
2. See Client and Family Teaching.

Procedure
1. Aerosolized therapy before sputum collection may stimulate sputum production and produce a better specimen.

2. When tuberculosis is suspected, collect three daily, early-morning sputum, deep-cough specimens in a sterile container.
3. When leprosy is suspected, obtain smear from nasal scrapings or biopsy from lesions and place in sterile container.

Postprocedure Care
1. Provide mouth care.

Client and Family Teaching
1. Perform oral hygiene before giving specimens to reduce chances of contamination.
2. Deep coughs are necessary to produce sputum, rather than saliva. To produce the proper specimen, take several breaths in, without fully exhaling each, and then expel sputum with a "cascade cough."

Factors That Affect Results
1. Antituberculous drug therapy may cause negative results because of inhibition of growth of *M. tuberculosis*.
2. A high–carbon dioxide atmosphere for growth may increase the number of positive cultures.
3. Culture medium containing glycerin accelerates growth.

Other Data
1. Culture results may take 3-8 weeks.
2. The most prevalent intestinal parasites in cancer clients diagnosed by acid-fast stain are *Entamoeba histolytica/Entamoeba dispar* (8.5%), *Giardia lamblia* (3.1%), *Strongyloides stercoralis* (0.6%), and *Cryptosporidium parvum* (0.3%).

Acid-Fast Stain, Nocardia Species—Culture

Norm. Negative.

Usage. Aids in diagnosis of Behçet's disease, mycetoma, *Nocardia brasiliensis*, and nocardiosis of the respiratory tract found in persons with systemic lupus erythematosus and nocardial thyroiditis.

Description. *Nocardia* is an aerobic, gram-positive, filamentous branching bacterium that segments into reproductive bacillary fragments. It is weakly acid fast; found outdoors in decayed matter, soil, grass, and straw; and enters the body primarily through inhalation of contaminated dust. The type species, *Nocardia asteroides*, and *N. brasiliensis, N. farcinica, N. otitidis-caviarum, N. nova,* and *N. transvalensis* cause a variety of diseases in both normal and immunocompromised humans and animals. The *N. asteroides* species causes primary skin lesions, visceral infections (most commonly abscesses of the lungs, brain, and subcutaneous tissue), and sometimes disseminated infections in humans.

Professional Considerations
Consent form NOT required.

Preparation
1. Obtain a sterile scalpel or spatula, or a sterile needle and syringe, and both anaerobic and aerobic culture media.

Procedure
1. Obtain a scraping from a skin lesion or an aspirate of an abscess using sterile technique.

2. Inoculate both aerobic and anaerobic culture media with the specimen.
3. Aerobic culture media of beef infusion broth or thioglycolate broth may be used.
4. Initial incubation at temperatures from 38 to 45 degrees C should be used.
5. Examine cultures for growth beginning at 48 hours and recheck daily for 2 weeks.

Postprocedure Care
1. Apply dry sterile dressing to site.

Client and Family Teaching
1. Avoid application of creams or lotions to sample site and allow site to remain open to air for healing.
2. At least 2-3 days are required for growth and results.

Factors That Affect Results
1. *Nocardia* growth may be mistaken for nontuberculous *Mycobacterium* when a *Mycobacterium* culture medium is used.

Other Data
1. Common specimens include pus, tissue, body fluid, and sputum.
2. Final reports may take 10 days.

Acid Hemolysin Test—Blood
See Ham's Test—Blood.

Acidified Serum Test—Blood
See Ham's Test—Blood.

Acid Phosphatase—Serum
Norm.

	Method	SI Units
Bodansky	0.5-2 U/L	2.7-10.7 IU/L
King-Armstrong	0.1-5 U/L	0.2-8.8 IU/L
Bessey-Lowery-Brock	0.1-0.8 U/L	1.7-13.4 IU/L
Gutman	0.1-2 U/L	

Increased. Bone fracture, cancer with bone metastasis, Gaucher disease, hairy cell leukemia (leukemic reticuloendotheliosis), hepatitis (viral), hyperparathyroidism, hypophosphatemia, idiopathic thrombocytopenic purpura (with bone marrow megakaryocytes), jaundice (obstructive), Laënnec's cirrhosis, leukemia (myelogenous), multiple myeloma, osteogenesis imperfecta, Paget's disease (advanced), partial translocation trisomy 21, prostate cancer, prostatic infarction, prostatic surgery or trauma, renal impairment (acute), sickle cell crisis, thrombocythemia, thrombocytosis, thromboembolism, and thrombophlebitis. Drugs include anabolic steroids.

A

Decreased. No clinical significance. Drugs include fluorides.

Description. Acid phosphatase is one of a group of enzymes located primarily in the prostate gland and prostatic secretions. Smaller amounts are found in the bone marrow, spleen, liver, kidneys, and blood components such as erythrocytes and platelets. Isoenzymes of acid phosphatase include prostatic isoenzyme and erythrocytic isoenzyme. Used in diagnosis of and monitoring for treatment response of prostate cancer.

Professional Considerations
Consent form NOT required.

Preparation
1. Tube: Red topped, red/gray topped, or gold topped.

Procedure
1. Collect a 4-mL blood sample.

Postprocedure Care
1. Send the specimen to the laboratory immediately.
2. Separate the serum, add 0.01 mL of 20% acetic acid per milliliter of serum, and refrigerate if the test is not performed immediately.

Client and Family Teaching
1. Results may not be available for several days.

Factors That Affect Results
1. Hemolysis or specimens received more than 15 minutes after collection invalidate results.
2. False-negative results may be attributable to use of a collecting tube containing fluorides, oxalates, or phosphates.
3. Drugs that cause false-positive results include clofibrate.
4. Elevated levels may be caused by rectal examination, prostatic massage, or urinary catheterization within 2 days before the test.

Other Data
1. This test is more helpful for diagnosis in advanced prostate cancer than in early prostate cancer.
2. Use of prostate-specific acid phosphatase as a tumor marker for prostate cancer is being replaced by Prostate-specific antigen—Serum.
3. See also Prostatic acid phosphatase—Blood.

Acid Phosphatase, Tartrate-Resistant—Blood

See Tartrate-Resistant Acid Phosphatase Stain—Specimen.

Acid Phosphatase—Vaginal Swab

Norm. Method: Dilution with a substrate of thymolphthalein monophosphate.

<5	Normal vaginal secretions
<7	Inconclusive
7-50	Highly suggestive of coitus within past 36 hours
≥50	Confirmation of recent coitus

Usage. Rape trauma workup.

Description. Acid phosphatase is one of a group of enzymes located primarily in the prostate gland and prostatic secretions, with smaller amounts found elsewhere in the body. Normal vaginal secretions contain only low levels of acid phosphatase. Because acid phosphatase is found in such high concentrations in semen, its isolation in high levels from vaginal fluid in cases of suspected rape is strong evidence that coitus occurred recently.

Professional Considerations
Consent form NOT required unless specimen may be used as legal evidence.

Preparation
1. Obtain speculum, cotton wool swab supplied in a sexual offense kit, and sterile container.

Procedure
1. If the specimen may be used as legal evidence, have the specimen collection witnessed.
2. Position the client in the dorsal lithotomy position and drape for privacy and comfort.

3. Gently scrape the walls of the vagina with a plain cotton wool swab until it is saturated.
4. Place the swab in a sterile container.

Postprocedure Care

1. Write the client's name, the date, the exact time of collection, and the specimen source on the laboratory requisition. Sign and have the witness sign the laboratory requisition.
2. Transport the specimen to the laboratory immediately in a sealed plastic bag marked as legal evidence. All clients handling the specimen should sign and mark the time of specimen receipt on the laboratory requisition.

Client and Family Teaching

1. Provide repeated and thorough explanation of the purpose and process of specimen collection.
2. Follow-up: Survivors of sexual assault should be referred to appropriate crisis counseling agencies as well as gynecologic follow-up. Facilitate referral if desired by client.
3. Referral for HIV testing should be reviewed and offered to all sexual assault victims.
4. Preventive treatment for *Chlamydia*, gonorrhea, and syphilis should be provided to all survivors of sexual assault.
5. The option of postcoital contraceptive should be reviewed with all survivors of sexual assault.

Factors That Affect Results

1. Vaginal swabs for acid phosphatase should be collected as soon as possible after the assault. Swabs have the highest chance of being positive when collected within 5 hours of the assault and are least likely to be positive after 12 hours. By 48 hours, normal vaginal levels are usually found.
2. Negative results may be obtained if the assailant was sexually dysfunctional or has had a vasectomy or if the client bathed, douched, or defecated after the assault.
3. This test cannot identify the perpetrator.
4. Contamination of the vagina or the specimen with substances other than semen or normal vaginal substances may cause false-positive results.

Other Data

1. Negative results caused by a long delay between the occurrence of the assault and collection of the vaginal specimen are sometimes used by defense attorneys as evidence that a rape did not occur.
2. Although swabs may also be taken of other body orifices for evidence of acid phosphatase, they rarely yield positive results when taken more than 5 hours after the sexual assault occurred.
3. A spot test, intended for field use outside of the lab, is currently being tested. A test swab is covered with the moistened specimen, and characteristic color changes in the swab indicate positive or negative presence of acid phosphatase. Vaginal washings should be evaluated within 24 hours of deposition. Results are independent of sperm count.
4. See also Blood group antigen of semen—Vaginal swab; Precipitin test against human sperm and blood—Vaginal swab.

Acoustic Immittance Tests—Diagnostic

Norm. Normal acoustic immittance.

Tympanogram. The tympanogram recording shows a symmetric, shallow upslope and downslope free of notches or peaks with middle ear pressure of −100 to +100 dPa.

Pure-Tone Reflex Threshold	
Transbrainstem	70-100 dB HL
Ipsilateral	3-12 dB HL
Reflex decay	< $\frac{1}{2}$ baseline/10 seconds

Usage. Assessment of middle ear and tympanic membrane functioning; identification of location of middle ear lesions; and differential diagnosis of brainstem lesions and hearing loss; evaluation of tinnitus or vertigo; and evaluation of Bell's palsy.

Description. The acoustic immittance tests measure middle ear functioning and locates abnormalities by tympanometry and measurement of acoustic reflexes and static acoustic impedance. Tympanometry assesses stiffness of the middle ear by measuring admittance (that is, how much impedance exists to the flow of sound into the ear). Lower than normal admittance can be caused by cerumen, the presence of fluid in the middle ear, or a perforated tympanic membrane. Higher than normal admittance results when ear scarring is present. Measurement of acoustic reflexes shows how well the stapedius muscle responds to the delivery of sound against it. Poor or no acoustic reflexes can indicate hearing loss, neurologic or stapedius muscle damage or lesions, otosclerosis, or absence of the stapes.

Professional Considerations
Consent form NOT required.

Risks
Infection.
Contraindications
May be contraindicated in clients with accidental head injuries or suspected labyrinthine fistula or in those who have recently undergone ear surgery.

Preparation
1. Obtain admittance meter; recorder; probe with tips, cuffs, and silicone putty; otoscope; and audiometer.
2. See Client and Family Teaching.

Procedure
1. Cleanse the bores of the ear probe with wire. Calibrate the admittance meter. Inspect the ear canal, and remove any impacted cerumen.
2. Lift the auricle up and out, and insert the admittance meter's cuffed probe into the external auditory canal until a pressure of −200 dPa is achieved, indicating an adequate seal.
3. Admittance measurement: Admittance recordings are made in response to air-pressure changes made by the meter.

4. Acoustic reflex measurement: Measure acoustic reflexes when a 500- to 4000-Hz tone is sent into either ear. Perform ipsilateral measurement in the stimulated ear. You may perform contralateral (transbrainstem) measurement by sending the tone into the opposite ear.
5. Reflex-threshold measurement: Measure the reflex threshold by sending progressively louder tones into the ear in 10-dB increments until a reflex occurs and then decreasing the decibels in smaller steps until the lowest level that elicits a reflex is identified.
6. Reflex-decay measurement: Measure the reflex decay by sending a 10-second tone equal to the reflex threshold plus 10 dB into the contralateral ear and comparing the degree of initial, 5-second, and 10-second reflexes.

Postprocedure Care
1. Cleanse the ear probe.

Client and Family Teaching
1. Avoid moving, talking, or swallowing during the test. The test involves transmitting loud tones into the ear, which may be uncomfortable but will not damage the ear.

Factors That Affect Results
1. The most accurate results are obtained when the air seal remains continuous. Silicone putty may be used around the circumference of the canal to help maintain the seal.
2. Cerumen or silicone putty clogging the probe may cause the tympanogram to show as a flat waveform.

Other Data
1. Incidence of hearing loss is 46% for persons more than 66 years of age, is greater in males than in females, and increases with age.

Acquired Immune Deficiency Syndrome (AIDS) Evaluation Battery—Diagnostic

Norm. Negative AIDS battery, nonreactive.

Antigen Detection by Serology. Negative for HIV antigens.

Antibody Detection. Negative for HIV antibodies.

Lymphocyte Subset Enumeration

Total	1500-4000/mL
B cells	65-475/mL
OKT-3 cells	875-1900/mL
OKT-4 cells (CD4)	450-1400/mL

Lymphocyte Subset Enumeration—cont'd

OKT-8 cells	190-725/mL
OKT-4:OKT-8 ratio	1-3.5
Beta$_2$-microglobulin	<2 mg/mL (<170 nmol/L, SI units)

Usage. Used often in combination with cultures and for confirmation of opportunistic infection to help diagnose acquired immune deficiency syndrome (AIDS). Included in well-woman screening recommendations from the American College of Obstetricians and Gynecologists for clients with any of the following risk factors: more than one sexual partner since their most recent HIV test or a sexual partner with more than one sexual partner since their most recent HIV test, diagnosed with a sexually transmitted disease in the past year, drug use by injection, invasive cervical cancer, and women seeking preconception evaluation.

Description. AIDS is caused by human immunodeficiency virus (HIV), a cytoplasmic retrovirus of the human T-cell leukemia and lymphoma virus family that reproduces and infects, even when antibodies against the virus are present. There are several strains. All attack a subgroup of T- lymphocytes known as "helper" T cells, which are important in cell-mediated immunity. AIDS causes immunosuppression and susceptibility to infection with opportunistic organisms such as *Pneumocystis carinii, Candida albicans, Cryptococcus neoformans, Mycobacterium, Toxoplasma gondii, Cryptosporidium,* and herpes simplex. The predominant modes of transmission of HIV are believed to be (1) direct contact between the blood of an uninfected person and the blood of an infected person and (2) sexual and body fluid transmission. The incubation period may be as short as 6 days and as long as several years.

HIV is now the leading cause of death in men 25-40 years of age, the sixth leading cause of death worldwide in adolescent males 15-24 years, and the fourth leading cause of death in women 25-44 years. It is estimated that 42 million people worldwide, including 980,000 North Americans, are HIV infected. In 2002 3.1 million people died of HIV/AIDS and AIDS-related diseases.

A person may be infected with the human immunodeficiency virus for several years without becoming symptomatic when the virus enters a non-replicating latent period. When the virus begins actively replicating, the person may develop AIDS. At 2-6 weeks after infection, clients may develop a viral-like illness consisting of fever, sweats, fatigue, malaise, lymphadenopathy, sore throat, and sometimes splenomegaly. Clients may remain asymptomatic for months to years, depending on the progression of the disease.

In 1993 the CDC expanded the AIDS surveillance case definition to include all HIV-infected persons who have <200 CD4+ T-lymphocytes/μL or a CD4+ T-lymphocyte percentage of total lymphocytes <14. This expansion includes the addition of three clinical conditions: pulmonary tuberculosis, recurrent pneumonia, and invasive cervical cancer. As the number of CD4+ T-lymphocytes decreases, the risk and severity of opportunistic illnesses increase. Measures of CD4+ T-lymphocytes are used to guide clinical and therapeutic management of HIV-infected persons. Antimicrobial prophylaxis and antiretroviral therapies have been shown to be most effective within certain levels of immune dysfunction.

The AIDS evaluation battery results are not usually performed unless a rapid screening test is preliminarily positive (see OraQuick rapid HIV tests—Specimen). The tests in this battery are often considered with other diagnostic tests for opportunistic infection such as body fluid culture and cytology, central nervous system tomography, bronchoscopy, and biopsy to complete the clinical picture description before diagnosis is made. The AIDS evaluation battery comprises the following tests: blood and body fluid cultures, antigen detection by serology, antibody detection, confirmatory antibody detection methods, and tests for immunologic status evaluation and beta$_2$-microglobulin. No test that by itself confirms HIV infection has yet been developed.

Blood and body fluid cultures have been found to show positive results in some persons soon after infection with HIV. Although difficult to do, isolation of HIV has been accomplished in concentrated peripheral blood lymphocytes and body fluids. However, a negative result does not rule out infection (see Blood culture—Blood; Body fluid, Routine—Culture).

Antigen detection by serology methods may be positive for the viral antigen (frequently p24 core protein, HIV core antigen) from 1-2 weeks up to about 1 month after infection with the virus. The antigen is detectable during acute (initial) infection, undetectable as the virus becomes latent, and again detectable as the infection progresses. The enzyme-linked immunosorbent assay (ELISA) is used for screening for HIV. Detection of HIV antibody by ELISA must be confirmed by Western blot. Alternative diagnosis may be made by viral culture, by antigen detection, or by HIV DNA or RNA polymerase chain reaction (PCR). Quantitative virology using quantitative RNA PCR or branched-chain DNA (bDNA) has become a popular method to access viral load in staging clients or for therapeutic monitoring. Maternal antibodies may be present in infants until 18 months of age; therefore CD4 counts, viral culture, or PCR followed by antibody detection after 18 months must be performed to diagnose HIV in infants.

Studies indicate that the frequency of false-positive tests in a low-prevalence population with both the ELISA and Western blot is about 0.0007%, and the frequency of false-negative results in a high-prevalence population is about 0.3%. The usual cause of false-negative tests is testing in the time between transmission and seroconversion, a period that rarely lasts longer than 3 months. When the results are positive, it is recommended that repeat testing be done for those with no likely risk factors, and those who report positive results from an anonymous test site. Periodic tests are suggested for clients with negative results who continue to practice high-risk behaviors.

Confirmatory antibody detection methods include the Western blot, immunofluorescence, radioimmunoprecipitation, and ELISA tests that detect antibodies to genetically engineered HIV proteins. The Western blot and immunofluorescence methods have similar sensitivities. Immunofluorescence results are obtained more quickly but are less reliable than those of the Western blot. Radioimmunofluorescence is more sensitive than the Western blot but is not widely used because of the technical

difficulty of the procedure. Newer ELISA tests are able to pinpoint the specific HIV antibody present in serum when one incubates the serum first with specific HIV proteins and then a tagged, anti-immunoglobulin enzyme and measures the amount of substrate hydrolyzed by the antigen-antibody reaction.

Quantitative testing for HIV p24 antigen may provide a surrogate marker for disease progression: however, this antigen usually disappears from the blood during the asymptomatic phase. The PCR for the detection of HIV DNA or RNA has been extensively used in the research setting and proven extremely valuable.

A few alternative detection methods are actively being studied. Two home test kits for HIV detection (Direct Access Diagnostics and ChemTrak) are under review by the FDA. There are currently two FDA-licensed rapid tests: SUDS (Murex) and Recombigen latex agglutination assay (Cambridge Biotech). These tests are attractive for use in areas such as emergency departments, autopsy areas, and STD clinics.

Tests for immunologic status evaluation include lymphocyte subset enumeration, T-lymphocyte and B-lymphocyte subset assays, and skin tests with known antigens for persons with infections such as *Candida* or mumps; these often demonstrate normal results until the later stages of infection. As T-lymphocyte helper cells (OKT-4 cells) become infected by the human immunodeficiency virus, their numbers decrease. Levels of suppressor T cells (OKT-8 cells) may remain normal or increase as virus activity progresses. Lymphocyte counts decrease as immune function decreases. False-negative results from known antigen skin tests indicate that the client's immune function is compromised.

Beta$_2$-microglobulin is an amino acid peptide component of lymphocyte HLA complexes that increases in the serum in inflammatory conditions and when lymphocyte turnover increases, as when T-lymphocyte helper (OKT-4) cells are attacked by HIV. Rising levels may also be caused by conditions other than HIV. Although beta$_2$-microglobulin levels usually rise with HIV infection, the levels do not always correlate with the stages of the infection (see Beta$_2$-microglobulin—Blood and 24-hour urine).

CD4+ T-lymphocyte test results alone should not be used as a surrogate marker for HIV or AIDS. A low CD4+ T-lymphocyte count without a positive HIV test result will not be reportable, since other conditions may be the cause. Health care providers must ensure that persons who have a CD4+ T-lymphocyte count of <200/μL are HIV-infected before initiating treatment for HIV disease.

Professional Considerations

Consent form IS required because of area-specific legal regulations. Testing should be voluntary with appropriate counseling before and after informed consent.

Preparation

1. Clarify the type of tube needed for lymphocyte subset enumeration if the Becton Dickinson Immunocytology Systems method is not used.
2. Tube: Red topped, red/gray topped, gold topped, or lavender topped.

Procedure

1. Antigen detection by serology, antibody detection, and confirmatory antibody detection method: Draw a 5-mL venous blood sample.
2. Lymphocyte subset enumeration (Becton Dickinson Immunocytology Systems method): Completely fill two lavender topped tubes with venous blood. Label one tube for complete blood count and the other tube for lymphocyte subset enumeration.
3. Beta$_2$-microglobulin: Draw a 10-mL venous blood sample in a lavender topped tube.

Postprocedure Care

1. Either leave reusable equipment in the client's room or dispose of the equipment in the room.

Client and Family Teaching

1. Explain the purpose of the test, the procedure for collection, and the results to the client.
2. Two days are required for the Western blot.
3. Assess client understanding of safe sex practices and provide counseling as needed.
4. CDC National AIDS hotline: 1-800-342-AIDS.

Factors That Affect Results

1. Antibody results may be negative up to 35 months after infection because of viral latency.
2. False-positive ELISA results may be caused by HLA antibody reaction with specific proteins in certain test kits. False-negative ELISA results may occur in a small proportion of clients with HIV-1 infection and in some children infected with HIV in utero.
3. Falsely depressed lymphocyte counts may be caused by steroids and general anesthetics.
4. Beta$_2$-microglobulin results are invalidated if the person has undergone a scan involving the administration of radioactive dyes within 1 week before the test.

Other Data

1. Legal restrictions exist and vary regarding HIV testing and reporting of results.
2. Demonstration of homogeneous B or T-lymphocytes is helpful in prognosis and therapeutic planning of malignant lymphoproliferative disorders.
3. In a recent study at the National Institute of Allergy and Infectious Diseases, in a small number of HIV-infected clients, infusions of an immune system protein significantly increased levels of the infection-fighting white blood cells normally destroyed during HIV infection.
4. Begin antiretroviral therapy before CD4 cells drop below 200/μL.
5. Progression of cytomegalovirus retinitis occurs in 17% with low CD4 cell count.
6. The Genie assay is faster, less costly, and yields fewer indeterminate results in detecting HIV-1 antibodies than the Western blot method.
7. Independent predictors to progression include CD4 <50 cells/mm^3, *pneumocystis carinii* pneumonia prophylaxis, low hemoglobin levels, and high virus load.
8. Total viral load can sometimes be assessed to help monitor the impact of treatment.
9. HIV testing should be performed at baseline, 4, 12, and 24 weeks.
10. See also T- and B-lymphocyte subset assay—Blood; Beta$_2$-microglobulin—Blood and 24-hour urine; Oral mucosal transudate—Specimen; and OraQuick rapid HIV test—Specimen.

A

ACTH Stimulation Test—Diagnostic

Norm. 17-Hydroxycorticosteroid (17-OHCS) levels increase by two to four times between the first and second 24-hour urine collection.

Usage. Definitive diagnosis of Addison's disease and adrenal adenoma.

Description. Adrenocorticotropic hormone (ACTH) is secreted by the pituitary gland and acts on the adrenal cortex to cause release of adrenal hormones. This test measures blood cortisol and urinary 17-OHCS levels before and after an infusion of ACTH. It is diagnostic of Addison's disease in a client with hypocortisolism when an infusion of ACTH fails to cause an increase in cortisol or 17-OHCS, urinary metabolites of plasma cortisol. A small response occurs in those with high mortality in the ICU and in older clients.

Professional Considerations
Consent form NOT required.

Preparation
1. To prevent hypersensitivity reactions when using biologic rather than synthetic ACTH, give 0.5 mg of dexamethasone orally before the test.
2. Obtain a 3-L container with 10 mL of concentrated hydrochloric acid (HCl) preservative.
3. Write starting time of collection on the laboratory requisition.
4. The test can be performed at any time of the day.

Procedure
1. Discard the first morning-urine specimen.
2. Save all urine voided for 24 hours in a refrigerated, clean, 3-L container to which

10 mL of concentrated HCl has been added. Document the quantity of urine output during the collection period. Include urine voided at the end of the 24-hour period.
3. Begin a second 24-hour urine collection.
4. During the second collection, infuse 24 units of ACTH in 500 mL of normal saline intravenously over 8 hours.

Postprocedure Care
1. Record the total 24-hour output on the laboratory requisition and send the entire specimen to the laboratory.

Client and Family Teaching
1. Save all urine voided in the 24-hour period, and urinate before defecating to avoid loss of urine. If any urine is accidentally discarded, discard the entire specimen and restart the collection the next day.

Factors That Affect Results
1. Maintenance steroids that must be given during the testing period should be in the form of small doses of dexamethasone to avoid false elevation of 17-OHCS in the urine.

Other Data
1. The test should be repeated in 24 hours if pituitary deficiency is suspected. Pituitary insufficiency would be evident by a gradual but small response to the ACTH stimulation test during the second test.
2. The ACTH stimulation test is useful for identifying adrenal insufficiency; however, it is not sensitive or specific for clients suspected of having secondary adrenal insufficiency or those with recent pituitary injury.

Actinomyces—Culture

Norm. Negative.

Positive. Abscess, actinomycosis, pelvic inflammatory disease, and root canal infection.

Description. A slow-growing, gram-positive, non–acid-fast, bacillus that is anaerobic to microaerophilic and appears in variable lengths and shapes on a Gram stain.

Actinomyces israelii is a part of the normal oral flora in many people. Possibly because of mouth trauma or infection, it sometimes becomes invasive, forms draining sinus tracts, and becomes a chronic, suppurative disease called "actinomycosis" that spreads by direct extension. The characteristic lesion is a hard, red, nontender nodule that eventually begins draining. The *Actinomyces* organisms are also found in the vaginal smears of a small percentage of women in whom intrauterine devices have been inserted.

Professional Considerations
Consent form NOT required.

Preparation
1. Obtain a sterile cotton swab and culture media.

Procedure
1. Swab the drainage (pus from lesion, sinus tract, or fistula; or sputum; or tissue biopsy material).
2. Inoculate the drainage into thioglycolate medium and streak it onto brain-heart infusion agar plates.
3. Incubate anaerobically for 2 weeks or more.

Postprocedure Care
1. Apply a dry sterile dressing as needed.
2. Send the specimen to the laboratory immediately.

Client and Family Teaching
1. Results will not be available for at least 14 days.
2. Treatment for actinomycosis usually includes drainage of lesions and penicillin or tetracycline drug therapy.

Factors That Affect Results
1. Do NOT refrigerate or store the specimen.

Other Data
1. Some tissue damage from actinomycosis is irreversible.

Activated Coagulation Time (ACT), Automated—Blood

Norm. Varies, depending on the type of system in use and the type of test reagent or activator. There are currently two commercially available systems for analyzing ACT by automation: ACT II by Medtronic Hemotec Inc. and Hemochron by International Technidyne Corporation.

Usage. Commonly used for heparin anticoagulation monitoring during bypass surgery, percutaneous transluminal coronary angioplasty (PTCA), interventional radiology, neonatal extracorporeal membrane oxygenation (ECMO), hemofiltration, hemodialysis, and critical and telemetry care.

Increased. Afibrinogenemia, circulating anticoagulants, dysproteinemia, factor deficiency (V, VIII, IX, X, XI, or XII), fibrinolysis, hemophilia, hemorrhagic disease of the newborn, hypofibrinogenemia, hypoprothrombinemia, leukemia, and liver disease. Drugs include antithrombin III, aprotinin, heparin calcium, heparin sodium (including blood obtained from an introducer with a heparin-coated pulmonary artery catheter), and warfarin.

Hemochron System

Tube	Range in Seconds	ACT II
TCA510 and FTCA510	105-167	Multiple methods are available for measuring ACT values; thus values should be evaluated according to reference levels of the individual machine and test tube used. The ACT II machine has an overall range of 0-999.
K-ACT and FTK-ACT	91-151	
P214/215	110-182	
S412	186-306	

Description. Measures the ability of blood to clot. Fresh whole blood is added to a test tube containing an activator (diatomaceous earth, glass particles, or kaolin) and timed for the formation of a clot. The ACT is more sensitive to the effects of factor VIII deficiency and heparin than is whole-blood clotting time. The ACT test has become a mainstay in monitoring heparin anticoagulation during invasive procedures and is the preferred method for monitoring high-level anticoagulation. The ACT is quick, reliable, and easy and can be performed at the bedside. Disadvantages of the ACT are operator variability and differences between the two commercially available systems.

Professional Considerations

Consent form NOT required.

Preparation

1. Obtain a tube with a designated activator for the specific ACT test. May be drawn from indwelling venous blood line, extracorporeal blood line port, direct venipuncture, or vacuum draw. Do not obtain blood from a heparinized access line, an indwelling heparinized lock, or a hemodialysis line.
2. Obtain two 5-mL syringes.

Procedure (if using the ACT II system, see instructions below before obtaining client sample):

1. *Indwelling venous line sampling*: With the first syringe, withdraw and discard 5 mL of blood. Attach the second syringe and withdraw a 3-mL blood sample.
2. *Venipuncture sampling*: With the first syringe, withdraw and discard 2 mL of blood. Attach the second syringe and withdraw a 3-mL sample.

Hemochron System

1. Dispense exactly 2 mL of blood into the test tube (NOTE: tubes P214/P215 require only 0.4 mL of blood). At the same time, depress the start-button timer on the machine. Close the tube and agitate it briskly 10 times.
2. Insert the test tube into the Hemochron machine port and rotate clockwise until the green indicator light is visible. Await the result, which will be displayed as the number of seconds required to obtain coagulation on the Hemochron screen.

Act II System

1. Prewarm the cartridge in the ACT heat block for 3 minutes.
2. Gently tap or shake the cartridge to resuspend the activator.
3. Inject the client sample into channel 2 and then channel 1 of the cartridge, filling to between the lines (<1 mL).
4. Place the cartridge in the instrument and pull the actuator cover forward. The instrument will sound an audible alert when the end point is reached. (NOTE: The instrument has two readout displays. The channel 1 result is of ACT without heparin; the channel 2 result is of ACT with the influence of heparin.)

Postprocedure Care

1. If the test is performed at the client's bedside, document on the client's medical record the result of the test, time, date, machine number, tube type or number, site of draw, and rate of infusion in units per hour if the client is receiving IV heparin.

Client and Family Teaching

1. Results are normally available within a few minutes.

Factors That Affect Results

1. Tests may be affected by hemodilution, poor operator technique, inadequate reagent-to-specimen mixture, improper storage of test kits, cardioplegic solutions, hypothermia, platelet dysfunction, hypofibrinogenemia, other coagulopathies, and certain medications.
2. In acute coronary conditions, such as unstable angina and acute myocardial infarction, baseline ACTs may be lower and heparin requirements higher, reflecting a thrombogenic state.
3. Heparinase-I (Neutralase) restores activated coagulation time in clients undergoing coronary artery surgery, as an alternative to protamine.

Other Data

1. Test cartridges available for the ACT II system: LR ACT, RACT, HR ACT, PT, GPC, and HTC. Test cartridges available for the Hemochron system are listed previously under Norms.
2. Heparin requirements as well as baseline ACTs vary from client to client, and so ACT determinations allow a quick titration of the effective heparin dose.
3. Therapeutic ACT values depend on several factors: type of ACT system, type of test tube and reagent, type of procedure being performed, clinical condition of client, and clinical preference of physician.
4. HemoTec and Hemochron ACT measurements cannot be used interchangeably.

Activated Partial Thromboplastin Substitution Test—Diagnostic

Norm. Normal factors VIII, IX, X, XI, and XII.

Usage. Helps identify single factor deficiencies causing prolonged partial thromboplastin time, including factors VIII, IX, XI, and XII.

Description. A differential activated partial thromboplastin time (APTT) method that identifies which factor deficiency or deficiencies are present when APTT is prolonged. Known reagents for each factor are systematically added to the client's blood sample. A factor is determined to be deficient when the substitution produces a normal APTT.

Professional Considerations
Consent form NOT required.

Preparation
1. Tubes: Red topped and blue topped.
2. Preschedule the test with the laboratory.

Procedure
1. Draw 2-3 mL of blood into a red topped tube and discard. Completely fill a blue topped tube with the blood sample.

Postprocedure Care
1. Apply pressure over the venipuncture site for 5 minutes if the client is receiving heparin therapy. Observe the site closely for development of a hematoma.

2. Write the collection time on the laboratory requisition.
3. Refrigerate the specimen until the test is completed.

Client and Family Teaching
1. Results are normally available within 24 hours.

Factors That Affect Results
1. Failure to discard the first few milliliters of blood drawn may contaminate the specimen with tissue thromboplastin, which can activate coagulation.
2. Failure to completely fill the tube with blood may cause falsely prolonged results.
3. Hematocrit >50% may cause falsely prolonged results, and hematocrit <20% may cause falsely decreased results.
4. Drawing the sample from a line being kept open with a heparin flush will cause falsely prolonged results.
5. Reject hemolyzed specimens and specimens received more than 2 hours after collection.
6. Anticoagulant therapy within 2 weeks before the test invalidates results.

Other Data
1. Useful only with single-factor deficiencies.
2. See also Activated partial thromboplastin time and partial thromboplastin time—Plasma.

Activated Partial Thromboplastin Time (APTT) and Partial Thromboplastin Time (PTT)—Plasma

NOTE: Activated partial thromboplastin time (APTT) is the current method of this test, which is still commonly referred to as "PTT."

Norm. Standardized times should be reported by each laboratory because results depend on the type of activator used. In general, standards are less than 35 seconds and vary by 20-36 seconds.

Premature infants	<120 seconds
Newborn	<90 seconds
Infants	24-40 seconds
Children	24-40 seconds
Adult panic level	>70 seconds

Therapeutic Heparin Therapy Levels

Acute coronary artery disease	50-80 seconds
Peripheral vascular disease with embolism	50-80 seconds

Panic Level Symptoms and Treatment
Symptoms. Prolonged bleeding, hematoma at venipuncture site, cerebrovascular accident, hemorrhage, shock.

Treatment
NOTE: Treatment choice(s) depend(s) on client's history and condition and episode history.

1. Assess heparin therapy.
2. Administer protamine sulfate (usual dose of 1 g of protamine sulfate for every 100 units of heparin).
3. Monitor vital signs.
4. Monitor for neurologic changes every hour until levels are within desired range.

Increased. *Major causes:* Genetic or acquired deficiency of blood clotting factors IX, X, XI, or XII and with factor V or II deficiencies.

These deficiencies usually must be below 30%-40% of normal levels for clotting factors to produce increased APTT and bleeding tendencies as seen in hemophilia A. Longer times are associated with deficiencies of high molecular weight (HMW) kininogen and Fletcher factor (prekallikrein). Longer times also occur with abruptio placentae, afibrinogenemia, cardiac surgery, hypothermia, cirrhosis, disseminated intravascular coagulation, dysfibrinogenemia, fibrinolysis, Fitzgerald factor deficiency (severe), hemorrhagic disease of the newborn, hypofibrinogenemia, liver disease, hypoprothrombinemia, presence of circulating anticoagulants, lupus anticoagulant, and von Willebrand's disease and in clients receiving hemodialysis.

Drugs include alcohol, antistreplase (a thrombolytic agent), bishydroxycoumarin (excess therapy), chlorpromazine, codeine, eptifibatide, heparin calcium, heparin sodium, methotrexate, phenothiazines, salicylates, warfarin administration, and valproic acid.

Decreased. Shortened times occur with abnormalities of Fletcher factor, which are not associated with bleeding and in which thromboemboli may occur. A shortened APTT (less than or equal to control) on presentation in clients with chest pain is associated with increased risk of acute MI.

Description. Partial thromboplastin time (PTT) evaluates how well the coagulation sequence is functioning by measuring the amount of time it takes for recalcified, citrated plasma to clot after partial thromboplastin is added to it. The PTT is abnormal in 90% of coagulation defects and screens for deficiencies and inhibitors of all factors except VII and XIII. This test is most commonly used to monitor effectiveness of heparin therapy and to screen for disorders of coagulation. When commercial activating materials are used to standardize the test, the PTT is called the APTT, or "activated partial thromboplastin time."

Professional Considerations
Consent form NOT required.

Preparation
1. For intermittent heparin dosing, the sample should be drawn 1 hour before the next dose. A baseline APTT may not be needed before heparin therapy unless disease is suspected.
2. Tube: 2.7- or 4.5-mL blue topped tube, a control tube, and a waste tube or syringe.
3. Do NOT draw specimens during hemodialysis.
4. Do NOT draw specimens from a closed-loop blood sampling system in an arterial line that uses heparin flush solution.

Procedure
1. Withdraw 2 mL of blood into a discard syringe or vacuum tube. Remove the syringe or tube, leaving the needle in place. Attach a second syringe, and draw a blood sample quantity of 2.4 mL for a 2.7-mL tube, or 4.0 mL for a 4.5-mL tube. Collect the sample without trauma.

Postprocedure Care
1. If the test cannot be performed within 2 hours after specimen collection, separate and freeze the plasma.
2. Transport the specimen to the laboratory immediately.

Client and Family Teaching
1. Surgery may be postponed if the results are prolonged.
2. Bleeding precautions for prolonged values include the following: use a soft toothbrush; use an electric razor; avoid aspirin or aspirin products; avoid constipation; wear loose clothing; avoid intramuscular injections.
3. Watch for and report signs of bleeding: bruising, petechiae, blood in stool/urine/sputum, bleeding from invasive lines, bleeding gums, abnormal or excessive vaginal bleeding.
4. Many herbs can cause bleeding effects. For this reason, do not take any herbal preparations or natural remedies without receiving your doctor's approval.

Factors That Affect Results

1. Do NOT draw samples from an arm into which heparin is infusing.
2. Failure to completely fill the tube will alter the results.
3. If you are drawing samples from an arterial line with a heparin-flush pressure bag, at least 10 mL of blood must be withdrawn before the PTT sample is drawn.
4. Failure to discard the first 1 to 2 mL of traumatic venous draw may result in a falsely decreased APTT.
5. A false-normal PTT may occur if factor levels are deficient but not less than 25% to 30% of normal.
6. Factor I (fibrinogen) deficiency may not be detectable unless levels are <100 mg/dL.
7. Hematocrit >55% may cause falsely prolonged results. The test should be redrawn in a tube furnished by the laboratory that has had the concentration or amount of citrate adjusted for the elevated hematocrit level.
8. Freezing the sample will decrease the test sensitivity to lupus anticoagulant and to deficiencies of XII, XI, HMW kininogen, and prekallikrein.
9. Herbs or natural remedies that may increase PTT include *dan shen* (redginseng, *Salvia miltiorrhiza*), *dang gui* [variants: tangkuei, dong quai] (*Angelica sinensis*) (in clients receiving warfarin concurrently), feverfew (*Tanacetum parthenium*), *ginkgo biloba*, ginger, and ginseng.

Other Data

1. 1 mg of protamine sulfate will reverse the effects of 100 units of heparin.
2. Hemophilia A causes increased APTT with normal PT and bleeding time.
3. Hemophilia B is diagnosed by increased APTT with normal or increased PT and direct assay of levels of factor IX.
4. APTT is not helpful in the diagnosis of hemophilia type.
5. APTT and PT are both increased with prothrombin and HMW kininogen and prekallikrein deficiencies.
6. Age, sex, and ABO blood group may have an influence on the APTT in normal clients.
7. Acceptable alternatives to APTT monitoring of direct anticoagulation thrombin inhibitors (DTIs) include the ecarin clotting time (ECT) and the thrombin inhibitor management (TIM) test.

Activated Protein C Resistance Test

See **Protein C**—Blood.

Acute Abdominal Series—Diagnostic

Norm. Requires individual interpretation.

Usage. Differential diagnosis of the cause of an acute condition of the abdomen. Some examples are abdominal aortic aneurysm dissection, abscess, acute cholecystitis, acute ischemia, acute pancreatitis, appendicitis, bile duct obstruction, bowel strangulation, choledocholithiasis, gastric outlet obstruction, perforated abdominal viscus, peritonitis, pyelonephritis, ruptured ectopic pregnancy, *Salmonella* enterocolitis, and ureteral obstruction. Also useful for identifying the presence and location of (a) foreign body(ies).

Description. An acute abdominal condition is characterized by the abrupt onset of abdominal pain, distention, diminished or absent bowel sounds, and, sometimes, guarding. There may be many causes of these symptoms, and the disorder within the abdomen is hidden. In addition to a routine external physical assessment, seven routes of diagnostic work-up are used. Less invasive testing is usually performed initially.

Laboratory studies include coagulation studies, hemoglobin and hematocrit tests, and blood volume determinations to rule out internal bleeding, leukocyte differential to determine whether an infectious or inflammatory process is present, amylase level to rule out pancreatic and other pathologic conditions, liver panels to rule out a

A

hepatic disorder, blood urea nitrogen and creatinine determinations and urinalysis to rule out urinary tract infection, and stool examination to rule out *Salmonella*. Fine-needle aspiration cytologic testing provides clues to the type of process occurring.

Plain-film radiography is taking a radiograph without the use of an injected radiopaque agent. Plain-film radiography of the abdomen may identify compression fractures, intestinal obstruction, metastasis, perforated abdominal viscus, pancreatic calcification, and renal calculi.

Contrast radiography involves injection of a radiopaque agent into the vascular space. The contrast agent enhances the appearance of organ and vascular lumens and is more likely to reveal a pathologic condition than is plain film radiography. Vascular contrast examinations of the abdominal area, such as intravenous pyelography, help identify lumbar aortic aneurysms, urinary tract trauma, lesions, or other disorders.

Intestinal contrast examinations such as barium enema, oral cholecystogram, and upper gastrointestinal series may identify colonic lesions or perforation but should not be performed when obstruction is suspected. They may also rule out appendicitis.

Ultrasonography may help diagnose acute abscesses, cholecystitis, Crohn's disease, dilated bile duct, hepatic cancer, hepatic or splenic hematoma, hydronephrosis, intussusception, pancreatitis, pancreatic pseudocyst, pancreatic carcinoma, splenomegaly, urinary tract obstruction, and the presence of foreign bodies.

Computed tomography helps identify, differentiate, and evaluate hepatic, pancreatic, renal, and retroperitoneal abscesses, fluid accumulations, masses and cysts, and pancreatitis.

Nuclear medicine studies help identify intra-abdominal abscesses, sites of gastrointestinal bleeding, hematoma, and areas of abnormal tissue metabolism. Nuclear medicine scans may also help to rule out cholecystitis.

In extremely acute situations and when findings from any combination of the above tests are inconclusive, surgical exploration of the abdomen may be required.

Professional Considerations
Consent form NOT required for the noninvasive studies. See individual listings for the invasive studies.

Risks
Allergic reaction to radiographic dye or nuclear medicine radiopharmaceutical for applicable tests (itching, hives, rash, tight feeling in the throat, shortness of breath, bronchospasm, anaphylaxis, death); renal toxicity.

Contraindications
Previous allergy to radiographic dye, iodine, or seafood or radionuclide for those tests involving injections; renal insufficiency.

Precautions
During pregnancy, risks of cumulative radiation exposure to the fetus from this and other previous or future imaging studies must be weighed against the benefits of the procedure. Although formal limits for client exposure are relative to this risk-benefit comparison, the United States Nuclear Regulatory Commission requires that the cumulative dose equivalent to an embryo/fetus from occupational exposure not exceed 0.5 rem (5 mSv). Radiation dose to the fetus is proportional to the distance of the anatomy studied from the abdomen and decreases as pregnancy progresses. For pregnant clients, consult the radiologist/radiology department to obtain estimated fetal radiation exposure from this procedure.

Preparation
1. No preprocedural care is required for plain-film radiography.
2. Intestinal contrast examinations often require clear liquids the day before the test and cathartics with or without cleansing enemas before the test. However, this requirement may be waived for a client with acute abdominal symptoms.
3. Have emergency equipment readily available for tests involving injection of radionuclide or dye.

Procedure
1. Plain-film radiography: The client is positioned in supine, upright, oblique, and lateral decubitus positions, and radiographic films are taken from various

angles. The best results are not obtained from portable films, especially in obese clients. The films should be taken in the radiology department, where the most powerful radiography is available, whenever possible. The lateral decubitus position is used for clients who are unable to stand, and the radiograph is taken horizontally across the table. A "kidneys, ureters, bladder film (KUB)" includes the majority of the abdomen and is taken from an anteroposterior angle. An anteroposterior scout film is used both before an intravenous pyelogram and in combination with an upright abdominal film for suspected intestinal obstruction. Subdiaphragmatic free air from a perforated abdominal viscus may be identified with an upright abdominal film or an upright chest film.

2. Vascular contrast examinations: Radiographic dye is injected into an arm vein, and oblique films of the abdomen are taken 15 minutes later. A left posterior oblique position may help identify a lumbar aortic aneurysm because the position enhances visualization by rotating the aorta off of the spine. Arteriography and venography may also help identify blood vessel abnormalities such as aneurysm, hemorrhage, or occlusion.

3. Intestinal contrast examination: The client is placed in a Sims' position. Barium, with or without air, is instilled into the lower gastrointestinal tract, and radiographic films are taken. In upper gastrointestinal series, the client must swallow barium, and radiographic films are then taken.

4. Ultrasonography: The client is positioned on the side or supine, and a series of high-frequency sound waves are transmitted into the abdomen. The echoes reflected from the differing tissue densities are converted by a gel-coated transducer to form patterns of the abdominal structures on an oscilloscope screen.

5. Computed tomography: The client is placed in a supine position on a platform table that moves the client through a circular computed tomography scanner. As several transverse films are taken, differing tissue densities are calculated based on varying absorption of the x-rays. Findings may indicate the need for further computed tomography after the administration of contrast medium.

6. Nuclear medicine studies: At varying intervals after the intravenous injection of a radioactive tracer, scintigraphic scans, which detect areas of increased concentration of the tracer at sites of a pathologic condition, are taken of the abdominal area.

Postprocedure Care

1. Fluids should be encouraged after studies involving the administration of radiopaque dyes or barium.

2. Cathartics may be prescribed after studies involving the administration of barium.

Client and Family Teaching

1. Explain the purpose of each test as appropriate, the procedure for the test, and the results. See individual test listings for specific client teaching.

Factors That Affect Results

1. The presence of gastrointestinal barium negates the value of plain-film radiography, vascular contrast examinations, ultrasonography, computed tomography, and nuclear medicine scintigraphy and so should be performed last.

Other Data

1. See also Barium enema—Diagnostic; Flat-plate radiography of the abdomen—Diagnostic; Intravenous pyelography—Diagnostic; Upper gastrointestinal series—Diagnostic; Computed tomography of the body—Diagnostic.

2. Health care professionals working in a nuclear medicine area must follow federal standards set by the Nuclear Regulatory Commission. These standards include precautions for the handling of the radioactive material and the monitoring of potential radiation exposure.

3. Some extra-abdominal conditions that may cause acute abdominal pain include pneumonia, pulmonary or myocardial infarction, and pericarditis. Other conditions that may cause symptoms of an acute abdominal condition include acute intermittent porphyria, diabetic neuropathy, heavy-metal poisoning, sickle cell disease, and tabes dorsalis.

A

Addis Count—12-Hour Urine

Norm.

Erythrocytes	0-5,000/mm³
Leukocytes	0-500,000/mm³
Casts	1,000,000/mm³

Increased. Glomerulonephritis and hematuria.

Description. When subclinical glomerulonephritis is suspected, an Addis count on a 12-hour urine specimen may demonstrate increased erythrocytes and leukocytes and increased rates of cast excretion in amounts too small to be detected in a random urine specimen examined microscopically. The count is performed on the sediment from a portion of the 12-hour collection.

Professional Considerations
Consent form NOT required.

Preparation
1. Obtain a 1- or a 2-L bottle that has been rinsed in formalin.

Procedure
1. The clean-catch urine technique must be used to decrease the risk of specimen contamination. See clean-catch collection instructions in Body fluid, Routine—Culture.

2. Keep the specimen container refrigerated during and after specimen collection. For catheterized specimens, keep the drainage bag on ice and empty it into the collection container hourly.

Postprocedure Care
1. Send the entire 12-hour urine specimen to the laboratory.

Client and Family Teaching
1. Do not drink any fluids throughout the collection period.
2. Collect a clean-catch urine sample according to the technique described previously if this collection method is used.

Factors That Affect Results
1. Hematuria, pyuria, or a contaminated specimen will cause falsely elevated results.

Other Data
1. This test is not usually necessary when a thorough history and renal work-up are done.
2. An approximate Addis count can be performed on a first-morning voided specimen after a 16-hour fast from fluids and food.

Adenovirus Antibody Titer—Serum

Norm. Negative. Results require interpretation with consideration of the site of the specimen correlated with clinical symptoms.

Current Adenovirus Infection. Fourfold rise in titer.

Increased. Adenovirus infection, respiratory failure, or graft failure in lung-transplanted clients. Gene therapy with replication-deficient adenoviral vector-mediated herpes simplex virus-thymidine kinase.

Description. A group of virus types responsible for upper respiratory tract disease, hemorrhagic cystitis, and epidemic keratoconjunctivitis. The mode of transmission is by direct or indirect contact. Measurement of adenovirus antibody titers is the test of choice for detection of current adenovirus infections. Results are reported as the highest dilution of serum that completely neutralizes the virus.

Professional Considerations
Consent form NOT required.

Preparation
1. Tube: Red topped, red/gray topped, or gold topped.

Procedure
1. Draw a 2-mL blood sample no later than 5-7 days after onset of symptoms.
2. After allowing the specimen to clot at room temperature, centrifuge and separate the serum into a separate vial.
3. Draw a convalescent sample in 14-21 days.

Postprocedure Care
1. Mark the tube label and laboratory requisition with "acute phase" or "convalescent

phase" for the first and second specimens, respectively.

Client and Family Teaching
1. Return in 2-3 weeks to have the convalescent sample drawn.

Factors That Affect Results
1. Reject hemolyzed or frozen specimens.

2. Specimens may be stored several weeks at 4 to 6 degrees C.
3. Antibody titers for both specimens should be performed by the same laboratory.

Other Data
1. This test is nonspecific for the type of adenovirus present.

Adrenocorticotropic Hormone (ACTH, Corticotropin)—Serum

Norm.

		SI Units
0800 hours, peak	25-100 pg/mL	25-100 ng/L
1800 hours, trough	0-50 pg/mL	0-50 ng/L
Random		
Adult Male	7-69 pg/mL	7-69 ng/L
Adult Female	6-58 pg/mL	6-58 ng/L
Adolescent (10-18 yr)	6-55 pg/mL	6-55 ng/L
Child (up to 10 yr)	5-46 pg/mL	5-46 ng/L

Increased. Addison's disease, ectopic ACTH syndrome, pituitary adenoma, pituitary Cushing's syndrome, primary adrenal insufficiency, and stress. Drugs include amphetamine sulfate, calcium gluconate, corticosteroids, estrogens, ethanol, lithium carbonate, and spironolactone.

Decreased. Primary adrenocortical hyperfunction (caused by tumor or hyperplasia) and secondary hypoadrenalism. Drugs include CPH 82—a nonsteroid antirheumatic drug.

Description. ACTH is an anterior pituitary hormone that stimulates cortisol and androgen production by the adrenal gland. Diurnal variations of ACTH are typical, with peak levels occurring from 0600 to 0800 and trough levels occurring from 1800 to 2300.

Professional Considerations
Consent form NOT required.

Preparation
1. Tube: Plastic or siliconized glass pink topped (containing K_2 EDTA) or plastic lavender topped, and ice-water slush.
2. See Client and Family Teaching.

Procedure
1. Draw a 3-mL blood sample at 0600. Repeat the sampling at 1800 if trough levels are needed.
2. Place the specimen in ice-water slush.

Postprocedure Care
1. Write the collection time on the laboratory requisition.
2. Transport the specimen to the laboratory immediately. The specimen should be frozen within 15 minutes if it will not be spun and tested within the first hour.

Client and Family Teaching
1. Consume a low-carbohydrate diet for 48 hours before the test.
2. Avoid physical and emotional stress for 12 hours before the test.
3. For peak and trough levels, two samples are required at different times of the day because the blood levels fluctuate throughout the day.
4. Results may take several days.

Factors That Affect Results
1. Reject specimens received more than 60 minutes after collection.
2. Values increase within 90 seconds of traumatic, repeated, or prolonged venipuncture.
3. Menstruation cycle, pregnancy, and radioactive scanning within 7 days affect ACTH levels.
4. This test may not detect certain types of synthetic ACTH.

Other Data
1. The ACTH stimulation test must be performed to confirm the diagnosis of Addison's disease.

ADT

See **Respiratory Antigen Panel**—Specimen.

AFB Smear

See **Sputum, Mycobacteria**—Culture and Smear.

AFP

See **Alpha-Fetoprotein**—Blood.

African Trypanosomiasis—Blood

Norm. Negative. No parasites identified.

Positive. African trypanosomiasis (African sleeping sickness).

Description. Also known as sleeping sickness, African trypanosomiasis is a vector-borne parasitic infection indigenous to tropical Africa caused in humans by the bite of a tsetse fly of the genus *Glossina*. Symptoms include a chancre at the site of the bite, progressing to headache, fever, insomnia, anemia, rash, and lymph node swelling. After inoculation, trypanosomes invade all body organs. CNS symptoms appear in disease stage II. The course of the disease may run months to years and is frequently fatal with treatment and always fatal without treatment.

Professional Considerations

Consent form NOT required.

Preparation

1. Obtain an alcohol wipe, lancet, and capillary tube.

Procedure

1. Perform this procedure in the early afternoon, again at night, and when fever spikes occur.
2. Cleanse the pad of the index or second finger with the alcohol wipe and allow the fingerpad to dry.
3. Perform a finger stick and fill the capillary tube completely with blood. Quickly seal the capillary tube.

Postprocedure Care

1. Write on the laboratory requisition the name of the parasite suspected and the place(s) and date(s) of recent travel.

Client and Family Teaching

1. Results are normally available within 24 hours.

Factors That Affect Results

1. Reject clotted specimens.
2. Transport the capillary tube to the laboratory immediately for thick and thin smears to be performed before blood clots form.

Other Data

1. Person-to-person transmission of African trypanosomiasis is possible either by direct contact with infected blood or from mother to fetus. Pentamidine and suramin are used for early-stage disease, depending on the causative organism. Melarsoprol is the drug of choice for late-stage treatment. Eflornithine is better tolerated but difficult to administer, and Nifurtimox is inexpensive and can be administered orally but is not fully validated yet for use in humans.
2. African trypanosomiasis may cause myocarditis in some clients.
3. See also Trypanosomiasis serologic test—Blood; Parasite screen—Blood.

AHI

See **Polysomnography**—Diagnostic.

AIDS Evaluation Battery

See Acquired Immune Deficiency Syndrome Evaluation Battery—Diagnostic; T- and B-Lymphocyte Subset Assay—Blood.

Air Tonometry

See Tonometry Test for Glaucoma—Diagnostic.

ALA

See Antiphospholipid Antibodies—Serum.

Alanine Aminotransferase (ALT, Alanine Transaminase, SGPT)—Serum

Norm.

Adult	5-57 mU/mL
Adult Female	4-19 U/L or 10-30 Karmen U/mL or 317 nKat/L
Adult Male	7-30 U/L or 14-50 Karmen U/mL or 500 nKat/L
Children	
<12 months	≤54 U/L
1-2 years	3-37 U/L
2-8 years	3-30 U/L
8-16 years	3-28 U/L

Increased. Anorexia nervosa, biliary tract obstruction, brain tumor, cerebrovascular accident (increased after 1 week), cirrhosis, congestive heart failure (with liver damage), delirium tremens, dermatomyositis, dysrhythmias, eating disorders (with liver impacted), Gaucher disease, hepatic cancer, hepatic damage, hepatitis (viral, toxic), hypercholesterolemia, hyperglycemia, hyperlipidemia, hypertension, hypertriglyceridemia, infectious mononucleosis, intramuscular injections, intestinal infarction, iron depletion, liver passive congestion, local irradiation injury, muscle injury (caused by electroshock, infection, seizure, or trauma), muscular dystrophy, myocardial infarction, myoglobinuria, Niemann-Pick disease, obesity, pancreatitis (acute), polymyositis, postoperatively (intestinal surgery), pulmonary infarction, renal infarction, Reye's syndrome, rhabdomyolysis, and shock with liver damage. Drugs include allopurinol, ampicillin, anabolic steroids, aspirin, barbiturates, bromocriptine mesylate, captopril, chlordiazepoxide, chlorpromazine hydrochloride, cinchophen, deferiprone, diphenylhydantoin, fosinopril, heparin (bovine, porcine) and statins. Herbal or natural remedies include chaparral tea (or misspelled chapparel tea, *Larrea tridentata*), *Echinacea*, pennyroyal. Herbal or natural remedies that have the potential to cause hepatotoxicity and elevate values include akee fruit (ackee, *Blighia sapida*), *Atractylis gummifera*, *Azadirachta indica (neem tree, margosa)*, *Berberis vulgaris* (barberry), *Callilepis laureola* (blazing star, *Liatris spicata*), chaparral tea (*Larrea tridentata*), cocaine, comfrey ("knitbone," *Symphytum officinale*), *Crotalaria* (bush tea), cycasin (a toxin from a *Cycas* species of sago palm of Guam), *Echinacea*, germander (genera *Teucrium* and *Veronica*; do not confuse with "safe skullcap," a name often falsely used in selling germander), *Heliotropium* (germander, valerian), *jin bu huan* ("gold-inconvertible", Jin Bu Huan Anodyne Tablets, patent medicine with misidentified constituents: essence of *t'ienchi [tianqi] flowers*, "Notoginseng"; also *kombucha*; also *Lycopodium serratum*, or club moss), *m huang* (Ephedra), *margosa* (Melia azadirachta, *Azadirachta indica*), maté tea (*Ilex paraguayensis*), mistletoe, pennyroyal, sassafras, *Senecio*, skullcap (*Scutellaria*; do not confuse with "unsafe germander"), syo-saiko-to (xiao chai *hu* tang, "minor

Bupleurum combination"), *Teucrium polium* (golden germander), and valerian (*Valeriana officinalis*, garden heliotrope).

Decreased. Steatosis in clients with hepatitis C and weight loss. Herbal or natural remedy is Chinese fructus schizandrae sinensis (wu wei zi, "five flavors herb," *Schisandra chinensis* [Turcz.] Baill.).

Description. Alanine aminotransferase (ALT) is an enzyme primarily produced by the liver and found in certain body fluids (such as bile, cerebrospinal fluid, plasma, and saliva) and in the heart, liver, kidneys, pancreas, and skeletal muscle. It acts as a catalyst in the transamination reaction that is necessary for amino acid production. This test is most commonly used to evaluate liver injury, where levels may rise to as much as 50 times normal range. The ALT levels are analyzed with aspartate aminotransferase (AST) levels to evaluate the degree of liver injury and to confirm a hepatic cause of AST increase. After the early stage of liver injury, ALT levels surpass AST levels. Serial measurements help track the course of hepatitis. This test may also be used by blood banks to screen for hepatitis in samples of donor blood.

Professional Considerations
Consent form NOT required.

Preparation
1. Tube: Red topped, red/gray topped, or gold topped.

2. List medications taken by the client within the last 3 days on the laboratory requisition.
3. Do NOT draw during hemodialysis.

Procedure
1. Draw a 4-mL blood sample.

Postprocedure Care
1. The specimen may be refrigerated but not frozen.

Client and Family Teaching
1. Results are normally available within 12 hours.

Factors that Affect Results
1. Hemolysis causes unreliable results.
2. Drugs that may cause falsely increased results include erythromycin, opiates, oxacillin sodium (Prostaphlin), and ampicillin (Polycillin).
3. Falsely decreased results may occur in beriberi, diabetic ketoacidosis, hemodialysis (chronic), liver disease (severe), and uremia or with coffee ingestion.
4. Herbal or natural remedies that may cause falsely decreased results include coffee (*Coffea*).
5. Serial norms generally vary by less than 10 U/L in the same healthy client.

Other Data
1. Older names for this test were glutamate-pyruvate transaminase and glutamic pyruvic transaminase.

Albumin–Serum, Urine, and 24-Hour Urine

Norm. Nephelometric, calorimetric, and (combined) nephorimetric.

		SI Units
Serum		
Adult	3.5-5.0 g/dL	35-50 g/L
>60 years	3.4-4.8 g/dL	34-48 g/L
Average at rest	0.3 g/dL	3 g/L
Urine		
Adult at rest	2-80 mg/24 hours	0.002-0.08 g/day
Adult, ambulatory	<150 mg/24 hours	<0.15 g/day
Child, <10 years	<100 mg/24 hours	<0.10 g/day

Increased in Serum. Dehydration, diarrhea, Hodgkin's disease, meningitis, metastatic carcinomatosis, multiple myeloma, myasthenia, neoplasms, nephrosis, nephrotic syndrome, non–Hodgkin's lymphoma, osteomyelitis, peptic ulcer, pneumonia, polyarteritis nodosa, pregnancy, protein-losing enteropathy, rheumatic fever, rheumatoid arthritis, sarcoidosis, scleroderma, sprue, steatorrhea, stress, systemic lupus erythematosus, trauma, tuberculosis, ulcerative colitis, uremia, vomiting, and water intoxication. Drugs include sulfobromophthalein (Bromsulphalein), cytotoxic agents, and oral contraceptives.

Increased in Urine. Acute tubular necrosis, amyloid disease, anemia (severe), Bartter syndrome, Butler-Albright syndrome, Bright's disease, cardiac disease, central nervous system lesions, cerebrovascular accident, convulsions, cystitis, diabetes insipidus (nephrogenic), diabetic nephropathy, diphtheria, drug reaction, epididymitis, exercise, Fanconi syndrome, fever, galactosemia, glomerular lesion, glomerulonephritis, glomerulosclerosis, Goodpasture's syndrome, heavy-metal poisoning, hyperthyroidism, idiopathic thrombocytopenic purpura, intestinal obstruction, leukemia, liver disease, membranous nephropathy, multiple myeloma, nephritis, nephrosclerosis, nephrotic syndrome, pneumonia, poisoning (arsenic, carbon tetrachloride, ether, lead, mercury, mustard, opiates, phenol, phosphorus, propylene glycol, sulfosalicylic acid, turpentine), polycystic kidney disease, prostatitis, pyelonephritis (bacterial, chronic, hypertensive), renal radiation, renal tubular acidosis, renal vein thrombosis, scarlet fever, septicemia, streptococcal infection, subacute bacterial endocarditis, systemic lupus erythematosus, toxemia of pregnancy, tumor (abdominal, bladder, renal pelvis), typhoid fever, and Wilson's disease. Drugs include amphotericin B, ampicillin, ampicillin sodium, aspirin, bacitracin, barbiturates, cephaloridine, corticosteroids, gentamicin sulfate, gold, kanamycin, mercurial diuretics, neomycin sulfate, phenylbutazone, and polymyxin B.

Decreased in Serum. Acute infection, alcoholism, ascites, atherosclerosis (advanced), beriberi, bone fractures, brucellosis, burns, cholecystitis, cirrhosis, congenital analbuminemia, congestive heart failure, Crohn's disease, cystic fibrosis, dementia, diabetes mellitus, edema, essential hypertension, glomerulonephritis, hemorrhage, hepatitis (viral), Hodgkin's dementia and disease, hyperthyroidism, infection, liver diseases, systemic lupus erythematosus (SLE), leukemia (lymphatic, monocytic, and myelogenous), lymphoma, macroglobulinemia, malabsorption syndrome, malnutrition,

meningitis, metastatic carcinomatosis, multiple myeloma, myasthenia, myocardial infarction, neoplasms, nephrosis, nephrotic syndrome, osteomyelitis, peptic ulcer, pneumonia, polyarteritis nodosa, pregnancy, protein-losing enteropathy, rheumatic fever, rheumatoid arthritis, sarcoidosis, scleroderma, sepsis, sprue, steatorrhea, stress, stroke (with poor outcome), surgery, trauma, tuberculosis, ulcerative colitis, uremia, and water intoxication. Drugs include ampicillin, asparaginase, fluorouracil, and oral contraceptives.

Decreased in Urine. Not clinically significant.

Description. Albumin is one of the two main protein factions of blood. It functions in maintaining oncotic pressure and in transportation of bilirubin, fatty acids, drugs, hormones, and other substances that are insoluble in water. Protein is normally almost completely reabsorbed by the kidneys and undetectable in the urine. Therefore the presence of detectable albumin, or protein, in urine is indicative of abnormal renal function.

Professional Considerations
Consent form NOT required.

Preparation
1. Tube: Red topped, red/gray topped, or gold topped for serum albumin.
2. Do NOT draw specimen during hemodialysis.
3. Obtain a 3-L specimen container without preservative for 24-hour urine albumin and write the beginning time of specimen collection on the container.
4. Obtain a clean specimen container for the spot urine specimen.
5. See Client and Family Teaching.

Procedure
1. *Serum:* Draw a 4-mL blood sample from an extremity that does not have intravenous fluids infusing into it (to avoid hemodilution and falsely low results). Avoid prolonged application of the tourniquet.
2. *24-hour urine:* Collect all urine voided in a 24-hour period and refrigerate. For catheterized clients, keep the collection bag on ice, and empty it hourly into the collection container.
3. Spot urine collection may also be collected.

Postprocedure Care

1. Document the quantity of urine output and the ending time for the collection period on the laboratory requisition.

Client and Family Teaching

1. Consume a low-fat diet the day of the test.
2. Empty the bladder before starting 24-hour urine collection.
3. Save all urine voided in the 24-hour period, and urinate before defecating to avoid loss of urine. If any urine is accidentally discarded, discard the entire specimen and restart the collection the next day.

Factors That Affect Results

1. The results are invalid if the measurement is performed on plasma rather than serum.
2. Bromsulphalein testing within 2 days before specimen collection invalidates serum results.
3. Values are higher when upright or ambulatory. Serum values are higher after hemodialysis caused by fluid overload.

4. Falsely elevated urine results may be caused by contamination of the specimen with pus, menstrual blood, or vaginal discharge.
5. One study found a diurnal variation in urinary albumin levels in clients with insulin-dependent diabetes. Levels significantly increased between 2400 and 0800.

Other Data

1. A 24-hour urine collection for measuring protein loss may be helpful in clients with low serum albumin levels.
2. Increased levels in conjunction with a low glomerular filtration rate has been found through a 2011 meta-analysis (Gansevoort et al) to be associated with increased risk for renal problems such as acute and chronic kidney disease and end-stage renal disease.
3. Microalbuminuria in conjunction with metabolic syndrome is suggested to be a predictor for chronic kidney and heart disease (Gobal et al, 2011).

Alcohol (Ethanol)—Blood

Norm. Negative.

		SI Units
Negative	0 mg/dL	0 mmol/L
Intoxication	>100 mg/dL	>22 mmol/L
Coma	>300 mg/dL	>65.1 mmol/L
Panic level	350-800 mg/dL	76.0-174.0 mmol/L

Ethyl Alcohol (Ethanol) Poisoning Overdose Symptoms and Treatment

Symptoms

<50 mg/dL	Muscular incoordination
50-100 mg/dL	Worsening incoordination of movement
100-150 mg/dL	Mood and behavior changes
150-200 mg/dL	Delayed reactions
200-300 mg/dL	Ataxia, double vision, nausea, vomiting
300-400 mg/dL	Amnesia, dysarthria, hypothermia
400-700 mg/dL	Respiratory failure, coma, death possible

Treatment

NOTE: Treatment choice(s) depend(s) on client's history and condition and episode history.

1. Support oxygenation and protect airway.
2. Monitor for dehydration. Administer fluids as needed.
3. Hemodialysis WILL remove ethanol but is seldom necessary unless levels rise above 300 mg/dL. During hemodialysis, levels drop an average of 62 mg %/hour.

Increased. Alcohol ingestion; concomitant use of alcohol and certain drugs (antihistamines, barbiturates, chlordiazepoxide, cyproheptadine, diazepam, glutethimide, guanethidine, isoniazid, meprobamate, opiates, phenytoin, tranquilizers); ethylene glycol poisoning; and ingestion of liniments, shaving lotion, astringents, elixirs, fluid extracts, tinctures, and cough medicines.

Description. Alcohol (ethanol) is a central nervous system depressant with anesthetic and diuretic effects that is taken orally by clients. Ethanol is also used to treat methanol poisoning, and may be used prophylactically to prevent the occurrence of alcohol withdrawal symptoms.

Professional Considerations

Consent form NOT required unless the specimen may be used as legal evidence.

Preparation

1. Tube: Red topped, red/gray topped, gold topped, black topped, or lavender topped.
2. Do NOT draw during hemodialysis.
3. If a specific type of alcohol measurement is desired (methanol, isopropanol, ethylene glycol), list the specific alcohol on the laboratory requisition.
4. Screen client for the use of herbal preparations or natural remedies such as kava-kava (*Piper methysticum*) or ginseng.

Procedure

1. If the specimen is being collected for legal evidence, have the collection witnessed.
2. Cleanse the venipuncture site with povidone-iodine solution and allow it to dry.
3. Draw a 3-mL blood sample.

Postprocedure Care

1. If the specimen may be used for legal evidence, include the exact time of specimen collection on the tube label and sign and have the witness sign the laboratory requisition.
2. Transport the specimen to the laboratory in a sealed plastic bag labeled as legal evidence.
3. Each person handling the specimen should sign and record the time of receipt on the laboratory requisition.

Client and Family Teaching

1. Results are normally available within 24 hours.
2. Refer clients with intentional overdose for crisis intervention.
3. Referrals to appropriate rehabilitation centers and therapeutic community programs should be offered to all addicted clients who may be interested.

Factors That Affect Results

1. Cleansing the venipuncture site with an alcohol wipe may cause false-positive results.
2. Ginseng (*Panax* spp.) increases alcohol clearance by increasing the activity of alcohol dehydrogenase and aldehyde dehydrogenase.

Other Data

1. Tolerance to alcohol's effects may develop in chronic alcoholics. Therefore, normally lethal levels may not lead to death in these clients.
2. Positive blood alcohol is associated with higher trauma severity in road accidents.
3. In hypothermia, the degree of ketosis is inversely proportional to blood ethanol concentration.
4. Men have significantly higher alcohol elimination rates compared to women.
5. Food intake increases alcohol elimination rates.
6. Only blood alcohol (rather than urine alcohol) levels are acceptable as legal evidence in most countries.
7. Postmortem alcohol levels may differ from sites including hematomas, blood, urine, and stomach contents.
8. Kava-kava (*Piper methysticum*), an herbal or natural remedy anxiolytic, potentiates the effects of ethanol.
9. The American College of Obstetricians and Gynecologists recommends annual blood alcohol screening women during the first trimester of pregnancy.
10. See also Toxicology, Volatiles group by GLC—Blood or urine.

Aldolase—Serum

Norm.

Adult

Ambulatory	1.0-7.5 U/L (30° C)
Bed rest	0.3-3.0 U/L (30° C)

Children

Newborn to 30 days	6.0-32.0 U/L
Age 1 month to 6 years	3.0-12.0 U/L
Age 7-17 years	3.3-9.7 U/L

Increased. Anemia (megaloblastic, hemolytic), burns, cancer, cirrhosis, congestive heart failure, crushing injury, dermatomyositis, Duchenne muscular dystrophy (early stages), eosinophilic fasciitis, erythroblastosis fetalis, hepatic necrosis, hepatitis (acute viral), hepatoma, jaundice (obstructive), lead intoxication, leukemia (chronic granulocytic), liver metastasis, lymphoma, metastasis, mononucleosis (infectious), muscle trauma, myocardial infarction (acute), myopathy, myositis, Niemann-Pick disease, pancreatitis (acute), pericarditis (hemorrhagic), polycythemia vera, polymyositis, prostate cancer, psychotic disorder, pulmonary infarction, skeletal muscle disease, surgical trauma, and trichinosis. Drugs include aminocaproic acid (large doses), carbenoxolone, chlorinated insecticides, clofibrate, corticotropin, cortisone acetate, cyclophosphamide (high dose), labetalol, organophosphorus insecticides, and thiabendazole.

Decreased. Not clinically significant. Drugs include phenothiazines (when aldolase values are initially high in schizophrenics).

Description. A group of isoenzymes (A, B, C) found throughout the body but in highest concentrations in skeletal muscle tissue, where aldolase is manufactured by myocytes. Because aldolase rises during active skeletal muscle disease, its measurement can help track the progress of diseases such as progressive muscular dystrophy, in which increases are seen in early stages, but levels fall as the disease progresses, reflecting lack of muscle ability to synthesize the aldolase enzyme. For most other muscle diseases, there are more specific tests available such as Creatine kinase—Serum; Alanine aminotransferase—Serum; and Aspartate aminotransferase—Serum. Norms for the isoenzymes are not established.

Professional Considerations
Consent form NOT required.

Preparation
1. Tube: Red topped, red/gray topped, or gold topped.
2. See Client and Family Teaching.

Procedure
1. Draw a 2-mL blood sample.

Postprocedure Care
1. Place the sample on ice for immediate transport to the laboratory.

Client and Family Teaching
1. Avoid strenuous exercise for 12 hours before sampling.
2. Results are normally available within 24 hours.

Factors That Affect Results
1. Reject hemolyzed specimen to avoid falsely elevated results.
2. Recent intramuscular injections may elevate results.

Other Data
1. This test replaced by creatine kinase (CK) in muscular dystrophy.

Aldosterone—Serum and Urine

Norm. Norms assume an average sodium diet (3 g/day).

Peripheral Blood	Serum <16	SI Units <44.8
Supine	<16 ng/dL	<44.8 nmol/L
Upright		
Adult Female		
Pregnant	18-100 ng/dL	0.5-2.8 nmol/L
Nonpregnant	5-30 ng/dL	0.14-0.8 nmol/L
Adult male	6-22 ng/dL	0.17-0.61 nmol/L
Adrenal Vein	200-800 ng/dL	5.54-2.22 nmol/L
Child		
<7 days	5-102 ng/dL	0.14-2.86 nmol/L
7-21 days	6-179 ng/dL	0.17-5.01 nmol/L
1-11 months	7-99 ng/dL	0.20-2.77 nmol/L
1-2 years	7-93 ng/dL	0.20-2.60 nmol/L

Peripheral Blood	Serum <16	SI Units <44.8
3-10 years	4-44 ng/dL	0.11-1.23 nmol/L
>10 years	<31 ng/dL	<0.86 nmol/L
Urine		
Normal-sodium diet (100-200 mEq)	6-25 µg/24 hours	16.8-70.0 nmol/day
Low-sodium diet (<25 mEq)	17-44 µg/24 hours	4.76-123.3 nmol/day
High-sodium diet (>200 mEq)	0-6 µg/24 hours	0-16.8 nmol/day

Increased in Serum and Urine. Adrenal tumor (aldosterone-producing adenoma), aldosteronism (primary, secondary), bilateral adrenal hyperplasia, cirrhosis, congestive heart failure, Conn's syndrome, hemorrhage, hypertension (essential, >140/90 mm Hg), hyponatremia, hypovolemia, idiopathic cyclic edema, nephrosis (lower nephron), nephrotic syndrome, and renovascular hypertension. Drugs that increase serum levels include angiotensin-converting enzyme (ACE) inhibitors, corticotropin, diuretics that promote sodium excretion, estrogens, laxatives that are abused, some oral contraceptives, and potassium. Drugs that increase urine levels include angiotensin, deoxycorticosterone, diuretics (loop, thiazide), etiocholanolone, oral contraceptives, and steroids.

Decreased in Serum and Urine. Addison's disease, preeclampsia, primary hypoaldosteronism, salt-wasting syndrome, septicemia, stress, and toxemia of pregnancy. Herbal or natural remedy is licorice. Drugs that decrease serum levels include aminoglutethimide, ACE inhibitors, deoxycorticosterone, etomidate, fludrocortisone, heparin (after several days of continuous therapy), indomethacin, methyldopa, and saralasin. Drugs that decrease urine levels include aminoglutethimide, clonidine, deoxycorticosterone, fludrocortisone, glucocorticoids, labetalol, heparin, methyldopa, metyrapone, and propranolol.

Description. Aldosterone is a mineralocorticoid secreted by the adrenal cortex that functions in blood pressure and body fluid regulation. It acts on the renal distal tubules, causing increased resorption of sodium and water and increased excretion of potassium.

Professional Considerations
Consent form NOT required.

Preparation
1. The client should rest in a supine position for 8-12 hours. The sample should be drawn before noon.
2. Tube: Red topped, red/gray topped, gold topped, lavender topped, or green topped for serum collection.
3. For urine test, obtain a 3-L container (to which 10 g of boric acid has been added) and a 100-mL specimen container for urinary sample.
4. See Client and Family Teaching.

Procedure
Serum Test
1. Collect 2.5-mL blood sample for serum aldosterone.

Urine Test
1. Discard the first morning-urine specimen.
2. Collect all urine voided in a 24-hour period in a refrigerated container to which 10 g of boric acid has been added. Include urine voided at the end of the 24-hour period. For catheterized clients, keep the drainage bag on ice and empty the urine into the collection container hourly.
3. At the end of 24 hours, mix the urine gently and collect a 100-mL aliquot in a clean container.

Postprocedure Care
1. Note total 24-hour urine volume on the laboratory requisition and the aliquot container label.
2. Transport the 24-hour and aliquot samples to the laboratory immediately.

Client and Family Teaching
1. Follow a 3-g/day sodium diet for 2 weeks if not contraindicated by medical condition.
2. Avoid physical or psychologic stress throughout the collection period.
3. Save all urine voided in the 24-hour period, urinate before defecating to avoid

loss of urine, and avoid contaminating the specimen with feces or soiled tissue. If any urine is accidentally discarded, discard the entire specimen and restart the collection the next day.

4. Results may not be available for several days.

Factors That Affect Results

1. Radioactive scans within 7 days before urine collection invalidate the results.
2. Hemolysis invalidates the serum results.

3. Decreased kidney perfusion may cause increased aldosterone and renin values.
4. Levels may be suppressed in clients with insulin-dependent diabetes mellitus.
5. An upright client position for serum collection invalidates the results. Changes in urine aldosterone are not affected by body position.

Other Data

1. Serum electrolyte and renin levels should be measured before this test.

Aldosterone Suppression Test—Diagnostic

Norm. <5 ng/dL (<0.14 nmol/L SI units).

Primary Aldosteronism. >10 ng/dL (>0.2777 nmol/L SI units).

Usage. Definitive diagnosis of primary aldosteronism, which is also common in clients with essential hypertension.

Description. Aldosterone is a mineralocorticoid secreted by the adrenal cortex that functions in blood pressure and body fluid regulation. It acts on the renal distal tubule, where it increases resorption of sodium and water at the expense of increased potassium excretion. Levels are affected by body position and sodium and potassium levels. The aldosterone suppression test measures aldosterone levels before and after an infusion of saline. In primary aldosteronism, the saline infusion fails to suppress aldosterone levels as much as it suppresses the levels in a normal client.

Professional Considerations

Consent form NOT required.

Risks

Volume overload, hypertension, myocardial ischemia, congestive heart failure.

Contraindications

The serum test is contraindicated in clients with congestive heart failure.

Preparation

1. The client should be positioned upright for 2 hours and then lie in a recumbent position from the onset of the test until the second specimen is drawn at the completion of the infusion.
2. Tubes: Two red topped, red/gray topped, gold topped, green topped, or lavender topped for blood test.

3. Obtain 2 L of 0.9% saline and a 24-hour urine collection container to which 10 g of boric acid has been added.

Procedure

Serum Collection

1. Draw a 2.5-mL blood sample for the baseline aldosterone level.
2. Infuse 2 L of normal saline intravenously over a 4-hour period to the recumbent client.
3. Draw a final 2.5-mL blood sample for aldosterone level.

Urine Collection

1. Discard the first morning-urine specimen.
2. Collect all urine voided in a 24-hour period in a refrigerated container to which 10 g of boric acid has been added. Include urine voided at the end of the 24-hour period. For catheterized clients, keep the drainage bag on ice and empty the urine into the collection container hourly.
3. At the end of 24 hours, mix the urine gently and collect a 100-mL aliquot in a clean container.

Postprocedure Care

1. Note the collection site and the time on all laboratory requisitions and blood tubes. For the urine sample, write the total 24-hour urine volume on the laboratory requisition and the aliquot container label.
2. Transport each specimen to the laboratory immediately after collection.

Client and Family Teaching

1. The test takes several hours. Bring reading material or other diversional item.

2. Results are normally available within 24 hours.

Factors That Affect Results
1. Reject hemolyzed specimens.
2. Radioactive scans within 7 days before urine collection invalidate results.

3. Cimetidine, but not omeprazole, inhibits test results.

Other Data
1. Insulin resistance occurs with primary hyperaldosteronism.

Alkaline Phosphatase, Heat Stable—Serum

Norm. Interpreted by laboratory. Results are reported as the percentage of alkaline phosphatase that is heat stable. Residual activity <30% favors hepatic origin and >30% favors bone origin

Usage. Aids in differentiation of the source of increased alkaline phosphatase activity. Decreased in premature uterine contractility in women in second trimester. Diagnosis and treatment monitoring for breast cancer, squamous cell carcinoma of the head and neck, and leukemia.

Description. Alkaline phosphatase is an enzyme normally found in bone, liver, intestine, and placenta that rises during periods of bone growth (osteoblastic activity), liver disease, and bile duct obstruction. It is made up of bone, liver, and placental and intestinal isoenzymes that can be separated by heat fractionation. Liver and placental alkaline phosphatase isoenzymes are heat stable, and bone isoenzyme is inactivated by heat. Greater than 30% of the alkaline phosphatase being heat stable is suggestive of activity of liver origin, whereas <30% being heat stable is suggestive of activity of bone origin.

Professional Considerations
Consent form NOT required.

Preparation
1. Tube: Red topped, red/gray topped, or gold topped.
2. Do NOT draw during hemodialysis.

Procedure
1. Draw a 4-mL blood sample.

Postprocedure Care
1. Transport the specimen to the laboratory immediately for testing or for spinning and refrigeration.

Client and Family Teaching
1. The client may be asked to fast for 10-12 hours.
2. Results may take several days.

Factors That Affect Results
1. Reject hemolyzed specimens.
2. Hepatotoxic drugs within 12 hours before specimen collection invalidate the test.
3. Failure to fast before the test may result in falsely elevated levels.
4. Specimens left at room temperature may result in falsely elevated levels.

Other Data
1. Postmenopausal females have slightly increased total alkaline phosphatase levels and a low percentage of heat-stable fraction, indicating osseous origin.

Alkaline Phosphatase, Isoenzymes

See Alkaline Phosphatase—Serum.

Alkaline Phosphatase—Serum

Norm.

Total Alkaline Phosphatase		SI Units
King-Armstrong Method		
Adults, 20-60 years	4.5-13 U/dL or 39-117 mU/mL	32-92 U/L
Elderly	Slightly higher	
Newborn	5-15 U/dL	36-107 U/L

A

Total Alkaline Phosphatase		SI Units
Premature newborn: 1.5-2 times adult value		
Children: Values remain high until epiphyses close		
1 month	10-30 U/dL	71-213 U/L
3 years	10-20 U/dL	71-142 U/L
10 years	15-30 U/dL	107-213 U/L
Bodansky Method		
Adults, 20-60 years	2-4 U/dL	10.7-21.5 U/L
Elderly	Slightly higher	
Children	5-14 U/dL	27-75 U/L
Bessey-Lowry-Brock Method		
Adults, 20-60 years	0.8-2.3 U/dL	13.3-38.3 U/L
Elderly	Slightly higher	
Bowers and McComb Method		
Females		
1-12 years	<350 U/L	<5.95 µKat/L
Puberty: Values may triple		
>15 years	25-100 U/L	0.43-1.70 µKat/L
Males		
1-12 years	<350 U/L	<5.95 µKat/L
12-14 years	<500 U/L	<8.50 µKat/L
Puberty: Values may triple		
>20 years	25-100 U/L	0.43-1.70 µKat/L

Isoenzyme Norms (Isoenzyme Inactivated after 16 Minutes at 55 degrees C)

Heat Inactivation Method	Percentage	Fraction
Liver isoenzyme	50-700	0.50-0.70
Bone isoenzyme	90-100	0.90-1.00
Intestinal isoenzyme	50-600	0.50-0.60
Placental isoenzyme: Trimester 1 to 1 month postpartum	50% of total	

Increased Biliary Isoenzyme. Biliary cirrhosis, biliary duct obstruction, cholangiohepatitis, and cholestasis.

Increased Bone Isoenzyme. Bone cancer accompanied by bone formation, bone growth or healing, familial hyperphosphatemia, familial osteoectasia, Gaucher disease, growth hormone overproduction, hyperparathyroidism, hyperthyroidism, leukemia of bone marrow, lymphoma, malabsorption, myositis ossificans, Niemann-Pick disease, osteoblastic metastases, osteogenesis imperfecta, osteomalacia, osteoporosis, osteogenic sarcoma, Paget's disease, polyostotic fibrous dysplasia, renal osteodystrophy, and rickets.

Increased Intestinal Isoenzyme. Gastrointestinal disease, clients with blood type O or B (some), pancreatic duct obstruction, pancreatic cancer, splenic infarction, steatorrhea (idiopathic), and ulcer (perforated).

Increased Liver I Isoenzyme. Impaired enzyme metabolism, liver congestion, hepatic carcinoma, hepatotoxic drugs, jaundice (obstructive), pregnancy, and vasculitis.

Increased Liver II Isoenzyme. Hepatitis (infectious, viral), parenchymal cell damage.

Increased Placental Isoenzyme. Pregnancy (late).

Increased Total Alkaline Phosphatase. May also be caused by alcoholism, carbohydrate ingestion (large quantities), children known to have increased values, cholelithiasis in persons with sickle cell disease, diabetes mellitus, Fanconi syndrome, fat ingestion, fibrous dysplasia, histiocytosis, Hodgkin's disease, hyperalimentation, hyperparathyroidism (with bone disease), hyperthyroidism, hypophosphatemia, kidney tissue rejection, liver abscess, liver disease, lung cancer, lymphoma, mononucleosis (infectious), multiple myeloma, myocardial infarction, osteosarcoma, primary biliary cirrhosis, pulmonary infarction, renal infarction, rheumatoid arthritis, rickets, sarcoidosis, and sickle cell crisis. Drugs include acetaminophen, acetohexamide, acyclovir, albumin, allopurinol, aluminum nicotinate, amiodarone, amitriptyline, ampicillin, anabolic steroids, androgens, asparaginase, aspirin, aurothioglucose, azathioprine, baclofen, barbiturates, bromocriptine mesylate, carbamazepine, carmustine, cephalexin, cephaloridine, chlordiazepoxide, chlorpromazine hydrochloride, chlorpropamide, cholestyramine resin, cimetidine, cinchophen, clindamycin, clonazepam, colchicine, diltiazem, ergosterol, erythromycin, estrogens, floxuridine, flurazepam, fosinopril, gold sodium, N-hydroxyacetamide, imipramine, imipramine pamoate, indomethacin, isoniazid, lincomycin, meclofenamate sodium, methotrexate, methyldopa, methyldopate hydrochloride, methyltestosterone, metoprolol tartrate, minoxidil, mithramycin, naproxen sodium, niacin, nifedipine, nitrofurantoin, novobiocin, oral contraceptives, oxacillin sodium, oxyphenisatin, papaverine hydrochloride, penicillamine, pertofrane, phenobarbital, phenothiazines, phenylbutazone, phenytoin, procainamide hydrochloride, propranolol, propylthiouracil, rifampin, salicylates, sildenafil, sulfamethoxazole, sulfisoxazole, sulfisoxazole acetyl, sulfobromophthalein sodium, tetracycline, thiomalate, thiothixene, thyroid hormone replacement, tolazamide, tolbutamide, tolmetin sodium, valproic acid, and vitamin D. Herbal or natural remedies include *Echinacea* (taken for 8 weeks or longer).

Decreased. Anemia (pernicious), blood transfusions (massive), celiac disease, cretinism, hypophosphatasia, hypothyroidism, malnutrition, milk-alkali syndrome (Burnett's syndrome), nephritis (chronic), osteolytic sarcoma, scurvy, vitamin D intoxication, and zinc depletion. Drugs include aminobisphosphonates (Neridronate), edetate disodium, fluorides, oxalates, phosphates, and propranolol.

Description. Alkaline phosphatase is an enzyme found in bone, liver, intestine, and placenta that rises during periods of bone growth (osteoblastic activity), liver disease, and bile duct obstruction. It is made up of bone, liver, placental, biliary, and intestinal isoenzymes that can be separated by electrophoresis. Alkaline phosphatase isoenzymes should be measured for any client who has an elevated alkaline phosphatase level.

Professional Considerations
Consent form NOT required.

Preparation
1. Tube: Red topped, red/gray topped, or gold topped.
2. See Client and Family Teaching.

Procedure
1. Draw a 4-mL blood sample.

Postprocedure Care
1. Transport the specimen to the laboratory for immediate testing or for spinning and refrigeration.

Client and Family Teaching
1. Client may be asked to fast for 10-12 hours.
2. Results are normally available within 24 hours.

Factors That Affect Results
1. Reject hemolyzed specimens.
2. Hepatotoxic drugs within 12 hours before collection invalidate the test.
3. Falsely elevated results may be caused by failure to fast before the test or by specimens left at room temperature.
4. *Echinacea* taken for 8 weeks or longer may cause hepatotoxicity.

Other Data
1. Isoenzymes are required to interpret the contributing source (liver, bone, placenta) of elevated total alkaline phosphatase.
2. At least 2 days are required for isoenzyme results.
3. Differentiation of bone and liver isoenzymes is difficult, because both are derived from a single gene. A monoclonal antibody assay that may aid in differentiation of liver and bone isoenzymes is being tested.
4. Studies have shown that some statins have been shown to decrease bone-specific alkaline phosphatase, but results are not yet conclusive.

Allergen-Specific IgE—Serum

Norm. <2% of serum immunoglobulins.

Adults	<41 U/mL
Children	
Neonate	<12 U/mL
1-3 years	<10 U/mL
4-6 years	<24 U/mL
7-8 years	<46 U/mL
9-12 years	<116 U/mL
13-14 years	<63 U/mL

Increased. Allergic rhinitis, anaphylaxis, asthma (exogenous), atopic dermatitis, atopic eczema, *Echinococcus* infestation, eczema, hay fever, hookworm disease, latex allergy, schistosomiasis, and visceral larva migrans. Drugs include aminophenazone, anticonvulsants, asparaginase, hydralazine hydrochloride, oral contraceptives, and phenylbutazone.

Decreased. Asthma (endogenous), pregnancy, and radiation therapy. Drugs include methotrexate.

Description. Immunoglobulin E (IgE) is a protein produced in the bone marrow that functions as an antibody in response to antigen stimulation in hypersensitivity reactions. IgE levels are influenced by the nature of the allergen, length of exposure to the allergen, symptomatic responses, and hyposensitization treatments. The test is performed by radioimmunoassay.

Professional Considerations

Consent form NOT required.

Preparation

1. Tube: Red topped, red/gray topped, or gold topped.
2. List vaccinations, immunizations, and tetanus antitoxin received within the previous 6 months on the laboratory requisition.
3. List the blood products the client received within 6 weeks before the test on the laboratory requisition.

Procedure

1. Draw a 3-mL blood sample.

Postprocedure Care

1. Transport the specimen to the laboratory immediately.

Client and Family Teaching

1. Fast, except for water, for 12-14 hours before the test.
2. Results are normally available within 24 hours.
3. Refer the client with elevated IgE levels and allergic symptoms to an allergist for more specific testing and guidance on potential treatments and environmental reduction of allergens.

Factors That Affect Results

1. A delay in testing invalidates results.
2. Results are invalidated if the client has undergone a scan using a radioisotope within 1 week before the test.

Other Data

1. This test is often used to accompany a negative radioallergosorbent test (RAST) to assess for reactivity to untested allergens.
2. A newer serum test under investigation to determine its sensitivity is the multiple antigen simultaneous test (MAST), which can simultaneously detect allergies to up to 3.5 allergens in one serum sample.
3. See also Allergen-Specific IgE antibody—Serum; Skin test for hypersensitivity—Diagnostic.

Allergen-Specific IgE Antibody (RAST Test, Radioallergosorbent Test, Allergy Screen)—Serum

Norm. Negative.

ImmunoCAP FEIA method. <0.35 kU/L.

Pharmacia CAP system

	Asymptomatic Clients	Symptomatic Allergy
Perennial allergens	≤10.7 kU/L	>10.7 kU/L
Seasonal allergens	≤8.4 kU/L	>8.4 kU/L
All allergens	≤11.7 kU/L	>11.7 kU/L

A

Results Reported by Allergen Scores on 0-4 Scale

0	No IgE detected
1	Borderline
2-4	Increasing levels of IgE

Modified RAST

Class	Counts	Significance
	0-749	No specific IgE activity
1	750-1,600	Borderline activity
2	1,601-3,600	Low positive
3	3,601-8000	Moderate positive
4	8,001-18,000	High positive
5	18,001-40,000	Very high positive
6	>40,000	Extreme high positive

Usage. Helps with differential diagnosis of allergies (especially food allergies of the immediate type), atopic asthma, natural rubber latex allergies, and psoriasis; monitoring of treatment for specific allergies.

Description. This test measures the amount of IgE directed against specific allergens by binding a specific antigen to a carrier substance and allowing it to react with a specific IgE antibody in the client's blood sample. The amount of bound IgE is then measured. The test is used to identify allergies to foods, grasses, weeds, trees, molds, epidermals, insects, and miscellaneous substances such as house dust, insulin, latex, and silk. An advantage of this test is that one can obtain the information without causing an allergic reaction because the allergen is introduced into the blood sample rather than into the body.

Professional Considerations
Consent form NOT required.

Preparation
1. Tube: Red topped, red/gray topped, or gold topped.

Procedure
1. Draw a 2-mL blood sample.

Postprocedure Care
1. Transport the specimen to the laboratory for immediate spinning, serum separation, and refrigeration of serum.

Client and Family Teaching
1. Results may take several days.

Factors That Affect Results
1. IgE levels are influenced by the nature of the allergen, length of exposure to the allergen, symptomatic responses, and hyposensitization treatments.
2. Results are invalidated if the client received radioactive dyes within 7 days before the test.
3. False-positive results may be caused by high IgE levels (>3000 U/mL) attributable to parasitic infection.

Other Data
1. This test correlates 80% to 85% with subcutaneous skin testing and is more specific.
2. A total IgE level should also be obtained. If the RAST test is negative but total IgE level is elevated, the allergen may not be one for which the RAST test can be used.
3. See also Allergen-Specific IgE—Serum; Skin test for hypersensitivity—Diagnostic.

Allergy Screen
See AllergenSpecific IgE Antibody—Serum.

Allergy Skin Test
See Skin Test for Hypersensitivity—Diagnostic.

Alpha₁-Antitrypsin—Serum

Norm. 85-215 mg/dL (15.64-39.56 μmol/L, SI units.)

Increased. Alzheimer's disease, cholangiocarcinoma, emphysema, hepatitis, hepatocholangiocarcinoma, hyaline membrane disease, hypercholesterolemia, infection, inflammation (acute, chronic), liver disease (chronic), neoplasm, pregnancy, sepsis, systemic lupus erythematosus, and ulcerative colitis. Drugs include estrogens, oral contraceptives, and steroids.

Decreased. Congenital alpha$_1$-antitrypsin deficiency, chronic obstructive pulmonary disease, emphysema, and liver disease (chronic) and in newborns (transient).

Description. A major faction of alpha$_1$-globulin protein detected by serum protein immunoelectrophoresis. Alpha$_1$-antitrypsin is a serine proteinase inhibitor that functions in protection of body fluids by inactivating neutrophil elastase, a byproduct of lung inflammatory or infectious processes. The test is used to screen for clients at high risk for emphysema and liver disease associated with a congenital absence of the protein. Clients who have symptoms of cough, dyspnea or wheezing, in conjunction with a smoking history, should be evaluated for COPD using this test and spirometry. Other

uses for this test include nonspecific detection of inflammatory, infectious, and necrotic processes.

Professional Considerations
Consent form NOT required.

Preparation
1. Tube: Red topped, red/gray topped, or gold topped.
2. See Client and Family Teaching.

Procedure
1. Draw a 4-mL blood sample.

Postprocedure Care
1. Freeze the specimen.

Client and Family Teaching
1. The client with hypercholesterolemia or hyperlipemia should fast 8-10 hours.
2. Results are normally available within 24 hours.

Factors That Affect Results
1. Reject hemolyzed specimens.

Other Data
1. Levels may also be measured in amniotic fluid.

Alpha-Fetoprotein (AFP)—Blood

Norm. Tumor marker <8.5 ng/mL.
(See also Amniocentesis and Amniotic fluid analysis—Diagnostic, for fetal values)

		SI Units
Nonpregnant Female	0-15 ng/mL	0-15 µg/L
Pregnant		
2 months	<75 ng/mL	<75 µg/L
3 months	<130 ng/mL	<130 µg/L
4 months	<210 ng/mL	<210 µg/L
5 months	<300 ng/mL	<300 µg/L
6 months	<400 ng/mL	<400 µg/L
7 months	<450 ng/mL	<450 µg/L
8 months	<450 ng/mL	<450 µg/L
9 months	<400 ng/mL	<400 µg/L
Immediately postpartum	<375 ng/mL	<375 µg/L
Adult Males	0-15 ng/mL	0-15 µg/L
Children		
Premature Infant	Up to 158,000 ng/mL	Up to 158,000 µg/L
Full-term Infant		
0-14 days	5000-105,000 ng/mL	5000-105,000 µg/L
2 weeks–1 month	100-10,000 ng/mL	10-10,000 µg/L
2 months	40-1000 ng/mL	40-1000 µg/L
3 months	11-300 ng/mL	11-300 µg/L

		SI Units
4 months	5-200 ng/mL	5-200 µg/L
5 months	0-90 ng/mL	0-90 µg/L
≥6 months	0-15 ng/mL	0-15 µg/L

Increased. Ataxia telangiectasia, Beckwith-Wiedemann syndrome (child), cirrhosis, gonadal teratoblastoma, cancer (embryonal, hepatoblastoma, hepatocellular [primary], lung, pancreatic with liver metastases, malignant teratoma of ovary or testes, gastric with liver metastases, biliary system, germ cell tumors), hemangioendothelioma, hepatitis (viral) (acute, chronic, neonatal), liver metastasis from gastric cancer, pregnancy (with fetal neural tube defects, multiple fetuses, fetal distress, fetal death, intrauterine death, duodenal atresia, omphalocele), pure seminoma, spontaneous abortion, spontaneous preterm birth in pregnant women 24-28 weeks of gestation, tetralogy of Fallot (or Turner's syndrome), tyrosinemia, and ulcerative colitis.

Decreased. Has been associated with Down syndrome when less than 0.25 times the normal median, associated with high birth weight with very low second-trimester levels. Drugs include protease inhibitors in females infected with human immunodeficiency virus.

Description. A globulin protein secreted by liver cells during hepatic cell multiplication and found in high amounts in fetal plasma. Highest adult amounts are found during pregnancy and in primary hepatic cancer. Maternal levels should be measured initially at 15-18 weeks of gestation as a screening method for fetal neural tube defects. Confirmatory testing (for levels greater than 0.5-2.5 times the normal median) should be repeated in 7 days. For positive confirmatory test, ultrasonography and amniotic fluid AFP measurement should be performed. Used as a tumor marker, the AFP level is most specific when concentrations are >1000 ng/mL.

Professional Considerations
Consent form NOT required.

Preparation
1. Tube: Red topped, red/gray topped, or gold topped.
2. List on the laboratory requisition: maternal weight, maternal race, weeks of gestation, and any history of diabetes mellitus.

Procedure
1. Draw a 4-mL blood sample from the mother.

Postprocedure Care
1. Apply a dry, sterile dressing over the amniocentesis site.

Client and Family Teaching
1. Results may take several days.

Factors That Affect Results
1. Normal levels are affected by the mother's age, weight, and number of fetuses present.
2. Reject hemolyzed specimens.
3. Results are invalid if the client has undergone a radioisotope scan within the previous 2 weeks.
4. Protease inhibitors are associated with lower AFP levels in women who are infected with HIV.

Other Data
1. AFP testing may also be performed on amniotic fluid to detect neurologic congenital defects and Down syndrome. Serum AFP measurement is believed to increase accuracy of antenatal detection of Down syndrome from 35% to 67%, but its accuracy can be affected by maternal weight, smoking history, and diabetes mellitus and by whether the gestational age of the fetus is correctly estimated.
2. AFP is not a screening test for cancer.
3. AFP is insensitive for the diagnosis of hepatocellular carcinoma in African-Americans.

ALT

See **Alanine Aminotransferase**—Serum.

Alternate Pathway Factor B

See **C3 Proactivator**—Serum.

AMA

See **Antimitochondrial Antibody**—Blood.

Amikacin Sulfate—Blood

Norm.

		SI Units
Therapeutic peak	20-25 mg/L or μg/mL	34-43 μmol/L
Toxic peak	>35 mg/L or μg/mL	>60 μmol/L
Therapeutic trough	5-10 mg/L or μg/mL	9-17 μmol/L
Toxic trough (adult)	>10 mg/L or μg/mL	>17 μmol/L
Toxic trough (child)	>5 ng/mL	>9 μmol/L

Toxic Level Symptoms and Treatment

Symptoms. Ototoxicity, nephrotoxicity.

Treatment

NOTE: Treatment choices depend on client's history and condition and episode history.

1. Stop drug.
2. Monitor amikacin levels.
3. Monitor serum urea nitrogen and creatinine levels every day.
4. Perform eighth cranial nerve assessments every day.
5. Both hemodialysis and peritoneal dialysis WILL remove amikacin.

Increased. Aminoglycoside toxicity and impaired renal function.

Decreased. Subtherapeutic levels in client treated with aminoglycoside.

Description. Amikacin is a semisynthetic aminoglycoside antibiotic derived from kanamycin and effective against gram-negative and gram-positive organisms. It is excreted by glomerular filtration, with a half-life of 1.9-2.8 hours. Peak and trough levels should be monitored throughout therapy. Toxicity is possible at trough levels. Steady-state levels are reached after 10-15 hours. Effective in gram-positive bacteremia in childhood and the treatment of ventilator-associated pneumonia.

Professional Considerations

Consent form NOT required.

Preparation

1. Tube: Red topped, red/gray topped, or gold topped.
2. Do NOT draw during hemodialysis.
3. Write the time, dose, and route of the most recent dose on the laboratory requisition.

Procedure

1. Draw a 4-mL blood sample.

Postprocedure Care

1. None.

Client and Family Teaching

1. Results are normally available within 24 hours.

Factors That Affect Results

1. Cross-reactivity may occur with concomitant antibiotic therapy (cephalosporin, chloramphenicol, clindamycin, kanamycin, penicillin, tetracycline, tobramycin).

Other Data

1. Potentially nephrotoxic, irreversibly ototoxic, and neurotoxic.
2. Creatinine clearance should be monitored every day for clients receiving amikacin.
3. Hypoalbuminemia correlates strongly with amikacin nephrotoxicity.

Amino Acid Screen

See **Dinitrophenylhydrazine Test**—Diagnostic.

A

Aminophylline

See **Theophylline**—Blood.

Amiodarone—Plasma or Serum

Norm. Negative.

		SI Units
Therapeutic	0.5-2.5 µg/mL	0.8-3.9 µmol/L level
Panic level	>2.5 µg/mL	>3.9 µmol/L

For samples tested >24 hours after collection, see Factors That Affect Results.

Panic Level Symptoms and Treatment

Symptoms. Bronchial asthma, heart failure, hepatic dysfunction, hyponatremia, jaundice, pulmonary fibrosis (irreversible), syndrome of inappropriate antidiuretic hormone, thyrotoxicosis.

Treatment

NOTE: Treatment choice(s) depend(s) on client's history and condition and episode history.
1. Provide respiratory and hemodynamic support.
2. Discontinue medication.
3. Provide continuous ECG monitoring to identify reappearing dysrhythmias and bradycardia.
4. Use a transcutaneous pacemaker (prophylactically for sinus arrest).
5. Induce emesis (cautiously) soon after ingestion.
6. Tap water or warm saline lavage may be added.
7. Administer activated charcoal, saline, or sorbitol cathartic.
8. Hemodialysis and peritoneal dialysis will NOT remove amiodarone.

Usage. Monitoring for therapeutic levels during amiodarone therapy.

Description. Amiodarone is a fat-soluble, Class III antidysrhythmic, with several mechanisms of action, including (weak) negative inotropic activity coupled with compensatory vasodilatation, prolongation of cardiac tissue refractory period, depression of sinus node automaticity, and slowing of atrioventricular node conduction. It is used to treat clients with a history of life-threatening dysrhythmias that are not controllable by other drugs and after a myocardial infarction for symptomatic or sustained ventricular dysrhythmias. Because amiodarone is fat soluble, with a long half-life, it takes up to 4 weeks to reach steady-state levels and will remain in the fat-storage sites of the body long after it is discontinued. Amiodarone is metabolized and excreted primarily by the liver. This drug's potentially life-threatening side effects (acute hepatitis, pulmonary toxicity, bronchiolitis obliterans, pulmonary fibrosis) necessitate close monitoring of blood levels as well as clear and specific client teaching about side effects.

Professional Considerations

Consent form NOT required.

Preparation

1. Tube: Red topped, red/gray topped, or gold topped.
2. MAY be drawn during hemodialysis.

Procedure

1. Draw the specimen before the dose, or at least 12 hours after the last dose.
2. Draw a 4-mL blood sample.

Postprocedure Care

1. None.

Client and Family Teaching

1. Results may not be available for several days.

2. If activated charcoal was given for elevated levels, the client should drink 4-6 glasses of water each day for 2 days to prevent constipation. Activated charcoal will also cause stools to be black for a few days.

Factors That Affect Results

1. Height and weight have not been shown to affect plasma concentrations.
2. Amiodarone levels in stored specimens decrease over time. One study recommends the following correction factors for stored values:

Time Sample Stored Before Testing	Correction Factor
24 hours	Add 8% to obtained value
48 hours	Add 16% to obtained value

Time Sample Stored Before Testing	Correction Factor
72 hours	Add 19% to obtained value
7 days	Add 23% to obtained value
14 days	Add 32% to obtained value

Other Data

1. Amiodarone minor side effects include (usually reversible) corneal and skin micro deposits of the drug, causing grayish coloring of the sclera and skin, photosensitivity, and neuromuscular weakness. Side effects may take several months to appear.
2. Any concurrent digoxin dose should be reduced during amiodarone therapy.
3. Increases in serum creatinine may be related to the drug itself.

Amitriptyline

See Tricyclic Antidepressants—Plasma or Serum.

Ammonia (NH₃)—Blood and Urine

Norm. Norms vary by specific laboratory.

		SI Units
Plasma		
Adult	9.5-49 µg/dL	7-35 µmol/L
Newborn	90-150 µg/dL	64-107 µmol/L
First 2 weeks	79-129 µg/dL	56-92 µmol/L
Child	40-80 µg/dL	28-57 µmol/L
Urine		
Spot	36-750 µg/dL	20-500 µmol/L
24-hour		
Adult	140-1500 mg/N/24 hours	10-107 mmol/N/24 hours
Infant	560-2900 mg/N/24 hours	40-207 mmol/N/24 hours

Arterial Blood in Uremic Clients

Adult before hemodialysis	98.32 mg/dL
Adult after hemodialysis	63.18 mg/dL

Venous Blood in Uremic Clients

Adult before hemodialysis	71.70 mg/dL
Adult after hemodialysis	58.05 mg/dL

Hepatic Encephalopathy Symptoms and Treatment

Symptoms. (Symptoms do not correlate well with blood levels.) Asterixis, ataxia, coma, confusion, drowsiness, seizures, sluggish speech, somnolence, stupor.

Treatment

NOTE: Treatment choice(s) depend(s) on client's history and condition and episode history.

1. Administer lactulose nasogastrically or rectally.
2. Both hemodialysis and peritoneal dialysis WILL remove NH_3.

Increased. Alzheimer's disease, azotemia, carbamoyl phosphate synthetase I deficiency (CPSID), cirrhosis, coma (diabetic, hepatic), congestive heart failure, erythroblastosis fetalis, esophageal varices (hemorrhagic), exercise, hepatic encephalopathy, hepatitis (acute), pneumonia, portacaval shunt, premature infant (with neurologic abnormalities), Reye's syndrome, and shock. Drugs include acetazolamide, ammonium salts, asparaginase, chlorothiazide, heparin calcium, heparin sodium, methicillin sodium, neomycin, thiazide diuretics, urea, and valproic acid.

Decreased. Hypertension (essential, malignant) and renal failure.

Description. Ammonia is a waste product from nitrogen breakdown during protein metabolism. It is metabolized by the liver and excreted by the kidneys as urea. Elevated levels caused by hepatic dysfunction may lead to encephalopathy.

Professional Considerations
Consent form NOT required.

Preparation
1. Tube: Refrigerated gray topped, lavender topped, or heparinized green topped.
2. Do NOT draw during hemodialysis.
3. See Client and Family Teaching.
4. Notify laboratory personnel that a blood sample for ammonia level will be arriving.

Procedure
Samples should preferably be taken from arterial or earlobe capillary blood because ammonia metabolism in muscle causes increased levels in venous blood.
1. *Arterial sampling*: Draw a 4-mL blood specimen.
2. *Capillary sampling*: Using a lancet, completely fill a capillary tube with blood from the earlobe.
3. *Venous sampling*: Leaving a tourniquet in place no more than 15 seconds, draw a 4-mL blood specimen. If a syringe is used for blood collection, uncap the tube and transfer the blood into it without using the needle. Tilt the tube back and forth to mix the contents.

Postprocedure Care
1. Place the specimen in an ice-water bath.
2. Transport the specimen to the laboratory immediately.

Client and Family Teaching
1. Fast, except for water, and refrain from smoking for 8-10 hours before sampling.
2. Avoid stress and strenuous exercise for several hours before sampling.

Factors That Affect Results
1. Green topped tubes containing ammonium-heparin should not be used.
2. Reject hemolyzed specimens.
3. A delay in processing the specimen may cause falsely elevated results.
4. A high-protein diet may increase levels.

Other Data
1. Ammonia levels are NOT reliable indicators of impending hepatic coma.
2. Liver transplant corrects hyperammonemia.

Amniocentesis and Amniotic Fluid Analysis—Diagnostic Routine Analysis

Color: Colorless, straw-colored, or clear to milky-colored.

	SI Units
Acetylcholinesterase	Negative
Alpha-fetoprotein:	
12 weeks of gestation	≤42 µg/mL
14 weeks of gestation	≤35 µg/mL
16 weeks of gestation	≤29 µg/mL
18 weeks of gestation	≤20 µg/mL
20 weeks of gestation	≤18 µg/mL

Continued

		SI Units
22 weeks of gestation	≤14 µg/mL	
30 weeks of gestation	≤3 µg/mL	
35 weeks of gestation	≤2 µg/mL	
40 weeks of gestation	≤1 µg/mL	

(Normal values may also be reported in multiples of the median [MOM] or 0.5-3.0 MOM.)

Bilirubin		
Trimesters 1 and 2	≤0.074 mg/dL	≤1.2 µmol/L
40 weeks of gestation	≤0.024 mg/dL	≤0.4 µmol/L
Calcium	4 mEq/L	4 mmol/L
Carbon dioxide	16 mEq/L	16 mmol/L
Chloride	102 mEq/L	102 mmol/L
Creatinine		
≤27 weeks of gestation	0.8-1.1 mg/dL	71-97 µmol/L
30-34 weeks of gestation	1.1-1.8 mg/dL	97-159 µmol/L
35-40 weeks of gestation	1.8-4.0 mg/dL	159-354 µmol/L
Estriol		
Trimesters 1 and 2	≤9 µg/dL	≤309 nmol/L
Term	<59 µg/dL	<2023 nmol/L
Glucose	30 mg/dL	2 mmol/L
Lecithin		
<35 weeks of gestation	6-9 mg/dL	
≥35 weeks of gestation	15-20 mg/dL	
Lecithin/sphingomyelin (L/S) ratio		
Immaturity	≤1:1	<1:1
Borderline maturity	1:1-2:1	1:1-2:1
Maturity	>2:1	>2:1
After maturity	≥4:1	≥4:1
Meconium	Negative	
Osmolality	Equals serum osmolality	
pCO_2		
Trimesters 1 and 2	33-55 mm Hg	4.4-7.3 kPa
Term	42-55 mm Hg	5.6-7.3 kPa
pH		
Trimesters 1 and 2	7.12-7.38	7.12-7.38
Term	6.91-7.43	6.91-7.43
Potassium	4.9 mEq/L	4.9 mmol/L
Protein, total		
Trimesters 1 and 2	0.36-0.84 g/dL	0.36-0.84 g/dL
Term	0.07-0.45 g/dL	0.07-0.45 g/dL
Sodium	7-10 mEq/L lower than serum sodium	7-10 mmol/L lower than serum sodium
Sphingomyelin	4-6 mg/dL	
Total protein	2.5 g/dL	25 g/L
Urea		
Trimesters 1 and 2	12-24 mg/dL	1.2-4 mmol/L
Term	19-42 mg/dL	3.2-7 mmol/L
Uric acid		
Trimesters 1 and 2	2.76-4.68 mg/dL	0.17-0.28 mmol/L
Term	7.67-12.13 mg/dL	0.46-0.72 mmol/L

Abnormalities That May Be Found on Routine Analysis

Abnormal Color	Possible Cause
Yellow	Caused by fetal bilirubin, erythroblastosis fetalis
Green	Caused by meconium, breech presentation, fetal death, defecation, distress, hypoxia, intrauterine growth restriction, status post
Red	Caused by presence of blood, intrauterine hemorrhage maturity, vagal stimulation
Port wine	Acute fetal distress, abruptio placentae
Brown	Oxidized hemoglobin, maternal tissue trauma, fetal death, fetal maceration

			SI Units
Abnormal Bilirubin			
Fetal involvement	0.10-0.28 mg/dL	= 1+	1.6-4.5 µmol/L
Later fetal involvement	0.29-0.36 mg/dL	= 2 +	4.7-5.8 µmol/L
Fetal distress	0.47-0.95 mg/dL	= 3 +	7.6-15.4 µmol/L
Fetal death	>0.95 mg/dL	= 4 +	>15.4 µmol/L
Abnormal Creatinine			
35-40 weeks of gestation			
Large muscle mass, possible diabetes		>4 mg/dL	>354 µmol/L
Low birth weight		<2 mg/dL	<177 µmol/L

Increased Alpha-fetoprotein. Anencephaly, cleft lip and palate, cystic fibrosis, duodenal atresia, esophageal atresia, fetal bladder neck obstruction with hydronephrosis, fetal death, meningomyelocele, multiple pregnancy, nephrosis (congenital), neural tube defects, spina bifida, omphalocele, and Turner's syndrome.

Increased Bilirubin. Anencephaly, erythroblastosis fetalis, hemolytic disease of the newborn, hydrops fetalis, intestinal obstruction, and Rh sensitization.

Increased Lamellar Bodies in Amniotic Fluid. Respiratory distress syndrome.

Positive Acetylcholinesterase. Neural tube abnormalities that allow cerebrospinal fluid (which contains acetylcholinesterase) to leak into the amniotic sac.

Positive Meconium. Fetal distress.

Decreased Alpha-fetoprotein. Not applicable.

Decreased Bilirubin. Not clinically significant.

Decreased Creatinine. Fetal lung immaturity.

Chromosome Analysis. Interpretation required.

Description. Detection of fetal jeopardy or genetic disease and determination of fetal maturity. Amniocentesis is a 20- to 30-minute procedure in which an aspiration of amniotic fluid is taken transabdominally and is usually performed after week 12 of gestation. In routine analysis, amniotic fluid is examined for levels of calcium, chloride, carbon dioxide, creatinine, estriol, glucose, pH, potassium, sodium, protein, urea, uric acid, and culture and for genetic defects, chromosomal studies, detection of fetal jeopardy or distress (by color, bilirubin), and to measure lung maturity (by L/S ratio) and age (by creatinine of the fetus). Alpha₁-fetoprotein is a globulin protein secreted by the yolk sac and by fetal liver cells during hepatic cell multiplication. The highest amounts are found during pregnancy and in hepatic cancer. Measurement is usually performed from week 16 to 20 to help identify fetal neural abnormalities, gastroesophageal atresia, and nephrosis. Chromosome analysis of amniotic fluid cells is performed by examination of karyotyped cells for genetic abnormalities such as Down syndrome, Tay-Sachs disease, and other inborn errors of metabolism. Amniotic fluid is examined for color and bilirubin level for detection of fetal jeopardy or distress caused by hemolysis of fetal red blood cells. Erythroblastosis fetalis occurs when maternal antibodies attack fetal red blood cells, causing fetal anemia. This occurs when the mother's blood contains the Rh factor that reacts with fetal erythrocyte antigens. The test is usually performed at gestation week 24 or later and can help determine the need for intrauterine fetal blood transfusion. After the 35th week of pregnancy, the phospholipid levels of lecithin and sphingomyelin change in a predictable pattern that indicates the level of maturity of fetal lungs. Lecithin rises and sphingomyelin decreases as the fetal lungs mature.

Professional Considerations

Informed consent is recommended for genetic testing and for the procedure itself.

Risks

Bleeding, intrauterine death, premature labor, spontaneous abortion.

Contraindications

Abruptio placentae, incompetent cervix, placenta previa, and a history of premature labor.

Preparation

1. Obtain an amniocentesis tray, surgical scrub solution, a light-protected container, and povidone-iodine solution. Also obtain RhoGAM for Rh-negative mothers.
2. Obtain maternal vital signs. Auscultate baseline fetal heart tones.
3. Note the estimated date of conception and week of gestation on the laboratory requisition.
4. Procedure should be performed in a darkened room if the specimen will be tested for bilirubin.
5. See Client and Family Teaching.
6. Just before beginning the procedure, take a "time out" to verify the correct client, procedure, and site.

Procedure

1. The position of the fetus and a pocket of amniotic fluid are determined using ultrasound and palpation, with the mother in a supine position.
2. The mother's abdominal area is cleansed with surgical scrub solution and povidone-iodine and allowed to dry.
3. The aspiration site is draped to demarcate a sterile field.

4. The mother is instructed to place her hands behind her head, and the aspiration site is anesthetized with 1 mL of 1% or 2% lidocaine intradermally and subcutaneously.
5. A 20- to 22-gauge, 5-inch-long spinal needle with a stylet is inserted through the abdominal wall into the intrauterine cavity, and the stylet is withdrawn.
6. About 7-15 mL of amniotic fluid is aspirated through the spinal needle into a syringe, and the needle is withdrawn. Use a 20-mL amniotic fluid sample for direct genetic analysis for the four most common mutations responsible for Tay-Sachs disease.

Postprocedure Care

1. Apply a dry, sterile dressing to the aspiration site.
2. Inject 2-5 mL of amniotic fluid into a light-protected (foil-covered or amber) test tube to test for bilirubin. Inject 5-10 mL of amniotic fluid into a sterile, siliconized glass container or a polystyrene container for culture and genetic and other studies (AFP). Specimens to be transported to another site for testing should be packed in a cool, insulated container to maintain a temperature of 2-5 degrees C. Freezing temperatures should be avoided.
3. Obtain the mother's vital signs. Auscultate fetal heart tones for changes from the baseline value.
4. The mother should rest on her right side for 15-20 minutes after the procedure.
5. RhoGAM may be prescribed for Rh-negative mothers.
6. Transport the amniotic fluid specimen to the laboratory immediately and refrigerate.

Client and Family Teaching

1. Empty your bladder immediately before the procedure if gestation is 21 weeks or more. You must have a full bladder during the procedure if gestation is 20 weeks or less.
2. It is important to lie motionless throughout the procedure. You may experience a strong contraction with the needle insertion.
3. Chromosome analysis results may take up to 4 weeks.

4. After the procedure, notify the physician for cramping, abdominal pain, unusual vaginal drainage/fluid loss, fever, chills, dizziness, or more or less than the usual amount of fetal activity.
5. Inform the client with abnormal genetic findings of choices regarding pregnancy and pregnancy termination. Also refer the client for genetic counseling before future attempts to become pregnant. Refer to section in this book on "Informed Consent for Genetic Testing".

Factors That Affect Results

1. Reject frozen or clotted specimens.
2. Inadvertent aspiration of maternal urine can be ruled out by testing the specimen for blood urea nitrogen (BUN) and creatinine. Urine BUN is >100 mg/dL, whereas amniotic fluid is well under 100 mg/dL. Urine creatinine is usually >80 mg/dL, whereas amniotic fluid creatinine is usually ≤4 mg/dL.
3. Nonsiliconized glass containers for routine analysis may result in cell adherence on the sides of the container.
4. Amniotic fluid testing must be performed within 3 days of collection.
5. Amniocentesis should be performed between weeks 24 and 28 when one is checking for hemolytic disease of the newborn and Rh sensitization.
6. Falsely low bilirubin levels may result from failure to protect the specimen from light.
7. Specimens contaminated with blood should be tested for fetal hemoglobin to determine whether the blood is of maternal or fetal origin. Fetal blood contamination results in falsely high bilirubin levels. Fetal or maternal blood will interfere with measurements of fetal lung maturity and amniotic fluid constituents that are also constituents of plasma, such as protein, potassium, and glucose.
8. Creatinine levels are affected by maternal creatinine clearance and maternal creatinine levels. A concurrent maternal serum creatinine should be drawn. Maternal serum to amniotic fluid creatinine ratio should be about 2:1.
9. Elevated AFP results may be caused by contamination of the specimen with fetal blood.
10. Small and closed neural tube defects may not cause elevated AFP levels.
11. Accurate L/S ratio measurement is not possible if the specimen is contaminated with blood (fetal or maternal) or meconium.

Other Data

1. Direct karyotyping of placental villi samples obtained by needle aspiration has been found to yield faster results than amniotic fluid chromosome analysis. (See Chorionic villi sampling—Diagnostic.)
2. Chromosomal aberration has been found in 4.6% of fetuses in women >38 years of age, the most common being trisomy 21 (62%), Klinefelter's syndrome (11%), and Edward's syndrome (trisomy 18) (11%).
3. For diamniotic twin pregnancies, each amniotic sac should be sampled.
4. Early amniocentesis is feasible from 11 weeks of gestation and can be performed for the usual indications as an alternative to chorionic villus sampling. Results are available in less than 1 week using cytogenetic techniques.
5. Prenatal cystic fibrosis profile may be performed by polymerase chain reaction (PCR) for mutations (F508, R553X, g551D, g542X, n1303K, and w1282X).
6. Amniotic fluid neuron-specific enolase is useful as a marker for neonatal neurologic injury.
7. Genetic testing of cell free fetal DNA using real-time quantitative polymerase chain reaction is available and used as an alternative to amniocentesis in some countries. This test can identify fetal gender and some inherited disorders from a maternal blood sample. Disorders identified include disorders where a single gene is involved, and X-linked conditions. Findings are unreliable at less than 7 weeks gestation and have 94.8% sensitivity and 98.9% specificity at 7-12 weeks, and 95.5% sensitivity and 99.1% specificity at 13 through 20 weeks, and the most optimal results 99.0% specificity and 99.6% sensitivity after 20 weeks of gestation.
8. The Genetic Information Nondiscrimination Act of 2008 prohibits health plans from using genetic family history or genetic test results from influencing eligibility or premiums for health insurance. It also prohibits employers from using

this information to influence decisions about hiring, terminating employment, or employment pay, promotions or privileges.

Amniotic Fluid, Alpha-Fetoprotein

See Amniocentesis and Amniotic Fluid Analysis—Diagnostic.

Amniotic Fluid, Chromosome Analysis

See Amniocentesis and Amniotic Fluid Analysis—Diagnostic.

Amniotic Fluid, Erythroblastosis Fetalis

See Amniocentesis and Amniotic Fluid Analysis—Diagnostic.

Amniotic Fluid Analysis

See Amniocentesis and Amniotic Fluid Analysis—Diagnostic.

Amoxapine

See Tricyclic Antidepressants—Plasma or Serum.

Amphetamines—Blood

Norm. Negative

Drug	ng/mL	µg/mL	mg/L	SI Units, nmol/L
Amphetamine sulfate	20-120	0.02-0.12		150-900
Toxic level	>200		>2	>1500
Chlorphentermine	100-400	0.10-0.40		750-3000
Diethylpropion	1-10	0.001-0.010		7.5-75
Ephedrine	50-100	0.05-0.10		375-750
Fenfluramine	30-300	0.03-0.30		225-2250
Methamphetamine	10-50	0.01-0.05		75-375
Toxic level	>500		>5	>3750
p-Methoxyamphetamine	<200	<0.2		<1500
Methylenedioxyamphetamine	<400	<0.4		<3000
Toxic level	>400		>4	>3000
Phendimetrazine	30-250	0.03-0.25		225-1875
Phenmetrazine	60-250	0.06-0.25		450-1875
Toxic level	>400		>4	>3000
Phentermine	30-90	0.03-0.09		225-675
Phenylpropanolamine	50-100	0.05-0.10		375-750
Tranylcypromine	10-100	0.01-0.10		75-750

Toxic Levels Symptoms and Treatment

Symptoms. Psychoses, tremors, convulsions, insomnia, tachycardia, dysrhythmias, impotence, cerebrovascular accident, and respiratory collapse.

Treatment

NOTE: Treatment choice(s) depend(s) on client's history and condition and episode history.

1. Use gastric lavage or induce vomiting (with extreme caution) if within 4 hours of ingestion. (Induction of vomiting is contraindicated in clients with no gag reflex or with central nervous system depression or excitation.)
2. Give a slurry of activated charcoal 1 g/kg (minimum 30 g), followed by a magnesium citrate cathartic.
3. Amphetamine excretion may be accelerated by acidification of the urine with ammonium chloride 1-2 g intravenously or ascorbic acid 0.5-1.5 g orally every 4-6 hours to keep urine pH <5.5.
4. Increase fluids to keep urine output at 3-6 mL/kg/hour.
5. Consider using mannitol or furosemide to force diuresis (efficacy of acid diuresis has not been clearly established).
6. Both hemodialysis and peritoneal dialysis WILL remove amphetamines.
7. Barbiturates may counteract amphetamine stimulant effects and chlorpromazine (Thorazine) may help control the symptoms of an overstimulated central nervous system.

Increased. Stimulant drug abuse or use.

Description. Amphetamines are sympathomimetic amines that act on the cortex and reticular activating system of the brain to stimulate the release and block the reabsorption of norepinephrine and dopamine. They cause mood elevation and wakefulness and decrease the perception of fatigue through stimulation of the heart and central nervous system. They are rapidly absorbed from the gastrointestinal tract and reach all tissues but concentrate in the central nervous system and are excreted by the kidneys. Half-lives vary depending on the individual drug. Synonyms include bennies, crystal, ice, pep pills, speed, uppers, and wake-ups. Side effects include multiple visceral aneurysms, cognitive deficits, hypertension, hyponatremia, jaw clenching, lack of appetite, loss of sexual interest, impaired gait, inability to concentrate, hepatic toxicity, memory problems, renal failure, and disseminated intravascular coagulation (DIC) (especially from MDMA/Ecstasy). Blood amphetamine levels are used for monitoring the appropriateness of dosage regimen and for detection of amphetamine abuse.

Professional Considerations

Consent form NOT required.

Preparation

1. Tube: Lavender topped.
2. Assess for a history of drug abuse.
3. Do NOT draw during hemodialysis.

Procedure

1. Draw a 5-mL blood sample.

Postprocedure Care

1. None.

Client and Family Teaching

1. Results are normally available within 4 hours.
2. If activated charcoal was given for elevated levels, drink 4-6 glasses of water each day for 2 days to prevent constipation. Activated charcoal will also cause stools to be black for a few days.
3. Referrals to appropriate rehabilitation centers and therapeutic community programs should be offered to all addicted clients.

Factors That Affect Results

1. High concentrations of beta-phenethylamine, a blood product formed from the decomposition of protein, may mask a low amphetamine level.

Other Data

1. Toxicity in children occurs over a wide range of doses.
2. Abrupt discontinuation may cause psychotic symptoms.
3. See also Toxicology drug screen—Blood or urine.

Amsler Grid Test—Screen

Norm. The lines are clearly visualized and appear straight. A black dot is visualized in the center of the grid. No distortions of the lines are seen. No spots are seen other than within each square.

Usage. Detection of macular edema, macular blind spots, scotoma. A component of visual field testing for diagnosing glaucoma.

Description. An optical screening test using a grid of intersecting lines with a black dot in the center. The visual acuity of the macular portion of the retina can be affected by macular edema, causing distortions of the lines, or by scotomas, causing blind spots, which make the grid appear to the client as having blank areas.

Professional Considerations

Consent form NOT required.

Preparation

1. Obtain an Amsler grid and an eye occluder (eye patch, hand held, or occluding eyeglasses).

Procedure

1. With one eye being covered, have the client view the Amsler grid at his or her usual reading distance.
2. Ask whether the black dot is visible, whether the complete square grid is visible when looking at the dot, whether the lines are perfectly straight, and whether any of the lines are blurred or look as though they are moving.
3. Ask if there are any blank areas on the grid, other than within each square. Have the client draw what he or she sees if the answer to any of the questions is yes.
4. Repeat the test for the other eye.

Postprocedure Care

1. Refer the client to a specialist if necessary.

Client and Family Teaching

1. The test takes less than 30 minutes.

Factors That Affect Results

1. Performing this test before retinal examination with an ophthalmoscope and fundus examination or refraction test avoids falsely abnormal results caused by retinal bleaching from the bright light or loss of focusing ability.

Other Data

1. An abnormal test indicates the need for more specific testing such as fluorescein angiography.
2. Amsler grid reports have poor validity and cannot be accurately interpreted for use in the clinical diagnosis of retinal defects or overall ocular disease.

Amylase—Serum and Urine and Amylase Clearance

Norm.

Serum Amylase		SI Units
Adults		
18-70 years	30-110	30-110 U/L U/L
>70 years	20-160 U/L	20-160 U/L
Children		
0-3 months	0-30 U/L	0-30 U/L
3-6 months	7-40 U/L	7-40 U/L
7-8 months	7-57 U/L	7-57 U/L
9-11 months	11-70 U/L	11-70 U/L
12-17 months	11-79U/L	11-79 U/L
18-35 months	19-92 U/L	19-92 U/L
3-4 years	26-106 U/L	26-106 U/L
5-12 years	30-119 U/L	30-119 U/L
13-18 years	30-110 U/L	30-110 U/L

Urine Amylase	
Mayo Clinic method	10-80 amylase U/hour
Somogyi method	26-950 U/24 hours
Beckman method	1-17 U/hour
Amylase clearance	1%-4%
Macroamylasemia	Decreased (usually <1%) or normal clearance
Pancreatitis	Increased clearance

Increased. Abdominal aortic aneurysm (ruptured), acute exacerbation of chronic pancreatitis, ampulla of Vater obstruction, cerebral trauma, cholecystitis (acute), choledocholithiasis, common bile duct obstruction, diabetic ketoacidosis, eating disorders (vomiting, pancreatitis), ectopic pregnancy, empyema (gallbladder), fructose malabsorption, hyperthyroidism, intestinal obstruction with strangulation, intra-abdominal abscess, lung cancer, macroamylasemia, mesenteric thrombosis, mumps, pancreatic duct obstruction, pancreatic cancer, pancreatitis (acute), perforated intestine, perforated ulcer, peritonitis, salivary gland disease (acute, duct obstruction, suppurative inflammation), spasm of sphincter of Oddi, surgery (postoperative upper abdominal, peripancreatic), trauma (pancreas, spleen), tuberculosis. Drugs include aspirin, opiates, propofol, radiographic dyes, and thiazides. Herbs or natural remedies include vinho abafado (augmented Port wine, Brazil).

Decreased. Alcoholic liver disease, alcoholism, burns (severe), cachexia, cirrhosis, cystic fibrosis (advanced), hepatic abscess, hepatic cancer, hepatitis, pancreatic cancer, pancreatitis (acute fulminant, advanced chronic), poisoning, renal dysfunction, thyrotoxicosis (severe), and toxemia of pregnancy. Drugs include glucose and fluorides.

Description. An enzyme produced by the pancreas and salivary glands that aids digestion of complex carbohydrates. It is excreted by the kidneys. In acute pancreatitis, serum amylase levels start rising at about 2 hours after the onset, peak at about 24 hours, and return to normal in 2-4 days after the onset. Urine amylase levels will be elevated from several hours after the onset until 7-10 days after the onset. Because urine amylase levels remain elevated longer than serum amylase levels, they are useful for providing evidence of pancreatitis after serum amylase has returned to normal levels.

Amylase clearance is reported as a ratio in proportion to creatinine clearance. This amylase clearance/creatinine clearance ratio helps determine whether hypermacroamylasemia is secondary to pancreatitis (see Norms):

Amylase clearance =
(urine amylase concentration)×
(serum creatinine concentration)/
(serum amylase concentration)×
(urine creatinine concentration)

Amylase concentration rises and falls in tandem with lipase concentration in acute pancreatitis but is a less specific marker than lipase for this condition.

Professional Considerations
Consent form NOT required.

Preparation
1. Obtain a urine container without preservatives, including toluene or acetic acid preservatives, in sizes as follows: 1-L size, 2- or 6-hour collection; 2-L size, 8- or 12-hour collection; 3-L size, 24-hour collection.
2. Tube: Red topped, red/gray topped, or gold topped.
3. List medications taken in the past 24 hours on the laboratory requisition.
4. Screen client for the use of herbal preparations or natural remedies such as vinho abafado.

Procedure
1. Discard the first morning-voided urine specimen.
2. Collect a timed urine specimen over 2, 6, 8, 12, or 24 hours in a refrigerated or iced container without preservatives or to which toluene or acetic acid has been added. For catheterized clients, keep the drainage bag on ice and empty the urine into the collection container hourly.
3. Encourage fluid intake throughout the collection period if not contraindicated.

4. For serum collection, draw a 4-mL sample at least 2 hours after a meal and before treatment has begun.

Postprocedure Care

1. Check pH of specimen. If pH is <6, add 2 mL of 5% NaOH to the container and mix well.
2. Send a well-mixed 10-mL aliquot to the laboratory and refrigerate.
3. List the beginning and ending times of urine specimen collection on the laboratory requisition, as well as total volume of the 24-hour specimen.

Client and Family Teaching

1. For the urine test, save all urine voided in the 2-, 6-, 8-, 12-, or 24-hour period. Urinate before defecating to avoid loss of urine and to avoid contaminating the specimen with feces or toilet tissue. If any urine is accidentally discarded, discard the entire specimen and restart the collection the next day.
2. Do not drink alcohol for 24 hours before sampling.

Factors That Affect Results

1. Urine amylase determinations should not be performed on females during menstruation.
2. Results reported in U/mL give an inaccurate picture because they are influenced by the varying urine volumes, depending on the length of the collection period.
3. Reject hemolyzed specimens.
4. Drugs that may falsely elevate results of serum amylase include aminosalicylic acid, asparaginase, azathioprine, bethanechol, bethanechol chloride, chloride salts, cholinergics, corticosteroids, corticotropin, cyproheptadine hydrochloride, ethacrynic acid, ethyl alcohol (large quantities), fluoride salts, furosemide, indomethacin, loop diuretics, mercaptopurine, methacholine, narcotic analgesics, oral contraceptives, pancreozymin, rifampin, sulfasalazine, and thiazide diuretics.
5. Falsely decreased results of serum amylase may be caused by citrates and oxalates.
6. pH of sample of <6 may cause up to a 30% decreased result.
7. Massive hemorrhagic pancreatic necrosis may cause so much pancreatic cell destruction that amylase cannot be produced, resulting in no elevation in serum amylase.
8. Contamination of the serum specimen with saliva will cause falsely elevated results.
9. Serum lipemia (hyperlipidemia) or hypertriglyceridemia may result in falsely low or spuriously normal serum amylase results.
10. Results are invalidated if the specimen is drawn less than 72 hours after cholecystography with radiopaque dyes.
11. Falsely high serum amylase results may be caused by renal failure.
12. There can be pronounced fluctuation in serum amylase levels, ranging from 115% to 1160% in clients with macroamylasemia, and this fluctuation may cause confusion in differentiating macroamylasemia from other causes of hyperamylasemia.
13. Baseline levels increase during pregnancy.

Other Data

1. Macroamylasemia causes a high serum but normal urine amylase concentration.
2. Urine amylase does not produce falsely high results with renal failure as serum amylase does.
3. Normal serum amylase may occur in pancreatitis, especially chronic pancreatitis and severe necrotizing pancreatitis.

ANA

See **Antinuclear Antibody**—Serum.

Anaerobic Culture

See **Body Fluid**—Anaerobic Culture.

ANCA
See Antineutrophil Cytoplasmic Antibody Screen—Serum.

A

Androstenedione—Serum
Norm.

		SI Units
Adult female	85-275 ng/dL	3.0-9.6 nmol/L
Postmenopausal	30-140 ng/dL	1.0-4.8 nmol/L
Adult male	70-205 ng/dL	2.6-7.2 nmol/L
Cord blood	30-150 ng/dL	1.0-5.2 nmol/L
Premature newborn	80-446 ng/dL	2.8-15.6 nmol/L
Newborn	20-290 ng/dL	0.7-10.1 nmol/L
Female Children		
1-3 months	15-25 ng/dL	0.5-0.9 nmol/L
3-5 months	10-15 ng/dL	0.3-0.5 nmol/L
Male Children		
1-3 months	20-45 ng/dL	0.7-1.6 nmol/L
3-5 months	10-40 ng/dL	0.3-1.4 nmol/L
Panic level (all ages)	>1000 ng/dL	>34.9 nmol/L

Usage. Nonspecific evaluation of androgen production in female hirsutism.

Increased. Alzheimer's disease, congenital adrenal hyperplasia, Cushing's syndrome, hirsutism, recurrent miscarriages, Stein-Leventhal disease (polycystic ovarian syndrome), and tumor (adrenal, ovarian). Herbs or natural remedies include Siberian ginseng.

Decreased. Decreases with age in men and potential factor in pathogenesis of bone loss.

Description. A metabolite of dehydroepiandrosterone sulfate (DHEA-S) produced in the ovaries and the adrenal gland that is converted to testosterone in peripheral tissues. Peak levels occur in the early morning and low levels in the late afternoon. After puberty, levels rise and peak around 20 years of age. Elevation is one of several causes of female hirsutism, which is characterized by a male hair-growth pattern. Very elevated levels are suggestive of the presence of a virilizing tumor.

Professional Considerations
Consent form NOT required.

Preparation
1. Schedule the test at least 7 days before or after a female client's menstruation.

2. Tube: Red topped, red/gray topped, or gold topped.
3. Screen client for the use of herbal preparations or natural remedies, such as Siberian ginseng.
4. See Client and Family Teaching.

Procedure
1. Draw a 2-mL blood sample. Draw between 0600 and 0900 for peak levels.

Postprocedure Care
1. Place the specimen on ice.
2. Transport the specimen to the laboratory immediately for spinning and freezing of serum.

Client and Family Teaching
1. Fast for 8 hours before sampling.
2. Test must be drawn 1 week before or after menstruation to avoid falsely elevated values.

Factors That Affect Results
1. Results are invalidated if the client has undergone a scan involving radioactive dyes within 1 week before specimen collection.

Other Data
1. Plasma levels do not correlate well with the severity of symptoms.

A

Angel Dust

See Phencyclidine, Qualitative—Urine.

Angiocardiography Procedure

See Cardiac Catheterization—Diagnostic.

Angiogram (Angiography)

See Arteriogram—Diagnostic; Cardiac Catheterization—Diagnostic; Cerebral Angiogram—Diagnostic; Pulmonary Angiogram—Diagnostic; or Renal Angiogram—Diagnostic.

Angiography

See Cerebral Angiogram—Diagnostic.

Angiotensin-Converting Enzyme (ACE)—Blood

Norm.

		SI Units
Adults	9-67 U/L	153-1139 µKat/L
Children		
0-6 years	18-90 U/L	306-1530 µKat/L
7-14 years	24-121 U/L	408-2057 µKat/L
15-17 years	18-101 U/L	306-1717 µKat/L

Increased. Arthritis (rheumatoid), bronchitis, cervical adenitis, cirrhosis (nonalcoholic), connective tissue disease, fungal diseases, Gaucher disease, histoplasmosis, Hodgkin's disease, hypercalcemia, hyperthyroidism (untreated), Langerhans cell histiocytosis, leprosy, myeloma, non-Hodgkin's lymphoma, pulmonary embolus, pulmonary fibrosis, sarcoidosis (active), and scleroderma.

Decreased. Acute respiratory distress syndrome, coccidioidomycosis, diabetes mellitus, farmer's lung, hypothyroidism, pulmonary neoplasm (advanced), severe illness, and tuberculosis. Drugs include cadmium, captopril, estrogen (replacement therapy), L-arginine, and steroids.

Description. An enzyme found mainly in lung epithelial cells and in smaller amounts in blood vessels and renal tissue that converts angiotensin I to angiotensin II—a vasopressor that also stimulates the adrenal cortex to produce aldosterone. High levels of ACE are strongly correlated with pulmonary sarcoidosis and levels drop to normal when spontaneous remission occurs.

Professional Considerations
Consent form NOT required.

Preparation
1. Write the client's age on the laboratory requisition.
2. Tube: Red topped, red/gray topped, gold topped, or green topped.
3. See Client and Family Teaching.

Procedure
1. Draw a 4-mL blood sample.

Postprocedure Care
1. Transport the specimen to the laboratory immediately. Freeze the specimen and store it in dry ice if the test is not performed immediately.

Client and Family Teaching
1. Fast for 12 hours before sampling.

Factors That Affect Results
1. Reject hemolyzed or lipemic specimens.
2. A delay in testing or failure to freeze the specimen if not tested immediately may cause falsely low results.

3. In clients with sarcoidosis, levels may be normal if clients have been treated with corticosteroids.

Other Data
1. ACE is useful in evaluating the effectiveness of therapy and in confirming clinical status.

ANH

See **Natriuretic Peptides**—Plasma.

Animals and Rabies

See **Fluorescent Rabies Antibody**—Specimen.

Animals and Rabies Negri Bodies, Brain Tissue—Specimen

Norm. Negative.

Positive. Rabies.

Description. A postmortem histologic examination of the brain tissue of an animal suspected to have rabies, usually performed after the animal has bitten a human. Rabies produces Negri bodies, a specific and diagnostic lesion of the central nervous system that contains inclusion bodies in the cytoplasm of the nerve cells. Animal specimen examination is the only method to identify rabies because there is no laboratory or diagnostic test to identify the disease in humans until after symptoms appear (listed below). Diagnosis in humans is based on history and symptoms. Symptoms may appear 10 days to a year after the bite but more commonly appear in humans 2-8 weeks later.

Professional Considerations
Consent form NOT required.

Preparation
1. Obtain a container and ice or dry ice.
2. Prepare for the examination by wearing protective clothing, a face shield, and heavy rubber gloves.

Procedure
1. The animal is killed and decapitated. The head is sealed in a watertight metal container and refrigerated as follows: with regular ice if the specimen will be examined within 24 hours; with dry ice if the specimen will be examined after 24 hours.
2. Thin-tissue impressions are made from the medulla, the cerebellum, and Ammon's horn of the hippocampus; immersed for 5 seconds in Seller's stain and then in tap water; and examined under high magnification. Negri bodies appear as cherry red, sharply defined, spherical, oval, or elongated bodies containing dark blue staining granules.

Postprocedure Care
1. Include a detailed history of the date of human exposure, the method of exposure, the names and addresses of the client(s) exposed, the animal's owners, the species and breed of animal, whether it died or was killed, and its vaccination history, if known.
2. The bitten human should be monitored for the development of signs of rabies, which include laryngeal spasm when drinking water, restless behavior, hyperreactivity or convulsions with increased sensory input, neuromuscular twitching, tachypnea/hyperventilation, hydrophobia, and excess salivation.

Client and Family Teaching
1. Client and family should observe for signs of rabies (listed above) for the next 12 months. Notify the physician immediately if symptoms appear.

2. Have pets vaccinated against rabies.
3. If a bite occurs, clean the wound quickly with a disinfectant to kill any rabies virus in the wound.
4. The family should follow universal precautions in handling any items from the client that have been contaminated with saliva until a year has passed without symptoms.

Factors That Affect Results

1. Inability to obtain animal or brain tissue.

Other Data

1. The likelihood of Negri body development increases with the length of time the animal lives after acquiring rabies. Therefore Negri bodies may not always be present.
2. Results should be confirmed by mouse inoculation intracerebrally with the animal's brain tissue.
3. The only method of preventing rabies is animal vaccination.
4. Rabies is a reportable disease in most areas, as are animal bites.

Anion Gap—Blood

Norm.

		SI Units
With K^+ in the equation	12-20 mEq/L	12-20 mmol/L
Without K^+ in the equation		
Adults	8-16 mEq/L	8-16 mmol/L
Child < age 3	10-14 mEq/L	10-14 mmol/L
Child ≥ age 3	10-18 mEq/L	10-18 mmol/L
Norm using Beckman E4A or CX5 analyzer	3-11 mEq/L	3-11 mmol/L

Increased. Acidosis, cancer, carbon monoxide poisoning, chronic renal failure, cyanide poisoning, dehydration, ethyl alcohol ketoacidosis, ethylene glycol poisoning, heart disease, heatstroke, hypertension, hypocalcemia, hypomagnesemia, lactic acidosis, metabolic acidosis caused by diabetic ketoacidosis (because of acetone, beta-hydroxybutyrate ketone content), methanol poisoning, multiple acyl-CoA dehydrogenase deficiency, renal failure, salicylate overdose, and uremia. Drugs include acetaminophen (alone or in combination with oxycodone), acetazolamide, ammonium chloride, antihypertensives, carbenicillin, corticosteroids, 5% dextrose in water (prolonged infusion), diazoxide, dimercaprol, ethacrynic acid, ethyl alcohol (ethanol), ethylene glycol, formaldehyde, fructose, furosemide, hippuric acid, hydrogen sulfide, iodine, iron, isoniazid, metformin, methenamine mandelate, nalidixic acid, nitrates, nitrites, oral phospho soda, oxalic acid, paraldehyde, penicillins, phenformin, propofol (infusion 100 μg/kg/min), salbutamol, salicylates, sodium bicarbonate, sodium nitroprusside, sorbitol, streptozotocin, sulfur (elemental), thiazides, ticarcillin, toluene, xylitol, and any drug that may result in hypotension with reduced tissue perfusion or renal failure.

Decreased. Bromism (from cough medications, very low to negative anion gap caused by halide ion falsely measured as chloride), hyperdilution, hypercalcemia, hypermagnesemia, hypoalbuminemia (causes a decrease in amount of anions not measured) (1 g/dL drop in serum albumin correlation with a 2.5 mEq/L decrease in anion gap), hyponatremia, hypophosphatemia, ingestion (of salicylate, ethanol, ethylene glycol, formaldehyde/methanol, paraldehyde, toluene, or sulfur), multiple myeloma (causes abnormal cations called paraproteins), polyclonal gammopathy, proteinuric hypertension from pregnancy, Waldenström's macroglobulinemia. Drugs include alkalis, ammonium chloride, boric acid, bromides, chlorpropamide, cholestyramine, corticotropin, cortisone acetate, hypercalcemia, hyperkalemia, hypermagnesemia, lithium carbonate (toxicity) (causes very low to negative anion gap because of excess unmeasured cation), magnesium-containing antacids, oxyphen-butazone, phenylbutazone, polymyxin B, sodium chloride (large amounts intravenously), tromethamine, and vasopressin. Herbal or natural remedies include licorice.

Description. A calculation of the difference between the major cations and the major anions in the blood that helps determine the cause of metabolic acidosis. The two formulas used to determine the anion gap are:

$$\text{Anion gap} = ([Na^+]) - ([Cl^-] + [HCO_3^-])$$

or

$$\text{Anion gap} = ([Na^+] + [K^+]) - ([Cl^-] + [HCO_3^-])$$

Anion gap is simply a term used to signify the amount of unmeasured anions in the blood plasma. The anion "gap" is created on paper because the formula excludes some anions (such as proteins, organic acids, phosphates, sulfates, and cations) (such as calcium and magnesium and, sometimes, potassium). If all possible types of anions and cations were used in the formula, instead of only those above, the answer would be zero, because the body's homeostatic mechanisms ensure electrochemical balance in the plasma. The formula's result has different implications depending on whether the answer is positive or negative. A negative anion gap is less common than an elevated anion gap.

Professional Considerations
Consent form NOT required.

Preparation
1. Tube: Red topped, red/gray topped, or gold topped.
2. Do NOT draw during hemodialysis.

Procedure
1. Draw a 10-mL blood sample.

Postprocedure Care
1. None.

Client and Family Teaching
1. Not applicable.

Factors That Affect Results
1. Metabolic acidosis may exist with a normal anion gap, as when bicarbonate is lost in body fluids and chloride is retained in the following conditions: hyperchloremic acidosis, renal tubular acidosis, biliary or pancreatic fistulas, and ileal loop hypofunctioning.
2. Iodine absorption from wounds packed with povidone-iodine solution may cause falsely low results.
3. Reject hemolyzed specimens.

Other Data
1. Normal anion gap can occur with diarrhea, hyperalimentation, ketoacidosis, renal tubular acidosis, ureterostomies, ingestion of ammonium chloride or ethanol, or infusion of total parenteral nutrition.
2. Treatment for an anion gap acidosis is to correct the cause. Sodium bicarbonate 1-2 mEq/kg has been used in some cases.
3. See also Ketone bodies—Blood; Beta-hydroxybutyrate—Blood.

Ankle-Brachial Index (ABI)—Diagnostic

Norm.

Pressure Index	Interpretation
≥0.86	Normal
0.75-0.85	Mild occlusive disease
0.50-0.75	Intermittent claudication
0.30-0.50	Severe disease: rest pain may occur; pregangrenous state
0.20-0.30	Poor probability for tissue healing or limb viability unless compensation by collateral blood flow occurs
<0.20	Ischemic or gangrenous extremities

Usage. Assessment of arterial blood flow in clients with peripheral vascular disease; monitoring postoperative flow in the lower extremities after vascular surgery such as femoral bypass or after aortofemoral bypass from iliac occlusion; assessment of severity of peripheral vascular disease; predicting carotid artery stenosis. Cilostazol (Pletal) increases ABI at rest.

Description. The ABI is a mathematically calculated ratio of the systolic pressure at a pulse point in a lower extremity with peripheral vascular disease as compared to the systolic pressure of the brachial artery. The index provides a quick, noninvasive assessment of how much arterial blood is perfusing the extremity. Typically an ABI that increases by at least 0.15 (15%) after vascular surgery indicates that the surgery was successful. A baseline in women with an ABI of <0.60 indicates significantly higher probability of developing severe disability for walking specific outcomes (such as walking a quarter of a mile).

Professional Considerations
Consent form NOT required.

Preparation
1. Obtain a dual-frequency Doppler ultrasonograph, a marker, two sphygmomanometers, and ultrasonic gel.

Procedure
1. Client is positioned supine.
2. The femoral, popliteal, dorsalis pedis, and posterior tibial pulse points in both lower extremities are palpated and identified with a marker.
3. The sphygmomanometer cuff is placed proximally to the marked site. If the flow is being assessed at the knee, the cuff is placed proximally to the popliteal pulse. If the flow is being assessed at the ankle, the cuff is placed proximally to the ankle.
4. Ultrasonic gel is placed over the marked site (popliteal, posterior tibial, or dorsalis pedis), and the Doppler flow signal is identified.
5. With the Doppler in place, the sphygmomanometer cuff is inflated until the Doppler flow signal disappears.
6. The cuff is slowly deflated, and the pressure at which the Doppler tone is again audible is noted and recorded.

7. The brachial systolic blood pressure in both arms is measured with a Doppler scanner, and the highest pressure is selected for use in the ABI calculation.
8. The ABI ratio is calculated with the following equation:

ABI ratio =
[Lower extremity pressure from step 6]/ [Brachial Doppler systolic pressure]

Postprocedure Care
1. Wipe the ultrasonic gel from the skin and remove the sphygmomanometer cuff.
2. If performing serial ABI measurements postoperatively, notify the physician for a decrease in ABI of at least 0.15 (15%) or for the loss of a previously palpable pulse or audible Doppler tone.

Client and Family Teaching
1. This test is painless.
2. This measurement helps estimate how much blood is flowing to the leg and foot.

Factors That Affect Results
1. Values may be inconsistent if the same arm is not used for every brachial pressure measurement.
2. Immediate postoperative hypotension and low body temperature may necessitate use of a Doppler scanner to locate pulse tones because pulses may not be palpable.

Other Data
1. The ABI is a good predictor of survival in clients with peripheral vascular disease. Those with ABIs less than 0.30 have significantly poorer survival than clients with ABIs of 0.31-0.91.
2. The transfer function index (TFI) has been shown to be superior to ABI in detecting vascular grafts at risk for failing. See Pulse volume recording of peripheral vasculature—Diagnostic.
3. See also Doppler ultrasonographic flow studies—Diagnostic.

ANP
See Natriuretic Peptides—Plasma.

Antegrade Pyelography—Diagnostic

Norm. The selected ureter fills from the renal pelvis to the urinary bladder. Normal renal pelvic, ureteral, and urinary bladder contours are demonstrated radiographically after the injection of radiopaque contrast material.

Usage. Most commonly requested in clinical scenarios where ureteral obstruction is suspected but cannot be diagnosed effectively by intravenous pyelography (IVP) or cystoscopy and retrograde pyelography. Used for detection of synchronous tumor of the upper urinary tract, ureteropelvic laceration after blunt body trauma, or ileal conduit stenosis. Frequently performed with the placement of percutaneous nephrostomy tubes in the treatment of urinary tract obstruction and analysis of ureteral stent placement.

Description. Antegrade pyelography is an invasive radiographic procedure in which radiocontrast material is injected percutaneously into the renal pelvis. The flow of the contrast material is then observed as it progresses into the ureter and urinary bladder. Hydronephrosis or obstruction of the flow of the radiocontrast material into the urinary bladder is diagnostic of urinary tract obstruction and may be suggestive of the need to place a percutaneous nephrostomy tube.

Professional Considerations
Consent form IS required.

Risks
Allergic reaction to the radiocontrast material or anesthetic agents, bleeding (bladder clots, hematuria, perinephric hematoma), bowel perforation, infection, laceration of the renal collecting system with resulting urine leaks, pneumothorax.

Contraindications
Allergy to radiocontrast material, hemorrhagic diathesis.

Precautions
During pregnancy, risks of cumulative radiation exposure to the fetus from this and other previous or future imaging studies must be weighed against the benefits of the procedure. Although formal limits for client exposure are relative to this risk-benefit comparison, the United States Nuclear Regulatory Commission requires that the cumulative dose equivalent to an embryo/fetus from occupational exposure not exceed 0.5 rem (5 mSv). Radiation dose to the fetus is proportional to the distance of the anatomy studied from the abdomen and decreases as pregnancy progresses. For pregnant clients, consult the radiologist/radiology department to obtain estimated fetal radiation exposure from this procedure.

Preparation
1. This test is generally performed by a urologist or an interventional radiologist in an area equipped with fluoroscopy or ultrasound equipment.
2. A formal assessment to rule out hemorrhagic diathesis (PT, PTT, bleeding time, platelet count) as well as baseline determination of hematocrit and hemoglobin is advisable. A baseline urinalysis is also often obtained. It is useful to determine if the client will permit transfusion in the event of hemorrhage. If not, it may be necessary to reconsider the procedure.
3. Orders may include a 4-hour fast from food and a sedative.
4. Vital signs (blood pressure reading, pulse rate, respiratory rate) immediately before the procedure are indicated.
5. Just before beginning the procedure, take a "time out" to verify the correct client, procedure, and site.

Procedure
1. In the fluoroscopy or sonography suite, the position of the renal pelvis is demonstrated radiographically. A posterior vertical approach to the kidney is usually selected.
2. The flank over the renal pelvis is prepped with an iodine solution, and sterile drapes are applied to create a sterile field.
3. A 22-gauge needle is advanced into the renal pelvis under fluoroscopic or ultrasonographic guidance. Once within the collecting system, urine samples can be obtained and radiocontrast material injected to confirm the location of the needle tip within the renal pelvis.

4. At this point, a guidewire is advanced through the needle, allowing placement of larger introducer needles or urostomy catheters, or both types. Further radiocontrast material can be injected to complete the antegrade pyelogram procedure.

Postprocedure Care

1. Frequent determination of the vital signs is indicated in the immediate postprocedure period. Vital signs are generally obtained at 15-minute intervals for the first hour after the procedure and then at frequent intervals as specified by the physician performing the test.
2. Close monitoring of the urine output and observation for the development of hematuria are important. The client may have a nephrostomy bag as well as a Foley catheter bag after the pyelography, so separate records of each output source may be necessary.
3. Serial determinations of hematocrit, hemoglobin, creatinine, and serum electrolytes may be indicated.
4. If nephrostomy tubes have been placed, dressing checks and changes may be needed.
5. New fluid and antibiotic orders may need to be executed after the pyelography procedure.

Client and Family Teaching

1. The need to frequently monitor vital signs and urine output should be discussed.

2. Gross hematuria is not unusual after this procedure, and a relatively small amount of blood will produce red urine. The client should be reassured that this development generally is to be expected and does not necessarily indicate an unfavorable outcome.
3. Special positioning of the client may be required because of the nephrostomy tubes, and this should be explained to the client.

Factors That Affect Results

1. Postprocedure bleeding or infection.
2. Hematuria resulting in clotting of nephrostomy tubes.
3. Formation of bladder clots causing pain and diminished urine output.
4. Accelerated urine output after nephrostomy tube placement (post obstructive diuresis), resulting in volume depletion (hypotension, tachycardia, electrolyte abnormalities).

Other Data

1. Intravenous pyelography, CT scan, and nuclear magnetic resonance scanning are noninvasive alternative diagnostic modalities useful in the evaluation of urinary tract obstruction.
2. Renal insufficiency is a relative contraindication for the administration of intravenous radiocontrast material but is not a contraindication for antegrade or retrograde pyelography.
3. See also Retrograde pyelography—Diagnostic.

Anthrax

See **Blood Culture**—Blood.

Antibody Identification, Red Cell—Blood

Norm. Requires interpretation.

Usage. Identification of the specific nature of antibodies detected with more general antibody screens (indirect Coombs' testing). Found in clients who are homozygous for sickle cell disease.

Description. Irregular antibodies are usually detected in clients who have had prior exposure to foreign antigens through blood transfusions or pregnancy. The presence of these irregular antibodies may cause transfusion reactions and hemolytic disease of the newborn. The exact antibody is identified when the client's serum is combined with a panel of red blood cell samples, each containing a known antigen. This test is typically performed in a blood bank or transfusion services department.

Professional Considerations
Consent form NOT required.

Preparation

1. Tube: One lavender topped or pink topped and one red topped, red/gray topped, or gold topped.
2. Note the client's age, medications, past transfusions of blood products, and number of pregnancies on the laboratory requisition.

Procedure

1. Draw a 5-mL blood sample in the lavender topped or pink topped tube.
2. Draw a 10-mL blood sample in the red topped, red/gray topped, or gold topped tube.

Postprocedure Care

1. None.

Client and Family Teaching

1. Results are normally available within 24 hours.

Factors That Affect Results

1. Reject hemolyzed specimens.

Other Data

1. Identification of cold-reacting antibodies reactive at −30 degrees C may require the use of a blood warmer during transfusion.
2. Anti-D and anti-C antibodies are associated with most neonatal morbidity.

Anticardiolipin Antibody

See **Antiphospholipid Antibodies**—Serum.

Antideoxyribonuclease B Antibody Titer (Anti-DNase B Antibody, Streptodornase)—Serum

Norm.

Adult	85 Todd U/mL or <1:85
Child <7 years	<60 Todd U/mL or <1:60
Child ≥7 years	<170 Todd U/mL or <1:170

A fourfold increase between acute and convalescent specimens indicates infection with group A streptococci.

Increased. Anorexia nervosa, glomerulonephritis (poststreptococcal), pharyngitis (streptococcal), poststreptococcal reactive arthritis (PSReA), pyodermic skin infections, rheumatic fever (acute), Tourette's syndrome.

Description. Deoxyribonuclease B is an antigen produced by group A streptococci. The anti-DNase B test detects antibodies to deoxyribonuclease B, which appear when a client has a poststreptococcal infection. The levels increase after a client recovers from a group A streptococcal infection and thus are a reliable indicator of recent hemolytic streptococcal infection.

Professional Considerations

Consent form NOT required.

Preparation

1. Tube: Red topped, red/gray topped, or gold topped.
2. List drug therapy and previous vaccinations on the laboratory requisition.
3. Transport the specimen to the laboratory immediately. Spin and refrigerate the specimen if not tested immediately.

Procedure

1. Draw a 4-mL blood sample. Label this as the acute sample.
2. Draw a repeat titer in 2 weeks.

Postprocedure Care

1. None.

Client and Family Teaching

1. Results are normally available within 48 hours.
2. Return in 2 weeks for collection of a convalescent sample.

Factors That Affect Results

1. Reject hemolyzed specimens.
2. False-negative results may occur in hemorrhagic pancreatitis.

Other Data

1. This test is more sensitive to streptococcal pyoderma than the antistreptolysin-O (ASO) test.
2. Anti–zymogen antibody titers are a better marker for streptococcal infection associated with acute glomerulonephritis.

Antidiuretic Hormone (ADH)—Serum

Norm.

Serum Osmolarity (mOSm/L)	ADH Level (pg/mL)	SI Units (pmol/L)
270-280	<1.5	<1.4
280-285	<2.5	<2.3
285-290	1-5	0.9-4.6
290-295	2-7	1.9-6.5
295-300	4-12	3.7-11.1

Increased. Acute intermittent porphyria, cancer (brain, intrathoracic nonpulmonary cancer, gastrointestinal cancer, gynecologic cancer, breast cancer, prostate cancer, sarcoma), cerebral infection, cerebrovascular disease, diabetes insipidus (nephrogenic), ectopic production from neoplasm, Guillain-Barré syndrome, meningitis (tuberculous), pneumonia, syndrome of inappropriate antidiuretic hormone secretion (SIADH) (caused by malignant tumors, CNS disorders, intrathoracic infections, positive-pressure ventilation), and tuberculosis (pulmonary). Drugs include anesthetics, antipsychotics, barbiturates, carbamazepine, chlorothiazide, chlorpropamide, cisplatin, clofibrate, cyclophosphamide, desmopressin, furosemide, estrogens, lithium, melphalan, morphine sulfate and other narcotic analgesics, oxytocin citrate, oxytocin injection, psychotropic drugs, thiazides, tolbutamide, tricyclic antidepressants and vidarabine, vinblastine, and vincristine sulfate.

Decreased. Enuresis, nephrotic syndrome, pituitary diabetes insipidus, and psychogenic polydipsia. Drugs include alcohol, demeclocycline, ethyl alcohol, lithium carbonate, and phenytoin sodium.

Description. A hormone produced by the hypothalamus and stored and released from the posterior lobe of the pituitary gland in response to increased serum osmolarity. Acts to maintain body water balance through regulation of sodium and potassium levels and vascular smooth muscle control. Release of ADH is inhibited by decreased serum osmolarity.

Professional Considerations
Consent form NOT required.

Preparation
1. See Client and Family Teaching.
2. Tube: Lavender topped, made of plastic rather than glass.
3. Notify laboratory personnel that a specimen for ADH measurement will be arriving shortly.

Procedure
1. Draw a 5-mL blood sample.

Postprocedure Care
1. Write the collection time on the laboratory requisition.
2. Transport the specimen to the laboratory for spinning within 10 minutes of collection.

Client and Family Teaching
1. Fast and refrain from stress and strenuous activity for 12 hours before the test.
2. Results are normally available in about 5 days.

Factors That Affect Results
1. Reject specimens received more than 10 minutes after collection.
2. Elevated ADH levels may be caused by physical and psychologic stress and positive-pressure mechanical ventilation. Highest levels are obtained at night. Pain, stress, exercise, and elevated blood osmolality will each cause increased secretion.
3. Decreased ADH levels may be caused by negative-pressure mechanical ventilation, recumbent position, hypoosmolar blood, and hypertension.
4. Results are invalidated if the specimen is drawn within 1 week after the client has undergone a scan using radioactive dye.
5. Glass causes degradation of ADH.

Other Data
1. None.

Anti-DNA—Serum

Norm.

Negative	0-0.9 mg of native DNA/ mL of plasma or <70 IU/mL
Borderline SLE	70-200 IU/mL

Increased. Autoimmune disorder (1-2.5 mg/mL), myasthenia gravis, rheumatoid arthritis, sclerosis (systemic), Sjögren's syndrome, systemic lupus erythematosus (SLE) nephritis, SLE (active = 10-15 mg/mL; remission = 1-2.5 mg/mL), and non-Hodgkin's lymphoma. Drugs include estrogen.

Description. Detects the presence of antibodies to native deoxyribonuclease that indicate autoimmune activity. The test may be used to monitor the progression (increasing levels) and remission (decreasing levels) of SLE.

Professional Considerations

Consent form NOT required.

Preparation

1. Tube: Red topped, lavender topped, or gray topped (depending on specific laboratory requirements).

Procedure

1. Draw a 2-mL blood sample.

Postprocedure Care

1. None.

Client and Family Teaching

1. Results may not be available for several days if testing is not performed on site.

Factors That Affect Results

1. Results are invalid if the specimen is drawn less than 1 week after the client received a scan using radioactive dye.
2. Procainamide and hydralazine can induce anti-DNA antibodies.

Other Data

1. In the past it was unnecessary to test clients with negative antinuclear antibodies (ANAs). However, there exists a group of ANA-negative lupus clients who have elevated anti-DNA levels.
2. In SLE, immune complexes of anti-DNA may be deposited in the brain, heart, kidneys, and synovial tissue.

Anti-DNase B Antibody

See Antideoxyribonuclease B Antibody Titer—Serum.

Antigen Detection Test

See Respiratory Antigen Panel—Specimen.

Antihemophilia Factor

See Factor VIII—Blood.

Antihyaluronidase (AH) Titer—Serum

Norm. <128 U/mL.

A fourfold increase between acute and convalescent samples is significant, regardless of the magnitude of the titer.

Increased. Recent group A streptococcal disease, glomerulonephritis (acute), and rheumatic fever (acute).

Description. Hyaluronidase is an extracellular enzyme antigen produced by group A beta-hemolytic streptococci. This test measures levels of antibodies to hyaluronidase that appear in clients who are recovering from group A beta-hemolytic streptococcal infections. Levels increase after a client recovers from a group A beta-hemolytic streptococcal infection (about the second week of infection) and decrease 3-5 weeks after infection. Levels are thus a reliable indicator of recent group A beta-hemolytic streptococcal infection.

Professional Considerations
Consent form NOT required.

Preparation
1. Tube: Red topped, red/gray topped, or gold topped.
2. List drug therapy and all previous vaccinations on the laboratory requisition.

Procedure
1. Draw a 5-mL blood sample.

Postprocedure Care
1. Transport the specimen to the laboratory immediately. Spin and refrigerate the specimen if not tested immediately.

Client and Family Teaching
1. Return in 1-3 weeks for convalescent samples to be drawn.

Factors That Affect Results
1. Reject hemolyzed specimens.
2. Drugs that may cause falsely suppressed results include antibiotics and corticosteroids.
3. Falsely elevated results may occur in the presence of hyperlipoproteinemia.

Other Data
1. A better test than the antistreptolysin-O (ASO) test for detecting antibodies in acute glomerulonephritis, which follows a streptococcal pyoderma.

Anti-La/SS-B Test—Diagnostic

Norm. Negative.

Usage. Differential diagnosis of systemic lupus erythematosus (SLE), Sjögren's syndrome, and mixed connective tissue disease.

Positive. Antinuclear antibody (ANA)–negative lupus, congenital heart block, neonatal lupus, Sjögren's syndrome. Drugs include terbinafine.

Description. Anti-La/SS-B is an autoantibody characteristically found in high titers in clients with primary Sjögren's syndrome or Sjögren's syndrome with SLE. The SS-B(La) are antibodies directed against ribonucleic acid (RNA) protein particles that are a cofactor in RNA polymerase III. Although electrophoresis is the most sensitive method for detecting anti-La/SS-B, immunodiffusion is the method most commonly used.

Professional Considerations
Consent form NOT required.

Preparation
1. Tube: Red topped, red/gray topped, or gold topped.

Procedure
1. Draw a 4-mL blood sample.

Postprocedure Care
1. Transport the specimen to the laboratory for immediate spinning.

Client and Family Teaching
1. Results may not be available for several days if testing is not performed on site.

Factors That Affect Results
1. None found.

Other Data
1. This test is less sensitive but more specific for primary Sjögren's syndrome than the anti-Ro/SS-A test.
2. The presence of both anti-La/SS-B and anti-Ro/SS-A antibodies is generally associated with a milder form of SLE.
3. Clients who are positive for antinuclear antibody and who have SS-A, but not SS-B, are likely to have nephritis.

Antimicrosomal Antibody
See **Thyroid Peroxidase Antibody**—Blood.

Antimitochondrial Antibody (AMA)—Blood

Norm. Negative at 1:5 to 1:10 dilution.
    <1.0 Units = Negative.
    1.0-1.3 Units = Inconclusive.
    >1.3 Units = Positive.

Suggestive of primary biliary cirrhosis	>1:20
Probable primary biliary cirrhosis; biopsy recommended	>1:80
Diagnostic of primary biliary cirrhosis	>1:160

Increased. Acute cholestatic hepatitis, autoimmune diseases, carbon monoxide poisoning, chronic active hepatitis (20% of clients), cryptogenic cirrhosis, gastric adenocarcinoma, hepatitis C, jaundice (drug induced), myasthenia gravis, and primary biliary cirrhosis.

Decreased or Absent. Autoimmune cholangitis, drug-induced cholestatic jaundice, extrahepatic obstructive biliary disease, status post liver transplantation for primary biliary cirrhosis, sclerosing cholangitis, and viral hepatitis.

Description. An immunofluorescent test that detects and measures autoimmune immunoglobulins of the IgG type (antibodies) to mitochondria that attack organs, which then expend large amounts of energy. A majority of clients with primary biliary cirrhosis have antimitochondrial antibodies. This test is usually performed with the test for anti–smooth muscle antibodies to aid in differentiating primary biliary cirrhosis and chronic active hepatitis from diffuse, extrahepatic biliary obstruction and other liver diseases.

Professional Considerations

Consent form NOT required.

Preparation

1. See Client and Family Teaching.
2. Tube: Red topped, red/gray topped, or gold topped.

Procedure

1. Draw a 4-mL blood sample.

Postprocedure Care

1. Transport the specimen to the laboratory for immediate spinning.

Client and Family Teaching

1. Fast for 8 hours before sampling.
2. Results may not be available for several days if testing is not performed on site.

Factors That Affect Results

1. Reject hemolyzed or visibly lipemic specimens.
2. Results are unreliable for clients using oxyphenisatin.
3. False-positive results may occur in clients with syphilis.

Other Data

1. AMA may be profiled into serologic subtypes.

Antimyocardial Antibody—Serum

Norm. Negative.

Positive. Cardiomyopathy (idiopathic), Dressler's syndrome, fibrosis (endomyocardial), status after myocardial infarction, myocarditis, pericarditis (idiopathic), pleural fluid analysis, postcardiac injury syndrome (PCIS), postpericardiotomy syndrome, postthoracotomy syndrome, rheumatic fever, rheumatic heart disease, systemic lupus erythematosus, and thoracic injury.

Description. Antimyocardial antibody is an antibody to an organ-specific antigen in myocardial tissue that causes autoimmune damage to the heart and may be detected in serum before the appearance of clinical symptoms. The myocardial antigenic determinant is also believed to be a characteristic of streptococci because the antibodies may appear in rheumatic fever or after a streptococcal infection. This test uses an indirect immunofluorescence method by treatment of extracts of animal cardiac tissue with the client's serum and observation for the development of antigen-antibody immune complexes. Positive results are reported in titers of the lowest dilution at which the immune complexes can be detected, and decreasing titers correlate with response to treatment. This test is used in the detection of an autoimmune cause for the above-listed conditions and for monitoring therapeutic response to treatment for the above-listed conditions.

Professional Considerations
Consent form NOT required.

Preparation
1. Tube: Red topped, red/gray topped, or gold topped.

Procedure
1. Draw a 5-mL blood sample.

Postprocedure Care
1. Transport the specimen to the laboratory for immediate spinning.

Client and Family Teaching
1. Results are normally available within 48 hours.

Factors That Affect Results
1. No factors known to affect results.

Other Data
1. Myocardial antibodies do not usually occur in clients with coronary insufficiency alone, but do occur in clients who also have had a myocardial infarction.
2. Pleural fluid can be analyzed for antimyocardial antibody to determine postcardiac injury syndrome (PCIS) and help exclude other diagnoses.

Antineutrophil Cytoplasmic Antibody Screen (ANCA, Cytoplasmic Neutrophil Antibodies)—Serum

Norm.

	Screen	Titer
p-ANCA	Negative	<1:20
c-ANCA	Negative	<1:20

Increased c-ANCA. Human immunodeficiency virus, microscopic polyangiitis, Wegener's granulomatosis.

Increased p-ANCA. Churg-Strauss syndrome, Crohn's disease, Felty's syndrome, hepatitis (50% to 80% of clients, chronic), systemic lupus erythematosus (SLE), microscopic polyangiitis, primary sclerosing cholangitis (72% to 80% of clients), rheumatoid arthritis, ulcerative colitis (72% to 80% of clients).

Description. Neutrophils are very active in the body's immune defenses by releasing proteolytic enzymes to phagocytose bacteria. In conditions characterized by necrotizing vasculitis, antineutrophil cytoplasmic antibodies (ANCAs) are present. ANCAs are autoimmune antibodies directed against the lysosomal enzymes in neutrophil granules. ANCAs occur in two staining patterns. The p-ANCA stains in a perinuclear pattern, similar to that of the antinuclear antibodies. The c-ANCA demonstrates a classical granular cytoplasmic staining pattern. p-ANCA and c-ANCA are present in most (>90%) clients with systemic necrotizing vasculitis and in few clients with collagen-type vascular disease. Thus this test helps diagnose vasculitis. p-ANCA is also used to help diagnose inflammatory bowel or liver disease.

Professional Considerations
Consent form NOT required.

Preparation
1. Tube: Red topped.

Procedure
1. Collect a 3-ml blood sample.

Postprocedure Care
1. Deliver specimen to the laboratory. Separate and refrigerate serum until testing.
2. Specimens are tested by staining and then examining the slide for characteristic C and P patterns. When samples stain positive, they are then serially diluted to determine the titer.

Client and Family Teaching
1. Results are not usually available for 3-5 days.

Factors That Affect Results
1. Both IgM and IgG antibodies must be tested to avoid a false-negative result.
2. Results are unreliable if formalin is used to fix the slides.
3. Immunofluorescence titers usually, but do not always, decrease with remission.
4. Reject hemolyzed lipemic specimen.

Other Data
1. The c-ANCA sensitivity and specificity for Wegener's granulomatosis are 90% and 80%, respectively.
2. p-ANCA is also known as "UC-ANCA" and "X-ANCA."

Antinuclear Antibody (ANA)—Serum

Norm. Negative at 1:20 dilution.

Positive. Autoimmune pancreatitis, autoimmune thyroid disease, cancer (hepatic or pulmonary), dermatopolymyositis, hepatitis (chronic active, lupoid), mixed connective tissue disease, myasthenia gravis, polymyositis, pulmonary fibrosis (idiopathic), Raynaud's syndrome, rheumatoid arthritis, scleroderma, some healthy older adults, systemic lupus erythematosus (SLE), systemic sclerosis, and Sjögren's syndrome. Drugs include beta-adrenergic blockers, carbamazepine, lovastatin, methyldopa, nitrofurantoin sodium, penicillamine, and tocainide.

Description. Antinuclear antibodies are antibodies the body produces against its own DNA and nuclear material that cause tissue damage and characterize autoimmune diseases. Highest titers occur in SLE. The immunofluorescent procedure results in four characteristic staining patterns, which help differentiate the type of connective tissue disease. These patterns and their specificities include the homogeneous pattern specific for SLE and other connective diseases; the peripheral pattern specific for SLE; the speckled pattern specific for mixed connective disease, SLE, Sjögren's syndrome, polymyositis, dermatomyositis, and scleroderma; and the nucleolar pattern specific for scleroderma and Sjögren's syndrome. These patterns, however, are not diagnostic of the various diseases. If positive results are obtained, the anti-DNA test should be performed to aid differentiation of SLE.

Professional Considerations
Consent form NOT required.

Preparation
1. Tube: Red topped, red/gray topped, or gold topped.
2. List drug therapy on the laboratory requisition.
3. See Client and Family Teaching.

Procedure
1. Draw a 2-mL blood sample.

Postprocedure Care
1. Transport the specimen to the laboratory for immediate spinning.

Client and Family Teaching
1. Fast for 8 hours before sampling.
2. Results may not be available for several days if testing is not performed on site.

Factors That Affect Results
1. Reject hemolyzed specimens.
2. False-negative results may be caused by drug therapy with corticosteroids.
3. Drugs that may cause false-positive results from a drug-induced syndrome resembling SLE include acetazolamide, aminosalicylic acid, carbidopa, chlorothiazide, chlorpromazine, clofibrate, diphenylhydantoin, ethosuximide, gold salts, griseofulvin microsize, griseofulvin ultramicrosize, hydralazine hydrochloride, hydroxytryptophan, isoniazid, mephenytoin, methyldopa, methyldopate hydrochloride, methylthiouracil, methysergide maleate, oral contraceptives, penicillin, phenylbutazone, phenytoin, primidone, procainamide hydrochloride, propylthiouracil, quinidine gluconate, quinidine polygalacturonate, quinidine sulfate, reserpine, streptomycin sulfate, sulfadimethoxine, sulfonamides, tetracyclines, thiouracil, and trimethadione.
4. Pregnancy or therapeutic exposure to UV radiation can increase ANA levels.

Other Data
1. The peroxidase method may be used, but patterns are not obtained.
2. In children with musculoskeletal or dermatologic disease, the prognosis of children who have positive ANA test results in the absence of autoimmune conditions is excellent.
3. Persons more than 60 years of age have a 20% chance of a positive test.
4. Up to one third of first-degree relatives of clients with SLE have a positive ANA, though they are healthy.

Anti-Parietal Cell Antibody
See Parietal Cell Antibody—Blood.

Antiphospholipid Antibodies (APAs)—Serum

Norm. Negative.

Positive. Anticardiolipin syndrome (primary, secondary), antiphospholipid (Hughes syndrome), Behçet's disease, cerebral palsy, chorea, diabetic muscle infarction, epilepsy, essential thrombocythemia, giant cell arteritis, human immunodeficiency virus (HIV), in vitro fertilization and embryo transfer failures, moyamoya, polymyalgia rheumatica, preeclampsia, renal allograft failure, retinal occlusive vasculopathy, syphilis, temporal arteritis, thrombosis (systemic venous), varicella zoster virus infection. Drugs include minocycline.

Description. Antiphospholipid antibodies (APAs) constitute a family of immunoglobulins active against phospholipids. Phospholipids are complex triglyceride esters containing long-chain fatty acids, phosphoric acid, and nitrogenous bases. The group includes fatty compounds, such as lecithin, found in animal and plant cells. The APA family is composed of the anticardiolipin antibodies (ACAs), lupus anticoagulant (LA), and antibodies that cause biologic false-positive results in syphilis serologic tests. ACA and LA have been described as occurring in thromboses, autoimmune disease, infectious diseases, and neoplastic disease. An APA syndrome that occurs during pregnancy includes loss of the fetus, systemic thromboses, and thrombocytopenia. The pathophysiology of fetal loss is not clearly known, but several theories have been suggested. Clients with APA syndrome are treated with long-term oral anticoagulation therapy.

Professional Considerations
Consent form NOT required.

Preparation
1. Tube: Red topped, red/gray topped, or gold topped.

Procedure
1. Draw a 4-mL blood sample.

Postprocedure Care
1. None.

Client and Family Teaching
1. Results are normally available within 48 hours.
2. This test detects antibodies that bind to fatty substances in your body. It helps identify an illness called "antiphospholipid syndrome" or "anticardiolipin syndrome," in which the blood clots faster than normal. It is important to identify and treat this syndrome because it can lead to a greater risk for fetal death and a higher incidence of stroke, heart attack, and blindness.

Factors That Affect Results
1. Levels vary, depending on which commercial kit is used for this test, because the assays are not yet standardized.

Other Data
1. In women with previous fetal loss who have received prophylactic treatment during subsequent pregnancy, the live birth rate is 70%. Treatment has included antiplatelet drugs, immunosuppressives, and/or anticoagulants including combination therapy with aspirin and heparin.
2. Antiphospholipid antibodies are found in pediatric clients with SLE who have thrombotic events.

Antiplatelet Antibody

See Platelet Antibody—Blood.

Antiribonucleoprotein Test

See Anti-RNP Test—Diagnostic.

Anti-RNP Test (Antiribonucleoprotein Test, Extractable Nuclear Antigen)—Diagnostic

Norm. Negative or <20 units.

Inconclusive. 20-49 units.

Positive. ≥50 units.

Usage. Assists in differentiating the type of autoimmune disease occurring. Highest titers (≥1:10,000) are suggestive of mixed connective tissue disease such as Raynaud's phenomenon. Positive in cytomegalovirus infection, neonatal lupus erythematosus, Sjögren's syndrome, systemic lupus erythematosus.

Description. An antinuclear antibody present in over 94% of mixed connective tissue autoimmune disease detected by an immunofluorescent procedure. Immuno-fluorescence results in characteristic staining patterns that help differentiate the type of connective tissue disease occurring. Anti-RNP antibodies are associated with a speck-led pattern and occur in almost all clients with mixed connective tissue syndrome and about one fourth of clients with scleroderma and discoid and systemic lupus erythemato-sus. High titers are usually accompanied by clinical symptoms of mixed connective tissue disease. A positive test is specific for mixed connective tissue disease when results of other autoantibody testing are negative.

Professional Considerations
Consent form NOT required.

Preparation
1. Tube: Red topped, red/gray topped, or gold topped.
2. See Client and Family Teaching.

Procedure
1. Draw a 4-mL blood sample.

Postprocedure Care
1. Transport the specimen to the laboratory for immediate spinning.

Client and Family Teaching
1. Fast for 8 hours before sampling.
2. Results may not be available for several days if testing is not performed on site.

Factors That Affect Results
1. Reject hemolyzed, lipemic, or contami-nated specimens.
2. False-negative results may be caused by drug therapy with corticosteroids.
3. Drugs that may cause false-positive results because of a drug-induced syndrome resembling systemic lupus erythematosus (SLE) include acetazolamide, aminosalicylic acid, carbidopa, chlorothiazide, chlorprom-azine, clofibrate, diphenylhydantoin, etho-suximide, gold salts, griseofulvin microsize, griseofulvin ultramicrosize, hydralazine, hydrochloride, hydroxytryptophan, isonia-zid, mephenytoin, methyldopa, methyldo-pate hydrochloride, methyl-thiouracil, methysergide maleate, oral contraceptives, penicillin, phenylbutazone, phenytoin, primidone, procainamide hydrochloride, propylthiouracil, quinidine gluconate, quinidine polygalacturonate, quinidine sulfate, reserpine, streptomycin sulfate, sul-fadimethoxine, sulfonamides, tetracyclines, thiouracil, and trimethadione.

Other Data
1. Titer is determined by counterimmuno-electrophoresis (CIE).

Anti-Ro/SS-A Test—Diagnostic

Norm. Negative or <20 units.

Inconclusive. 20-49 units.

Positive. ≥50 units.

Positive. ANA-negative lupus, complete congenital heart block, neonatal lupus, polymyositis/dermatomyositis, and Sjögren's syndrome.

Description. Anti-Ro/SS-A is an autoanti-body to the cytoplasmic RNA Ro antigen characteristically found in high titers in clients with primary Sjögren's syndrome or Sjögren's syndrome with systemic lupus ery-thematosus (SLE). Although electrophoresis is the most sensitive testing method for detection of these antibodies, the most common method used is immunodiffusion. This test is used in the differential diagnosis of SLE, Sjögren's syndrome, and mixed connective tissue disease. The antibody is present in over 70% of Sjögren's syndrome, 30%-40% of SLE, and only 5%-10% of progressive systemic sclerosis.

Professional Considerations
Consent form NOT required.

Preparation
1. Tube: Red topped, red/gray topped, or gold topped.

Procedure
1. Draw a 4-mL blood sample.

Postprocedure Care
1. Send the specimen to the laboratory for immediate spinning.

Client and Family Teaching
1. Results may not be available for several days if testing is not performed on site.

Factors That Affect Results
1. Reject lipemic, hemolyzed, or contaminated specimens.

Other Data
1. This test is more sensitive but less specific for primary Sjögren's syndrome than the anti-La/SS-B test.
2. The presence of both anti-La/SS-B and anti-Ro/SS-A antibodies is generally associated with a milder form of SLE.
3. Clients who are positive for antinuclear antibody and who have SS-A, but not SS-B, are likely to have nephritis.
4. African-Americans are at increased risk for the presence of anti-Ro antibodies and SLE.

Anti-Sm Test (Extractable Nuclear Antigen)—Diagnostic

Norm. Negative.

Usage. Assists in differentiating the type of autoimmune disease occurring. The presence of antibodies specific against Sm is strongly suggestive of systemic lupus erythematosus (SLE) when other autoantibodies are negative. Increases in Sm antibody levels are seen in arthritis, heart-related diseases, Raynaud's phenomenon, and SLE.

Description. An antinuclear antibody active against acidic nuclear proteins, present in autoimmune disease detected by an immunofluorescent procedure. Immunofluorescence results in characteristic staining patterns that help differentiate the type of connective tissue disease occurring. Anti-Sm antibodies are associated with a speckled pattern and occur in clients with mixed connective tissue syndrome and in about one fourth of clients with scleroderma, discoid lupus erythematosus, and SLE.

Professional Considerations
Consent form NOT required.

Preparation
1. Tube: Red topped, red/gray topped, or gold topped.
2. See Client and Family Teaching.

Procedure
1. Draw a 4-mL blood sample.

Postprocedure Care
1. Send the specimen to the laboratory for immediate spinning.

Client and Family Teaching
1. Fast for 8 hours before sampling.
2. Results may not be available for several days if testing is not performed on site.

Factors That Affect Results
1. Reject hemolyzed, lipemic, or contaminated specimens.
2. False-negative results may be caused by drug therapy with corticosteroids.
3. Drugs that may cause false-positive results arising from a drug-induced syndrome resembling SLE include acetazolamide, aminosalicylic acid, carbidopa, chlorothiazide, chlorpromazine, clofibrate, diphenylhydantoin, ethosuximide, gold salts, griseofulvin microsize, griseofulvin ultramicrosize, hydralazine hydrochloride, hydroxytryptophan, infliximab, isoniazid, mephenytoin, methyldopa, methyldopate hydrochloride, methylthiouracil, methysergide maleate, oral contraceptives, penicillin, phenylbutazone, phenytoin, primidone, procainamide hydrochloride, propylthiouracil, quinidine gluconate, quinidine polygalacturonate, quinidine sulfate, reserpine, streptomycin sulfate, sulfadimethoxine, sulfonamides, tetracyclines, thiouracil, and trimethadione.

Other Data

1. There is a clinical association of this antibody titer with vasculitis.

2. Not useful as a screening test for lupus because results must be interpreted in consideration of other antibody testing.

Anti–Smooth Muscle Antibody—Serum

Norm. Negative at titer <1:20.

Increased. Asthma (intrinsic) (positive at titer <1:10), autoimmune hepatitis, biliary cirrhosis (positive at titer 1:10 to 1:40), chronic active (lupoid) hepatitis (majority of clients) (positive at titers of 1:80 to 1:320), cryptogenic cirrhosis (rare), hepatocellular carcinoma, malignancies, mononucleosis (infectious with liver damage), pancreatitis (autoimmune), tumors (infiltrative), viral hepatitis (acute) (positive at titers <1:10), yellow fever, and in clients 50 to 70 years of age. Drug includes minocycline.

Description. An immunofluorescent test that detects and measures autoimmune immunoglobulins (antibodies) in smooth muscle that occur in chronic active hepatitis and also in response to damaged liver cells. This test is usually performed with the test for antimitochondrial antibodies as an aid in differentiating primary biliary cirrhosis and chronic active hepatitis from diffuse, extrahepatic biliary obstruction and other liver diseases.

Professional Considerations

Consent form NOT required.

Preparation

1. Tube: Red topped, red/gray topped, or gold topped.
2. See Client and Family Teaching.

Procedure

1. Draw a 4-mL blood sample.

Postprocedure Care

1. Send the specimen to the laboratory for immediate spinning.

Client and Family Teaching

1. Fast for 8 hours before sampling.
2. Results may not be available for several days if testing is not performed on site.

Factors That Affect Results

1. Reject hemolyzed specimens.
2. Antinuclear antibody impairs interpretation of results.

Other Data

1. This test is not diagnostic. A liver biopsy is recommended.
2. Low titers may occur with infectious mononucleosis, rheumatoid arthritis, liver disease, and malignancies.

Antisperm Antibodies

See Infertility Screen—Specimen.

Antistreptococcal Enzyme

See Antistreptolysin-O Titer—Serum.

Antistreptolysin-O (ASO) Titer—Serum

Norm.

Adults	<330 IU/mL
Children	
<2 years	<200 IU/mL
2-5 years	<240 IU/mL
5-19	<330 IU/mL

A fourfold rise in titer between acute and convalescent specimens is diagnostically significant.

Increased. Acute poststreptococcal endocarditis, acute poststreptococcal glomerulonephritis (500-5000 Todd U/mL), pediatric autoimmune neuropsychiatric disorders associated with streptococcal infections (PANDAS), reactive arthritis, rheumatic fever (inactive is <250 Todd U/mL; active is 500-5000 Todd U/mL), scarlet fever, recent streptococcal disease (small elevations), Sydenham's chorea, Tourette's syndrome.

Decreased. Not clinically significant. Levels may decrease with antibiotic therapy.

Description. Antibody to the streptolysin-O enzyme produced by Lancefield group A beta-hemolytic streptococci. These titers rise about 7 days after infection, peak at 3-5 weeks, and then gradually return to baseline level over the next 6-12 months. Because ASO titers remain elevated in clients with post-streptococcal infections, the test is used to determine whether symptoms such as joint pains, rheumatic fever, or glomerulonephritis are of a poststreptococcal disease origin.

Professional Considerations
Consent form NOT required.

Preparation
1. Tube: Red topped, red/gray topped, or gold topped.

Procedure
1. Draw a 4-mL blood sample.
2. Draw a repeat titer in 10-14 days.

Postprocedure Care
1. Send the specimen to the laboratory for immediate spinning.

Client and Family Teaching
1. Repeated ASO titers every 10-14 days are recommended. When poststreptococcal

disease occurs, titers begin to rise 1 week after the initial streptococcal infection and peak 2-4 weeks later; 6 months to 1 year is required for postinfection levels to return to the baseline level.
2. Results may not be available for several days if testing is not performed on site.

Factors That Affect Results
1. Reject hemolyzed specimens.
2. Falsely suppressed results may be caused by nephrotic syndromes, antibody deficiency syndromes, or drug therapy with corticosteroids or antibiotics.
3. Falsely elevated results may be caused by contaminated serum, hyperbetalipoproteinemia, hypercholesterolemia, hyperglobulinemia, lipemic serum, or liver disorders.
4. The persistent presence of an antibody from a previous but not recent infection may mildly increase titers. Only very high titers are indicators of recent infection (such as adult, >250 Todd U; child, >333 Todd U).

Other Data
1. Up to 20% of clients with poststreptococcal glomerulonephritis may have normal titers. The anti-DNase-B test is recommended to improve specificity.
2. Increased C-reactive protein and ASO are some of the key factors in the development of chronic gingivitis.
3. See also Antihyaluronidase titer—Serum; Streptozyme—Blood.

Antithrombin III (AT-III) Test—Diagnostic

Norm.

		SI Units
Plasma	21-30 mg/dL	210-300 mg/L
	85-115% of standard >50% of control value	
Serum	15-35% lower than plasma values	0.85-1.15
Immunologic	17-30 mg/dL	
Functional	80-130%	

Increased. Factor deficiency (V, VII), hemophilia (A, B), hepatitis (acute), inflammation, jaundice (obstructive), menstruation, nephrotic syndrome, renal transplantation, vitamin K deficiency. Drugs include anabolic steroids, androgens, bishydroxycoumarin, gemfibrozil, oral contraceptives (containing progesterone), progesterone, and warfarin sodium.

Decreased. Alcoholic liver disease, arteriosclerosis, burns, carcinoma, cardiovascular disease, cerebrovascular accident, cirrhosis, congenital antithrombin III deficiency, deep vein thrombosis, dengue shock syndrome, diabetes mellitus (type II), disseminated intravascular coagulation, hepatic disease (abscess, hepatitis), homocystinuria, hyper-coagulation, liver failure (chronic), liver transplantation, malignancy (extensive), malnutrition, nephrotic syndrome, status post partial hepatectomy, postoperatively, postpartum, preeclampsia, pulmonary embolism, septicemia, thromboembolism, veno-occlusive disease (VOD). Drugs include estrogens, fibrinolytics, gestodene, heparin calcium, heparin sodium, L-asparaginase, methylprednisolone, and oral contraceptives (containing estrogen).

Description. A naturally occurring protein, IgG (immunoglobulin G), probably synthesized by the liver, that inhibits coagulation through inactivation of thrombin and other factors. The action of AT-III is catalyzed by heparin. Hereditary AT-III deficiency is an autosomal dominant disease that predisposes clients to venous thrombosis and heparin resistance.

Professional Considerations
Consent form NOT required.

Preparation
1. Tube: 2.7 or 4.5-mL blue topped.
2. See Client and Family Teaching.

Procedure
1. Draw 2.4 mL of blood for a 2.7-mL tube or 4.0 mL of blood for a 4.5-mL tube.

Postprocedure Care
1. Send the specimen to the laboratory for immediate spinning.

Client and Family Teaching
1. Fast, except for water, for 10-12 hours before testing.

Factors That Affect Results
1. Reject hemolyzed, lipemic, or contaminated specimens.
2. Results are normally available within 3-5 days.

Other Data
1. Levels of 50% to 75% indicate moderate risk for thrombosis, whereas levels under 50% indicate significant risk for thrombosis.
2. A low level in clients taking warfarin indicates that the warfarin is not working effectively.
3. AT-III is positively correlated to hematoma volume in hypertensive intracerebral hemorrhage (HICH).

Antithyroglobulin Antibody
See Thyroid Antithyroglobulin Antibody—Serum.

Antithyroid Microsomal Antibody
See Thyroid Peroxidase Antibody—Blood.

Apexcardiography (ACG)—Diagnostic

Norm. Normal a wave, c point, e point, o point, rf wave, f point, sf wave, and stasis.

Cardiac Abnormalities	Changes That May Be Found in Apexcardiographic Recording
Aortic valve stenosis	Large a wave; apical impulse occurring late in systole
Atrial fibrillation	Absent a wave; steepened slope of rf wave
Cardiac failure	Apical impulse occurring late in systole
Coronary artery disease	Apical impulse occurring late in systole
Mitral regurgitation	Steepened slope of rf wave
Mitral stenosis	Absent a wave; shallow slope of rf wave
Hypertension	Large a wave; apical impulse occurring late in systole

Continued

Cardiac Abnormalities	Changes That May Be Found in Apexcardiographic Recording
Idiopathic hypertrophy	Large a wave subaortic stenosis
Left ventricular aneurysm	Apical impulse occurring late in systole
Myocardial ischemia or pericarditis	Apical impulse occurring late in systole infarction; steepened slope of rf wave

Usage. Helps diagnose heart abnormalities and arterial hypertension. In conjunction with phonocardiography, helps to identify heart sounds.

Description. Apexcardiography is a method to transfer cardiac movement and pulsations into electrical energy by a transducer and produce a graphic recording of waveforms that characterize the status of the heart. The test takes less than $\frac{1}{2}$ hour to perform.

Professional Considerations
Consent form NOT required.

Preparation
1. Remove jewelry and any metal objects.
2. The client should disrobe above the waist.

Procedure
1. The client is placed in a left oblique position, and electrocardiographic limb leads are applied. The transducer tip, covered with electroconductive gel, is strapped in place in contact with the point of maximum impulse at the apex of the heart.
2. Apexcardiographic recordings are made as the client lies motionless and performs

isometric hand-clenching exercises, which increase systemic vascular resistance.

Postprocedure Care
1. Remove transducer and limb leads. Cleanse the electroconductive gel off the transducer and off the client's chest.

Client and Family Teaching
1. The test is painless.
2. Slow, even respirations promote the most accurate test results. You should not talk or move during the procedure.
3. You will be asked to isometrically clench your fists, which means clenching them and then squeezing them and holding them tightly shut.

Factors That Affect Results
1. Implantable metal devices in the chest wall, such as venous access devices, do not interfere with the test as long as leads are not placed directly over the metal device.

Other Data
1. This test is rarely used due to the availability of echocardiogram and nuclear medicine testing.

Apnea Hypopnea Index

See **Polysomnography**—Diagnostic.

Apnea Test—Diagnostic

Negative test (absence of brain death). Spontaneous respiratory effort occurs after mechanical ventilation is stopped.

Positive test (presence of brain death). Absence of spontaneous respiratory effort throughout test (up to 8 minutes for adults and up to 15 minutes for pediatrics), $Paco_2$ ≥60 mm Hg or 20 mm Hg higher than baseline value.

Usage. Determination of the absence (or presence) of spontaneous breathing when one is testing for brain death; evaluation of the intracranial hemodynamic status in carotid occlusive disease.

Description. The apnea test is part of a neurologic evaluation that tests for the respiratory reflex in clients suspected of having brain death. It is performed with a full neurologic examination, clinical history that includes a central nervous system event, and other confirmatory tests to determine brain death. Brain death is the term used when the entire brain, including the brainstem, has irreversibly stopped functioning. Brain death cannot be determined in clients receiving neuromuscular blockers, or with low core-body temperatures (such as ≤32.2 degrees C).

Professional Considerations
Consent form recommended from spokesperson for the client.

Risks
Cardiac arrest, pneumoperitoneum, pneumothorax.

Contraindications
Use for purposes other than those described in the previous discussion is contraindicated.

Preparation
1. Obtain and document baseline $Paco_2$ value.
2. Determine if client meets requirements for apnea testing:
   i. $Pco_2 = 40$ mm Hg
   ii. Mean arterial pressure (MAP) >54 mm Hg
   iii. Positive fluid balance in previous 6 hours
   iv. Absence of the possibility of acute drug or alcohol intoxication
   v. Absence of the presence of any centrally acting drugs that could depress respiration
3. Obtain a pulse oximeter, ice, oxygen T-piece, and arterial blood gas kit.

Procedure
1. Position pulse oximetry probe on client. Set heart rate, blood pressure, and respiratory rate alarms. Monitor all throughout the test.
2. Preoxygenate client with 100% oxygen for 10 minutes.
3. Remove client's gown or clothing from the chest and abdominal area to allow visualization of respiratory muscle efforts.
4. Discontinue mechanical ventilation. Apply oxygen through a T-piece at 6 L/min. Monitor for spontaneous respiratory effort.
   i. If no respiratory effort is noted after 5-8 minutes, obtain an arterial blood gas sample and restart mechanical ventilation.
   ii. Observe chest for spontaneous respirations or any respiratory effort.
   iii. Discontinue the test if any of the following occur:
      (1) Presence of spontaneous respiratory effort
      (2) Hemodynamic instability
5. Test is repeated at least 6-12 hours later.

Postprocedure Care
1. Document procedure, including methodology, length of apneic time, baseline and ending $Paco_2$ values, stability of vital signs, and apneic status.
2. For positive tests, request organ donation, as and when appropriate.

Client and Family Teaching
1. Organ and tissue donation rates are higher when families or significant others receive a careful and thorough explanation of the concept of brain death.

Factors That Affect Results
1. $Paco_2$ rises approximately 3 mm Hg each minute while the client is apneic and not receiving mechanical ventilation.
2. Results must be interpreted with extreme caution in clients with brain injury. Caution should be used in determining brain death when the cause of the brain injury is not known and in high cervical spine fracture in which there is damage to the spinal cord.
3. Posturing may make detection of respiratory effort impossible.

Other Data
1. The neurologic examination in brain death reveals the absence of spontaneous reflexes, absence of response to pain, and absence of brainstem reflexes, including the respiratory reflex.

Apolipoprotein A-I (Apoprotein-A, Apo-A)—Plasma

Norm. Values are 5% to 10% higher in African-Americans.

	Female		Male	
Age	mg/dL	SI Units (g/L)	mg/dL	SI Units (g/L)
Adult				
20-29 years	80-184	0.80-1.84	81-153	0.81-1.53
30-39 years	83-187	0.83-1.87	79-155	0.79-1.55
40-49 years	93-181	0.93-1.81	100-140	1.00-1.40
50-59 years	76-204	0.76-2.04	81-169	0.81-1.69
60-65 years	122-214	1.22-2.14	86-166	0.86-1.66
Child				
Birth	38-106	0.38-1.06	41-93	0.41-0.93
0.5-4 years	60-148	0.60-1.48	67-163	0.67-1.63
5-7 years	90-151	0.90-1.51	92-151	0.92-1.51
8-9 years	94-151	0.94-1.51	96-151	0.96-1.51
10-11 years	92-151	0.92-1.51	96-151	0.96-1.51
12-13 years	83-146	0.83-1.46	88-151	0.88-1.51
14-15 years	96-146	0.96-1.46	85-139	0.85-1.39
16-17 years	96-151	0.96-1.51	83-146	0.83-1.46

	Apolipoprotein B/A Ratio	
Coronary Atherosclerotic Risk	Female	Male
Average risk	0.6	0.7
Two times average risk	0.9	0.9
Three times average risk	1.0	1.0

Increased. Not clinically significant. Familial hyperalphalipoproteinemia. Drugs include carbamazepine, chlorinated hydrocarbons, clofibrate, deflazacort, estrogen, ethyl alcohol, exercise, gemfibrozil, hormone replacement therapy of conjugated estrogen and medroxyprogesterone or 17-beta-estradiol/desogestrel, lovastatin, niacin, oral contraceptives (containing estrogen), phenobarbital, phenytoin, pravastatin, simvastatin, weight-reduction diet. Ingestion of beef increases apolipoprotein A-I.

Decreased. Alzheimer's disease, atherosclerosis, cholestasis, coronary artery disease, diabetes mellitus (poorly controlled), hepatectomy, hepatocellular abnormalities, hypertriglyceridemia, hypoalphalipoproteinemia, ischemic coronary disease, lipoprotein lipase cofactor deficiency, myocardial infarction, nephrotic syndrome, polycystic ovary syndrome (PCOS), renal failure (chronic), stroke. Drugs include androgens, beta-adrenergic receptor blocking agents, diuretics, probucol, progestins, and Synthroid.

Description. An inherited alpha$_1$-globulin that is the major protein component (70%) of high-density lipoprotein (HDL). It is synthesized in the liver and small intestine and is essential for the transport of peripheral cholesterol to the liver for eventual excretion. Variants of the APOA1 gene have been linked to several types of amyloidosis. Calculation of the ratio of apolipoprotein A-I to apolipoprotein B and plasma levels of apo A-I are the strongest predictors, more useful than HDL cholesterol level, for identifying clients at risk for coronary artery disease.

Professional Considerations
Consent form NOT required.

Preparation
1. Tube: Red topped, red/gray topped, or gold topped.
2. Several testing methods are used to measure apolipoprotein A-I. Clarify the proper blood-drawing procedure with the individual laboratory.
3. See Client and Family Teaching.

Procedure
1. Draw a 4-mL blood sample.

Postprocedure Care
1. None.

Client and Family Teaching
1. Fast for 12 hours before testing.
2. Refrain from smoking for 4 hours before testing.
3. A ratio of apolipoprotein A to apolipoprotein B is sometimes used to predict risk of coronary heart disease.

Factors That Affect Results
1. Reject hemolyzed or lipemic specimens.
2. Apolipoprotein A-I levels rise during acute illness.
3. Levels are decreased in smokers and in clients who consume high-carbohydrate or high–polyunsaturated fat diets.

Other Data
1. Apolipoprotein levels remain stable after acute ischemic stroke.

Apolipoprotein B (Apoprotein B, Apo B)—Plasma

Norm.

	Female		Male	
Age	mg/dL	SI Units (g/L)	mg/dL	SI Units (g/L)
Adult	86-159	0.86-1.59	96-174	0.96-1.74
Child				
Birth	11-31	0.11-0.31	11-31	0.11-0.31
0.5-4 years	23-75	0.23-0.75	23-75	0.23-0.75
5-7 years	49-110	0.49-1.10	47-106	0.47-1.06
8-9 years	53-132	0.53-1.32	49-105	0.49-1.05
10-11 years	54-121	0.54-1.21	52-110	0.52-1.10
12-13 years	46-110	0.46-1.10	46-113	0.46-1.13
14-15 years	41-108	0.41-1.08	44-103	0.44-1.03
16-17 years	41-96	0.41-0.96	48-139	0.48-1.39

	Apolipoprotein B/A Ratio	
Coronary Atherosclerotic Risk	Female	Male
Average risk	0.6	0.7
Two times average risk	0.9	0.9
Three times average risk	1.0	1.0

Increased. Acute illness, Alzheimer's disease, angina pectoris, anorexia nervosa, cigarette smokers, coronary heart disease (premature), Cushing's syndrome, diabetes mellitus, dysglobulinemia, hepatic disease and obstruction, hypercalcemia (infantile), hyperlipemia (familial combined), hypothyroidism, myocardial infarction, nephrotic syndrome, porphyria, pregnancy, renal failure, sexual ateliotic dwarfism, sphingolipodystrophies, stress (emotional), and Werner's syndrome.

Decreased. Alpha-lipoprotein deficiency, anemia (chronic), hepatocellular dysfunction, heterozygous hypobetalipoproteinemia, hyperlipoproteinemia (type I), hyperthyroidism, joint inflammation, lecithin-cholesterol acyltransferase deficiency, lipoprotein lipase cofactor deficiency, malabsorption, malnutrition, myeloma, pulmonary disease (chronic), Reye's syndrome, stress (acute physical), weight-reduction diet. Drugs include orlistat (Xenical), levothyroxine (Synthroid).

Description. A beta-globulin that is the major protein component of low-density lipoprotein (LDL) and is also found in very-low-density lipoprotein (VLDL). Functions in cholesterol synthesis and is required for the secretion into plasma of intestinal and hepatic triglyceride-rich lipoproteins. There are two Apo B glycoproteins, Apo B-48 and

Apo B-100, which have different molecular weights. Apo B-48 is produced in the small intestine and Apo B-100 is produced in the liver. Calculation of the ratio of apolipoprotein A-I to apolipoprotein B is believed to be more useful than LDL cholesterol level for identifying clients at risk for atherosclerosis.

Professional Considerations
Consent form NOT required.

Preparation
1. Tube: Red topped, red/gray topped, or gold topped.
2. Several testing methods are used to measure apolipoprotein B. Clarify the proper blood-drawing procedure with the individual laboratory.
3. See Client and Family Teaching.

Procedure
1. Draw a 4-mL blood sample.

Postprocedure Care
1. None.

Client and Family Teaching
1. Fast for 12 hours before testing.
2. A ratio of apolipoprotein A to apolipoprotein B is sometimes used to predict coronary risk of heart disease.

Factors That Affect Results
1. Reject hemolyzed or lipemic specimens.
2. Apolipoprotein B levels rise during acute illness.

Other Data
1. Garlic has no effect on apolipoprotein levels.

Apolipoprotein E-4 (Apo E-4) Genotyping—Plasma

Norm. Apo E-4 allele is not present.

Usage. Helps identify risk for, but cannot confirm, Alzheimer's disease, because the disease also occurs in those not carriers or homozygotes. Genotyping more recently piloted for determination of risk of developing Alzheimer's disease through the National Institutes of Health. NOT useful for monitoring disease progression.

Description. Alzheimer's disease, the most common form of dementia, is characterized by the presence of senile plaques and neurofibrillary tangles. Two forms of Alzheimer's disease are known to exist. The majority (90% to 95%) are termed "late onset," with the remaining 5% to 10% termed "early onset." Human apolipoprotein E is a gene involved in lipoprotein, triglyceride, and cholesterol metabolism and its lipid transport protein helps to repair membranes of central and peripheral nervous system cells. Apolipoprotein E has several genetic variations, one being the apolipoprotein (Apo) E-4 allele. The Apo E4 allele is an important genetic risk factor for late-onset Alzheimer's disease, occurring more than twice as often in those with Alzheimer's disease as in control groups. The exact mechanism by which the Apo E-4 allele contributes to the development of Alzheimer's disease is not known, but there is some evidence that its action contributes to the development of plaques and neurofibrillary tangles, as well as to the loss of brain tissue volume. Carriers of the Apo E-4 allele can have up to 2.9 times greater chance and homozygotes can have up to 15 times greater chance than noncarriers of developing Alzheimer's disease. This test has low sensitivity and specificity.

Professional Considerations
Informed consent is recommended for genetic testing.

Preparation
1. Tube: Green topped.

Procedure
1. Draw a 4-mL blood sample.

Postprocedure Care
1. None.

Client and Family Teaching
1. Results are normally available in 1-2 weeks.
2. Refer the client with abnormal results for genetic counseling. Refer to section in this book on "Informed Consent for Genetic Testing".

Factors That Affect Results
1. Heparin in the specimen collection tube must be sodium heparin.

Other Data
1. This test is currently available for research and experimental purposes.

2. The Genetic Information Nondiscrimination Act of 2008 prohibits health plans from using genetic family history or genetic test results from influencing eligibility or premiums for health insurance. It also prohibits employers from using this information to influence decisions about hiring, terminating employment, or employment pay, promotions or privileges.

APTT

See Activated Partial Thromboplastin Time and Partial Thromboplastin Time—Plasma.

Arsenic—Blood, Hair, Nails or Urine

Norm.

		SI Units
Whole Blood		
Normal	2-23 µg/L	0.03-0.31 µmol/L
Chronic poisoning	100-500 µg/L	1.33-6.65 µmol/L
Acute poisoning	>600 µg/L	>7.98 µmol/L
Serum	1.7-1.54 µg/L	0.02-0.20 µmol/L
Hair		
Normal levels	20-60µg/100g	<8.7 nmol/g
Chronic poisoning	>100µg/100g	>13.4 nmol/g
Nails		
Normal levels	20-60µg/100g	<8.7 nmol/g
Chronic poisoning	90-180µg/100g	12-24 nmol/g
Urine		
Normal 24 hours	0-35 µg/L or µmol/day	5-50 µg/L or 0-50 ug/day
Chronic poisoning	0.67-66.50 µmol/L	50-5000 µg/L
Acute poisoning	>13.3 µmol/L	>1000 µg/L

Acute Poisoning Symptoms and Treatment

Symptoms. Abdominal pain, nausea, vomiting, bloody diarrhea, thirst progressing to dehydration and fluid and electrolyte imbalance, hematuria, metallic taste, pain (gastrointestinal), renal failure, jaundice, hypoxia, convulsions, coma, and respiratory and cardiovascular collapse. May lead to death.

Treatment

NOTE: Treatment choice(s) depend(s) on client's history and condition and episode history.

1. Induce emesis.
2. Lavage GI tract.
3. Administer saline cathartic.
4. Administer penicillamine chelation.
5. Administer dimercaprol (BAL).
6. Support hemodynamic status.
7. Replace blood lost to GI hemorrhage.
8. Both hemodialysis and peritoneal dialysis WILL remove arsenic.

Chronic Poisoning Symptoms and Treatment

Symptoms. Abnormal erythropoiesis and myelopoiesis, alopecia (thinning of hair), anemia, basophilic stippling, delirium, diarrhea, gastrointestinal symptoms, hepatomegaly, hyperkeratosis of palms of hands and soles of feet, leukopenia, macular hypopigmentation, Mees' lines, metallic taste, peripheral neuropathy, rain drop–like skin pigmentation changes and scaling, and thrombocytopenia.

Treatment

NOTE: Treatment choice(s) depend(s) on client's history and condition and episode history.

1. Avoid exposure to arsenic.
2. Remove household sources of arsenic (described below).

Increased. Arsenic poisoning and heavy-metal poisoning/environmental exposure to arsenic, blackfoot disease, peripheral vascular disease. Herbs or natural remedies include Korean herbal medicines usually prescribed for hemorrhoids, powdered blend of folk remedies of Hmong people from Thailand, and Indian ethnic remedies for treatment of congenital retinoblastoma.

Decreased. Not clinically significant.

Description. Arsenic is a trace element found in all human tissues. It is also a common heavy-metal poison that combines with intracellular proteins and is rapidly removed from the blood. It may become elevated when occupational (treated wood), environmental (coal burning), or intentional usage occurs. Sixty-three percent of ingested arsenic is excreted in the urine. Arsenic is found environmentally in well water and as an ingredient of pesticides, paints, treated wood, cosmetics, and antiprotozoal medications. Arsenic inhibits sulfhydryl enzyme systems required for cellular metabolism. Workplace exposure or chronic ingestion is associated with skin, lung and other cancers

Blood specimens are used for rapid confirmation of acute poisoning and blood levels are transitory. Because it can be found in keratin, specimens of hair and nails are used to pinpoint chronic exposure to arsenic. Urine specimens are used for rapid confirmation of acute poisoning and monitoring ongoing exposure.

Professional Considerations

Consent form NOT required unless the specimen may be used for legal evidence.

Preparation

1. For blood test: Tube: Black topped or green topped (whole blood) or red topped, red/gray topped, or gold topped (serum). Also obtain a blue topped tube containing Na_2 EDTA.
2. Do NOT draw during hemodialysis.
3. For hair or nails specimen collection: Obtain scissors or nail clippers and metal-free container.
4. Screen client for the use of herbal preparations or natural remedies such as Korean red or white ginseng (Panax).

Procedure

1. The specimen should be collected and labeled in the presence of a witness if it may be used for legal evidence.
2. Draw a 10-mL blood sample. Draw a second sample in the blue topped tube to use for confirmatory testing of trace elements.
3. Hair: Collect 0.5 g of hair from the area below the posterior crown of the head. Cut a ¼-inch-wide section close to the scalp. Trim off the proximal ½ inch into the metal-free container.
4. Nails: Clip the ends of all 10 toenails. Collect a total of 1 g of nails (preferably toenails) in a heavy, metal-free plastic container.
5. Urine: Collect a 24-hour urine sample in a 3-L container without preservatives.
   a. Discard the first morning-urine specimen. Save all urine voided in the 24-hour period, and urinate before defecating to avoid loss of urine. If any urine is accidentally discarded, discard the entire specimen and restart the collection the next day.
   b. Document the quantity of urine output during the collection period. Include urine voided at the end of the 24-hour period. For catheterized clients, keep the drainage bag on ice and empty the urine into the collection container hourly.

Postprocedure Care

1. Note the exact time of specimen collection, along with the client's name, date, contents, and your signature on the tube label and laboratory requisition.
2. Have the witness sign the laboratory requisition.
3. Transport the specimen to the laboratory in a sealed plastic bag labeled as legal evidence if that is the case. Have each person handling the specimen write his or her name and time of receipt of the specimen on the laboratory requisition.

Client and Family Teaching

1. For intentional poisoning, refer the client and family for crisis intervention.
2. For chronic poisoning, the client should be taught to remove household sources of arsenic (described above).
3. Hair or nails test results are normally available after several days.

Factors That Affect Results

1. A diet rich in seafood may elevate the blood level and may show elevated concentration levels in the urine as high as 500-1500 mg/L with no apparent signs of toxicity.
2. Arsenic in toenails represents deposition of arsenic for 6 months.
3. The earliest detection of excess arsenic in hair is 2 weeks after a dose of arsenic and may persist for months or years.
4. A 10-fold increase in well water concentrations is reflected in a 2-fold increase in toenail concentration.

5. Hyperbilirubinemia and increased serum ALP are found in conjunction with arsenic in the urine.

Other Data

1. Arsenic is easily transferred to a fetus.
2. Symptoms of chronic toxicity include fatigue, weakness, diarrhea, weight loss, dermatitis, and nausea progressing to paralysis, encephalopathy, renal and hepatic damage, and respiratory tract inflammation.
3. Children exposed to high levels of arsenic in drinking water have a health risk.

ART

See **Automated Reagin Test**—Diagnostic.

Arterial Blood Gases

See **Blood Gases, Arterial**—Blood.

Arteriogram—Diagnostic

Norm. Even filling of the arteries with radiographic dye. The artery walls show progressive narrowing without abrupt occlusions, isolated bulging, or narrow areas. No evidence of leakage of the dye into tissues, which would indicate hemorrhage. No evidence of vascular anomalies. No displacement of vessels.

Usage. Aids diagnosis of arterial occlusion, aneurysm, abnormal vascular development, hemorrhage and transient ischemia attacks (TIAs). Helps identify areas of arterial narrowing caused by plaque buildup, degree of stenosis after myocardial infarction (MI), tumor, or vascular abnormalities. Useful preoperatively to help identify potential failing arterial bypass grafts.

Description. An arteriogram is a radiographic examination of arteries through which radiographic contrast medium is flowing. The arteries are assessed for abnormalities in blood flow, such as narrowing or outpouching of the walls, and for collateral circulation.

Professional Considerations

Consent form IS required.

Risks

Aphasia, cerebrovascular accident, dysrhythmias, embolus, endocarditis, hematoma, hemiplegia, hemorrhage, infection, MI, paresthesia, allergic reaction to dye (itching, hives, rash, tight feeling in the throat, shortness of breath, bronchospasm, anaphylaxis, death), renal toxicity.

Contraindications

Anticoagulant therapy, bleeding disorders, thrombocytopenia, dehydration, uncontrolled hypertension, previous allergy to radiographic dye, iodine, or shellfish, renal insufficiency, and pregnancy (if iodinated contrast medium is used, because of radioactive iodine crossing the blood-placental barrier).

Preparation

1. See Client and Family Teaching.
2. Obtain baseline CBC, PT, and APTT values.
3. Remove all jewelry and metal objects.
4. The client should void just before the procedure.
5. Obtain baseline vital signs, and mark peripheral pulses.

6. Have emergency equipment readily available for anaphylaxis and cardiac arrest.
7. Just before beginning the procedure, take a "time out" to verify the correct client, procedure and site.

Procedure

1. Client is placed supine on the radiograph table.
2. A maintenance intravenous line is started.
3. The peripheral pulses are marked, and the extremity is immobilized.
4. The femoral or brachial artery area is located and cleansed with povidone-iodine solution and allowed to dry, and the surrounding area is covered with a sterile drape.
5. A local anesthetic (1% to 2% lidocaine) is injected intradermally and subcutaneously over the artery.
6. The femoral or brachial artery is punctured with a large-bore needle. A wire is passed through the needle and the needle removed over the guidewire.
7. The catheter is then inserted into the artery over the guidewire, and placement is confirmed by fluoroscopy.
8. The catheter is advanced under fluoroscopy to a location depending on the area to be examined, and radiographic dye is injected.
9. Several rapid radiographic pictures are taken of the artery and its branches during and after dye injection.
10. The catheter is removed, and sterile gauze is applied immediately, with pressure, to the site for at least 15 minutes.

Postprocedure Care

1. Apply pressure dressing to arterial puncture site.
2. The client remains on bed rest with the affected extremity immobilized for 12 hours.
3. Assess the site and dressing for hematoma or bleeding; the distal pulses for presence and strength; and color, motion, temperature, and sensation of the affected extremity every 15 minutes × 4, every half hour × 4, then every hour × 4, and then every 4 hours.
4. Apply pressure for at least 15 minutes if bleeding occurs.
5. Encourage oral intake of fluids if not contraindicated.

Client and Family Teaching

1. If the abdominal vasculature is to be examined, a cathartic may be administered 1 day before the test and a tap-water enema may be given on the morning of the test.
2. Consume clear liquids only for 24 hours and fast from food and fluids for 8 hours before the test.
3. It is normal to experience a brief flushing sensation and possibly nausea when the dye is injected, but the feeling will pass quickly.
4. It is important to lie still throughout the procedure.
5. Bed rest and frequent site and extremity checks are performed as standard postprocedure care.
6. In women who are breast-feeding, formula should be substituted for breast milk for 1 or more days after the procedure.

Factors That Affect Results

1. Movement of the client during filming may obscure the pictures.

Other Data

1. Clients with cardiomegaly need to be monitored carefully during this procedure or assessed to see if this procedure is fundamentally necessary.
2. Odds of receiving this test are lower for Hispanics when compared to non-Hispanic Caucasian counterparts.
3. See also Cardiac catheterization—Diagnostic; Cerebral angiogram—Diagnostic; Pulmonary angiogram—Diagnostic; or Renal angiogram—Diagnostic.

Arthrography—Diagnostic

Norm. Intact soft-tissue structures of the joint. Absence of lesions, fractures, or tears.

Usage. Detection of damage to joint connective tissue and structures (that is, adhesions, tears, fractures). Specific for full-thickness triangular fibrocartilage tears, rotator cuff tears, and ankle ligament visualization. Ganglion cyst.

Description. Arthrography involves fluoroscopic and radiographic examination of a joint after an injection into the joint of air or radiographic dye. Arthrography provides better visualization of the connective tissue of joints than routine radiography. It is most commonly used to view the knees and shoulders but may also be performed on other joints such as the ankle, hip, wrist, or temporomandibular joint.

Professional Considerations
Consent form IS required.

Risks
Allergic reaction to dye (itching, hives, rash, tight feeling in the throat, shortness of breath, bronchospasm, anaphylaxis, death), renal toxicity; bleeding, hematoma, or infection at injection site.

Contraindications
Previous allergy to iodine, seafood, or radiographic dye; pregnancy; active rheumatoid arthritis; infection of the joint to be studied; pregnancy (if iodinated contract medium is used, because of crossing the blood-placental barrier).

Preparation
1. Obtain a sterile arthrography tray, povidone-iodine solution, and 1% to 2% lidocaine.
2. Have emergency equipment readily available.
3. See Client and Family Teaching.
4. Just before beginning the procedure, take a "time out" to verify the correct client, procedure, and site.

Procedure
1. The skin is cleansed with povidone-iodine solution and allowed to dry.
2. A local anesthetic (1%-2% lidocaine) is injected subdermally and subcutaneously around the site to be punctured.

3. A needle is inserted into the joint space, and a small amount of contrast dye is injected through it as placement is checked under fluoroscopy.
4. After correct placement is confirmed, the remainder of the dye is injected and the needle withdrawn.
5. The extremity may be moved briefly through a range of motion, and then several fluoroscopic films are taken of the joint in different positions.

Postprocedure Care
1. Minimize use of the joint for 12 hours.
2. For knee arthrography, an elastic wrap should be worn over the knee for 3-4 days.

Client and Family Teaching
1. Fast from food and fluids for 8 hours before the procedure.
2. Some mild pain and pressure will be felt during the procedure, but local anesthesia will be used to keep these sensations tolerable.
3. Postarthrography edema and tenderness occur frequently for 1-2 days and may be treated with ice packs and mild analgesia. Symptoms lasting more than 2 days necessitate a physician's assessment.
4. If air injection was used, it is normal to feel crepitus in the joint for up to 2 days, because air remains in the joint space until it dissolves into the tissues. The air causes a popping or cracking sensation when the joint moves.

Factors That Affect Results
1. Fluid in the joint space decreases the quality of the films caused by dilution of the dye. If present, it should be aspirated before dye injection.

Other Data
1. Arthrography is 100% specific and 85% sensitive for detection of full-thickness triangular fibrocartilage tears.
2. MRI and arthrography have similar diagnostic values.

Arthropod Identification—Specimen

Norm. Requires interpretation.

Usage. Insect bites.

Description. There are over 1 million species in the phylum Arthropoda, including flies, mosquitos, fleas, lice, itch mites (producing scabies), mites, maggots, bedbugs, spiders, cockroaches, termites, ticks, bees, wasps, and scorpions. Specimens are usually presented for identification after a human

A

has been bitten by or infested with them. Arthropod bites may cause a variety of wheals, rashes, or anaphylactic reactions in humans.

Professional Considerations
Consent form NOT required.

Preparation
1. Obtain alcohol wipes, tweezers, and a container of 70% alcohol.

Procedure
1. Capture and preserve the arthropod in a sealed container of 70% alcohol. If the arthropod is a tick, rub the tick and site with an alcohol wipe. Then, holding the tick close to the skin with tweezers, pull the tick straight out and apply gentle pulling, without twisting, until the tick lets loose from the skin.
2. Wash fly larvae in water and then boil for a few minutes before placing in 70% alcohol.

Postprocedure Care
1. Transport the specimen to the laboratory.

Client and Family Teaching
1. For an arthropod bite or sting, swelling and itching can be controlled by placement of a cold washcloth or towel over the site for 20 minutes once per hour. Change to warm washcloths after 1-2 days.
2. Pain can be reduced by application of a paste of water and baking soda to the site for 5-10 minutes.
3. Itching can be controlled with calamine lotion.
4. Use insect repellent whenever venturing into grassy or wooded areas.
5. The main concern with flea bites is secondary infection. Therefore keep fingernails short to avoid scratching. Bathe in a tub of water filled with 1 kg of starch, apply calamine lotion to skin, and take antihistamines as prescribed. If an infection develops, antibiotics such as neomycin or polymyxin may be prescribed.
6. For head lice:
   i. To avoid transmitting head lice:
      a. Do not allow your head to come into close proximity with that of another person.
      b. During active infestation, rinse hairbrushes and combs off after use,

to wash away any lice. Avoid sharing hairbrushes or combs, because they may forcibly remove healthy head lice, which can reinfest for up to 24 hours.
   ii. It is not necessary to wash or "disinfest" clothing or linen. This advice is common, but mistaken, and applies only to clothing lice, which are found only on clothes and not on the body. Healthy head lice do not disperse except when scraped off (such as by combing) or when moving directly to another person's head. Shedding on linen occurs only when they are dying.

Factors That Affect Results
1. None.

Other Data
1. Spiders: Two venomous spiders are the brown recluse and the black widow spiders, which are more common in the southern United States. The redleg spider of Florida may also produce symptoms of poisoning. Treatment includes slow intravenous administration of 10 mL of 10% calcium gluconate and a muscle relaxant such as diazepam. A commercially prepared antivenom for the black widow, though rarely needed, is available in vials of 6000 U diluted in 2.5 mL of sterile water and given intramuscularly or intravenously.
2. A generalized systemic reaction to bee, wasp, and ant stings is believed to be IgE mediated. Treatment includes epinephrine hydrochloride 1:1000, 0.3-0.5 mL for an adult and 0.01 mL/kg for a child, prednisone orally to reduce swelling, and diphenhydramine hydrochloride, 25-50 mg orally, to relieve itching. "Killer bees" envenomation can cause acute tubular necrosis and death.
3. Lice or itch mites (producing scabies), frequently found in hair on the head or on the hands, feet, and pubic hair, require a thorough application of gamma-benzene hexachloride (Kwell, GBH) cream or lotion. Because GBH is toxic, it is questionable whether it should be used for young children or pregnant women. Some references recommend treatment only if a live louse is found.

4. The puss caterpillar, found in the southeastern United States, especially Texas and Florida, can cause shocklike signs and symptoms, as well as skin necrosis, edematous infiltration, and major fibrinogenolysis. Treatment includes immediate removal of the stinger. This may be followed by slow intravenous administration of 10 mL of 10% calcium gluconate and a muscle relaxant such as diazepam.

5. Mosquitoes are known carriers of yellow fever.

6. Dust mites are retained, thereby increasing allergy symptoms, by larger carpet surfaces, fluorocarbon-treated fibers, and carpets with low pile.

Arthroscopy—Diagnostic

Norm. Internal anatomy of the joint space is undisturbed. Synovial fluid is clear. Synovial membranes are not erythematous. There are no free-floating materials within the joint space.

Usage. Diagnostic use of the procedure is mainly to determine the cause of chronic arthritic complaints that cannot be established with serologic tests. The therapeutic use of the procedure involves the treatment of various acute and chronic arthritic conditions (including the management of septic arthritis and the treatment of torn ligaments) that would otherwise require arthrotomy.

Description. A diagnostic and therapeutic procedure involving the insertion of an arthroscope into a joint that provides direct visualization of the joint space to the physician without the requirement of surgical exposure of the joint (arthrotomy). In addition to the arthroscope, an irrigation cannula and various small resection instruments can be introduced into the joint space during the procedure. Total intravenous anesthesia with propofol and alfentanil or remifentanil does not affect the risk of postoperative nausea and vomiting. Joints that are frequently studied with this procedure include the knee, shoulder, wrist, and (occasionally) the temporomandibular joint. Neurovascular complications are the most serious and devastating complications of this procedure.

Professional Considerations
Consent form IS required.

Risks
Bleeding (hemarthrosis), infection, allergic reaction to the local or general anesthetic agent(s) to be used during the procedure.

Contraindications
History of bleeding diathesis, history of allergic reaction to anesthetic agents to be used during the procedure, severe arthritis resulting in narrowing of the joint space that would preclude insertion of the required instruments, cellulitis over the joint to be studied.

Preparation
1. Preoperative determination of the vital signs is indicated.
2. The surface over the joint to be studied is shaved and prepped with an iodine solution.
3. If the procedure is to be performed with the client under general anesthesia, anesthetic premedication may be given and the client is taken to the operating room where a general anesthetic agent is administered.
4. If the procedure is to be performed with the client under local anesthesia, the client may need to be properly positioned. (As an example, arthroscopy of the knee is at times performed with the client in a sitting position.)
5. Just before beginning the procedure, take a "time out" to verify the correct client, procedure, and site.

Procedure
1. If the procedure is to be performed with the client under local anesthesia, infiltration of the skin over the joint is performed with a local anesthetic agent (lidocaine).
2. The joint space is infiltrated with the local anesthetic agent.
3. If the joint to be studied is located in an extremity, a proximal tourniquet is occasionally applied.

4. A small incision is made, and the irrigation cannula is passed into the joint space. The joint space is irrigated and distended with irrigation solution (saline).
5. The arthroscope is placed into the joint space through a second incision. The internal structures of the joint are visualized.
6. If arthroscopic surgery is to be performed, insertion of various arthroscopic surgical cannulae can be performed through a third incision.
7. At the end of the procedure the instruments are removed from the joint, and the incisions are closed with sutures or Steri-strip tape.
8. Various dressings are applied. In the case of knee arthroscopy, an Ace wrap is often used.
9. The pneumatic cuff is then deflated.

Postprocedure Care
1. Postoperative determination of the vital signs and a dressing check are indicated.
2. Neurovascular assessment of distal extremity for color, temperature, movement and sensation.
3. Frequent reevaluation of the dressing and the joint may be needed. The physician supervising the care of the client should be informed if bleeding, swelling of the joint, or leakage of synovial fluid is noted.
4. Postoperative analgesic medications and antibiotic agents may be ordered by the physician supervising the test.
5. A program of physical therapy may be required, although frequently the client may resume normal activity within 24 hours of the procedure.

Client and Family Teaching
1. A general preoperative orientation to the procedure and postoperative care plan is indicated.

2. The client and family will need instruction in any physical therapy routines or mobility limitations imposed by the procedure.
3. Orientation as to the nature and prognosis of the disease process diagnosed by the arthroscopy may be indicated.
4. An ice pack may help ease postprocedure pain. Use a towel between the ice pack and the joint.
5. Give instructions for crutch walking, including going up and down stairs.
6. Do not exercise the joint more than normal activity for 5-6 weeks after the procedure if surgery was performed.
7. Contact the physician if edema continues more than 3 days or if fever over 101 degrees F (38.3 degrees C) or increased knee pain develops.

Factors That Affect Results
1. Client cooperation during arthroscopy performed with the client under local anesthesia is essential.
2. Severe arthritis-producing deformity of the joint space may limit the effectiveness of the procedure.
3. Postoperative complications such as bleeding or infection may limit the effectiveness of arthroscopic surgical procedures.

Other Data
1. Wrist arthroscopy is ideal for evaluating intra-articular soft tissue injuries.
2. The cause of various types of chronic arthritis can frequently be determined with radiographic or serologic tests without the need to perform arthroscopy.
3. The increasing availability of smaller arthroscopic instruments has resulted in a growing trend to perform these procedures with the client under local anesthesia and in an office (rather than a hospital) setting.

ASA

See **Salicylate**—Blood.

ASA

See **Infertility Screen**—Specimen.

Ascorbic Acid

See **Vitamin C**—Plasma or Serum.

ASC-US

See **Pap Smear**—Diagnostic.

Ashkenazi Jewish Genetic Carrier Screening Profile

Norm. Negative.

Usage. Pre-conception screening for autosomal recessive carrier status.

Description. Clients whose families have Jewish ancestors from Eastern or Central Europe (Ashkenazi) carry a genetically higher risk for conceiving a child with certain autosomal recessive inherited diseases when both parents carry the abnormal gene. Screening for these abnormal genes associated with Canavan disease, cystic fibrosis, familial dysautonomia, Fanconi anemia, Gaucher disease, Riley-Day syndrome and Tay-Sachs disease may be done as part of genetic counseling prior to conception (Kalman, Wilson, Buller, 2009).

Professional Considerations

Informed consent is recommended for genetic testing.

Preparation

1. Collect required screening questionnaires regarding client history, including those for cystic fibrosis and Tay-Sachs disease.
2. Tube: Lavender topped EDTA and yellow topped ACD tube.

Procedure

1. Collect 10 ml whole blood.

Postprocedure Care

1. Keep lavender topped tube at room temperature. Refrigerate yellow topped tube.
2. Transport to testing laboratory within 48 hours.

Client and Family Teaching

1. Genetic counseling is recommended. Refer to section in this book on "Informed Consent for Genetic Testing".
2. If the first person tested is negative for any of the autosomal recessive conditions, testing of the partner is not needed.
3. Rare variants of the diseases may not be identified by this test.

Factors That Affect Results

1. Hemolysis or frozen state of the specimen invalidates results

Other Data

1. Test not indicated for those of non-Ashkenazi ancestry.
2. The Genetic Information Nondiscrimination Act of 2008 prohibits health plans from using genetic family history or genetic test results from influencing eligibility or premiums for health insurance. It also prohibits employers from using this information to influence decisions about hiring, terminating employment, or employment pay, promotions or privileges.

ASM Antibody

See **Anti–Smooth Muscle Antibody**—Serum.

ASO Titer

See **Antistreptolysin-O Titer**—Serum.

Aspartate Aminotransferase (AST, Aspartate Transaminase, SGOT)—Serum

Norm.

		SI Units
Adult Females		
<61 years	13-45 mU/mL or 8-20 U/L	0.14-0.34 µKat/L
	10-40 Karmen U/mL	8-20 U/L
>60 years	10-20 U/L	0.17-0.34 µKat/L
Adult Males		
<61 years	13-45 mU/mL or 8-20 U/L	0.14-0.34 µKat/L
	10-40 Karmen U/mL	8-20 U/L
>60 years	11-26 U/L	0.19-0.44 µKat/L
Children		
Newborn	25-75 U/L	0.43-1.28 µKat/L
Infants	15-60 U/L	0.26-1.02 µKat/L
2-5 months	20-50 U/L	0.34-0.85 µKat/L
1 year	16-35 U/L	0.27-0.60 µKat/L
5 years	19-28 U/L	0.32-0.48 µKat/L
8-12 years	15-40 U/L	0.26-0.68 µKat/L
12-14 years	15-35 U/L	0.26-0.60 µKat/L
14-16 years	15-30 U/L	0.26-0.51 µKat/L

Increased. Acute myocardial infarction (increases 6-12 hours after injury, peaks at 18-24 hours, and returns to normal within 1 week; average increases are about 4-fold; large infarcts may cause increases up to 15-fold), alcoholism, anorexia nervosa (emaciated multiorgan disorders), calcium dust inhalation, cerebral infarction, cirrhosis, diabetes mellitus, eating disorders (with liver impacted), hepatitis (viral preicteric phase), HELLP syndrome, intestinal injury, intramuscular injections, irradiation injury, Lassa fever, lead, lipemia, liver disease, liver necrosis post laparoscopic cholecystectomy, metal poisoning, musculoskeletal diseases, myoglobinuria, pancreatitis (acute), polymyositis/dermatomyositis, pulmonary infarction, renal infarction, toxic shock syndrome, trauma. Drugs include allopurinol, aluminum nicotinate, amantadine, ampicillin, anabolic steroids, androgens, ascorbic acid, asparaginase, aspirin (value returns to normal within 48 hours of ingestion), azaserine, baclofen, barbiturates, bethanechol chloride, bromocriptine mesylate, captopril, carbenicillin, carbon tetrachloride, cardiotonic glycosides, carmustine, cephalothin sodium, chlordiazepoxide, chloroquine, chlorpromazine hydrochloride, cholestyramine resin, cholinergics, cinchophen, clindamycin, clofibrate, cloxacillin, codeine, colchicine, cortisone, cyclacillin, cycloserine, desipramine, dicumarol, digitalis, diphenylhydantoin, disopyramide phosphate, erythromycin, ethionamide, ethyl biscoumacetate, floxuridine, flurazepam, flutamide, fosinopril, gentamicin sulfate, griseofulvin, guanethidine analogs, hydralazine, N-hydroxyacetamide, ibufenac, isoniazid, lincomycin, lorazepam, meperidine, methotrexate, methyldopa, metoprolol tartrate, mithramycin, morphine, nafcillin, nalidixic acid, narcotics, niacin, nifedipine, nitrofurantoin, oral contraceptives, oxacillin, para-aminosalicylic acid, phenothiazines, placebo, Polycillin, procainamide hydrochloride, propranolol, propylthiouracil, Prostaphlin, pyrantel pamoate, pyrazinamide, pyridoxine, rifampin, salicylates, statins, sulfamethizole, sulfamethoxypyridazine, tetracycline, theophylline, thiabendazole, thiothixene, thyroid hormone, tolbutamide, tolmetin sodium, troleandomycin, valproic acid, vitamin A, and vitamin B_6. Herbal or natural remedies include chaparral tea (or misspelled chapparel tea, *Larrea tridentata*), *Echinacea*, pennyroyal. Herbal or natural remedies that have the potential to cause hepatotoxicity and elevate values include akee fruit (ackee, *Blighia sapida*), *Atractylis gummifera*, *Azadirachta indica* (*Neem tree, margosa*), *Berberis vulgaris* (barberry), *Callilepis laureola* (blazing star, *Liatris spicata*), chaparral tea (*Larrea tridentata*), cocaine, comfrey ("knitbone," *Symphytum*), *Crotalaria* (bush tea), cycasin (a toxin from a *Cycas* species of sago palm of Guam), *Echinacea*, germander (genera *Teucrium* and *Veronica*; do not confuse with safe skullcap, a name often falsely used in selling germander), *Heliotropium* (germander, valerian), jin bu huan ('gold-inconvertible,' Jin Bu Huan Anodyne Tablets, patent medicine with misidentified constituents: essence of t'ienchi [tianqi] flowers, "Noto-ginseng"; also kombucha; also *Lycopodium serratum*, or club moss; but with plant alkaloid levotetrahydropalmatine, a potent neuroactive substance), ma huang (*Ephedra*), margosa (*Melia azadirachta, Azadirachta indica*), maté tea (*Ilex paraguayensis*), mistletoe, pennyroyal, sassafras, skullcap (*Scutellaria*; do not confuse with unsafe germander), syosaiko-to (xiao chai hu tang, "minor Bupleurum combination"), *Teucrium polium* (golden germander), and valerian (*Valeriana officinalis*, garden heliotrope).

Decreased. Beriberi, diabetic ketoacidosis, hemodialysis (chronic), liver disease, and uremia (all conditions cause false decreases). Drugs include metronidazole and trifluoperazine. Herbal or natural remedies include Chinese *fructus schizandrae sinensis* (*wu wei zi*, coffee (*Coffea*) [in alcoholics], "five flavors herb," *Schisandra chinensis* [Turcz.] Baill.).

Description. A catalytic enzyme found primarily in the heart, liver, and muscle tissue.

AST is found in two distinct forms or isoenzymes. c-AST is located in cytoplasm, and m-AST is found in mitochondria. Increases in the serum total AST level occur any time there is serious damage to cells. In addition, AST may be found in complex with IgA in hepatic cancer. AST is also evaluated in comparison with alanine aminotransferase (ALT) to serially monitor liver damage.

Professional Considerations
Consent form NOT required.

Preparation
1. Tube: Red topped, red/gray topped, or gold topped.
2. Do NOT draw during hemodialysis.

Procedure
1. Draw a 4-mL, nontraumatic blood sample.

Postprocedure Care
1. Handle the specimen carefully, avoiding hemolysis.

Client and Family Teaching
1. Results are normally available within 12 hours.

Factors That Affect Results
1. Hemolysis of specimen and recent IM injections may cause falsely elevated values.
2. *Echinacea* taken for 8 weeks or longer may cause hepatotoxicity.

Other Data
1. There are no conditions that result in a true decrease in AST. All decreases listed are false decreases.
2. Bloodletting reduces serum aminotransferase in persons with chronic hepatitis C and iron overload.

Aspergillus Antibody

Norm. Negative <1:8. Suspicious infection: Fourfold rise in paired serum specimens. (Isolation does not prove pathogenesis for opportunistic fungi.)

Increased. Allergic bronchopulmonary aspergillosis, hypersensitivity to *Aspergillus*, immunodeficiency, leukemia, and pulmonary aspergilloma.

Description. *Aspergillus* species are saprophytic, opportunistic fungi that can grow on soil and organic materials and often become airborne in large numbers. More than 200 strains exist and may colonize the human body (respiratory tract, skin, nails, ear canal, burns) and become pathogenic when they invade immunosuppressed clients, when they invade human tissue, or when a client becomes sensitized to the organism. In this test, an indirect Coombs' test is performed to identify the presence of *Aspergillus* antibody.

Professional Considerations
Consent form NOT required.

Preparation
1. Verify whether the client received antifungal skin testing within the last few weeks. Write the dates and names of such tests on the laboratory requisition.
2. Tube: Red topped, red/gray topped, or gold topped.

Procedure
1. Collect a 10-mL blood sample as soon as possible after infection is suspected. Label the specimen as the acute sample.
2. Repeat the test in 2-3 weeks and label the specimen as the convalescent sample.

Postprocedure Care
1. Transport the specimen to the laboratory promptly and refrigerate at 25 degrees C for no longer than 9 hours.

Client and Family Teaching
1. Return in 2-3 weeks for the convalescent sampling.

2. Amphotericin B is used to treat aspergillosis.

Factors That Affect Results
1. False-negative results may occur in immunosuppressed clients.
2. False-positive results may be caused by recent fungal antigen skin tests.

Other Data
1. Five percent of clients without pulmonary aspergillosis or *Aspergillus* allergy will have *Aspergillus* antibodies.
2. Identification requires that *Aspergillus* be directly identified in body tissues or fluids, be isolated in multiple specimens, and be identified by microscopic observation of characteristic conidial formation.
3. The lysis-centrifugation method of culturing is the most sensitive method for detecting molds that cause fungemia. Blood cultures for *Aspergillus* are helpful in diagnosing an *Aspergillus* infection only when repeated lysis-centrifugation tests can distinguish between specimen contamination and pathogenesis based on the number of colonies appearing.
4. A biopsy is required to diagnose invasive aspergillosis.

Aspirin
See **Salicylate**—Blood.

Aspirin Tolerance Test (ASA Tolerance Test, Bleeding Time Aspirin Tolerance Test)—Diagnostic

Norm. Requires interpretation. Normal baseline Ivy bleeding time is 2-7 minutes. One study demonstrated bleeding time in normal clients to increase from 2.5 to 4.2 minutes at 2 hours after aspirin ingestion. Bleeding time should return to baseline level by 96 hours after aspirin ingestion.

Increased. Bernard-Soulier syndrome, collagen vascular disease, Cushing's disease, disseminated intravascular coagulation, Glanzmann's thrombasthenia, gray platelet syndrome, hypersplenism, thrombocytopenia with immunosuppression, and von Willebrand's disease. Drugs include anticoagulants (oral), indomethacin, phenylbutazone, and platelet aggregation inhibitor drugs (aspirin, clopidogrel, eptifibatide). Herbs or natural remedies that may inhibit platelet activity include feverfew (*Tanacetum parthenium*), garlic, ginger, *Ginkgo biloba*, ginseng.

Decreased. Drugs include 1-deamino-8-D-arginine vasopressin (DDAVP).

Description. The Ivy bleeding time test is performed before and after aspirin ingestion to evaluate the drug's effect on platelet function. In normal clients, aspirin ingestion has minimal influence on bleeding time.

Professional Considerations
Consent form NOT required for most laboratories.

Risks
Bleeding, ecchymoses, hematoma.
Contraindications
In clients who require upper-extremity restraints, have edematous or very cold arms, or are prone to keloid formation. This test should not be performed if there are contraindications to placing or inflating a blood pressure cuff on the arm (casts, rash, arteriovenous fistula). Other contraindications include platelet count <50,000/mm^3, severe bleeding disorders, skin infectious diseases, senile skin changes, or medications containing acetyl groups, such as those containing aspirin, within the previous 5 days.

Preparation
1. See Client and Family Teaching.
2. Obtain povidone-iodine solution, a blood pressure cuff, a lancet, a stopwatch, and filter paper.

Procedure
1. Cleanse the volar aspect of the forearm with povidone-iodine and allow it to dry completely.
2. Place the blood pressure cuff on the upper arm and inflate to 40 mm Hg.
3. Make two small incisions 2-3 mm deep on the prepared site. Start timing with the stopwatch.
4. Remove blood from the wound with filter paper every 15 seconds until bleeding stops. Stop timing with the stopwatch.
5. If bleeding time is more than 10 minutes, do not proceed further because this test would be contraindicated.
6. Administer 10 grains (adults) or 5 grains (children weighing less than 32 kg) of aspirin orally.
7. Repeat steps 1 through 5 after 2 hours.

Postprocedure Care
1. If bleeding time is normal, apply a Band-Aid to the site. If bleeding time is prolonged, apply a pressure bandage to the site.
2. Assess the site(s) for bleeding every 5 minutes for ½ hour. Observe for signs of site infection until healed.

Client and Family Teaching
1. Do not take aspirin for 5 days before this test.
2. Bring reading material or some other diversion because the test takes 2-3 hours.

Factors That Affect Results
1. The most sensitive and reproducible measurements may be those taken from a horizontal incision.

Other Data
1. The depth of the puncture with the lancet is difficult to standardize and results in poorly reproducible bleeding times.

AST
See Aspartate Aminotransferase—Serum.

AT-III Test
See Antithrombin III Test—Diagnostic.

A

Atrial Natriuretic Hormone

See **Natriuretic Peptides**—Plasma.

Atrial Natriuretic Peptide

See **Natriuretic Peptides**—Plasma.

Audiometry Test (Pure Tone Audiometry and Speech Audiometry, Vestibular Evoked Myogenic Potential)—Diagnostic

Norm.

Adult	0-25 dB HL hearing sensitivity
Child	0-15 dB HL hearing sensitivity
Word-discrimination score	Client is able to repeat list of spoken words with 90% accuracy
VEMP	Positive steady results

Usage. Delineation of type and amount of hearing loss (that is, conductive, sensorineural, or mixed), rehabilitation monitoring post cochlear implant or post stapedectomy, diagnosis of glue ear (otitis media with effusion). Vestibular evoked myogenic potential (VEMP) is used to help evaluate clients experiencing symptoms of dizziness and/or suspected of having vestibulocochlear disorders, as well as to help differentiate sudden deafness from the beginning stage of Ménière's disease. Higher peak amplitudes (VEMP) are seen in clients with endolymphatic hydrops or multiple sclerosis and in clients with distended saccular hydrops seen in the early stage of Ménière's disease.

Description. *Pure tone audiometry* is a hearing test using an audiometer that sends tones into the client's ear and vibrations through the bone. It measures the frequencies at which the client is able to hear 50% or more of the tones. The test is able to detect defects in air conduction (conductive hearing loss) through the use of tones or defects in air and bone conduction (sensorineural hearing loss) through the use of vibrations to help identify the amount and type of hearing loss present. *Speech audiometry* is a hearing test that determines the client's speech-reception threshold and word-discrimination score by measuring the number of words the client can repeat after they are heard when delivered through earphones at precise decibel intensities. Speech audiometry helps differentiate between conductive and sensorineural hearing loss. *Vestibular evoked myogenic potential* is a reflex conducted via the inferior vestibular nerve that indicates the integrity of the vestibular response. Measurement is performed via skull taps with recording of resultant muscular responses.

Professional Considerations

Consent form NOT required.

Preparation

1. See Client and Family Teaching.
2. Ensure that the external auditory canal is free of impacted cerumen.
3. Obtain an audiometer, earphones, a vibrator for bone-conduction testing, and an otoscope.

Procedure

1. A plastic tube may be inserted into the external auditory canal to maintain the canal's patency during testing with earphones.
2. The earphones are placed over the ears and fastened in place.
3. A preliminary tone is demonstrated for the client to become familiar with the test.

A

4. The ear not being tested is masked with audiometer noise to prevent crossover interference and subsequent inaccurate estimation of hearing loss.

5. *Air conduction testing*: The better ear is tested first. The client is instructed to give a signal each time a tone is heard. Starting with 1000 Hz, tones are delivered to the ear, decreasing by increments of 10 dB until a negative response is obtained. Tone levels are then increased in smaller increments and then decreased until the air conduction threshold level is obtained. The air conduction threshold level is the lowest hertz level at which the client is able to hear two out of three tones. This procedure is then repeated several times, starting with a different tone level each time (such as 2000, 4000, 8000, 1000, 500, and finally 250 Hz). The second ear is then tested in the same way. Finally, retesting is performed on each ear to determine test/retest reliability. Acceptable variation for retesting for each ear must be within 5 dB above or below the initial test result. Graphic recordings are made of the threshold levels.

6. *Bone conduction testing*: The better ear is tested first. After removal of the earphones, the bone conduction vibrator is held on the mastoid process of the ear. Starting from 250 Hz, tones are delivered to the ear, with decrements at 10 dB until a negative response is obtained. Tone levels are then increased in smaller increments and then decreased until the bone conduction threshold level is obtained. The bone conduction threshold level is the lowest hertz level at which the client is able to hear two out of three tones. This procedure is then repeated several times, starting with a different tone level each time (500, 1000, 2000, and finally 4000 Hz). The second ear is then tested in the same way. Finally, retesting is performed on each ear to determine test/retest reliability. Acceptable variation for retesting for each ear must be within 5 dB above or below the initial test result. Graphic recordings are made of the threshold levels.

7. *Speech reception threshold measurement*: Two-syllable, familiar, spoken words are delivered through the earphones. The client is asked to repeat each word. The speech reception threshold is the decibel level at which the client is able to restate correctly at least half the words.

8. *Word discrimination score*: One-syllable, familiar, phonetically balanced words are delivered through the earphones at 30 dB higher than the client's own speech reception threshold. The client is asked to repeat each word. Clients with conductive hearing loss will have a normal word discrimination score. Those with sensorineural hearing loss will have a lower than normal score.

9. *Amount-of-hearing-loss calculation:* The amount of hearing loss, called the "pure tone average" (PTA), is calculated by averaging the air conduction threshold levels. Mild hearing loss demonstrates a PTA of 26-40 dB. Moderate hearing loss demonstrates a PTA of 41-55 dB. Moderately severe hearing loss demonstrates a PTA of 56-70 dB. Severe hearing loss demonstrates a PTA of 71-90 dB. Profound hearing loss demonstrates a PTA of >90 dB.

10. *Type-of-hearing-loss calculation:* The type of hearing loss is interpreted by examination of the relationship between the air conduction threshold levels and the bone conduction threshold levels at the different frequencies. In sensorineural hearing loss, both thresholds are depressed to about the same degree. In conductive hearing loss, only the air conduction thresholds are depressed. In mixed hearing loss, both thresholds are depressed, but air conduction threshold levels are more depressed than bone conduction threshold levels.

11. *Vestibular evoked myogenic potential*: Skin electrodes are placed over both sternocleidomastoid muscles. Light skull taps over each ear and on the middle of the forehead are manually applied. Alternatively, loud clicks are produced externally to each ear. The responses evoked by these taps that travel through the sternocleidomastoid muscles are measured through the electrodes and recorded as waveforms.

Postprocedure Care

1. Cleanse the earphones and otoscope with antiseptic.

Client and Family Teaching

1. Stay in an environment free of extremely loud noises for 16 hours before the test.

Factors That Affect Results

1. Testing should be performed in a very quiet environment for the most accurate results.
2. The client should not be able to see the examiner because changes in tone level are made. Signals should be delivered in a nonrhythmic pattern.
3. The client must be able to distinguish between the pure tones and tinnitus or vibrotactile stimulation.
4. Test/retest differences of more than 10 dB may be caused by unreliable equipment.

5. The use of plastic tubes to maintain external auditory canal patency should be noted on the audiogram.
6. Low levels of serum estradiol can impede hearing sensitivity in pure tone audiometry results in postmenopausal women.

Other Data

1. See also Acoustic immittance tests—Diagnostic.
2. There is higher prevalence of age-related hearing impairment in persons with high body mass index, history of high triglyceride levels, and history of smoking. Therefore efforts directed toward modifiable risk factors for cardiovascular disease could also impact or slow the development of age-related hearing loss.

Automated Reagin Testing (ART)—Diagnostic

Norm. Negative.

Titer	Interpretation
Nonreactive	Negative
≤1:8	False positive
1:9 to 1:32	Primary-stage syphilis (requiring interpretation)
>1:32	Secondary-stage syphilis

Positive. Syphilis. (See Factors That Affect Results for biologic false-positive results.)

Description. A nonspecific, nontreponemal test used for syphilis screening and monitoring of response to therapy in the post chancre period of the primary stage and in the secondary stage when treponemal antibodies are more difficult to detect. When *Treponema pallidum*, the causative agent of syphilis, invades human tissue, reagin is produced and can be isolated from 7 to 21 days after the appearance of the chancre. Results are reported as the highest titer that produces a positive reaction.

Professional Considerations

Consent form NOT required.

Preparation

1. Tube: Red topped, red/gray topped, or gold topped.
2. See Client and Family Teaching.

Procedure

1. Draw a 5-mL blood sample.

Postprocedure Care

1. None.

Client and Family Teaching

1. Do not drink alcohol for 24 hours before testing.
2. Weekly testing for 2 months is recommended before syphilis can be ruled out.
3. If testing positive:
   i. Notify all sexual contacts from the last 90 days (if early stage) to be tested for syphilis.
   ii. Syphilis can be cured with antibiotics. These may worsen the symptoms for the first 24 hours.
   iii. Do not have sex for 2 months and until after repeat testing has confirmed that the syphilis is cured. Use condoms after that for 2 years. Return for repeat testing every 3-4 months for the next 2 years to make sure the disease is cured.
   iv. Do not become pregnant for 2 years because syphilis can be transmitted to the fetus.
   v. If left untreated, syphilis can damage many body organs, including the brain, over several years.

Factors That Affect Results

1. Reject hemolyzed specimens.
2. False-negative results may occur before the appearance of the chancre in the initial stage of syphilis or during the tertiary stage.
3. False-negative results may be caused by ingestion of alcohol within 24 hours before specimen collection.
4. Biologic false-positive results lasting up to 6 months may be caused by bejel, chickenpox, DPT immunization, hepatitis (infectious), malaria, measles, mononucleosis (infectious), pneumonia (atypical, pneumococcal), scarlet fever, smallpox vaccination, subacute bacterial endocarditis, or tuberculosis.
5. Biologic false-positive results lasting more than 6 months may be caused by hyperglobulinemia, leprosy, leptospirosis, periarteritis nodosa, pinta, rheumatic fever, rheumatoid arthritis, systemic lupus erythematosus, thyroiditis, *Vaccinia*, or yaws.

Other Data

1. Suspected false-positive results should be followed by repeat testing at 3, 6, and 9 months.

Autoprothrombin IIA

See **Protein C**—Blood.

Autopsy—Diagnostic

Norm. Requires interpretation.

Usage. Determination of cause and manner of death, reporting of contagious diseases, quality assurance, teaching, and legal purposes.

Description. A postmortem examination and dissection of a corpse. The procedure is usually performed by two pathologists and an assistant.

Professional Considerations

Consent form IS required.

Preparation

1. After death, determination should be made whether the circumstances of death require that the coroner be notified. Coroner's cases usually include unexpected death, death within 24 hours of admission to a hospital, death while under anesthesia, suspected homicides or suicides, accidental or violent deaths, deaths of clients with contagious disease, or any death occurring under unusual circumstances or involving the public interest. If any of these conditions apply, the coroner should be called by the physician for a determination of the need for an autopsy. If the coroner determines that an autopsy is required, the family should be notified, but next-of-kin permission is not needed.
2. Autopsy may also be performed without next-of-kin permission when it is necessary to complete the death certificate or when the deceased client has given consent before death.
3. When the need for an autopsy is determined, other than for coroner's cases, next-of-kin permission must be obtained by means of a signature on the consent form or possibly by a witnessed telephone conversation between the physician and the next of kin. Guidelines vary depending on area laws and institution.
4. All invasive lines, tubes, and devices should be left intact in the body.
5. Obtain an autopsy knife with a blade, a scalpel with a disposable blade, toothed forceps, forceps with serrated tips, a medium-long knife with a blade, a long knife with a blade, scissors with one pointed and one blunt blade, scissors with two blunt blades, scissors for cutting bones, intestinal scissors (enterotome), scissors with long curved blades, a 1-mm probe, a metal metric rule, a costotome, rib shears, intestinal clamps, a vibratory saw with large blades, an amputating saw, a band saw, a hammer with a hook, a chisel, bone-cutting forceps, a meter stick, a body scale, an organ scale, balances, a ladle, a graduate, sea sponges, pans with fixative, pan and pail containers, a large container for fixation of gross organs in solution, fixing solution, string, needles, abrasive whetstone and oil, and a slicing machine.

6. Obtain containers for the samples for toxicologic studies, culture, or cytologic tests.
7. Make sure that the autopsy-permit name and identification number correspond to the name and identification number on the client's body. If there are no tags on the body, have the nurse, physician, or relative identify the body.
8. Wear a mask, an eye or face shield, gloves, and a plastic apron.

Procedure

1. *Recording*: The sequence of events and findings of autopsy are recorded either by concurrently written notes or by a foot-operated dictation machine. Descriptions of the body and organs, including condition, arrangement, and weight of the organs, are made and recorded as the dissection is performed.
2. *Sequence*: The sequence of the autopsy may vary. In cases in which a specific cause of death is suspected, the appropriate body cavity for that cause may be opened first. A usual autopsy proceeds in the following order: external examination; incision of the skin, ribs, and sterno-clavicular joints; examination of thoracic and abdominal cavities; removal and examination of the organs of the trunk (thymus, heart, lungs, mediastinal lymph nodes, spleen, intestines, diaphragm, liver, gallbladder, pancreas, stomach, duode-num, rectum, spermatic cords, testes, adrenals, uterus, ovarian tubes, ovaries, bone marrow [sternal, vertebral, femoral], neck organs, bones, joints, and muscles); and removal and examination of the organs of the cranium and spine (brain, eyes, ears, paranasal sinuses, pituitary gland, spinal cord, and spinal root ganglia).
3. *Content of assessment*: In the external examination, the body is observed and palpated, and the length, size, and weight are measured. Rigor mortis, edema, and jaundice are noted. The head, lymph nodes, and genitalia are assessed. A Y incision is then made on the torso, and the thoracic and abdominal cavities are assessed. The arrangement and status of the organs and the presence of adhe-sions, excess fluid, or gas are noted. As they are excised, the weight, size, and

contents of the organs and blood vessels are assessed. Biopsy specimens, sections, and smears may be taken throughout the process. The organs of the cranium and spine are then assessed. An incision is made from ear to ear over the vertex of the cranium, and the scalp is separated from the skull with a scalpel. The anterior portion of the scalp is pulled down over the forehead and face. After the skull is opened with a saw and the top portion removed, the brain is removed and placed in 10% formalin. Biopsy specimens of the brain are taken if a virus is suspected. The remainder of the head organs are removed and examined. Formalin is injected into the eyes before removal. The spinal cord is then removed and exam-ined for lesions. Complete organs or por-tions of organs may be fixed in solution for later reference. An alternative method is to remove the trunk organs in one block, with examination of organs on a dissecting table.

Postprocedure Care

1. The body is cleansed, and the incisions are sewn. The body may or may not be embalmed at this point.

Client and Family Teaching

1. Autopsy incisions will not be visible should an open-casket wake be held.
2. Durable Power of Attorney for Health Care does NOT apply after death.

Factors That Affect Results

1. A routine hospital autopsy should be interrupted and the coroner notified if any unexpected findings that may be of traumatic origin are encountered.

Other Data

1. The order of authority for granting per-mission for an autopsy is normally spouse, adult child, parent, adult sibling, other relative, and any other person accepting responsibility for burial of the body. This order may vary by area laws.
2. Be aware of religious considerations con-cerning autopsy.
3. There is a 44% discordance rate between clinical and autopsy diagnosis of malig-nant neoplasms.

B2M

See Beta₂-Microglobulin—Blood and 24-Hour Urine.

Bacterial Inhibition Assay

See Guthrie Test for Phenylketonuria—Diagnostic.

BAEP

See Brainstem Auditory Evoked Potential—Diagnostic.

Banding in Genetic Disorders—Diagnostic

Norm. Cytogenic techniques with numerical designations map each chromosome for abnormalities.

Female	44 autosomes + 2X chromosomes Karyotype: 46, XX
Male	44 autosomes + 1X and 1Y chromosomes Karyotype: 46, XY

Usage. Assists in the diagnosis of genetic and neoplastic disorders.

Description. Banding techniques are used for chromosome identification. Human chromosomes are numbered in 23 pairs. Each chromosome pair has a unique pattern with intricate detail produced by different distributions of DNA in the chromosomes. Banding helps detect different regions of the same chromosome for use in identification of both the chromosome and the chromosomal abnormalities. R banding uses a reverse Giemsa stain called acridine orange, which produces reverse contrast to the light Q bands detected by quinacrine mustard and dark and light crossband G bands detected with trypsin and Giemsa stain. R dark bands are useful for observing the very dark ends of chromosomes. The chromosome count per cell and banded karyotype with interpretation is included in the testing.

Professional Considerations

Informed consent is recommended for genetic testing.

Preparation

1. Tube: Green topped.

Procedure

1. Draw a 4-mL blood sample.

Postprocedure Care

1. None.

Client and Family Teaching

1. Results are normally available in 1-2 weeks.
2. Refer the client with abnormal results for genetic counseling. Refer to section in this book on "Informed Consent for Genetic Testing".

Factors That Affect Results

1. Heparin in the specimen collection tube must be sodium heparin.

Other Data

1. This method is used widely in European countries, especially France.
2. See also Chromosome analysis—Blood.
3. The Genetic Information Nondiscrimination Act of 2008 prohibits health plans from using genetic family history or genetic test results from influencing eligibility or premiums for health insurance. It also prohibits employers from using this information to influence decisions about hiring, terminating employment, or employment pay, promotions or privileges.

Bands

See **Differential Leukocyte Count**—Peripheral Blood.

B

Barbiturates, Quantitative—Blood

Norm. Negative.

Levels During Barbiturate Therapy

Amobarbital	Trough	SI Units
Therapeutic	1-5 µg/mL	4.4-22.1 µmol/L
Toxic	>10 µg/mL	>44.2 µmol/L
Panic	>70 µg/mL	>309.4 µmol/L
Butabarbital		
Therapeutic	1-2 µg/mL	4.4-8.4 µmol/L
Toxic	10-40 µg/mL	44.2-176.8 µmol/L
Pentobarbital		
Therapeutic	1-5 µg/mL	4.4-22.1 µmol/L
Therapeutic coma	>10 µg/mL	88.4-221 µmol/L
Toxic	20-50 µg/mL	>44.2 µmol/L
Panic	>60 µg/mL	>265.2 µmol/L
Phenobarbital		
Therapeutic	15-40 µg/mL	66.3-176.8 µmol/L
Toxic	35-80 µg/mL	154.7-353.6 µmol/L
Panic	>100 µg/mL	>442 µmol/L
Secobarbital		
Therapeutic	1-2 µg/mL	4.2-8.4 µmol/L
Toxic	3-40 µg/mL	13.3-176.8 µmol/L
Panic	>50 µg/mL	>221 µmol/L

Panic Level Symptoms and Treatment

Symptoms. Central nervous system depression (ataxia, confusion, drowsiness) progressing to respiratory depression, hypotension, and coma. Death may occur with ingestion of 1 g of pentobarbital, 1.5 g of phenobarbital, or 2 g of secobarbital.

Treatment

NOTE: Treatment choice(s) depend(s) on client's history and condition and episode history.

1. Protect airway and provide oxygen.
2. Administer gastric lavage with tap water or saline up to 24 hours after ingestion.
3. Do NOT induce emesis.
4. Administer activated charcoal.
5. Diurese with urea if hemodynamically stable and adequate renal function is present.
6. Alkalinize urine.
7. Delay absorption by using subcutaneous or intramuscular routes and packing sites with ice or using tourniquets.

	Removed by Hemodialysis	Removed by Hemoperfusion	Removed by Peritoneal Dialysis
Amobarbital	Yes	Yes	No
Pentobarbital	No	Yes	
Phenobarbital	Yes	Yes	Yes
Secobarbital	No		No

B

Usage. Drug abuse, overdose, suicide attempt, and monitoring blood levels during barbiturate therapy, for example, in the treatment of catatonia.

Description. Barbiturates are a group of central nervous system depressants used as hypnotics, anticonvulsants, and sedatives and preoperatively. They are believed to act at the level of the reticular activating system. Barbiturates are metabolized in the liver and excreted by the kidneys. Overdose may lead to coma and death from respiratory arrest.

Professional Considerations
Consent form NOT required unless the specimen may be used as legal evidence.

Preparation
1. Tube: Red topped, red/gray topped, gold topped, lavender topped, or black topped.
2. Do NOT draw the sample for amobarbital or phenobarbital level during hemodialysis.
3. Sample for pentobarbital MAY be drawn during hemodialysis.
4. Screen client for the use of herbal preparations or natural remedies such as *Valeriana officinalis* and kava-kava (*Piper methysticum*).

Procedure
1. Collection should be witnessed if the specimen may be used as legal evidence.
2. Draw a 2-mL TROUGH blood sample.
3. Obtain serial measurements at the same time each day.

Postprocedure Care
1. If the specimen may be used as legal evidence, write the client's name, the exact time of the blood draw, and the contents of the tube on the tube label and the laboratory requisition. Sign and have the witness sign the laboratory requisition. Transport the specimen to the laboratory in a sealed plastic bag labeled as legal evidence.
2. Refrigerate the specimen if not tested immediately.

Client and Family Teaching
1. For intentional overdose, refer the client and family for crisis intervention.
2. Client with panic-level symptoms will require intensive care for at least 24 hours.
3. Physical and psychologic addiction occur in clients taking barbiturates over a long period of time. Serious withdrawal symptoms that may occur include severe headache, body pains, numbness or burning in the arms and legs, seizures, hallucinations, chest pain, sweating, and breathing difficulties. Seek medical treatment if any of these symptoms occur.
4. If activated charcoal was given for elevated levels, the client should drink 4-6 glasses of water each day for 2 days to prevent constipation. Activated charcoal will also cause stools to be black for a few days.

Factors That Affect Results
1. Reject hemolyzed specimens to avoid falsely decreased results.
2. Drugs that may cause falsely elevated results include atropine sulfate, dexchlorpheniramine maleate, ethotoin, glutethimide, meperidine hydrochloride, phenytoin, salicylamide, and theophylline.
3. Amobarbital cross-reactivity may occur with any of the other barbiturates. Pentobarbital cross-reactivity may occur with secobarbital or phenobarbital.
4. Barbiturates can decompose after embalming, and analysis then may lead to false negatives.

Other Data
1. Panic-level symptoms may occur with smaller doses if alcohol is also ingested.
2. Use of barbiturates increases the risk of nasopharyngeal carcinoma, congenital heart defects, and cleft palate.
3. Herbal or natural remedies that may cause excessive sedation when used with barbiturates include valerian and kava-kava (*Piper methysticum*). However, *Valeriana officinalis* (allheal, setwall, garden heliotrope, vandalroot) may reduce symptoms of benzodiazepine withdrawal.

Barium Enema (BE)—Diagnostic

Norm. Requires interpretation. Characteristics examined include filling, passage pattern of barium, and the contour, patency, position, and mucosal pattern of the colon.

Usage. Part of the diagnostic workup for bowel obstruction, celiac sprue, colorectal cancer, diverticulitis, diverticulosis, gastroenteritis, Hirschsprung's disease, intestinal cancer, intestinal polyps, intussusception, irritable bowel syndrome, rectal stenosis, stercoral appendicular fistula and ulcerative colitis.

Description. A fluoroscopic and radiographic examination of the large intestine after rectal instillation of barium sulfate with or without air for the purpose of identifying structural abnormalities or slowing of normal intestinal activity. The American Cancer Society recommends a screening double-contrast barium enema every 5 years beginning at age 50. Positive results should be followed with a colonoscopy.

Professional Considerations
Consent form NOT required.

Risks
Constipation, dizziness, infection, intestinal impaction, rectal or bowel perforation, rectovaginal perforation, and vasovagal reaction.

Contraindications
Severe active ulcerative colitis accompanied by toxicity and megacolon, perforated intestine, toxic megacolon, tachycardia.

Precautions
During pregnancy, risks of cumulative radiation exposure to the fetus from this and other previous or future imaging studies must be weighed against the benefits of the procedure. Although formal limits for client exposure are relative to this risk-benefit comparison, the United States Nuclear Regulatory Commission requires that the cumulative dose equivalent to an embryo/fetus from occupational exposure not exceed 0.5 rem (5 mSv). Risk of exposure to the uterus from a barium enema is 2-4 rad. Radiation dose to the fetus is proportional to the distance of the anatomy studied from the abdomen and decreases as pregnancy progresses.

Preparation
1. Laxatives or cathartic suppositories, or both, are usually indicated the day before and on the morning of the test to facilitate complete emptying of the intestines. However, they may be contraindicated for certain clients with conditions such as ulcerative colitis or intestinal obstruction. There is no difference between using Picolax or Fleet Phospho-Soda as laxatives except taste and Picolax provokes less nausea.
2. If the client is pregnant, notify the physician before examination preparation.
3. See Client and Family Teaching.

Procedure
1. After baseline abdominal radiographs are taken, the client lies in a Sims' position on a tilt table and receives a slow administration of barium sulfate or barium sulfate with air insufflation through a rectal tube.
2. As the client assumes different positions, the filling is monitored by fluoroscopy.
3. Spot films are taken during and after the filling.
4. The rectal tube is withdrawn, and the barium expelled, after which another film is taken to examine the pattern of the intestinal mucosa and to determine how well emptying has occurred.

Postprocedure Care
1. Where not contraindicated, the client should increase fluid intake for 24-48 hours.
2. Where not contraindicated, a mild cathartic may be prescribed to facilitate emptying of the barium from the intestine.
3. Stools should be inspected by the client/family or the health care professional for passage of barium for 48 hours. Barium stools will look chalky white in color.
4. Failure to have a bowel movement within 2 days after the test should be reported to the physician.

Client and Family Teaching
1. It is important to have the bowel emptied of stool before the procedure. A low-residue diet may be prescribed for 1-3 days before the test, although it does not offer any advantage over a normal diet in preparation for the test if purgatives are used.
2. A clear liquid diet is usually prescribed for 1 day before and on the morning of the test. A normal diet may be resumed after the procedure.
3. A laxative may be prescribed before and after the procedure.
4. The procedure takes about 60 minutes. It is important to hold your breath when you are asked to do so during the procedure.

5. Make sure all the barium empties from the intestinal tract after the procedure. Drinking fluids and taking laxatives or enemas after the procedure may be prescribed for this purpose.
6. See Postprocedure Care.
7. Call the physician if stomach or lower abdominal pain is experienced or if stools are much smaller than the normal diameter.

Factors That Affect Results

1. Failure to achieve complete emptying of the intestinal tract before the test may necessitate a repeated barium enema.

2. Improper adjustment of radiographic equipment to accommodate very thin or obese patients.

Other Data

1. The barium enema should be performed before a barium swallow.
2. There is evidence that occult stool testing reduces mortality from colon cancer. There is no similar current evidence regarding BE for screening of colon cancer.
3. Absorbed dose is 20-80 mGy to the embryo and 10-20 mGy to the fetus.

Barium Swallow—Diagnostic

Norm. Requires interpretation. Characteristics examined include filling of the pharynx and esophagus, mucosal patterns, and esophageal size, contour, and peristaltic motion.

Usage. Part of the diagnostic workup for achalasia, bronchoesophageal fistula, duodenal ulcer, dysphagia, esophageal diverticula, esophageal varices, head and neck cancer, hiatal hernia, hypertrophic pyloric stenosis, pharyngeal muscle disorders, piriform sinus fistula, Plummer-Vinson syndrome, polyps, strictures, stomach cancer, tracheoesophageal compression, and ulcers.

Description. A fluoroscopic and radiographic examination of the pharynx and esophagus as mixtures of barium sulfate are swallowed. The test takes 20-30 minutes.

Professional Considerations
Consent form NOT required.

Risks
Constipation, dizziness, intestinal impaction, vasovagal reaction.
Contraindications
During pregnancy; clients with upper tract dysphagia; those with a risk of barium aspiration; and clients with intestinal obstruction.
Precautions
During pregnancy, risks of cumulative radiation exposure to the fetus from this and other previous or future imaging studies must be weighed against the benefits of the procedure. Although formal limits for client exposure are relative to this risk-benefit comparison, the United States Nuclear Regulatory Commission requires that the cumulative dose equivalent to an embryo/fetus from occupational exposure not exceed 0.5 rem (5 mSv). Radiation dose to the fetus is proportional to the distance of the anatomy studied from the abdomen and decreases as pregnancy progresses. For pregnant clients, consult the radiologist/radiology department to obtain estimated fetal radiation exposure from this procedure.

Preparation
1. See Client and Family Teaching.

Procedure
1. The client is positioned on a tilt table.
2. After baseline fluoroscopic examinations of the heart, lungs, and abdomen, the client takes one swallow of a thick barium mixture while cineradiographic films are taken.
3. The client then takes several swallows of a thin barium mixture while its passage is recorded by fluoroscopy and radiography.
4. The process is repeated with the table tilted to various positions.
5. About 350-450 mL of barium is swallowed during the entire procedure.
6. For infants with pyloric stenosis, note the number of milliliters of barium given. This information is used at the end of the procedure when feeding tube should be inserted and used to aspirate out the same amount of barium.

Postprocedure Care

1. Where not contraindicated, the client should increase fluid intake for 24-48 hours after the test.
2. Where not contraindicated, a mild cathartic may be prescribed to facilitate emptying of barium from the gastrointestinal tract.
3. Failure to have a bowel movement within 2 days should be reported to the physician.

Client and Family Teaching

1. Fast from food and fluids for 8 hours before the procedure.
2. This procedure lasts approximately 15 minutes.
3. Make sure all of the barium empties from the intestinal tract after the procedure.

Drinking fluids and taking laxatives or enemas after the procedure may be prescribed for this purpose.
4. See Postprocedure Care.
5. Call the physician if stomach or lower abdominal pain is experienced or if stools are much smaller than the normal diameter.

Factors That Affect Results

1. Improper adjustment of radiographic equipment to accommodate very thin or obese patients.

Other Data

1. Barium swallow is not very sensitive as an aid in the diagnosis of proximal reflux in asthmatic children.

Barr Body Analysis Buccal Smear for Staining Sex Chromatin Mass—Diagnostic

Norm.

	Number of Barr Bodies
Normal female (XX)	1
Normal male (XY)	0
Turner's syndrome (female) (XO)	0
Klinefelter's syndrome (male) (XXY)	1
Klinefelter's syndrome (male) (48,XXXY)	2
Klinefelter's syndrome (male) (49,XXXYY)	2
Klinefelter's syndrome (male) (49,XXXXY)	3

Usage. Screening for sex chromosome abnormalities.

Description. A Barr body, or sex chromatin body, is a tightly coiled X chromosome lying against the nuclear membrane of female cells or any cell with more than one X chromosome. It appears as a dark-staining body in the shape of a half-moon and is absent in male cells. Barr bodies are believed to function in early embryonic development and later become inactivated to maintain gene balance of Xs to autosomes. The number of Barr bodies in a client is one less than the number of Xs.

Professional Considerations

Informed consent is recommended for genetic testing.

Preparation

1. Rinse the mouth with mouthwash.
2. Obtain a metal spatula, saline, two slides, and preservative.

Procedure

1. Gently scrape the buccal mucosa with the metal spatula dipped in saline.
2. Clean the spatula and repeat the procedure gently but firmly.
3. Smear the material on the two slides and place them in the preservative.

Postprocedure Care

1. Label the container of the slides with the client's name, the date, and the contents.

Client and Family Teaching

1. Refer the client with abnormal results for genetic counseling.

B

Factors That Affect Results
1. None known.
2. Refer to section in this book on "Informed Consent for Genetic Testing".

Other Data
1. Barr bodies do not give any information about Y chromosomes.
2. Human chromosome analysis, rather than buccal smears, should be used for evaluations of newborns with ambiguous genitalia.
3. The Genetic Information Nondiscrimination Act of 2008 prohibits health plans from using genetic family history or genetic test results from influencing eligibility or premiums for health insurance. It also prohibits employers from using this information to influence decisions about hiring, terminating employment, or employment pay, promotions or privileges.

Basal Gastric Secretion Test

See Hollander Test—Diagnostic.

Basic Metabolic Panel (BMP)—Blood

Norm. See individual test listings: Calcium, Chloride, Carbon dioxide, Creatinine, Glucose, Potassium, Sodium, and Urea nitrogen.

Usage. See individual test listings.

Description. The basic metabolic panel (BMP) is a term defined by The Centers for Medicare and Medicaid Services (CMS) in the United States to indicate a group of tests for which a bundled reimbursement is available. This panel is one of several that replaces the multichannel tests, such as SMA-7. The panel is disease oriented, meaning that payment through Medicare is available only when the test is used to diagnose and monitor a disease, and payment is not available when the test is used for screening purposes in clients who have no signs and symptoms that qualify for the test. All the tests in the panel must be carried out when a BMP is ordered.

Professional Considerations
Consent form NOT required.

Preparation
1. Tube: Red topped, red/gray topped, or gold topped.
2. Do NOT draw specimens during hemodialysis.

Procedure
1. Draw a 5-mL blood sample.

Postprocedure Care
1. None.

Client and Family Teaching
1. See individual test listings.

Factors That Affect Results
1. See individual test listings.

Other Data
1. The selection of tests approved for inclusion in this panel is updated periodically.
2. See individual test listings.

Basophils

See Differential Leukocyte Count—Peripheral Blood.

BASOS

See Differential Leukocyte Count—Peripheral Blood.

BE

See Barium Enema—Diagnostic.

B

Bence Jones Protein—Urine

Norm. Negative.

Positive. Amyloidosis (primary), benign monoclonal gammopathy, cryoglobuline-mia, Fanconi syndrome (adult), hyperparathyroidism, multiple myeloma (high levels indicate poor prognosis), osteomalacia, and Waldenström's macroglobulinemia.

Description. A low-molecular-weight, light-chain immunoglobulin synthesized by malignant plasma cells in the bone marrow and initially broken down and reabsorbed by the kidneys. In multiple myeloma, such a large amount of these proteins are produced that they exceed the kidneys' capacity to metabolize them. This causes them to spill into the urine. Prolonged production of Bence Jones protein eventually causes degeneration of the renal tubular cells, and the protein accumulates in the tubules, causing inclusions that may lead to renal failure. Subsequently, increasing amounts of the protein spill into the urine and can be detected by thermal coagulation and acid tests and confirmed by immunoelectrophoresis.

Professional Considerations

Consent form NOT required.

Preparation

1. Obtain a clean specimen container without preservatives.

Procedure

1. Obtain a 25-mL first morning-voided, random urine specimen in a clean container. A fresh specimen may be taken from a urinary drainage bag.

Postprocedure Care

1. Send the specimen to the laboratory and refrigerate.

Client and Family Teaching

1. Results are normally available within 24 hours.

Factors That Affect Results

1. Failure to refrigerate the specimen may result in false-negative results.
2. False-positive results may be caused by chronic renal insufficiency, connective tissue diseases (such as rheumatoid arthritis, systemic lupus erythematosus [SLE], scleroderma, polymyositis, or Wegener's granulomatosis), and other malignancies (leukemia, lymphoma, and metastatic cancer of the lung or of the gastrointestinal or genitourinary tracts).
3. Drugs that may cause false-positive results include aminosalicylic acid, cephaloridine, chlorpromazine, penicillin (high doses), promazine hydrochloride, sulfisoxazole, and tolbutamide.
4. False-negative results may be caused by very alkaline urine and severe urinary tract infections in which urea splitting occurs.

Other Data

1. In light-chain disease, pancytopenia is absent.

Bentiromide Test

See **Chymex Test for Pancreatic Function**—Diagnostic.

Benzodiazepines—Plasma and Urine

Norm. Blood and urine: negative.
Urine panic level: >200 ng/mL.

	Therapeutic Plasma Values	SI Units
Alprazolam	5-25 ng/mL	
High-dose therapy	25-55 ng/mL	
Panic level	>60 ng/mL	
Chlordiazepoxide	700-1000 ng/mL	2.34-3.34 μmol/L
Panic level	>5000 ng/mL	>16.70 μmol/L

	Therapeutic Plasma Values	SI Units
Clonazepam	15-60 ng/mL	48-190 nmol/L
Panic level	>80 ng/mL	>254 nmol/L
Diazepam	100-1000 ng/mL	0.35-3.51 µmol/L
Panic level	>5000 ng/mL	>17.55 µmol/L
Flurazepam		0.0005-0.280 µg/mL
Panic level	>0.2 µg/mL	>0.5 µmol/L
Lethal level	0.5-4.0 µg/mL	0.00125-0.07 µmol/L
Lorazepam	50-240 ng/mL	1.25-10 µmol/L
Midazolam	0.08-0.25 µg/mL	156-746 nmol/L
Oxazepam	0.15-1.4 µg/mL	
Panic level	>2 µg/mL	
Prazepam	0.12-1.0 µg/mL	0.4-3.1 µmol/L
Temazepam	0.4-0.9 µg/mL	
Triazolam	0.2 µg/mL	

Panic Level Symptoms and Treatment

Symptoms. Acute ingestion: Somnolence, confusion, ataxia, diminished reflexes, vertigo, slurred speech, respiratory depression, and coma.

Chronic ingestion: Confusion, disorientation, ataxia, dizziness, vertigo, impaired coordination, fatigue, and antegrade amnesia.

Treatment

NOTE: Treatment choice(s) depend(s) on client's history and condition and episode history.

1. Administer activated charcoal if within 4 hours of ingestion or if symptoms are present. Repeat as necessary, as benzodiazepines undergo hepatic recirculation.
2. Gastric lavage is not recommended, but should be considered if within 1 hour of ingestion and if ingestion of additional lethal substance is suspected. Use warm tap water or 0.9% saline.
3. Monitor for central nervous system depression.
4. Protect airway. Support breathing with oxygen and mechanical ventilation if necessary.
5. Flumazenil is not recommended for routine use in benzodiazepine overdose. Flumazenil has been used as a competitive antagonist to reverse the profound effects of benzodiazepine overdose. Use of flumazenil is contraindicated if concomitant tricyclic antidepressants were taken or in dependence states because of the risk of causing seizures from lowering the seizure threshold and because it may precipitate symptoms of benzodiazepine withdrawal. Flumazenil may not completely reverse benzodiazepine effects. Thus close monitoring for resedation is required and repeated doses may be needed.
6. Do NOT use barbiturates.
7. Do NOT induce emesis.
8. Forced diuresis or hemodialysis will NOT remove benzodiazepines. No information was found on whether peritoneal dialysis will remove these drugs.

Positive. Hepatic encephalopathy. Drugs include chlordiazepoxide, clonazepam, clorazepate dipotassium, diazepam, fluoxetine, flurazepam hydrochloride, lorazepam, midazolam, oxazepam, prazepam, sertraline, temazepam, and triazolam.

Usage. Suspected drug overdose and drug-use screening.

Description. Benzodiazepines are nonbarbiturate, sedative-hypnotic, and anticonvulsant schedule IV drugs used to treat anxiety and insomnia. They are strongly protein bound, metabolized in the liver, and excreted in urine and feces. Benzodiazepines have long half-lives of 30-200 hours. Overdose may lead to coma and death from respiratory arrest. Serum levels are used to determine therapeutic and toxic levels and the full range of benzodiazepines but are not generally helpful in gauging the effects of overdose.

Professional Considerations

Consent form NOT required.

B

Preparation

1. Blood test: Tube: Lavender topped. MAY be drawn during hemodialysis. Preserve with sodium fluoride.
2. Urine test: Obtain a clean specimen container.
3. Screen client for the use of herbal preparations or natural remedies such as kava-kava (*Piper methysticum*).

Procedure

1. Blood test: Draw a 10-mL blood sample.
2. Urine test: Collect a 30-mL, clean, voided urine sample. A fresh specimen may be taken from a urinary drainage bag.

Postprocedure Care

1. Refrigerate the urine specimen until tested.
2. Preserve blood with sodium fluoride, store at −20 degrees C, and assay within a week.

Client and Family Teaching

1. Offer substance abuse or crisis intervention counseling if applicable.
2. Referrals to appropriate rehabilitation centers and therapeutic community programs should be offered to all addicted clients who may be interested.
3. Results are normally available within 24 hours.

4. If activated charcoal was given for elevated levels, the client should drink 4-6 glasses of water each day for 2 days to prevent constipation. Activated charcoal will also cause stools to be black for a few days.

Factors That Affect Results

1. False-positive urine test results are seen with oxaprozin.
2. Nitrobenzodiazepines are stable in blood stored for up to 24 months at −20 degrees C.
3. Their 7-amino metabolites lose 29% stability at −20 degrees C after 2 months.
4. Benzodiazepine levels are not affected by the administration of flumazenil. The clinical effects of flumazenil occur because of selective displacement of benzodiazepines at receptor sites.

Other Data

1. The positive predictive value for detecting benzodiazepines in urine using the triage visual panel was 77%.
2. Withdrawal symptoms may occur after even a single large dose of benzodiazepines.
3. Urinalysis fails to identify 10% of coabuse of benzodiazepines in opiate addicts.
4. Kava-kava (*Piper methysticum*), a natural herbal remedy anxiolytic, potentiates the effects of benzodiazepines.

Beta Natriuretic Peptide

See **Natriuretic Peptides**—Plasma.

Beta-Amyloid Protein (ABeta, Aβ42)—CSF

Norm. 1250-2100 pg/mL
Alzheimer's disease <1138 pg/mL

Usage. A biomarker used to monitor the progression of Alzheimer's disease. Testing is done in conjunction with CSF testing for the hTau antigen.

Description. Alzheimer's disease, the most common form of dementia, is characterized by the presence of senile plaques and neurofibrillary tangles. The senile plaques contain 40/42-residue beta-amyloid protein (Aβ42), a proteolytic fragment of beta-amyloid precursor protein (APP). APP is present from a

very young age and functions in the development of neural stem cells. The abnormal fragment Abeta is thought to be a primary cause of Alzheimer's disease and floats freely in the cerebrospinal fluid (CSF). CSF levels generally drop the more the disease progresses because the fragments are being deposited from the CSF into the tissues of the brain, forming amyloid plaques. The neurofibrillary tangles of the plaques contain hTau protein that is abnormally phosphorylated. Some studies indicate that the dual findings of low CSF Aβ42 and high CSF hTau protein are useful in diagnosis of

Alzheimer's disease. Levels in plasma are normally 100 times less than those of CSF and also decrease with disease progression.

Professional Considerations

Consent form IS required for the procedure used to obtain the specimen.

Risks
See Lumbar puncture—Diagnostic.
Contraindications
See Lumbar puncture—Diagnostic.

Preparation
1. See Lumbar puncture—Diagnostic.
2. Obtain a sterile container for CSF fluid.

Procedure
1. Collect a 4-mL sample of CSF during the lumbar puncture procedure.

Postprocedure Care
1. See Lumbar puncture—Diagnostic.

Client and Family Teaching
1. See Lumbar puncture—Diagnostic.

Factors That Affect Results
1. Levels increase as the number of neurofibrillary tangles increases.
2. A study published in 2011 (Bayer-Carter et al), found that a low saturated fat, low glycemic index diet reduced CSF levels of Aβ42 in healthy adults.
3. Values may be low in early stages of Alzheimer's disease and earlier stages of dementia.

Other Data
1. The ELISA-based test for Aβ42 is available from Athena Neurosciences (http://www.athenadiagnostics.com).
2. This test is sometimes done in conjunction with hTau antigen testing. See Tau test—CSF.

Beta-1C

See **C3 Complement**—Serum.

Beta-Glucosidase—Diagnostic

Norm. Positive.

Usage. Screening for Gaucher disease, a sphingolipid storage disease.

Description. Beta-glucosidase deficiency is an autosomal recessive disease resulting in a gangliosidosis called "Gaucher disease," which is quickly fatal in infants but progresses more slowly in older children. Beta-glucosidase is an enzyme found in peripheral blood leukocytes that normally metabolizes the glycolipid glucocerebroside. In Gaucher disease, glucocerebroside accumulates and causes splenomegaly, hepatomegaly, anemia, thrombocytopenia, erosion of long bones and pelvic bones, and mental retardation (in infantile form).

Professional Considerations

Consent form NOT required.

Preparation
1. Tube: Green topped and container of ice.
2. If the specimen must be sent to an outside laboratory for processing, notify the in-house laboratory that a specimen will be drawn.

Procedure
1. Draw a 7-mL blood sample.
2. Place the specimen on ice.

Postprocedure Care
1. Transport the specimen to the laboratory immediately.
2. For transport to an outside laboratory, the specimen must be transported in an ice bath the same day.

Client and Family Teaching
1. Results are normally available within 72 hours.

Factors That Affect Results
1. Results are invalid for specimens not placed on ice.

Other Data
1. Anemia can be severe enough to cause respiratory difficulty.
2. Enzyme infusion therapy is recommended treatment in type 3 Gaucher disease.

Beta-Hydroxybutyrate (BHB, BHY, BOHB)—Blood

Norm.

Plasma	<1.2 mmol/L
Serum	<3 mg/dL or <0.3 mEq/L

Usage. Helps differentiate cause of metabolic acidosis with increased anion gap; monitoring effectiveness of therapy for acute diabetic ketoacidosis.

Description. Beta-hydroxybutyrate (BHB) is one of three types of ketone bodies occurring in diabetic ketoacidosis (DKA) and is responsible for the nausea and vomiting that occurs in this condition. When DKA occurs, BHB predominates and contributes significantly to the presence of an increased anion gap. BHB is also the predominant ketone that responds to treatment for acute DKA; thus this test is more useful than the ketone bodies test for assessing the effectiveness of treatment.

Professional Considerations
Consent form NOT required.

Preparation
1. Tube: Red topped, green topped, or gold topped; tube must be precooled in ice.

Procedure
1. Collect a 4-mL blood sample.

Postprocedure Care
1. Place specimen on ice and deliver to the laboratory immediately.

Client and Family Teaching
1. If elevated because of diabetic ketoacidosis, levels will decrease with treatment.

Factors That Affect Results
1. Increased values may be due to acetaminophen or propylene glycol toxicity, statin medications, thiamine deficiency, toluene poisoning.

Other Data
1. None.

Beta₂-Microglobulin (B₂M)—Blood and 24-Hour Urine

Norm.

		SI Units
Blood	<2 µg/mL	<170 nmol/L
Urine	<120 µg/24 hours	<10 mmol/day

Increased. Acquired immune deficiency syndrome (AIDS), aminoglycoside toxicity, Burkitt's lymphoma Daudi, cadmium poisoning (urine), Crohn's disease, hepatitis, leukemia (chronic lymphocytic), malignancies (some), mercury exposure, multiple myeloma, osteitis fibrosa cystica, preeclampsia, renal disease (glomerular, end stage), sarcoidosis, vasculitis, Wilson disease (urine), and Waldenström's microglobulinemia.

Description. A serum protein component found on the surface of nucleated cells throughout the body. It increases in inflammatory conditions and when lymphocyte turnover increases, as in lymphocytic leukemia, or when T-lymphocyte helper (OKT4) cells are attacked by human immunodeficiency virus. Beta₂-microglobulin is metabolized by the renal tubules, with over 99% being reabsorbed. Blood beta₂-microglobulin levels become elevated with malfunctioning glomeruli but drop with malfunctioning tubules. The test (both blood and urine) is most often used for evaluation of renal disease, chronic lymphocytic leukemia, and AIDS. Although beta₂-microglobulin levels rise with HIV infection, the levels do not always correlate with the stages of the infection.

Professional Considerations
Consent form NOT required.

Preparation
1. Tube: Lavender topped or 3-L urine collection container and toluene preservative.
2. Follow protective isolation precautions for clients with AIDS.
3. Write the exact beginning time of the 24-hour urine collection on the laboratory requisition.

Procedure
1. Draw a 4-mL blood sample.
2. For 24-hour urine, discard the first morning-urine specimen. Save all urine voided for 24 hours in a refrigerated, clean, 3-L container to which toluene preservative

has been added. Document the quantity of urine output during the specimen collection period. Include voiding at the end of the 24-hour period. For catheterized clients, keep the drainage bag on ice and empty the urine into the collection container hourly.

Postprocedure Care

1. Compare the quantity of urine in the specimen container with urinary output records. If the specimen contains less urine than was recorded as output, some of the sample may have been discarded, thus invalidating the results.
2. Document the quantity of urine output and the ending time for the 24-hour collection period on the laboratory requisition.

Client and Family Teaching

1. Save all urine voided in the 24-hour period. Urinate before defecating to avoid loss of urine. If any urine is accidentally discarded, discard the entire specimen and restart the collection the next day.
2. Results are normally available within 24 hours.
3. Offer support and referrals for AIDS, cancer, or Crohn's disease as appropriate. The national AIDS information Hotline is 1-800-HIV-0440, the NationalAIDS Hotline is 1-800-CDC-INFO and the telephone number for AIDS Treatment data Network is 1-800-734-7104.

Factors That Affect Results

1. Results are invalidated if the client has received radioactive dyes within 1 week before the test.

Other Data

1. Results can be normal in HIV infection.
2. See also Acquired immune deficiency syndrome (AIDS) evaluation battery—Diagnostic.

Betke-Kleihauer Stain (Fetal Hemoglobin Stain, Kleihauer-Betke Stain, K-B)—Diagnostic

Norm.

	HBF Cells
Adults	<2%
Children	
Newborn	60%-90%
6 months	<5%
1 year	<2%

Usage. Assessment of fetal-maternal hemorrhage in the newborn for determination of the amount of Rh immune globulin (RhoGAM) needed. Routinely performed on RhD-negative women after the birth of an RhD-positive child.

Increased. Anemia (aplastic, congenital hemolytic, myeloblastic, myelophthisic, untreated pernicious, refractory, sickle cell, sideroblastic, spherocytic), diabetes, erythroleukemia, Fanconi anemia, hereditary persistence of fetal hemoglobin (HPFH), hyperthyroidism, hypothyroidism, infants (small-for-gestational-age, with chronic intrauterine anoxia, with developmental abnormalities), leakage of fetal hemoglobin into maternal bloodstream, leukemia (all types, acute, chronic), myelofibrosis, paroxysmal nocturnal hemoglobinuria, pregnancy, thalassemia, thyrotoxicosis, and trisomy D syndrome. Drugs include anticonvulsants.

Description. This test measures the amount of hemoglobin present in the fetal form (HbF) compared to the adult form (HbA). When blood is present in the stool, emesis, or mucus of a newborn, this test differentiates "swallowed blood syndrome" as a result of maternal bleeding from infant gastrointestinal hemorrhage.

Professional Considerations

Consent form NOT required.

Preparation

1. Tube: Lavender topped, or obtain a clean container for the mucus specimen.

Procedure

1. Draw a 4-mL blood sample.
2. For gastrointestinal or mucus specimens from an infant, use a clean glass or plastic container to collect a small amount of emesis, stool, or mucus.

Postprocedure Care

1. None.

Client and Family Teaching

1. Cord blood may be sent as a positive control.
2. Results are normally available within 24 hours.

Factors That Affect Results

1. Reject hemolyzed specimens or specimens received more than 6 hours after collection.

2. Smears must be fixed within 1 hour after preparation.

Other Data

1. A newborn cord blood specimen is recommended as a source of fetal blood to be used as a positive control.
2. Flow cytometry is more precise than Kleihauer-Betke manual technique.

BGP

See **Osteocalcin**—Plasma or Serum.

BHB

See **Beta-Hydroxybutyrate**—Blood.

BHY

See **Beta-Hydroxybutyrate**—Blood.

BIA

See **Guthrie Test for Phenylketonuria**—Diagnostic.

Bicarbonate (HCO₃)—Blood

Norm.

		SI Units
Adult		
Normal venous range	17-23 mEq/L	17-23 mmol/L
Normal arterial range	22-31 mEq/L	22-31 mmol/L
Newborn		
Normal venous range	16-24 mEq/L	16-24 mmol/L
Panic venous range	≤15 mEq/L or >35 mEq/L	≤15 mmol/L or >35 mmol/L

Increased. Anoxia, burns (extensive), compensated respiratory acidosis, eating disorders, fat embolism, gastric lavage, gastric suction, hypokalemia, metabolic alkalosis, and vomiting. Drugs include barbiturates (causing respiratory depression), bicarbonate, corticosteroids (chronic use), diuretics (ethacrynic acid, furosemide, hydrochlorothiazide), laxative (abuse), opiates (causing respiratory depression), oral glutamine, and alkaline salts.

Decreased. Compensated respiratory alkalosis, diabetes mellitus, diarrhea, ethylene glycol poisoning, metabolic acidosis, and renal failure. Drugs include acid salts, ammonium chloride, acetazolamide, cholestyramine, cyclosporin A, methanol, metformin, nitrofurantoin, salicylate toxicity, and triamterene. Herbal or natural remedies include products containing aristolochic acids (*Akebia* spp., *Aristolochia* spp., *Asarum* spp., birthwort, *Bragantia* spp., *Clematis* spp., *Cocculus* spp., *Diploclisia* spp., Dutchman's pipe, Fang chi, Fang ji, Guang fang ji, Kan-Mokutsu, *Menispermum* spp., Mokutsu, Mu tong, *Sinomenium* spp., and *Stephania* spp.).

Description. Bicarbonate is part of the bicarbonate-carbonic acid buffering system and is mainly responsible for regulating the pH of body fluids. It also facilitates the transport of carbon dioxide from the body tissues to the lungs. In the digestive tract, bicarbonate is secreted by the pancreas and liver into the duodenum to neutralize the acid chyme entering from the stomach. Serum bicarbonate levels are approximated from the serum carbon dioxide level minus 1.2 mmol (the average concentration of carbonic acid). More accurate diagnoses regarding the buffering system can be determined by obtainment of an arterial blood sample for blood gas analysis.

Professional Considerations
Consent form NOT required.

Preparation
1. Tube: Green topped.

Procedure
1. Draw a 4-mL blood sample anaerobically.
2. Do NOT draw specimen during dialysis.

Postprocedure Care
1. None.

Client and Family Teaching
1. Results are normally available within 2 hours.

Factors That Affect Results
1. Ingestion of acidic or alkaline solutions may cause increased or decreased results, respectively.
2. Underfilling a Vacutainer tube lowers serum bicarbonate values.
3. Prolonged tourniquet application before phlebotomy increases serum bicarbonate levels.

Other Data
1. Bicarbonate does not improve the hemodynamic condition when lactic acidosis is present.
2. Not reliable in assessing fluid deficit in children.

Bile—Urine

Norm. Reagent screening test: Negative.

Quantitative. <0.2 mg/dL.

Increased or positive. Biliary tract obstruction, cirrhosis, hepatitis (acute, alcoholic, chronic, drug induced), hyperthyroidism, infectious mononucleosis, septicemia, and tumor (biliary tract, liver).

Description. This is a routine test used to detect unsuspected liver disease where jaundice is absent. The test is also used in the differential diagnosis of jaundice because plasma bilirubin present as a result of hemolytic disorders exists in a water-soluble form that cannot be filtered by the kidneys. Bilirubinuria is detected by a yellow foam that forms in a shaken specimen or by a yellow-orange to brown urine color. Serial levels can guide clinical management of liver and biliary disorders.

Professional Considerations
Consent form NOT required.

Preparation
1. Obtain a clean container and a paper bag.

Procedure
1. Obtain a 50-mL random urine specimen in a clean glass or plastic container. A fresh specimen may be taken from a urinary drainage bag.

Postprocedure Care
1. Write the collection time on the laboratory requisition.
2. Place the specimen in the paper bag and transport it to the laboratory immediately.
3. Refrigerate the specimen if the test will not be performed within 1 hour of collection.

Client and Family Teaching
1. Inform the nurse immediately after the specimen has been obtained.
2. Do not contaminate the urine specimen with stool.
3. Results are normally available within 24 hours.

Factors That Affect Results

1. Reject specimens received more than 1 hour after collection.
2. Drugs that may cause false-positive results include chlorpromazine, mefenamic acid, phenothiazines, and salicylates.
3. Drugs that may cause false-negative results include ascorbic acid, ethoxazene hydrochloride, and phenazopyridine.
4. False-positive results may be caused by contamination of the specimen with stool.
5. False-negative results may be caused by prolonged exposure of the specimen to room temperature or to light.

Other Data

1. Bilirubinuria is an insensitive indicator of liver disease.
2. Urinary bile acids are higher in formula-fed infants compared to breast-fed infants.
3. Doxorubicin hydrochloride (Adriamycin) chemotherapy and its metabolites are found in urine and bile.

Bilirubin, Direct (Conjugated)

See Bilirubin—Serum.

Bilirubin, Indirect (Unconjugated, Free)

See Bilirubin—Serum.

Bilirubin (Total, Direct [Conjugated] and Indirect [Unconjugated])—Serum

Norm.

		SI Units
Total Bilirubin		
1 Month to Adult	<1.5 mg/dL	1.7-20.5 µmol/L
Premature Infant		
Cord	<2.8 mg/dL	<48 µmol/L
24 hours	1-6 mg/dL	17-103 µmol/L
48 hours	6-8 mg/dL	103-137 µmol/L
3-5 days	10-12 mg/dL	171-205 µmol/L
Full-Term Infant		
Cord	<2.8 mg/dL	<48 µmol/L
24 hours	2-6 mg/dL	34-103 µmol/L
48 hours	6-7 mg/dL	103-120 µmol/L
3-5 days	4-6 mg/dL	68-103 µmol/L
Direct Bilirubin	0.0-0.3 mg/dL	1.7-5.1 µmol/L
Indirect Bilirubin	0.2-1.2 mg/dL	3.4-20.5 µmol/L

Increased Total Bilirubin. Alcoholism, anemia (pernicious), biliary calculi, biliary obstruction, biliary scar tissue, carcinoma of pancreas head, cholangitis, cirrhosis, Crigler-Najjar syndrome, eating disorders (with liver affected), Dubin-Johnson syndrome, erythroblastosis fetalis, fasting (prolonged), Gilbert disease, graft-versus-host disease (GVHD), hemolysis (autoimmune), hemorrhage, hepatic cryosurgery, hepatitis (alcoholic, infectious, toxic, viral, obstructive), hereditary spherocytosis, impaired liver function, malaria, mononucleosis (infectious), myocardial infarction, pancreatitis (biliary tract origin), pulmonary embolism, sickle cell anemia, toxic shock syndrome, transfusion reactions, and tumor. Drugs include acetaminophen, acetazolamide, acyclovir, aminophenol, amiodarone, amphotericin B, androgens, antimalarials, ascorbic acid, asparaginase, aspirin, barbiturates, carmustine, chlorambucil, chloramphenicol, chlordiazepoxide, chloroquine hydrochloride, chloroquine phosphate, chlorothiazide sodium, chlorpromazine hydrochloride, cholinergics, clindamycin, cyclophosphamide, dextran, diazoxide, dicumarol (dicoumarin), diethylstilbestrol, epinephrine bitartrate, epinephrine borate, epinephrine hydrochloride, erythromycin, ethyl alcohol (ethanol), ethoxazene hydrochloride, floxuridine, flurazepam, fosinopril, histidine, hydrochlorothiazide, hydroxychloroquine sulfate, imipramine, indican, indomethacin, iproniazid, iron, isoniazid, isoproterenol hydrochloride, levodopa, lincomycin, meclofenamate, methanol, methyldopa, methyltestosterone, morphine sulfate, niacin, novobiocin, novobiocin sodium, oral contraceptives, oxazepam, penicillin, phenazopyridine, phenelzine sulfate, phenothiazines, phenprocoumon, phenylbutazone, primaquine phosphate, probenecid, procainamide hydrochloride, protein, pyrazinamide, pyrimethamine, quinacrine hydrochloride, quinidine gluconate, quinidine polygalacturonate, quinidine sulfate, radiographic dyes, rifampin, streptomycin sulfate, tetracyclines, theophylline, thiazide diuretics, tyrosine, valproic acid, vitamin A, vitamin K, and warfarin sodium. Herbs and natural remedies that have the potential to cause hepatotoxicity and elevate values include akee fruit (ackee, *Blighia sapida*), *Atractylis gummifera, Azadirachta indica* (see margosa), *Berberis vulgaris* (barberry), *Callilepis laureola* (blazing star, *Liatris spicata*), chaparral tea (*Larrea tridentata*), cocaine, comfrey ("knitbone," *Symphytum*), *Crotalaria* (bush tea), cycasin (a toxin from a Cycas species of sago palm of Guam), germander (genera *Teucrium* and *Veronica*; do not confuse with safe skullcap, a name often falsely used in selling germander), *Heliotropium* (germander, valerian), *jinbuhuan* ("gold-in-convertible," Jin Bu Huan Anodyne tablets, patent medicine with misidentified constituents: essence of *t'ienchi or tien chi [tianqi]* flowers, "Notoginseng"; also *kombucha*; also *Lycopodium serratum*, or club moss; but with plant alkaloid levo-tetrahydropalmatine, a potent neuroactive substance), mahuang (*Ephedra*), margosa (*Melia azadirachta, Azadirachta indica*), yerba maté or erva maté tea (*Ilex paraguariensis*), mistletoe, pennyroyal, sassafras, skullcap (*Scutellaria*; do not confuse with unsafe germander), syo-saiko-to (*xiao chai hu tang*, "minor Bupleurum combination"), *Teucrium polium* (golden germander), and valerian (*Valeriana officinalis*, garden heliotrope).

Increased Direct Bilirubin. Biliary obstruction, carcinoma of head of the pancreas, cirrhosis, Dubin-Johnson syndrome, hepatitis (acute, alcoholic, infectious, viral, toxic), and rotor syndrome. Also drugs that increase total bilirubin levels: vinho abafado ("augmented Port wine," Brazil), *chuan lian* (*huanglian*, Cantonese *ch'uen lin, Coptis chinensis/japonica*, goldenthread, Huang Lian), tonic, *yinchen* (*Artemisia scoparia, A. capillaris*, mugwort, wormwood).

Increased Indirect Bilirubin. Anemia (pernicious), autoimmune hemolysis, Bartter syndrome, cirrhosis (acute, alcoholic, nonalcoholic), Crigler-Najjar syndrome, erythroblastosis fetalis, Gilbert's disease, hepatitis (all types), hereditary spherocytosis, intracavitary and soft-tissue hemorrhage, malaria, myocardial infarction, septicemia, sickle cell disease, and transfusion reaction (hemolytic). Also, drugs that increase total bilirubin levels.

Decreased Total, Direct, and Indirect Bilirubin. Phototherapy. Drugs include barbiturates, caffeine, chlorine, citrate, corticosteroids, dicophane, eating disorders (with impaired RBC mass), ethyl alcohol (ethanol), fat emulsion, penicillin, protein, salicylates, sulfonamides, thioridazine, and urea.

Description. Bilirubin is produced in the liver, spleen, and bone marrow and is also a by-product of hemoglobin breakdown. Total bilirubin levels can be broken down into direct (conjugated) bilirubin, which is primarily excreted through the intestinal tract, and indirect (free) bilirubin, which circulates primarily in the bloodstream. Total bilirubin levels rise with any type of jaundice, whereas direct and indirect levels rise depending on the cause of the jaundice. Direct (conjugated) bilirubin is that portion of bilirubin that is normally excreted primarily by the gastrointestinal tract, with only small amounts entering the bloodstream. When obstructive or hepatic jaundice occurs, increasing amounts of conjugated bilirubin enter the bloodstream, rather than the gastrointestinal tract, and they are filtered and excreted by the kidneys. Indirect bilirubin (free or unconjugated bilirubin) is the portion of bilirubin that normally circulates in the bloodstream. When hemolytic jaundice occurs, increasing amounts of free bilirubin accumulate in the bloodstream as a result of increased hemoglobin breakdown. There is no direct laboratory test for indirect bilirubin; rather, it is a calculation of total bilirubin minus direct bilirubin.

Professional Considerations
Consent form NOT required.

Preparation
1. See Client and Family Teaching.
2. Tube: Red topped, red/gray topped, or gold topped or a lancet and capillary tube for heelstick specimens. Also obtain foil.
3. Do NOT draw blood during hemodialysis.

Procedure
1. Draw a 4-mL blood sample.
2. For babies, collect heel-stick blood in a capillary tube. Pre-warming the heel is not necessary. Cleanse the lateral curvature of the heel with an alcohol wipe and allow it to dry. Puncture the lateral curvature of the heel with a lancet and collect blood in a capillary tube. Avoid puncturing the posterior curvature of the heel.

Postprocedure Care
1. Leave the heel-stick site open to air.
2. Protect the sample from light. Wrap it in foil or place it in a darkened refrigerator if the test will not be run immediately.

Client and Family Teaching
1. Eat a diet low in yellow foods (such as carrots, yams, yellow beans, pumpkin) for 3-4 days before sampling.
2. Fast for 4 hours before sampling.
3. Serum levels will be elevated with the use of alcohol, morphine, theophylline, ascorbic acid, and aspirin.
4. Results are normally available within 24 hours.

Factors That Affect Results
1. Reject hemolyzed or grossly lipemic specimens.
2. Results are invalidated if the client received a radioactive scan within 24 hours before the test.
3. Cord blood values may be elevated.
4. Drugs that may cause falsely elevated values include acetazolamide, androgens, chlordiazepoxide, chlordiazepoxide hydrochloride, chlorpromazine, erythromycin, erythromycin ethylsuccinate, indomethacin, isoniazid, methanol, nitrofurantoin, nitrofurantoin sodium, oxacillin sodium, oxyphenbutazone, phenothiazines, phenylbutazone, salicylates, sulfinpyrazone, sulfonylureas, sulfonamides, and vitamin A.

Other Data
1. Indirect bilirubin levels may increase in hemolytic disease of the newborn to >20 mg/dL.
2. Neonate treatment for serum bilirubin >15 mg/dL may include exchange transfusion or phototherapy. Phototherapy converts bilirubin into a colorless compound that has no effects on the neonate.
3. Biliary atresia can be differentiated from infantile hepatitis using bilirubin conjugates with MicroMed chromatography.

Bilirubin, Total
See Bilirubin—Serum.

Bilirubin—Urine

Norm. Negative≤0.02 mg/dL (≤0.34 μmol/L, SI units).

Positive or Increased. Arsenic ingestion, cirrhosis, hepatitis (alcoholic, chronic, acute, drug induced), hyperthyroidism, malignancy (hepatic or biliary tract), mononucleosis (infectious), and septicemia. Herbal or natural remedies that have the potential to cause hepatotoxicity and elevate values include akee fruit (ackee, *Blighia sapida*), *Atractylis gummifera, Azadirachta indica* (margosa), *Berberis vulgaris* (barberry), *Callilepis laureola* (blazing star, *Liatris spicata*), chaparral tea (*Larrea tridentata*), cocaine, comfrey ("knitbone," *Symphytum*), *Crotalaria* (bush tea), cycasin (a toxin from a *Cycas* species of sago palm of Guam), germander (genera *Teucrium* and *Veronica*; do not confuse with safe skullcap, a name often falsely used in selling germander), *Heliotropium* (germander, valerian), *jinbuhuan* ("gold-inconvertible," Jin Bu Huan Anodyne tablets, patent medicine with misidentified constituents: essence of *t'ienchi [tianqi]* or tien chi flowers, "Notoginseng"; also *kombucha*; also *Lycopodium serratum*, or club moss; but with plant alkaloid levo-tetrahydropalmatine, a potent neuroactive substance), *mahuang* (Ephedra), margosa (*Melia azadirachta, Azadirachta indica*), yerba maté tea (*Ilex paraguayensis*), mistletoe, pennyroyal, sassafras, skullcap (*Scutellaria*; do not confuse with unsafe germander), *Syo-saiko-to* (*xiao chaihu tang*, "minor Bupleurum combination"), *Teucrium polium* (golden germander), and valerian (*Valeriana officinalis*, garden heliotrope).

Description. Screens for the presence of conjugated bilirubin in the urine. Bilirubin is a by-product of hemoglobin breakdown that is normally excreted by the gastrointestinal tract. When obstructive or hepatic jaundice occurs, conjugated bilirubin enters the bloodstream, rather than the gastrointestinal tract, and is filtered and excreted by the kidneys.

Professional Considerations
Consent form NOT required.

Preparation
1. Obtain Ictotest tablets, N-Multistix, or Chemstrips for urine samples, and a clean container.

Procedure
1. Collect a 20-mL fresh random urine sample in a clean container.
2. Follow package directions exactly for either Ictotest tablets, N-Multistix, or Chemstrips for urine samples.

Postprocedure Care
1. None.

Client and Family Teaching
1. Phenothiazines and ascorbic acid may affect results.
2. Results are normally available within 24 hours.

Factors That Affect Results
1. Drugs that may cause false-positive results with Ictotest tablets include salicylates.
2. Drugs that may cause false-negative results with Ictotest tablets include ascorbic acid.
3. Drugs that may cause false-positive N-Multistix or Chemstrip bilirubin results include phenazopyridine, phenothiazines, and etodolac (nonsteroidal antiinflammatory).
4. A delay in performing the test may result in false-negative results.

Other Data
1. Even trace amounts of bilirubin in the urine require further diagnostic investigation.
2. Pruritus associated with hepatic cholestasis can be improved with the use of phototherapy.
3. There is good agreement between the use of Multistix and Clinitek 200+ analyzer.

Biograph Imaging
See **Dual Modality Imaging**—Diagnostic.

Biopsy, Site-Specific—Specimen

Norm. Interpreted by pathologist.

Usage. Abscess (abscess wall), acute interstitial nephritis (kidney), adrenal feminization (testis), alcoholic myopathy (muscle), alveolar proteinosis (lung), amebiasis (rectum), amyloidosis (tissue), amyotrophic lateral sclerosis (muscle), arthritis (joint), bronchogenic carcinoma (lung, lymph node, pleura), brucellosis (spleen, tissue), carcinoma of pancreas head (pancreas), cardiac transplant rejection, cat-scratch disease (lymph node), cardiovascular disease (endomyocardial), Chagas disease (lung, lymph node), chancroid (lymph node), celiac disease (small intestine), cholesterol ester storage disease (liver), chromoblastomycosis (tissue), chronic inflammatory splenomegaly (spleen), cirrhosis (liver), coccidioidomycosis (joint), coccidiosis (small intestine), colon cancer (colon), de Quervain's thyroiditis (thyroid), Dubin-Johnson syndrome (liver), esophageal cancer (biopsy diagnoses 95% of these) farmer's lung (lung), fatty liver (liver), female infertility, filariasis (lymph node), galactosemia (liver), Gaucher disease (skin), germinal aplasia (testis), glucuronyltransferase deficiency (liver), goiter (thyroid), Goodpasture's syndrome (kidney), glycogenesis (liver), gonorrhea (rectum), Hamman-Rich syndrome (lung), Hashimoto's thyroiditis (thyroid), hemochromatosis (liver), hepatitis (liver), Hirschsprung's disease (rectum), histiocytosis (spleen), Hodgkin's disease (lymph node, spleen), Hurler's syndrome (skin), hypertension (endomyocardium), hyperthyroidism (muscle), hypophosphatemia (bone), immunodeficiency (lymph node), infectious mononucleosis (lymph node), jaundice (liver), kidney transplant rejection (kidney), Kimmelstiel-Wilson syndrome (kidney), Klinefelter's syndrome (testis), legionnaires' disease (lung), leprosy (nasal scrapings, lepromatous lesion), leukemia (spleen), lymphangitis (lymph node), lymphatic leukemia (lymph node), lymphogranuloma venereum (lymph node), lymphoma (lymph node), malabsorption (small intestine), male infertility (testicle), McArdle syndrome (muscle), menstrual irregularities (endometrium), metabolic diseases (muscle, skin), metachromatic leukodystrophy (nerve), metastasis (liver, lymph node), mitochondrial myopathy (muscle), muscular dystrophy (muscle), myasthenia gravis (muscle), myotonia congenita (muscle), myotubular myopathy (muscle), narcotic addiction (liver), nemaline myopathy (muscle), Niemann-Pick disease (rectum, skin), osteomalacia (bone), osteopenia (bone), parasitic infections (spleen), pelvic inflammatory disease (endometrium), pleural tumor (pleura), pneumoconiosis (lung, lymph node), Pneumocystis pneumonia (lung), polyarteritis nodosa (tissue), polymyalgia rheumatica (muscle, temporal artery), polymyositis (muscle), poststreptococcal glomerulonephritis (kidney), proctitis (rectum), rat-bite fever (joint fluid), renal disease (kidney tissue), Reye's syndrome (liver), rheumatoid pleurisy (pleura), Riedel's thyroiditis (thyroid), Rocky Mountain spotted fever (skin), sarcoidosis (lung, lymph node, tissue), schistosomiasis (bladder, rectum), scleroderma (tissue), septic pyelophlebitis (liver), Sjögren's syndrome (kidney), Stein-Leventhal syndrome (ovary), stiff-man syndrome (muscle), stomach carcinoma (bone marrow, liver, lymph node), systemic lupus erythematosus (full-thickness skin, tissue), temporal arteritis (temporal artery), toxemia of pregnancy (kidney), trichinosis (muscle), tuberculosis (bone marrow, lung, lymph node, spleen), tularemia (lymph node), Turner's syndrome (ovary, testis), ulcerative colitis (liver, rectum), villous adenoma (rectum), visceral larva migrans (liver), Wegener's granulomatosis (kidney), Whipple's disease (lymph node, small intestine), Wilson's disease (liver), and yellow fever (liver).

Description. Excisional biopsy (remove entire lump), incisional biopsy (remove part of lump), pinch biopsy (using forceps), snare excision (for large polyps) or needle punch or fine-needle aspiration (FNA) (a small sample is withdrawn through a 22- to 25-gauge needle) done under sterile technique and examined for cell morphology and tissue abnormalities. The procedure takes 15-30 minutes. Each specimen is evaluated by gross examination, by microscopic examination, and through tissue processing (staining and preserving). Adjunct brush cytology is helpful for diagnosing gastric malignancy of infection.

Professional Considerations
Consent form IS required for most specimens and is specific to the institution.

Risks
Allergic reaction to local anesthetic (itching, hives, rash, tight feeling in the throat, shortness of breath, bronchospasm, anaphylaxis, death). Infection, hematoma, mild to severe bleeding, organ damage, and hemorrhage. Vasovagal reaction. Death is possible from biopsies of internal organs.

Contraindications

Previous allergy to local anesthetic. Cutaneous infection at site, platelet count of less than 100,000/mm^3, prothrombin time longer than 15 seconds.

Preparation

1. Obtain the baseline PT/PTT or ACT.
2. Type and crossmatch may be prescribed 24 hours before the biopsy.
3. Obtain sterile containers: one with 10% formaldehyde, the other with sterile saline. For anaerobic culture, obtain a sterile petri dish with premoistened sterile gauze or an anaerobic culture container.
4. Just before beginning the procedure, take a "time out" to verify the correct client, procedure, and site.

Procedure

1. Decubiti should be debrided before the biopsy.
2. Surface wounds, skin, and mucosal surfaces should be cleansed with an alcohol wipe and allowed to dry just before the biopsy.
3. Obtain 20-500 mg of tissue by needle aspiration, excision, or needle-punch using an aseptic technique. Do not contaminate the specimen with other tissue in the area.
4. Place the biopsied material in a sterile container of 10% formaldehyde and in another with sterile saline. Transport the specimens to the laboratory immediately.
5. Anaerobic culture specimens:
   a. For anaerobic culture specimens, a biopsy of the tissue is obtained by the physician, with care being taken to avoid contamination of the specimen with other area organisms and to minimize exposure of the specimen to air.
   b. After it is obtained, the biopsied material is quickly placed on premoistened sterile gauze in a sterile, 100-mm petri dish or in a sterile container with the cap loosened.
   c. An anaerobic transport container such as the Bio-Bag type A Anaerobic Culture Set (Marion) may be used. It consists of a gas-impermeable plastic bag and two ampules: one that generates hydrogen and the other that releases resazurin indicator.
   d. Place the container or petri dish inside the plastic bag with both ampules and seal the bag with a heat sealer.
   e. Crush the gas-generator ampule. Hydrogen from the gas-generator ampule should combine with oxygen in the presence of a catalyst to produce water vapor condensation inside the bag. (See Body fluid—Anaerobic culture for instructions for liquid specimens.)

Postprocedure Care

1. Specific to site and surgery. A dry, sterile dressing is placed over the site.
2. Write the collection time on the laboratory requisition.
3. Assess vital signs and the site for bleeding or hematoma formation every 15 minutes × 4 and then every 30 minutes × 2.
4. Observe for signs of infection (fever, chills, hypotension, tachycardia) every 24-48 hours.

Client and Family Teaching

1. Fast from food, and drink only clear liquids after midnight and before the biopsy.
2. Report signs of infection at the operative site to the physician: increasing pain, redness, swelling, purulent drainage, or temperature >101 degrees F (>38.3 degrees C).
3. Check temperature every 6 hours for 24 hours, and notify the physician if fever, chills, faintness, weakness, or dizziness occurs. Place pressure over the site for 10 minutes if bleeding is noted.
4. Results are normally available within 72 hours. The full report may take up to 5 days.

Factors That Affect Results

1. Taking multiple samples and using a combination of biopsy sampling techniques can increase the accuracy of resulting diagnosis(es).
2. Do not refrigerate the specimen.

Other Data

1. The use of endomyocardial biopsy for evaluation of cardiovascular disease can be controversial due to the risks posed by the procedure. A task force in 2007 identified 14 specific indications for endomyocardial biopsy that can be found at

http://content.onlinejacc.org/cgi/reprint/ 50/19/1914.pdf (Cooper et al).

2. See also Sentinel lymph node biopsy— Diagnostic (specific for breast cancer).

Bladder Tumor—Associated Antigen
See **BTA Test for Bladder Cancer**—Diagnostic.

Blastomycosis (Gilchrist's) Skin Test—Diagnostic

Norm. Negative.

Usage. Diagnosis of *Blastomyces dermatitidis.*

Description. Blastomycosis, a chronic granulomatous and suppurative fungal disease of the lungs and skin, occurs primarily in 20- to 40-year-old males in rural areas throughout the world. There is no evidence of transmission from one client to another, and there is usually no epidemic. The mode of transmission is believed to be inhalation of spores from soil. The spores then disseminate by invading the blood and lymphatic systems. Blastomycosis skin lesions may be erythematous nodes or papular lesions, which can break down, ulcerate, drain, and spread. ARDS can develop from pulmonary blastomycosis and has a death rate of 89%.

Professional Considerations
Consent form NOT required.

Preparation
1. Obtain a sterile container for the biopsy specimen.

Procedure
1. Using a sterile technique, a biopsy specimen is taken from the periphery of a skin lesion where pus and yeast cells are found. A wet mount of the specimen shows broadly attached buds on thick-walled cells.

Postprocedure Care
1. Apply a dry, sterile dressing to the site if bleeding occurs.

Client and Family Teaching
1. Report signs of infection at the biopsy site to the physician: increasing pain, redness, swelling, purulent drainage, or temperature >101 degrees F (>38.3 degrees C).
2. Results are normally available within 72 hours.

Factors That Affect Results
1. Treatment with amphotericin B may cause false-negative results.

Other Data
1. Blastomycosis is a general term used in parts of the world to refer to any infection caused by budding yeasts in the tissue.
2. Endemic areas in the United States include northeast Tennessee, Vilas County (Wisconsin), Mississippi, and the Ohio River valley.

Bleeding Time, Duke—Blood

Norm. 1-5 minutes.

Increased. Anemia (aplastic, pernicious), collagen diseases, congenital heart disease, disseminated intravascular coagulopathy, drug sensitivity, ethyl alcohol ingestion along with aspirin ingestion, factor deficiency (I, II, V, VII, VIII, IX, XI), fibrinolytic activity, Glanzmann's disease, hemorrhagic disease of the newborn, Hodgkin's disease, hypothyroidism, idiopathic thrombocytopenic purpura, infections (measles, mumps, streptococcal), leech bite, leukemia (acute), liver disease (severe), mononucleosis (infectious), multiple myeloma, purpura hemorrhagica, scurvy, thrombasthenia, thrombocytopathy, thrombocytopenia purpura (secondary caused by allergy), von Willebrand's disease, and uremia. Drugs include anticoagulants (oral), indomethacin, non-sterile anti-inflammatory agents (NSAIDS), phenylbutazone, and platelet aggregation inhibitor drugs (aspirin, clopidogrel, eptifibatide). Herbs or natural remedies that may inhibit platelet activity include feverfew (*Tanacetum parthenium*), *Ginkgo biloba*, garlic, ginger, and ginseng.

Decreased. Not clinically significant.

Description. The duration of active bleeding from a standardized superficial puncture wound of the skin is measured. It is most helpful as an indicator of platelet abnormality, either in their number or from their function.

Professional Considerations
Consent form NOT required.

Risks
Bleeding, hematoma, infection, ecchymoses.
Contraindications
This test is contraindicated in clients with a platelet count <50,000/mm³, in clients with severe bleeding disorders, or in clients who have taken medications containing aspirin within 7 days before the test.

Preparation
1. Obtain alcohol wipes, a lancet, a stopwatch, and filter paper.
2. Screen client for the use of herbal preparations or natural remedies such as feverfew (*Tanacetum parthenium*), *Ginkgo biloba*, garlic, ginger, ginseng.

Procedure
1. Cleanse the site for puncture with an alcohol wipe and allow it to dry completely.
2. Make a small lancet puncture in the fingertip or earlobe and simultaneously start the stopwatch.

3. Remove blood from the wound by gently blotting with filter paper, without exerting pressure on the wound, every 30 seconds.
4. When blood flow ceases, stop timing with the stopwatch. If bleeding continues for more than 20 minutes, discontinue the test and apply pressure to the site.

Postprocedure Care
1. Apply a dry, sterile dressing to the site after bleeding stops.

Client and Family Teaching
1. Do not take aspirin for 7 days before the test.
2. Call the physician if there are signs of infection at the test site: increasing pain, bleeding, redness, swelling, purulent drainage, or temperature >101 degrees F (>38.3 degrees C).
3. Results are normally available within 24 hours.

Factors That Affect Results
1. A uniform incision is difficult to make without considerable skill.
2. Pressing too hard on the blood with the filter paper disturbs the platelet plug and prolongs bleeding time.

Other Data
1. The depth of the puncture with the lancet is difficult to standardize and results in difficulty reproducing bleeding times.
2. In one study, daily administration of 75 mg of aspirin for 2 weeks in healthy pregnant women yielded results of Duke bleeding time within normal limits.

Bleeding Time, Ivy—Blood

Norm. 1-9 minutes. Panic range: >15 minutes. Shorter in men than in women, and shorter in persons more than 50 years of age.

Increased. Anemia (aplastic, pernicious), collagen diseases, congenital heart disease, disseminated intravascular coagulopathy, drug sensitivity, ethyl alcohol ingestion along with aspirin ingestion, factor deficiency (I, II, V, VII, VIII, IX, XI), fibrinolytic activity, Glanzmann's disease, hemorrhagic disease of the newborn, Hodgkin's disease, hypothyroidism, idiopathic thrombocytopenic purpura, infections (measles, mumps, streptococcal), leech bite, leukemia (acute), liver disease (severe), mononucleosis (infectious), multiple myeloma, purpura hemorrhagica, scurvy, thrombasthenia, thrombocytopathy, thrombocytopenia purpura (secondary because of allergy), von Willebrand's disease, and uremia. Drugs include anticoagulants (oral), indomethacin, ketorolac, non-sterile anti-inflammatory agents (NSAIDS), phenylbutazone, and platelet aggregation inhibitor drugs (aspirin, clopidogrel, eptifibatide). Herbs or natural remedies that may inhibit platelet activity include feverfew (*Tanacetum parthenium*), *Ginkgo biloba*, garlic, ginger, and ginseng.

Decreased. Not clinically significant.

Description. The duration of active bleeding from superficial incisions of the skin is measured. It is most helpful as an indicator of platelet abnormality, either in their number or from their function. This method is more sensitive than the Duke bleeding time because a blood pressure cuff is used to increase venous pressure and ensure capillary filling without interfering with venous return.

Professional Considerations
Consent form NOT required for most labs.

Risks
Bleeding, hematoma, infection, ecchymoses, scar, or keloid formation.
Contraindications
This test is contraindicated in clients who require upper-extremity restraints, have edematous or very cold arms, or are prone to keloid formation. It should not be performed if there are contraindications to placing or inflating a blood pressure cuff on the arm (casts, rash, dressings, arteriovenous fistula). Other contraindications include platelet count <50,000/mm^3, severe bleeding disorders, skin infectious diseases, and senile skin changes or if the client has taken medications containing acetyl groups within 7 days before the test.

Preparation
1. See Client and Family Teaching.
2. Obtain a blood pressure cuff, a manometer, alcohol wipes, a stopwatch, a lancet, and filter paper.
3. Screen client for the use of herbal preparations or natural remedies such as feverfew (*Tanacetum parthenium*), *Ginkgo biloba*, garlic, ginger, and ginseng.

Procedure
1. Cleanse the volar aspect of the forearm with an alcohol wipe and allow it to dry completely. Choose a site with no superficial veins.
2. Place the blood pressure cuff on the upper arm and inflate it to 40 mm Hg.
3. Make two small incisions or puncture wounds 2-3 mm deep with the lancet on the site that was cleansed with alcohol. Start timing with the stopwatch.
4. Remove blood from the wounds by gently blotting with filter paper, without exerting pressure on the wound, every 30 seconds.
5. When the blood flow ceases, stop timing with the stopwatch. If bleeding continues for more than 20 minutes, discontinue the test and apply pressure to the site.
6. Calculate the bleeding time by averaging the bleeding time of both incisions.

Postprocedure Care
1. If the bleeding time is normal, apply a dry dressing to the site. If the bleeding time is prolonged, apply a pressure bandage to the site.

Client and Family Teaching
1. Do not take aspirin for 7 days before the test.
2. Call the physician if there are signs of infection at the test site: increasing pain, bleeding, redness, swelling, purulent drainage, or temperature >101 degrees F (>38.3 degrees C).
3. Results are normally available within 24 hours.

Factors That Affect Results
1. A uniform incision is difficult to make without considerable skill.
2. Pressing too hard on the blood with the filter paper disturbs the platelet plug and prolongs bleeding time.

Other Data
1. The depth of the puncture with the lancet is difficult to standardize and results in difficulty reproducing bleeding times.
2. Healthy pregnant women given 75 mg of aspirin for 2 weeks have an increased bleeding time by Ivy tests.
3. Nitric oxide does not affect IV bleeding time.

Bleeding Time, Mielke—Blood

Norm. 2.5-8 minutes.

Increased. Anemia (aplastic, pernicious), collagen diseases, congenital heart disease, disseminated intravascular coagulopathy, drug sensitivity, ethyl alcohol ingestion along with aspirin, factor deficiency (I, II, V, VII, VIII, IX, XI), fibrinolytic activity, Glanzmann's disease, hemorrhagic disease of the newborn, Hodgkin's disease, hypothyroidism, idiopathic thrombocytopenic purpura, infections (measles, mumps, streptococcal), leech bite, leukemia (acute), liver disease (severe), mononucleosis (infectious), multiple myeloma, purpura hemorrhagica, scurvy, thrombasthenia, thrombocytopathy, thrombocytopenia purpura (secondary because of allergy), von Willebrand's disease, and uremia. Drugs include anticoagulants (oral), indomethacin, non-sterile anti-inflammatory agents (NSAIDS), phenylbutazone, and platelet aggregation inhibitor drugs (aspirin, clopidogrel, eptifibatide). Herbs or natural remedies that may inhibit platelet activity include feverfew (*Tanacetum parthenium*), *Ginkgo biloba*, garlic, ginger, and ginseng.

Decreased. Not clinically significant.

Description. The duration of active bleeding from a standardized superficial incision of the skin is measured. It is particularly helpful as an indicator of platelet abnormality, either in the number or from the function of the platelets. This method is more sensitive than the Duke bleeding time because a blood pressure cuff is used to increase venous pressure and ensure capillary filling without interfering with venous return. Because the template standardizes the length and depth of the incision, this is the most accurate manual method for measuring bleeding time. An automated Surgicutt instrument is available to further standardize the incision.

Professional Considerations

Consent form NOT usually required.

Risks

Bleeding, hematoma, infection, ecchymoses, scar, or keloid formation.

Contraindications

In clients who require upper-extremity restraints, have edematous or very cold arms, or are prone to keloid formation. The test should not be performed if there are contraindications to placing or inflating a blood pressure cuff on the arm (casts, rash, dressings, arteriovenous fistula). Other contraindications include platelet count <50,000/mm³, severe bleeding disorders, skin infectious diseases, and senile skin changes, or if the client has taken medications containing acetyl groups within 7 days before the test.

Preparation

1. See Client and Family Teaching.
2. Obtain a blood pressure cuff and a manometer, alcohol wipes, a stopwatch, a template, and filter paper.
3. Screen client for the use of herbal preparations or natural remedies such as feverfew (*Tanacetum parthenium*), *Ginkgo biloba*, garlic, ginger, and ginseng.

Procedure

1. Cleanse the volar aspect of the forearm with an alcohol wipe and allow it to dry completely. Choose a site with no superficial veins.
2. Place the blood pressure cuff on the upper arm and inflate to 40 mm Hg.
3. *Manual incision:* Using a specially calibrated template to pass the scalpel blade through, make two incisions 9 mm long and 1 mm deep on the site that was cleansed with alcohol. Start timing with the stopwatch.
4. *Automated incision:* Place the Surgicutt instrument on the site that was cleansed with alcohol and start the stopwatch at the same time as the device is triggered. The device will make a standardized puncture incision 5 mm long by 1 mm deep. Repeat at a second site.
5. Remove the blood from the wound by gently blotting with the filter paper, without exerting pressure on the wound, every 30 seconds.
6. When the blood flow ceases, stop timing with the stopwatch. If bleeding continues

for more than 20 minutes, discontinue the test and apply pressure to the site.
7. Calculate the bleeding time by averaging the bleeding times of both incisions.

Postprocedure Care
1. If the bleeding time is normal, apply the dressing to the site. If the bleeding time is prolonged, apply a pressure bandage to the site.
2. A butterfly closure may be required for 24 hours.

Client and Family Teaching
1. Do not take aspirin for 7 days before the test.
2. Call the physician if there are signs of infection at the test site: increasing pain, bleeding, redness, swelling, purulent drainage, or temperature >101 degrees F (>38.3 degrees C).
3. Results are normally available within 24 hours.

Factors That Affect Results
1. With standardized incisions, one incision yields as much information as two non-standardized incisions.
2. Pressing too hard on the blood with the filter paper disturbs the platelet plug and prolongs the bleeding time.

Other Data
1. This procedure is not widely used because the scalpel and template require sterilization after each use and the procedure may produce a small scar.

Bleeding Time Aspirin Tolerance Test
See Aspirin Tolerance Test—Diagnostic.

Blood Biopsy
See Bone Marrow Aspiration Analysis—Specimen and Circulating Tumor Cell Test—Blood.

Blood Culture—Blood

Norm. Negative or no growth.

Positive. Anthrax, bacteremia, and septicemia (common in low-birth-weight infants).

Description. Blood is inoculated in aerobic and anaerobic laboratory culture media and observed for growth of pathogenic organisms. Blood cultures may be positive in either bacteremia or septicemia. Bacteremia is a localized infection, as in a particular organ or area of tissue, in which a small portion of the infectious bacteria escapes into the bloodstream. It may occur transiently, without infection after tooth brushing or specialized procedures such as dental surgery, bronchoscopy, tonsillectomy, endoscopy, cystoscopy, and transurethral resection. Septicemia occurs when a large amount of pathogenic microorganisms are dispersed throughout the bloodstream and is usually accompanied by systemic shock symptoms. Blood cultures are generally drawn as the fever is spiking, from two different sites at the same time (one immediately after the other) and again 3 hours later. The number and frequency may vary by institution and practitioner, although more than 2 or 3 is neither helpful nor cost-effective in assessment of persons with endocarditis. For clients in whom antimicrobial therapy has preceded blood cultures, the number of times cultured may be doubled (that is, double cultures drawn four different times). Results are reported as the amount of growth after a specific number of days.

Professional Considerations
Consent form NOT required.

Preparation
1. Obtain alcohol, a sterile gauze, povidone-iodine, two needles, two 30-mL syringes, and two anaerobic and two aerobic culture bottles.
2. MAY be drawn during hemodialysis.

Procedure
1. Palpate the vein to determine location. Do not touch the site after cleansing.

2. Cleanse the site for culture with an alcohol wipe and allow it to dry.
3. Cleanse the site with povidone-iodine and allow it to dry completely or for at least 1 minute.
4. Draw 10-20 mL of blood into a syringe. Avoid aspirating air into the syringe. If bacteremia is suspected, increase the volume of blood drawn to 30 mL.
5. Place a fresh needle on the syringe.
6. Remove the caps from the vacuum culture bottles and inject 5-10 mL into a vacuum bottle containing an anaerobic culture medium and 5-10 mL into a vacuum bottle containing an aerobic culture medium. If bacteremia is suspected, inject at least 15 mL into each bottle. Depending on the size of the bottle, more blood may be required to obtain at least a 1:10 dilution. Mix both bottles gently.
7. Immediately repeat the above procedure at a different site.

Postprocedure Care

1. Cleanse the puncture site with antiseptic and apply pressure.
2. Write the collection time on the laboratory requisition.
3. Write the presumptive diagnosis and the recent antimicrobial therapy on the laboratory requisition.
4. Transport the specimens to the laboratory for incubation within 1 hour.

Client and Family Teaching

1. Call the physician if there are signs of infection at the culture site: increasing pain, redness, swelling, purulent drainage, or temperature >101 degrees F (>38.3 degrees C).
2. Antibiotic or antifungal treatment will begin after the cultures are taken and before the final results.
3. The first results are normally available in 24 hours and continue for up to 2 weeks.

Factors That Affect Results

1. Reject specimens received more than 1 hour after collection.
2. Increasing the volume of blood cultured in suspected bacteremia may yield more positive cultures.
3. False-negative results or delayed growth may be obtained when blood cultures are drawn after antimicrobial therapy has begun.
4. Some common skin flora that may contaminate blood cultures include *Staphylococcus epidermidis*, diphtheroids, and *Propionibacterium*.
5. There is a higher incidence of positive blood cultures in clients receiving hyperalimentation.

Other Data

1. Pathogenic species most often cultured include *Actinobacter, Bacteroides, Brucella, Citrobacter, Clostridium, Enterobacter, Escherichia coli, Francisella, Haemophilus, Klebsiella, Leptospira, Listeria, Mycobacterium, Neisseria, Nocardia, Pseudomonas, Salmonella, Serratia, Staphylococcus, Streptococcus*, and *Vibrio*.
2. The contamination rate for blood cultures collected using an iodophor (povidone-iodine) is greater than when iodine tincture is used.
3. Clients on antimicrobial therapy have an enhanced yield for staphylococci using a FAN bottle compared to the standard aerobic BacT/Alert bottle.
4. Eleven percent of blood cultures are negative in infective endocarditis.
5. Instillation of 1.5 mL of taurolidine 2% into a central line daily decreases catheter-related bloodstream infections.
6. Use of chlorhexidine and silver sulfadiazine coated catheters reduces the risk of catheter colonization.

Blood, Fungus—Culture

Norm. Negative or no growth.

Usage. Definitive diagnosis of systemic fungal infections.

Description. Fungi are slow-growing, eukaryotic organisms that can grow on living and nonliving organic materials and are subdivided into yeasts and molds. Factors that predispose clients to fungal infections by lowering the normal host defense mechanisms include administration of broad-spectrum antibiotics or chemotherapy, history of severe trauma or burns, invasive lines, poor nutritional status, parenteral nutrition, surgery, trauma, and long-term use of steroids. Some fungi may be inhaled or introduced by traumatic inoculation into deep tissue spaces and cause serious infections. Although tentative identification of fungi can be made quickly with staining techniques, culture of the organism in special fungal culture media is required to confirm a diagnosis of a fungal infection. Fungal cultures are generally inoculated on at least three media to facilitate recovery of all etiologic agents.

Professional Considerations
Consent form NOT required.

Preparation
1. Obtain alcohol wipes, sterile gauze, povidone-iodine, two needles, two 20-mL syringes, and two fungal culture bottles.

Procedure
1. Palpate the vein to determine the location. Do not touch the site after cleansing.
2. Cleanse the site for culture with an alcohol wipe and allow it to dry.
3. Cleanse the site with povidone-iodine and allow it to dry completely or for at least 1 minute.
4. Remove the caps from two fungal culture vacuum bottles, cleanse the rubber stoppers with an alcohol wipe and 2% iodine, and allow them to dry.
5. Draw a 10-mL blood sample into a syringe.
6. Place a fresh needle on the syringe and inject the 10 mL of blood into a vacuum bottle containing a blood culture medium specific for fungi. Mix the bottle gently.
7. Immediately repeat the above procedure at a different site.

Postprocedure Care
1. Wipe the venipuncture site with an antimicrobial agent.

2. Write the collection time on the laboratory requisition.
3. Write the presumptive diagnosis and recent antifungal therapy on the laboratory requisition.
4. Incubate the culture bottles at 25-30 degrees C in the laboratory.

Client and Family Teaching
1. Preliminary results will be available within 72 hours and final results in 30 days.
2. Treatment for potential infection will begin before results are obtained and may include macrophage colony-stimulating factor, amphotericin B, itraconazole, or fluconazole.

Factors That Affect Results
1. Some common skin floras that may contaminate blood cultures include *Staphylococcus epidermidis*, diphtheroids, and *Propionibacterium*.

Other Data
1. Fungal cultures of blood must be incubated at least 30 days before being reported as negative.
2. Fungi most often cultured from blood include *Blastomyces dermatitidis*, *Coccidioides immitis*, *Cryptococcus neoformans*, *Histoplasma capsulatum*, *Histoplasma duboisii*, *Paracoccidioides brasiliensis*, *Candida albicans*, *Aspergillus fumigatus*, and *Pseudallescheria boydii*.
3. The BacT/Alert system may miss some fungi growth. This problem can be overcome by prolonged incubation and terminal subculture when fungal infection is considered to be likely.
4. Detection of amphotericin B resistance of yeast isolates (*Candida species*, *Torulopsis glabrata*, *Saccharomyces cerevisiae*, *Cryptococcus neoformans*) within 12-14 hours after inoculation of the test medium is possible.

Blood Gases, Arterial (ABG)—Blood

Norm. Must be corrected for body temperature.

		SI Units
pH		
Adults	7.35-7.45	7.35-7.45
Panic values	≤7.2 and >7.6	≤7.2 and >7.6

		SI Units
Children		
Birth to 2 months	7.32-7.49	7.32-7.49
2 months to 2 years	7.34-7.46	7.34-7.46
>2 years	7.35-7.45	7.35-7.45
PaCO$_2$	35-40 mm Hg	4.7-5.3 kPa
Panic values	<20 mm Hg	<2.7 kPa
	>70 mm Hg	>9.4 kPa
PaO$_2$	80-100 mm Hg	10.7-13.3 kPa
Panic values	<40 mm Hg	<5.3 kPa
HCO$_3^-$	22-31 mEq/L	22-31 mmol/L
Panic values	<10 mEq/L	<10 mmol/L
	>40 mEq/L	>40 mmol/L
O$_2$ Saturation	96%-100%	0.96-1.00
Panic value	<60%	<0.60
Oxyhemoglobin Dissociation Curve		No shift

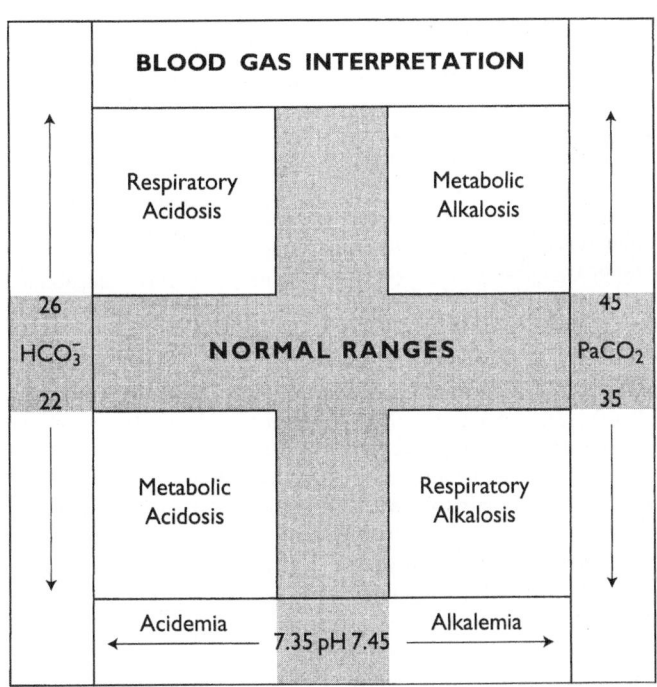

Increased pH. Alkali ingestion, Cushing's disease, diarrhea, fever, high altitude, hyperventilation, hysteria, intestinal obstruction (pyloric, duodenal), metabolic alkalosis, peptic ulcer therapy, renal disease, respiratory alkalosis, salicylate intoxication, and vomiting (excessive). Drugs include sodium bicarbonate.

Increased PaCO$_2$. Acute intermittent porphyria, aminoglycoside toxicity, asthma (late stage), brain death, coarctation of the aorta, congestive heart failure, electrolyte disturbance (severe), emphysema, empyema, hyaline membrane disease, hyperemesis, hypothyroidism (severe), hypoventilation (alveolar), metabolic alkalosis, near drowning, pleural effusion, pleurisy, pneumonia, pneumothorax, poisoning, pulmonary edema, pulmonary infection, renal disorders, respiratory acidosis, respiratory failure, shock, tetralogy of Fallot, transposition of the great vessels, and vomiting. Drugs include aldosterone, ethacrynic acid, metolazone, prednisone, sodium bicarbonate, and thiazides.

Increased PaO₂. Hyperbaric oxygenation and hyperventilation.

Increased HCO₃⁻. Anoxia, metabolic alkalosis, and respiratory acidosis.

Increased O₂ Saturation. High altitudes, hyperbaric oxygenation, hypocapnia, hypothermia, increased cardiac output, increased oxygen affinity for hemoglobin, oxygen therapy, positive end-expiratory pressure (PEEP) added to mechanical ventilation, respiratory alkalosis.

Decreased pH. Addison's disease, asthma, cardiac disease, diabetic ketoacidosis, diarrhea, emphysema, dysrhythmias, hepatic disease, hypercapnia, hypoventilation, malignant hyperthermia, metabolic acidosis, myocardial infarction, nephritis, nephrosis, pneumonia, pulmonary edema, pulmonary embolism, pulmonary infection, pulmonary malignancy, pulmonary obstructive disease, renal disease, respiratory acidosis (also caused by large volumes of lactated Ringer's), respiratory failure, sepsis, and shock.

Decreased PaCO₂. Dysrhythmias, asthma (early stage), diabetic ketoacidosis, diabetes mellitus, fever, high altitude, hyperventilation, metabolic acidosis, respiratory alkalosis, and salicylate intoxication. Drugs include acetazolamide, dimercaprol, methicillin sodium, nitrofurantoin, nitrofurantoin sodium, tetracycline, and triamterene.

Decreased PaO₂. Acute respiratory distress syndrome, anesthesia, anoxia, aortic valve stenosis, arteriovenous shunt, asthma, atelectasis, atrial septal defect, berylliosis, carbon monoxide poisoning, cerebrovascular accident, coarctation of the aorta, emphysema, flail chest, Hamman-Rich syndrome, head injury, hyaline membrane disease, hypercapnia, hypoventilation, lung resection, lymphangitic carcinomatosis, near drowning, pain causing restricted diaphragmatic breathing, phrenic nerve paralysis,

pickwickian syndrome, pleural effusion, pneumonia, pneumothorax, poisoning, poliomyelitis (acute), pulmonary adenomatosis, pulmonary embolism, pulmonary hemangioma, pulmonary infection, pulmonic stenosis, respiratory failure, sarcoidosis, shock, smoke inhalation, status epilepticus, tetanus, transposition of the great vessels, tricuspid atresia, and ventricular septal defect.

Decreased HCO₃⁻. Hypocapnia, metabolic acidosis, and respiratory alkalosis.

Decreased O₂ Saturation. Acute respiratory distress syndrome, anesthesia, anorexia, anoxia, aortic valve stenosis, arteriovenous shunt, asthma, atelectasis, atrial septal defect, berylliosis, carbon monoxide poisoning, cerebrovascular accident, coarctation of the aorta, congenital heart defects, decreased cardiac output, decreased oxygen affinity for hemoglobin, emphysema, fever, flail chest, Hamman-Rich syndrome, head injury, hyaline membrane disease, hypercapnia, hypoventilation, hypoxia, lung resection, lymphangitic carcinomatosis, near drowning, pain causing restricted diaphragmatic breathing, phrenic nerve paralysis, pickwickian syndrome, pleural effusion, pneumonia, pneumothorax, poisoning, poliomyelitis (acute), pulmonary adenomatosis, pulmonary embolism, pulmonary hemangioma, pulmonary infection, pulmonic stenosis, respiratory acidosis, respiratory failure, sarcoidosis, shock, smoke inhalation, status epilepticus, tetanus, transposition of the great vessels, tricuspid atresia, and ventricular septal defect.

Oxyhemoglobin Dissociation Curve. See diagram.

Shift to Left. 2,3-DPG deficiency, high altitude, hypocapnia, hypothermia, and respiratory alkalosis.

Shift to Right. Cluster headaches, emphysema, fever, hypercapnia, increased production of 2,3-DPG, and respiratory acidosis.

Description. The arterial blood gas test measures the dissolved oxygen and carbon dioxide in the arterial blood and reveals the acid-base state and how well the oxygen is being carried to the body. The pH is the measurement of free H⁺ ion concentration in circulating blood. Intracellular metabolism results in the continuous production of

NORMAL OXYHEMOGLOBIN DISSOCIATION CURVE

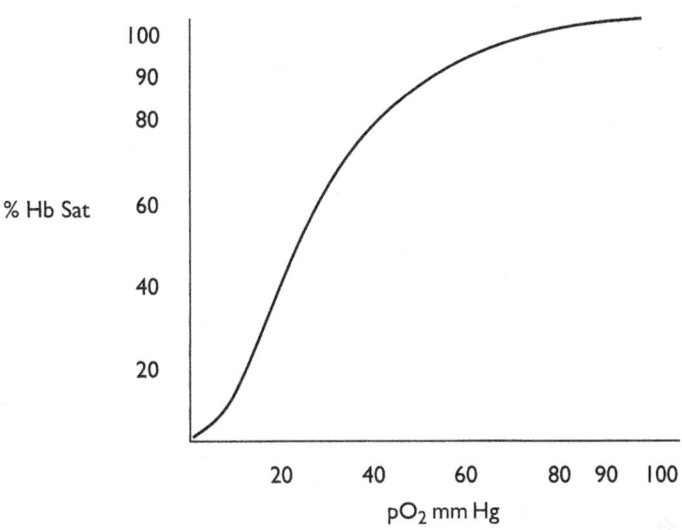

hydrogen ions, which are buffered as either an acid (HCO_3^-) or a base (H_2CO_3). The body demands that pH remain constant. The kidneys and lungs regulate pH by preserving the ratio of acid to base. Any alteration in the ratio between bicarbonate and carbonic acid will cause a reciprocal change in release or uptake of free H^+, thereby altering pH value. Significant deviations in pH can be life threatening. Both bicarbonate (HCO_3^-) and carbonic acid (H_2CO_3) are components of the body's acid-base system that influence pH. The partial pressure of carbon dioxide (pCO_2, $PaCO_2$) is the amount of carbon dioxide in the blood based on the pressure it exerts in the bloodstream and represents the degree of alveolar ventilation occurring. When pH decreases, more CO_2 dissociates from carbonic acid and is exhaled through the lungs, counteracting the pH reduction and increasing the breathing rate. The partial pressure of oxygen (pO_2, PaO_2) is the amount of oxygen dissolved in plasma and represents the status of alveolar gas exchange with inspired air. Oxygen saturation (O_2Sat) is the amount of oxygen actually bound to hemoglobin (as a percentage of the maximum amount that could be bound) and available for transport throughout the body. SaO_2 applies to arterial hemoglobin saturation:

Oxygen saturation =
    Oxygen content × (100/Oxygen capacity)

The oxyhemoglobin dissociation curve represents the affinity of hemoglobin for oxygen by demonstrating the normal levels of arterial oxygen saturation (O_2Sat, SaO_2) of hemoglobin at varying partial pressures of oxygen. P-50 is the partial pressure of oxygen at which the given hemoglobin sample is 50% saturated. The Hem-O-Scan machine analyzes and plots the hemoglobin-oxygen dissociation on a curve. When the curve is shifted to the left, more oxygen is delivered to the tissues for a given partial pressure of oxygen; when the shift is to the right, less oxygen is delivered to the tissues. Generally, decreased oxygen saturation to less than 90%-92% must be addressed by thorough assessment of the client and clinical status.

Professional Considerations
Consent form NOT required.

Risks
Two percent overall complication rate with brachial artery puncture. Prolonged bleeding, hematoma, infection, or nerve damage near puncture site. Arterial occlusion.
Contraindications and Precautions
In clients with bleeding disorders or anticoagulated states, repeated sampling from an invasive arterial catheter is preferred over arterial punctures.

B

Preparation

1. A modified Allen's test should be performed on both wrists before radial artery specimens are drawn. This test is performed to ensure adequate ulnar artery blood flow to the hand, in the event that the radial artery becomes occluded as a procedural complication. Occlude both the ulnar and the radial arteries with two fingers for 10 seconds. Then release the pressure over the ulnar artery and observe the hand. If the pink coloring does not return to the hand within 15 seconds, this extremity should NOT be used for arterial puncture.
2. Obtain a blood gas syringe, a 23-gauge needle, a povidone-iodine swab, alcohol wipes, sterile gloves, sterile gauze, and a container of ice.
3. The client should rest for 30 minutes before specimen collection.

Procedure

1. The site for arterial puncture may be anesthetized with 1%-2% lidocaine.
2. Attach a 1-inch-long, 23-gauge needle to a plastic or glass blood gas syringe containing 0.5 mL of lithium heparin (1000 U/mL). Rotate the syringe to coat the inside surface with heparin (1000 U/mL) and eject the heparin through the needle into the sterile gauze.
3. Cleanse the site for puncture with povidone-iodine solution and then with alcohol and allow it to dry.
4. While wearing a sterile glove, palpate the artery and puncture the skin at a 30-45-degree angle (for radial artery), a 45-60-degree angle (for brachial artery), or a 45-90-degree angle (for femoral artery) with the bevel of the needle turned up.
5. Advance the needle until the artery is punctured, and allow the syringe to self-fill with at least 0.6 mL of arterial blood.
6. Remove the syringe and needle and apply pressure to the sterile gauze over the site while discarding the needle, expelling the air from the syringe, and quickly capping the syringe with a rubber stopper and gently mixing the specimen.
7. Immediately place the specimen in an ice bath.

Postprocedure Care

1. Record the client's body temperature and the mode and amount of oxygen delivery on the laboratory requisition.

2. Transport the specimen to the laboratory for processing within 15 minutes.
3. If the specimen was obtained by means of direct arterial puncture, hold pressure over the site for 5-10 minutes.

Client and Family Teaching

1. Results are normally available within 30 minutes.
2. The client's temperature is necessary for calculation and interpretation of the results.
3. Results are interpreted according to the disease or condition and compared to previous blood gas results.

Factors That Affect Results

1. Reject clotted specimens.
2. If the client is receiving endotracheal suctioning or respiratory therapy treatments, the specimen should be drawn at least 20 minutes after either procedure.
3. Failure to expel all air from the blood gas syringe will result in a falsely elevated PaO_2 and a falsely decreased $PaCO_2$.
4. Failure to place the specimen in an ice bath may result in a decreased pH, PaO_2, and oxygen saturation.
5. Failure to expel the heparin from the syringe before specimen collection may result in decreased pH, $PaCO_2$, and PaO_2.
6. Specimen storage at room temperature accelerates the fall in pH.
7. Elevated body temperature decreases the oxygen saturation result.
8. Clients with a history of cigarette smoking can have decreased arterial oxygen saturation after anesthesia.
9. Elevated WBC causes a rapid pH drop.
10. Sodium fluoride can cause either an increase or a decrease in pH.
11. A prolonged time lapse between collection and testing may result in a decreased pH.
12. Herbs or natural remedy effects: In one study, people who received 20 mg of ginseng twice each day for 3 months demonstrated improved arterial blood oxygen and walking distance, as well as pulmonary function test measurements (FVC, FEV1, and PEFR).

Other Data

1. If arterial blood is not practical to obtain, venous blood may be obtained by

venipuncture, but accuracy is evident only for monitoring pH, PaCO$_2$, and base excess.

2. Evaluation of pH should take into consideration alterations in electrolyte, carbon dioxide, oxygen, and bicarbonate levels.

3. Samples of cord blood stored in heparinized syringes for more than 30 minutes result in significant changes in pH and pCO$_2$.

4. Earlobe gas analysis is an accurate substitute for arterial sampling.

5. In anemia, oxygen saturation may be normal, but hypoxia may still be present because of decreased oxygen-carrying capacity.

6. Continuous oxygen saturation monitoring by pulse oximetry is useful during cardiac catheterization in conjunction with intracardiac pressure measurement in the detection of intracardiac abnormalities.

7. A base deficit of less than or equal to −6 indicates a high mortality in trauma.

8. See also Oximetry—Diagnostic.

Blood Gases, Capillary—Blood

Norm. Must be corrected for body temperature.

		SI Units
pH		
Adults	7.35-7.45	7.35-7.45
Panic values	<7.2 or >7.6	<7.2 or >7.6
Children (arterialized capillary sample)		
Birth to 2 months	7.32-7.49	7.32-7.49
2 months to 2 years	7.34-7.46	7.34-7.46
>2 years	7.35-7.45	7.35-7.45
pCO$_2$	26.4-41.2 mm Hg	3.5-5.4 kPa
Panic values	<20 mm Hg	<2.7 kPa
	>70 mm Hg	>9.4 kPa
pO$_2$	75-100 mm Hg	10.0-13.3 kPa
Panic values	<40 mm Hg	<5.3 kPa
HCO$_3^-$	22-26 mEq/L	22-26 mmol/L
Panic values	<10 mEq/L	<10 mmol/L
	>40 mEq/L	>40 mmol/L
O$_2$ Saturation	96%-100%	0.96-1.00
Panic value	<60%	<0.60

Increased pH. See Blood gases, Arterial—Blood.

Increased pCO$_2$. See Blood gases, Arterial—Blood.

Increased pO$_2$. See Blood gases, Arterial—Blood.

Increased HCO$_3^-$. See Blood gases, Arterial—Blood.

Increased O$_2$ Saturation. See Blood gases, Arterial—Blood.

Decreased pH. See Blood gases, Arterial—Blood.

Decreased pCO$_2$. See Blood gases, Arterial—Blood.

Decreased pO$_2$. Capillary po$_2$ interpretation is limited to assessment for hypoxia.

Decreased HCO$_3^-$. See Blood gases, Arterial—Blood.

Decreased O$_2$ Saturation. See Blood gases, Arterial—Blood.

Description. A method for determining acid-base status from a heel stick for capillary blood. Used mostly in infants to assess pH and pCO$_2$. (See Blood gases,

Arterial-Blood, for complete description of the test components.)

Professional Considerations
Consent form NOT required.

Preparation
1. Warmth may be applied to the heel for 15 minutes before collection but is not necessary.
2. Obtain alcohol wipes, a lancet, sterile gauze, two capillary tubes with a metal stirrer, and a magnet.

Procedure
1. Cleanse an area on the medial or lateral plantar surface of the heel with an alcohol wipe and allow it to dry.
2. Using a 2.5-mm lancet, puncture the heel until a free flow of blood is obtained.
3. Wipe away the first drop of blood.
4. Completely fill two heparinized, 250-mL capillary tubes without air bubbles and add a heparinized metal stirrer. Quickly seal them and mix well by maneuvering a magnet around the tubes.

Postprocedure Care
1. Place the capillary tubes in an ice bath.
2. Write the client's temperature, mode and amount of oxygen delivery, and the type and site of specimen collection on the laboratory requisition.
3. Place pressure on the heel for 5-10 minutes and leave the site open to air to heal.
4. Transport the specimens to the laboratory within 15 minutes.

Client and Family Teaching
1. The client's temperature is important in evaluating results.
2. Results are normally available within 30 minutes.
3. Results are interpreted according to disease or condition and compared to previous gases.

Factors That Affect Results
1. Avoid milking the heel.
2. Reject hemolyzed or clotted specimens.
3. Storage at room temperature accelerates the drop in pH.
4. Elevated white blood cell counts cause a rapid pH drop.
5. Sodium fluoride can cause either an increase or a decrease in pH.
6. A prolonged time lapse between collection and testing may result in decreased pH.
7. Capillary blood gas specimens are contraindicated in low cardiac output, vasoconstriction, shock, and hypotension because the results will not be valid.

Other Data
1. Avoid puncturing over previous puncture sites.
2. Avoid puncturing the posterior curvature of the heel.
3. Specimens may also be taken from the earlobe in adults.
4. Evaluation of pH should take into consideration alterations in electrolyte, carbon dioxide, oxygen, and bicarbonate levels.
5. Capillary blood gases accurately reflect arterial pH and pCO_2 in pediatric clients.

Blood Gases, Umbilical Cord Analysis—Blood

Norm.

	Umbilical Vein	Umbilical Artery
pH	7.26-7.49	7.15-7.43
pO_2	15.4-48.2 mm Hg	10-33.8 mm Hg
pCO_2	23.2-61.7 mm Hg	31.1-74.3 mm Hg
HCO_3^-	16.3-24.9 mEq/L	13.3-27.5 mEq/L
Base excess	−5.1 to 0.1 mEq/L	−6.1 to −3.9 mEq/L

Usage. Evaluation of fetal oxygen status at birth and to examine the acid-base balance of the neonate. See also Blood gases, Arterial—Blood.

Description. The analysis of umbilical blood gases measures and records the pH, pO_2, pCO_2, bicarbonate, and base excess of the neonate after delivery. These assessments of both arterial and venous blood provide immediate feedback of the adequacy of fetal oxygenation for energy production. This method may be used to correlate diagnosis of respiratory acidosis, metabolic acidosis, or mixed respiratory-metabolic acidosis. The value of base excess helps differentiate between respiratory and metabolic acidosis, providing an indication as to whether the fetus has sufficient buffer reserves to neutralize hydrogen ions and acids. (See Blood gases, Arterial—Blood for a complete description of each test component.)

Professional Considerations
Consent form NOT required.

Preparation
1. Obtain two prepackaged, heparinized blood gas syringes, or aspirate 0.2 mL of a 100 U/mL heparin solution into two 3-mL syringes.
2. Obtain two 18- or 20-gauge needles and two caps for the syringes.
3. Obtain a segment of umbilical cord that is 10 to 20 cm (4 to 8 inches) in length.

Procedure
1. Connect needles to syringes.
2. Using a 45-degree angle, insert the needle, bevel down into the umbilical artery and withdraw 1-3 mL of blood into the syringe. Repeat this technique on the umbilical vein.
3. Discard needles. Aspirate air from syringes and cap the syringes. Label them with the mother's name, date and time of collection, and source of blood, specifying whether the sample is arterial or venous cord blood.

Postprocedure Care
1. Place samples on ice and transport to the lab immediately.
2. Discard samples if not tested within 1 hour.

Client and Family Teaching
1. Results should be available within 1 hour.
2. Results are interpreted according to maternal history, intrapartum management, delivery information, and neonate status.

Factors That Affect Results
1. Hemolysis affects results.
2. Improper capping or prolonged exposure of the specimen to air invalidates results.

Other Data
1. Umbilical blood gas testing does not provide definitive diagnosis. Alterations in maternal and neonate status must be assessed and taken into consideration to confirm any medical diagnosis.

Blood Gases, Venous—Blood

Norm. Must be corrected for body temperature.

		SI Units
pH	7.32-7.43	7.32-7.43
Panic value	<7.2 or >7.6	<7.2 or >7.6
pCO_2	35-45 mm Hg	4.6-6.0 kPa
pO_2	20-49 mm Hg	2.6-6.5 kPa
HCO_3^-	17-23 mEq/L	17-23 mmol/L
Panic values	<10 mEq/L	<10 mmol/L
	>40 mEq/L	>40 mEq/L
O_2 Saturation	60%-80%	0.60-0.80

Increased pH. See Blood gases, Arterial—Blood.

Increased pCO_2. See Blood gases, Arterial—Blood.

Increased pO_2. Interpretation of oxygen levels is not appropriate on venous blood specimens.

Increased HCO_3^-. See Blood gases, Arterial—Blood.

Increased O_2 Saturation. Interpretation of oxygen saturation is not appropriate on venous blood specimens.

Decreased pH. See Blood gases, Arterial—Blood.

Decreased pCO$_2$. See Blood gases, Arterial—Blood.

Decreased pO$_2$. Interpretation of oxygen levels is not appropriate on venous blood specimens.

Decreased HCO$_3^-$. See Blood gases, Arterial—Blood.

Decreased O$_2$ Saturation. Interpretation of oxygen saturation is not appropriate on venous blood specimens.

Description. A method for assessing acid-base status and for cellular hypoxia without performing an arterial puncture. Venous blood gases may be used in situations where assessment of oxygenation is unnecessary. (See Blood gases, Arterial—Blood for complete descriptions of the test components.)

Professional Considerations
Consent form NOT required.

Preparation
1. The client should rest quietly for 30 minutes before specimen collection.
2. Obtain alcohol wipes, a tourniquet, a needle, a syringe or Vacutainer, heparin, and a green topped tube.

Procedure
1. Draw 1 mL of heparin (1000 U/mL) into a 3-mL syringe and coat the inside of the syringe with heparin. Eject the heparin.
2. Draw a 2-mL venous blood sample into the syringe, taking care to avoid getting air bubbles mixed with the blood.
3. Inject blood from the syringe into the tube.
4. Alternatively, perform a Vacutainer collection directly into a heparinized, green topped tube and remove the tube from the Vacutainer before removing the needle from the vein.

5. The specimen may be obtained from cord blood.

Postprocedure Care
1. Place the specimen on ice.
2. Write the client's temperature and the type of specimen on the laboratory requisition.
3. Write the mode and amount of oxygen delivery on the laboratory requisition.

Client and Family Teaching
1. Do not pump your fist during collection.
2. The client's temperature is needed to interpret results.
3. Results are normally available within 30 minutes.
4. Results require interpretation depending on disease or condition and compared to previous gases.

Factors That Affect Results
1. Avoid using a tourniquet, if possible. If one is used, it should be left in place while the sample is being drawn.
2. Reject clotted specimens or specimens not received on ice.
3. Storage at room temperature accelerates the fall in pH.
4. Elevated white blood cell counts cause a rapid pH drop.
5. Sodium fluoride can cause either an increase or a decrease in pH.
6. A prolonged time lapse between collection and testing may result in decreased pH.

Other Data
1. For data on oxygenation, arterial blood is required.
2. Evaluation of pH should take into consideration alterations in electrolyte, carbon dioxide, oxygen, and bicarbonate levels.

Blood Group Antigen of Semen—Vaginal Swab

Norm. Blood group antigens may be identified in 80% of the population. Blood group matches the victim's where coitus has not occurred or where the perpetrator's blood group matches the blood group of the victim. Blood group differs from the victim's where coitus has occurred with a perpetrator of a different ABO blood group.

Usage. Rape trauma investigation.

Description. Approximately 80% of the population (both males and females) is classified as having a dominant secretor gene that causes them to secrete their ABO blood group antigen in their body fluids. Samples of vaginal fluid are analyzed for soluble A, B, and O blood group substances for the purpose of identifying the blood group of the perpetrator of a sexual assault. Although the results can be compared with the blood group antigen obtained from body fluid of the suspected assailant, this test cannot confirm this client as the perpetrator. However, it can rule out a suspect if the blood group antigens are different.

Professional Considerations
Consent form NOT required unless results may be used for legal evidence.

Preparation
1. Obtain a speculum, a cotton wool swab supplied in a sexual offense kit, glass slides, and a Coplin jar of 95% ethyl alcohol (ethanol).

Procedure
1. If the specimen may be used as legal evidence, have the specimen collection witnessed.
2. Position the woman in a lithotomy position and drape her for privacy and comfort.
3. Gently scrape the walls of the vagina with a plain cotton wool swab until it is saturated.
4. Roll the swab onto two glass slides and place the slides in a Coplin jar of 95% ethyl alcohol (ethanol).

Postprocedure Care
1. Write the client's name, the date, the exact time of collection, and the specimen source on the laboratory requisition. Sign and have the witness sign the laboratory requisition.
2. Transport the specimen to the laboratory immediately in a sealed plastic bag marked as legal evidence. All persons handling the specimen should sign and mark the time of receipt on the laboratory requisition.

Client and Family Teaching
1. Offer the client and family immediate counseling or crisis intervention and support. Survivors of sexual assault should be referred to appropriate crisis-counseling agencies as well as gynecologic follow-up study. Facilitate the connection if desired by the client.
2. Referral for HIV testing should be reviewed and offered to all sexual assault victims.
3. Preventive treatment for chlamydiosis, gonorrhea, and syphilis should be provided to all survivors of sexual assault.
4. The option of postcoital contraceptive should be reviewed with all survivors of sexual assault.
5. Results will be available within 5 days.

Factors That Affect Results
1. Results are inconclusive if the blood groups of the victim and the suspect are the same.
2. Vaginal swabs for blood group antigen detection should be collected as soon as possible after the rape. Semen is rarely detected in the vagina more than 72 hours after coitus.
3. Negative results may be obtained if the assailant was sexually dysfunctional or has had a vasectomy or if the woman bathed, douched, or defecated after the rape.

Other Data
1. Vaginal swabs can be examined by use of an MHS-5-ELISA (SEMA kit), which is sensitive to cases of azoospermia or aspermia.
2. See also Acid phosphatase—Vaginal swab; Precipitin test against human sperm and blood—Vaginal swab.

Blood Indices—Blood

Norm.

Mean Corpuscular Hemoglobin (MCH)		SI Units
Adults	26-34 pg	1.61-2.11 fmol
Children		
Newborn		
1 day old	1-38 pg	2.36 fmol
2-3 days	37 pg	2.30 fmol
4-8 days	36 pg	2.23 fmol
9-13 days	33 pg	2.05 fmol
2-8 weeks	30 pg	1.86 fmol

Continued

Mean Corpuscular Hemoglobin (MCH)		SI Units
3 months	28 pg	1.73 fmol
4-5 months	27 pg	1.67 fmol
6-11 months	26 pg	1.61 fmol
1-2 years	25 pg	1.55 fmol
3 years	26 pg	1.61 fmol
4-10 years	27 pg	1.67 fmol
11-15 years	28 pg	1.73 fmol

Mean Corpuscular Hemoglobin Concentration (MCHC)		
Adults	31%-38%	19.2-23.58 mmol/L
Children		
Newborn		
1-3 days	36%	22.34 mmol/L
2-8 days	35%	21.72 mmol/L
9-13 days	34%	21.10 mmol/L
2-8 weeks	33%	20.48 mmol/L
3-5 months	34%	21.10 mmol/L
6-11 months	33%	20.48 mmol/L
1-2 years	32%	19.86 mmol/L
3 years	35%	21.72 mmol/L
4-15 years	34%	21.10 mmol/L

Mean Corpuscular Volume, Mean Cell Volume (MCV)		
Adults	82-98 μm^3	82-98 fL
Children		
Newborn		
1 day	106 μm^3	106 fL
2-3 days	105 μm^3	105 fL
4-8 days	103 μm^3	103 fL
9-13 days	98 μm^3	98 fL
2-8 weeks	90 μm^3	90 fL
3 months	82 μm^3	82 fL
4-5 months	80 μm^3	80 fL
6-11 months	77 μm^3	77 fL
1 year	78 μm^3	78 fL
2 years	77 μm^3	77 fL
3 years	79 μm^3	79 fL
4-10 years	80 μm^3	80 fL
11-15 years	82 mm^3	82 fL

Increased MCV. Alcoholism (chronic), anemia (acquired hemolytic, aplastic, immune hemolytic, macrocytic induced by megaloblastic anemias, pernicious [early]), benzene exposure, cigarette smokers, cirrhosis, chronic lymphocytic leukemia, cytomegalovirus, diabetic ketoacidosis, diabetes mellitus, DNA synthesis disorders (inherited), folate deficiency, hepatic disease, infants, leukocytosis (pronounced), methanol poisoning, newborns, obesity, pancreatitis, peripheral arterial disease, preleukemia, reticulocytosis, sprue, and vitamin B_{12} deficiency. Drugs include capecitabine, hydroxyurea, zidovudine (AZT).

Increased MCH. Anemia (macrocytic, pernicious), cold agglutinin conditions, cigarette smokers, dysproteinemia, infants, newborns, and presence of monoclonal blood proteins. Drugs include heparin calcium and heparin sodium.

Increased MCHC. High titer of cold agglutinins, dehydrated hereditary stomatocytosis, hereditary spherocytosis, infants, intravascular hemolysis, lipemia, newborns, obese. Drugs include heparin calcium, heparin sodium, and chemical components from smoking.

Decreased MCV. Anemia (chronic, dyserythropoietic, hypochromic, iron deficiency, microcytic, pyridoxine responsive, sickle cell), alpha- or beta-thalassemia, Brunner's gland hamartoma, chlorosis, chronic disease, colorectal cancer, diverticulitis, diverticulosis, endocarditis, G6PD deficiency, gangrene, hemoglobin E, hemoglobin H, leukocytosis (pronounced), malaria, myocarditis, nephropathy (nonimmune), pruritus, radiation therapy, red blood cell fragmentation, subacute bacterial endocarditis, and warm autoantibodies. Drugs include stavudine.

Decreased MCH. Anemia (iron deficiency, microcytic, normocytic), cyanotic congenital heart disease. Drugs include blood stored at room temperature more than 2 days, enalaprilat (Vasotec).

Decreased MCHC. Aluminum intoxication, anemia (iron deficiency, chronic, hypochromic, megaloblastic, microcytic, sideroblastic), benzene exposure, colorectal cancer.

Description. Blood indices encompass a group of six different blood tests—the MCH, MCHC, MCV, RBC, Hct, and Hb—that are used to establish the characteristics and hemoglobin content of the red blood cells. (See Red blood cell—Blood; Hematocrit—Blood; Hemoglobin—Blood.) They assist in the diagnosis and differentiation of compensated and uncompensated anemias. A stained blood smear is prepared to study the shape and size of the red blood cell. Combined with staining, the indices assist in determinations of red blood cell morphology. This visual or electronic counting of erythrocytes is regarded as the most reliable index for distinguishing and differentiating erythrocyte morphology. MCH is the average weight of the hemoglobin of each red blood cell, expressed in picograms.

MCHC is a calculated value of the amount of hemoglobin present in the red blood cell compared to its size. A ratio of weight to volume is expressed as a percentage. MCV is a calculated value, expressed in cubic micrometers, of the average volume of an erythrocyte.

Professional Considerations
Consent form NOT required.

Preparation
1. Tube: Lavender topped.

Procedure
1. Draw a 7-mL blood sample. A stained blood smear is prepared.

Postprocedure Care
1. The collection tube should be filled completely, inverted, and gently rotated to thoroughly mix the anticoagulant.
2. The serum sample is stable at room temperature for 10 hours, may be refrigerated for up to 18 hours, and should not be frozen.

Client and Family Teaching
1. Results are normally available within 24 hours.
2. All results must be available to make an accurate interpretation associated with the diagnosis or condition.

Factors That Affect Results
1. Reject hemolyzed specimens.
2. High altitude affects MCV (standard deviation [SD] =.810 fL), MCH (SD =.583 pg), and MCHC (SD =.630 g/dL).
3. Results are falsely elevated in blood stored at room temperature more than 2 days.

Other Data
1. Bone marrow suppression in the chronically ill can be a frequent cause of anemia.
2. Production of macroreticulocytes is an early sign of engraftment after bone marrow transplantation.
3. Hemoglobin E trait is common in Bengali, Burmese, Khmer, Malay, Thai, and Vietnamese groups.
4. See also Red blood cell morphology—Blood.

Blood Sugar

See **Glucose**—Blood.

B

Blood Type

See ABO Group and Rh Type—Blood.

Blood Urea Nitrogen

See Urea Nitrogen—Plasma or Serum.

Blood Urea Nitrogen/Creatinine Ratio—Blood

Norm.

Normal	10:1 to 15:1
Diminished urea concentration	<10:1
Inadequate renal function	>15:1

Increased. Azotemia, burns, cachexia, catabolic states, Cushing's disease, dehydration, delirium, excessive protein intake, fever, gastrointestinal bleeding, glomerular disease, heart failure, hemorrhage, hypercalcemia, hypertension, impaired renal blood flow, ileal conduit, infection, muscle or tissue destruction, prerenal azotemia, shock, surgery, swallowing of food into the upper airway, thyrotoxicosis, urinary reabsorption (ureterocolostomy), and urinary tract obstruction (rare). Drugs include tetracyclines and steroids.

Decreased. Diarrhea, diet (inadequate protein intake), hemodialysis, hepatic insufficiency, hyperammonemias (genetic), intravenous therapy (prolonged), ketosis, malnutrition, marasmus, pregnancy, renal failure (muscular people, chronic), rhabdomyolysis, syndrome of inappropriate antidiuretic hormone secretion (SIADHS), and vomiting. Drugs include phenacemide. Drugs that increase only the creatinine and not the blood urea nitrogen (BUN) include cephalosporins, cimetidine, tetracyclines, and trimethoprim.

Description. The BUN/creatinine ratio assists in the interpretation of laboratory values in assessing renal failure and in the evaluation of an elevated BUN level. This test is a more sensitive indicator of the relationship between BUN and creatinine than each separate test because BUN rises at a greater rate than creatinine in renal disease.

Professional Considerations
Consent form NOT required.

Preparation
1. Tube: Red topped, red/gray topped, or gold topped.
2. Do NOT draw specimen during hemodialysis.

Procedure
1. Draw a 5-mL blood sample.

Postprocedure Care
1. None.

Client and Family Teaching
1. Assess knowledge and provide information about adequate dietary protein.

Factors That Affect Results
1. Low-protein diet lowers BUN value.

Other Data
1. Before a change in BUN is significant, there exists approximately 60% renal impairment.
2. See also Urea nitrogen—Plasma or serum.

Blood Volume—Blood

Norm.

Blood Volume	
	8.5%-9% of body weight
Adult female	54.01-63.89 mL/kg
Adult male	52.95-70.13 mL/kg
Erythrocyte Volume	
Adult female	21.65-26.83 mL/kg
Adult male	24.16-32.38 mL/kg

Plasma Volume

Adult female	31.53-38.01 mL/kg
Adult male	28.27-38.63 mL/kg

Usage. Anemia, differentiation of relative polycythemia from absolute polycythemia, preoperative or postoperative evaluation to estimate need for replacement blood, and unexplained hypotension. Decreased in preeclampsia but normal in gestational hypertension.

Description. Blood volume comprises plasma and cellular components and varies with body weight, muscle mass, height, age, sex, environment, and physical activity. This nuclear medicine test uses a dilution technique that measures blood volume after radiolabeled albumin and radiolabeled red blood cells are injected intravenously. A tagged sample of the client's blood is then measured for blood volume, erythrocyte volume, and plasma volume with a scintillation well counter. This test is based on the principle of adding a known quantity of tracer substance to an unknown quantity of diluent (blood). The final tracer concentration should be inversely proportional to the volume of blood. Radiolabeled albumin is used to measure plasma volume, and the radiolabeled red blood cells are used to measure volume of the cellular component of blood. This test is helpful in differentiating between fluid shifts or other causes of decreased plasma volume (relative polycythemia) and increased red blood cell mass (absolute polycythemia).

Professional Considerations
Consent form NOT required.

Risks
Allergic reaction to radiolabeled albumin (itching, hives, rash, tight feeling in the throat, shortness of breath, bronchospasm, anaphylaxis, death), hematoma, or infection at injection site.

Contraindications
Previous allergy to radioactive dyes, iodine, or shellfish; during pregnancy; while breastfeeding; hypersensitivity to iodine; extended clotting times; in edematous or hemorrhaging clients.

Preparation
1. Have emergency equipment readily available.
2. Obtain alcohol wipes, a tourniquet, a 19-gauge needle, five syringes, one glass green topped tube, two plastic green topped tubes, a centrifuge bag, a sterile glass beaker of 3 mL Strumia formula solution, chilled sterile 0.9% saline solution, and centrifuge.
3. Draw a 25-mL blood sample and inject into a sterile centrifuge bag to which 3 mL of Strumia formula solution has been added. Add 50-100 mCi of ^{51}Cr (sodium chromate) to the container and gently agitate it for 3 minutes. Then fill the bag with sterile, chilled 0.9% saline and centrifuge it at a 45-degree angle for 7 minutes. Remove the supernatant fluid and resuspend the cells in 10 mL of sterile 0.9% saline solution.
4. Obtain a mixture of 5 mL of ^{125}I-albumin in 20 mL of sterile normal saline solution for plasma volume measurement.
5. Lugol's solution may be used to prevent uptake of ^{125}I-albumin by the thyroid gland.

Procedure
1. Draw an 8-mL blood sample in a heparinized green topped tube and label it as the baseline sample.
2. *Injection for red blood cell volume measurement:* Draw 2-3 mL of the 51Cr-labeled red blood cell solution into a syringe with a 19-gauge needle. Note the exact amount in the syringe. Inject the mixture directly into a vein in the right arm of the client.
3. *Injection for plasma volume measurement:* Draw 2-3 mL of the ^{125}I-albumin at 2 mCi/mL into a syringe. Note the exact amount in the syringe. Inject the mixture directly into a vein in the right arm of the client.
4. *Recovery of tagged blood for blood volume determination:* At 10 and 20 minutes after the two tracer injections, draw an 8-mL blood sample from the left arm in a

heparinized plastic, rather than glass, green topped tube. Label each sample with the time drawn.

5. Using the multidose vials from which the ^{51}Cr-tagged red blood cells and ^{125}I-albumin were drawn as controls, measure blood volume, red blood cell volume, and plasma volume of the samples with a scintillation well counter.

Postprocedure Care
1. None.

Client and Family Teaching
1. This test involves injection of a nuclear medicine tracer, followed by two timed blood sample collections. Total test time is less than 1 hour.
2. Results are normally available within 24 hours.

Factors That Affect Results
1. Blood volume is usually highest in the morning.
2. Glass tubes used for the tagged sample may cause falsely low plasma volume results because glass absorbs energy from ^{125}I-albumin.
3. The ^{51}Cr rate of tagging red blood cells varies with pH, type of anticoagulant, and

body temperature. In general, tagging should be complete by 5 minutes after injection.

4. If the client has recently taken polyvitamins or antibiotics, ^{51}Cr may not label the client's own red blood cells. Blood bank ^{51}Cr-labeled group O-Rh-negative blood should be substituted.
5. Injection through intravenous tubing or tissue extravasation of tracer will cause falsely decreased results.
6. Two post–tracer injection blood samples are required both to establish that mixing of ^{51}Cr-labeled red blood cells is complete and to determine the rate of loss of the ^{125}I-albumin tracer.
7. If the 10- and 20-minute sample results vary by more than 3%, a third sample should be drawn 60-90 minutes after the initial injection.

Other Data
1. No isolation of the client is necessary.
2. Furosemide (Lasix) has no effect on blood volume, shape, or viscosity.
3. Ringer's solution expands blood volume by 20%-25% in awake individuals and by 60% during general anesthesia.

Blood Volume Determination Studies—Diagnostic

Norm. Requires interpretation.

Usage. Differential diagnosis of pericardial effusion from pericardial cysts or tumors, diagnosis of peripheral vascular disease, and thrombophlebitis.

Description. A nuclear medicine study of circulation dynamics in which a tracer is circulated in the blood for a period of time. Measures of diluted radioactivity are used to calculate the volume distribution of compartments and regions of the circulation. Pericardial effusions are detected by examination of the blood volumes in and around the heart. Peripheral vascular disease and thrombophlebitis are detected by examination of the rates at which the venous pools of the legs change in volume with exercise and posture changes.

Professional Considerations
Consent form IS required.

Risks
Allergic reaction to radiolabeled albumin (itching, hives, rash, tight feeling in the throat, shortness of breath, bronchospasm, anaphylaxis, death), hematoma, or infection at injection site.

Contraindications
Previous allergy to iodine, radiographic dye, seafood, or a nuclear medicine radiolabeled albumin tracer.

Precautions
During pregnancy, risks of cumulative radiation exposure to the fetus from this and other previous or future imaging studies must be weighed against the benefits of the procedure. Although formal limits for client exposure are relative to this risk-benefit comparison, the United States Nuclear Regulatory Commission requires that the cumulative dose equivalent to an embryo/fetus from occupational exposure not

exceed 0.5 rem (5 mSv). Radiation dose to the fetus is proportional to the distance of the anatomy studied from the abdomen and decreases as pregnancy progresses. For pregnant clients, consult the radiologist/radiology department to obtain estimated fetal radiation exposure from this procedure.

Preparation

1. Have emergency equipment readily available.
2. Establish intravenous access in an arm vein.
3. Just before beginning the procedure, take a "time out" to verify the correct client, procedure, and site.

Procedure

1. A tracer of labeled albumin, red blood cells, or substances bound by plasma proteins is injected intravenously and allowed to circulate. The circulatory compartment to be studied is scanned, and a scintillation well counter is used to compare the diluted radioactivity of the compartment with a standard. This is followed by calculation of the volume distribution of the compartment.

Postprocedure Care

1. Encourage the oral intake of fluids.

Client and Family Teaching

1. The risk of radioactivity from this test is less than that of a regular radiograph.

Factors That Affect Results

1. Blood volume is highest in the morning.

Other Data

1. No isolation of the client is necessary.
2. Health care professionals working in a nuclear medicine area must follow federal standards set by the Nuclear Regulatory Commission. These standards include precautions for handling the radioactive material and monitoring of potential radiation exposure.

Blue Light Test

See **Tonometry Test for Glaucoma**—Diagnostic.

B-Lymphocytes—Blood

Norm.

		SI Units
Adults	270-640/mm³ or 270-640/μL	270-640 cells x 10⁶/L
	5%-15% of circulating lymphocytes or 25%-35% of	0.05-0.15
	total lymphocytes	0.25-0.35
Children		
Newborn	61% of total lymphocytes	0.61
Infants	60% of total lymphocytes	0.60
6 years	42% of total lymphocytes	0.42
12 years	38% of total lymphocytes	0.38

Increased. Active antibody formation in young children, agranulocytosis, bacterial infections (acute, chronic), brucellosis, Burkitt's lymphoma, carcinoma, chickenpox, cytomegalovirus, DiGeorge syndrome, hepatitis (viral), hyperthyroidism, influenza, leukemia (lymphocytic), leukosarcoma, lymphocytosis (infectious), lymphoma (non-Hodgkin's), measles, malnutrition, mononucleosis (infectious), multiple myeloma, multiple sclerosis, mumps, parathyroid fever, pertussis, pneumonia (viral), polyneuropathy, scurvy, syphilis, thyrotoxicosis, tuberculosis, tularemia, typhoid fever, typhus, and Waldenström's macroglobulinemia.

Decreased. Anemia (aplastic), burns, cardiac failure, Cushing's syndrome, Hodgkin's disease, immunoglobulin deficiency, leukemia (chronic granulocytic, monocytic), lymphatic irradiation, stress reactions, systemic lupus erythematosus (SLE), terminal carcinoma, thymic hypoplasia (children), trauma, uremia, and X-linked agammaglobulinemia. Drugs include corticotropin, cortisone acetate, epinephrine bitartrate, epinephrine borate, epinephrine hydrochloride, intravenous immunoglobulin, and nitrogen mustard.

Description. B-lymphocytes are white blood cells with a short life span that are produced by bone marrow and are responsible for humoral immunity and production of immunoglobulin and specific antibodies. They are found in the lymph nodes, spleen, bone marrow, and blood and are a primary defense against virulent, encapsulated, bacterial pathogens. When stimulated by an antigen, they transform themselves into plasma cells that rapidly secrete antibodies. These antibodies neutralize viruses, interfere with the absorption of foreign proteins, and detoxify other proteins. B-lymphocytes lose their ability to respond to antigenic or mutagenic stimulation with age.

Professional Considerations
Consent form NOT required.

Preparation
1. Tube: Green topped.

Procedure
1. Draw a 5-mL blood sample.

Postprocedure Care
1. None.

Client and Family Teaching
1. Inform the physician of 6-month history of colds and infections.

Factors That Affect Results
1. Medications containing epinephrine cause unreliable results.

Other Data
1. Plasma cells seldom appear in the blood, but they may appear in increased numbers in severe infections, especially in children, to reinforce immunity when sufficient antibodies are not available.

BMD

See **Bone Densitometry**—Diagnostic.

BMP

See **Basic Metabolic Panel**—Blood.

BNP

See **Natriuretic Peptides**—Plasma.

Body Fluid, Amylase—Specimen

Norm. Negative.

Positive. Benign ovarian cyst fluid, esophageal rupture, necrotic bowel, pancreatic ascites, pancreatic duct trauma, pancreatitis (with or without pseudocyst), perforated peptic ulcer, and malignant pleural effusions in the presence of cancer of the lung, breast, gastrointestinal tract, ovary, and lymphoma.

Small cell lung carcinoma metastasis to the liver resulting in necrosis.

Description. Amylase is produced in large quantities by the pancreas, salivary glands, and certain malignant tumors. It is produced in lesser quantities by the fallopian tubes and lungs. Amylase from the pancreas and salivary glands is normally contained in the gastrointestinal tract. The presence of a significant amount of amylase in a body fluid specimen indicates a pathologic process.

Professional Considerations

Consent form NOT required. See individual procedures for procedure-specific risks and contraindications.

Preparation

1. Obtain a pleural or peritoneal aspiration tray and a clean container or red topped tube. Sterile 0.9% saline is needed for peritoneal lavage.

Procedure

1. Obtain a body fluid specimen by needle aspiration of pleural or peritoneal fluid, or by catheter irrigation and aspiration of the peritoneum, and inject it into a clean container or red topped tube.

Postprocedure Care

1. Apply a dry, sterile dressing to the site.

Client and Family Teaching

1. Results are normally available within 72 hours.

Factors That Affect Results

1. When ascitic fluid is being collected, the location of the collection site or of the catheter tip will likely affect the level of amylase that may be present. For example, a catheter directed to the left upper quadrant may produce a false-negative specimen.

Other Data

1. A common finding of lung carcinoma with pleural effusion.
2. Amylase levels indicative of saliva can be obtained on penile swabs, vaginal swabs, and breast swabs in sexual assault cases.

Body Fluid—Anaerobic Culture

Norm. Negative. No growth.

Positive. Aspiration pneumonia; biliary tract infections; bite wounds; bronchiectasis; chronic osteomyelitis; chronic sinus infection; dental and mouth infections; deep tissue infection or necrosis; gastrointestinal infections (especially of the colon); gynecologic intraabdominal or extraabdominal infections; immunodeficiency states; immunosuppressive therapy; infections caused by *Actinomyces, Arachnia, Bacteroides fragilis, Bacteroides melaninogenicus, Bifidobacterium, Clostridium, Coccidioides, Eubacterium, Fusobacterium, Lactobacillus, Peptostreptococcus, Propionibacterium, Veillonella,* and others; malignancy; and trauma (accidental, surgical). Drugs include aminoglycosides.

Description. The test identifies anaerobic bacterial infections in body fluids, including ascitic fluid, bile, cerebrospinal fluid, pleural fluid, and synovial fluid, and from wounds and abscesses. Anaerobes live and grow where there is no free oxygen and obtain energy for growth and metabolism from fermentation reactions rather than from oxygen. Anaerobes are part of the normal flora of the skin, oral cavity, lower gastrointestinal tract, urethra, and the female external genital tract. When displaced from their location into other body tissues or spaces,

they become pathogenic, causing localized abscesses in oxygen-poor body cavities and specific body organs. Untreated anaerobic infections may lead to bacteremia. Special collection methods are necessary for isolation of anaerobes. Anaerobic cultures are grown on complex media, and identification is made by means of colony morphology, pigmentation, fluorescence, and gas-liquid chromatography.

Professional Considerations

Consent form IS required for some of the procedures used to obtain the specimen. See specific procedures for risks and contraindications.

Preparation

1. Notify laboratory personnel that an anaerobic specimen will be arriving.
2. For the needle and syringe method, obtain a needle, a syringe, a sterile "gassed-out" tube (a tube flushed with oxygen-free carbon dioxide or nitrogen gas), and a double stopper.
3. For the two-tube swab method, obtain several sterile swabs prepared and stored in oxygen-free carbon dioxide tubes and tubes containing prereduced transport media with a methylene blue indicator as needed.

B

4. Just before beginning the procedure, take a "time out" to verify the correct client, procedure, and site.

Procedure

1. *Needle and syringe method*: Expel all air from the syringe. Aspirate the specimen directly into the syringe. Carefully expel any air from the syringe. Immediately inject the specimen into a sterile "gassed-out" tube, preferably with a double stopper to prevent the introduction of air when the specimen is injected. If this anaerobic transport tube is not available, the needle can be tightly capped or embedded in a sterile rubber stopper. Because the specimen must be centrifuged, the volume should be more than 2 mL. In the presence of extensive wounds involving large amounts of tissue or multiple lesions, several samples should be taken.

2. *Two-tube swab method*: Collect the specimen on at least two sterile swabs that have been prepared and stored in oxygen-free tubes. Expose the swabs to air as briefly as possible. Keeping the methylene blue transport tube upright, quickly place the swabs in the tubes and close them tightly. Never let the swab samples dry out.

3. Alternatively, an anaerobic transport container may be used.

Postprocedure Care

1. Apply a sterile dressing over the aspiration site.

2. Keep the specimen at room temperature and transport it to the laboratory within 30 minutes for immediate processing. Some anaerobes survive for only a short time after collection.

3. Write the specimen source, any recent antibiotic therapy, and the client's diagnosis and symptoms on the laboratory requisition.

Client and Family Teaching

1. Results are normally available within 72 hours.

2. Report signs of infection at the aspiration site to the physician: increasing pain, redness, swelling, purulent drainage, or temperature >101 degrees F (>38.3 degrees C).

3. Treatment of the condition may begin before the results are obtained.

Factors That Affect Results

1. Reject small specimens (a few drops) in a syringe received more than 10 minutes after collection.

2. Reject larger specimens (>1 mL) in a syringe received more than 1 hour after collection.

3. Reject specimens in anaerobic oxygen-free vials or tubes received more than 3 hours after collection.

4. Exposure of the specimen to air may cause false-negative results.

5. Failure to use anaerobic transport specimen containers may cause false-negative results.

6. Do not use methylene blue indicator tubes if the ring of blue extends beyond the top surface of the tube.

7. Letting the specimens dry out invalidates the results.

8. The client's symptoms, condition, and type of organism suspected determine the specific type of anaerobic culture medium selected.

Other Data

1. Malignancy, immunosuppressive deficiency states, immunosuppressive therapy, and some types of antibiotic therapy favor the multiplication of endogenous anaerobes.

2. The use of swabs to obtain anaerobic cultures is not recommended. When necessary, commercial anaerobic swab sets consisting of two containers must be used.

Body Fluid, Fungus—Culture

Norm. Negative. No growth.

Positive. *Aspergillus fumigatus, Aspergillus flavus, Blastomyces dermatitidis, Candida albicans, Candida tropicalis, Coccidioides immitis, Cryptococcus neoformans, Histoplasma capsulatum, Sporothrix schenckii,* and others.

Description. Fungi are slow-growing, eukaryotic organisms that can grow on living and nonliving organic materials and are subdivided into yeasts and molds. Normal human host defense mechanisms limit the damage they cause superficially. Some fungi can be inhaled or introduced by traumatic inoculation into deep tissue spaces and cause serious infections. Factors that predispose a client to a fungal infection include immunosuppression, treatment with corticosteroids or broad-spectrum antibiotics, or debilitated states. Although tentative identification of fungi can be made quickly with staining techniques, culture of the organism on special fungal culture media is required to confirm a diagnosis of a fungal infection.

Professional Considerations

Consent form NOT required for the culture but may be required for the procedure used to obtain the specimen.

Preparation

1. Obtain a sterile specimen container, sterile gloves, a needle, a syringe, and any necessary aspiration trays, depending on the site to be cultured.
2. For urine collection, obtain a sterile container and povidone-iodine wipes. If the client will be collecting the specimen independently, instructions should include a demonstration.
3. Obtain the specimen early in the day so that it may be processed promptly.

Procedure

1. Use an aseptic technique to collect a specimen of the body fluid to be cultured.
2. The specimen should be examined for yeast cells at the bedside whenever possible or placed in a sterile container and transported promptly to the laboratory.
3. Urine collection:
   a. Instruct the client to void and discard the urine.
   b. Thirty minutes later, while holding the labia open or foreskin back, cleanse the urethral meatus in an outward circular motion with each of three povidone-iodine wipes. Allow the iodine to dry while protecting the urethral meatus from contamination.
   c. Instruct the client to void a small amount and then stop the stream of urine.
   d. Place the sterile specimen container under the urethral meatus and have the client void into it, filling it no more than halfway before again stopping the stream of urine. Cap the specimen container.

Postprocedure Care

1. Apply an appropriate dressing as needed.
2. Write the collection date and time, specimen source, suspected disease, and any recent antibiotic or antifungal therapy on the laboratory requisition.
3. Transport the specimen to the laboratory immediately.
4. Do not refrigerate.

Client and Family Teaching

1. Preliminary results are normally available within 72 hours; final results in about 30 days.
2. Treatment is usually begun before final results.

Factors That Affect Results

1. Best results are obtained if cultures are inoculated immediately. Other than noted above, the maximum time allowed between specimen collection and inoculation is 3 hours.

Other Data

1. Four to six weeks are required for fungal culture results.
2. More yeast is acquired using Fan bottles.
3. *Sporothrix schenckii* infection is on the increase in HIV-positive clients.
4. Coccidioidomycosis can be associated with hypercalcemia.

Body Fluid, Glucose—Specimen

Norm.

Cerebrospinal Fluid

Lags behind blood glucose levels by 2-4 hours. Fasting to 4 hours postprandially
   50%-80% of serum glucose

Continued

		SI Units
Adult	40-80 mg/dL	2.2-4.4 mmol/L
Premature infant	24-63 mg/dL	1.3-3.5 mmol/L
Full-term infant	34-119 mg/dL	1.9-6.6 mmol/L
Child	35-75 mg/dL	1.9-4.1 mmol/L
Peritoneal Fluid	70-100 mg/dL	3.8-5.5 mmol/L
Pleural Fluid	Same as blood glucose level, with a time lag of 2-4 hours or no less than 40 mg/dL below blood glucose	No less than 2.2 mmol/L below blood glucose
Fasting	60-110 mg/dL	3.3-6.1 mmol/L
Synovial Fluid	No more than 10 mg/dL lower than blood glucose level	No more than 0.6 mmol/L lower than blood glucose level

Increased CSF Glucose. Brain tumor, cerebral hemorrhage, cerebral trauma, diabetic coma, hyperglycemia, hypothalamic lesions, increased intracranial pressure, and uremia.

Increased Peritoneal, Pleural, or Synovial Fluid Glucose. Hyperglycemia and primary and symptomatic diabetes.

Decreased CSF Glucose. Brain abscess, brain tumor, cancer, central nervous system sarcoidosis, choroid plexus tumor, coccidioidomycosis, encephalitis (mumps or herpes simplex origin), hypoglycemia, increased intracranial pressure, leukemic infiltration, lupus myelopathy, lymphocytic choriomeningitis, lymphoma, melanomatosis, meningeal carcinomatosis, meningitis (acute pyogenic, aseptic, chemical, cryptococcal, fungal, granulomatous, pyogenic, rheumatoid, tuberculous, viral), neurosyphilis, rheumatoid arthritis, subarachnoid hemorrhage, toxoplasmosis, and tuberculoma of brain.

Decreased Peritoneal Fluid Glucose. Peritoneal carcinomatosis, peritonitis (tuberculous), and hypoglycemia.

Decreased Pleural Fluid Glucose. Infection (bacterial), effusion (malignant, neoplastic, rheumatoid, septic, tuberculous), and hypoglycemia.

Decreased Synovial Fluid Glucose. Arthritis (inflammatory, noninflammatory, rheumatoid, septic, tuberculous) and hypoglycemia.

Description. Body fluid glucose content is similar to blood serum glucose content. Most abnormalities result in decreased body fluid glucose levels caused by increased use of glucose by the pathogenic process. This test is interpreted when a blood glucose level is compared to the body fluid glucose level.

Professional Considerations

Consent form IS required for the procedure used to obtain the specimen. See specific procedures for risks and contraindications.

Risks
See appropriate procedure being performed.
Contraindications
See appropriate procedure being performed.

Preparation

1. Tube: Red topped, red/gray topped, or gold topped for blood glucose specimen.
2. Obtain a sterile specimen container, a tube, or an evacuated glass bottle, and a sterile tray (arthrocentesis, lumbar puncture, paracentesis, thoracentesis) depending on the procedure being performed.
3. Just before beginning the procedure, take a "time out" to verify the correct client, procedure, and site.

Procedure

1. Draw a 5-mL blood sample for glucose in a red topped tube.
2. Collect the appropriate specimen as follows:
   a. *Cerebrospinal fluid (CSF):* Collect 3-5 mL of cerebrospinal fluid in a sterile glass tube by means of a spinal tap no more than 4 hours postprandially.
   b. *Peritoneal fluid:* Collect 5 mL of peritoneal fluid in a sterile glass tube by a paracentesis immediately after blood glucose specimen collection.

c. *Pleural fluid*: Collect 5 mL of pleural fluid in a sterile glass tube by thoracentesis 2-4 hours after blood glucose specimen collection.

d. *Synovial fluid*: Collect 3-5 mL of synovial fluid in a sterile gray topped tube containing sodium fluoride by arthrocentesis immediately after blood glucose specimen collection.

Postprocedure Care

1. Apply a sterile dressing to the sites.
2. Write the specimen source and collection time on the laboratory requisition.
3. Transport the specimens to the laboratory immediately. Analysis must be performed promptly on freshly collected specimens to avoid erroneous results caused by glycolysis.

4. For CSF collection, see Lumbar puncture—Diagnostic.

Client and Family Teaching

1. Report to the physician if there are signs of infection at the collection site: increasing pain, redness, swelling, purulent drainage, or temperature >101 degrees F (>38.3 degrees C).
2. Results are normally available within 24 hours.

Factors That Affect Results

1. This method provides the least reliable diagnosis of bacterial peritonitis.

Other Data

1. None.

Body Fluid, Mycobacteria—Culture

Norm. No growth after 8 weeks.

Usage. Diagnose the presence of *Mycobacterium* in body fluid.

Description. Mycobacteria are nonmotile, non–spore-forming, straight, or slightly curved rods that resist staining by Gram's method or by acid solutions because of their high-lipid-containing cell walls. They grow slowly, with colonies developing after 2 days to 8 weeks of incubation. Some species are found in soil and water. Others are obligate parasites. The most common mycobacteria causing human disease are *Mycobacterium asiaticum, M. avium-scrofulaceum complex, M. fortuitum, M. haemophilum, M. kansasii, M. leprae, M. malmoense, M. marinum, M. simiae, M. szulgai, M. tuberculosis complex, M. ulcerans,* and *M. xenopi.* These organisms may attack any organ, but the primary site of infection is usually the lungs. Tubercle bacillus is the most common *Mycobacterium* infection in the United States, except in clients with AIDS. The bacilli are usually inhaled and are small enough to be carried into the alveoli without being expelled.

Professional Considerations

Consent form NOT required for the culture but may be required for the procedure used to obtain the specimen.

Risks

Complications of nasogastric tube insertion include bleeding, dysrhythmias, esophageal perforation, laryngospasm, and decreased mean pO_2.

Contraindications

For nasogastric tube insertion: esophageal varices.

Preparation

1. Obtain a sterile specimen container.
2. For gastric lavage, obtain a nasogastric tube, lubricant, sterile water, a sterile 50-mL syringe, and a sterile specimen container.
3. For paracentesis, thoracentesis, pericardiocentesis, or arthrocentesis, obtain the appropriate sterile procedure tray.

Procedure

1. *Sputum specimen*: Collect an early morning sputum specimen of 5-10 mL on 3 separate days. Label the specimens sequentially.
2. *Gastric lavage*: Used for clients who cannot produce sputum. The specimen should be obtained in the early morning after an 8-hour fast from food and fluids. Insert a nasogastric tube into the stomach. Instill 20-50 mL of sterile water into the stomach through the nasogastric tube

with a sterile syringe and then aspirate the fluid out of the stomach with the syringe. Remove the nasogastric tube.

3. *Peritoneal fluid*: Collect 5-10 mL of peritoneal fluid in a sterile syringe by paracentesis using an aseptic technique.

4. *Pleural fluid*: Collect 5-10 mL of pleural fluid in a sterile syringe by thoracentesis using an aseptic technique.

5. *Pericardial fluid*: Collect 5-10 mL of pericardial fluid in a sterile syringe by pericardiocentesis using an aseptic technique.

6. *Synovial fluid*: Collect 5-10 mL of synovial fluid in a sterile syringe by arthrocentesis using an aseptic technique.

7. *Urine*: Collect first morning-voided specimens by the clean-catch technique or by aspiration from an indwelling urinary catheter or suprapubic puncture on 3 separate days. Label the specimens sequentially. See clean-catch collection instructions in procedure section of the test Body fluid, Routine—Culture.

Postprocedure Care

1. Apply a dry, sterile dressing to the aspiration site. Observe the site for drainage or bleeding hourly × 4.

2. For specimens obtained by pericardiocentesis or thoracentesis, assess vital signs every 15 minutes × 4, then every 30 minutes × 2, and then hourly × 4. Observe for dysrhythmias for 24 hours.

3. Write the specimen source, collection time, current antibiotic or antifungal therapy, and clinical diagnosis on the laboratory requisition. The request to culture the specimen for *Mycobacterium* must be specified on the laboratory requisition.

4. Transport the specimen to the laboratory promptly. Refrigerate urine specimens if not cultured immediately.

Client and Family Teaching

1. *Needle aspiration*: Call the physician if there are signs of infection at the procedure site: increasing pain, redness, swelling, purulent drainage, or temperature >101 degrees F (>38.3 degrees C).

2. *Sputum*: Deep coughs are necessary to produce sputum rather than saliva. To produce the proper specimen, take in several breaths without fully exhaling each and then expel sputum with a "cascade cough."

3. Results are normally available within 72 hours.

Factors That Affect Results

1. Specimens are best if collected in the early morning upon arising and before eating or drinking.

Other Data

1. Sputum induction by respiratory therapy may be required.

2. Povidone-iodine solution 0.02% inactivates *Mycobacterium tuberculosis, M. avium,* and *M. kansasii* within 30 seconds.

Body Fluid, Routine—Culture

Norm. No growth.

Usage. Identification and isolation of aerobic infectious organisms.

Positive Urine Culture. Titers >100,000/mL indicate urinary tract infection (viral [cytomegalovirus] or bacterial [frequently *Escherichia coli, Klebsiella, Proteus, staphylococcus,* or *Streptococcus*]).

Negative Urine Culture. Titers >1000/mL are not considered clinically significant but more likely result from contamination caused by poor collection technique.

Description. Routine body fluid culture is an aseptic collection of an aerobic culture that may be performed on ascitic, pericardial, pleural, or synovial fluids and on bone marrow or urine. For urine specimens collected by suprapubic puncture, anaerobic culture may be performed.

Professional Considerations

Consent form NOT required for the culture but may be required for the procedure used to obtain the specimen.

Preparation

1. Obtain povidone-iodine solution, sterile towels, and an appropriate sterile tray (paracentesis, thoracentesis, arthrocentesis, bone marrow aspiration).

2. For the clean-catch urine culture, obtain povidone-iodine wipes and a sterile specimen container.

3. For the urine culture for indwelling urinary catheter, obtain alcohol wipes, a needle, and a 10-mL syringe.

4. For the urine culture from suprapubic puncture, force fluids (200 mL/hour for 6 hours), and instruct the client not to void. The bladder must be full and distended for puncture. Obtain a sterile red topped tube (or an anaerobic culture container for recovery of anaerobic organisms), povidone-iodine, and an aspiration tray.

5. Cultures should be obtained before antibiotic or antifungal therapy is started whenever possible.

Procedure

1. *Ascitic, pericardial, pleural, or synovial fluid:*
   a. Cleanse the collection site with povidone-iodine and allow it to dry.
   b. The physician uses an aseptic technique to collect a minimum of 2 mL of fluid by paracentesis, pericardiocentesis, thoracentesis, or arthrocentesis and transfers it into a closed, sterile container or petri dish that is free of preservative.

2. *Bone marrow:*
   a. The physician uses an aseptic technique to collect a small amount of bone marrow via bone marrow aspiration and transfers it into a petri dish that is free of any preservative.
   b. See Bone marrow aspiration analysis—Specimen for procedural details.

3. *Urine culture from clean-catch specimen (also known as Urine culture, Routine—Specimen):* The clean-catch urine technique must be used to decrease the risk of specimen contamination.
   a. Have the client void to empty the bladder of long-standing urine. Thirty minutes later, obtain a 10-mL clean-catch urine specimen or sample from a straight or indwelling catheter in a sterile container.
   b. *Female:* While holding the labia minora apart, cleanse the mucous membranes surrounding the periphery of the urethral meatus by using antiseptic-moistened cotton balls. Use the first cotton ball to wipe from front to back on one side, followed by the same procedure with the second cotton ball on the opposite side; then cleanse directly over the meatus with the third cotton ball. Discard each cotton ball after one use.
   c. *Male:* Retract the foreskin and cleanse the glans of the penis with soap and water. Then cleanse the glans with antiseptic-moistened cotton balls, using a circular motion from the urethral meatus outward and discarding each cotton ball after one use.
   d. Have the client void a small amount of urine and discard. Then stop the stream and place the specimen container in the urine path and void 30-90 mL (1-3 ounces) of urine into the container. Avoid contaminating the container by touching the inside of the container to the body.

4. *Urine culture from indwelling catheter:*
   a. Clamp the tubing for 15 minutes to allow the urine to accumulate in the upper portion of the tubing.
   b. Cleanse the needle port of the rubber catheter with an alcohol wipe and allow it to dry.
   c. Insert a sterile needle attached to a syringe through the port and withdraw 10 mL of urine. Collect only fresh urine as it drains. Do not collect urine that has already passed the collection point.
   d. Remove the syringe and discard the needle. Expel the syringe contents into a sterile specimen cup and cap tightly. Remove the clamp from the tubing.

5. *Urine culture from suprapubic puncture:*
   a. Cleanse the skin around the aspiration site with povidone-iodine and allow it to dry.
   b. Drape the aspiration site with sterile towels.
   c. The physician performs the suprapubic puncture into the bladder and withdraws at least 10 mL of urine.
   d. For aerobic culture, the needle is removed from the syringe after withdrawal, and the urine is expelled into a sterile container.
   e. For anaerobic culture, a fresh needle is placed on the syringe, and the urine is quickly injected into an anaerobic culture container.

6. Body fluids and bone marrow aspirates may be inoculated into blood culture media.

Postprocedure Care

1. Apply a dry, sterile dressing to the aspiration site. Observe the site for drainage or bleeding hourly × 4.
2. For specimens obtained by pericardiocentesis or thoracentesis, assess vital signs every 15 minutes × 4, then every 30 minutes × 2, and then hourly × 4. Observe for dysrhythmias for 24 hours.
3. Write the specific collection site, date, time, client's age, diagnosis, and recent antibiotic or antifungal therapy on the laboratory requisition. Requests for anaerobic culture must be specified on the requisition.
4. Send the specimen to the laboratory immediately. Urine specimens should be refrigerated if not cultured immediately. Specimens from other sites should not be refrigerated.

Client and Family Teaching

1. Call the physician if signs of infection appear at the procedure site: increasing pain, redness, swelling, purulent drainage, or temperature >101 degrees F (>38.3 degrees C).
2. Results are usually available within 5 to 30 days.
3. Treatment may begin before culture results.

Factors That Affect Results

1. Reject specimens not tightly sealed.
2. Refrigeration decreases the accuracy of results for all except urine specimens.
3. Antibiotic or antifungal therapy initiated before specimen collection may produce false-negative results.
4. The most frequent interference with urine culture results is improper collection technique, which results in specimen contamination.
5. An early-morning urine specimen yields the highest concentration of microorganisms.

Other Data

1. Preliminary results are reported in 24 hours. At least 48 hours is required for the isolation of organisms in the presence of pathogens. Fungi and mycobacteria may take several weeks. Gram stains should be available within 1 hour.
2. *Mycobacterium* and *Chlamydia* infections of the urinary tract are not diagnosed by this test.
3. If cytomegalovirus is suspected, several urine specimens are recommended because the virus is shed intermittently.
4. Urine for culture should be sent on infants suspected of UTI because 4%-6% would otherwise be misdiagnosed.

Body Fluid Analysis—Specimen

Norm.

Pericardial Fluid	
Appearance	Clear to pale yellow
Glucose	
Transudate	Approximates whole blood levels (whole blood adult norm, 60-89 mg/dL; whole blood child norm, 51-85 mg/dL)
Exudate	Lower than whole blood levels
Lactate dehydrogenase	
Transudate	≤Client's serum LD (serum adult norm, 45-90 U/L; serum child norm, 60-170 U/L)
Other	
Interleukin-1 beta >45 pg/ml indicates ischemic heart disease.	

Peritoneal Fluid		SI Units
Appearance	Clear or pale yellow	
Albumin	Negative	
Alkaline phosphatase		
Adult female	76-250 U/L	
Adult male	90-239 U/L	
Ammonia	<50 g/L	
Cholesterol		
Transudate	<46 mg/dL	<1.19 mmol/L
Exudate	≥46 mg/dL	≥1.19 mmol/L
Glucose		
Transudate	60-110 mg/dL	3.3-6.1 mmol/L
Exudate	Lower than whole blood levels (whole blood adult norm, 60-89 mg/dL; child norm, 51-85 mg/dL)	
Lactic acid	10-20 mg/dL	1.1-2.3 mmol/L
Lactate dehydrogenase		
Transudate	≤Client's serum LD serum (adult norm, 45-90 U/L; child norm, 60-170 U/L)	
Exudate	>Client's serum LD	
pH	7.4	7.4
Specific gravity		
Transudate	<1.016	<1.016
Exudate	≥1.016	≥1.016
Total protein		
Transudate	<2.5 g/dL	<25 g/L
Exudate	>3 g/dL	>30 g/L
Volume	<100 mL	
White blood cells		
Transudate	<100/mm^3	<100 x 10^9/L
Exudate	>1000/mm^3	>1000 x 10^9/L
Other		

Interleukin-8 and macrophage migration inhibitory factor (MIF) are elevated in women with endometriosis.

Matrix metalloproteinases (MMP)-2 and MMP-9 are overexpressed in ovarian cancer in peritoneal fluid.

Dendritic cells in peritoneal fluid are significantly higher than in peripheral blood in infertile women.

Pleural Fluid		SI Units
Appearance	Clear, slightly amber	
Cholesterol		
Transudate	<60 mg/dL	<1.55 mmol/L
Exudate	≥60 mg/dL	≥1.55 mmol/L
Glucose		
Transudate	Approximates whole blood levels (whole blood adult norm, 60-89 mg/dL; child norm, 51-85 mg/dL)	
Exudate	Lower than whole blood levels	

Continued

Pleural Fluid		SI Units
Lactate dehydrogenase		
Transudate	≤Client's serum LD (serum adult norm, 45-90 U/L; child norm, 60-170 U/L)	
Exudate	>Client's serum LD	
Pleural fluid LD > 7500 IU/L may indicate *Streptococcus pneumoniae.*		
pH	7.4	
Specific Gravity		
Transudate	<1.016	<1.016
Exudate	≥1.016	≥1.016
Total Protein		
Transudate	<2.5 g/dL	<25 g/L
Exudate	>3 g/dL	>30 g/L
Volume	<25 mL	
White Blood Cells		
Transudate	<100/mm³	<100 × 10⁹/L
Exudate	>1000/mm³	>1000 × 10⁹/L
Other		
Amylase-rich pleural effusion (ARPE) common in lung cancer, adenocarcinoma, and mesothelioma.		

Synovial Fluid		SI Units
Appearance	Clear or colorless to pale yellow	
Crystals	Absent	
Glucose		
Transudate	≤10 mg/dL lower than blood glucose (whole blood adult norm, 60-89 mg/dL; child norm, 51-85 mg/dL)	
Exudate	Lower than whole blood levels	
Lactate Dehydrogenase		
Transudate	≤Client's serum LD (serum adult norm, 45-90 U/L; child norm, 60-170 U/L)	
Exudate	>Client's serum LD	
pH	7.4	
Specific Gravity		
Transudate	<1.016	<1.016
Exudate	>1.016	>1.016
Total Protein		
Transudate	1-3 g/dL	10-30 g/dL
Exudate	>3 g/dL	>30 g/dL
Volume	<4 mL	
Viscosity	High	
White Blood Cells		
Transudate	<100/mm³	<100 x 10⁹/L
Exudate	>1000/mm³	>1000 x 10⁹/L

Causes of Increased Volume

Pericardial Fluid	Peritoneal Fluid
Cardiac tamponade	Abscess
Constrictive pericarditis	Ascites
Central venous catheter insertion	Hepatic disease
Pericardial effusion	Peritonitis
	Portal hypertension

Pleural Fluid	Synovial Fluid
Bacterial pneumonia	Amyloidosis
Bronchogenic carcinoma	Aseptic necrosis
Chronic hepatic disease	Bacterial infection
Congestive heart failure	Charcot's joint
Constrictive pericarditis	Connective tissue disease
Hypertrophic pulmonary osteoarthropathy	Crystal-induced arthritis
Hypoproteinemia	Epiphyseal dysplasia
Lymphoma	Gout
Metastatic carcinoma	Hemochromatosis
Neoplasm	Osteoarthritis
Nephrotic syndrome	Osteochondritis dissecans
Pulmonary infarct	Paget's disease
Rheumatoid disease	Polymyositis
Systemic lupus erythematosus	Psoriasis
Trauma	Regional enteritis
Tuberculosis	Reiter's disease
Viral pneumonia	Rheumatic arthritis
	Sarcoidosis
	Scleroderma
	Sickle cell disease
	Subacute bacterial endocarditis
	Systemic lupus erythematosus
	Traumatic arthritis
	Ulcerative colitis
	Villonodular synovitis

Causes of Turbidity

Pericardial Fluid	Peritoneal Fluid
Abscess	Abscess

Pleural Fluid	Synovial Fluid
Abscess	Abscess
Bacterial infection	Floating cartilage fragments
	Inflammation
Rheumatic fever	Leukocytes
Rheumatoid disease	Pseudogout
Tuberculosis	Rheumatoid arthritis
	Septic arthritis
	Systemic lupus erythematosus
	Tuberculous arthritis

Causes of Milky Color

Synovial Fluid
Gouty arthritis
Lymphatic drainage
Rheumatoid arthritis
Systemic lupus erythematosus
Tuberculous arthritis

B

B

Causes of Pink or Red Color

Pericardial Fluid	Peritoneal Fluid
Hemorrhage	Hemorrhage
Trauma	Trauma
Traumatic tap	Traumatic tap

Pleural Fluid	Synovial Fluid
Congestive heart failure	Hemophilic arthritis
Hemorrhage	Hemorrhage
Pancreatitis	Joint fracture
Pneumonia	Neurogenic arthropathy
Postmyocardial infarction syndrome	Osteoarthritis
Pulmonary infarction	Pigmented villonodular synovitis
Trauma	Recent hemarthrosis
Traumatic tap	Rheumatoid arthritis
	Septic arthritis
	Trauma
	Traumatic arthritis
	Traumatic tap
	Tumor

Increased Lactic Acid. Infection (pleural, peritoneal) and malignancy.

Causes of Decreased Glucose

Pericardial Fluid	Peritoneal Fluid
(Not applicable)	Rheumatoid effusion

Pleural Fluid	Synovial Fluid
Bacterial infection	Inflammatory arthritis
Malignancy	Noninflammatory arthritis
Neoplastic effusion	Rheumatoid arthritis
Septic effusion	Rheumatoid effusion
Tuberculous effusion	Septic arthritis
	Tuberculous arthritis

Causes of Decreased pH

Pleural Fluid	Peritoneal Fluid
Empyema	Peritoneal effusion
Esophageal rupture	
Loculated effusion	
Parapneumonic effusion	
Tuberculous effusion	

Decreased Synovial Fluid Viscosity. Gout, inflammatory joint disease, rheumatic fever, rheumatoid arthritis, sepsis, septic arthritis, and trauma.

Increased Synovial Fluid Viscosity. Hashimoto's thyroiditis, hypothyroidism.

Description. A sample of body fluid is obtained for analysis of its various components and for detection of the presence of abnormal constituents that may be caused by pathogenic processes. Some conditions that may cause abnormalities include neoplasm, infection, inflammation, leakage of gastrointestinal tract contents or secretions, trauma, and hemorrhage.

Professional Considerations

Consent form IS required for the procedure used to obtain the specimen. See specific procedures for risks and contraindications.

Preparation

1. Obtain sterile tubes or evacuated glass bottles for the specimens.
2. Obtain a sterile specimen container, a tube, or an evacuated glass bottle, and a sterile tray (arthrocentesis, pericardiocentesis, paracentesis, thoracentesis) depending on the procedure being performed.
3. Obtain alcohol wipes, a tourniquet, a needle, a syringe, and a gray topped tube for blood glucose and a red topped tube for lactate dehydrogenase comparisons to body fluid levels.
4. Just before beginning the procedure, take a "time out" to verify the correct client, procedure, and site.

Procedure

1. A sample of body fluid is obtained by needle aspiration under sterile conditions.
2. The amount collected varies based on the purpose of the procedure and type of specimen.
3. Draw a 7-mL blood sample in the gray topped tube for whole blood glucose and a 7-mL blood sample in the red topped tube for lactate dehydrogenase levels.

Postprocedure Care

1. Apply a sterile dressing to site.

Client and Family Teaching

1. Report signs of infection at the collection site to the physician: increasing pain, redness, swelling, purulent drainage, or temperature >101 degrees F (>38.3 degrees C).

2. Results are normally available within 72 hours.

Factors That Affect Results

1. Lack of aseptic technique will alter cultures results.

Other Data

1. Ascitic fluid collection versus fluid from an overdistended bladder can be differentiated with a urea nitrogen analysis. Urine urea nitrogen should be greater than 12 g/dL, whereas ascitic fluid should be less.
2. A pleural fluid pH >7.30 and glucose concentration >60 mg/dL predict decreased survival from neoplastic metastasis to the lung.
3. See also Body fluid, Glucose—Specimen; Body fluid analysis, Cell count—Specimen; Body fluid, Amylase—Specimen.

Body Fluid Analysis, Cell Count—Specimen

Norm.

		SI Units
Pericardial Fluid		
Red blood cells	None	
White blood cells	<500/mm³	
Polymorphonuclear leukocytes	0%-25%	0-0.25
Peritoneal Fluid		
Cell count	<500/mm³	
Red blood cells	None	
Transudate	Few	
Exudate	Variable	
White blood cells	<300/μL	0-0.30 × 10⁹/L
Polymorphonuclear leukocytes	0%-25%	0-0.25
Pleural Fluid		
Cell count		
White blood cells		<1000/mm³
Transudate	Few	
Exudate	Many	
Eosinophils	0%-10%	0-0.10
Lymphocytes	0%-50%	0-0.50
Neutrophils	0%-50%	0-0.50
Polymorphonuclear leukocytes	0%-25%	0-0.25
Synovial Fluid		
Red blood cells	None	
White blood cells	0-200/μL	0-0.20 × 10⁹/L
Neutrophils	0%-25%	0-0.25
Lymphocytes	0%-78%	0-0.78
Monocytes	0%-71%	0-0.71

Continued

		SI Units
Macrophages (clasmatocytes)	0%-26%	0-0.26
Polymorphonuclear leukocytes	0%-25%	0-0.25
Synovial cells	0%-12%	0-0.12
Unclassified	0%-21%	0-0.21

Increased Leukocytes. Acute gouty arthritis, carcinoma (pleural fluid), chylothorax (pleural fluid), congestive heart failure (pleural fluid), empyema (pleural fluid), gonorrheal arthritis, inflammation (pleural fluid), lymphatic leukemia, lymphocytic leukemia (pleural fluid), lymphomas (pleural fluid), parapneumonic effusion (pleural fluid), postpneumonic effusion (pleural fluid), rheumatic fever, rheumatoid arthritis, septic arthritis, tuberculosis (pleural fluid), tumors, and uremia (pleural fluid).

Increased Polymorphonuclear Cells. Bacterial inflammation, bacterial peritonitis, and infectious processes (acute).

Increased Eosinophils. Infarcts, parasites, pneumothorax, postpneumonic effusions, rheumatic fever, rheumatoid arthritis, and tumors.

Increased Plasma Cells. Chronic inflammation, Hodgkin's disease, and lymphoma. Atypical plasma cells may be associated with multiple myeloma.

Decreased Glucose. Rheumatoid effusion (synovial fluid).

Description. The specific body fluid is tested for white blood count and differential, total red blood cell count, protein, lactate dehydrogenase, and other tests. The various cell counts of body fluids assist in the differentiation of exudate from transudate. Body fluid analysis may be performed on the following body fluids: ascitic, cyst, joint, pericardial, peritoneal, pleural, and synovial.

Professional Considerations

Consent form IS required for the procedure used to obtain the specimen. See specific procedures for risks and contraindications.

Preparation

1. The client should be properly positioned and the specimen site cleaned and prepped.
2. Obtain heparin 1000 U/mL concentration.

3. Obtain a sterile specimen container, a tube or an evacuated glass bottle, and a sterile tray (arthrocentesis, pericardiocentesis, paracentesis, thoracentesis) depending on the procedure being performed.
4. Just before beginning the procedure, take a "time out" to verify the correct client, procedure, and site.

Procedure

1. A sample of body fluid is obtained by needle aspiration under sterile conditions.
2. The amount collected varies based on the purpose of the procedure and the type of specimen.

Postprocedure Care

1. Apply a small dressing to the aspiration site.
2. To each 100 mL of body fluid add 1 mL of heparin 1000 U/mL concentration. Additional heparin will not alter results.
3. Write the specimen source on the laboratory requisition.
4. Transport the specimen to the laboratory immediately.

Client and Family Teaching

1. Report signs of infection at the operative site to the physician: increasing pain, redness, swelling, purulent drainage, or temperature >101 degrees F (>38.3 degrees C).
2. See individual procedure listings for procedure-specific teaching.
3. Results are normally available within 72 hours.

Factors That Affect Results

1. Reject contaminated or hemolyzed specimens.

Other Data

1. Ascitic fluid collection versus fluid from an overdistended bladder can be differentiated with a urea nitrogen analysis. Urine urea nitrogen should be greater than 12 g/dL, whereas ascitic fluid should be less.

Body Fluid Cytology

See **Bronchial Washing**—Specimen, Diagnostic; **Brushing Cytology**—Specimen, Diagnostic; **Cerebrospinal Fluid, Routine, Culture and Cytology**; **Cytologic Study of Breast Cyst, Effusions, Gatrointestinal Tract, Nipple Discharge, Respiratory Tract, or Urine**—Diagnostic; **Oral Cavity Cytology**—Specimen.

BOHB

See **Beta-Hydroxybutyrate**—Blood.

Bone Densitometry (Dual-Energy X-Ray Absorptiometry, DXA, DEXA Scan)—Diagnostic

Norm.

Bone by mineral density (BMD)	Percentage within range of standard deviations from the norm provided the manufacturer of the device used for the test. Each manufacturer provides a database of BMDs from many persons for comparison to those with similar age, race, sex, and ethnicity. Low BMD indicates androgen deprivation in prostate cancer, cystic fibrosis, or osteoporosis.
Z-score	(Percent young adult) within range of manufacturer's norms.
T-score (per WHO definitions)	(Age-matched) within range of manufacturer's norms.
	Normal: Better than -1 g cm^{-2}
	Osteopenia: -1 to -2.5 g cm^{-2}
	Osteoporosis: Lower than -2.5 g cm^{-2}

Usage. Measurement of bone mass or bone mineral density in estrogen deficient women or in clients with vertebral abnormalities or roentgenographic osteopenia, clients receiving glucocorticoids on a long-term basis, and those with asymptomatic primary hyperparathyroidism. Most commonly used for diagnosing osteoporosis and predicting risk of fracture, skeletal morphometry, and body-composition analysis (less common). Bone densitometry is one of the diagnostic criteria for osteoporosis established by the World Health Organization (WHO). Included in well woman screening recommendations from the American College of Obstetricians and Gynecologists for postmenopausal women younger than 65 years, history of prior fracture as an adult, family history of osteoporosis, Caucasian, dementia, poor nutrition, smoking, low weight and body mass index, estrogen deficiency, low lifelong calcium intake, alcoholism, impaired eyesight, history of falls, inadequate physical activity, and medical conditions and certain drugs associated with an increased risk for osteoporosis.

Description. Considered the standard of comparison often used for diagnosis of osteoporosis, bone densitometry, approved by the FDA in 1988, is also known as dual-energy x-ray absorptiometry (DEXA). The procedure is carried out using an x-ray device that scans the heel, finger, lumbar spine, and nondominant proximal femur or forearm and determines bone mineral density (BMD). The site selected for scanning is determined by the purpose of the test. The BMD measurement at one site can allow prediction of the risk of fracture at another site of the body. For assessment of general fracture risk, either the spine or the neck of the femur is measured. This test is not indicated if treatment decisions will not be affected by the results. In addition to the BMD, results are also often reported as a "Z-score" and a "T-score." The Z-score represents a comparison to the peak bone mass scores in other persons of similar age, sex, and ethnicity, and helps one to predict the risk of future fracture. The T-score represents a comparison to the person's bone density to that of the average 30-year old of the same sex and ethnicity. See Other Data for screening and monitoring recommendations.

Professional Considerations

Consent form NOT required.

Precautions

During pregnancy, risks of cumulative radiation exposure to the fetus from this and other previous or future imaging studies must be weighed against the benefits of the procedure. Although formal limits for client exposure are relative to this risk-benefit comparison, the United States Nuclear Regulatory Commission requires that the cumulative dose equivalent to an embryo/fetus from occupational exposure not exceed 0.5 rem (5 mSv). Radiation dose to the fetus is proportional to the distance of the anatomy studied from the abdomen and decreases as pregnancy progresses. For pregnant clients, consult the radiologist/radiology department to obtain estimated fetal radiation exposure from this procedure.

Preparation

1. Notify radiologist if client is pregnant.
2. Remove any metal items, such as buckles, jewelry, or buttons, from the area to be scanned.

Procedure

1. The client is positioned for the radiograph. For spinal or femoral densitometry, the client lies on a radiograph table. For peripheral densitometry, the client may sit upright in a chair and place the foot, finger, or forearm on a smaller device designed for peripheral densitometry. A square cushion may be placed under the client's knees and lower legs to decrease back pain, especially in those with osteoporosis.
2. The scan is taken.

Postprocedure Care

1. None.

Client and Family Teaching

1. The procedure is painless and uses minimal radiation.
2. The scan takes only a few minutes.
3. It is important to lie as still as possible during the scan.

4. Low DXA results may indicate need to increase calcium and vitamin D intake as well as increase impact activity, if tolerated.

Factors That Affect Results

1. The trabecular area of the spine is the preferred site for repeated testing because it has a high rate of bone turnover and thus will show the greatest magnitude of change with treatment for osteoporosis.
2. Spinal abnormalities such as scoliosis can impair accuracy of results. An additional method of evaluation of bone density should be used in these persons.
3. High doses of levothyroxine replacement therapy are associated with reduced bone quality and density.
4. Falsely elevated results are caused by crushed vertebrae.

Other Data

1. 2011 recommendations from the United States Preventive Services Task force include:
   a. Men: Recommended via rating of "B", but notes that evidence is lacking regarding benefits of screening in men.
   b. Women 65 and over: Recommended bone density screening
   c. Women under age 65: Calculate fracture risk assessment using the World Health Organization Fracture Risk Assessment Tool (FRAX) calculator; then compare the result to that of a healthy 65-year old white woman with no additional risk factors (using the same calculator) to determine the "Threshold Fracture Risk".
   d. Carry out bone density testing if the fracture risk of the client is equal to or greater than the 65-year old value (9.3%).
2. The American Association of Clinical Endocrinologists recommends for clients undergoing osteoporosis treatment that they be monitored with a repeat DXA every 1-2 years until findings are stable.
3. Contributors to low bone mineral density include type I diabetes, and low body weight, including that achieved via eating disorder.
4. Oral bisphosphonates taken for more than 5 years by women aged 68 and older reduce the risk for osteoporotic hip

fracture in women, but have been found to increase the risk for atypical femoral fractures.

5. Other techniques used to measure bone density include the following: single x-ray absorptiometry (SXA), quantitative computed tomography (QCT), and quantitative ultrasonography (QUS).

6. See also Bone ultrasonometry—Diagnostic.

Bone GLA Protein

See **Osteocalcin**—Plasma or Serum.

Bone Marrow Aspiration Analysis—Specimen (Biopsy, Bone Marrow Iron Stain, Iron Stain, Bone Marrow)

Norm. Red marrow contains connective tissue, fat cells, and hematopoietic cells. Yellow marrow contains connective tissue and fat cells. Interpretation of cell count and histopathology by a hematologist, pathologist, or oncologist is required.

Response to Staining. Iron stain for hemosiderin: 2+.

Periodic Acid–Schiff (PAS) Glycogen Reactions. Negative.

Sudan Black B (SBB) Granulocyte. Negative.

Differential Cell Count

	Adult (%)	Child (%)	Infant (%)
Basophils	0.1	0.06	0.07
Eosinophils	3.1	3.6	2.6
Hemocytoblasts	0.1-1.0		
Lymphocytes (all stages)	2.7-24	16	49
Megakaryocytes	0.03-0.5	0.1	0.05
Plasmacytes	0.1-1.5	0.4	0.02
Promyelocytes	0.5-8.0	1.4	0.76
Reticulum cells	0.1-2.0		
Undifferentiated cells	0.0-0.1		
Neutrophils, total	56.5	57.1	32.4
Metamyelocytes	9.6-24.6	23.3	11.3
Neutrophilic	10-32		
Eosinophilic	0.3-3.7		
Basophilic	0-0.3		
Monocytes (all stages)	0-2.7		
Myeloblasts	0.1-5.0	1.2	0.62
Myelocytes	4.2-15	18.4	2.5
Neutrophilic	5.0-20		
Eosinophilic	0.1-3.0		
Basophilic	0-0.5		
Segmented granulocytes	6.0-12.0	12.9	3.6
Neutrophilic	7.0-30		
Eosinophilic	0.2-4.0		
Basophilic	0-0.7		
Band cells	9.5-15.3	0	14.1
Neutrophilic	10-35		
Eosinophilic	0.2-2.0		
Basophilic	0-0.3		

Continued

Differential Cell Count—cont'd

	Adult (%)	Child (%)	Infant (%)
Erythroid series			
Normoblasts, total	25.6	23.1	8.0
Pronormoblasts	0.2-4.0	0.5	0.1
Basophilic normoblasts	1.5-5.8	1.7	0.34
Polychromatophilic normoblasts	5.0-26.4	18.2	6.9
Orthochromic normoblasts	3.6-21	2.7	0.54
Promegaloblasts	0		
Basophilic megaloblasts	0		
Polychromatic megaloblasts	0		
Orthochromic megaloblasts	0		

M:E Ratio. The myeloid:erythroid ratio is the ratio of white blood cells to nucleated red blood cells.

Adult	6:1 to 2:1
Birth	1.85:1
2 weeks	11:1
1-2 months	5.5:1
1-20 years	2.95:1

Usage. Helps to distinguish primary and metastatic tumors. Assists in the identification, classification, and staging of neoplasias. Aids evaluation of the progress or response to the treatment of neoplasias. Assists in the definitive diagnosis of blood disorders. Culture of an aspirated sample can aid in the identification of infections such as histoplasmosis or tuberculosis. Histologic examination aids in the diagnosis of carcinoma, granulomas, lymphoma, or myelofibrosis. Iron stain showing decreased hemosiderin levels may indicate iron deficiency or malnutrition from anorexia nervosa, and SBB stain differentiates acute granulocytic leukemia from acute lymphocytic leukemia.

Increased Eosinophils. Bone marrow carcinoma, eosinophilic leukemia, hypereosinophilic syndrome, lymphadenoma, myeloid leukemia, and pernicious anemia (relapse).

Increased Lymphocytes. Aplastic anemia, hypoplasia of the bone marrow, infectious lymphocytosis or mononucleosis, lymphatic leukemoid reactions, lymphocytic leukemia (B-cell and T-cell), lymphoma, macroglobulinemia, myelofibrosis, and viral infections.

Increased Megakaryocytes. Acute hemorrhage, aging, chronic myeloid leukemia, hypersplenism, idiopathic thrombocytopenia, infection, megakaryocytic myelosis, myelofibrosis, pneumonia, polycythemia vera, and thrombocytopenia.

Increased Plasma Cells. Agranulocytosis, amyloidosis, aplastic anemia, carcinomatosis, collagen disease, hepatic cirrhosis, Hodgkin's disease, hypersensitivity reactions, infection, irradiation, macroglobulinemia, malignant tumor, multiple myeloma, rheumatic fever (acute), rheumatoid arthritis, serum sickness, syphilis, and ulcerative colitis.

Increased Granulocyte. Hypoplasia of the bone marrow, infections, myelocytic leukemia, myelocytic leukemoid reaction, and myeloproliferative syndrome.

Increased Normoblasts. Anemia (iron deficiency, hemolytic, megaloblastic), blood loss (chronic), erythema, erythroid-type myeloproliferative disorders, hypoplasia of the bone marrow, and polycythemia vera.

Increased M:E Ratio Above 7:1. Decreased hematopoiesis, erythroid hypoplasia, infection, leukemoid reactions, and myeloid leukemia.

Increased Diffuse Bone Marrow Hyperplasia. Myeloproliferative syndromes and pancytopenia reactions.

Decreased Megakaryocytes. Anemia (aplastic, pernicious), bone marrow hyperplasia (with carcinomatous or leukemic deposits), cirrhosis, irradiation (excessive), and thrombocytopenia purpura. Drugs include benzene, chlorothiazides, and cytotoxic drugs.

Decreased Granulocyte. Agranulocytosis, barbiturate coma, hyperplasia of the bone marrow, and ionizing radiation.

Decreased Normoblasts. Anemia (aplastic, hypoplastic), folic acid, or vitamin B_{12} (cyanocobalamin) deficiency.

Decreased M:E Ratio Below 2:1. Agranulocytosis, anemia (iron deficiency, normoblastic, pernicious, posthemolytic, posthemorrhagic), erythroid activity (increased), hepatic disease, myeloid formation (decreased), polycythemia vera, sprue, and steatorrhea.

Decreased Diffuse Bone Marrow Hypoplasia. Aging, cellular infiltrations, dengue fever, hepatitis C virus, myelofibrosis, myelosclerosis, myelotoxic agents, osteoporosis, rubella, and viral infections.

Description. Bone marrow is the soft, organic, spongelike material contained in the medullary cavities, long bones, and some haversian canals and within the spaces between trabeculae of cancellous bone. It is composed of red and yellow marrow, with the chief function being production of erythrocytes, leukocytes, and platelets. Only the rusty, red marrow produces blood cells. The yellow marrow is formed of connective tissue and fat cells, which are inactive. During infancy and childhood, bone marrow is primarily red marrow, but in the adult, 50% is red marrow. The bone marrow aspiration procedure is a way to obtain a sample of bone marrow by needle. A stained blood smear of the sample is evaluated for bone marrow morphology and examination of blood cell erythropoiesis, cellularity, differential cell count, bone marrow iron stores, and M:E ratios. This test is used mainly in the diagnosis and management of anemia, fever, leukemia, lymphoma, pancytopenia, and thrombocytopenia.

Professional Considerations
Consent form IS required.

Risks
Bleeding, heart damage (with sterna biopsy), hemorrhage, infection, and meningitis.

Contraindications
Bone marrow aspiration is contraindicated in haemophilia, hemostasis, and coagulation defects; also contraindicated in clients receiving anticoagulants.

Preparation
1. Obtain a bone marrow aspiration tray, laboratory slides and stains, and a lavender topped or green topped tube.

2. Obtain a sterile container of Zenker's acetic acid solution if a bone marrow biopsy is to be performed.
3. Pain medication may be given to lessen procedure discomfort.
4. Just before beginning the procedure, take a "time out" to verify the correct client, procedure, and site.

Procedure
1. The most common sites for bone marrow aspiration include the sternum (preferred for bone marrow biopsy), the posterior superior iliac spine (for needle biopsy), and the anterior iliac crest and vertebral spinous process in the adult. For infants under 18 months, the anterior tibia site is used, and for children, the iliac crest is preferred.
2. The designated site is prepped, shaved, and draped. After a local anesthetic is injected and under sterile technique, a $\frac{1}{8}$-inch stab wound is made. A Jamshidi needle with the stylet in place is inserted until the outer surface of the bone is impinged. The needle guard is engaged, and the outer needle is inserted with a boring motion, about 3 mm deep, into the bone marrow cavity.
3. *For bone marrow aspiration:* The stylet is removed, and a 10-mL syringe is attached to the needle. When aspiration of 0.2 to 0.5 mL of bone marrow has entered the syringe, it is removed and given to a technician for preparation of a stained blood smear. A second syringe may be attached and a 2-mL sample of bone marrow withdrawn and placed into a lavender topped tube containing EDTA or a heparinized green topped tube.
4. *For bone marrow biopsy:* The stylet is removed, and a biopsy or inner needle with a trephine tip is inserted. A tissue plug is removed and placed into a container of Zenker's acetic acid solution.
5. The needle is withdrawn.

Postprocedure Care
1. Apply a pressure dressing to the bone marrow aspiration site.
2. Observe the aspiration site for bleeding.

Client and Family Teaching
1. Bone marrow aspiration is painful, but only for a few moments. Preprocedure pain medicine may be used to lessen the

discomfort. It is also normal to experience a deep pressure feeling as the bone marrow is withdrawn.

2. It is important to lie very still during the procedure.

3. Results are normally available within 24-72 hours.

4. Call the physician if there are signs of infection at the procedure site: increasing pain, redness, swelling, purulent drainage, or temperature >101 degrees F (>38.3 degrees C).

Factors That Affect Results

1. Cytotoxic drugs, folic acid, iron, liver or vitamin B_{12} agents, and recent blood transfusions should be noted before the biopsy.

2. Chloramphenicol causes higher frequency (90%) of marrow hypocellularity.

3. Send the specimen to the laboratory immediately.

Other Data

1. The presence of normal bone marrow at one site does not eliminate the possibility of disease elsewhere in the bone marrow.

2. Normal M:E ratio may be associated with aplastic anemia, myeloma, and myelosclerosis.

Bone Marrow Biopsy

See **Bone Marrow Aspiration Analysis—Specimen.**

Bone Marrow Iron Stain

See **Bone Marrow Aspiration Analysis—Specimen.**

Bone Marrow Scan—Diagnostic

Norm. Even concentration of the radionuclide throughout the reticuloendothelial system, red blood cells, and bone marrow.

Usage. Assists in the diagnosis of defects in bone marrow or bone marrow depression after chemotherapy or radiation, in the differential determinations of myeloproliferative disorders, and with increased pulmonary uptake consideration of *Pneumocystis carinii pneumonia*. Differentiates acute from chronic hemolysis and bone infarction from osteomyelitis in sickle cell disease. Aids in the selection of bone marrow biopsy sites and in the staging of Hodgkin's disease, lymphomas, and metastatic diseases of the bone marrow. Assists in evaluation of hyperplasia of the bone marrow associated with chronic hemolytic anemia and polycythemia vera.

Description. The bone marrow scan is a nuclear medicine study in which the radionuclide indium chloride is administered intravenously and followed by radiographic imaging of the entire body. This scan can be nonspecific in conditions of diffuse disease such as osteomyelitis and tumor. However, areas of increased vascularity and hyperproliferation of bone marrow can be demonstrated much earlier with a bone marrow scan than by conventional radiography.

Professional Considerations

Consent form IS required.

Risks

Hematoma at injection site.

Precautions

During pregnancy, risks of cumulative radiation exposure to the fetus from this and other previous or future imaging studies must be weighed against the benefits of the procedure. Although formal limits for client exposure are relative to this risk-benefit comparison, the United States Nuclear Regulatory Commission requires that the cumulative dose equivalent to an embryo/fetus from occupational exposure not exceed 0.5 rem (5 mSv). Radiation dose to the fetus is proportional to the distance of the anatomy studied from the abdomen and decreases as pregnancy progresses. For pregnant clients, consult the radiologist/radiology department to obtain estimated fetal radiation exposure from this procedure.

Contraindications

Pregnancy or during breast-feeding.

Preparation

1. The client should void before the procedure.
2. Have emergency equipment readily available.
3. Just before beginning the procedure, take a "time out" to verify the correct client, procedure, and site.

Procedure

1. The radionuclide indium chloride is administered intravenously.
2. Whole-body imaging is planned for 48 hours after intravenous injection.
3. If the radioisotope ^{99m}Tc-sulfur colloid is given, the scan can be completed 1 hour after the intravenous injection.

Postprocedure Care

1. None.

Client and Family Teaching

1. Notify the physician for previous reaction to radionuclide.
2. An IV tube may be inserted for the scan and removed after the scan is complete. Some technicians may use direct venipuncture for the injection.
3. Results are normally available within 24 hours.
4. In women who are breast-feeding, formula should be substituted for breast milk for 1 or more days after the procedure.

Factors That Affect Results

1. None found.

Other Data

1. Health care professionals working in a nuclear medicine area must follow federal standards set by the Nuclear Regulatory Commission. These standards include precautions for handling the radioactive material and monitoring of potential radiation exposure.
2. Indium scan is positive in 20%-30% of clients after other imaging methods failed to detect metastasis.

Bone Radiography—Diagnostic

Norm. Negative.

Usage. Identification of abnormal growth patterns by serial radiography. Detection of ankylosing spondylitis, congenital abnormalities, fractures, healing fractures, hyperparathyroidism, infection, joint destruction, osteomalacia, osteomyelitis, osteoporosis, the presence of joint fluid, rickets, and tumors.

Description. Specific bones are radiographed in several positions for visualization of the bone from all angles. Kiuru et al (2002) found magnetic resonance imaging superior to bone radiography for detecting bone stress injuries in the early phase of damage.

Professional Considerations

Consent form NOT required.

Precautions

During pregnancy, risks of cumulative radiation exposure to the fetus from this and other previous or future imaging studies must be weighed against the benefits of the procedure. Although formal limits for client exposure are relative to this risk-benefit comparison, the United States Nuclear Regulatory Commission requires that the cumulative dose equivalent to an embryo/fetus from occupational exposure not exceed 0.5 rem (5 mSv). Radiation dose to the fetus is proportional to the distance of the anatomy studied from the abdomen and decreases as pregnancy progresses. For pregnant clients, consult the radiologist/radiology department to obtain estimated fetal radiation exposure from this procedure.

Preparation

1. Handle injured parts carefully.
2. Shield the client's testes, ovaries, or pregnant abdomen.

Procedure

1. The client is placed on the radiography table in several positions, with a radiograph taken in each position.
2. The client must lie still for the radiograph.

Postprocedure Care

1. The client remains in the radiology department until it is determined that the films are satisfactory.

Client and Family Teaching

1. The amount of exposure to radiation is minimal and not dangerous.
2. It is important to stay still during the radiograph.
3. Results are normally available within 24 hours.

Factors That Affect Results

1. Movement results in an unsatisfactory radiograph.
2. Too little or too much exposure results in a radiograph that is too light or too dark and may need to be repeated for interpretation.

Other Data

1. Wear a lead apron if remaining in the room with the client during radiography.

Bone Scan (Bone Scintigraphy)—Diagnostic

Norm. Even concentration of radioactive isotope throughout the osseous tissues.

Usage. Detection, staging, and evaluation of osseous metastatic disease. Detection of pathologic conditions that cause increased uptake, including acute hematogenous osteomyelitis (AHOM), aseptic necrosis, bone fractures, bone infarction, bone infection, bone metastasis, bone necrosis, bone trauma, bone tumors, osseous metastatic disease, osteoarthritis, osteoid osteoma, osteomyelitis, Paget's disease, renal osteodystrophy, temporomandibular joint disease, transient osteoporosis, tuberculosis, and soft-tissue calcification. Differentiation of cellulitis from osteomyelitis. Monitoring of degenerative bone disorders, bone grafts, and prosthetic joint replacements. Aids in the selection of a biopsy site in the abnormal bone, in the evaluation of the effectiveness of arthritides, and in suspected abuse of a child.

Description. A nuclear medicine radioactive isotope study that will show bone changes from a few weeks up to 6 months before conventional radiographs will show such changes. Diagnostic sensitivity is 95.2% and accuracy 78.7%. The radioactive isotope ^{99m}Tc-diphosphonate (technetium diphosphate) is administered intravenously. As the entire body is scanned, images from the low-level radioactive isotope in the bony tissues are recorded on paper or film, creating two-dimensional images of the skeletal outlines. The epiphyses of growing bones or new bone formation shows up as areas of high metabolism, or concentration, and are called "hot spots," whereas areas of low concentration, associated with ischemia or tumor displacement, are referred to as "cold spots." Increased uptake of the isotope by bone tissue indicates an abnormality in that area. There is a phenomenon called bone scan flare, which shows an increase in bone lesions with improvement while the client is receiving chemotherapy for either breast or small-cell lung or non–small-cell lung cancers. Bone scintigraphy is especially important in detecting metastatic tumors and fractures not immediately seen on radiograph, especially in the spine, ribs, face, and small bones of the hands and feet. This test is invaluable in evaluating clients with osteomyelitis. Its disadvantage is that when it shows an abnormality, it is nonspecific as to the pathologic process present.

Professional Considerations

Consent form NOT required.

Risks
Hematoma at injection site.
Contraindications
Clients who cannot lie still for an extended period of time.
Precautions
During pregnancy, risks of cumulative radiation exposure to the fetus from this and other previous or future imaging studies must be weighed against the benefits of the procedure. Although formal limits for client exposure are relative to this risk-benefit comparison, the United States Nuclear Regulatory Commission requires that the cumulative dose equivalent to an embryo/fetus from occupational exposure not exceed 0.5 rem (5 mSv). Radiation dose to

the fetus is proportional to the distance of the anatomy studied from the abdomen and decreases as pregnancy progresses. For pregnant clients, consult the radiologist/radiology department to obtain estimated fetal radiation exposure from this procedure.

Preparation

1. The client should not drink unnecessary fluids for 2-4 hours.
2. Obtain an alcohol wipe, a tourniquet, a needle, a syringe, and a radioactive isotope.
3. Remove all jewelry and metal objects.
4. Sedatives are used only if the client is unable to lie still for the scan.
5. The client should void before the intravenous radioisotope is administered.

Procedure

1. ^{99m}Tc-diphosphonate (technetium diphosphate) is administered intravenously into a vein of the arm.
2. During the next 2-3 hours, the client must drink 32 ounces of water to promote renal filtering of excess tracer.
3. The client should void just before the scan to remove any tracer not picked up by bone that was filtered by the kidney.
4. For 1-3 hours after the injection, the client is placed in a supine position on the scanning table and instructed to lie still while the entire body is scanned and two-dimensional images of the skeleton are recorded.

Postprocedure Care

1. If deep sedation was used, follow institutional protocol for postsedation monitoring. Typical monitoring includes continuous ECG monitoring and pulse oximetry, with continual assessments (every 5-15 minutes) of airway, vital signs, and neurologic status until the client is lying quietly awake, is breathing independently, and responds appropriately to commands spoken in a normal tone. The client should not operate a motor vehicle for 24 hours after receiving sedation.
2. Check the injection site for redness or swelling. If a hematoma is present, apply warm soaks.
3. Encourage oral fluid intake.

Client and Family Teaching

1. The radioisotope delivers less radiation than a regular radiograph, and the scanning machine is detecting the injected isotope, rather than exposing the client to radiation.
2. Do not drink fluids for 4 hours before the scan.
3. The radioisotope will be injected intravenously before the scan.
4. Most of the radioactive material will be excreted from the body through urine and stool within 48 hours and is not harmful to other people nearby.
5. Results are normally available within 24 hours.
6. In women who are breast-feeding, formula should be substituted for breast milk for 1 or more days after the procedure.

Factors That Affect Results

1. Failure to void before the test may cause an overdistended urinary bladder, which can interfere with pelvic imaging.

Other Data

1. Health care professionals working in a nuclear medicine area must follow federal standards set by the Nuclear Regulatory Commission. These standards include precautions for handling the radioactive material and monitoring of potential radiation exposure.
2. 32% of bone scans give false-positive results for persons with T1 or T2 breast cancer.
3. Routine bone scans are not warranted in clients with squamous cell carcinoma of the head and neck.

Bone Scintigraphy

See **Bone Scan**—Diagnostic.

Bone Ultrasonometry—Diagnostic

Norm.

The lower the T-score, the greater the risk for fracture.

T-score ≤1.0 = low bone mass, at increased risk for fracture.

Usage. This test is used to determine a qualitative ultrasound measurement of the calcaneus. This along with clinical factors is used to assist in determining osteoporosis, primary hyperparathyroidism, risk for fracture, and type 1 Gaucher disease.

Description. This procedure uses an ultrasonometer to measure bone density of the heel and identify bone fragility and risk for osteoporosis. The ultrasonometer is an ultrasound device that measures the speed of sound and broadband ultrasonic attenuation of an ultrasound beam passed through the heel. The process determines a quantitative ultrasound index (QUI), expressed as a T-score and an estimate of the bone mineral density (BMD in g/cm^2) of the heel. Ultrasonographic bone densitometry of the heel is most useful as a screening tool. It is not recommended for frequent monitoring of response to osteoporosis treatment because the heel does not respond quickly to treatment. A 3-year interval is recommended by the manufacturer as necessary to identify improvement. Other methods of bone density testing should be used if more frequent monitoring is needed. (The test described below is based on information available for the Sahara Clinical Bone Sonometer. At least 15 commercial systems are available.)

Professional Considerations

Consent form NOT required.

Risks

None.

Contraindications

The Sahara should not be used in clients whose skin is abraded or have an open sore in an area that comes in contact with the system.

Preparation

1. The client must remove shoes and socks or stockings.

Procedure

1. If the test has been performed in the past, select the same foot for testing.
2. The client's heel is covered with Sahara Coupling Gel and then rested against the ultrasonometer.

Postprocedure Care

1. Remove gel from heel.

Client and Family Teaching

1. The test takes only a few seconds, and results are available during the same visit.
2. No x-rays or radiation is involved.
3. *T-Score −2.5 to − 4.0:*
   a. Treatment is usually indicated in this range.
   b. Treatment is almost always indicated if there has been an osteoporotic fracture.
4. *T-Score −0.5 to −2.5*
   Treatment may be indicated in this range if:
   a. There is a family history of osteoporosis.
   b. There is a history of smoking.
   c. The client is underweight or has experienced a weight loss.
   d. The range is close to a −2.5 T-score.
   e. There is a likelihood of bone loss.
5. *T-Score +1.0 and above:*
   a. Values in this range are good. Continue to maintain a healthy lifestyle, exercise, and eat a good diet.
6. With extra risk factors consider a baseline DEXA scan.

Factors That Affect Results

1. Sahara Coupling Gel should be used as directed, and no other gels should be substituted because water-based gels have been associated with coupling delays.
2. Avoid measuring bone density on a foot or limb that has had a recent reduction because of immobilization or fracture, for example.

Other Data

1. Although ultrasound bone sonometry allows one to predict the risk of hip fracture in elderly females almost as well as

dual-energy x-ray absorptiometry (DEXA), the latter is considered the standard of comparison often used for measuring bone density.

2. Testing can be done in a physician's office. Medicare reimbursement is not available for this test because of its designation as a screening test.

Bordetella pertussis—Culture

Norm. No growth.

Usage. Diagnosis of pertussis (whooping cough).

Description. Pertussis is a highly communicable, acute bacterial infection of the tracheobronchial tree caused by *Bordetella pertussis*, a gram-negative coccobacillus. The disease occurs commonly in children throughout the world and can be prevented in 99.8% of cases by vaccination of 3 doses of DTaP (diphtheria, tetanus, and acellular pertussis) vaccine. Mode of transmission is believed to be either by direct contact with the respiratory discharges of infected clients or by inhalation of airborne droplets. It is most communicable in the early stages, before the paroxysmal cough appears. Pertussis is characterized by an explosive cough followed by a "whooping" sound on inspiration and may include respiratory distress and apnea as symptoms. Pertussis can lead to CNS encephalopathy and pulmonary hypertension, and there are known cases of reinfection up to 12 years after initial diagnosis.

Professional Considerations

Consent form NOT required.

Preparation

1. Wear mask and gloves when collecting the specimen.
2. Obtain a culture tube, flexible wire swab, penlight, and tongue blade or "cough plate."

Procedure

1. Obtain a sterile swab of the nasopharynx or have the client cough onto a cough plate held in front of his or her mouth.
2. To obtain nasopharyngeal swab:
   a. With the client's head tilted back, use a penlight and tongue depressor to visualize the nasopharynx.
   b. Gently pass the swab through the nostril and into the nasopharynx, keeping the swab near the septum and floor of the nose.
   c. Rotate the swab quickly and remove it carefully, making sure it does not touch the tongue or the sides of the nostril.

Postprocedure Care

1. Hand-deliver the specimen to the laboratory immediately.
2. Inform laboratory personnel if pertussis is suspected because a special growth medium is required.

Client and Family Teaching

1. Observe for signs of pertussis in other children who were in contact with the infected child and who were not immunized.
2. Therapy may begin before culture results are supplied.
3. In the absence of antibiotic therapy, the period of communicability is considered to be from 7 days after exposure to 3 weeks after the paroxysmal cough appears. With erythromycin treatment, the period of communicability extends 7 days after the treatment is initiated.
4. Results are normally available within 72 hours.

Factors That Affect Results

1. An insufficient specimen or current antibiotic therapy may cause false-negative results.
2. Most uncomplicated pertussis does not lead to serious complications.

Other Data

1. Immunization is available for pertussis prevention. Oral administration of rotavirus vaccine can be given with DTaP and oral administration of polio vaccine without interference to children at 2, 4, and 6 months of age.
2. Resistance to erythromycin can occur, and alternatives for treatment include clarithromycin, azithromycin, trimethoprim sulfamethoxazole, or the newer fluoroquinolones, such as gatifloxacin.
3. A preliminary report should be available in 24 hours.
4. Azithromycin is used to treat *Bordetella* infection.

Borrelia burgdorferi C6 Peptide Antibody—Serum

Norm.

≤0.90 LI	Negative	No presence of C6 peptide antibody to *Borrelia burgdorferi*
0.91-1.09 LI	Equivocal	Repeat test in 14 days
≥1.09 LI	Positive	C6 peptide antibody to *Borrelia burgdorferi* is present

Usage. Definitive testing for active Lyme disease; should be used in place of Lyme disease IgG and IgM antibody testing for those who are suspected of recurrent Lyme disease, or who have been vaccinated for Lyme disease in the past. Differentiation of symptoms of Lyme disease from *B. burgdorferi* vaccine—related side-effects.

Description. See Lyme disease antibody—Blood for a description of Lyme disease. This blood test identifies the C6 glycoprotein, a newly discovered peptide, which is part of the variable antigen VlsE[1,2]. C6 is important because it can definitively confirm active infection with *Borrelia burgdorferi*, the causative agent of Lyme disease, even in those who have previously had the disease or been vaccinated for it. In this group of people, the active disease could be present, but traditional IgG and IgM antibody testing could indicate immunity. This is because the antibodies can remain present for up to 20 years after the acute disease resolves in those who previously had Lyme disease, yet the person can become reinfected. In addition, 25% of people vaccinated for Lyme disease fail to develop enough OpsA antibodies for active immunity. It is the OpsA antibodies that cause the false-positive results on traditional tests. Because the C6 peptide does not target OpsA antibodies for measurement, it is ideal for definitive testing.

Professional Considerations
Consent form NOT required.

Preparation
1. Tube: Red topped, red/gray topped, or gold topped.

Procedure
1. Draw a 3-mL blood sample.

Postprocedure Care
1. Separate serum and freeze until testing.

Client and Family Teaching
1. No fasting or special preparation is required.

Factors That Affect Results
1. None.

Other Data
1. The trade name for this test is the *Borrelia burgdorferi* C6 Peptide Antibody DetectR.
2. See also Lyme disease antibody—Blood.

Botulism, Diagnostic Procedures—Stool

Norm. Negative culture.

Usage. To diagnose the presence of *Clostridium botulinum* or *Clostridium baratii* in the culture of feces.

Description. The three main naturally occurring types of botulism are food-borne, intestinal, and wound botulism. Botulism food poisoning is a severe condition resulting from the ingestion of the bacterial endotoxins of *Clostridium botulinum* or *Clostridium baratii*. The exotoxin from *C. botulinum* exerts central nervous system actions and may lead quickly to death if an antidote is not administered before the onset of neurologic symptoms. Botulism most frequently occurs in home-canned food that has not been sufficiently heated during the canning process or in food left at room temperature for several days (such as foil-wrapped baked potatoes). It is often acquired in infants from ingestion of soil or honey.

Professional Considerations
Consent form NOT required.

Botulism Symptoms and Emergency Treatment
Symptoms. Afebrile, diarrhea, dizziness, double or blurred vision, dysarthria, dysphagia, fatigue, gastrointestinal pain,

headache, hypotonia, nausea, vomiting, weakness. Cardiac and respiratory paralysis is possible.

Treatment

NOTE: Treatment choice(s) depend(s) on client's history and condition and episode history.

1. Establish IV access.
2. Administer trivalent botulism antitoxin (Connaught Laboratories, Ltd, also known as Aventis Pasteur). (Note: Anaphylaxis is possible if the antitoxin is given to clients with asthma, hay fever, horse or horse serum allergies, or past exposure to horse serum.)
3. Follow package insert instructions for sensitivity testing before antitoxin administration.
4. Induce vomiting (with extreme caution) with syrup of ipecac, if the syrup can be given soon after the ingestion of the contaminated food. (Induction of emesis is contraindicated in clients with no gag reflex or with central nervous system depression or excitation.)
5. Use gastric lavage if emesis does not produce the contaminated food.
6. Give activated charcoal slurry.
7. Give saline cathartic solution if no ileus is present.
8. Monitor for respiratory decompensation, which may occur suddenly in clients with botulism. Elective intubation is advisable for large ingestions.
9. Notify the state health department and the Centers for Disease Control and Prevention (CDC) (770-488-7100).

Preparation

1. Obtain a sterile specimen container.

Procedure

1. Collect a stool specimen directly into a sterile, wide-mouthed, waxed container with a tight-fitting lid. Be sure there is no urine or paper in the specimen.

2. If a stool specimen is not readily available, a rectal swab may be substituted. Insert a sterile microbiologic swab into the rectum and leave in place for 10 seconds. Remove the swab and send it to the laboratory in a culture container.

Postprocedure Care

1. Properly seal the container to avoid leakage and contamination.
2. Refrigerate the specimen if it cannot be sent immediately to the laboratory.

Client and Family Teaching

1. Avoid contaminating the stool with urine or toilet paper.
2. Botulism may be prevented by cooking foods sufficiently to inactivate the toxins.
3. An antitoxin is available for botulism.
4. If activated charcoal was given for elevated levels, the client should drink 4-6 glasses of water each day for 2 days to prevent constipation. The activated charcoal will also cause stools to be black for a few days.
5. Results are normally available within 72 hours.

Factors That Affect Results

1. Specimens not refrigerated invalidate the results.

Other Data

1. In infant botulism, the organism and the toxin can be found in the bowel contents but not in serum. The presence of the toxin can be demonstrated by injection of mice with 0.4 mL of the suspected food, the client's fecal extract, and the client's serum. The presence of toxin results in flaccid paralysis within 24 hours and death within 3 days.
2. The treatment for botulism is to give an antitoxin. However, the antitoxin inactivates only unbound toxins.
3. See also Clostridial toxin—Serum.

Brain Biopsy—Diagnostic

Norm. Normal tissue.

Usage. Confirmation of Alzheimer's disease, cerebral amyloid angiopathy, cerebral blastomycosis, cerebral Whipple's disease, Creutzfeldt-Jakob disease, encephalitis, granulomatous angiitis, HIV complications,

identification and classification of tumors of the brain or metastasis to the brain, neuronal ceroid lipofuscinosis.

Description. Specimens of brain tissue are obtained during a craniotomy and sent to the pathology laboratory. The electron microscope is used to identify and classify tumors for more accurate diagnosis, on which proper therapy and prognosis depend. The pathologist may also examine the specimen for antigen localization, which identifies the cell of origin of the antigen. This identifies the origin of metastatic carcinoma.

Professional Considerations
Consent form IS required for the procedure used to obtain the biopsy sample.

Risks
Blindness, cerebrovascular accident, headache, hemorrhage (silent after stereotactic brain biopsy), infection, meningitis, paralysis.
Contraindications
Anticoagulant therapy, bleeding disorders, increased intracranial pressure.

Preparation
1. Obtain a specimen container.
2. Arrange for immediate handling of the specimen in the pathology department.
3. Just before beginning the procedure, take a "time out" to verify the correct client, procedure, and site.

Procedure
1. A fresh specimen of brain tissue is placed into a plastic container with saline-moistened, sterile gauze and given to the pathologist, who is in the operating room or waiting in the laboratory for the immediate delivery of the specimen.
2. If immediate preparation of the specimen by the pathologist is not possible, the specimen is immediately cut into 1-mm cubes and placed into a vial of 2%-4% phosphate, cacodylate-buffered glutaraldehyde, paraformaldehyde, or other fixative, according to the policy of the institution.

Postprocedure Care
1. Tailor care to the procedure used to gain access to the brain tissue.

Client and Family Teaching
1. Results are normally available within 24 hours.

Factors That Affect Results
1. The specimen must be fresh.
2. Placing the specimen in formalin or in the wrong fixative or taking more than 2-3 minutes to place it in the fixative after collection invalidates the results.
3. If antigen localization is done, the antisera must be available.

Other Data
1. Brain scans are usually performed before surgery to assist in specific localization of the tumor for biopsy.

Brain Echogram

See **Brain Ultrasonography**—Diagnostic.

Brain Natriuretic Peptide

See **Natriuretic Peptides**—Plasma.

Brain Scan, Cerebral Flow and Pathology—Diagnostic

Norm. Negative.

Usage. Abscess of the brain, brain ischemia, brain tumors, contusions, cerebral vascular accidents, hematomas, and causes of seizures. Posttraumatic stress disorder.

Description. A nuclear medicine scan of the brain after the intravenous injection of a radioactive isotope. An immediate scan after the injection will show changes in the cerebral blood flow from one side of the brain compared to the other side. A later scan will show pathogenic tissue, which has a greater concentration of the isotope present than does normal tissue. This method of brain scanning has largely been replaced by newer, faster, and better quality SPECT scanning.

Professional Considerations
Consent form IS required.

Risks
Infection.

Contraindications
Pregnancy and in clients who cannot lie still for an extended length of time.

Preparation
1. Potassium chloride capsules are given 2 hours before the isotope injection to prevent an inordinate amount of isotope uptake in the choroid plexus. Too much uptake in the choroid plexus would simulate a pathologic condition in the cerebrum.
2. Just before beginning the procedure, take a "time out" to verify the correct client, procedure, and site.

Procedure
1. The client is placed in a supine position on the scanning table with the isotope scanner in position over the head.
2. The radioactive isotope is injected into a vein in the arm, and the scan is started immediately for the study of cervical flow.

3. The scan is repeated 1 hour later to detect the presence of pathogenic tissue.

Postprocedure Care
1. Encourage the oral intake of fluids.

Client and Family Teaching
1. Most of the radioactive material will be excreted from the body through urine and stool within 48 hours and is not harmful to other persons nearby.
2. Venous access will be necessary.
3. Results are normally available within 24 hours.

Factors That Affect Results
1. None found.

Other Data
1. Health care professionals working in a nuclear medicine area must follow federal standards set by the Nuclear Regulatory Commission. These standards include precautions for handling the radioactive material and monitoring of potential radiation exposure.
2. See also Single-photon emission computed tomography (SPECT scan), Brain—Diagnostic.

Brain Ultrasonography (Brain Echogram, Brain Ultrasound, Echoencephalogram)—Diagnostic

Norm. Normal position of the brain's midline structures and normal blood-flow velocity.

Usage. Diagnosis of brain deformities in newborns and infants, Leigh disease, space-occupying lesions, and structural shifts caused by cerebral edema, subdural hematoma, or extradural hematoma. Determination of viability of brain tissue based on the sequential measurement of blood flow velocity. Brain ultrasonograms can also be used for early detection of cerebral ischemia during a carotid endarterectomy while cerebral blood flow is interrupted. Ventriculomegaly.

Description. An ultrasound beam is transmitted through the skull. The time required for the beam to be reflected back to the transducer is converted to an electrical impulse displayed on an oscilloscope screen and measured to determine the structure, position, and blood flow of the brain. A shift in the third ventricle of more than 3 mm from midline is abnormal. An enlargement of the third ventricle of more than 10 mm in the adult or more than 7 mm in the child is abnormal.

Professional Considerations
Consent form NOT required.

Preparation
1. Remove jewelry and metal objects from the client's head and neck.
2. Obtain ultrasonic gel or paste.

Procedure
1. The client is placed in a supine position.
2. A small transducer, with water-soluble paste applied to it, is placed on the side of the head over the temporoparietal region.
3. Ultrasonic beams are sent into the head, and their reflection is recorded on the oscilloscope and photographed.

Postprocedure Care
1. Cleanse the paste from the scalp.

Client and Family Teaching

1. Do not drink hot or cold caffeine-containing beverages on the morning of the test.
2. It is normal to hear an echo that sounds like repetitious humming or a musical note as the brain structures reflect the ultrasonic beam.
3. This procedure takes approximately 1 hour.
4. Results are normally available within 24 hours.

Factors That Affect Results

1. Failure to remove jewelry and metal objects from the head and neck will interfere with the clarity of the oscilloscope pictures.

Other Data

1. Follow-up studies using a computed tomographic scan or radionucleotides may be indicated.
2. An enlarged fourth ventricle is a physiologic variant in early fetal life of 14-16 weeks.

Brain Ultrasound

See Brain Ultrasonography—Diagnostic.

Brainstem Auditory-Evoked Potential (BAEP)—Diagnostic

Norm. Morphologically normal waveform activity generated by electrical response to auditory stimulation.

Usage. Employed as an adjunct in the diagnosis of neurologic hearing deficits or children with language impairments; in the diagnosis and treatment of migraines, acoustic neuromas, chronic renal failure, and tuberculous meningitis; and in the determination of brain death versus reversible coma.

Adults. May be prescribed to test the time required for nerve signals to travel from the ear to the brainstem.

Description. A series of rapid clicks is delivered through earphones applied to the client. The brainstem response (electrical potential activity) is recorded through electrodes applied to the client's head. This recording (a series of waveform activities) is then interpreted by a physician skilled in electroencephalography.

Professional Considerations

Consent form NOT required.

Preparation

1. The test is generally performed in a neurology clinic or neurology diagnostic area even though portable test equipment is available and the test can be performed at the bedside.
2. No pretest medication or preparation is required. The rationale behind the test should be explained to the client or family before the procedure.

Procedure

1. An electrode is placed on the scalp at the vertex, and a reference electrode is placed on the earlobe.
2. Headphones, which mask the auditory responses of the outer ear, are applied.
3. Auditory stimulation occurs, and the brainstem response is recorded as waveform activity.

Postprocedure Care

1. Electrodes and headset are removed. The client may require transport from the test area back to the nursing unit.
2. The test results are interpreted by the appropriate physician.
3. No other special postprocedure care is required.

Client and Family Teaching

1. Occasionally this test is used to determine brain death or the possible reversibility of coma. In this situation, close contact with the family by all members of the health care delivery team and the provision of emotional and educational support are essential.

2. Parental teaching is important when the test is used to determine the presence of neural hearing loss in infants and children.

Factors That Affect Results
1. Experience of the physician interpreting the results.

2. Proper function of the acoustic and recording equipment.

Other Data
1. A variation of this technique has been developed in which direct application of the recording electrodes to the brainstem is accomplished during neurosurgery to direct certain neurosurgical procedures.

Brazelton Neonatal Behavioral Assessment Scale—Diagnostic

Norm. Normal reflexes and responses to stimulation in the newborn. Girls show higher levels of functioning when compared to boys in newborn infants of optimal health.

Usage. Evaluation of the newborn-caretaker unit to assess infant's behavior and responses to the environment and to provide recommendations for caregiving and interactions. This test has been primarily used in the research arena, although it has been applied clinically to assess neurobehavioral functioning in full-term infants who were exposed to cocaine and to assess tactile-kinesthetic stimulation in preterm infants.

Description. The newborn is administered the Neonatal Behavioral Assessment Scale (NBAS) multiple times in the first 10 days of life to study four levels of function of the neonate: physiologic, motor, state, and attentional/ interactional. Function is determined by assessment of the response to 28 behavioral items with 7 supplementary items, all scored on a 9-point scale, and 18 reflex items, scored on a 4-point scale. The hypothesis is that a newborn's behavior is dependent on not only genetics but also intrauterine nutrition, infection, drug abuse, and perinatal events. All these factors contribute to a child's temperament and may explain why different babies respond to touch, sound, or visual stimuli in different ways. Once the child has been assessed, Brazelton believes that recommendations can be made how best to interact with that child by describing the behavioral strengths and weaknesses.

Professional Considerations
Consent form NOT required.

Preparation
1. If the scale is to be used for research, training is required. Training takes up to several months, with renewal certification every 3 years. This is necessary for reliability of the test.
2. Obtain a manual, training handbook, examination video, and testing kit, which are available from the Brazelton Institute, 1295 Boylston St., Suite 320, Boston, MA 02215 (857) 355-4959.
3. Obtain needed equipment: light, rattle, and bell.
4. Provide a quiet environment and dim lighting.

Procedure
1. Using the scoring manual, the baby and caregiver are evaluated, and a score is given.

Postprocedure Care
1. None.

Client and Family Teaching
1. The test is more accurate if a caretaker is available to interact with the neonate during the test.
2. The test takes about 30 minutes to perform.
3. Repetition improves the reliability of the test.

Factors That Affect Results
1. The tester must be appropriately trained.
2. If the neonate is crying, hungry, or sleepy, assessment may not be accurate.

Other Data
1. None.

BRCA Tumor Suppressor Genes 1 and 2—Blood

Norm. Negative.

Usage. BRCA testing is completed to determine a client's genetic risk for breast or ovarian cancer.

Positive. Presence of *BRCA1* or *BRCA2* gene mutation(s).

Negative. Absence of *BRCA1* or *BRCA2* gene mutation(s).

Description. *BRCA1* and *BRCA2* are inherited breast cancer tumor suppressor genes that can be recognized on the human genome. *BRCA1* and *BRCA2* help stabilize cells to prevent overgrowth. They are found on chromosomes 17 and 13, respectively. Inherited mutations of these genes have been found to be associated with an 82% increased risk of familial breast cancer and a 44% increased risk of ovarian cancer occurrences in women and an increased risk of breast cancer in men. In addition, individuals experiencing breast cancer, who have these gene mutations have up to a 4.5-fold increased risk of developing cancer in the contralateral breast. Carriers of *BRCA1* mutations have an increased risk of ovarian cancer (epithelial or transitional cell) and microglandular adenosis, and carriers of *BRCA2* are at increased risk for Fanconi anemia, pancreatic cancer, and prostate cancer. Manual direct sequencing or automated fluorescent sequencing of DNA can detect mutations of these genes.

Professional Considerations

Informed consent is recommended for genetic testing.

Preparation

1. Tube: Lavender topped.

Procedure

1. Draw a 10-mL blood sample.
2. Send sample immediately to the laboratory.

Postprocedure Care

1. None.

Client and Family Teaching

1. Refer to section in this book on "Informed Consent for Genetic Testing". Genetic counseling is to be completed before and after testing.
2. A complete family history, including first- and second-degree relatives, should be taken before the test.
3. Test results will be available in 1 to 4 weeks. Testing for Ashkenazi mutation takes less time than *BRCA1* and *BRCA2* sequencing.
4. Affected relative(s) should be tested first to determine whether the mutation exists.
5. Clients should be informed of any test limitations, possibilities for discovery of unrelated DNA findings including nonpaternity, treatment options, cost, and other emotional, legal, or insurance consequences of testing.
6. Clients whose families have had multiple members with breast cancer, or both breast and ovarian cancer, or members with primary cancers from more than one site, or those who have Jewish ancestors from Eastern or Central Europe (Ashkenazi) should be provided with education for prevention and early detection of breast or ovarian cancer regardless of their decision to undergo genetic testing for *BRCA1* and *BRCA2* gene mutation.

Factors That Affect Results

1. Clients receiving chemotherapy or radiation treatment should not be concurrently tested for *BRCA1* or *BRCA2*. (Chemotherapy and radiation may alter DNA transcription.) The recommended waiting period for testing is 3-4 weeks after discontinuation of these treatment modalities or immediately before the next chemotherapy or radiation treatment course.
2. In clients with a history of blood transfusion, a waiting period of 3 months after transfusion is suggested before testing.

Other Data

1. Screening cost for *BRCA1* and *BRCA2* mutations is $2100 to $2600.
2. Smoking does not appear to be a risk factor for breast cancer among carriers of the BRCA mutation.
3. The cost of this test ranges from $300 to $3000, depending on how much of the gene is sequenced.
4. The Genetic Information Nondiscrimination Act of 2008 prohibits health plans

from using genetic family history or genetic test results from influencing eligibility or premiums for health insurance. It also prohibits employers from using this information to influence decisions about hiring, terminating employment, or employment pay, promotions or privileges.

Breast Ultrasonography (Breast Echogram, Breast Ultrasound)—Diagnostic

Norm. Normal breast tissue boundaries demonstrate bright echo reflections. The nipple and skin reflections are higher than the areola echo reflection. Fat demonstrates low reflectivity, with a mixture of low and strong echoes, whereas connective tissue and ligaments are bright. Tumors and cysts are absent. The breasts of young women have less fatty tissue than the breasts of older women.

Usage. Detection of tiny breast tumors, differentiation of breast cysts from breast tumors less than $\frac{1}{4}$ inch in diameter; screening for breast abnormalities in low-risk clients or where mammography is not readily available; helpful for clients with radiographically dense breasts or breast prostheses or with extensive nodal involvement; and evaluation of symptomatic clients with breast inflammation or who are pregnant or lactating.

Description. A noninvasive test, with a sensitivity of 98.3% and specificity of 91.7%, in which a picture of breast tissue is produced on a screen by the beaming of high-frequency sound waves into the breast and the computer processing of the signals received back through a transducer. The time required for the ultrasonic beam to be reflected back to the transducer from differing densities of tissue is converted by a computer to an electrical impulse displayed on an oscilloscopic screen to create a three-dimensional picture of the breast. An advantage of this test is that it can display all breast tissue, whereas radiography cannot. In clients with fibrocystic breast disease, the water-path method of ultrasonography may be used.

Professional Considerations
Consent form NOT required.

Preparation
1. Obtain ultrasonic gel or paste.

Procedure
1. The client is positioned supine and obliquely and rolled 35 degrees toward the side of the breast that will be examined. A sponge, blanket roll, or folded towel may be used to support the shoulders and hips. The client's arm on the same side to be examined should be placed behind the head.
2. A greasy, conductive paste is applied to the 5.0- or 7.5-MHz, small-diameter, high-frequency transducer.
3. The transducer is passed methodically over all the skin of the breast. Any known breast mass is identified, and the surrounding area in a 3-cm square is marked on the breast. The breast and marked area are scanned transversely from the inferior margin toward the head in small intervals, followed by sagittal scans moving medially to laterally. Scanning is performed with light pressure.
4. Photographs are taken of the oscilloscopic display.
5. Dedicated water-path breast instrumentation:
   a. The client is positioned either prone on a special bed, with the breast suspended over and into water, or supine with a bag of water overlying the breast.
   b. Scanning is performed in 1- to 2-mm intervals through the water path with a transducer. Any lesions are identified in two axes.

Postprocedure Care
1. Cleanse the skin of the ultrasonic paste.

Client and Family Teaching
1. Wear a two-piece outfit to facilitate breast exposure for exam (if the test is performed on an outpatient basis).
2. Some facilities request that no deodorants, powders, or perfumes be worn the day of the test.
3. The procedure will take approximately 30 minutes.

4. A breast ultrasonogram may improve the accuracy of the diagnosis when used as an adjunct to mammography.
5. Results are normally available in 1-2 days.

Factors That Affect Results
1. Compression of the breast may be used to eliminate nipple shadows, enable the use of high-frequency transducers, and improve delineation of the tissue.

However, compression causes a misrepresentation of the breast anatomy.

Other Data
1. Negative ultrasonographic results should not be used to conclude a lesion is benign.
2. Ultrasonography of the breast should not be used as a screening method for breast cancer because of its high rates of false-positive and false-negative outcomes.

Breath Hydrogen Analysis—Diagnostic

Norm. <20 ppm elevation over fasting level.

Usage. Assessment of orocecal transit time; determination of bronchiectasis, irritable bowel syndrome, lactose intolerance, hypolactasia; screening for early diagnosis of necrotizing enterocolitis; and evaluation of peptic ulcer disease before and during treatment with ranitidine.

Description. This test measures the hydrogen exhaled at specific intervals during the first 3 hours after ingestion of the carbohydrate (such as lactose, lactulose, fructose, or sucrose) being studied. In the normal client, hydrogen is produced exclusively by the bacterial metabolism of carbohydrates. Clients who are unable to digest or absorb carbohydrates in the small intestine have an increased volume of carbohydrates reaching the colon. These carbohydrates are metabolized in the colon, producing hydrogen, which is absorbed in the colon and exhaled by the lungs. The hydrogen breath test detects higher than normal levels and abnormal timing of peak releases of exhaled hydrogen. Ranitidine inhibits the action of histamine on the H_2-receptors of the parietal cells of the stomach, thus reducing hydrochloric acid production. The breath test can be used to evaluate hydrogen release after administration of the ranitidine.

Professional Considerations
Consent form NOT required.

Preparation
1. See Client and Family Teaching.
2. Obtain a syringe or balloon.

Procedure
1. After measurement of a basal breath hydrogen level, an oral dose of lactose, 1 g/kg of body weight, is given.

2. End-alveolar air is expired into a 30-mL glass syringe or a special plastic balloon.
3. The breath sample is injected into an analyzer to determine H_2 and CO_2 concentrations.
4. A rise of 720 ppm in exhaled hydrogen is diagnostic for lactose malabsorption.
5. Clients with bacterial overgrowth of the small intestine will have an increased production of hydrogen, with an early peak (within 3 hours) of hydrogen release after carbohydrate ingestion.
6. Clients with disease of the small intestine and carbohydrate malabsorption have a later peak of hydrogen release.

Postprocedure Care
1. Resume normal diet.

Client and Family Teaching
1. Fast after midnight the day of the test. A carbohydrate-controlled diet the day before the test affects the fasting breath hydrogen levels and may improve the test accuracy.
2. Do not use laxatives or enemas for 3 days before being tested.
3. Do not smoke for at least 15 minutes before being tested.

Factors That Affect Results
1. Diarrhea within 3 days before the test invalidates the results.
2. Storage of the samples allows for leakage of the gases. A glass syringe stored on its side with the barrel lubricated with mineral oil will have negligible leakage over a 2-week period. Upright storage may result in leakage of mineral oil and loss of the barrel seal.
3. High-fiber diet increases results.

Other Data
1. Hydrogen content increases as carbohydrate malabsorption increases.

Breath Test (Carbon-13 or Carbon-14 Urea Breath Test)

See Urea Breath Test—Diagnostic.

Bromides—Serum

Norm. Negative.

		SI Units
Reference range	0-11.7 mg/dL	0-1.46 mmol/L
Panic levels	>120 mg/dL	
Bromide ion	>150 mg/dL	
Sodium bromide	>15 mEq/L	>15 mmol/L

Panic Level Symptoms and Treatment

Symptoms. Abdominal pain, ataxia, central nervous system depression (coma), cyanosis, eye irritation (if inhaled), gastrointestinal tract corrosion (if swallowed), increased cerebrospinal fluid pressure, mental disturbance (confusion, hallucinations, irritability, mania), rash, tachycardia, respiratory irritation (if inhaled), shock, vertigo, vomiting.

Treatment

NOTE: Treatment choice(s) depend(s) on client's history and condition and episode history.

For bromide poisoning caused by inhalation:

1. Give oxygen.
2. Maintain patent airway and support breathing.
3. Monitor for and treat pulmonary edema.
   For bromide poisoning from ingestion:
1. Induce vomiting with syrup of ipecac. (Induction of vomiting is contraindicated in clients with no gag reflex or with central nervous system depression or excitation.)
2. Perform gastric lavage.
   General intervention:
1. Administer 1 g of NaCl in water orally every hour until serum bromide level is less than 50 mg/dL.
2. Monitor for and treat shock symptoms.
3. Monitor liver and kidney function.
4. Hydrate and provide mild diuresis.
5. Both hemodialysis and peritoneal dialysis WILL remove bromides.

Usage. Screening for bromide toxicity.

Increased. Exposure to vapors in photography and chemical industries, exposure to bromides in pesticides, and ingestion of over-the-counter medications such as Bromo-Seltzer or nonsteroidal antiinflammatory drugs (NSAIDs).

Description. The element bromine is a reddish brown, nonvolatile liquid that gives off suffocating vapors that are highly toxic and severely irritating to the skin. Bromine replaces chlorine in the body tissues, resulting in sedation and depression of the central nervous system. For this reason, it was used in the past as a medication to sedate clients until more effective, less toxic medications became available.

Professional Considerations

Consent form NOT required.

Preparation

1. Tube: Red topped, red/gray topped, gold topped, or green topped.
2. Do NOT draw during hemodialysis.

Procedure

1. Draw a 5-mL blood sample.

Postprocedure Care

1. Monitor closely for signs of bromide toxicity.

Client and Family Teaching

1. Bromide poisoning rarely causes death.

Factors That Affect Results

1. Falsely elevated levels may occur in clients receiving iodine therapy.
2. Age over 45 years and female sex indicate high normal levels.

Other Data

1. Alcoholics are especially susceptible to bromide intoxication.

Bronchial Aspirate, Fungus—Culture

Norm. Negative. No growth.

Usage. Diagnosis of the presence and type of potentially pathogenic fungi in the bronchi.

Positive. *Aspergillus fumigatus, Aspergillus flavus, Blastomyces dermatitides, Candida albicans, Candida tropicalis, Coccidioides immitis, Cryptococcus neoformans, Histoplasma capsulatum,* and *Sporothrix schenckii.*

Description. Fungi are slow-growing, eukaryotic organisms that can grow on living and nonliving organic materials and are subdivided into yeasts and molds. Normal human host defense mechanisms limit the damage they cause superficially. Some fungi can be inhaled or introduced by traumatic inoculation into deep tissue spaces and cause serious infections. Although tentative identification of fungi can be made quickly with staining techniques, culture of the organism on special fungal culture media is required to confirm a diagnosis of a fungal infection.

Professional Considerations

Consent form is NOT required unless a bronchoscopy is used to obtain the specimen.

Preparation

1. Obtain a sterile container or suction trap, suction tubing, sterile suction catheter, and gloves.
2. Prepare a suction machine or a wall suction.
3. See Bronchoscopy—Diagnostic (Preparation) if this method is used.

Procedure

1. A specimen trap is inserted into the suctioning line of a flexible, fiberoptic bronchoscope or between the suctioning catheter and a regular suctioning line. When the bronchoscope is in place or the suction catheter is completely inserted into a bronchus, suction is applied, and a specimen is obtained while the suction trap is held upright.
2. Specimens obtained by expectoration should be collected early in the morning after the client has removed any dentures and gargled and rinsed the mouth with water. A deep cough is required to deliver a good specimen, and the specimen should be expectorated directly into a sterile cup.

Postprocedure Care

1. Write the collection time on the laboratory requisition.
2. Write any current antibiotic or antifungal therapy on the laboratory requisition.
3. Transport the specimen to the laboratory immediately.
4. See Bronchoscopy—Diagnostic if this method is used.

Client and Family Teaching

1. See Bronchoscopy—Diagnostic if this method is used.
2. To produce a specimen by coughing, take several breaths in without fully exhaling in between. When you feel you cannot breathe any more air in, cough out forcefully and catch the sputum in a specimen cup.
3. 4-6 weeks are required for a final fungal culture report.

Factors That Affect Results

1. The specimen should be obtained with the first suctioning.
2. A break in the sterile technique invalidates the results.
3. The best results are obtained if the cultures are inoculated immediately. The maximum time allowed between specimen collection and inoculation is 3 hours.

Other Data

1. None.

Bronchial Aspirate, Routine—Culture

Norm. No growth or growth of only normal upper respiratory tract flora.

Usage. Diagnosis of infections of the tracheobronchial tree.

Description. Sputum obtained by bronchoscopy, routine tracheal suctioning, or coughing is cultured and Gram-stained. Suctioned samples may be obtained nasotracheally, endotracheally, or through a tracheostomy.

B

Professional Considerations
Consent form NOT required.

Preparation
1. Obtain a sterile container or suction trap, suction tubing, a sterile suction catheter, and gloves.
2. Prepare the suction machine or wall suction.
3. See Bronchoscopy—Diagnostic (Preparation) if this method is used.

Procedure
1. A specimen trap is inserted into the suctioning line of a flexible, fiberoptic bronchoscope or between the suctioning catheter and a regular suctioning line. When the bronchoscope is in place or the suction catheter is completely inserted into the bronchi, suction is applied, and a specimen is obtained while the suction trap is held upright.
2. Specimens obtained by expectoration should be collected early in the morning after the client has removed any dentures and gargled and rinsed the mouth with water. A deep cough is required to deliver a good specimen, and the specimen should be expectorated directly into a sterile cup.

Postprocedure Care
1. Write the collection time on the laboratory requisition.
2. Write any current antibiotic or antifungal therapy for the client on the laboratory requisition.
3. See Bronchoscopy—Diagnostic if this method is used.

Client and Family Teaching
1. To produce a specimen by coughing, take several breaths in, without fully exhaling in between. When you feel you cannot breathe any more air in, cough out forcefully and catch sputum into a specimen cup.
2. See Bronchoscopy—Diagnostic if this method is used.
3. Cultures with no growth can be reported in 48 hours. Results take up to 10 days.

Factors That Affect Results
1. The specimen should be obtained with the first suctioning.
2. Reject specimens more than 4 hours old.

Other Data
1. Pulmonary nocardiosis is best treated with a combination of imipenem and amikacin.

Bronchial Challenge Test
See Methacholine Challenge Test—Diagnostic.

Bronchial Washing (Bronchoalveolar Lavage)—Specimen

Norm. Negative for culture and cytologic testing.

Usage. Diagnosis of infections, for example, *Mycobacterium szulgai* and *Bipolaris hawaiiensis*, and pathologic processes in the lungs.

Description. Procedure useful to obtain respiratory tract specimens for culture and cytologic testing when very few secretions are present. Specimens are obtained from a normal saline wash, which is instilled into the bronchi and then suctioned out. Saline may be instilled through a bronchoscope, an endotracheal tube, or a tracheal tube. A bronchoalveolar wash will provide a specimen from the alveoli and is done by insertion of the flexible fiberoptic bronchoscope as far into the bronchiole as possible and instillation of the saline at that point. This procedure is used when adequate deep sputum specimens cannot be obtained and is often helpful in the diagnosis of *Pneumocystis* pneumonia.

Professional Considerations
Consent form is NOT required unless the washing is done by bronchoscopy. See Bronchoscopy—Diagnostic for risks and contraindications if bronchoscopy is used to obtain the specimen.

Preparation
1. Obtain a specimen trap, suction tubing, a sterile suction catheter, and sterile gloves.

2. Prepare a wall suction or a suction machine.
3. If the washing is performed during bronchoscopy, obtain sterile specimen containers for the bronchoscope.
4. See Bronchoscopy—Diagnostic, if this procedure is used.

Procedure

1. A specimen trap is inserted into the suctioning line from the bronchoscope, or between the suctioning catheter and the suctioning line.
2. Up to 20 mL of normal saline is instilled into the respiratory tract through the bronchoscope, the endotracheal tube, or the tracheal tube, and the specimen is obtained when suction is applied to the bronchoscope catheter or suction catheter.

Postprocedure Care

1. Write the time of specimen collection and any current antibiotic or antifungal therapy on the laboratory requisition.
2. See Bronchoscopy—Diagnostic if this procedure is used.

Client and Family Teaching

1. See Bronchoscopy—Diagnostic if this procedure is used.
2. Results are normally available within 1-2 days.

Factors That Affect Results

1. Bronchial washing specimens must be collected using a sterile technique.

Other Data

1. May be used to diagnose *Pneumocystis carinii* in clients with AIDS.
2. High number of neutrophils found in bronchial washing fluid of COPD clients.

Bronchoalveolar Lavage

See Bronchial Washing—Specimen.

Bronchoscopy—Diagnostic

Norm. Normal larynx, trachea, and bronchi.

Usage. Used to examine the bronchi for abscesses, aspiration pneumonia, hemoptysis, unresolved pneumonias, strictures, and tumors; for removal of foreign objects; and to obtain deep sputum specimens and tissue biopsy specimens.

Description. Direct visual examination of the larynx, trachea, and bronchi with a rigid bronchoscope or a flexible fiberoptic bronchoscope.

Professional Considerations

Consent form IS required.

Risks

Bleeding, bronchospasm, cardiopulmonary arrest, dysrhythmias, hypotension, hypoxia, pneumothorax.

Contraindications

Pregnancy; clients with severe shortness of breath who cannot tolerate interruption of high-flow oxygen. Such clients may be intubated for the procedure to ensure optimal oxygenation. Sedatives are contraindicated in clients with central nervous system depression.

Preparation

1. Obtain vital signs, activated partial thromboplastin time, platelet count, and prothrombin time.
2. Remove any dentures or eyeglasses.
3. Sedation may be prescribed. Sedation includes benzodiazepines in 63% of cases, opioid in 14%, and both in 12% of cases (Smyth & Stead, 2002).
4. Prepare suctioning equipment.
5. Have emergency resuscitation equipment readily available.
6. Just before beginning the procedure, take a "time out" to verify the correct client, procedure, and site.

Procedure

1. The nasopharynx and oropharynx are anesthetized with a local anesthetic.
2. The client is placed in a sitting or supine position.

3. After the tube is passed through the mouth or nose into the larynx, more local anesthetic is sprayed into the trachea to inhibit the cough reflex.
4. If the client has a large endotracheal tube in place, the flexible bronchoscope can be inserted through it.
5. The trachea and bronchi are visually examined for abnormal color, structure, or lesions.
6. Mucus is then suctioned until clear, bronchial washings are performed and the specimens are collected, and biopsy specimens are obtained if the flexible tube is used.
7. The rigid bronchoscope is used to retrieve foreign bodies and excise lesions.
8. The client is observed for impaired respirations or laryngospasms throughout the procedure.

Postprocedure Care

1. No food or fluids are given until the gag reflex has returned, about 2 hours after the procedure.
2. The client should not attempt to swallow saliva until the gag reflex has returned. Saliva should be expectorated into an emesis basin. Observe the client's sputum for blood if a biopsy was performed. If a tumor is suspected, collect post bronchoscopy sputum specimens for cytologic examination.
3. Observe postanesthesia precautions if a sedative was given. If deep sedation was used, follow institutional protocol for post sedation monitoring. Typical monitoring includes continuous ECG monitoring and pulse oximetry, with continual

assessments (every 5-15 minutes) of airway, vital signs, and neurologic status until the client is lying quietly awake, is breathing independently, and responds appropriately to commands spoken in a normal tone.
4. Observe closely for postprocedure complications, including bronchospasm, bacteremia, bronchial perforation (indicated by facial or neck crepitus), cardiac dysrhythmias, fever, hemorrhage from the biopsy site, hypoxemia, laryngospasm, pneumonia, and pneumothorax.

Client and Family Teaching

1. Fast after midnight the day of the procedure. Your diet will be restarted a few hours after the procedure.
2. Arrange for transportation home after the procedure because you will not be permitted to drive for 24 hours after receiving sedation.
3. Notify the physician if you are experiencing fever or difficulty in breathing during the next 48-72 hours.
4. You can begin drinking or eating approximately 2 hours after the procedure.

Factors That Affect Results

1. The procedure should be stopped if the client becomes uncooperative or if impaired respiratory function is noted.

Other Data

1. Intermittent negative-pressure ventilation is safe during interventional rigid bronchoscopy.
2. Virtual bronchoscopy (use of computed tomography) has shown promise for assessing complications of lung transplantation.

Brucellosis Agglutinins—Blood

Norm. Negative or less than 1:80. Titers of 1:20 to 1:80 are normal in farmers with cattle, swine, goats, or sheep, or in endemic areas without clinical manifestations.

Positive. Brucellosis caused by *Brucella abortus, B. canis,* or *B. melitensis.* Titers ≥1:160 indicate past or present infection. A fourfold increase in the titer within 2 weeks indicates an acute infection.

Description. Brucellosis (Bang's disease, Malta fever, Mediterranean fever, undulant fever) is a systemic disease acquired from animals that lasts days to years. It is found with greatest frequency in Europe, North Africa, Asia, Mexico, and South America. *Brucella* is an obligate parasite on animals. The mode of transmission to humans is through direct body tissue contact with fluids, milk, and dairy products of infected animals or by transmission to infants by breast-feeding. Onset may be acute or insidious, and symptoms may include arthralgia, body aches, chills, diaphoresis, depression, fever(s), headache, weakness, pneumonitis, and nonpurulent meningitis. In this test, *Brucella* antigens are mixed with a client's serum and observed for an agglutination reaction. The sample is heated and observed for clumping and unclumping. A sample that clumps upon warming and unclumps upon cooling is considered a positive test. A positive reaction is followed by serial dilutions of serum and retesting. The results are expressed as the highest titer showing agglutination. Agglutination at a titer greater than 1:80 indicates the presence of antibodies generated by any of three closely related *Brucella* species and is used in the indirect diagnosis of human brucellosis.

Professional Considerations
Consent form NOT required.

Preparation
1. Tube: Red topped, red/gray topped, or gold topped. Cool the tube in the refrigerator or on ice before specimen collection.

Procedure
1. Draw a 5-mL venous blood sample.

Postprocedure Care
1. Send the specimen to the laboratory for immediate testing.

Client and Family Teaching
1. Serial testing is recommended for clients with positive titers. Titers usually begin rising 5-30 days after exposure and peak in 1-2 months.

Factors That Affect Results
1. Reject hemolyzed specimens.
2. Falsely elevated titers may occur in clients who have received *Brucella* skin testing.
3. Falsely elevated titers may occur from cross-reactions of the *Brucella* test antigens with agglutinins produced by clients who have tularemia, cholera, and *Proteus vulgaris* Ox-19 infections, and in clients recently vaccinated against cholera.
4. Falsely depressed titers may occur in immunosuppressed clients or clients receiving antibiotic therapy.

Other Data
1. Isolation of the organism is necessary to confirm the diagnosis.
2. Brucellosis is a reportable disease in most areas.
3. Serum calcium levels are >2.35 mmol/L in persons with brucellosis.
4. See also Febrile agglutinins—Serum.

Brushing Cytology—Specimen

Norm. Negative. Requires interpretation.

Positive. Allergic reaction, asbestosis, Barrett's esophagus, cryptosporidiosis, echinococcosis, Goodpasture's syndrome, infection (herpes virus, cytomegalovirus, measles virus, fungus), legionnaires' disease, neoplasm (primary or metastatic), paragonimiasis, pneumonia (lipoid, *Pneumocystis carinii*), pulmonary infection (anaerobic), and strongyloidiasis.

Description. A brushing is taken (usually by means of endoscopy, bronchoscopy, cystoscopy, or gastroscopy) from a particular body site, smeared onto a slide, stained, examined microscopically, and possibly cultured. The specimens may be examined for bacterial and tumor antigens. Possible sites may be the bronchus, colon, esophagus, stomach, oropharynx, small bowel, trachea, or urethra.

Professional Considerations
Consent form NOT required.

Preparation
1. Obtain a brush, a glass slide, and a fixative container.
2. Label the slide with the client's name.

Procedure
1. Obtain a brushing from a body site or a lesion.
2. Gently roll the brush over the slide and immediately fix in 95% ethyl alcohol (ethanol).
3. For bronchial brushings, omit the slide and transport the disposable brush immediately to the laboratory.

4. The specimens for the culture require a double-sheathed brush sealed with the sheath after specimen collection.

Postprocedure Care

1. Write on the laboratory requisition the date, the site brushed, and the client's diagnosis, age, and history pertinent to this test.
2. Transport the fixative container or brush to the laboratory.

Client and Family Teaching

1. The test is painless.
2. Results are normally available within 24 hours.

Factors That Affect Results

1. Do NOT allow the slide to dry before fixing in alcohol.

Other Data

1. May be used to diagnose *Pneumocystis carinii* in clients with AIDS.

BTA Test for Bladder Cancer—Diagnostic

Norm. Bladder tumor–associated antigen negative.

Usage. Used in the diagnosis of superficial transitional cell carcinoma of the urinary bladder. Has a 61% sensitivity, 74% specificity, 64% accuracy, 88% positive predictive value, and 38% negative predictive value for bladder carcinoma (Lokeshwar et al, 2002).

Positive. Presence of bladder tumor–associated antigen in urine sample.

Negative. Absence of bladder tumor–associated antigen in urine sample.

Description. BTA test is a noninvasive tumor-marker quantitative enzyme immunoassay. The tumor marker is an antigen named "human complement factor H–related protein" (hCFHrp). hCFHrp is not detectable in healthy epithelial cells but has been identified in bladder cancer cells. hCFHrp is similar to human complement factor (hCFH), which plays a role in the prevention of cell lysis through interruption of a complement pathway. hCFH causes lysis of foreign cells in a host by inhibiting the development of a membrane attack complex. Cancer cells are believed to be protected from lysis by hCFHrp, which also interrupts a complement pathway, thereby facilitating invasion to the host.

Professional Considerations

Consent form NOT required.

Preparation

1. Urine specimen suggested amount is 35 mL (minimum of 2 mL).

Procedure

1. Collect voided or catheterized urine sample in clean urine specimen container without additives. Urine specimens cannot be collected in foam or paper cups.
2. Transport to lab on ice.

Postprocedure Care

1. None.

Client and Family Teaching

1. Obtain complete medical history (including current medical state).
2. Use a dipstick urine to verify absence of hematuria before test.
3. Inform client that a positive bladder tumor antigen test will be confirmed by biopsy of bladder tissue.

Factors That Affect Results

1. False-positive tests occur in 9% of cases (Friedrich et al, 2002) including any condition that causes hCFHrp to be present in the bladder. These conditions are renal lithiasis, nephritis, renal neoplasm, urinary tract infections, cystitis, history or presence of urinary stents or nephrostomy tubes, genitourinary cancer, bowel interposition segment, and trauma to the urinary system. A false-negative test occurs in 2% of those tested and is associated with tumor recurrence.
2. Hematuria may yield false-positive tests, and therefore urine samples should first be tested for the presence of blood.
3. If blood is detected in urine sample, urine cytologic testing is suggested.

Other Data

1. None.

B

Buccal Smear for Sex Chromatin Evaluation

See Barr Body Analysis, Buccal Smear for Staining Sex Chromatin Mass—Diagnostic.

BUN

See Blood Urea Nitrogen/Creatinine Ratio—Blood; Urea Nitrogen—Plasma or Serum.

BUN/Creatinine Ratio

See Blood Urea Nitrogen/Creatinine Ratio—Blood.

C1q Immune Complex Detection—Serum

Norm. None detected.

Increased or Positive. Arthritis, glomerulonephritis (acute), hepatitis (serum), IgA nephropathy, infectious disease, inflammatory bowel disease, neoplasms, primary biliary cirrhosis, rheumatic disease, subacute bacterial endocarditis, systemic lupus erythematosus, thrombotic thrombocytopenic purpura, and vasculitis.

Description. *Complement* is a term describing 20 specific serum globulin proteins that, in combination with antigen-antibody complexes, cause lysis of erythrocytes sensitized to the antibody contained in the complex. The nine major complement components are labeled C1 to C9. C1q immune complex is a component of C1 complement that is bound into a circulating immune complex (CIC) when foreign antigens react with IgG or IgM antibodies in the body. It is very important because immune complex reactions involving the C1q component activate the classic pathway of the complement cascade. Many tests for circulating immune complexes are based on C1q-binding properties. Exacerbations of immune complex disease cause elevated CICs because the lymphoreticular system is unable to clear the immune complex effectively. This test is used in serial monitoring of the progress of immune complex disease that activates the classic pathway of the complement cascade.

Professional Considerations
Consent form NOT required.

Preparation
1. Tube: Red topped, red/gray topped, or gold topped.

Procedure
1. Draw a 3-mL venous blood sample.

Postprocedure Care
1. Send the specimen to the laboratory immediately because complement is very unstable.

Client and Family Teaching
1. Serial measurements are recommended.
2. Results are normally available within 24 hours.

Factors That Affect Results
1. The presence of serum cryoglobulins may cause false-positive results.
2. Recent heparin therapy may interfere with accurate results.
3. Reject hemolyzed specimens.

Other Data
1. False-negative results occur about 10% of the time; therefore a negative result does not rule out disease.
2. See also Complement components—Serum; Complement fixation—Serum; and Complement Total—Serum.

C3 Activator

See C3 Proactivator—Serum.

C3 Complement (Beta-1c Globulin)—Serum

Norm.

C3 Complement		SI Units
Adult	88-201 mg/dL	0.88-2.01 g/L
Child		
Cord blood	65-113 mg/dL	0.65-1.13 g/L
Birth-1 month	59-121 mg/dL	0.59-1.21 g/L
Between 1-2 months	55-129 mg/dL	0.55-1.29 g/L
Between 2-3 months	61-155 mg/dL	0.61-1.55 g/L
Between 3-4 months	67-136 mg/dL	0.67-1.36 g/L
Between 4-5 months	65-182 mg/dL	0.65-1.82 g/L
Between 5-6 months	67-174 mg/dL	0.67-1.74 g/L
Between 6-7 months	77-179 mg/dL	0.77-1.79 g/L
Between 7-9 months	78-173 mg/dL	0.78-1.73 g/L
Between 9-11 months	76-187 mg/dL	0.76-1.87 g/L
Between 1-2 years	87-181 mg/dL	0.87-1.81 g/L
Between 2-3 years	84-177 mg/dL	0.84-1.77 g/L
Between 3-5 years	80-178 mg/dL	0.80-1.78 g/L
Between 5-11 years	89-203 mg/dL	0.89-2.03 g/L
Between 12-18 years	88-201 mg/dL	0.88-2.01 g/L

Increased. Acute-phase plasma protein response such as infection, dermatomyositis, inflammation, keratoconus, malignancy with metastasis, necrotizing disorders, rheumatic fever, and rheumatoid arthritis.

Decreased. Anemia (pernicious, folic acid deficiency), anorexia nervosa, arthralgias, celiac disease, cirrhosis, congenital C3 deficiency, disseminated intravascular coagulation, glomerulonephritis (acute), membranoproliferative, poststreptococcal hepatitis (chronic active), hypocomplementeric nephritis, immune complex disease, infection (recurrent pyogenic), liver disease (chronic), malnutrition (protein), multiple myeloma, multiple sclerosis, renal transplant rejection, septicemia (gram negative), serum sickness, subacute bacterial endocarditis, systemic lupus erythematosus (active, with renal involvement), and uremia.

Description. *Complement* is a term describing 20 specific serum globulin proteins that, in combination with antigen-antibody complexes, cause lysis of erythrocytes sensitized to the antibody contained in the complex. The nine major complement components are labeled C1 to C9. C3 complement is one of the nine major components of total complement protein and is involved in both the classic and alternative pathways of the complement cascade that function in humoral immunologic responses. Activation of the complement cascade functions in phagocytic activity, destruction of foreign bacteria, and the inflammatory response. This test evaluates the integrity of the cascade and is increased during acute-phase responses and inflammatory processes. Serial C3 levels may reflect the progress of such conditions based on the return of values to normal levels.

Professional Considerations
Consent form NOT required.

Preparation
1. Tube: Red topped, red/gray topped, or gold topped.

Procedure
1. Draw a 4-mL venous blood sample.

Postprocedure Care
1. None.

Client and Family Teaching
1. Serial measurements are recommended.
2. Results are normally available within 24 hours.

Factors That Affect Results
1. Complement is heat sensitive and deteriorates rapidly. Send the specimen to the laboratory immediately.

2. Reject hemolyzed specimens or specimens received more than 1-2 hours after collection.
3. Freeze serum if not tested within 2 hours.

Other Data

1. See also C3 proactivator—Serum; Complement components—Serum; Complement fixation—Serum; Complement total—Serum.

C3 Proactivator (Alternate Pathway Factor B, C3 Activator)—Serum

Norm. 20-42 mg/dL, or 0.20-0.42 g/L (2.16-4.54 mmol/L, SI units).

Increased. Burns, childhood nephrotic syndrome, diffuse intravascular coagulation, inflammation, subacute bacterial endocarditis, bacteremia (with shock symptoms), paroxysmal nocturnal hemoglobinuria, rheumatoid arthritis, and sickle cell disease.

Decreased. Chronic liver disease, glomerulonephritis (acute), and systemic lupus erythematosus.

Description. Used in serial monitoring of the progress of immune complex diseases. A factor involved in the alternate pathway of the complement cascade, which is involved in the humoral immune response. Polysaccharides, bacterial endotoxins, or aggregated IgA or IgG immunoglobulins reacting with factor B produce an enzyme that activates the C3 component of complement and initiation of the alternative pathway of the complement cascade.

Professional Considerations
Consent form NOT required.

Preparation
1. Tube: Red topped, red/gray topped, or gold topped.

Procedure
1. Draw a 4-mL venous blood sample.
2. Allow the specimen to clot at room temperature for 30 minutes.
3. Refrigerate the specimen at 4 degrees C for 1 hour.
4. Remove the specimen from the refrigerator.

Postprocedure Care
1. Send the specimen to the laboratory after refrigerating, as described above.

Client and Family Teaching
1. Serial measurements are recommended.

Factors That Affect Results
1. Reject hemolyzed specimens or specimens received more than 2 hours after collection.
2. Freeze the serum if the test cannot be performed within 2 hours after collection.

Other Data
1. See also C3 complement—Serum; Complement components—Serum; Complement fixation—Serum; Complement total—Serum.

C4 Complement—Serum

Norm.

C4 Complement		SI Units
Adult	15-45 mg/dL	0.15-0.45 g/L
Child		
Cord blood		
Birth-1 month	8-30 mg/dL	0.08-0.3 g/L
Between 1 and 2 months	9-33 mg/dL	0.09-0.33 g/L
Between 2 and 3 months	9-37 mg/dL	0.09-0.37 g/L
Between 3 and 4 months	10-35 mg/dL	0.1-0.35 g/L
Between 4 and 5 months	10-49 mg/dL	0.1-0.49 g/L
Between 5 and 6 months	9-48 mg/dL	0.09-0.48 g/L
Between 6 and 7 months	12-55 mg/dL	0.12-0.55 g/L
Between 7 and 9 months	13-48 mg/dL	0.13-0.48 g/L

C4 Complement		SI Units
Between 9 and 11 months	16-51 mg/dL	0.16-0.51 g/L
Between 1 and 2 years	16-52 mg/dL	0.16-0.52 g/L
Between 2 and 5 years	12-47 mg/dL	0.12-0.47 g/L
Between 5 and 11 years	12-52 mg/dL	0.12-0.52 g/L
Between 12 and 18 years	10-40 mg/dL	0.10-0.40 g/L

Increased. Cancer, chronic urticaria, dermatomyositis, juvenile rheumatoid arthritis, keratoconus, and rheumatoid spondylitis.

Decreased. Chronic bronchitis, cigarette smoking, congenital C4 complement deficiency, cryoglobulinemia, glomerulonephritis, Henoch-Schönlein purpura, hepatitis (chronic active), hereditary angioedema, hypergammaglobulinemic state, immune complex disease, lupus nephritis, pesticide workers exposed to pyrethroids, renal transplant rejection, serum sickness, subacute bacterial endocarditis, systemic lupus erythematosus (active), and tubulointerstitial nephritis and uveitis (TINU syndrome).

Description. *Complement* is a term describing 20 specific serum globulin proteins that, in combination with antigen-antibody complexes, cause lysis of erythrocytes sensitized to the antibody contained in the complex. The nine major complement components are labeled C1 to C9. C4 complement is one of the nine components of total complement protein and is involved in only the classical pathway of the complement cascade that functions in humoral immunologic responses and is normally present in human colostrum. C4 complement deficiency is an inherited autosomal recessive trait and results in decreased resistance to infection. Activation of the complement cascade functions in phagocytic activity, destruction of foreign bacteria, and the inflammatory response. C3 and C4 levels are helpful in distinguishing the cause of glomerulonephritis, because C3 is decreased but C4 is usually normal when the cause is poststreptococcal.

Professional Considerations
Consent form NOT required.

Preparation
1. Tube: Red topped, red/gray topped, or gold topped.

Procedure
1. Draw a 3-mL blood sample.

Postprocedure Care
1. Allow the specimen to clot for 15-30 minutes at room temperature and then refrigerate.
2. Freeze the serum if not processed immediately.

Client and Family Teaching
1. Serial measurements are recommended.

Factors That Affect Results
1. Complement is heat sensitive and deteriorates rapidly. Send the specimen to the laboratory immediately.
2. Reject hemolyzed specimens or specimens received more than 1-2 hours after collection.

Other Data
1. See also C3 complement—Serum; Complement components—Serum; Complement fixation—Serum; Complement total—Serum.

C6 Peptide
See *Borrelia burgdorferi* C6 Peptide Antibody—Serum.

CA 15-3 (Carbohydrate Antigen 15-3, Cancer Antigen 15-3)—Serum

Norm. <31 U/mL.

Increased. Breast cancer (prebiopsy increases are associated with 14% 5-year survival rate), liver cancer, lung cancer, ovarian cancer, prostate cancer, pregnancy (higher in third trimester), during lactation, systemic lupus erythematosus, hepatitis, benign gynecologic tumors, chronic pelvic inflammatory disease, cirrhosis, tuberculosis, sarcoidosis.

Usage. Used to monitor response to treatment in breast cancer clients. A prognostic marker in node-negative breast cancer with risk of relapse increasing from 10 U/mL.

Decreased. Positive response to therapy.

Description. The MUC1 gene is a high-molecular-weight glycoprotein found in specific tissues throughout the body (see Mucin-like carcinoma-associated antigen—Blood). The MUC1 gene has many varieties of carbohydrate chains that are termed mucin-like antigens, and one of these is the carbohydrate antigen 15-3 (CA 15-3) that circulates in the bloodstream when cancer is present. Approximately 80% of clients with metastatic breast cancer have elevated CA 15-3 levels and 36% of cases show elevations in relapse. Approximately 50% of clients with ovarian carcinoma have increased values (95% specificity and 92% predictive value), although CA 15-3 is not routinely used to monitor ovarian cancer clients. CA 125 levels are used preferentially to monitor ovarian cancer clients. Clients with high concentrations of CA 15-3 have a significantly worse prognosis than clients with low CA 15-3 concentrations. Preoperative concentrations of CA 15-3 may have a role in the selection of clients for adjuvant treatment and may serve as independent prognostic indicators in breast cancer. Preoperative levels >40 U/mL correlate well with large tumor size, metastasis, and higher grade. Postoperative levels >86 U/mL are indicative of metastatic disease, but normal levels do not exclude metastasis. Transient elevations of CA 15-3 often occur in the first weeks of therapy and should not be confused with treatment failure. Although individual levels may not be useful in monitoring

disease status, trends are useful, and a change of 25%, whether a decrease or an increase, is good evidence for either response to therapy or recurrence, respectively. Because of its low detection rate in early disease and in micrometastatic disease, CA 15-3 is not a useful screening test and is also not likely to detect early recurrent disease. CA 15-3 levels are measured via monoclonal antibody immunoassay.

Professional Considerations
Consent form NOT required.

Preparation
1. Tube: Red topped or serum separator (red/gray or gold topped).

Procedure
1. Collect a 4-mL blood sample.
2. Refrigerate specimen.

Postprocedure Care
1. None.

Client and Family Teaching
1. CA 15-3 is not a useful screening test for early carcinoma, but it is the most widely used serum marker for breast cancer.
2. Results are normally available within 3 working days.

Factors That Affect Results
1. Persons with benign breast or ovarian disease may have elevated levels.
2. Results are invalid if the client has received radioisotopes within the past 30 days.

Other Data
1. Results >25 U/mL are found in women with metastatic breast carcinoma.
2. CA 15-3 when used with CA 125 can improve the management of women presenting with a pelvic mass.
3. According to a study of 120 breast cancer clients, the median survival of clients with increased CA 15-3 was less than 13 months.

CA 19-9 (Carbohydrate Antigen 19-9, GICA, Gastrointestinal Cancer Antigen)—Blood

Norm.

		SI Units
Norm	<37 AU/mL	<37 kU/L
Metastasis	>1000 AU/mL	>1000 kU/L

Usage. Used to monitor gastrointestinal, pancreatic, and colorectal malignancies. Concurrent measurement of CA 19-9 with carcinoembryonic antigen is useful when clients are being monitored for possible recurrence of gastric carcinoma.

Increased. Gastrointestinal, pancreatic, hepatobiliary, lung, testicular, and colorectal malignancies; acute pancreatitis; cholangitis; cirrhosis; echinococcus infection; hydronephrosis; and hypothyroidism.

Description. The *MUC1* gene is a high-molecular-weight glycoprotein found in specific tissues throughout the body (see Mucin-like carcinoma-associated antigen—Blood). The *MUC1* gene has many varieties of carbohydrate chains that are termed mucin-like antigens, and one of these is the carbohydrate antigen 19-9 (CA 19-9) that circulates in the bloodstream when cancer is present. CA 19-9 is a glycoprotein present on a wide variety of adenocarcinomas of the gastrointestinal and hepatobiliary systems. CA 19-9 is produced in excess by the adenocarcinomas and released into the blood, enabling measurement. CA 19-9 is considered the standard of comparison often used marker for pancreatic cancer, along with CT, to differentiate from benign pancreatic disease. A total of 70%-80% of pancreatic cancers, 60% of hepatobiliary cancers, and 50%-60% of gastric carcinomas have elevated CA 19-9 levels. In pancreatic adenocarcinoma, 96% of tumors with CA 19-9 levels >1000 U/mL are considered unresectable. Serial elevated postoperative CA 19-9 levels often predict relapse of pancreatic carcinoma before clinical or radiographic findings, but the CA 19-9 levels are not often monitored because of the paucity of effective treatment for relapsed pancreatic carcinoma. The CA 19-9 glycoprotein is not expressed in Lewis (a- b-) individuals (nonsecretors), who account for approximately 7% of the U.S. population and approximately 20% of the population of Japan, leading to the possibility of false-negative results when CA 19-9 levels are being obtained. Because of the lack of high sensitivity and specificity of CA 19-9, it has not previously been considered useful as a screening test for early pancreatic cancer. However it is currently being studied in conjunction with endoscopic ultrasound as a possible method for early detection. Of note, CA 19-9 is measured using a double monoclonal immunoassay.

Professional Considerations
Consent form NOT required.

Preparation
1. Tube: Red topped, serum-separator (red/gray or gold topped) for serum samples, lavender topped for plasma samples.

Procedure
1. Collect a 4-mL blood sample.
2. Specimen should be refrigerated or frozen immediately.

Postprocedure Care
1. None.

Client and Family Teaching
1. CA 19-9 is not useful as a screening test.
2. Results are usually available within 3 working days.

Factors That Affect Results
1. Reject hemolyzed specimens or specimens left at room temperature.
2. Nonsecretor client. Individuals who are Lewis (a–b–) phenotype (6% of the population) cannot synthesize CA 19-9, CA 50, and CA 195, and this inability may account for the lesser diagnostic value of these markers.
3. Specimen left at room temperature invalidates results.
4. Results are invalidated if the client has received radioisotopes within the past 30 days.

Other Data
1. Elevated levels are found in cystic fibrosis clients and in human seminal fluid.

CA 50 (Carbohydrate Antigen 50, Cancer Antigen 50)—Blood

Norm. <17 U/mL.

Increased. Gastrointestinal (GI) tract tumors, biliary tract tumors, cholangiocarcinoma, oral cancer, pancreatic cancer, transitional cell carcinoma, non–small-cell lung cancer, benign extrahepatic jaundice, cirrhosis, cystic fibrosis.

Usage. Used with other tumor markers to determine prognosis, monitor response to therapy, and monitor for relapse.

C

Decreased. Positive response to therapy.

Description. The *MUC1* gene is a high-molecular-weight glycoprotein found in specific tissues throughout the body (see Mucin-like carcinoma-associated antigen—Blood). The *MUC1* gene has many varieties of carbohydrate chains that are termed mucin-like antigens, and one of these is the carbohydrate antigen 50 (CA 50) that circulates in the bloodstream when cancer is present. CA 50 is found in the blood of clients with GI tumors and biliary tract tumors and appears to be a more sensitive marker for disease progression than that for regression. Although studies have shown relatively high specificity and sensitivity when CA 50 levels are used to aid in diagnosing pancreatic cancer, the specificity is high only when combined with specific signs and symptoms of pancreatic cancer. CA 50 is not a widely used marker in the evaluation of clients with GI tumors because other markers are more reliable and more readily available.

Professional Considerations
Consent form NOT required.

Preparation
1. Tube: Red topped, red/gray or gold topped.

Procedure
1. Collect a 7-mL blood sample.

Postprocedure Care
1. Evaluate other antigen tests and liver function studies.

Client and Family Teaching
1. This test is not used as a screening test for early carcinoma. It is used to monitor the progress of your cancer and treatment.
2. Results are normally available within 7 working days.

Factors That Affect Results
1. False-positive results occur in benign liver disease.
2. Results are invalid if the client has received radioisotopes within the past 30 days.
3. Splenic cysts may produce an elevated CA 50 serum level.

Other Data
1. CA 50 is higher for more undifferentiated and advanced-stage bladder tumors.
2. CA 50 cannot be used as a tumor marker in cirrhotic clients because cytolysis increases this test result.

CA 72-4 (Carbohydrate Antigen 72-4, Cancer Antigen 72-4, Tumor-Associated Glycoprotein 72, Tag 72)—Blood

Norm. Negative.

Usage. Can be used in combination with tumor M2-PK for detection of gastric cancer. CA 72-4 is specific (100%) for esophageal, gastric, and colorectal cancer, but not very sensitive (18%, 32%, and 56%, respectively) when tested alone. When used in combination with M2-PK, there is increased sensitivity for gastric cancer up to 81% and increased sensitivity for esophageal cancer to 74% (Schneider et al, 2005). The test is more sensitive than CA 125 for ovarian cancer and has been found to be most elevated in mucinous type of ovarian cancer; it is less sensitive than CA 19 for pancreatic cancer.

Description. The *MUC1* gene is a high-molecular-weight glycoprotein found in specific tissues throughout the body (see Mucin-like carcinoma-associated antigen—Blood). The *MUC1* gene has many varieties of carbohydrate chains that are termed mucin-like antigens, and one of these is the carbohydrate antigen 72-4 (CA 72-4) that circulates in the bloodstream when cancer is present. CA 72-4 is elevated in several types of gastrointestinal cancer and in ovarian cancer, and levels are most useful when evaluated in combination with other carbohydrate antigens. CA 72-4 is not helpful in detecting micrometastasis of colorectal cancer, but is positive in advanced metastatic tumors. It is being investigated for its usefulness as a prognostic indicator of survival in gastric cancer. CA 72-4 levels are determined using a monoclonal antibody immunoassay.

Professional Considerations
Consent form NOT required.

Preparation
1. Tube: Red topped, serum-separator (red/gray or gold topped) for serum samples, lavender topped for plasma samples.

Procedure
1. Collect a 4-mL blood sample.
2. Specimen should be refrigerated or frozen immediately.

Postprocedure Care
1. None.

Client and Family Teaching
1. Results are usually available within 3 working days.

Factors That Affect Results
1. Reject hemolyzed specimen or specimen left at room temperature.
2. Results are invalid if the client has received radioisotopes within the past 30 days.
3. Positive tests may occur in 85% of invasive ductal breast carcinomas, more than 85% of gastrointestinal adenocarcinomas (gastric, colon, pancreatic, and esophageal), and in ovarian and endometrial adenocarcinomas. Specificity can be improved with concurrent testing for other tumor markers.

Other Data
1. None.

CA 125 (Carbohydrate Antigen 125, Cancer Antigen 125)—Blood

Norm. <21 U/mL (<21 kU/L, SI units).

Usage. Used to aid in the management of clients with malignancies that produce the CA 125 glycoprotein; especially useful in monitoring ovarian carcinoma and breast cancer.

Increased. Abdominal inflammation, cirrhosis, endometriosis, luteal phase of menstrual cycle, menses, neoplasms (breast, cervix, colon, endometrium, fallopian tube, gastrointestinal tract, liver, lung, lymphoma, non–Hodgkin's lymphoma, ovary, pancreas), nonmucinous ovarian epithelial neoplasms, ovarian abscess, pancreatitis (acute), pelvic inflammatory disease, pelvic or peritoneal tuberculosis, peritonitis (acute), polyarteritis nodosa, pregnancy (higher in first and third trimesters with median 23 U/mL), serosal (pericardial, pleural, peritoneal) inflammation, Sjögren's syndrome, and systemic lupus erythematosus.

Description. The *MUC1* gene is a high-molecular-weight glycoprotein found in specific tissues throughout the body (see Mucin-like carcinoma-associated antigen—Blood). The *MUC1* gene has many varieties of carbohydrate chains that are termed mucin-like antigens, and one of these is the carbohydrate antigen 125 (CA 125) that circulates in the bloodstream when cancer is present. The CA 125 epitope is present on most adult tissues derived from the coelomic epithelium. The CA 125 level is used to aid in the management of clients with malignancies that produce the glycoprotein in amounts large enough to be measured in the blood. It is rarely found in normal ovarian tissue but is found in 80% of epithelial ovarian cancers. Twenty-six percent of women with benign ovarian tumors also have an elevated CA 125 level. Although CA 125 cannot distinguish benign from malignant tumors, levels >65 U/mL are associated with malignancy in 90% of pelvic masses. Clients with very high CA 125 levels (>450 U/mL) have poor median survival, whereas clients with levels less than 55 U/mL tend to do somewhat better. CA 125 is used to monitor response to chemotherapy and to monitor for recurrence. Because a normal CA 125 level does not exclude the presence of disease, serial CA 125 levels, in combination with second-look surgery, are recommended for monitoring clients for disease recurrence. It is preferable not to perform the assay until 3 weeks after primary chemotherapy and at least 2 months after abdominal surgery. In endometrial carcinoma, an elevated CA 125 level correlates well with higher grade, higher stage, increased myometrial invasion, and reduced survival. CA 125 levels are obtained by means of a CA 125 II immunoassay, which uses monoclonal antibodies.

Professional Considerations
Consent form NOT required.

Preparation

1. Tube: Red topped, red/gray, or gold topped.

Procedure

1. Draw a 4-mL blood sample.
2. Specimen may remain at room temperature for up to 7 days but must be refrigerated if assay not performed within 7 days.

Postprocedure Care

1. None.

Client and Family Teaching

1. This test is to monitor the progress of your cancer.
2. Results should be available within 3 working days.

Factors That Affect Results

1. Antineoplastic therapy may lower results.
2. An increased CA 125 level may be seen in clients with congestive heart failure.
3. Results are invalidated if the client has received radioisotopes within the past 30 days.

Other Data

1. Sensitivity of this test to ovarian cancer is 75%-80%.
2. See also Human epididymis protein 4 ovarian cancer monitoring test—Blood
3. See also Prostasin—Serum. Combining serum prostasin levels and CA 125 levels as a marker for ovarian cancer reveals a sensitivity of 94% (compared with a sensitivity of 64.9% for CA 125 and of 51.4% for prostasin).

CA 549 (Carbohydrate Antigen 549, Cancer Antigen 549)—Blood

Norm. <10-15.5 U/mL (cutoff = 12.6 U/mL).

Usage. Monitoring for breast cancer disease response to treatment; monitoring for early detection of breast cancer recurrence.

Increased. Breast cancer (low sensitivity [0.51] early in the disease, but high specificity [0.93]). In advanced breast cancer, sensitivity is about 0.70 alone, and 0.79 in combination with other markers, such as carcinoembryonic antigen (CEA) or CA 15-5.

Decreased. Positive response to therapy.

Description. The *MUC1* gene is a high-molecular-weight glycoprotein found in specific tissues throughout the body (see Mucin-like carcinoma-associated antigen—Blood). The *MUC1* gene has many varieties of carbohydrate chains that are termed mucin-like antigens, and one of these is the carbohydrate antigen 549 (CA 549) that circulates in the bloodstream when cancer is present. One of the newest serum markers, CA 549 is present in the serum of clients with moderate to advanced breast cancer. Levels increase as the disease progresses, and decrease as the disease goes into remission. CA 549 is also increased when breast cancer metastasizes. It can be used as a marker alone or in combination with other tests such as CA 15-5 or CEA. However, because CEA is elevated in a variety of other conditions and types of cancer, it is less sensitive than CA 549 for breast cancer. Because of its low detection rate in early disease, CA 549 is not a useful screening test and is also not likely to detect early recurrent disease. CA 549 levels are determined using a monoclonal antibody immunoassay.

Professional Considerations

Consent form NOT required.

Preparation

1. Tube: Red topped or serum-separator (red/gray or gold topped).

Procedure

1. Collect a 4-mL blood sample.
2. Refrigerate specimen.

Postprocedure Care

1. None.

Client and Family Teaching

1. This test is used to monitor the response of your cancer to treatment and to screen for recurrence of your cancer.
2. Results are normally available within 3 working days.

Factors That Affect Results

1. CA 549 is normal in clients with benign breast disease.

2. CA 549 can be normal in early breast cancer.
3. False-positive results are possible, but infrequent in other types of cancer, such as liver, colon, lung, and prostate cancer, and in healthy persons.
4. Results are invalid if the client has received radioisotopes within the past 30 days.

Other Data

1. Because CA 549 is commonly found on immunohistochemical staining of biopsies of a variety of carcinomas, the immunohistochemical method of CA 549 detection is not useful for differentiating breast cancer. Sensitivity can be improved if other cancer markers are also tested.

CAC

See Circulating Anticoagulant—Blood.

Cadmium—Serum and 24-Hour Urine

Norm.

		SI Units
Serum		
Nonsmoker	0.1-0.50 μg/dL	0.89-4.45 nmol/L
Excess exposure	>10 μg/dL	>89 nmol/L
Panic level	>41 μg/dL	>365 nmol/L
Urine		
Nonsmoker	0.5-4.7 μg/L	4.4-41.8 nmol/L
Excess exposure	>10 μg/L	>88.97 nmol/L

Panic Level Symptoms and Treatment

Symptoms. Abdominal cramps, acute renal failure, diarrhea, exhaustion, headache, nausea, pulmonary edema (when cadmium dust or fumes are inhaled), shock, vertigo, vomiting.

Treatment

NOTE: Treatment choice(s) depend(s) upon client's history and condition and episode history.

1. Give demulcents.
2. Use gastric lavage with milk or water.
3. Induce vomiting with a saline cathartic or syrup of ipecac if within ½ hour of exposure. (Induction of vomiting is contraindicated in clients with no gag reflex or with central nervous system depression or excitation.)
4. Give saline or sorbitol cathartic.
5. Closely monitor and support respiratory and hemodynamic status.
6. Activated charcoal is NOT helpful.
7. Monitor for liver and kidney damage.
8. CaNa$_2$-EDTA will enhance cadmium removal for acute exposure only.

Increased. Bladder cancer, early delivery because of maternal exposure, industrial exposure to cadmium dust and fumes such as in torch cutters, ingestion of contaminated water or food stored in cadmium-plated containers, lung cancer. Drugs include traditional Indian or Croatian remedies, herbal remedies from Lublin's drugstores (Poland).

Decreased. Not clinically significant.

Description. Cadmium is a heavy metal with a half-life of 15-20 years in humans that is obtained from zinc ores and is used in the manufacture of alloys, in storage batteries, and in electroplating. The general population is exposed to small amounts daily through fertilizers, food, water, air, and cigarette smoke. Cadmium is a respiratory tract irritant that can produce fatal pulmonary edema, proliferative interstitial pneumonia, and cardiovascular collapse if inhaled as dust or fumes. Cadmium ingestion poisoning produces a sudden onset of severe gastrointestinal symptoms within 30 minutes. Chronic exposure can produce osteomalacia and renal, lung, and hepatic disorders and can also cause severe gastroenteritis. Cadmium is not metabolized in the body. It accumulates in tissue, concentrating primarily in the kidneys and the liver. More than 95% of the blood cadmium is contained in the erythrocytes. Serum levels are used for diagnosis of acute cadmium intoxication. Urine cadmium levels are measured to detect chronic exposure. It is believed that urine cadmium levels >10 mg/L (>88.97 nmol/L, SI units) are indicative of renal tubular damage.

Professional Considerations
Consent form NOT required.

Preparation
1. *Serum*: Tube: green topped or black topped.
2. *Urine*: Obtain a 3-L, metal-free container without a preservative.

Procedure
1. *Serum*: Draw a 5-mL blood specimen in a metal-free tube.
2. *Urine*:
   a. Discard the first morning urine specimen.
   b. Save all the urine voided for 24 hours in a refrigerated, clean, metal-free, 3-L container without preservatives. Include the urine voided at the end of the 24-hour period. For catheterized clients, keep the drainage bag on ice and empty urine into the collection container hourly.

Postprocedure Care
1. Send the serum specimen to the laboratory immediately.

2. *Urine*:
   a. Compare urine quantity in the specimen container with the urinary output record for the test. If the specimen contains less urine than was recorded as output, some urine may have been discarded, thus invalidating the test.
   b. Document the quantity of urine output for the collection period on the laboratory requisition.
   c. It is best to send the entire specimen to the laboratory so that it can be measured and mixed well before being tested.

Client and Family Teaching
1. *Urine*: Save all the urine voided in the 24-hour period and urinate before defecating to avoid loss of urine. If any urine is accidentally discarded, discard the entire specimen and restart the collection the next day.
2. A client with elevated levels should identify and reduce sources of cadmium exposure and see the physician regularly for monitoring of the effects of chronic cadmium exposure.

Factors That Affect Results
1. Reject hemolyzed specimens.
2. Urine levels increase with aging.
3. Cadmium levels normally increase with aging.

Other Data
1. Death may occur if pulmonary edema, shock, or renal failure is caused by cadmium poisoning.

Calcitonin (Thyrocalcitonin)—Serum
Norm.

		SI Units
Serum		
Adult female	<4.6 pg/mL	<4.6 ng/L
Adult male	<11.5 pg/mL	<11.5 ng/L
Adult, stimulated	<100 pg/mL	<100 ng/L
6 months to 3 years	<15 pg/mL	<15 ng/L
<6 months	<40 pg/mL	<40 ng/L
Term newborn, cord blood	30-240 pg/mL	30-240 ng/L
Neonate, 2 days old	91-580 pg/mL	91-580 ng/L
Neonate, 7 days old	77-293 pg/mL	77-293 ng/L

		SI Units
Diagnostic of MCT		
Female, stimulated test	>120 pg/mL	>120 ng/L
Male, stimulated test	>265 ng/mL	>265 ng/L

Usage. Calcitonin measurements are useful as a screening tool for medullary thyroid carcinoma (MCT) or multiple endocrine neoplasia with a family history of these conditions. The test is also used to detect residual or recurrent MCT.

Increased. Anemia (pernicious), cancer (breast, lung, thyroid), chronic renal failure, Cushing's disease (type II), ectopic calcitonin production, Hashimoto's thyroiditis, hypercalcemia, islet cell tumors, leukemia, medullary cancer of the thyroid (MCT), myeloproliferative disorders, parafollicular C cell hyperplasia, parathyroid adenoma, pheochromocytoma, renal failure (chronic), sepsis, thyroiditis, uremia, and Zollinger-Ellison syndrome.

Decreased. Chronic autoimmune thyroiditis.

Description. Calcitonin (thyrocalcitonin) is a thyroid gland polypeptide hormone that helps maintain normal serum calcium and phosphorus levels. It is secreted by parafollicular C cells in response to hypercalcemia. Its functions include inhibition of calcium absorption from the gastrointestinal tract, inhibition of calcium resorption from the bone and soft tissues by osteoclasts and osteocytes, and increasing the amount of renal calcium excretion. Calcitonin functions in calcium homeostasis by antagonizing parathyroid hormone and vitamin D to lower serum calcium levels.

Professional Considerations
Consent form NOT required.

Preparation
1. For a stimulated test, insert a saline lock.
2. Tube: Green topped tube, or chilled red topped or chilled red/gray topped tube, or gold topped tube.

3. Notify laboratory personnel that a specimen for calcitonin measurement will be delivered.

Procedure
1. Random test:
   a. Draw a 4-mL venous blood sample.
2. Stimulated test:
   a. Draw a 4-mL baseline venous blood sample for calcitonin and calcium levels.
   b. Give 2 mg/kg of calcium gluconate slow IV push over 1 minute.
   c. Draw a 4 mL blood sample for calcitonin at 1, 3, 5, and 10 minutes after completion of the calcium gluconate infusion. Label tubes with time drawn.

Postprocedure Care
1. Send the specimen to the laboratory immediately for immediate serum separation into a plastic tube, followed by freezing.

Client and Family Teaching
1. Fast (except for sips of water) for 8 hours before sampling.
2. Up to 1 month is required for completion of this test in the laboratory.

Factors That Affect Results
1. Reject hemolyzed specimens.

Other Data
1. Calcitonin levels do not differ significantly by race.
2. A study of 65 postoperative medullary thyroid carcinoma clients revealed that calcitonin doubling times may be superior to initial clinical staging and one of the most powerful prognostic indicators of medullary thyroid carcinoma.

Calcium, Calculated Ionized—Serum

Norm. 46%-50% of total calcium.

Increased. See Calcium, Ionized—Blood.

Decreased. See Calcium, Ionized—Blood.

Description. Calcium is a cation that is absorbed into the bloodstream from dietary sources. Calcium functions in bone formation, nerve impulse transmission, contraction of myocardial and skeletal muscles, and in blood clotting by converting prothrombin to thrombin. Calcium is stored in the teeth and bones, and circulating calcium is filtered by the kidneys, with most being reabsorbed when serum calcium levels are normal. Calculated ionized calcium is an indirect method for calculating the amount of ionized (biologically active) calcium based on serum protein levels. Normally, 46%-50% of total calcium is ionized, and most of the remainder (40%) is bound to proteins. The remaining 8%-10% is complexed with anions such as bicarbonate and lactate and is biologically inactive. Of the portion bound to proteins, 80% is bound to albumin, and 20% is bound to globulin. Calculated ionized calcium is also called protein-corrected total calcium and is used as a formula to calculate the amount of protein-bound calcium and to deduct that from the total calcium level to derive an estimate of the biologically active ionized calcium. This method is often imprecise and unreliable, especially in clients with low or high protein levels, and is being replaced by newer laboratory methods for ionized calcium measurement.

Professional Considerations
Consent form NOT required.

Preparation
1. See Calcium, Total—Serum; Albumin—Serum, Urine, and 24-Hour urine; and Protein, total—Serum for instructions on drawing the blood for the results needed for the calculation.

Procedure
1. Obtain total calcium, albumin, and globulin levels and calculate the amount of ionized calcium with the following formulas:
   Step 1: Percent of protein-bound Ca^{++} = 8(albumin g/dL) + 2(globulin g/dL) + 3
   Step 2: Percent of ionized Ca^{++} = total calcium mg/dL − % of protein-bound Ca^{++}

Postprocedure Care
1. Not applicable.

Client and Family Teaching
1. None.

Factors That Affect Results
1. Results are unreliable for hypoproteinemic or hyperproteinemic states. The ion-selective electrode procedure should be used for these clients.
2. Serum ionized calcium concentration is significantly decreased in the elderly.

Other Data
1. Other formulas exist for calculation of ionized calcium. Many of these formulas have been disputed, which makes the reliability of this calculation questionable.
2. There is a negative correlation between serum calcium and triglycerides in young and elderly hypertensives.
3. See also Calcium, Ionized—Blood; Calcium, Total—Serum.

Calcium, Ionized (Free Calcium, Dialyzable Calcium)—Blood

Norm. 46%-56% of total serum calcium.

		SI Units
Serum		
Adults	4.45-5.30 mg/dL	1.10-1.30 mmol/L
Newborn	2.24-2.46 mEq/L	1.12-3.20 mmol/L
Cord blood	5.2-6.40 mg/dL	1.30-1.60 mmol/L
2 hours old	4.84-5.84 mg/dL	1.21-1.46 mmol/L
1 day old	4.40-5.44 mg/dL	1.10-1.36 mmol/L
3 days old	4.60-5.68 mg/dL	1.15-1.42 mmol/L
5 days old	4.88-5.92 mg/dL	1.22-1.48 mmol/L
Children, teens	4.80-5.52 mg/dL	1.20-1.38 mmol/L
Capillary Blood		
6-36 hours old	4.20-5.48 mg/dL	1.05-1.37 mmol/L
60-84 hours old	4.40-5.68 mg/dL	1.10-1.42 mmol/L
108-132 hours old	4.80-5.92 mg/dL	1.20-1.48 mmol/L

		SI Units
Whole Blood		
Adults		
18-60 years	4.48-5.28 mg/dL	1.10-1.30 mmol/L
60-90 years	4.64-5.16 mg/dL	1.16-1.29 mmol/L
>90 years	4.48-5.28 mg/dL	1.12-1.32 mmol/L
Plasma		
Adults	4.12-4.92 mg/dL	1.03-1.23 mmol/L

Increased. Acidemia, hyperparathyroidism (primary), hypervitaminosis D, malignancy, tumors that produce or elevate parathyroid hormone, varicose veins. Drugs include hydrochlorothiazide (chronic use), lithium compounds, and rilmenidine.

Decreased. Alkalemia, burns, after citrate-containing blood transfusions, hyperosmolar states, hypoparathyroidism (primary), magnesium deficiency, multiple organ failure, pancreatitis, postoperatively, pseudohypoparathyroidism, sepsis, trauma, and vitamin D deficiency. Drugs include anticonvulsants, danazol, foscarnet, furosemide, and hyperosmolar solutions.

Description. Calcium is a cation that is absorbed into the bloodstream from dietary sources. Calcium functions in bone formation, nerve impulse transmission, contraction of myocardial and skeletal muscles, and in blood clotting by converting prothrombin to thrombin. Calcium is stored in the teeth and bones, and circulating calcium is filtered by the kidneys, with most being reabsorbed when serum calcium levels are normal. Ionized calcium is a cation that circulates freely in the bloodstream and constitutes 46%-50% of all circulating calcium. Levels increase and decrease directly with increases and decreases in blood pH. For every 0.1 pH unit decrease, ionized calcium increases 1.5%-2.5%. Ionized calcium is sometimes considered a more sensitive and reliable indicator of primary hyperparathyroidism for clients with low levels of albumin than total serum calcium because ionized calcium is not affected by changes in serum albumin concentrations. Total serum calcium values increase and decrease directly with serum albumin levels, but ionized calcium levels do not (see Calcium, Total—Serum).

Professional Considerations
Consent form NOT required.

Preparation
1. The client should lie supine for 30 minutes.
2. Tube: Red topped, red/gray topped, gold topped, or green topped tube that does not contain zinc heparin. Also obtain ice.
3. Do NOT draw during hemodialysis.

Procedure
1. Completely fill the tube with blood without using a tourniquet. Use a Vacutainer to collect the specimen directly into the tube without removing the tube stopper.
2. Capillary tubes from heelstick specimens are also acceptable.
3. Place the specimen immediately on ice.

Postprocedure Care
1. Deliver the specimen to the laboratory immediately and refrigerate.

Client and Family Teaching
1. Results are normally available within 4 hours.
2. For chronic hypocalcemia, food sources high in calcium include milk, egg yolks, cheese, beans, cauliflower, chard, kale, and rhubarb.

Factors That Affect Results
1. Prolonged exposure of the serum to air causes an increase in pH that in turn causes an increased ionized calcium level. Collect the specimen anaerobically.
2. The test must be performed within 48 hours of specimen collection.
3. A diurnal variation exists, with the lowest values occurring in the early morning

C

hours (0200-0400) and the highest values occurring at mid evening.
4. Levels may decrease from baseline in women taking oral contraceptives, and may increase from baseline in women taking injectable contraceptives.

Other Data
1. This is the most reliable test for diagnosing hyperparathyroidism in clients with low albumin.
2. See also Calcium, Total—Serum; Calcium, Calculated ionized—Serum.

Calcium, Total—Serum

Norm.

		SI Units
Adults		
18-60 years	8.2-10.7 mg/dL	2.10-2.70 mmol/L
60-90 years	8.8-10.2 mg/dL	2.20-2.55 mmol/L
>90 years	8.2-9.6 mg/dL	2.05-2.40 mmol/L
Children		
Cord blood	8.2-11.2 mg/dL	2.05-2.80 mmol/L
Premature infant	6.2-11.0 mg/dL	1.55-2.75 mmol/L
<10 days	7.6-10.4 mg/dL	1.90-2.60 mmol/L
10 days–2 years	9.0-11.0 mg/dL	2.25-2.75 mmol/L
2-12 years	8.8-10.8 mg/dL	2.20-2.70 mmol/L
12-18 years	8.4-10.2 mg/dL	2.10-2.55 mmol/L
Panic Levels		
Tetany	<7 mg/dL	<1.75 mmol/L
Coma	>12 mg/dL	>2.99 mmol/L
Possible death	≤6 mg/dL	≤1.50 mmol/L
	≥14 mg/dL	≥3.49 mmol/L

Panic Level Symptoms and Treatment
NOTE: Treatment choice(s) depend(s) on client's history and condition and episode history.

Symptoms of hypercalcemia
Constipation, ECG changes (shortened ST segment), lethargy, muscle weakness, nausea, neurologic depression (headache, apathy, reduced level of consciousness) progressing to coma, vomiting.

Treatment of hypercalcemia panic levels
1. Correct the cause.
2. Give normal saline and diuretics to speed renal calcium excretion.
3. Administer calcitonin or steroids to move calcium intracellularly.
4. Hemodialysis WILL remove calcium.

Symptoms of hypocalcemia
Convulsions, carpopedal spasm (positive Trousseau's sign), dysrhythmias, ECG changes (prolonged ST segment and QT interval), facial spasm (positive Chvostek's sign), muscle cramps, numbness, tetany,

tingling, and muscle twitching, spasms of the larynx.

Treatment of hypocalcemia panic levels
1. Implement seizure precautions.
2. Maintain continuous ECG monitoring.
3. Correct the cause.
4. Give calcium, magnesium, and vitamin D replacement.
5. Administer IV calcium chloride or calcium gluconate (100 mg of elemental calcium) or 4-7 mL of 10% calcium chloride mixed in 50-100 mL of solution over 20 minutes. Follow with calcium infusion at 1-2 mg/kg/hour.

Increased. Acidosis (respiratory), acromegaly, acute tubular necrosis (recovery phase), Addison's disease, bacteremia, berylliosis, coccidioidomycosis, diet (high calcium), ectopic neoplasms that produce parathyroid hormone, familial hypocalciuric hypercalcemia, hepatic disease (chronic advanced), histoplasmosis, hyperparathyroidism (primary, tertiary renal),

C

hyperthyroidism, hypervitaminosis (vitamin D or A intoxication), immobility (prolonged), infants (idiopathic), leukemia, lymphoma, malignancy (bladder, breast, kidney, lung), metastatic bone cancer, milk-alkali (Burnett's) syndrome, multiple endocrine neoplasia, multiple myeloma, mycoses, osteoporosis, Paget's disease, peptic ulcer diet, pheochromocytoma, polycythemia vera, porphyria, renal calculi, renal osteomalacia (induced by aluminum), renal transplantation, respiratory disease, rhabdomyolysis, sarcoidosis, and tuberculosis. Drugs include anabolic steroids, androgens, antacids (alkaline), calciferol, calcium gluconate, calcium salts, calusterone, chlorothiazide sodium, chlorthalidone, danazol, diethylstilbestrol, dihydrotachysterol, diuretics, ergocalciferol, estrogens, hydrochlorothiazide, indomethacin, isotretinoin, lithium carbonate, magnesium salts, parathyroid hormone, phenobarbital, progesterone, secretin, tamoxifen, testolactone, theophylline (toxicity), thiazide diuretics, thyroid hormones, vitamin A, and vitamin D.

Decreased. Alkalosis, bacteremia, blood transfusions (excessive without replacement of calcium), burns, cachexia, celiac disease, chronic renal disease, cystic fibrosis of pancreas, diarrhea, eating disorders (slight decrease), Fanconi syndrome (with renal tubular acidosis), hypomagnesemia, hypoparathyroidism, hypoproteinemia, infection (severe), malabsorption, malaria (uncomplicated), Milkman syndrome, nephritis, nephrosis, nephrotic syndrome, obstructive jaundice, osteomalacia, pancreatitis (acute), parathyroidectomy, pregnancy (late), pseudohypoparathyroidism, renal failure, renal insufficiency, renal tubular acidosis, rickets, sprue, starvation, toxic shock syndrome, thyroidectomy with accidental removal of parathyroid gland, and vitamin D deficiency. Drugs include acetazolamide, albuterol, alprostadil, aminoglycosides, antacids, anticonvulsants, asparaginase, aspirin, barbiturates (in elderly), calcitonin, carbamazepine, carbenoxolone, carboplatin, citrates, corticosteroids, cholestyramine resin, ethacrynic acid, fluorides, furosemide, gastrin, gentamicin, glucagon, glucose, heparin, hydrocortisone, indapamide, insulin, iron, isoniazid, laxatives (excessive), magnesium salts, mercurial diuretics, mestranol, methicillin, mithramycin, phenobarbital, phenytoin, phosphates, plicamycin, saline (in hypercalcemic state), tetracycline (during pregnancy), and thiazide diuretics.

Description. Calcium is a cation that is absorbed into the bloodstream from dietary sources and functions in bone formation, nerve impulse transmission, contraction of myocardial and skeletal muscles, and in blood clotting by converting prothrombin to thrombin. Calcium is stored in the teeth and bones, and circulating calcium is filtered by the kidneys, with most being reabsorbed when serum calcium levels are normal. To maintain a normal calcium balance and counteract any excreted calcium, at least 1 g of calcium must be ingested daily. Normally, 46%-50% of total calcium is ionized and most of the remainder (40%) is bound to proteins. Only ionized calcium can be used by the body. The remaining 8%-10% is complexed with anions such as bicarbonate and lactate and is biologically inactive. Total serum calcium values increase and decrease directly with serum albumin levels, but ionized calcium levels do not. For every 1 g/dL decrease in albumin, total serum calcium decreases by 0.8 mg/dL. When acidosis is present, more calcium is ionized. In alkalosis, most is bound to protein and cannot be used by the body.

Professional Considerations
Consent form NOT required.

Preparation
1. Tube: Red topped, red/gray topped, or gold topped.
2. Do NOT draw during hemodialysis.

Procedure
1. Leaving the tourniquet in place less than 1 minute, draw a 4-mL venous blood sample.

Postprocedure Care
1. Send the specimen to the laboratory for spinning within 1 hour.

Client and Family Teaching
1. Eat a diet with normal calcium levels, 800 mg/day (15-20 mmol/day, SI units), for 3 days before sampling.
2. Fast, except for water, for 8 hours (only for multichannel tests).
3. For elevated levels, avoid foods high in calcium, ambulate when possible,

and increase fluid intake unless contraindicated.

Factors That Affect Results
1. Reject hemolyzed specimens.
2. Falsely elevated values may be caused by hemolysis, dehydration, or hyperproteinemia.
3. Falsely decreased values may be caused by dilutional hypervolemia, by administration of intravenous sodium chloride, or by the administration of sulfobromophthalein sodium (Bromsulphalein) dye within 2 days before specimen collection.
4. Serum calcium should be corrected for the serum albumin. For every gram below 4 mg/dL, add 0.8 to the calcium level.
5. Phosphate drugs may cause falsely decreased results if test is performed by emission flame method.

Other Data
1. Hypercalcemia can induce digoxin toxicity and decreased neuronal permeability.
2. The impact of calcium supplementation has been the focus of several studies and meta-analyses. Some findings include increased risk of cardiovascular events and lack of additional protection from bone fracture with high calcium intake.
3. See also Calcium, Calculated ionized—Serum; Calcium, Ionized—Blood.

Calcium—Urine

Norm. Semiquantitative Sulkowitch test: 1+ to 2+

Quantitative Tests		SI Units
Random specimen	<40 mg/dL	<1.0 mmol/L
24-hour specimen		
Low-calcium diet	<150 mg/day	<3.7 mmol/day
Normal-calcium diet	100-250 mg/day	2.5-6.2 mmol/day
High-calcium diet	250-300 mg/day	6.2-7.5 mmol/day

Increased. Acromegaly, amyotrophic lateral sclerosis, bone metastasis, cancer (primary) of the breast or lung, Crohn's disease, diabetes mellitus, diet (high calcium or high sodium chloride), ectopic hyperparathyroidism, Fanconi syndrome (with renal tubular acidosis), glucocorticoid excess, hypercalcemia, hyperparathyroidism, hyperthyroidism, hypervitaminosis D, hypocitraturia, idiopathic hypercalciuria, immobility (long term), leukemia, lymphoma, metastasis, medullary sponge kidney, multiple myeloma, nephrolithiasis, osteoporosis, Paget's disease, renal tubular acidosis, sarcoidosis, ulcerative colitis, and Wilson's disease. Drugs include ammonium chloride, androgens, anabolic steroids, antacids, calcipotriol, cholestyramine, EB 1089 (vitamin D analog), furosemide, mercurial diuretics, parathyroid hormone, potassium citrate, and vitamin D.

Decreased. Chronic renal failure, familial hypocalciuric hypercalcemia, hypocalcemia, hypoparathyroidism, malabsorption, milk-alkali syndrome, metastatic carcinoma of the prostate, nephrosis, osteomalacia, preeclampsia, pseudohypoparathyroidism, renal insufficiency, renal osteodystrophy, rickets (vitamin D resistant), steatorrhea, and vitamin D deficiency. Drugs include aspirin, indomethacin, oral contraceptives, sodium phytate, thiazide diuretics, and viomycin.

Description. Calcium is a cation that is absorbed into the bloodstream from dietary sources and that functions in bone formation, nerve impulse transmission, contractility of muscles, and blood clotting. Calcium is stored in the bones and circulating calcium is filtered by the kidneys, with most being reabsorbed when serum calcium levels are normal. When serum calcium levels rise above normal, the kidneys reabsorb less calcium, and elevated levels of calcium appear in the urine. Whereas quantitative tests must be performed by a laboratory, the Sulkowitch test is a semiquantitative test suitable for home use.

Professional Considerations
Consent form NOT required.

Preparation

1. Note daily dietary level of calcium intake for the previous 3 days on the laboratory requisition.
2. Obtain a 3-L container with hydrochloric acid (HCl) additive or an acid-washed glass bottle for 24-hour collection. Write the starting date and the time on the container.
3. Obtain a small container to collect a random sample.

Procedure

1. 24-hour collection (quantitative):
   a. Discard the first morning urine specimen.
   b. Begin to time a 24-hour urine collection.
   c. Save all the urine voided for 24 hours in a clean, plastic, 3-L container to which 10 mL of 6 N HCl has been added or in an acid-washed glass bottle. Include the urine voided at the end of the 24-hour period.
2. Random specimen collection (quantitative):
   a. When evaluating for hypocalciuria, collect a postprandial specimen. When evaluating for hypercalciuria, collect an early-morning specimen before breakfast. Obtain a 100-mL random urine specimen in a clean container. A fresh specimen may be taken from a urinary drainage bag.
3. Sulkowitch test (semiquantitative):
   a. Obtain a 20-mL random urine specimen.
   b. Follow the package instructions.

Postprocedure Care

1. Compare the urine quantity in the specimen container with the urinary output record for the test. If the specimen contains less urine than what was recorded as output, some urine may have been discarded, thus invalidating the test.
2. Document the quantity of urine output for the collection period on the laboratory requisition.
3. Send the specimen to the laboratory within 1 hour.

Client and Family Teaching

1. The client should consume a diet with normal calcium levels, 600-800 mg/day (15-20 mmol/day, SI units), for 3 days.
2. Save all the urine voided in the 24-hour period and urinate before defecating to avoid loss of urine. If any urine is accidentally discarded, discard the entire specimen and restart the collection the next day.
3. Clients with elevated levels should be told to notify the physician for symptoms of renal calculi (flank or abdominal pain, severe dysuria).

Factors That Affect Results

1. Failure to add HCl to the collection container before the collection is started will result in falsely decreased results.
2. All the urine voided for the 24-hour period must be included to avoid a falsely low result.
3. For a random specimen, a delay in processing may cause falsely decreased results.
4. Elevated urine phosphate may cause decreased results.

Other Data

1. 20%-25% of clients who form calcium stones have hyperuricosuria.
2. See also Calcium, Total—Serum.

Calcium Disodium EDTA Mobilization Test

See Lead Mobilization Test, 24-Hour—Urine.

California Encephalitis Virus Titer (La Crosse Virus Titer)—Serum

Norm. Less than a fourfold increase in titer in paired sera (acute and convalescent sera).

Usage. Supports the diagnosis of viral encephalitis.

Description. The California encephalitis virus commonly produces aseptic meningitis, which occurs in the summer and is clinically indistinguishable from enteroviral disease. Encephalitis is an inflammation of the brain caused by an arbovirus infection transmitted by infected mosquitoes and tics. It causes an abrupt onset of severe frontal headache, fever of 38-40 degrees C, stiff neck, sore throat, aphasia, loss of consciousness and sometimes lethargy, bronchitis, pneumonia, meningitis, convulsions, and coma. Incidence is highest in children and in the inhabitants of tundra, taiga, and leafy forest and the north central states of the United States including Indiana, Tennessee, North Carolina, and West Virginia. Risk increases with number of hours spent outdoors and living residence with one or more tree holes within 100 meters.

Professional Considerations
Consent form NOT required.

Preparation
1. Tube: Red topped, red/gray topped, or gold topped.
2. MAY be drawn during hemodialysis.

Procedure
1. Draw a 15-mL venous blood sample.

2. Repeat the test for a convalescent serum specimen in 10-14 days.

Postprocedure Care
1. Send the specimen to the laboratory within 2 hours.

Client and Family Teaching
1. Return in 10 days to 2 weeks for repeat testing.

Factors That Affect Results
1. Reject hemolyzed specimens.
2. The serum should be separated from the clot within 2-3 hours.

Other Data
1. The virus can rarely be isolated from blood or spinal fluid in the acute phase.
2. Serologic diagnosis can be made by demonstration of rising antibody titers between the acute and convalescent specimens.
3. Specific serologic diagnosis may be complicated by cross-reactions in clients with prior exposure to dengue or other flaviviruses.

---

cAMP

See Cyclic Adenosine Monophosphate—Serum and Urine.

Campylobacter-like-Organism (CLO) Test (Rapid Urease Test)—Specimen

Norm. Negative (CLO test gel turns yellow 24 hours after specimen insertion).

Positive. Presence of *Helicobacter pylori* (amount present is decided by deepening in color of the specimen).

Description. This is a simple test used to determine the presence of *H. pylori* in gastric mucosal biopsy specimens. *H. pylori* has been implicated as a primary etiologic factor in duodenal ulcer disease, gastric ulcer, and nonulcer dyspepsia. By causing chronic inflammation, *H. pylori* may weaken mucosal defenses and allow acid and pepsin to disrupt the epithelium. *H. pylori* produces large amounts of urease enzyme, which can be found in 83% of dental plaque scrapings and 59% of tongue scrapings. Although urease primarily allows *H. pylori* to use urea as a nitrogen source, the breakdown of urea also

produces high local concentrations of ammonia, which enables the organism to tolerate a low pH. Simple tests such as the CLO test enable a rapid diagnosis. The CLO test is a sealed plastic slide holding an agar gel that contains urea, a pH indicator, phenol red, buffers, and bacteriostatic agents that help prevent false color changes that could lead to false-positive readings. If the urease enzyme of *H. pylori* is present in an inserted tissue sample, the resulting degradation of urea causes the pH to rise, and the color of the gel turns from yellow to a bright magenta color.

Professional Considerations
Consent form NOT required but IS required for the endoscopy procedure used to obtain the specimen. See Esophagogastroduodenoscopy—Diagnostic for risks and contraindications.

Preparation

1. See Client and Family Teaching.
2. Inspect the CLO test slide to make sure that the well is full and is a yellow color. If a CLO test slide has an orange color, it should be used with caution because it may give a false-positive result.
3. See also Esophagogastroduodenoscopy— Diagnostic.

Procedure

1. Immediately before endoscopy, place the CLO test on a warming plate at 30 to 40 degrees C. Warming helps to speed the chemical reaction.
2. Obtain a tissue sample from the gastric mucosa by endoscopy. Place the sample immediately in the well of the CLO test slide.

Postprocedure Care

1. Be certain that the tissue specimen is completely immersed so that it will have maximum contact with the urea and bacteriostat in the gel.
2. Reseal the CLO test container.
3. Keep the CLO test in a warm place for the next 3 hours.
4. See also Esophagogastroduodenoscopy— Diagnostic.

Client and Family Teaching

1. Do not take antibiotics or bismuth salts for at least 3 weeks before the test.

2. This test will help identify whether the *H. pylori* bacterium is present in your stomach. The bacterium is believed to be a cause of ulcers and gastritis.
3. Since *H. pylori* therapy is only 50%-75% effective, it is important that you return for retesting 28 days after completing therapy to confirm complete eradication of *H. pylori*.
4. See also Esophagogastroduodenoscopy— Diagnostic.

Factors That Affect Results

1. False-negative results may occur when very low numbers of *H. pylori* are present or when the bacterium has a patchy distribution.
2. The CLO test will be less sensitive if the client has recently been taking antibiotics or bismuth.

Other Data

1. The CLO test has proved to be an accurate test with few false-negative results.
2. Treatment for *H. pylori* eradication may include pantoprazole, clarithromycin, and amoxicillin
3. Clients receiving Carburazepam therapy may have a higher total cholesterol, HDL, and LDL, and therefore should be monitored closely for hyperlipidemia.

Campylobacter Pylori

See *Helicobacter pylori* Quick Office Serology, Serum and Titer—Blood; or Campylobacter-like Organism Test—Specimen.

C-ANCA

See Antineutrophil Cytoplasmic Antibody Screen—Serum.

Cannabinoids, Qualitative—Blood or Urine

Norm. None present. Negative.

Usage. Testing for use of marijuana.

Description. Marijuana is derived from an Asiatic herb, *Cannabis sativa*, and contains many biologically active chemicals, with most of the pharmacologic effects resulting from 9-tetrahydrocannabinol (THC). THC has an unusual high lipid solubility; therefore it is widely distributed in the body, with a high affinity for brain tissue. THC affects mood, memory, motor coordination, cognitive ability, sensorium, time sense, and self-perception. THC also significantly increases cortical and cerebellar blood flow and suppresses immunologic function of macrophages. The effects are dose related and are three to four times more potent when smoked than when ingested or injected. THC is metabolized to numerous active and inactive metabolites called cannabinoids. Seventy percent of the dose from smoking THC is excreted within 72 hours in the urine and feces. Because of slow release of THC from tissue storage sites, urine may test positive for 2-5 days after marijuana use by infrequent smokers. The primary psychoactive metabolite, which is also the most abundant and inactive, is 11-hydroxy-THC. Most immunoassay tests use antibodies directed at 11-hydroxy-THC. Immunoassays are also available to measure the drug THC, which can be used in the treatment of persistent nausea and vomiting associated with cancer chemotherapy or to decrease the pain of glaucoma.

Professional Considerations

Consent form NOT required but is usually obtained for preemployment testing or for medicolegal specimens.

Preparation

1. Tube: Red topped, red/gray topped, or gold topped. Also obtain a sterile plastic urine collection container.
2. Do NOT draw during hemodialysis.

Procedure

1. If specimens are being obtained for medicolegal purposes, the collection, transportation, and processing should be performed in the presence of a witness.
2. Draw a 5-mL venous blood sample.
3. Obtain a random 50-mL urine specimen in a sterile plastic container.

Postprocedure Care

1. Write the exact time of the specimen collection and the source, date, and client's name on the laboratory requisition.
2. If the specimen may be used as legal evidence, sign and have the witness sign the laboratory requisition. Transport the specimen to the laboratory in a sealed plastic bag labeled as legal evidence. Each client handling the specimen should sign and write the time of specimen receipt on the laboratory requisition.

Client and Family Teaching

1. The long-term effects of marijuana use include impaired lung structure, chromosomal mutation, higher incidence of birth defects, mononucleic white blood cells, memory impairment, flashbacks, and impairment of fertility.
2. Offer substance abuse counseling referral to all clients using cannabinoids without a medical prescription.

Factors That Affect Results

1. Serum levels of THC peak within 10-30 minutes of inhalation and within 3 hours of ingestion depending on the dosage.
2. Urine levels peak from 2 to 6 hours after THC has entered the system.
3. Urine levels are detectable for 4-6 days in acute users and for 20-77 days in chronic users.
4. Urine loss is 23% if stored at room temperature for 10 days and 8%-20% if frozen for up to 3 years.
5. The use of an adulterant in the urine sample will cause negative results in a positive sample. Commercially available urine adulterants include Stealth, Urine Aid, Urineluck, and Clean Add-it-ive.

Other Data

1. Because of the cardiac stimulant effects, cannabinoids may pose a threat to clients with cardiovascular disease.
2. Marijuana is the most widely used illicit drug in the United States.
3. The signs and symptoms of *Cannabis* intoxication are tachycardia, conjunctival infection, hypotension, muscle weakness, tremors, unsteadiness, increased deep tendon reflexes, psychologic and cognitive impairments, hallucinations, loss of consciousness, and, rarely, death.
4. Common street names for marijuana include Acapulco gold, bhand, blunts, chronic (or "the chronic"), Colombian, ganja, grass, hash, hash oil, hay, herb, J, jay, jive stick, joint, loco weed, Mary Jane, Panama red, pot, reefer, rope, smoke, stick, tea, and weed.

Captopril Renography

See **Renocystogram**—Diagnostic.

Carbamazepine—Blood

Norm. Negative.

	Trough	SI Units
Therapeutic value	4-12 µg/mL	17-51 µmol/L
Value for persons taking concurrent antiepileptic medications	4-8 µg/mL	17-34 µmol/L
Panic level	>20 µg/mL	>84 µmol/L

Panic Level Symptoms and Treatment

Symptoms

Stage I	Levels >25 µg/mL—stupor, coma up to 24 hours, seizures, respiratory depression
Stage II	Levels 15-25 µg/mL—adventitial choreiform movements, combativeness, hallucinations, moderate stupor
Stage III	Levels 11-15 µg/mL—mild drowsiness
Stage IV	Levels <11 µg/mL—ataxia and nystagmus with otherwise normal neurologic status; relapse to earlier stages may recur unexpectedly; ataxia, blurred vision, CNS depression, coma, diplopia, dizziness, drowsiness, dysrhythmias (conduction defects, right bundle branch block, sinus tachycardia), dystonic reaction, hallucination, hypotension, nystagmus, pulmonary edema, reduced myocardial contractility, respiratory depression, seizures (when levels exceed 20 g/mL), vomiting

Treatment

NOTE: Treatment choice(s) depend(s) on client's history and condition and episode history.

1. Do NOT induce emesis.
2. Perform gastric lavage if the drug has been recently ingested (most effective mechanism to reduce absorption).
3. Maintain and protect airway.
4. Give activated charcoal unless ileus is present.
5. Treat hypotension with fluids and vasopressors.
6. Treat seizures with diazepam, phenobarbital, or phenytoin.
7. Monitor for cardiovascular toxicity (ECG, vital signs, renal function, electrolytes, CBC).
8. Carbamazepine CANNOT be hemodialyzed out of the body.
9. Hemoperfusion for at least 4 hours WILL remove 50 mg to 2.4 g of carbamazepine in most clients.

Increased. Drug abuse, glossopharyngeal neuralgia, renal failure (increases metabolite 10,11-epoxide), tic douloureux, and trigeminal neuralgia. Drugs include calcium-channel blockers, cimetidine, erythromycin, fluoxetine, influenza vaccine, isoniazid, verapamil, and vigabatrin.

Decreased. Convulsions, epilepsy, and seizures. Drugs include phenobarbital, primidone, and phenytoin.

Description. Carbamazepine (CBZ) is an anticonvulsant, anticholinergic sedative, antidepressant, and muscle relaxant that is used alone or with other anticonvulsants to treat seizures. This drug is metabolized in the liver, with a half-life of 10-30 hours in adults and 8-19 hours in children. Steady-state levels occur in 2-6 days. This drug is affected by circadian rhythm and therefore should be ingested at a consistent time of day. CBZ crosses the placenta and appears in breast milk. For rapid detection, the fluorescence polarization assay method can be used.

Professional Considerations
Consent form NOT required.

Preparation
1. Serum should be drawn before the morning dose is given.
2. Tube: Green topped, red topped, red/gray topped, or gold topped.
3. MAY be drawn during hemodialysis.

Procedure

1. Draw a 7-mL TROUGH venous blood sample.
2. Obtain serial measurements at the same time each day.

Postprocedure Care

1. Reject hemolyzed specimens.

Client and Family Teaching

1. Early toxic signs include fever, sore throat, oral ulcers, easy bruising, unusual bleeding, and joint pain.
2. Levels should be checked weekly x 12 during initiation of therapy and then monthly for 2-3 years.
3. If activated charcoal was given for elevated levels, the client should drink 4-6 glasses of water each day for 2 days to prevent constipation. Activated charcoal will also cause stools to be black for a few days.

Factors That Affect Results

1. Absorption of the drug is enhanced with the eating of food.
2. Therapeutic values should be toward the lower norms when both CBZ and other anticonvulsants are taken.
3. Peak levels occur 2-4 hours after oral dosage.

Other Data

1. Side effects include bone marrow depression, eosinophilia, hepatic dysfunction, and urticaria.
2. CBZ can be responsible for testing positive on a tricyclic antidepressant immunoassay.
3. Serum levels of breast-fed infants are 20% of maternal CBZ values.
4. Antemortem serum concentration of CBZ is not significantly different from whole blood concentrations 72 hours after death.
5. The trade name for CBZ is Tegretol.

Carbohydrate Antigen 19-9

See CA 19-9.

Carbohydrate Antigen 50

See CA 50.

Carbohydrate Antigen 72-4

See CA 72-4.

Carbohydrate Antigen 125

See CA 125.

Carbohydrate Antigen 549

See CA 549.

Carbon-13 or Carbon-14 Urea Breath Test

See Urea Breath Test—Diagnostic.

Carbon Dioxide, Partial Pressure (pCO₂)—Blood

Norm.

		SI Units
Arterial sample	35-45 mm Hg	4.7-6.0 kPa
Panic level	<20 mm Hg	<2.6 kPa
	>70 mm Hg	>9.2 kPa
Arterialized capillary sample (<2 years of age)	26.4-41.2 mm Hg	3.5-5.4 kPa
Venous sample	38-50 mm Hg	5.0-6.7 kPa

Increased. Acute intermittent porphyria, aminoglycoside toxicity, asthma (late stage), brain death, coarctation of the aorta, congestive heart failure, cystic fibrosis, electrolyte disturbance (severe), emphysema, empyema, extubation after coronary artery bypass graft, hyaline membrane disease, hyperemesis, hypothyroidism (severe), hypoventilation (alveolar), metabolic alkalosis, near drowning, pleural effusion, pleurisy, pneumonia, pneumothorax, poisoning, pulmonary edema, pulmonary infection, renal disorders, respiratory acidosis, respiratory failure, shock, tetralogy of Fallot, transposition of the great vessels, and vomiting. Drugs include aldosterone, bicarbonate (HCO_3^-), ethacrynic acid, glucose-insulin-kalium mixture, hydrocortisone, laxatives, metolazone, morphine, prednisone, thiazides, tromethamine, and viomycin.

Decreased. Asthma (early stage), diabetic ketoacidosis, diabetes mellitus, dysrhythmias, epileptic spike waves, fever, high altitude, hyperventilation, metabolic acidosis, respiratory alkalosis, and salicylate intoxication. Drugs include acetazolamide, dimercaprol, dimethadione, methicillin sodium, nitrofurantoin, nitrofurantoin sodium, phenformin, tetracycline, and triamterene.

Description. Carbon dioxide gas present in air and also occurring as a nutritional metabolite is essential to the body's regulation of acid-base buffer system. This test measures the partial pressure exerted by carbon dioxide (pCO_2) dissolved in the blood and reflects the body's ability to produce carbonic acid and the efficiency of lung alveoli to excrete carbon dioxide. Laboratory measurement of pCO_2 assists in differentiating respiratory from metabolic causes of acidosis and alkalosis.

Professional Considerations

Consent form NOT required.

Preparation

1. The client should rest for 30 minutes before specimen collection.
2. Obtain a 22-gauge needle, a green topped tube, a glass syringe, heparin, 2% lidocaine, sterile gauze, and ice.
3. Do NOT draw during hemodialysis.

Procedure

1. Brachial, femoral, and radial arteries are choice sites for obtaining blood specimens. If an arterial site is selected, anesthetize surrounding tissue.
2. Draw a 5-mL anaerobic arterial or mixed venous blood sample into a heparinized, green topped tube or glass syringe.
3. To maintain the blood specimen anaerobically, completely fill syringe or green topped tube with blood. If using a syringe, place the needle in a rubber stopper or apply a rubber cap immediately. Avoid pulling back on the syringe plunger. When using a green topped vacuum tube, remove it from the adapter before removing the needle from the artery or vein and do not remove the stopper from the tube.
4. Place the specimen immediately in an ice bath and send the specimen to the laboratory while maintaining anaerobic integrity.

Postprocedure Care

1. Hold direct pressure over the site for 3-5 minutes.
2. Write the time of collection on the requisition.

Client and Family Teaching

1. Results are normally available within 4 hours.

Factors That Affect Results

1. Reject specimens containing air bubbles, not packed in ice, or received more than 15 minutes after collection. Test results are more accurate if performed within 15-20 minutes after specimen collection.

Other Data

1. The pCO_2 level must be analyzed with consideration given to electrolyte and pH levels.
2. See also Carbon dioxide, Total content—Blood, because pCO_2 is only a measure of the pressure exerted by carbon dioxide present in the blood.

Carbon Dioxide (CO₂) Total Content—Blood

Norm.

		SI Units
Adult	22-30 mEq/L	22-30 mmol/L
	38-50 mm Hg	
Panic level	<15 mEq/L	<15 mmol/L
	>50 mEq/L	>50 mmol/L
Neonates to 2 years	32-44 mm Hg	
Child >2 years	22-26 mEq/L	22-26 mmol/L

Increased. Adrenal cortex hormone imbalance, airway obstruction, alcoholism, aldosteronism, bradycardia, cardiac disorders, emphysema, fat embolism, hypoventilation, metabolic alkalosis, pneumonia, prolonged nasogastric tube drainage, pulmonary dysfunction, pyloric obstruction, renal disorders, respiratory acidosis, respiratory disease, and vomiting (severe). Drugs include antacids, corticotropin, cortisone acetate, mercurial diuretics, sodium bicarbonate, and thiazide diuretics.

Decreased. Alcoholic ketosis, dehydration, diabetic ketoacidosis, diarrhea (severe), drainage of intestinal fluid (gastric suction), head trauma, hepatic disorders, high fever, hyperventilation, lactic acidosis, malabsorption syndrome, metabolic acidosis, renal disorders, renal failure (acute), respiratory alkalosis (compensated), salicylate intoxication, starvation, and uremia. Drugs include acetazolamide, ammonium chloride, aspirin, chlorothiazide diuretics, dimercaprol, methicillin, nitrofurantoin, paraldehyde, and tetracycline.

Description. Carbon dioxide (CO_2) gas is present in air and also occurs as a nutritional metabolite. Total carbon dioxide level reflects the total amount of carbon dioxide in the body (that is, in solution bound to proteins and bound as bicarbonate, carbonate, and carbonic acid) and is a general guide to the body's buffering capacity. Total CO_2 content is a bicarbonate and base solution that is regulated by the kidneys. CO_2 gas is acidic and is regulated by the lungs. Because more than 80% of CO_2 is present in the form of bicarbonate, this test is a good reflection of bicarbonate level. Elevated or decreased levels indicate an acid-base imbalance and are related to hyperventilation or hypoventilation from a variety of causes as well as a metabolic cause. Total CO_2 is generally measured with electrolytes in the SMA-6 test but may be measured alone.

Professional Considerations

Consent form NOT required.

Preparation

1. Tube: Green topped. Obtain a container of ice for the arterial samples.
2. Do not allow the client to clench-unclench the hand before blood drawing.
3. Do NOT draw during hemodialysis.

Procedure

1. Collect the specimen without a tourniquet or quickly after tourniquet application, to prevent stasis.
2. Completely fill a heparinized green topped tube with venous blood to prevent diffusion of CO_2 into the tube. Collect the specimen directly into the tube without exposing to the air.
3. In the newborn, blood may be drawn from the heel, fingertips, or toes.
4. Write the body temperature on the laboratory requisition.

Postprocedure Care
1. Place the arterial sample on ice immediately.
2. Transport the specimen to the laboratory within 15 minutes.

Client and Family Teaching
1. Results are normally available within 4 hours.

Factors That Affect Results
1. Pumping the fist before venipuncture may cause falsely elevated results.

2. High altitudes require a decrease in values of 5 mm Hg/mile (3 mm Hg/km).
3. A clotted sample or air bubbles in the sample invalidate the results.
4. Hyperthermia causes an increased CO_2 level. Values must be corrected for temperature abnormalities.

Other Data
1. See also Carbon dioxide, Partial pressure—Blood.

Carbon Monoxide (CO)—Blood

Norm.

	% of Total Hemoglobin
Rural environment, nonsmoker	0.05-2.5
Heavy smoker	5-10
Acute toxicity	>25
Newborn	10-12

Panic Level Symptoms and Treatment
Symptoms. Symptoms correlate poorly with blood levels. Levels >10% cause dizziness, headache, dyspnea on exertion, and impaired judgment. Levels >30% additionally cause nausea, syncope, tachycardia, tachypnea, and vomiting. Deep coma, convulsions, respiratory failure, and death may occur at levels >50%.

Treatment
NOTE: Treatment choice(s) depend(s) on client's history and condition and episode history.
1. Administer 100% oxygen by high-flow mask until CO level is less than 10%.
2. Provide continuous ECG monitoring.
3. Laboratory work should include arterial blood gas, electrolytes, creatine kinase, and urinalysis. Repeat blood carbon monoxide measurements every 2-4 hours until results are <15%.
4. Treat metabolic acidosis only if pH is <7.15. Acidosis increases the availability of oxygen to the tissues from a right shift in the oxyhemoglobin dissociation curve. Acidosis will resolve as the CO levels normalize.
5. Cerebral edema is possible. Observe for and treat seizures with diazepam,

phenobarbital, or phenytoin. Perform frequent neurologic checks.
6. Use hyperbaric oxygen for severely elevated levels (e.g., >40% or when symptoms continue after 4 hours of treatment) and in all clients who are pregnant.
7. Both hemodialysis and peritoneal dialysis WILL remove carbon monoxide.

Increased. Accidental or intentional inhalation of fumes from combustion of carbon-containing fuels (caused by smoking or exposure to passive smoke, automobile exhaust fumes, or gas-burning appliances).

Decreased. Not clinically significant.

Description. Carbon monoxide (CO) is a chemical asphyxiant found in the fumes of automobile exhaust, improperly functioning furnaces, and defective gas-burning appliances. When inhaled, it combines with the hemoglobin in the red blood cells with an affinity 200 times greater than oxygen. This produces a hemoglobin derivative, carboxyhemoglobin, that is unable to transport or release oxygen throughout the body, resulting in hypoxia. CO induces toxicity according to level and duration of exposure.

Professional Considerations
Consent form NOT required.

Preparation
1. Tube: Lavender topped or green topped.
2. Do NOT draw during hemodialysis.

Procedure
1. If specimen will be tested immediately, draw a 5-10-mL blood sample as soon as

C

possible after exposure. Prevent contamination of the specimen with room air.
2. If specimen will not be tested immediately, draw a specimen as described previously but completely fill a heparinized, green topped tube.

Postprocedure Care
1. Deliver the specimen to the blood gas laboratory immediately.

Client and Family Teaching
1. For accidental inhalation, refer the client or family for crisis intervention.
2. CO cannot be seen, tasted, or smelled. It can be emitted by gas fireplaces; poorly vented gas clothes' dryers; charcoal, wood, gas, or coal stoves; cars; and kerosene heaters. An in-home CO detector is an inexpensive safety essential that can provide early warning of rising levels.

Factors That Affect Results
1. Draw a sample before administering oxygen, if possible.
2. Newborn levels are higher than adult levels because fetal hemoglobin has a higher affinity for CO than does adult hemoglobin.

Other Data
1. The results are most accurate if tested immediately, but the specimen may be stored in the refrigerator for several hours if the tube is completely filled and tightly stoppered.
2. The expired breath carbon monoxide (COHbe) is correlated with clinical severity in carbon monoxide poisoning.
3. An increase in exposure to carbon monoxide during the first trimester may result in a reduction in birth weight.

Carboxyhemoglobin
See **Carbon Monoxide**—Blood.

Carcinoembryonic Antigen (CEA)—Serum

Norm.

		SI Units
Nonsmoker	<3.0 ng/mL	<3.0 mg/L
Smoker	<5.0 ng/mL	<5.0 mg/L

Usage. CEA is a helpful marker in establishing prognosis, determining effectiveness of therapy, and recognizing recurrent disease in clients with adenocarcinoma, especially those arising in the colon or stomach (elevated in 25% of cases). CEA is the marker of choice for monitoring colorectal carcinoma, and levels above 15 ng/ml indicate high-risk clients and the need for adjuvant or neoadjuvant chemotherapy.

Increased. Adenocarcinoma of the colon, rectum, breast cancer metastasis, lung, pancreas, and stomach; bronchitis; cholangitis; cholelithiasis; chronic hepatitis; cirrhosis; COPD; emphysema; hepatocellular carcinoma; inflammatory bowel disease; liver abscess; medullary carcinoma of the thyroid; obstructive jaundice.

Decreased. Not clinically significant.

Description. CEA is a glycoprotein that functions as a homotypic intercellular adhesion molecule that promotes aggregation of human colorectal carcinoma cells. It is likely that CEA facilitates metastasis of colorectal carcinoma cells to the liver and lung. Moderately differentiated tumors usually secrete more CEA than either poorly or well-differentiated tumors. Measurement of the CEA level is useful in establishing prognosis, monitoring effectiveness of therapy, and recognizing recurrent disease. CEA is the marker of choice for monitoring colorectal cancer. High preoperative levels are associated with metastatic disease and poorer prognosis. CEA levels should return to normal 4-6 weeks after surgery, and elevated postoperative levels signal early recurrence or incomplete resection. CEA is measured preoperatively and every 2 months for at least 2 years. Progressive elevations of CEA are often the first evidence of recurrent tumor, many times present 3 to 36 months before clinical symptoms and often before CT-evident lesions. Transient elevations of

CEA may be noticed after chemotherapy or radiation therapy secondary to tumor cell necrosis or membrane damage, permitting the escape of CEA into the circulation. CEA is the most frequently used tumor marker in pleural fluid, where an elevated CEA level is highly suggestive of malignancy but may be elevated in complicated parapneumonic effusions and empyema. An elevated CSF/serum CEA ratio is found in 90% of leptomeningeal cancers. Because the liver is the major site of clearance of CEA, single measurements of CEA may not be useful in clients with liver disease, but progressively rising CEA levels are highly suggestive of disease. CEA levels are obtained by means of an immunoreactive assay using double monoclonal antibodies.

Professional Considerations
Consent form NOT required.

Preparation
1. Tube: Red topped or serum-separator for serum. Lavender topped for plasma.
2. May be drawn during hemodialysis.

Procedure
1. Draw a 4-mL venous blood sample without hemolysis.
2. Specimen may be kept at room temperature or refrigerated for 24 hours but should be frozen if assay not performed within 24 hours after collection.

Postprocedure Care
1. None.

Client and Family Teaching
1. Results are usually available in 1-3 working days.

Factors That Affect Results
1. Hemolysis of specimen.
2. Thawing of frozen specimen.
3. Recently administered isotopes.
4. Specimen not separated within 6 hours of collection.
5. CEA results obtained with a different assay method and different specimen type cannot be used interchangeably. It is recommended that only one assay method and specimen type be used consistently.

Other Data
1. Cells must be separated from the plasma or serum within 6 hours. The specimen is then stable at room temperature for 3 days or in a refrigerator for 1 week.
2. Levels may exceed 10 ng/mL (10 mg/L, SI units) in acute inflammatory disorders and 12 ng/mL (12 mg/L, SI units) in the presence of neoplasm.

Carcinogenic Antigen 15-3
See CA 15-3—Serum.

Cardiac Calcium Scoring (Coronary Artery Calcium Scoring)—Diagnostic

Norm. No evidence of plaque in the coronary arteries.

Calcium Score	Presence of Coronary Artery Plaque	Chance That Heart Disease Is Present	Implication
0	No evidence of plaque	<5% (low)	Look further for non-angina causes of chest pain.
1-10	Minimal evidence of plaque	<10% (low)	Offer CT angiography
11-100	Mild evidence of plaque	Moderate	Offer CT angiography
101-400	Moderate evidence of plaque	Moderate to high	Offer CT angiography
>400	Extensive evidence of plaque	>90% (high)	Offer invasive coronary angiography

C

Usage. Helps assess for the presence of plaque in the coronary arteries in clients with some risk factors for heart disease. This CT scan of the heart can provide an early indication of the presence and severity of heart disease. May also be used to help predict risk of coronary artery disease. Not recommended for use in clients with known heart disease or clients with no risk factors for heart disease. Indicated for clients where there is a low likelihood that their chest pain is caused by angina.

Description. Cardiac calcium scoring is a term used to describe an assessment of the quantity of calcified plaque in the coronary arteries using electron beam tomography (EBT). Because detection of calcium with EBT can be affected by heart motion, newer techniques add the use of multislice computed tomography or the use of ECG-gated multidetector tomography, which helps provide additional accuracy.

Professional Considerations
Consent form NOT required

Risks
While the test is an x-ray, the risk from radiation is minimal.
Contraindications
Pregnancy.

Preparation
1. For clients with atrial fibrillation or tachycardia, a negative inotropic drug may be ordered before the test.
2. Client must disrobe and wear a gown. Remove jewelry present on the client's chest.

Procedure
1. ECG electrodes are applied to monitor heart rate during the test.
2. The client is positioned supine, with his or her head secured and resting on a headrest on a motorized handling table.
3. The client must lie motionless as the table slowly advances through the circular opening of the scanner.
4. The table will slide into the scanner; the scanner may make some noises, which are

normal. The client may be asked to hold his or her breath at times.
5. The test should take between 10 and 30 minutes.

Postprocedure Care
1. None, as this is a noninvasive test.

Client and Family Teaching
1. Do not smoke and avoid caffeine for 4 hours before the test.
2. You must lie motionless during the scan. Because this can be a frightening test, it should be described carefully to the client before he or she enters the CT room.
3. A radiology technician will be in the control room monitoring you closely throughout the scan.
4. Sometimes a medication may need to be given to slow the heart rate if the heart rate is faster than 90 beats per minute.
5. If the scoring is high, the client will need to take steps to lower the risk of heart attack. These can include reducing risk factors such as smoking and high blood pressure, losing weight, and exercising, all of which should be discussed with the health care professional.

Factors That Affect Results
1. Caffeine, smoking, and rapid heart rate reduce the accuracy of the results because they cause motion artifact. Combination scans as described previously can help improve the accuracy of the results when a great deal of motion artifact occurs.
2. False-negative results may occur if the type of coronary artery plaque present has not been present long enough to harden and be detected by the scan.
3. Results indicate only the amount of calcified plaque present, but cannot reveal the stability of the plaque.

Other Data
1. This test should be used in combination with physical examination and other diagnostic tests to determine a client's heart disease status; it is not the definitive test for heart disease and should not be used alone.

Cardiac Catheterization (Angiocardiography, Cardioangiography, and Coronary Angiography)—Diagnostic

Norm. Normal heart anatomy with normal chamber volumes and pressures, normal wall and valve motion, and patent coronary arteries. Normal cardiac output and chamber pressures are listed below:

	Normal Pressures
Cardiac output (CO)	4-8 L/min
Right-Sided Heart Catheterization	
Right atrial (RA)	3-11 mm Hg
Right atrial mean	6 mm Hg
Right ventricular systolic	20-30 mm Hg
Right ventricular end-diastolic	<5 mm Hg
Pulmonary artery systolic (PAS)	20-30 mm Hg
Pulmonary artery end-diastolic pressure (PAEDP)	8-15 mm Hg
Pulmonary artery mean (PAM)	<20 mm Hg
Pulmonary artery wedge pressure (PAWP) or pulmonary capillary wedge pressure (PCWP)	4-12 mm Hg
Left-Sided Heart Catheterization	
Ascending aorta systolic	140 mm Hg
Ascending aorta diastolic	90 mm Hg
Ascending aorta mean	105 mm Hg
Left ventricle (LV) systolic	140 mm Hg
Left ventricular end-diastolic pressure (LVEDP)	8-12 mm Hg
Left atrium mean (LAM)	12 mm Hg

Usage. Identification, documentation, and quantitation of congenital disorders of the heart and diseases and disorders of the greater vessels of the heart; evaluation of cardiac muscle function; evaluation of coronary artery patency; identification of ventricular aneurysms; and identification and quantitation of the severity of acquired or congenital cardiac valve disease. This procedure is safe in morbidly obese clients.

Description. Cardiac catheterization involves passing a catheter through the brachial or femoral artery or antecubital or femoral vein into the left or right side of the heart through the aorta or vena cava, respectively. Angiographic films can be taken after radiopaque dye is injected from the catheter tip. The dye makes it possible to visualize chamber function, valve function, and chamber size. Measurements of oxygen content and pressure and flow rate of blood can be obtained in each chamber, along with the cardiac output and perfusion of the coronary arteries.

Professional Considerations
Consent form IS required.

Risks
Air embolism, allergic reaction to dye (itching, hives, rash, tight feeling in the throat, shortness of breath, bronchospasm, anaphylaxis, death), asystole, cardiac tamponade, cerebrovascular accident (left-sided heart catheterization), congestive heart failure, cerebrovascular accident, dysrhythmias, embolus (left-sided heart catheterization), endocarditis, hematoma, hemorrhage, hemothorax, hypovolemia, infection, myocardial infarction, pneumothorax, pulmonary edema, pulmonary embolism (right-sided heart catheterization), renal toxicity, retroperitoneal bleed, thrombophlebitis (right-sided heart catheterization with antecubital site), thrombus (left-sided heart catheterization), and vagal response (right-sided heart catheterization). This invasive procedure poses a 2% risk of complications.

Contraindications and Precautions
Pregnancy (because of radioactive iodine crossing the blood-placental barrier), severe cardiomyopathy, severe dysrhythmias, uncontrolled congestive heart failure.

This procedure should be performed with extreme caution on clients allergic to local anesthetics, iodine, shellfish, or radiopaque contrast material. Steroids and diphenhydramine should be given before the procedure to these clients.

Preparation

1. See Client and Family Teaching.
2. Routine cardiac medications may be given with a small sip of water.
3. Record the baseline height and weight for the calculation of dye dosage.
4. Sedation is usually prescribed for relaxation, but the client remains awake.
5. Assess peripheral pulses and mark them for easy location.
6. Assess baseline ECG and arterial blood pressure and monitor continuously because of the potential for occurrence of cardiac dysrhythmias during the procedure.
7. Have emergency cardiac medications and emergency equipment readily available.
8. Just before beginning the procedure, take a "time out" to verify the correct client, procedure, and site.

Procedure

1. *Left-sided heart catheterization*: In a cardiac catheterization laboratory under fluoroscopy, a long catheter is inserted through a percutaneously inserted sheath into the brachial or femoral artery retrograde through the aorta into the left ventricle or to the beginning of the coronary arteries. Radiopaque dye is then injected from the catheter tip, and the patency of the coronary arteries (coronary angiography, coronary arteriography, cineangiography, or angiocardiography), left ventricular function (contrast ventriculography), and bicuspid and aortic valve function are assessed and recorded radiographically.
2. *Right-sided heart catheterization*: In a cardiac catheterization laboratory under fluoroscopy, a long catheter is inserted through a percutaneously inserted sheath into an antecubital or femoral vein through the vena cava, right atrium, and right ventricle and into the pulmonary artery. Heart chamber and pulmonary artery pressures may be measured as well as cardiac output, tricuspid and

pulmonary valve function, and right ventricular function. Radiographic films of the procedure are made.

Postprocedure Care

1. Maintain bed rest for 4-6 hours.
2. Apply a pressure dressing to the arterial catheter insertion site and immobilize the extremity for 4-6 hours. A sandbag may be placed over an arterial site. Check the dressing and site for bleeding and hematoma formation along with vital sign and pulse checks. Bed rest and extremity immobilization may be extended in clients receiving heparin.
3. Check vital signs and peripheral pulses, color, skin temperature, and sensation of the procedural extremity every 15 minutes × 4, then every 30 minutes × 2, and then hourly for 8-12 hours. Also check for low back or flank pain, which may indicate a retroperitoneal bleed.
4. Assess for dysrhythmias, chest pain, or symptoms of cardiac tamponade.
5. An analgesic may be prescribed for catheterization site discomfort.
6. Encourage the oral intake of fluids if not contraindicated.
7. Resume diet.

Client and Family Teaching

1. Fast from food for 8 hours and from fluids for 3 hours before the procedure.
2. The procedure lasts 1-3 hours.
3. A momentary warm flush and metallic taste or racing pulse may be experienced when the dye is injected. It is also normal to feel a few skipped beats when the catheter is in the ventricle.
4. If coronary angiography will be performed, you might experience momentary chest pain while the dye is injected into the arteries, but no damage will result.
5. It is important to lie motionless throughout the procedure. Symptoms of more than momentary chest pain should be verbalized immediately.
6. Vital signs, pulse checks, and assessments for pain will be taken after the procedure at frequent intervals.
7. Report any difficulty breathing during and after the procedure.

Factors That Affect Results

1. Atherosclerosis of peripheral vessels prohibits easy passage of the catheter.

Other Data

1. The procedure should be stopped for severe chest pain, neurologic symptoms of a cerebrovascular accident, cardiac dysrhythmias, or hemodynamic changes.
2. Because of the risk of complete coronary artery occlusion from plaque disruption or coronary artery perforation, it is advisable (and legally required in many states) to have backup cardiothoracic surgery availability whenever a cardiac catheterization is performed.
3. African-Americans and females are less likely to be referred for cardiac catheterization (Shire, 2002).
4. Madsen et al (2009) found no correlation between the amount of contrast material used and the incidence of contrast-induced nephropathy.
5. Pre- and post-cath measurement of serum Cystatin C is a predictor of subsequent contrast-induced nephropathy in clients with moderate renal insufficiency (Ishibashi et al, 2010).

Cardiac Enzymes/Isoenzymes (CK, LD, ALT, AST)—Blood

Norm. Results are method dependent and should be compared with the reference values of the laboratory performing the test.

Creatine Kinase (CK)		SI Units
Adult female	<80 U/L	<1.33 mkat/L
Adult male	<90 U/L	<1.50 mkat/L
Newborn	<200 U/L	<3.33 mkat/L

CK Isoenzymes	% of Total CK	Fraction of Total CK
CK_1BB (brain)	0-3	0-0.03
CK_2MB (heart)	0-6	0-0.06
CK_3MM (muscle)	90-97	0.90-0.97

Lactate Dehydrogenase (LD)		SI Units
Wróblewski method 30 degrees C	150-450 U	72-217 IU/L
Adult		
≤60 years	45-90 U/L	45-90 U/L
>60 years	55-102 U/L	55-102 U/L
Child		
Newborn	160-500 U/L	160-500 U/L
Neonate	300-1500 U/L	300-1500 U/L
Infant	100-250 U/L	100-250 U/L
Child	60-170 U/L	60-170 U/L

Lactate Dehydrogenase Isoenzymes (Agarose, Electrophoresis)	% of Total LD	Fraction of Total CK
Fraction LD_1	14-26	0.14-0.26
Fraction LD_2	29-39	0.29-0.39
Fraction LD_3	20-26	0.20-0.26
Fraction LD_4	8-16	0.08-0.16
Fraction LD_5	6-16	0.06-0.16

Aspartate Aminotransferase (AST, SGOT)		SI Units
Adult female		
≤60 years	8-20 U/L	8-20 U/L
>60 years	10-20 U/L	10-20 U/L
Adult male		
≤60 years	8-20 U/L	8-20 U/L
>60 years	11-26 U/L	11-26 U/L
Child		
Newborn	16-72 U/L	16-72 U/L
Infant	15-60 U/L	15-60 U/L

Continued

Aspartate Aminotransferase (AST, SGOT)		SI Units
1 year	16-35 U/L	16-35 U/L
5 years	19-28 U/L	19-28 U/L

Alanine Aminotransferase (ALT, SGPT)		SI Units
Adult female		
≤60 years	8-20 U/L	8-20 U/L
>60 years	7-16 U/L	7-16 U/L
Adult male		
≤60 years	8-20 U/L	8-20 U/L
>60 years	6-24 U/L	6-24 U/L
Children		
Newborn	5-28 U/L	5-28 U/L
Infant	5-28 U/L	5-28 U/L

Increased. Patterns in myocardial infarction are generally as follows:

CK. Total CK levels may be normal in acute myocardial infarction, even when the CK-MB isoenzyme is elevated. CK levels begin rising before LD and AST levels. In general, CK begins rising at 4-8 hours, peaks at 12-24 hours, and returns to baseline level by 3-4 days after the onset of myocardial damage.

CK Isoenzymes. CK_2MB begins rising at 6 hours, peaks at 18 hours, and returns to baseline level by 72 hours after the onset of myocardial damage. CK-MB sub forms are a new test in which results are available within 1 hour.

LD. Total LD levels begin rising at 24 hours, peak at 3-4 days, and return to baseline level in 8-12 days.

LD Isoenzymes. LD_1 peaks with an LD_1:LD_2 ratio inversion 48 hours after onset of damage.

AST. AST initially rises at 6-10 hours, peaks at 12-48 hours, and returns to baseline by 4-6 days after the onset of myocardial damage.

AST/ALT Ratio. ≥3.1, or double that of the baseline level after myocardial damage.

Increases in Selected Other Conditions. Cardiomyopathy (total CK, CK_1BB, CK_2MB, total LD), congestive heart failure (CK_2MB [rare], total LD, AST, ALT), myocardial infarction (total CK, CK_2MB, CK_3MM, total LD, LD_1, LD_2, LD_1:LD_2 inversion, AST [pronounced], ALT [slight], AST/ALT ratio), myocarditis (total CK, CK_2MB), pericarditis (AST), pulmonary infarction (total CK, AST, total LD, LD_2, LD_3), and severe angina (total CK [rare], CK_2MB).

Decreased. See individual test listings. Decreases not applicable for myocardial infarction.

Description. Cardiac enzymes are a group of enzymes released by the heart as a result of myocardial injury. They aid in the differential diagnosis of myocardial infarction from congestive heart failure, pericarditis, pulmonary infarction, angina, and other conditions. CK is an enzyme found in specific body tissues, and lactate dehydrogenase is an enzyme present in many tissues. Both are composed of subcomponent isoenzymes that are released in fairly consistent patterns when myocardial injury occurs. Isoenzyme CK_2MB (found mainly in the heart) is normally absent in the serum but becomes present and increases in a specific pattern when released from damaged myocardial cells. Isoenzymes LD_1 and LD_2 (found mainly in the heart and red blood cells) are normally present in a fairly constant ratio of about 1:2 in the serum but begin rising after myocardial damage until the ratio reverses. Serial levels of CK and LD and isoenzymes of both are evaluated for demonstration of characteristic patterns of rise and fall when differentiating suspected acute myocardial infarction from other disorders that may cause similar symptoms. Serum AST is an enzyme found in several body organs, including large amounts in the heart, but is nonspecific for myocardial injury. It is sometimes compared to serum ALT levels, which are found mainly in the liver, with only small amounts in the heart and other organs. An AST level that rises much more than an ALT level can help identify whether the cause is cardiac injury. See also Creatine kinase—Serum; Lactate dehydrogenase—Blood; Alanine aminotransferase—Serum; and Aspartate aminotransferase—Serum, for discussion of abnormalities from causes other than cardiac.

Professional Considerations
Consent form NOT required.

Preparation
1. Tube: Red topped, red/gray topped, or gold topped.
2. MAY be drawn during hemodialysis.

Procedure
1. Draw a 5-mL venous blood sample without hemolysis.
2. Samples are drawn immediately with suspected myocardial infarction and serially at 12, 24, and 48 hours or every 8 hours for three samples.

Postprocedure Care
1. The serum should be separated and left at room temperature for LD and ALT measurement; the CK serum should be frozen if not tested within 24 hours of specimen collection.

Client and Family Teaching
1. Samples will be drawn in a set sequence to evaluate changes in laboratory results to facilitate the plan of care.

Factors That Affect Results
1. Reject hemolyzed specimens, which invalidate several values.
2. Drugs that may cause falsely elevated LD, AST, and ALT levels include heparin (porcine, bovine). See individual tests for a more detailed listing of drugs that affect the results.
3. Alcohol ingestion within 24 hours of specimen collection causes increased values.
4. If intramuscular injections must be given, they should be given after or at least 1 hour before this test.

Other Data
1. Previous terminology used for aspartate aminotransferase includes serum glutamic-oxaloacetic transaminase (SGOT). Previous terminology for alanine aminotransferase includes serum glutamic-pyruvic transaminase (SGPT) and glutamic-pyruvic transaminase (GPT). Previous terminology used for lactate dehydrogenase includes lactic acid dehydrogenase (LDH).
2. Echocardiography can diagnose ischemic heart disease before a rise in cardiac enzymes is detected.
3. CK-MB sub form results are available within the hour and are very reliable for determining if a person has had an MI. This should replace CK-MB in emergency departments.

Cardiac Natriuretic Hormones

See Natriuretic Peptides, Atrial, Pro-Brain, C-Type—Plasma.

Cardiac Output, Thermodilution—Diagnostic

Norm. 4-8 L/minute.

Usage. Evaluation of hemodynamic instability (heart failure, pulmonary hypertension) and shock states, determination of optimal myocardial function preoperatively by Starling curve, and evaluation of response to fluid administration and inotropic drugs. Cardiac output is performed to determine the amount of blood being propelled forward by the heart.

Description. Cardiac output (CO) is the product of heart rate (HR) and stroke volume (SV). It is the volume of blood ejected from the heart over a period of 1 minute. The determinants of cardiac output are preload, afterload, and heart rate in beats per minute and stroke volume in milliliters per beat ($CO = HR \times SV$). Stroke volume is the volume of blood ejected with each ventricular contraction and is the difference between the volume of the left ventricle at end diastole and the volume remaining in the ventricle at end systole. In an average-sized adult at rest, cardiac output is approximately 4-8 L/min. In diseased states, cardiac output is usually found to be less than normal and may be so low that an adequate blood supply to the body's tissues cannot be delivered. A low cardiac output may be the result of poor filling of the ventricle (reduced preload) or poor forward emptying of the ventricle (increased afterload). Some causes of low resting cardiac output are diminished myocardial function resulting from myocardial infarction, aortic stenosis, arterial hypertension, and cardiomyopathy. The thermodilution method of cardiac output determination measures the change in core temperature in the pulmonary artery before and after injection of a specific quantity of injectate of a known temperature. The change in temperature reflects the cardiac output in an inverse manner and is used to plot a cardiac output/thermodilution curve. A low cardiac output produces a greater change in temperature for a longer period of time than does a high cardiac output.

Professional Considerations

Consent form IS required for insertion of pulmonary artery catheter.

Risks

Pulmonary embolus from dislodgement of clot on catheter. See Pulmonary artery catheterization—Diagnostic for catheter-specific risks and contraindications.

Contraindications

None. Injections should be kept to the minimum volume needed for clients who are fluid overloaded.

Preparation

1. Client must have a pulmonary artery catheter in place.
2. Obtain cardiac output tubing, a 10-mL syringe, and injectate. Also obtain ice if injectate is less than 10 degrees C cooler than the client's core temperature. Iced injectate should also be used for hemodynamically unstable clients and hypothermic clients.
3. Just before beginning the procedure, take a "time out" to verify the correct client, procedure, and site.

Procedure

1. The client may be positioned up to 60 degrees of head-of-bed elevation but should be positioned similarly for each cardiac output measurement. Hemodynamically unstable clients should be positioned supine.
2. Cardiac output is performed through a 2- or 3-lumen pulmonary artery catheter. A 3-lumen catheter contains two lumens that exit into the right atrium for measurements of central venous pressure, cardiac output injection, and fluid infusions and one lumen that exits the pulmonary artery, plus a thermistor at the distal catheter tip in the pulmonary artery for measurement of core blood temperature.
3. A computation constant is selected for the specific injectate temperature and quantity, and the catheter in use is entered into the computer that will calculate cardiac output. The injectate used must be at least 10 degrees C cooler than the client's core temperature for the most accurate thermodilution curve.
4. After the catheter placement has been verified, a bolus of 5 or 10 mL of iced or room-temperature intravenous fluid (D_5W or NS) is injected into the external catheter port that exits into the right atrium. The injection should begin as the client begins exhalation and should be completed within 4 seconds.
5. As the fluid exits into the right atrium, it cools the blood that is in the right atrium. This volume of cooled blood moves into the right ventricle and then into the pulmonary artery.
6. In the pulmonary artery, the catheter thermistor senses the temperature change as the cooled blood passes over it. The thermistor will record a decrease in temperature followed by a gradual return to body temperature as the cold solution flows distally. The resulting temperature change is plotted on a temperature/time curve by the cardiac output computer.
7. Generally, three cardiac output readings are obtained and averaged to calculate cardiac output. However, the procedure may be stopped and the cardiac output calculated if the second measurement is within 10% of the first measurement.

Postprocedure Care

1. Resume slow flush infusion to maintain patency of the cardiac output lumen, if used before injection.

Client and Family Teaching

1. The client will not feel injections.

Factors That Affect Results

1. Too much or too little of injectate solution injected will produce erroneous values.
2. Injection not completed within 4 seconds will produce a falsely high value.
3. If the catheter is kinked, the cardiac output value will be falsely high.
4. If the catheter is not inserted far enough for the cardiac output port to be distal to the tip of the introducer (sheath, Cordis), retrograde injection into the Cordis will produce a falsely high cardiac output.
5. Changes in stroke volume resulting from dysrhythmias or changing heart rates can produce wide variations in serial cardiac output readings.
6. An incorrect catheter computation constant entered into the cardiac output calculation will produce an erroneous value.

Other Data

1. One single duration-controlled injection thermodilution measurement is as accurate as the mean of four phase-controlled measurements.

Cardioangiography

See **Cardiac Catheterization**—Diagnostic.

Cardiopulmonary Sleep Study

See **Polysomnography**—Diagnostic.

Carotene—Serum

Norm.

		SI Units
Adult	50-200 µg/dL	0.793-3.72 µmol/L
	50-300 IU/L	
High	>400 µg /dL	>7.44 µmol/L
Moderately high	300-399 µg /dL	5.58-7.42 µmol/L
Low	≤20 µg /dL	<0.37 µmol/L
Child	40-130 µg/dL	0.74-2.41 µmol/L
Infant	0-40 µg/dL	0.0-0.74 µmol/L

Increased. Amenorrhea, anorexia nervosa, diabetes mellitus, diarrhea, excessive dietary carotene intake, hypercholesterolemia, hyperlipidemia, hypervitaminosis A, hypothyroidism, myxedema, nephritis (chronic), nephrotic syndrome, and pancreatitis.

Decreased. Celiac disease, cystic fibrosis, fever, HIV, infectious hepatitis, jaundice (obstructive), kwashiorkor, liver disease, low-fat diet, malabsorption, pancreatic insufficiency, poor dietary intake, pregnancy, smokers, and steatorrhea. Drugs include contraceptives.

Description. Carotene is a fat-soluble precursor of vitamin A that exists in green and yellow vegetables. A small portion of carotene is absorbed from the intestines and contributes to the yellow serum color. The carotenes include β-Carotene, α-carotene and γ-carotene. β-Carotene from the diet, when reaching the small intestine, is broken down by fats and bile salts into retinal for use by the body; A portion is also stored in the liver until needed by the body. α-carotene is also obtained from the diet, particularly from vegetables that are yellow, orange, or green in color. Because low values indicate poor dietary intake or malabsorption, this test is most commonly used as a screening test for malabsorption syndrome. Carotenemia, or elevated carotene levels, is characterized by yellow skin pigmentation with no scleral color change. The client may also have malaise, itching, or weight loss. The condition is usually benign and treated with changes in diet.

Professional Considerations
Consent form NOT required.

Preparation
1. Tube: Red topped, red/gray topped, or gold topped; and a paper bag.
2. See Client and Family Teaching.

Procedure
1. Draw a 6-mL venous blood sample.
2. Place the specimen in a paper bag or otherwise protect it from light.

Postprocedure Care
1. Transport the specimen to the laboratory for immediate spinning and freezing in a plastic vial until carotene can be measured.
2. If results are low because of poor dietary intake, institute diet teaching.

Client and Family Teaching
1. You may have to eliminate carotene-rich foods for 2-3 days. A high-carotene diet may be prescribed for several days if the test purpose is to evaluate ability to absorb carotene.
2. Fast overnight before sampling.

Factors That Affect Results
1. Reject hemolyzed specimens.
2. Women have higher levels than men.

Other Data
1. This is a nonspecific test. There may be an overlap between carotene levels of normal clients and those with malabsorption syndromes. Dietary intake must be considered when one is interpreting results.
2. Increased intake of beta-carotene by lactating mothers increases the supply of milk beta-carotene to breast-fed infants.
3. High-dose beta-carotene may enhance lung tumorigenesis, thus lowering the risk of lung cancer.

Carotid Doppler
See **Doppler Ultrasonic Flow Studies**—Diagnostic.

Carotid Phonoangiography
See **Color Duplex Ultrasonography**.

CAT Scan
See **Cerebral Computed Tomography**—Diagnostic; **Computed Tomography of the Body**—Diagnostic; **Tomography of Paranasal Sinuses**—Diagnostic.

Catecholamines, Fractionation
See **Catecholamines**—Plasma.

Catecholamines, Fractionation Free
See **Catecholamines**—Plasma.

Catecholamines—Plasma
Norm. Values vary by laboratory.

		SI Units
Fractionation		
Standing		
Epinephrine	0-140 pg/mL	0-762 pmol/L
Norepinephrine	200-1700 pg/mL	1088-9256 pmol/L
Dopamine	0-30 pg/mL	0-163 pmol/L
Supine		
Epinephrine	0-110 pg/mL	0-599 pmol/L
Norepinephrine	70-750 pg/mL	381-4083 pmol/L
Dopamine	0-30 pg/mL	0-163 pmol/L
Fractionation Free		
Total	150-650 pg/mL	886-3843 pmol/L

Increased Epinephrine. Anger, electro-convulsive therapy, exercise (extreme), fear, ganglioblastoma (slight increase), ganglio-neuroma (slight increase), hypoglycemia, hypotension, hypothyroidism, ketoacidosis (diabetic), kidney disease, myocardial infarction (acute), neuroblastoma (slight increase), paragangliomas (slight increase), pheochromocytoma (continuous or intermittent increase), postoperatively, prolonged exposure to cold, shock, stress, thyrotoxicosis, and volume depletion. Drugs include epinephrine bitartrate, epinephrine borate, epinephrine hydrochloride, and ethyl alcohol (ethanol) (in large amounts).

Increased Norepinephrine. Anxiety, burns, exercise (extreme), ganglioblastoma (large increase), ganglioneuroma (large increase), hypoglycemia, hypotension, hypothyroidism, ketoacidosis (diabetic), kidney disease, myasthenia gravis, myocardial infarction (acute), neuroblastoma (large increase), paragangliomas (large increase), pheochromocytoma (slight increase), postoperatively, progressive muscular dystrophy, shock, thyroid disease, thyrotoxicosis, and volume depletion. Drugs include ethyl alcohol (ethanol) (in large amounts) and norepinephrine bitartrate.

Increased Dopamine. Ganglioneuroma and neuroblastoma. Drugs include dopamine hydrochloride.

Increased Catecholamines (Any). Drugs include aspirin, decongestants, sympatho-mimetics, and tricyclic antidepressants.

Decreased Epinephrine. Alzheimer's disease.

Decreased Norepinephrine. Anorexia nervosa, autonomic nervous system dysfunction, and orthostatic hypotension.

Decreased Dopamine. Parkinson's disease.

Decreased Catecholamines (Any). High-altitude exposure. Drugs include barbiturates, clonidine, and reserpine.

Description. The catecholamines (epinephrine, norepinephrine, and dopamine) are found in the adrenal medulla, neurons, and the brain. This test is used to help rule out the presence of catecholamine-secreting tumors such as pheochromocytoma.

Epinephrine is a hormone and neurotransmitter synthesized from tyrosine and secreted after the splanchnic nerve is stimulated because of hypoglycemia, stress, fear, or anger. Epinephrine acts during the body's fight-or-flight response to dilate the bronchioles, increase the heart rate, increase glycogenolysis to provide more glucose for body fuel, and decrease peripheral resistance and blood flow to the skin and kidneys.

Norepinephrine is the predominant catecholamine hormone and neurotransmitter secreted by the adrenal medulla in response to splanchnic nerve stimulation and is also secreted by certain neurons in the peripheral nervous system. Synthesized from dopamine and in the presence of tyramine, norepinephrine acts to increase blood pressure through constriction of the peripheral vasculature, dilate the pupils, and relax the gastrointestinal system. It also functions as an intermediary in epinephrine synthesis.

Dopamine is a neurotransmitter found in the brain, sympathetic ganglia, liver, lungs, intestines, and retina. A product of dopa decarboxylation, dopamine acts to dilate renal arteries, increase the heart rate, and constrict the peripheral vasculature.

In a fractionated test, total catecholamines are differentiated into the portions comprising epinephrine, norepinephrine, and dopamine. Plasma levels reveal the balance between synthesis, release, uptake, catabolism, and excretion of catecholamines. In pheochromocytoma, the tumor secretes increased amounts of catecholamines, causing paroxysmal or persistent hypertension. Therefore, catecholamine levels are most helpful when drawn during or just after a hypertensive episode. Total catecholamine levels exceeding 1000 pg/mL are suggestive of pheochromocytoma, and levels greater than 2000 pg/mL are presumptive of this condition. In normal clients, epinephrine and norepinephrine results should be higher when the clients are standing than when they are supine. Absence of this difference may indicate autonomic nervous system dysfunction.

Professional Considerations
Consent form NOT required.

Preparation
1. See Client and Family Teaching.
2. Insert heparin lock 24 hours before the test.
3. Tubes: Two chilled lavender topped or green topped.
4. Notify laboratory personnel that a specimen for plasma catecholamine levels will be drawn and must be spun and frozen immediately upon arrival in the laboratory.

Procedure
Baseline-level specimens should be collected between 0600 (6 am) and 0800 (8 am) as follows:
1. The client should relax in a recumbent position before the procedure for 40-60 minutes.
2. Withdraw and discard 3 mL of heparin and blood from the heparin lock. Draw a 10-mL venous blood sample from the heparin lock and inject it into a chilled green topped or lavender topped tube, depending on laboratory requirements. Once the specimen is collected, relock the site according to institutional protocol.
3. Follow Postprocedure Care instructions and have the specimen transported to the laboratory immediately.
4. Have the client stand for 10 minutes and draw a second specimen as in step 2 above. Remove or flush the heparin lock according to institutional protocol.

Postprocedure Care
1. Mix the specimen well by gently inverting several times, but avoid agitation. Place the specimen in an ice bath and transport it to the laboratory immediately. Write the body position (supine or standing) and the collection time on the laboratory requisition.

Client and Family Teaching
1. Explain test and guidelines thoroughly, because without the client's compliance the results are unreliable.
2. Do not eat foods high in amines within 48 hours before the test. These foods include avocados, bananas, beer, cheese, chocolate, cocoa, fava beans, grains, tea, vanilla, walnuts, and wine.
3. Do not consume the herb coffee (*Coffea*) within 48 hours before the test.
4. Medications that increase catecholamines may be withheld for 48 hours. Diuretics, antihypertensives, and sympathomimetics (including nonprescriptive cold and allergy medications) must be withheld for 5-14 days.
5. Follow a normal sodium diet for 3 days and fast from food and fluids for 10-12 hours before sampling.
6. Avoid strenuous exercise and tobacco smoking immediately before testing.
7. Evaluate the client's understanding of the importance of following pretest instructions to ensure accuracy of the results.
8. Results may not be available for at least 1 week.

Factors That Affect Results
1. Reject specimens received in the laboratory more than 5 minutes after collection. Plasma catecholamine levels drop quickly if the red blood cells are not separated within 5 minutes of specimen collection. The specimen should be spun in a refrigerated centrifuge or chilled carrier. Plasma should be separated from the red blood cells and frozen upright in a plastic vial at minus 70 degrees C.
2. The trauma of direct venipuncture may increase the amount of catecholamines in the specimen.
3. Stressors such as a cold or hypoglycemia may cause elevated results.
4. The results may be invalid if the client has undergone a radioactive scan within 1 month before specimen collection.

5. The results of this test are unreliable in clients taking ascorbic acid, chloral hydrate, chlorpromazine, decongestants, hydralazine, Isuprel, levodopa, methenamine mandelate, methyldopa, phenothiazines, quinidine, quinine, theophylline, or tricyclic antidepressants.
6. Drugs that may cause falsely elevated results include amphetamines, bronchodilators, isoproterenol hydrochloride, and vasodilators.
7. Drugs that may cause falsely decreased results include anticonvulsants, antidysrhythmics, and barbiturates.

8. A diet high in amines may elevate the results.

Other Data
1. Because plasma catecholamine levels are difficult to measure, urine catecholamine measurements are more often used.
2. This test is often used in conjunction with urinary levels and VMA determinations to diagnose pheochromocytoma or neuroblastoma.
3. The complete analysis may take up to 1 week.

Catecholamines—Urine

Norm.

		SI Units
Random Urine		
Total Catecholamines	0-18 µg/dL	0-103 nmol/dL
Daytime Specimen		
Total Catecholamines	1.4-7.3 µg/day	8-43 nmol/24 hr
24-Hour Urine		
Total Catecholamines	0-135 µg/day	0-796 nmol/24 hr
Panic level	>200 µg/day	>1180 nmol/24 hr
Epinephrine		
Adult	0-15 µg/day	0-82 nmol/24 hr
Children		
1-4 years	0-6 µg/day	0-33 nmol/24 hr
4-10 years	0-10 µg/day	0-55 nmol/24 hr
10-15 years	0.5-20 µg/day	2.7-110 nmol/24 hr
Epinephrine panic level	>50 µg/day	>295 nmol/24 hr
Norepinephrine		
Adult	0-100 µg/day	0-590 nmol/24 hr
Children		
1-4 years	0-29 µg/day	0-170 nmol/24 hr
4-10 years	8-65 µg/day	47-380 nmol/24 hr
10-15 years	15-80 µg/day	89-470 nmol/24 hr
Dopamine		
4 years to adult	65-400 µg/day	384-2364 nmol/24 hr
4 years or less	40-260 µg/day	236-1535 nmol/24 hr

Increased. Adrenocortical adenoma, burns, exercise (strenuous), ganglioneuroma, neuroblastoma, pheochromocytoma, seizures (tonic-clonic epileptic), and other catecholamine-secreting tumors and stress (severe anger, anxiety). Drugs include caffeine, ethyl alcohol (ethanol) (large amounts), reserpine (short-term use), and sympathomimetics.

Decreased. Anorexia nervosa, familial dystonia, and idiopathic orthostatic hypotension. Drugs include guanethidine sulfate, phenothiazines, and reserpine (chronic use).

Description. Catecholamines are a group of hormones that are secreted from the adrenal medulla (epinephrine and

C

norepinephrine) and are also released from nerve endings (epinephrine, norepinephrine, and dopamine). These hormones function in the fight-or-flight response, sympathetic nervous system functioning, blood pressure and hemodynamic controls, and response to stressors. Catecholamines are degraded and excreted by the kidneys and can be measured in random urine samples. In pheochromocytoma, the tumor secretes increased amounts of catecholamines, causing paroxysmal or persistent hypertension. Therefore 24-hour urine catecholamine levels are helpful in detecting paroxysmal secretion that occurs throughout the day and may be missed by random plasma levels.

Professional Considerations
Consent form NOT required.

Preparation
1. Obtain a clean container for random urine.
2. For 24-hour collections, obtain a clean 3-L container to which hydrochloric acid (HCl) preservative has been added.

Procedure
1. *Random collection*: Collect a 50-mL random urine specimen in a clean container.
2. *24-hour collections*:
   a. Discard the first morning urine specimen.
   b. Begin to time a 24-hour urine collection.
   c. Save all the urine voided for 24 hours in a refrigerated 3-L container to which HCl preservative has been added. Include the urine voided at the end of the 24-hour period.
   d. For catheterized clients, keep the drainage bag on ice and empty the urine into the acidified collection container hourly.

Postprocedure Care
1. Compare the urine quantity in the specimen container with the urinary output record for the test. If the specimen contains less urine than was recorded as output, some of the sample may have been discarded, invalidating the test.

2. Document the 24-hour urine quantity on the laboratory requisition.
3. Keep the specimen chilled until testing.

Client and Family Teaching
1. Save all the urine voided in the 24-hour period, and urinate before defecating to avoid loss of urine.

Factors That Affect Results
1. All the urine voided for the 24-hour period must be included to avoid a falsely low result.
2. The client should have a quiet environment and avoid strenuous exercise throughout the specimen collection period.
3. Foods that may cause falsely elevated levels include bananas, beer, cheese, Chianti wines, and walnuts.
4. An herb that may cause falsely elevated levels is coffee (*Coffea*).
5. Hypoglycemia may cause falsely elevated levels.
6. Drugs that may cause unreliable results as a result of interference with the laboratory fluorescence testing method include ampicillin, ampicillin sodium, ascorbic acid, chloral hydrate, epinephrine bitartrate, epinephrine borate, epinephrine hydrochloride, erythromycin, erythromycin ethylsuccinate, hydralazine hydrochloride, methenamine mandelate, methyldopa, methyldopate hydrochloride, niacin, quinidine gluconate, quinidine polygalacturonate, quinidine sulfate, riboflavin, salicylates, tetracyclines, and vitamin B complex.

Other Data
1. A random urine sample may be prescribed just after a hypertensive episode for pheochromocytoma diagnosis.
2. Urine samples are easier to study than plasma catecholamines and so are more frequently used for diagnosis.
3. Determination of urine levels of vanillylmandelic acid (VMA) (urinary metabolite of epinephrine), metanephrine (urinary metabolite of epinephrine and norepinephrine), and homovanillic acid (urinary metabolite of dopamine) is often prescribed with this test.
4. 24-hour urine catecholamines are more reliable than plasma catecholamines.

C

Cathepsin D—Specimen

Norm.

Normal reference range	<30 pmol/mg CP
Borderline positive	30-70 pmol/mg CP
Positive (high-risk)	>70 pmol/mg CP

Increased. Increased total antigen amounts of cathepsin D in breast tissue have been associated with increased disease recurrence, more frequent metastasis, and increased mortality in breast cancer clients; however, measurement of Cathepsin D is not recommended for management of clients with breast cancer, due to insufficient supportive data. Cathepsin D levels are increased in squamous cell carcinoma of the head and neck including laryngeal squamous carcinoma. The presence of cathepsin D in aortic aneurysm walls increases mechanical resistance of arteries.

Decreased. Not clinically significant.

Description. Cathepsin D is an independent prognostic factor associated with high risk for metastasis in breast cancer. It is an estrogen-inducible lysosomal protease that is believed to have a role in tumor invasion and metastasis. The overexpression of cathepsin D is associated with visceral and increased soft-tissue metastases and decreased overall survival. Current thought is that cathepsin D is more of a marker of increased metabolism rather than a specific marker for cancer.

Professional Considerations

Consent NOT required for the test but IS required for the procedure used to obtain the specimen. See the specific procedure for risks and contraindications.

Preparation

1. Obtain biopsy equipment.

Procedure

1. Specimen requirement: 0.5-1.0 g of solid tumor, trimmed of excess fat.
2. The tissue is cut into small pieces and then quick-frozen on dry ice in a cryostat or in liquid nitrogen within 20 minutes of excision.
3. The specimen is placed in a 60-mL biopsy bottle without formalin, with the cap secured.
4. Label the specimen bottle with the client's name, the date collected, and the client's identification number.
5. The tissue must remain frozen.

Postprocedure Care

1. Apply a dry, sterile dressing to the biopsy site.
2. Use a mild analgesic for site tenderness.

Client and Family Teaching

1. Use a mild analgesic for site tenderness.
2. Notify the physician for increased or purulent drainage, redness, or increasing tenderness at the site.
3. This test is investigational.

Factors That Affect Results

1. None found.

Other Data

1. Cathepsin D may be prescribed in combination with other prognostic tests. The test has been recommended for investigative use only and should not be used as a diagnostic procedure without confirmation of the diagnosis by another medically established diagnostic product or procedure.

CBC

See **Complete Blood Count**—Blood.

CBL

See **Vitamin B$_{12}$**—Serum.

CCCT™

See Circulating Tumor Cell Test—Blood

CD4

See Acquired Immune Deficiency Syndrome Evaluation Battery—Diagnostic.

C. difficile Amplified Probe—Stool

Norm. Negative.

Usage. Rapid identification of C. difficile toxin.

Description. A rapid method of identifying the C. difficile toxin using polymerase chain reaction (Goldenberg, 2010) that amplifies the presence of known nucleotides until there are enough copies present to be detectable by standard laboratory methods. This test provides more rapid results than standard enzyme immunoassay testing, and provides higher sensitivity, but comparable specificity. However, it is unclear whether accuracy of results is improved. This test is four times more expensive to perform than standard enzyme immunoassay testing, and evidence is lacking regarding whether the faster speed of obtaining results leads to better clinical outcomes.

Professional Considerations

Consent form NOT required.

Preparation

1. Obtain a dry, sterile stool collection container.

Procedure

1. Obtain a sample of liquid, soft, or formed stool in the collection container. Do not include toilet paper or other materials or liquids in the container.

Postprocedure Care

1. Label the container with the client's name and other pertinent identifiers.
2. Send specimen to the lab for testing.
3. Store the container between 2 and 25 degrees Centigrade. Avoid freezing or heat exposure. May be stored at room temperature for up to 48 hours.

Client and Family Teaching

1. Test may have to be repeated, if negative results are obtained.

Factors That Affect Results

1. This test should be repeated if results are negative, but clinical signs indicate possible infection with C. difficile. Indications include 3 or more unformed stools occurring on consecutive days and occurring within 72 hours of an inpatient admission, and negative testing for enteric pathogens.

Other Data

1. Brand names include "GeneOhm™ *C. diff* assay" (BD Diagnostics), "ProGastro™ Cd assay" (Prodesse Inc.), and "Xpert *C. difficile* assay" (Cepheid).

CDT

See Transferrin, Carbohydrate Deficient—Serum.

CEA

See Carcinoembryonic Antigen—Serum.

Cell Free Fetal DNA

See Amniocentesis and Amniotic Fluid Analysis—Diagnostic Routine Analysis.

C-*erb*-2

See HER-2/*neu* Oncogene—Specimen.

Cerebral Angiography (Cerebral Angiogram)—Diagnostic

Norm. Symmetric pattern of vascular circulation to the brain with no areas of absent vessels. The vessels are smooth, and there are no areas of pooling of the contrast dye (which would indicate bleeding from the vessels or aneurysm).

Usage. Suspected cerebral aneurysm or other cerebral vascular disease such as carotid occlusion in Behçet's disease, Churg-Strauss syndrome, Parry-Romberg syndrome, fistulas, spasms, atherosclerosis, or arteriovenous malformations; tumors of the brain; and work-up for transient ischemic attack or other neurologic signs and symptoms. The need for angiography may be suggested by brain scan findings.

Description. Cerebral angiography is a procedure performed in the radiology department using a special radiographic machine with a rapid biplane cassette changer. It involves a series of radiographic views of the cerebral circulation obtained after intra-arterial injection of a contrast medium and shows the patterns of circulation, any interruptions to circulation, or changes in vessel wall appearance.

Professional Considerations
Consent form IS required.

Risks
Allergy to contrast medium, aphasia, embolus, hematoma, hemiplegia, hemorrhage, infection, loss of consciousness, renal toxicity, transient ischemic attack.
Contraindications
Atherosclerosis; coagulopathy; dehydration; previous allergy to iodine, shellfish, or contrast medium; renal disease; hepatic disease; thyroid disease; during breast-feeding.
Precautions
During pregnancy, risks of cumulative radiation exposure to the fetus from this and other previous or future imaging studies must be weighed against the benefits of the procedure. Risk of exposure to the uterus from cerebral angiography is <10 mrad. Radiation dosage to the fetus decreases as pregnancy progresses.

Preparation
1. See Client and Family Teaching.
2. Have emergency equipment readily available.
3. Remove all jewelry and metal objects (such as hairpins) from the client's head area.
4. Obtain sterile gauze, tape, alcohol or other skin-cleansing agent, arterial catheter, razor, contrast medium, normal saline or heparinized normal saline, syringes, and automatic contrast injector.
5. For clients who are unable to cooperate and especially for children, a general anesthetic may be administered by an anesthesia professional.
6. Just before beginning the procedure, take a "time out" to verify the correct client, procedure, and site.

Procedure
1. The client is placed supine on a special radiographic table.
2. A site for intra-arterial injection is selected and prepared by cleansing of the skin with 70% alcohol or povidone-iodine solution and injection of a local anesthetic.
   a. Carotid artery: The client's neck must be hyperextended by placement of a rolled towel under the shoulders, and the client's head must be immobilized with tape.
   b. Femoral artery: The area must be shaved before cleansing. A long catheter is threaded through the femoral artery to the aortic arch.
   c. Brachial artery: The area may require shaving before cleansing. The brachial artery is the least common injection site. A blood pressure cuff is applied distal to the injection site and inflated

before the injection to prevent contrast medium flow to the lower arm.

3. Needle and catheter placement appropriate to the site is performed by the physician and verified by fluoroscopy.

4. Contrast medium is injected, and the client is carefully observed for signs of an allergic reaction such as hives, flushing, or stridor.

5. A series of radiographs of the head, both anterior and lateral views, are taken during the 5-15 seconds after the injection. Approximately another 6 seconds after the arteries appear, capillary and venous blood flow may be studied by radiographs.

6. The contrast injection may be repeated, and the views varied to complete the study, as indicated by the suspected abnormalities.

7. The artery catheter is kept open with continuous or intermittent flushing or with heparinized normal saline.

Postprocedure Care

1. The catheter is withdrawn and pressure is applied to the artery for at least 15 minutes.

2. Apply a dry, sterile or pressure dressing to the site and observe for bleeding or hematoma formation at the catheter insertion site.

3. Maintain bed rest for 12-24 hours.

4. Assess neurologic status and vital signs hourly for 4 hours and then every 4 hours for 20 hours.

5. For femoral or brachial approaches, immobilize the leg or arm straight for 12 hours. Check color, motion, temperature, sensation, and distal pulses of the immobilized extremity every 15 minutes for 4

hours, then every 30 minutes for 2 hours, then every 1 hour for 4 hours, and then every 4 hours for 12 hours.

6. For the carotid approach, observe for respiratory distress, dysphagia, or hoarseness, which may indicate extravasation of the dye.

7. If general anesthesia was used, continue the assessment of respiratory status and follow institutional protocol for post sedation monitoring. Typical monitoring includes continuous ECG monitoring and pulse oximetry, with continual assessments (every 5-15 minutes) of the airway, vital signs, and neurologic status until the client is lying quietly awake, is breathing independently, and responds appropriately to commands spoken in a normal tone.

Client and Family Teaching

1. Fast from food and fluids for 4-8 hours before the procedure.

2. It is important to lie still for this test. A sensation of burning may be felt because of the injection of the contrast medium, but this feeling lasts for only a few moments.

Factors That Affect Results

1. Head movement during the study obscures the clarity of the radiographs.

2. Radiopaque objects such as earrings obstruct the view of the internal vasculature.

Other Data

1. The femoral artery approach has the advantage of providing visualization of both carotid arteries and both vertebral arteries, extending the study to the supply vessels.

Cerebral Computed Tomography—Diagnostic

Norm. Normal-appearing skull and symmetry and size of cerebral or other brain tissue. Cerebrum appears with black-gray shadings, and bone or other very dense tissues appear white. There is normally no evidence of tumor, high-density to whitish hematoma, edema, or congenital abnormalities such as hydrocephalus.

Usage. Brain tumor (astrocytoma, meningioma, metastatic or primary lesions);

cerebral atrophy or infarction; cerebral edema; cerebrovascular accident (CVA); evaluation of neurologic symptoms; evaluation of effects of surgery, radiation, or chemotherapeutic treatment of intracranial tumors; head injury; hematoma (epidural, subdural); hydrocephalus; subarachnoid hemorrhage and other acute hemorrhage.

Description. Computed tomography (CT) uses special radiographic equipment and computers to produce a series of images (or tomographs) of cross sections of the brain tissues. Images may be "slices" taken of the skull and brain across anteroposterior, horizontal, sagittal, or coronal planes. Although contrast medium may be used, the test is often noninvasive and therefore provides a safe, effective diagnostic tool for the study of tumors of the brain, evaluation of neurologic clinical changes, evaluation of CVA or intracranial bleeds, and assessment of clients with possible head injury for hematoma before symptoms are evident. For evaluation of vascular malformations, high-resolution CT (HRCT) is preferred. HRCT improves upon traditional CT technology by providing optimized spatial resolution of body structures and better differentiation of normal from abnormal blood vessels. For rapid evaluation after stroke symptoms appear, spiral (helical) CT is the preferred method. (See also Computed tomography of the body—Diagnostic for further description of the different types of CT technology available.)

Professional Considerations

Consent form IS required when contrast medium is injected as part of the study.

Risks

Allergic reaction to contrast media (itching, hives, rash, tight feeling in the throat, shortness of breath, bronchospasm, anaphylaxis, death), dehydration, renal toxicity, vomiting.

Contraindications

Claustrophobia; dehydration; severe liver or kidney disease; previous allergy to contrast medium, iodine, or shellfish; pregnancy (relative contraindication); and renal insufficiency if CT with contrast will be performed. Weight >136 kg, or >300 pounds, may exceed the capabilities of some scanners.

Precautions

During pregnancy, risks of cumulative radiation exposure to the fetus from this and other previous or future imaging studies must be weighed against the benefits of the procedure. Although formal limits for client exposure are relative to this risk: benefit comparison, the United States Nuclear Regulatory Commission requires that the cumulative dose equivalent to an embryo/ fetus from occupational exposure not exceed 0.5 rem (5 mSv). Risk of exposure to the uterus from cerebral CT is <10 mrad. Radiation dosage to the fetus decreases as pregnancy progresses.

Preparation

1. Remove all jewelry, hairpins, wigs, or dentures.
2. Establish intravenous access if contrast medium will be used.
3. Have emergency equipment readily available for CT with contrast medium if necessary.
4. Just before beginning the procedure, take a "time out" to verify the correct client, procedure, and site.

Procedure

1. The client is placed on a movable radiographic table in a supine position. The table has a specialized headrest with straps that are positioned to immobilize the head.
2. The table head is moved into a circular CT scanner, which moves around the client's head, taking an extensive series of radiographs at each degree of a 180-degree arch.
3. The automated computer then produces a reconstruction of the images, which shows slices through the skull and the brain.
4. The study may then continue to include intravenous administration of contrast material. A second series of views is completed. The client is observed for rash or respiratory difficulty, which may indicate reaction to the contrast medium. Reactions develop within 30 minutes.

Postprocedure Care

1. None for CT without contrast.
2. For CT with contrast, observe for side effects such as headache, nausea, and vomiting and delayed hypersensitivity reaction.
3. Resume previous diet.

Client and Family Teaching

1. You must lie very still for this test.
2. If a contrast medium will be used, fast from midnight before the test.
3. Results are normally available the same day.
4. Inform CT personnel if you feel claustrophobic in enclosed spaces.

Factors That Affect Results

1. Movement of the client's head interferes with the quality of the films.
2. Metal objects such as jewelry or hairpins interfere with complete visualization.

Other Data

1. Intracerebral hemorrhage is higher among Hispanics as a result of chronic hypertension; therefore cerebral CT should be considered.

Cerebral Near-Infrared Spectroscopy

See Transcranial, Near-Infrared Spectroscopy—Diagnostic.

Cerebrospinal Fluid, Cytology

See Cerebrospinal Fluid, Routine, Culture and Cytology.

Cerebrospinal Fluid, Fungus

See Cerebrospinal Fluid, Routine, Culture and Cytology.

Cerebrospinal Fluid, Glucose—Specimen

Norm. (Fasting) 50%-80% of serum glucose.

		SI Units
Adult	40-80 mg/dL	2.2-4.4 mmol/L
Premature infant	24-63 mg/dL	1.3-3.5 mmol/L
Full-term infant	34-119 mg/dL	1.9-6.6 mmol/L
Child	35-75 mg/dL	1.9-4.1 mmol/L

Increased. Brain tumor, cerebral hemorrhage, cerebral trauma, diabetic coma, hyperglycemia, hypothalamic lesions, increased intracranial pressure, and uremia.

Decreased. Brain abscess, brain tumor, cancer, central nervous system sarcoidosis, choroid plexus tumor, coccidioidomycosis, encephalitis (mumps or herpes simplex origin), glut-1 deficiency syndrome, hypoglycemia, increased intracranial pressure, leukemic infiltration, lupus myelopathy, lymphocytic choriomeningitis, lymphoma, melanomatosis, meningeal carcinomatosis, meningitis (acute pyogenic, aseptic, chemical, cryptococcal, fungal, granulomatous, *Haemophilus influenzae*, pyogenic, rheumatoid, tuberculous, viral), neurosyphilis, rheumatoid arthritis, subarachnoid hemorrhage, toxoplasmosis, and tuberculoma of brain.

Description. Cerebrospinal fluid (CSF) glucose content is related to the blood serum glucose content of 1-4 hours earlier. Most abnormalities result in a decreased CSF glucose level because of increased use of glucose by the pathogenic process. This test is interpreted by comparison of a blood glucose level to a CSF glucose level.

Professional Considerations

Consent form IS required for the lumbar puncture, which is necessary to obtain the specimen. See Lumbar puncture—Diagnostic for procedure risks and contraindications.

Preparation

1. Obtain a lumbar puncture tray, sterile drapes, and 1%-2% lidocaine.
2. Tube: Red topped, red/gray topped, or gold topped.

Procedure

1. Draw a 4-mL blood sample.
2. 3-10 mL of CSF is collected by a physician in sequentially numbered sterile glass tubes through a spinal tap between L3-L4

or L4-L5 or from the ventricles of the brain during special procedures.

Postprocedure Care

1. Transport the specimens to the laboratory immediately. Analysis must be performed on a freshly collected specimen to avoid erroneous results from glycolysis.
2. Refrigerate the CSF if it is not analyzed promptly.

Client and Family Teaching

1. See Lumbar puncture—Diagnostic.

Factors That Affect Results

1. Falsely decreased levels may be caused by cellular and bacterial utilization if the test is not performed immediately.
2. See Lumbar puncture—Diagnostic.

Other Data

1. See Lumbar puncture—Diagnostic.

Cerebrospinal Fluid, Immunoglobulin G (Igg), Immunoglobulin G Ratios and Immunoglobulin G Index, Immunoglobulin G Synthesis Rate—Specimen

Norm.

IgG	0.5-5 mg/dL (5-50 mg/L, SI units), or <12% of CSF total protein
IgG/albumin ratio	22-28% of serum IgG/albumin ratio
IgG index	0.3-0.7
Immunoglobulin G synthesis rate	-9.9 to +3.3 mg/day or 0.0 to 0.8 mg/day

Increased. Brain tissue destruction, Claude's syndrome, CNS infection (chronic), CNS lupus erythematosus, CNS vasculitis, Guillain-Barré syndrome, Landau-Kleffner syndrome, Miller Fischer syndrome, multiple sclerosis, neurosyphilis, and Sjögren's syndrome (primary with CNS involvement).

Decreased Immunoglobulin G. Not applicable.

Decreased Immunoglobulin G Index. Contamination of cerebrospinal fluid (CSF) with blood from spinal tap, intracerebral hemorrhage, or disturbance of the blood-brain barrier.

Decreased Immunoglobulin G Synthesis Rate. Not applicable.

Description. IgG antibodies constitute a portion of immunoglobulin proteins secreted by beta-lymphocytes. They act as antibacterial and antiviral neutralizers of toxins produced by bacteria and viruses by activating phagocytic cells. Although slow to develop, they remain present in CSF long after the bacteria and viruses have disappeared and reappear rapidly on subsequent exposure to the antigens. IgG antibodies are identified by electrophoretic testing of the CSF that separates the protein into its component factors.

The IgG ratio and IgG index help rule out the possibility that blood has entered the CSF, bringing with it increased amounts of IgG antibodies. If this is the case, IgG and albumin will be present in about the same proportion in which they are present in the bloodstream, as evidenced by the IgG/albumin ratio of CSF compared to the IgG/albumin ratio of serum.

The IgG index measures CSF production of IgG by the following formula:

$$\frac{(\text{CSF IgG/CSF albumin})}{(\text{serum IgG/serum albumin})}$$

The elevation of either measure indicates the presence of CNS disease.

The IgG synthesis rate helps rule out the possibility that blood has entered the CSF, bringing with it increased amounts of IgG antibodies. If this is the case, IgG synthesis will be greater in CSF than in serum, indicating the presence of CNS disease. The rate is calculated according to the "formula of Tourtellotte":

IgG synthesis (mg/day) =
$$[(\text{IgG}_{\text{CSF}} - \text{IgG}_{\text{SERUM}}/369) - (\text{Alb}_{\text{CSF}} - \text{Alb}_{\text{SERUM}}/230) \times (\text{IgG}_{\text{SERUM}}/\text{Alb}_{\text{SERUM}})0.43] \times 5$$

Professional Considerations

Consent form IS required for the lumbar puncture, which is necessary to obtain CSF. See Lumbar puncture—Diagnostic for procedure risks and contraindications.

Preparation

1. A CT scan is typically performed to rule out increased intracranial pressure before lumbar puncture in critically ill clients or those with changed mental status.
2. Obtain a lumbar puncture tray, sterile drapes, and 1%-2% lidocaine. See Lumbar puncture—Diagnostic.
3. Tube: Red topped, red/gray topped, or gold topped.

Procedure

1. 3-10 mL of CSF is collected by a physician in sequentially numbered sterile glass tubes through a spinal tap between L3-L4 or L4-L5 or from the ventricles of the brain during special procedures.
2. Draw a 2-mL blood sample for IgG/albumin ratio (also known as IgG/albumin index) and comparison of the serum and CSF IgG.

Postprocedure Care

1. See also Lumbar puncture—Diagnostic.
2. Transport the specimens to the laboratory immediately.

3. Refrigerate the CSF if it is not analyzed promptly.

Client and Family Teaching

1. See Lumbar puncture—Diagnostic.

Factors That Affect Results

1. This test should be performed on tube 2 or higher to lessen the chance of contamination of the specimen with blood from a traumatic spinal tap.
2. The results are invalidated if the client has recently undergone a myelogram.
3. Immunoglobulin G synthesis rate norms vary by laboratory.
4. Protein >100 mg/dL results in yellow-tinged CSF.

Other Data

1. The possibility exists that CSF IgG may be elevated because of leakage of serum into the spinal canal during disruption of the blood-brain barrier. The CSF IgG ratios and IgG index test should be performed to rule out this possibility.
2. The IgG synthesis rate sensitivity is 70%-96%, which is slightly less sensitive and reproducible than the IgG index.
3. In one study, 55% of clients with multiple sclerosis had an elevated IgG synthesis rate.
4. See also Lumbar puncture—Diagnostic.

Cerebrospinal Fluid, Lactic Acid—Specimen

Norm.

	SI Units
9-26 mg/dL	1.13-3.23 mmol/L

Increased. Brain abscess, central nervous system carcinoma, cerebral infarct, cerebral ischemia, cerebral trauma, hydrocephalus, hypotension, increased cerebrospinal fluid (CSF) white blood cells, intracranial hemorrhage, low CSF glucose, meningitis (bacterial, fungal, tuberculous), multiple sclerosis, respiratory alkalosis, and seizures.

Decreased. Not clinically significant.

Description. Elevated CSF lactic acid levels indicate increased glucose utilization and anaerobic metabolism associated with decreased oxygenation of the brain or increased intracranial pressure. This test aids in the differentiation of meningitis and in identification of central nervous system disease processes.

Professional Considerations

Consent form IS required for the lumbar puncture, which is necessary to obtain CSF. See Lumbar puncture—Diagnostic for procedure risks and contraindications.

Preparation

1. A CT scan is typically performed to rule out increased intracranial pressure before the lumbar puncture in critically ill clients or those with changed mental status.
2. See Lumbar puncture—Diagnostic.
3. Obtain a lumbar puncture tray, sterile drapes, and 1%-2% lidocaine.

Procedure

1. 3-10 ml of CSF is collected by a physician in sequentially numbered sterile glass tubes through a spinal tap between L3-L4

or L4-L5 or from the ventricles of the brain during special procedures.

Postprocedure Care

1. See Lumbar puncture—Diagnostic.

Client and Family Teaching

1. See Lumbar puncture—Diagnostic.

Factors That Affect Results

1. Discard the first specimen because it is most likely to be contaminated with blood.

2. Lactic acid determination should be performed on tube 2 or higher to lessen the chance of blood contamination.
3. Refrigerate the CSF if it is not analyzed promptly.

Other Data

1. Cell counts and other chemical and serologic studies may also be performed on this sample.
2. See also Lumbar puncture—Diagnostic.

Cerebrospinal Fluid, Mycobacteria

See Cerebrospinal Fluid, Routine, Culture and Cytology—Specimen.

Cerebrospinal Fluid, Heparin Binding Protein, Myelin Basic Protein, Oligoclonal Bands, Protein, and Protein Electrophoresis—Specimen

Norm.

		SI Units
Heparin-binding Protein	2.4-8.7 ng/mL	2.4-8.7 mg/L
Myelin Basic Protein		
Negative	<4 ng/mL	<4 mg/L
Active demyelination	>6 ng/mL	>6 mg/L
Oligoclonal Bands	Absent	
Total Protein		
Adults		
20-40 years		
Lumbar	15-45 mg/dL	150-450 mg/L
Cisternal	15-25 mg/dL	150-250 mg/L
Ventricular	5-15 mg/dL	50-150 mg/L
40-50 years	20-50 mg/dL	200-500 mg/L
50-60 years	20-55 mg/dL	200-550 mg/L
>60 years	30-60 mg/dL	300-600 mg/L
Children		
Premature infant	400 mg/dL	4000 mg/L
Full-term newborn	20-170 mg/dL	200-1700 mg/L
1-4 weeks	30-150 mg/dL	300-1500 mg/L
4-12 weeks	20-100 mg/dL	200-1000 mg/L
3-6 months	15-50 mg/dL	150-500 mg/L
6 months-10 years	10-30 mg/dL	100-300 mg/L
10-20 years	15-45 mg/dL	150-450 mg/L
Protein Electrophoresis	Fraction of Total CSF Protein	
Prealbumin	2%-7%	0.02-0.07
Albumin	45%-76%	0.45-0.76
Alpha$_1$ globulin	1.1%-7%	0.01-0.07
Alpha$_2$ globulin	3%-12%	0.03-0.12
Beta globulin	7.5%-18%	0.07-0.18
Gamma globulin	3%-13%	0.03-0.13

Increased Heparin-binding Protein. Acute bacterial meningitis (Linder et al, 2011).

Increased Myelin Basic Protein. Cerebral infarcts, demyelinating diseases, and multiple sclerosis (acute).

Increased Oligoclonal Bands. CNS lesions (destructive), CNS lupus erythematosus, CNS vasculitis, diabetes mellitus, Guillain-Barré syndrome, multiple sclerosis, neurosyphilis, panencephalitis (progressive rubella, subacute sclerosing), polyneuropathy, Sjögren's syndrome (primary involving the CNS), and spinal arteriovenous malformation.

Increased Protein. Anesthetics (spinal), arteriosclerosis (cerebral), aseptic meningeal reaction, brain abscess, brain tumor, cerebral aneurysm (ruptured), coccidioidomycosis, cord tumor, diabetic neuropathy, encephalitis (postinfectious), Froin's syndrome, Guillain-Barré syndrome, head trauma (bloody), heavy-metal poisoning, hemorrhage (intracerebral, subarachnoid), herpes zoster, hyperproteinemia, infections (acute, coxsackievirus, echovirus), lead encephalopathy, measles, meningitis (acute pyogenic, bacterial, cryptococcal, fungal, tuberculous, viral), meningoencephalitis (bacterial, mycotic), multiple sclerosis, mumps, myxedema, neuropathy (retrobulbar), poliomyelitis (acute anterior), polyneuritis (ascending), sarcoidosis, syphilis (tabes dorsalis, general paresis, meningovascular), systemic lupus erythematosus, thrombosis (cerebral), and toxoplasmosis (congenital). Drugs that increase cerebrospinal fluid (CSF) protein at toxic levels include ethyl alcohol (ethanol), isopropanol, phenytoin, and phenytoin sodium.

Protein Electrophoresis
Increased Beta Globulin.
Cerebrovascular disease, meningitis (acute), neoplasms.

Increased Gamma Globulin. Multiple sclerosis, neurosyphilis, and subacute sclerosing leukoencephalitis.

Increased IgG. Guillain-Barré syndrome, meningoencephalitis (viral), multiple sclerosis, neurosyphilis, subacute sclerosing panencephalitis, and systemic lupus erythematosus of the CNS.

Decreased Myelin Basic Protein. Not applicable.

Decreased Oligoclonal Bands. Multiple sclerosis.

Decreased Protein. Not applicable.

Description. Myelin basic protein is a part of the myelin protein that composes the sheath surrounding myelinated nerves. The myelin sheath surrounds and insulates nerve axons and functions to speed nerve impulse conduction. In demyelinating diseases, the myelin sheath is broken down, resulting in the release of myelin basic protein into the CSF. The detection of myelin basic protein in CSF aids in the diagnosis and staging of demyelinating diseases.

Oligoclonal bands are identified by means of protein electrophoresis, which separates CSF protein into its component factors. They are present only in certain CNS diseases that cause the normally homogeneous gamma globulin to break up into specific bands called "oligoclonal bands." This signifies the presence of antibodies produced in the CNS. Oligoclonal bands help differentiate CNS diseases that produce similar signs and symptoms.

Elevated CSF protein levels provide a nonspecific indicator of serious disease. Protein levels normally remain constant and are elevated in CSF only during increased tissue catabolism or by a disturbance in the normal capillary impermeability to plasma proteins.

Electrophoretic testing of CSF separates the protein into its component factors. Synthesis of the immunocompetent cells contained in the CNS and small amounts of protein that diffuse from the bloodstream account for the protein content of the CSF. Under normal circumstances, CSF contains minute amounts of protein. Inflammation and infection increase the permeability of blood vessels, allowing all proteins to more easily cross the blood-brain barrier. Certain disease states produce characteristic changes in specific types of CSF protein, such as albumin, alpha globulin, beta globulin, and gamma globulin. Electrophoresis is a measurement of proteins, which under the influence of an electrical field, at a pH of 8.6, separate by charge, size, and shape. This separation produces homogeneous bands that are plotted on specially treated paper.

IgG immunoglobulin is the principal immunoglobulin represented with protein electrophoresis.

Professional Considerations

Consent form IS required for the lumbar puncture, which is necessary to obtain CSF. See Lumbar puncture—Diagnostic for procedure risks and contraindications.

Preparation

1. A CT scan is typically performed to rule out increased intracranial pressure before the lumbar puncture in critically ill clients or those with changed mental status.
2. See Lumbar puncture—Diagnostic.

Procedure

1. 3-10 mL of CSF is collected by a physician in sequentially numbered sterile glass tubes through a spinal tap between L3-L4 or L4-L5 or from the ventricles of the brain during special procedures.

Postprocedure Care

1. Apply a dry sterile dressing over the spinal tap site.
2. See also Lumbar puncture—Diagnostic.
3. Refrigerate the CSF if it is not analyzed promptly.
4. Monitor for headaches, dizziness, or change in level of consciousness.

Client and Family Teaching

1. See also Lumbar puncture—Diagnostic.

Factors That Affect Results

1. Discard the first specimen.
2. Myelin basic protein determination should be performed on tube 2.
3. Cell counts and other chemical and serologic studies may also be performed on this specimen.
4. Transport the specimens to the laboratory immediately. Analysis must be performed promptly on freshly collected specimens to avoid erroneous results from cell lysis and disintegration.
5. Falsely elevated protein levels may result from a traumatic spinal puncture.
6. Drugs that may cause falsely elevated CSF protein results include aspirin, chlorpromazine, phenacetin, salicylates, streptomycin sulfate, and sulfonamides.

Other Data

1. Serum electrophoresis should be performed if oligoclonal bands are found in the CSF. Oligoclonal bands would be considered abnormal only if they are absent in the serum.
2. Protein >100 mg/dL results in yellow-tinged CSF.
3. See also Lumbar puncture—Diagnostic.

Cerebrospinal Fluid, Oligoclonal Bands

See Cerebrospinal Fluid, Myelin Basic Protein, Oligoclonal Bands, Protein, and Protein Electrophoresis—Specimen.

Cerebrospinal Fluid, Protein

See Cerebrospinal Fluid, Myelin Basic Protein, Oligoclonal Bands, Protein, and Protein Electrophoresis—Specimen.

Cerebrospinal Fluid, Protein Electrophoresis

See Cerebrospinal Fluid, Myelin Basic Protein, Oligoclonal Bands, Protein, and Protein Electrophoresis—Specimen.

Cerebrospinal Fluid, Routine—Culture and Cytology

Norm.
Routine Culture. No growth.

Fungus Culture. No growth after several weeks.

Mycobacteria Culture. No growth after 8 weeks.

Cytology. Cerebrospinal fluid free of abnormal cells.

		SI Units
Adults and children	<5 cells/μL	<5 × 10⁶/L
Newborn	<30 cells/μL	<30 × 10⁶/L
Adults		
Neoplastic cells	Negative	Negative
Erythrocytes	<10/μL	<10 × 10⁶/L
Leukocytes	<10/μL	<10 × 10⁶/L
Differential lymphocytes	63%-99%	
Beta-lymphocytes	<4%	
T-lymphocytes	89%-97%	
Monoctyes	3%-37%	
Neutrophils	Absent	
Eosinophils	<5%	
Children		
Neoplastic Cells	Negative	Negative
Erythrocytes		
Newborn	<675/μL	<675 × 10⁶/L
Leukocytes		
Infants	<30/μL	<30 × 10⁶/L
1-4 years	<20/μL	<20 × 10⁶/L
5-20 years	<10/μL	<20 × 10⁶/L

Cytology Usage. Establish the presence of primary or metastatic neoplasm; diagnosis of cryptococcal meningitis, bacterial meningitis, cerebral hemorrhage, brain abscess, encephalitis (postinfection, tick borne), lead encephalopathy, medulloblastoma, neurosyphilis, sarcoidosis (meningeal); and study of CNS changes related to acquired immunodeficiency syndrome.

Positive Routine Culture. CNS infections, encephalitis, meningitis, and sepsis neonatorum.

Negative Routine Culture. Normal finding.

Positive Fungus Culture. Brain abscess, meningitis, and systemic fungal infections.

Negative Fungus Culture. Normal finding.

Positive Mycobacteria Culture. Mycobacterial meningitis. The most common mycobacteria causing human disease are *Mycobacterium asiaticum, M. avium-scrofulaceum* complex, *M. fortuitum, M. haemophilum, M. kansasii, M. leprae, M. malmoense, M. marinum, M. simiae, M. szulgai, M. tuberculosis* complex, *M. ulcerans*, and *M. xenopi*.

Negative Mycobacteria Culture. Normal finding.

Description. This test includes cultures for anaerobic, aerobic, and acid-fast organisms, bacteria, protozoa, fungi, or viruses. A culture of cerebrospinal fluid (CSF) for fungus is performed to detect systemic fungal infections and normally harmless fungi that become pathogenic in the presence of immunosuppressive conditions. Although tentative identification of fungi can be made quickly with staining techniques, a culture of the organism on a special fungal culture medium is required to confirm a diagnosis of a fungal infection. Cell count and cytologic examination (the number and character of cells) are performed to identify the presence of abnormal cells, infective organisms, or variations in the usually low numbers of red and white blood cells. Abnormalities include increases in the numbers of normal cells or the presence of neoplastic cells.

Professional Considerations
Consent form IS required for the lumbar puncture, which is necessary to obtain CSF. See Lumbar puncture—Diagnostic for procedure risks and contraindications.

C

Preparation

1. A CT scan is typically performed to rule out increased intracranial pressure before the lumbar puncture in critically ill clients or those with changed mental status.
2. Hand washing significantly decreases false-positive coagulase negative staphylococcal culture rates.
3. See also Lumbar puncture—Diagnostic.

Procedure

1. 3-10 mL of CSF is collected by a physician in sequentially numbered sterile glass tubes through a spinal tap between L3-L4 or L4-L5 or from the ventricles of the brain during special procedures.

Postprocedure Care

1. Write the specimen source, collection time, current antibiotic or antifungal therapy, and clinical diagnosis on the laboratory requisition.
2. Monitor for headaches, dizziness, or change in level of consciousness.
3. Transport the specimens to microbiology immediately. Analysis must be performed promptly on freshly collected specimens.
4. See also Lumbar puncture—Diagnostic.

Client and Family Teaching

1. See Lumbar puncture—Diagnostic.
2. Growth of fungi may take several weeks.

Factors That Affect Results

1. The results are invalid when the specimen stands over 1 hour at room temperature.

2. Previous radiation, intrathecal therapy, myelogram, or pneumoencephalogram may cause cytologic changes that produce false results.
3. Microbiologic studies should be performed on tube 3 or higher to lessen the chance of skin contamination.
4. At least 5 mL is necessary to detect fungal and mycobacterial infections.

Other Data

1. Glucose and protein determinations may also be performed on this specimen.
2. If CNS infection is strongly suspected but initial cell counts are normal, the test should be repeated a few hours later to detect rising white cell counts.
3. Store CSF for culture in a bacteriologic incubator when not tested promptly.
4. A portion of the sample should be frozen at −20 degrees C when viral meningitis is suspected.
5. For positive CSF cultures, sensitivity = 92%, specificity = 95%, false-positive = 5%, and false-negative = 8%. The results are most accurate when samples are obtained before the initiation of antibiotic therapy.
6. CSF specimens: most common organism for adults is *Cryptococcus* and most common diagnosis for children is medulloblastoma.
7. See also Lumbar puncture—Diagnostic.

Cerebrospinal Fluid, Routine Analysis—Specimen

Norm.

		SI Units
Appearance	Clear, colorless	
Specific gravity	1.006-1.008	1.006-1.008
Opening pressure		
Adults	50-180 mm H_2O	50-180 mm H_2O
Child up to 8 years of age	10-100 mm H_2O	10-100 mm H_2O
Child more than 8 years of age	60-200 mm H_2O	60-200 mm H_2O
pH	7.30-7.40	
AST	0-19 U	
Bicarbonate	22.9 mEq/L	
Calcium	2.1-2.7 mEq/L	1.05-1.35 mmol/L
	4.2-5.4 mg/dL	
Chloride	118-132 mEq/L	118-132 mmol/L
Cholesterol	0.2-0.6 mg/dL	
pCO_2	42-52 mm Hg	
Creatinine	0.4-1.5 mg/dL	

Continued

		SI Units
Glucose (fasting)	40-80 mg/dL	2.2-4.4 mmol/L
Glutamine	6-16 mg/dL	
Iron	1-2 mg/dL	
Lactate	10-18 mg/dL	
LD	1/10 of serum level	
Magnesium	2.0-3.1 mEq/L	
Phosphorus	1.2-2.1 mEq/L	
Potassium	2.7-3.9 mEq/L	0.15-0.45 g/L
Protein	15-45 mg/dL	150-450 mg/L
Sodium	138-154 mEq/L	
Urea	6-28 mg/dL	
Uric acid	0.5-4.5 mg/dL	
WBC	0-10 mg/L	

Increased. Acute anterior poliomyelitis (*protein, WBC*), alcoholism (*pressure [possibly]*), aseptic meningeal reaction (*protein, WBC*), brain abscess (*protein, neutrophils*), brain tumor (*pressure, protein, glucose*), cerebellitis (*protein*), cerebral hemorrhage (*RBC, pressure, protein*), cerebral thrombosis (*protein, lymphocytes*), cerebral trauma (*pressure, glucose*), coccidioidomycosis (*pressure, protein, WBC*), coma (*diabetic*) (*glucose*), cord tumor (*protein, WBC*), diabetes mellitus (*protein*), encephalitis (postinfectious) (*pressure, protein, lymphocytes*), Guillain-Barré (*protein*), head trauma (*pressure, protein*), herpes zoster (*protein, WBC*), infections (*protein*), hyperglycemia (*glucose*), hypothalamic lesions (*glucose*), lead encephalopathy (*pressure, protein, WBC*), leptomeningeal carcinomatosis (*malignant cells*), meningitis (acute pyogenic) (*pressure, protein, neutrophils*), meningitis (aseptic) (*pressure, protein, WBC*), meningitis (cryptococcal, fungal, tuberculous, viral) (*pressure, protein, lymphocytes*), meningoencephalitis (primary amebic) (*pressure, protein, WBC*), measles (*pressure [possibly], protein, WBC*), multiple sclerosis (*protein, lymphocytes*), mumps (*pressure [possibly], protein, WBC*), polyneuritis (*protein, lymphocytes*), pseudotumor cerebri (*pressure*), subarachnoid hemorrhage (*endothelin, pressure, protein*), subdural hematoma (*pressure, protein, lymphocytes*), syphilis (*protein, lymphocytes*), uremia (*pressure, protein, glucose*), and viral infections (coxsackievirus and echovirus) (*neutrophils*).

Decreased. Only decreased glucose is significant. See Cerebrospinal fluid, Glucose—Specimen.

Description. Analysis of cerebrospinal fluid (CSF) components is performed to aid diagnosis of a wide variety of CNS diseases, including infectious and malignant diseases.

Professional Considerations

Consent form IS required for the lumbar puncture, which is necessary to obtain CSF. See Lumbar puncture—Diagnostic for procedure risks and contraindications.

Preparation

1. A CT scan is typically performed to rule out increased intracranial pressure before the lumbar puncture in critically ill clients or those with changed mental status.
2. See Lumbar puncture—Diagnostic.

Procedure

1. 3-10 ml of CSF is collected by a physician in sequentially numbered sterile glass tubes through a spinal tap between L3-L4 or L4-L5 or from the ventricles of the brain during special procedures.

Postprocedure Care

1. Apply a dry sterile dressing over the spinal tap site.
2. See also Lumbar puncture—Diagnostic.
3. Transport specimens to the laboratory immediately.
4. Monitor for headaches, dizziness, or change in level of consciousness.

Client and Family Teaching

1. See Lumbar puncture—Diagnostic.

Factors That Affect Results

1. Discard the first specimen.

2. Cell counts, chemistry, and serology should be performed on tube number 2.
3. Microbiologic studies should be performed on tube 3 or higher to lessen the chance of skin contamination.
4. The analysis must be performed promptly on freshly collected specimens to avoid erroneous results from cell lysis, disintegration, and continued glycolysis.
5. Colored or very cloudy spinal fluid requires additional mixing with 0.5 mL of sterile sodium citrate per 5 mL of CSF to prevent clotting. This item is not applicable if tuberculous meningitis is suspected.

6. Withdraw at least 10.5 mL of CSF to avoid false-negative results for leptomeningeal carcinomatosis.

Other Data

1. Handle specimens cautiously to prevent self-contamination.
2. Refrigerate the CSF if it is not analyzed promptly.
3. Cloudy specimens may be caused by elevated white blood cells. Yellow specimens may be caused by elevated protein. Pink or red specimens may be caused by red blood cells.
4. See also Lumbar puncture—Diagnostic.

Ceruloplasmin (CP)—Serum

Norm.

		SI Units
Adult	14-40 mg/dL	0.93-2.65 µmol/L
Newborn	1-30 mg/dL	0.06-1.99 µmol/L
6-12 months	15-50 mg/dL	0.99-3.31 µmol/L
1-12 years	30-65 mg/dL	1.99-4.30 µmol/L

Increased. Cancer (breast), cardiovascular disease, cirrhosis, diabetes mellitus, epilepsy, hepatitis, infection, myocardial infarction, pregnancy, primary sclerosing cholangitis, rheumatoid arthritis, and thyrotoxicosis. Drugs include oral contraceptives, estrogens, phenytoin (Dilantin), and methadone.

Decreased. Aceruloplasminemia, hepatic disease, Klippel-Trénaunay syndrome, kwashiorkor, malabsorption (such as sprue), meningococcal sepsis, nephrosis, nephrotic syndrome, in early infancy, and Wilson's disease (<23 mg/dL).

Description. Ceruloplasmin is an alpha$_2$-globulin transport protein that transports copper and aids in mobilizing iron stores. It is an acute-phase reactant that becomes elevated during stress, pregnancy, and infection. This test is most often used to aid diagnosis of Wilson's disease, in which subnormal quantities of ceruloplasmin are manufactured by the liver. The resulting tissue deposition of copper causes brain and liver damage.

Professional Considerations
Consent form NOT required.

Preparation

1. Tube: Red topped, red/gray topped, or gold topped.

Procedure

1. Draw a 4-mL blood sample.

Postprocedure Care

1. None.

Client and Family Teaching

1. Results may not be available for several days.

Factors That Affect Results

1. Hemolysis invalidates the results.
2. The results are unreliable in infants under 3 months old.

Other Data

1. The serum level of ceruloplasmin is determined by electrophoresis.

Cervical Culture

Norm. Negative for pathogenic vaginal microorganisms.

Positive. The most common organisms recovered in positive cervical cultures include *Actinomyces, Candida, Chlamydia, Mobiluncus, Gardnerella,* herpes simplex, *Mycoplasma hominis, Neisseria gonorrhoeae, Trichomonas,* and *Ureaplasma urealyticum.*

Description. A cervical culture is included in routine gynecologic examinations or in cases of cervicitis, endometritis, leukorrhea, vaginitis, suspected infection, or rape. A smear is usually included as well. The specimen is obtained by means of a vaginal examination. Although cultures are considered the standard for diagnosis of cervical infections, because of their specificity they are difficult to collect. Newer nucleic acid and antigen/antibody detection methods are becoming available that can detect the organisms in a urine specimen.

Professional Considerations
Consent form NOT required.

Preparation
1. The client must disrobe below the waist.
2. Obtain a speculum, a sterile Culturette, glass slides, two spatuli, potassium hydroxide, and sterile 0.9% saline.

Procedure
1. Position the client in the dorsal lithotomy position and drape for privacy and comfort.
2. Insert a speculum into the vagina and expose the cervix and vaginal walls.
3. Collect exudate from the cervix or vagina or both on a sterile Culturette. The exudate may be expressed from the cervix by being gently pressed between two spatuli. Smear exudate onto two glass slides. Place one slide in the potassium hydroxide fixative and the other in the sterile 0.9% saline.

Postprocedure Care
1. Write the clinical data, specimen source, and any recent antibiotic therapy on the laboratory requisition.
2. Send the specimen to the laboratory within 2 hours. Do not refrigerate the specimen.

Client and Family Teaching
1. Do not douche for 24 hours before the test.
2. Several days may be required for growth in the culture. Empiric therapy is often begun while the client awaits culture results.
3. Instruct the client with a positive culture on the preventive measures appropriate to the grown organism, where applicable.
4. The client with a positive test for a sexually transmitted organism should inform all sexual partners of the infection, return for a follow-up culture 7-10 days after finishing the medication prescribed for the infection, and refrain from sexual activity with another person until negative follow-up cultures are received.

Factors That Affect Results
1. The test must be repeated if the Culturette is contaminated by touching the speculum or walls of the labia or if other contamination occurs during the procedure.
2. If *Actinomyces* is suspected, a special anaerobic culture container with a theocolate broth must be obtained.
3. *Chlamydia* is difficult to culture with this method.

Other Data
1. A fishy odor from a fresh slide treated with potassium hydroxide is a positive indication for *Gardnerella.*
2. Yeast vaginal infections, especially *Candida,* are easily noted microscopically when spores are stained with potassium hydroxide.
3. On saline-treated culture slides, the *Trichomonas* organism has a typical pear shape and flagella.
4. Wet vaginal swab PCR detects more *Chlamydia* and more gonorrhea than routine cervical culture.

Cervical Culture for *Neisseria gonorrhoeae*—Culture

Norm. No *Neisseria gonorrhoeae* is isolated.

Positive. Gonorrheal infection of the female genitalia.

Negative. No infection is detected.

Description. *N. gonorrhoeae* is a pyogenic, gram-negative, oxidase-positive coccus that is an obligate parasite of humans. It is the causative organism of the sexually transmitted infection called "gonorrhea." *N. gonorrhoeae* inhabits the mucous membranes of the genital tract and may also be found in the oral mucosa of clients who have engaged in oral sex with a partner infected with *N. gonorrhoeae*. The symptoms include dysuria, purulent urethral discharge, proctitis, and pharyngitis. Females are often asymptomatic. Left untreated, gonorrhea leads to skin lesions, arthritis, meningitis, and reproductive problems. The cervix is the best site for obtaining accurate culture specimens in females.

Professional Considerations
Consent form NOT required.

Preparation
1. The client should disrobe below the waist.
2. Obtain a special packaged culture swab with culture medium, a speculum, and warm water.

Procedure
1. Place the client in the dorsal lithotomy position.
2. Lubricate the speculum with warm water and insert it into the vagina to expose the cervix.
3. Clean off any mucus with a dry cotton swab.
4. Insert a sterile cotton-tipped swab into the endocervical canal and move the swab from side to side.
5. Hold the swab in place for several seconds and then withdraw it and place it in a special culture medium (Jembec or Mager-Martin).

6. Alternatively, gently compress the cervix between the speculum blades to express exudate onto the swab.
7. Cultures of the throat and the anus may also be taken to test for *N. gonorrhoeae*.

Postprocedure Care
1. Send the specimen to the laboratory immediately. Do not refrigerate the specimen.

Client and Family Teaching
1. Do not douche for 24 hours before the test.
2. Gonorrhea is a reportable disease.
3. If your test is positive, you should inform all your sexual partners of the infection, return for follow-up culture 7-10 days after finishing antibiotics, and refrain from sexual activity with another person until negative follow-up cultures are received.
4. Instruct the client with a positive culture on the preventive measures appropriate to a grown organism, where applicable.

Factors That Affect Results
1. A lubricant gel should not be used.
2. Care must be taken not to contaminate the culture tip by touching the sides of the vagina during the procedure.

Other Data
1. This test is often included in a rape-trauma workup.
2. Women with cervical *N. gonorrhoeae* or cervical *Chlamydia* trachomatis are at high risk for endometriosis.
3. For positive results, the client should also be serologically tested for syphilis.
4. See also *Neisseria gonorrhoeae* smear—Specimen.

Cervical/Vaginal Cytology
See Pap Smear—Diagnostic.

CFTR Mutation
See Cystic Fibrosis CFTR Mutations—Specimen

Chagas' Disease Serologic Test
See Trypanosomiasis Serologic Test—Blood.

Chem-6, -7, -12, -20
See **SMA-6, -7, -12, -20**—Blood.

Chemistry Profile—Blood
Norm.

		SI Units
Albumin (Nephelometric, Colorimetric)		
Adults	3.5-5.5 g/dL	35-55 g/L
>60 years	3.4-4.8 g/dL	34-48 g/L
Average at rest	0.3 g/dL	3 g/L
Alkaline Phosphatase		
Adults		
20-60 years		
Bodansky	2-4 U/dL	10.7-21.5 IU/L
King-Armstrong	4-13 U/dL	28.4-92.3 IU/L
Bessey-Lowrey-Brock	0.8-2.3 U/dL	13.3-38.3 IU/L
Elderly	Slightly higher	
Newborn	1-4 times adult values	
Children: Values remain high until epiphyses close.		
Females		
2-10 years	100-350 U/L	
10-13 years	110-400 U/L	
Males		
2-13 years	100-350 U/L	
13-15 years	125-500 U/L	
Aspartate Aminotransferase		
Adult females		
<60 years	8-20 U/L	8-20 U/L
≥60 years	10-20 U/L	10-20 U/L
Adult males		
<60 years	8-20 U/L	8-20 U/L
≥60 years	11-26 U/L	11-26 U/L
Children		
Newborn	16-72 U/L	16-72 U/L
Infant	15-60 U/L	15-60 U/L
1 year	16-35 U/L	16-35 U/L
5 years	19-28 U/L	19-28 U/L
Bilirubin		
1 month-adult	<1.5 mg/dL	1.7-20.5 μmol/L
Premature infant		
Cord	<2.8 mg/dL	<48 μmol/L
24 hours	1-6 mg/dL	17-103 μmol/L
48 hours	6-8 mg/dL	103-137 μmol/L
3-5 days	10-12 mg/dL	171-205 μmol/L
Full-term infant		
Cord	<2.8 mg/dL	<48 μmol/L
24 hours	2-6 mg/dL	34-103 μmol/L
48 hours	6-7 mg/dL	103-120 μmol/L
3-5 days	4-6 mg/dL	68-103 μmol/L

		SI Units
Calcium		
Adult	4.5-5.5 mEq/L	
	8.2-10.2 mg/dL	2.05-2.5 mmol/L
Child	4.5-5.8 mEq/L	
	9.0-11.5 mg/dL	2.24-2.86 mmol/L
Infant	5.0-6.0 mEq/L	
	8.6-11.2 mg/dL	2.15-2.79 mmol/L
Newborn	3.7-7.0 mEq/L	
	7.0-11.5 mg/dL	1.75-2.87 mmol/L
Panic levels		
Tetany	<7 mg/dL	<1.75 mmol/L
Coma	>12 mg/dL	>2.99 mmol/L
Possible death		
	≤6 mg/dL	=1.50 mmol/L
	≥14 mg/dL	≥3.49 mmol/L
Creatinine		
Jaffe, manual method	0.8-1.5 mg/dL	70-133 μmol/day
Jaffe, kinetic or enzymatic method		
Adults		
Female	0.5-1.1 mg/dL	44-97 μmol/L
Male	0.6-1.2 mg/dL	53-106 μmol/L
Elderly	May be lower	May be lower
Children		
Cord blood	0.6-1.2 mg/dL	53-106 μmol/L
Newborn	0.8-1.4 mg/dL	71-124 μmol/L
Infant	0.7-1.7 mg/dL	62-150 μmol/L
1 year of age, female	≤0.5 mg/dL	≤44 μmol/L
1 year of age, male	≤0.6 mg/dL	≤53 μmol/L
2-3 years, female	≤0.6 mg/dL	≤53 μmol/L
2-3 years, male	≤0.7 mg/dL	≤62 μmol/L
4-7 years, female	≤0.7 mg/dL	≤62 μmol/L
4-7 years, male	≤0.8 mg/dL	≤71 μmol/L
8-10 years, female	≤0.8 mg/dL	≤71 μmol/L
8-10 years, male	≤0.9 mg/dL	≤80 μmol/L
11-12 years, female	≤0.9 mg/dL	≤80 μmol/L
11-12 years, male	≤1.0 mg/dL	≤88 μmol/L
13-17 years, female	≤1.1 mg/dL	≤97 μmol/L
13-17 years, male	≤1.2 mg/dL	≤106 μmol/L
18-20 years, female	≤1.2 mg/dL	≤106 μmol/L
18-20 years, male	≤1.3 mg/dL	≤115 μmol/L
Lactate Dehydrogenase		
Wróblewski method	150-450 U	72-217 IU/L
30 degrees C		
Adult		
<60 years	45-90 U/L	45-90 U/L
≥60 years	55-102 U/L	55-102 U/L
Newborn	160-500 U/L	160-500 U/L
Neonate	300-1500 U/L	300-1500 U/L
Infant	100-250 U/L	100-250 U/L
Child	60-170 U/L	60-170 U/L

Continued

C

		SI Units
Phosphorus		
Adults <60 years	3.0-4.5 mg/dL	0.97-1.45 mmol/L
Females ≥60 years	2.8-4.1 mg/dL	0.90-1.30 mmol/L
Males ≥60 years	2.3-3.7 mg/dL	0.74-1.20 mmol/L
Children		
Cord blood	3.7-8.1 mg/dL	1.19-2.62 mmol/L
Premature infant	5.4-10.9 mg/dL	1.74-3.52 mmol/L
Newborn	3.5-8.6 mg/dL	1.13-2.78 mmol/L
Infant	4.5-6.7 mg/dL	1.45-2.16 mmol/L
Child	4.5-5.5 mg/dL	1.45-1.78 mmol/L
Protein, Total		
Adults	6.0-8.0 g/dL	60-80 g/L
Children		
Premature infant	4.3-7.6 g/dL	43-76 g/L
Newborn	4.6-7.4 g/dL	46-74 g/L
Infant	6.0-6.7 g/dL	60-67 g/L
Child	6.2-8.0 g/dL	62-80 g/L
Urea Nitrogen		
Young Adults (<40 Years)	5-18 mg/dL	1.8-6.5 mmol/L
Adults	5-20 mg/dL	1.8-7.1 mmol/L
Elderly (>60 Years)	8-21 mg/dL	2.9-7.5 mmol/L
Children		
Cord blood	21-40 mg/dL	7.5-14.3 mmol/L
Premature infant, first 7 days	3-25 mg/dL	0.1-0.9 mmol/L
Full-term newborn	4-18 mg/dL	1.4-6.4 mmol/L
Infant	5-18 mg/dL	1.8-6.4 mmol/L
Child	5-18 mg/dL	1.8-6.4 mmol/L
Mild Azotemia	20-50 mg/dL	7.1-17.7 mmol/L
Panic Level	>100 mg/dL	>35.7 mmol/L
Uric Acid		
Adult females	2.4-6.0 mg/dL	143-357 µmol/L
		0.17-0.45 mmol/L
Adult males	3.4-7.0 mg/dL	202-416 µmol/L
		0.21-0.51 mmol/L
Children	2.5-5.5 mg/dL	119-327 µmol/L
		0.15-0.33 mmol/L
Elderly	3.5-8.5 mg/dL	204-550 µmol/L
		0.21-0.51 mmol/L
Panic level	>12 mg/dL	>714 µmol/L

Increased. See individual test listings.

Decreased. See individual test listings.

Description. A chemistry profile is a group of several laboratory tests performed on one blood sample and measured on an automated instrument. It can be performed for routine screening on healthy populations or for the purpose of detecting specific changes for a client. This profile generally includes the following tests: Albumin—Serum; Alkaline phosphatase—Serum; Aspartate aminotransferase—Serum; Bilirubin—Serum; Calcium—Serum; Creatinine—Serum; Lactate dehydrogenase—Blood; Phosphorus—Serum; Protein, Total—Serum; Urea nitrogen—Plasma or serum; and Uric acid—Serum. See individual test listings for individual test descriptions.

Professional Considerations
Consent form NOT required.

Preparation
1. Tube: Red topped, red/gray topped, or gold topped.
2. Do NOT draw during hemodialysis.

Procedure
1. Draw a 5-mL blood sample.

Postprocedure Care
1. None.

Client and Family Teaching
1. See individual test listings.
2. Results are normally available within 24 hours.

Factors That Affect Results
1. Anabolic steroids increase AST, ALT, and CK levels.
2. See individual test listings.

Other Data
1. See individual test listings.

Chest Radiography (Chest X-Ray, CXR)—Diagnostic

Norm. Normal anatomy and no pathologic changes evident.

Usage. Chest radiography may be used as a general screening tool preoperatively or for general physical examinations or may be prescribed for a specific diagnostic purpose. Provides information regarding the anatomic location and abnormalities of the heart, great vessels, lungs, soft tissue of the chest and mediastinum, and the bones. Many types of pulmonary, cardiac, and orthopedic abnormalities may be seen on a chest radiograph, particularly if serial films are available for study. Pulmonary uses include abscess, acute respiratory distress syndrome (ARDS), atelectasis, Bethel myopathy, bronchitis, cystic fibrosis, emphysema, fibrosis bullae, hemothorax, malignancies of the lung, pleural effusion, pneumonia, pneumothorax, pulmonary edema, and tuberculosis calcific changes. Cardiac uses include congestive heart failure and determination of heart size. Uses in the great vessels include abnormalities of aortic arch (calcification), some aneurysms, and transposition. Orthopedic uses include bone tumors, fracture of clavicles, kyphosis, rib fractures, scoliosis, and spinal fractures. General uses include placement of central lines, endotracheal tubes, tracheostomy tubes, chest tubes, nasogastric tubes, pacemaker wires and intra-aortic balloon pumps, foreign bodies, lymph node enlargement, mediastinal changes, and pulmonary artery catheter placement.

Description. X-rays are passed through the chest and react on a special photographic plate. Normally the lungs are radiolucent. Bones and fluid-containing bodies such as the heart, the aorta, and any tumor or infiltrate are denser than the lungs and can be easily visualized. Chest radiographs can be performed with the client standing or sitting upright, during inhalation, and in anteroposterior, posteroanterior, and lateral views. Portable, in-bed, anteroposterior chest radiographs can be performed for clients too ill to transport to the radiology department.

Professional Considerations
Consent form NOT required.

Risks
Fetal teratogenicity, vasovagal response (hypotension, bradycardia) to breath-holding.

Contraindications
Screen the client for contraindications to performing the Valsalva maneuver (recent myocardial infarction, bradycardia). If these conditions are present, teach the client how to hold breath without bearing down.

Precautions
During pregnancy, risks of cumulative radiation exposure to the fetus from this and other previous or future imaging studies must be weighed against the benefits of the procedure. Although formal limits for client exposure are relative to this risk:benefit comparison, the United States Nuclear Regulatory Commission requires that the cumulative dose equivalent to an embryo/fetus from occupational exposure not exceed 0.5 rem (5 mSv). Radiation dosage to the fetus is proportional to the distance of the anatomy studied from the abdomen and decreases as pregnancy progresses. For pregnant clients, consult the radiologist/radiology department to obtain estimated fetal radiation exposure from this procedure.

Preparation

1. Remove from the chest area all jewelry, clothing with snaps, electrocardiographic patches (if not contraindicated), and other metal objects that may interfere with the interpretation of the results.
2. Females should be asked if they are pregnant or if there is any possibility that they may be pregnant.

Procedure

1. The client is positioned sitting or standing upright in front of the x-ray machine, with arms held slightly out from the sides, chest expanded, and shoulders pressed forward. The radiographic film is placed against the anterior chest.
2. For lateral views, the client stands with his or her arms elevated from the shoulders and with the forearms resting on the arm of the radiographic equipment, if necessary. The radiographic film is placed flush against the right or left side of the chest.
3. As the client holds very still and takes in a deep breath and holds it, one or more radiographs are taken.
4. For portable radiographs, the client is positioned sitting in a high-Fowler's position, and the portable x-ray machine is moved into place in front of the chest for the radiographic exposure onto the plate positioned behind the back and chest.

Postprocedure Care

1. Replace the electrocardiographic patches and wires if they have been removed.
2. Return personal belongings to the client and help him or her dress.
3. In the event of usage of a portable x-ray machine, help the client return to a comfortable position.

Client and Family Teaching

1. It is important to breathe in deeply, hold your breath, and remain motionless while the radiograph is taken.
2. A radiograph takes approximately 15 minutes to complete and verify that the images are properly exposed.
3. No restrictions are necessary on food or fluid intake.
4. No sedation is used for this procedure.
5. Views are taken in various positions on the table or chair.

Factors That Affect Results

1. Overall misinterpretation of a chest radiograph can occur because of tumor, post-op changes, massive pulmonary emboli, false ventricular aneurysm and esophageal varices. Knowledge of the client's history is essential to consider.
2. Clothing, jewelry, and metal objects cause shadows on the film.
3. Movement obscures the clarity of the picture.
4. Improper positioning makes radiographs difficult to interpret.
5. Portable radiographs are not as reliable as those performed in radiology departments. The anteroposterior position may cause the heart to appear larger than it is.
6. Overexposure or underexposure results in inadequate visualization.
7. The experience of the physician interpreting the films affects the accuracy of the findings.

Other Data

1. Chest radiography is not suggested as a first-line screening tool for tuberculosis or cancer because of possible dangers from frequent radiographic exposure.
2. Health care workers in areas near frequent usage of x-rays should wear an x-ray badge to track exposure level. They should wear a lead apron when remaining in the room with the client during exposure. For portable radiographs, health care workers should stand at least 5 feet from the x-ray source during exposure.

Chlamydia Culture and Group Titer—Specimen

Norm. No chlamydial inclusions on staining.

<1:8 = Normal titer or less than a fourfold increase in titer between the acute and the convalescent specimen. A fourfold elevation indicates recent infection.

>1:16 = Previous exposure to *Chlamydia*

1:32 in babies = Positive for *Chlamydia trachomatis*

1:16 in adults = Positive for *Chlamydia psittaci*

1:64 in adults = Positive for lymphogranuloma venereum, if clinical symptoms are also present.

Usage. Suspected *Chlamydia psittaci* or *C. trachomatis* infections, including lymphogranuloma venereum or trachoma eye infection. Also used as part of infertility workup.

Description. *Chlamydia* are intracellular parasites with the characteristics of bacteria and of viruses that cause psittacosis, pneumonia, eye infections, and lymphogranuloma venereum. The culture method is more widely used for diagnosis of *C. trachomatis* and the serologic group titer test is more often used for diagnosis of *C. psittaci* (because of danger to laboratory workers of inhalation transmission of the disease). *Chlamydia* group titer uses complement fixation or microimmunofluorescence to measure the amount of IgG antibodies to *Chlamydia*. It is a nonspecific, in vitro, antigen-antibody study that detects previous exposure to *Chlamydia* organisms. *Chlamydia* infection is confirmed by a fourfold increase in serial titers.

Professional Considerations
Consent form NOT required.

Preparation
1. Culture: Obtain sterile cotton-tipped culture swabs, a cytobrush, and a culture medium. If other culture samples are collected, collect this sample last.
2. Where *Chlamydia psittaci* is suspected, health care workers should wear a mask when obtaining a specimen to avoid inhalation of the microorganism.
3. Group titer test: Tube: red topped, red/gray topped, gold topped, or SST.

Procedure
1. Culture: The specimens for culture are obtained by vigorous scraping or swabbing of suspected sites. A cytobrush may be used. Purulent drainage does not provide accurate or adequate results; therefore, remove secretions and discharge from the site prior to obtaining the specimen. Obtaining two specimens is recommended, as *Chlamydia* lives inside normal cells and thus is difficult to diagnose. See Culture, Routine for collection instructions.
2. Serologic titer: Draw a 7-mL blood sample.
   a. For suspected lymphogranuloma venereum, return in 10-14 days to have convalescent sample drawn.
   b. For suspected psittacosis, paired samples are drawn during the acute phase and the convalescent phase 2 to 3 weeks apart.

Postprocedure Care
1. Transport the specimen to the laboratory immediately.

Client and Family Teaching
1. Several days may be required for titer results. Treatment is often started while you await the results. *Chlamydia* is curable with medication.
2. For elevated titer, your sexual partner(s) should subsequently be tested.
3. *Chlamydia trachomatis* infection may cause difficulties with conception in the future and in pregnancy may cause premature labor.

Factors That Affect Results
1. Reject hemolyzed specimens.
2. Serious illness, immune disorders, and immunosuppressive therapy may interfere with antigen-antibody reaction and show false-negative results.
3. Antibiotic therapy may cause false-negative results.
4. Other infections such as brucellosis and Q fever can cause false-positive results.

Other Data
1. *Chlamydia* titer is not used in neonatal infection diagnosis because the mother's autoantibodies to *Chlamydia* are present in the neonate for up to 9 months.
2. Lymphogranuloma venereum begins with a primary lesion characterized by a painless genital papule or ulcer and is followed by rapid swelling of regional lymph nodes, causing unilateral inguinal lymphadenopathy. When systemic, symptoms include a prolonged fever along with myalgias and headache.
3. Clients being evaluated for LGV should also be tested for gonorrhea, HIV, and syphilis, because of the common routes of transmission.
4. Diagnosis of *C. psittaci* should include a record of prior contact with sick birds (parrots) or employment in pet shops. Because laboratory recovery of *C. psittaci* is often difficult, diagnosis is made after a significant rise in the titer of antibodies

directed at the psittacosis-lymphogranu-loma group of *Chlamydia* is detected.

5. If a cough is present in the acute stage, psittacosis is communicable. The client must be placed on respiratory isolation, with close contacts wearing masks for protection. All body discharges must be disinfected.

6. Direct fluorescent test or ELISA on clinical specimens is now preferred over *Chlamydia* antibody titer. See *Chlamydia* screening—Specimen.

Chlamydia Screening—Specimen

Norm. *Chlamydia* Rapid Test: Negative
Direct fluorescent antibody: No *C. trachomatis* visualized
DNA probe: No luminescence
ELISA: No change in color noted
Leukocyte esterase: Negative
Nucleic acid amplification: Negative

Usage. Screening for and diagnosing *C. trachomatis* infection of the urogenital tract.

Description. *Chlamydia* are intracellular parasites with the characteristics of bacteria and of viruses that cause psittacosis, pneumonia, eye infections, and lymphogranuloma venereum. *C. trachomatis* infection in the lower genital tract of women causes mucopurulent cervicitis, and can lead to pelvic inflammatory disease, tubal occlusion, infertility, and, rarely, lymphogranuloma venereum. It can also be passed on to an infant via direct contact with the mother's cervix during birth, and cause neonatal infections such as conjunctivitis and pneumonia. In men, genital tract infection with *Chlamydia* causes urethritis and epididymitis. The tests that are most commonly used for screening and diagnosis of *Chlamydia trachomatis* infections are:

1. *Urine nucleic acid amplification* test, which has the highest sensitivity (82-100% for urine sample), but is expensive.

2. Less sensitive (75%-80%) is an *enzyme linked immunosorbent assay (ELISA)* performed on a cervical or urethral swab, or urine sample.

3. A *DNA probe* from cervical or urethral swabs is more commonly used in inpatient settings for *C. trachomatis* detection.

4. Testing a urine dipstick for *leukocyte esterase* can be used for urethritis in males, but a positive result must be confirmed by any of the more specific tests (see Urinalysis—Urine) because this test is prone to false positive results.

5. *Direct fluorescent antibody (DFA)* testing may also be done on either a cervical or urethral swab or urine sample. DFA is expensive, but has high specificity (~88%) and provides rapid results; thus it can be used to confirm other less specific findings, such as the leukocyte esterase test or ELISA.

6. *Point-of-care Chlamydia testing* is also available, but has lower sensitivity (52%-85%, depending on the brand) than the nucleic acid amplification test and is more expensive. However, compliance with repeat testing is higher because this test can be done at home. It is recommended that women undergoing treatment be re-tested after 3 months to detect re-infection from an infected partner.

Professional Considerations
Consent form NOT required.

Preparation
1. For swabs or brushings, see Culture, Routine.

Procedure
1. Urine sample: Obtain a clean container.
2. For urine collection, wait 1 hour after last void before collecting specimen.

Postprocedure Care
1. For swabs or brushings, see Culture, Routine.
2. For urine sample, collect at least 20 mL of a first-catch urine sample.
3. Refrigerate urine until testing.

Client and Family Teaching
1. *Chlamydia trachomatis* infection may cause difficulties with conception in the future and in pregnancy may cause premature labor.

Factors That Affect Results
1. ELISA is prone to having false-positive results when infection is caused by *Acinetobacter, Escherichia coli, Salmonella,*

Klebsiella, Gardnerella vaginalis, and *Streptococci* group A.
2. Nucleic acid amplification test may be falsely negative if ligase is present in the specimen or if the client is receiving a drug that inhibits DNA polymerase, such as rifampicin or its derivatives, actinomycin, aphidicolin, or novobiocin.

Other Data
1. See also *Chlamydia* culture and group titer—Specimen.

Chloramphenicol—Blood

Norm. Negative.

		SI Units
Therapeutic level	10-25 µg/mL	31-77 µmol/L
Trough level	<5 µg/mL	<15 µmol/L
Gray baby syndrome	40-100 µg/mL	124-309 µmol/L
Panic level	>50 µg/mL	>154 µmol/L

Panic Level Symptoms and Emergency Treatment

Symptoms. Hematopoietic toxicity, including reversible bone marrow suppression and irreversible aplasia, may occur; hemolysis; allergic reaction; and peripheral neuritis.

Treatment
NOTE: Treatment choice(s) depend(s) on client's history and condition and episode history.
1. Monitor closely.
2. Maintain peak serum levels below 25 mg/mL by dose adjustments.
3. Hemodialysis WILL remove the drug.
4. Peritoneal dialysis will NOT remove chloramphenicol.

Usage. Evaluation for appropriate dosing when chloramphenicol is used for treatment of *Chlamydia* or vancomycin-resistant *Enterococcus*, infants with severe anaerobic infections, *Haemophilus influenzae*, meningitis, *Mycoplasma, Rickettsias, Salmonella,* or typhoid fever.

Description. Chloramphenicol is a potent, broad-spectrum, synthetic antibiotic used for gram-negative, gram-positive, and anaerobic microorganisms when other antibiotics cannot be used or are ineffective. It is metabolized by the liver and excreted by the kidneys, with a half-life of 2.5-3.0 hours in clients with normal hepatic and renal function. Chloramphenicol levels, complete blood counts, and reticulocyte levels must be closely monitored during therapy because of the risk of bone marrow depression side effects.

Professional Considerations
Consent form NOT required.

Preparation
1. Tube: Red topped, red/gray topped, gold topped, or green topped or lavender topped.
2. Do NOT draw during hemodialysis.

Procedure
1. Draw a 4-mL blood sample. For a trough level, draw the specimen just before the next dose. For a peak level, draw the specimen 15 minutes after completion of the dose.

Postprocedure Care
1. Send the specimen to the laboratory for immediate separation of test sample. Freeze the sample after separation if not tested immediately.

Client and Family Teaching
1. Results are normally available within 24 hours.

Factors That Affect Results
1. Concurrent use of phenobarbital may reduce chloramphenicol levels.
2. Toxic levels are more likely to occur in clients with impaired renal or hepatic function.
3. Therapeutic levels may last for up to 8 hours after administration.

Other Data
1. Bone marrow suppression is most commonly dose related but may occur up to 2 months after completion of any dose of therapy and be irreversible.

2. Can cause gray baby syndrome in premature infants with impaired hepatic function and in newborns less than 3 weeks old, resulting in cardiovascular collapse and death.
3. Chloramphenicol-resistant bacterial isolates are also resistant to tetracycline.

4. *Streptococcus pneumoniae* and *Streptococcus pyogenes* are resistant to chloramphenicol in 3.9% and 2.2% of clients, respectively, and 26.1% are resistant to enterococci. *Salmonella typhi* and *Salmonella worthington* are also resistant to chloramphenicol.

Chlordiazepoxide (Librium)—Blood

Norm. Negative.

		SI Units
Therapeutic levels	700-1000 ng/mL	2.34-3.34 µmol/L
Panic level	>5000 ng/mL	>16.7 µmol/L

Panic Level Symptoms and Emergency Treatment

Symptoms. Drowsiness, dysarthria, ataxia, and confusion.

Treatment

NOTE: Treatment choice(s) depend(s) on client's history and condition and episode history.
1. Gastric lavage is not recommended, but should be considered if within 1 hour of ingestion and if ingestion of additional lethal substance is suspected. Use warm tap water or 0.9% saline.
2. Administer activated charcoal if within 4 hours of ingestion or if symptoms are present. Repeat as necessary, because benzodiazepines undergo hepatic recirculation.
3. Monitor for central nervous system depression.
4. Protect airway. Support breathing with oxygen and mechanical ventilation, if necessary.
5. Flumazenil is not recommended for routine use in benzodiazepine overdose. Flumazenil has been used as a competitive antagonist to reverse the profound effects of benzodiazepine overdose. Use of flumazenil is contraindicated if concomitant tricyclic antidepressants were taken or in dependence states because of the risk of causing seizures from lowering of the seizure threshold and because it may precipitate symptoms of benzodiazepine withdrawal. Flumazenil may not completely reverse benzodiazepine effects. Close monitoring for re-sedation

is required and repeated doses may be needed.
6. Do NOT use barbiturates.
7. Do NOT induce emesis.
8. Forced diuresis or hemodialysis will NOT remove benzodiazepines to any significant extent. No information was found on whether peritoneal dialysis will remove these drugs.

Usage. Drug abuse, ongoing monitoring for therapeutic dosage, and overdose. Also used in conjunction with clidinium for treatment of acute thrombocytopenic purpura.

Description. Chlordiazepoxide is a mild benzodiazepine used for relief of mild to severe anxiety and tension, withdrawal symptoms of acute alcoholism, preoperative apprehension, and anxiety. It is also used for the short-term treatment of insomnia, acute treatment for seizures, and management of alcohol withdrawal symptoms. Chlordiazepoxide is metabolized by the liver and excreted by the kidneys, with a half-life of 5-30 hours. Overdose may lead to respiratory depression and coma. Levels chronically more than the therapeutic range may cause renal dysfunction. Use is safe during pregnancy and lactation.

Professional Considerations
Consent form NOT required.

Preparation
1. Tube: Red topped, red/gray topped, or gold topped.
2. Do NOT draw during hemodialysis.

Procedure
1. Collect a 3-mL blood sample.

Postprocedure Care
1. None.

Client and Family Teaching
1. For the client who takes chlordiazepoxide regularly, watch for, and call the physician in the event of, early signs of overdose: drowsiness, unsteady gait, or confusion.
2. For an intentional overdose, refer the client and his or her family for crisis intervention.
3. Referrals to appropriate rehabilitation centers and therapeutic community programs should be offered to all addicted clients who may be interested.

4. If activated charcoal was given for elevated levels, the client should drink 4-6 glasses of water each day for 2 days to prevent constipation. The activated charcoal will also cause stools to be black for a few days.

Factors That Affect Results
1. Kidney disease elevates blood levels.

Other Data
1. The drug should be tapered off rather than abruptly withdrawn.
2. The drug is one of the most frequent inappropriately prescribed drugs for the elderly and is associated with an increased risk for injury in the elderly.
3. See also Benzodiazepines—Plasma and urine.

Chloride—Serum

Norm.

		SI Units
Children and adults	95-108 mEq/L	95-108 mmol/L
Premature infants	95-110 mEq/L	95-110 mmol/L
Full-term infants	96-106 mEq/L	96-106 mmol/L
Panic levels	<80 mEq/L	<80 mmol/L
	>115 mEq/L	>115 mmol/L

Panic Level Symptoms and Emergency Treatment
Symptoms. Impaired mentation, hypotension, and cardiac dysrhythmias.

Treatment
Correct the underlying disorder.

Increased. Acidosis (hyperchloremic, nephrotic), alcoholism, alkalosis (respiratory), hyperaldosteronism (primary), anemia, bromism, congestive heart failure, Cushing's disease, dehydration, diabetes insipidus, diarrhea (sodium loss > chloride loss), eating disorders (laxatives), eclampsia, fever, head trauma, hypercorticoadrenalism, hypernatremia, hyperparathyroidism, hyperventilation, hypoproteinemia, intestinal fistula (sodium loss > chloride loss), nephritis (acute), nephrosis, neurogenic hyperventilation, ostomies, prostatic obstruction, renal failure (acute), salicylate intoxication, seawater aspiration (severe),

serum sickness, uremia, ureterosigmoidostomy, and urinary obstruction. Drugs include acetazolamide, ammonium chloride, boracic acid, boric acid, chlorothiazide, cholestyramine, corticosteroids, cyclosporin A, glucocorticoids, guanethidine sulfate, imipenem-cilastatin sodium, methyldopa, oxyphenbutazone, phenylbutazone, saline infusions, sodium bromide, sodium chloride, and spironolactone. Herbal or natural remedies include products containing aristolochic acids (*Akebia* spp., *Aristolochia* spp., *Asarum* spp., birthwort, *Bragantia* spp., *Clematis* spp., *Cocculus* spp., *Diploclisia* spp., Dutchman's pipe, Fang chi, Fang ji, Guang fang ji, Kan-Mokutsu, *Menispermum* spp., Mokutsu, Mu tong, *Sinomenium* spp., and *Stephania* spp.).

Decreased. Acidosis (diabetic, diarrheal, lactic, metabolic, tubular, respiratory), Addison's disease, amyotrophic lateral sclerosis (indication of shorter survival), anesthesia, burns, CNS disorders, cholera, congestive heart failure, diabetic ketoacidosis, diaphoresis, diarrhea (severe), eating disorders (vomiting), edema, emphysema, fasting, fever, freshwater aspiration, heat exhaustion, heavy-metal poisoning, hypertrophic pyloric stenosis, hypokalemia, hyponatremia, hypoventilation, infections (acute), intestinal obstruction, nephritis, paralytic ileus, pneumonia, pyelonephritis (chronic), pyloric obstruction, pyloric stenosis (infants), renal failure (chronic), rickettsial diseases, suction (gastric), syndrome of inappropriate antidiuretic hormone secretion, typhus fever, ulcerative colitis, uremia, vomiting, Waterhouse-Friderichsen syndrome, and water intoxication. Drugs include aldosterone, amiloride hydrochloride, bicarbonate, bumetanide, corticotropin, corticosteroids, dextrose infusions (prolonged), ethacrynic acid, furosemide, mercurial diuretics, prednisolone, prednisolone acetate, prednisolone sodium phosphate, prednisolone tebutate, sodium bicarbonate, spironolactone, triamterene, and thiazide diuretics.

Description. Chloride, a hydrochloric acid salt, is the most abundant body anion in the extracellular fluid. It functions in counterbalancing cations such as sodium and also acts as a buffer during oxygen/carbon dioxide exchange in red blood cells. Chloride also aids in digestion, osmotic pressure, and water balance. It is measured in serum, along with other electrolytes, to evaluate electrolyte acid-base balance.

Professional Considerations
Consent form NOT required.

Preparation
1. Tube: Red topped, red/gray topped, or gold topped.
2. Do NOT draw during hemodialysis.

Procedure
1. Draw the specimen from an extremity that does not have saline infusing into it. Draw a 3-mL blood sample without a tourniquet if possible.
2. The sample may be taken from infants from a capillary heelstick.
3. Do NOT allow the client to clench-unclench the hand before blood drawing.

Postprocedure Care
1. None.

Client and Family Teaching
1. Results are normally available within 4 hours.

Factors That Affect Results
1. Reject hemolyzed specimens.
2. Any condition accompanied by prolonged vomiting or diarrhea will alter levels.
3. Potassium chloride, ammonium chloride, acetazolamide, methyldopa, diazoxide, and bromides may cause falsely elevated results.
4. Drugs such as ethacrynic acid, furosemide, thiazide diuretics, and bicarbonate may lead to decreased levels.

Other Data
1. In respiratory acidosis, chloride excretion is a necessary component of renal compensation.
2. Useful interpretation of the results requires clinical knowledge of the client.

Chloride, Sweat—Specimen

Norm.

		SI Units
Adults	10-70 mEq/L	10-70 mmol/L
Children	5-45 mEq/L	5-45 mmol/L

Increased. Cystic fibrosis (levels >60 mEq/L are indicative of cystic fibrosis in children under 20 years of age). Also Addison's disease, adrenal insufficiency, diabetes insipidus (hereditary nephrogenic), ectodermal dysplasia, fucosidosis, glucose-6-phosphate dehydrogenase deficiency, hypothyroidism, malnutrition, mucopolysaccharidosis, pseudohypoaldosteronism type 1, and renal failure.

Decreased. Hypoaldosteronism and sodium depletion. Drugs include mineralocorticoids.

Description. Chloride is an electrolyte normally excreted in sweat and urine combined chemically with sodium or other cations. It functions in the maintenance of acid-base balance and electrical neutrality of the body. Sweat chloride levels are found to be especially high in children with cystic fibrosis, a genetic disease that affects exocrine gland functioning, including the sweat glands of the skin, which secrete abnormally high levels of sodium, potassium, and chloride electrolytes. Sweat chloride levels are often high in genetic carriers of the cystic fibrosis genome as well. Genetic carriers have one recessive defective gene and one dominant normal gene and have no other manifestations of the disease. This test involves the stimulation of sweat production by iontophoresis, the painless delivery of a small amount of electric current to the skin. Results are considered diagnostic for cystic fibrosis when serial testing on two sequential days produce positive results AND when the client demonstrates at least one clinical sign of cystic fibrosis.

Risks

None.

Contraindications

In clients with dermatitis.

Professional Considerations

Preparation

1. Obtain equipment for the iontophoresis and preweighed gauze or filter paper, sterile water, normal saline, forceps, weighing bottle, tape, plastic, and pilocarpine.

Procedure Gibson-Cooke Technique

1. Wash and dry the right forearm or right thigh with distilled water.
2. Place a small amount of the pilocarpine-soaked gauze on the skin of the area to be studied and attach it to the positive electrode. Place a small amount of the saline-soaked gauze on the skin and attach it to the negative electrode.
3. Deliver 4 mA of current in 15- to 20-second intervals for 5 minutes.
4. Remove and discard the electrodes.
5. Place the preweighed, dry, sterile gauze or filter paper over the pilocarpine gauze site. Cover it with plastic and seal it with waterproof tape.
6. After 30-40 minutes, droplets visible beneath the plastic indicate an adequate accumulation of sweat. At least 100 mg of sweat is preferred.
7. Remove and discard the tape and plastic.
8. Remove the gauze or filter paper with forceps and place it directly into a weighing bottle, seal it tightly, and send it to the laboratory.

Postprocedure Care

1. It is normal for the studied area to remain reddened for several hours.

Client and Family Teaching

1. The test is not painful but does cause a minor tingling sensation.
2. Parents are able to stay with the child during the test to help provide distraction.
3. Skin erythema will fade within 24 hours.
4. If results are positive, refer the clients for genetic counseling.

Factors That Affect Results

1. Improper cleansing of the test area may cause unreliable results.
2. The hands have a higher sweat chloride content than arms or legs and thus should be avoided as a study site.
3. Hot weather could deplete sodium chloride stores and affect the results.
4. Poor or incomplete sealing of the test site could result in falsely increased chloride levels by allowing evaporation of sweat.
5. Falsely low values may occur in clients with edema or hypoproteinemia.
6. Increased levels may be caused by skin rashes or lesions over the testing site.
7. Results are invalid if less than 50 mg of sweat is tested.

Other Data

1. A positive sweat test in itself is not diagnostic of cystic fibrosis. The clinical picture and family history are important considerations.
2. Repetition of both borderline and positive tests is recommended.
3. See also Genetic carrier screening for cystic fibrosis—Blood.
4. The Genetic Information Nondiscrimination Act of 2008 prohibits health plans from using genetic family history or genetic test results from influencing eligibility or premiums for health insurance. It also prohibits employers from using this information to influence decisions about hiring, terminating employment, or employment pay, promotions or privileges.

C

Chloride—Urine

Norm.

		SI Units
24-Hour Urine		
Adult	110-250 mEq/24 hr	110-250 mmol/day
>60 years	95-195 mEq/24 hr	95-195 mmol/day
Spot Urine		
	15-115 mEq/L	15-115 mmol/L
Child		
Infant	2-10 mEq/L	2-10 mmol/L
12 months-6 years	15-40 mEq/L	15-40 mmol/L
6-10 years		
Female	18-74 mEq/L	18-74 mmol/L
Male	36-110 mEq/L	36-110 mmol/L
10-14 years		
Female	36-173 mEq/L	36-173 mmol/L
Male	64-176 mEq/L	64-176 mmol/L

Increased. Cushing's syndrome, dehydration, hypernatremia, salicylate toxicity, syndrome of inappropriate antidiuretic hormone secretion (SIADHS), and starvation. Drugs include chlorothiazide diuretics and mercurial diuretics.

Decreased. Addison's disease, congestive heart failure (prolonged), diaphoresis, diarrhea, emphysema, low-salt diet, malabsorption syndrome, nasogastric suction (prolonged), pyloric obstruction, and renal damage.

Description. Chloride is the most abundant extracellular anion. It is normally excreted by the kidney to help maintain the normal fluid and electrolyte and acid-base balance of the body. The amount of chloride excreted in the urine is an indication of the state of electrolyte balance.

Professional Considerations
Consent form NOT required.

Preparation
1. Obtain a clean 3-L specimen container without preservatives.
2. Write the beginning time of collection on the laboratory requisition and specimen container.

Procedure
1. Discard the first morning urine specimen.
2. Begin to time a 24-hour urine collection.
3. Save all the urine voided for 24 hours in a clean 3-L container without preservatives. Refrigeration is unnecessary. Include the urine voided at the end of the 24-hour period.

Postprocedure Care
1. Compare the urine quantity in the specimen container with the urinary output record for the test. If the specimen contains less urine than what was recorded as output, some of the sample may have been discarded, invalidating the test.
2. Document the quantity of the urine output for the 24-hour collection period on the laboratory requisition.
3. Send the specimen to the laboratory for refrigeration.

Client and Family Teaching
1. Save all the urine voided in the 24-hour period and urinate before defecating to avoid loss of urine. If any urine is accidentally discarded, discard the entire specimen and restart the collection the next day.

Factors That Affect Results
1. All the urine voided for the 24-hour period must be included to avoid a falsely low result.
2. Bromides may cause falsely elevated results.

Other Data
1. Dietary intake should be considered when results are being evaluated. This is a useful test for monitoring the effects of a low-salt diet.
2. Urine chloride levels are more precise than urine sodium levels for differentiating between saline responsiveness and saline-resistant conditions associated with metabolic alkalosis.

Chlorphentermine

See Amphetamines—Blood.

Chlorpromazine

See Phenothiazines—Blood.

Cholangiogram

See Endoscopic Retrograde Cholangiopancreatography—Diagnostic; Intravenous Cholangiography—Diagnostic; Percutaneous Transhepatic Cholangiography—Diagnostic; or T-Tube Cholangiography, Postoperative—Diagnostic.

Cholecystography Radiography

See Gallbladder and Biliary System Ultrasonography—Diagnostic

NOTE: Cholecystography is being replaced by ultrasonography, which is now the diagnostic test of choice, or by MRI/CT in selected situations.

Cholesterol (Total Cholesterol)—Blood

Norm. 100-200 mg/dL.
(NOTE: See Lipid profile—Blood for interpretation of findings related to risk of heart disease.)

Actual Ranges in a Population of Clients Consuming a Typical North American Diet

	Male		Female	
Age	mg/dL	SI Units mmol/L	mg/dL	SI Units mmol/L
Total Cholesterol				
Adult (10% Higher Levels for African-Americans)				
20-24 years	124-218	3.21-5.64	122-216	3.16-5.59
25-29 years	133-244	3.44-6.32	128-222	3.32-5.75
30-34 years	138-254	3.57-6.58	130-230	3.37-5.96
35-39 years	146-270	3.78-6.99	140-242	3.63-6.27
40-44 years	151-268	3.91-6.94	147-252	3.81-6.53
45-49 years	158-276	4.09-7.15	152-265	3.94-6.86
50-54 years	158-277	4.09-7.17	162-285	4.20-7.38
55-59 years	156-276	4.04-7.15	172-300	4.45-7.77
60-64 years	159-276	4.12-7.15	172-297	4.45-7.69
65-69 years	158-274	4.09-7.10	171-303	4.43-7.85
≥70 years	144-265	3.73-6.86	173-280	4.48-7.25
Child				
Cord blood	44-103	1.14-2.66	50-108	1.29-2.79
≤4 years	114-203	2.95-5.25	112-200	2.90-5.18
5-9 years	121-203	3.13-5.25	126-205	3.26-5.30
10-14 years	119-202	3.08-5.23	124-201	3.21-5.20
15-19 years	113-197	2.93-5.10	119-200	3.08-5.18

		SI Units
Cholesterol Esters	60-75% of total	0.60-0.75
	or <210 mg/dL	<5.43 mmol/L
Free Cholesterol	<50 mg/dL	<1.29 mmol/L
LDL:HDL Ratio	<3	<3

Increased Total Cholesterol. Anemia (aplastic), anorexia nervosa, atherosclerosis, bile duct blockage, carbon disulfide occupational exposure as in viscose rayon workers, celiac disease, cholestasis, cirrhosis (biliary), congestive heart failure, coronary heart disease, Cushing's disease, debrancher deficiency, diabetes mellitus (poorly controlled), eclampsia, Forbes' disease, glomerulonephritis, *Helicobacter pylori*, hepatic cholesterol ester storage disease, hepatic phosphorylase deficiency, hypercholesterolemia (idiopathic), hyperlipoproteinemia, hypothyroidism, jaundice (obstructive, cholestatic), leukemia, limit dextrinosis, lipid disorders, lipoidosis, malnutrition (early stages) nephrosis, nephrotic syndrome, Niemann-Pick C disease, obesity, pancreatectomy, pancreatitis (chronic), periodontal pockets, pregnancy, starvation (early), stress, type III glycogen deposition disease, type VI glycogen storage disease, and von Gierke's disease. Drugs include amiodarone, anabolic steroids, androgens, catecholamines, chenodeoxycholic acid, cinchophen, chlorpropamide, corticosteroids (glucogenic), cyclosporin A, diuretics, epinephrine, epinephrine bitartrate, epinephrine borate, epinephrine hydrochloride, epinephrine (racemic), ergocalciferol, isotretinoin, levodopa, miconazole, oral contraceptives, phenytoin, phenytoin sodium, sulfonamides, thiazides.

Decreased Total Cholesterol. Abetalipoproteinemia, acanthocytosis, amylopectinosis, Andersen's disease, anemia (pernicious, hemolytic, hypochromic), Bassen-Kornzweig syndrome, brancher deficiency, cancer, chromium-enriched diet, cirrhosis (Laënnec's, portal), depression, epilepsy, familial lecithin-cholesterol acyltransferase deficiency (absent cholesterol esters), gastric bypass surgery, Gaucher disease, Hansen's disease, hepatic disease, hepatitis (toxic, viral), hyperthyroidism, hypobetalipoproteinemia, infections (severe), intestinal obstruction, jaundice (hepatocellular), leprosy, liver cellular necrosis, malnutrition (later stages), pancreatic carcinoma, porphyria (acute, intermittent), premenstrual time phase, steatorrhea, suicidal behavior, Tangier disease, tuberculosis, type IV glycogen deposition disease, and uremia. Drugs include allopurinol, aminosalicylic acid, androgens, asparaginase, azathioprine, carbutamide, chlorpropamide, chlortetracycline, cholestyramine, clofibrate, clomiphene, colchicine, colestipol, cyproterone acetate, dextrothyroxine, doxazosin, erythromycin, estrogens, fenfluramine, gemfibrozil, glucagon, haloperidol, heparin sodium, hydralazine, interferon, isoniazid, kanamycin, ketoconazole, levothyroxine sodium, lovastatin, MAO inhibitors, neomycin, niacin, orlistat, phenformin, pravastatin, prazosin, probucol, simvastatin, tamoxifen, tetracyclines, thiazides, thyroxine, tolbutamide, trimethadione, and vitamin A. Herbs or natural remedies include *Coccinia indica,* guar gum, *meshasringi* (*Gymnema sylvestre, mesha shringi,* Indian milkweed vine), methi (fenugreek leaves), *tundika.*

Description. Cholesterol is a sterol compound synthesized exogenously in the liver from dietary fats and endogenously within cells. It is present in all body tissues and is a major component of low-density lipoproteins (LDLs), brain and nerve cells, cell membranes, and some gallstones. Hypercholesterolemia, combined with low levels of high-density lipoprotein (HDL), increases the risk for developing arteriosclerotic heart disease. Levels of total cholesterol less than 200 mg/dL (5.17 mmol/L, SI units) are desirable. Levels from 200 to 239 mg/dL (5.17 to 6.18 mmol/L, SI units) are classified as borderline high, and levels greater than 239 mg/dL (>6.18 mmol/L, SI units) are classified as high. Cholesterol levels tend to decrease temporarily with major illness or surgery. Total cholesterol levels are used for screening for hypercholesterolemia. When a full assessment of the risk for heart disease is desired, total cholesterol is measured along with components of the Lipid profile—Blood test.

Professional Considerations
Consent form NOT required.

Preparation
1. See Client and Family Teaching.
2. Tube: Red topped, red/gray topped, or gold topped.
3. Screen the client for the use of herbal preparations or natural remedies such as *dai-saiko-to* (Chinese: *da-chaihu-tang,* "major Bupleurum preparation": mixture of Pinellia, Scutellaria, Zizyphus, ginseng,

licorice, and ginger) and *saiko-ka-ryukotsu-boreito* (Chinese: *chaihu-jia-longgu-mul-itang*, "Bupleurum-with added- dragon bone-oyster-Preparation", composed of Bupleurum, Pinellia, ginger, Scutellaria, Zizyphus, cinnamon, China root fungus [fuling, hoelen, *Poria cocos, P. sclerotium*], Codonopsis, Chinese rhubarb, ginseng, oyster shell, and fossil bone for calcium).

Procedure
1. Leave the tourniquet on for as short a time as possible and no more than 2 minutes.
2. Draw a 4-mL blood sample.

Postprocedure Care
1. Transport the specimen to the laboratory immediately.

Client and Family Teaching
1. Consume a diet containing consistent levels of cholesterol for 3 weeks before this test.
2. If this test is performed as part of a full lipid profile, fast from food and liquids, except for water, for 12-14 hours and from alcohol for 24 hours before the test.
3. The evening meal before the test should be free of high-cholesterol foods and have less than 30% total fat content.
4. Drugs affecting the results should be withheld for 24 hours, whenever possible.
5. Desirable cholesterol levels and risk for coronary heart disease are listed in the test description. These may be used to identify and teach desirable levels to clients.

6. Screen the client for the use of herbal preparations or natural remedies such as *dai-saiko-to* and *saiko-ka-ryukotsuboreito* (see preceding Preparation paragraph).

Factors That Affect Results
1. Reject hemolyzed specimens.
2. Levels may be lower when collected with the client recumbent for 20 minutes or more than in those samples collected when the client is standing erect.
3. Cholesterol levels should always be drawn at the same time of day after the same type of diet the day before, with the client in the same position.
4. Drugs that may cause falsely elevated results include ascorbic acid, bromides, chlorpromazine, corticosteroids, iodides, viomycin, and vitamin A.
5. Drugs that may cause falsely decreased levels include nitrates, nitrites, and propylthiouracil.

Other Data
1. Total cholesterol specimen is stable for 7 days at room temperature when nonhemolyzed.
2. Cholesterol esters convert to free choles-terol when left at room temperature.
3. Chinese herbs or natural remedies (*dai-saiko-to and saiko-ka-ryukotsuboreito*) increase high-density lipoproteins.
4. Statins are the preferred drugs for the treatment of hypercholesterolemia and fibrates for hypertriglyceridemia
5. See also Lipid profile—Blood, Low-density lipoprotein cholesterol—Blood; High-den-sity lipoprotein cholesterol—Blood; Phos-pholipids—Serum; Triglycerides—Blood.

Cholinesterase II
See **Pseudocholinesterase**—Plasma.

Cholinesterase (Pseudo)
See **Pseudocholinesterase**—Plasma.

Chorionic Villi Sampling—Diagnostic

Norm. No detection of chromosome or genetic defects.

Usage. Detection of genetic defects, chro-mosomal abnormalities, and acquired disorders in fetuses in women who are at high risk. Disorders such as beta-glucuronidase deficiency, hemophilia (factor VIII or IX), cystic fibrosis, mental retardation, Down syndrome, chromosome abnormalities, fragile X syndrome, beta-thalassemia, and Duchenne's muscular dystrophy; infections.

Description. Chorionic villi sampling (CVS) consists of extracting a small amount of villous tissue directly from the chorion. This procedure can be performed at about 10 weeks of gestation and does not require in vitro culturing of cells because sufficient numbers are directly available in the extracted tissue. The procedure allows prenatal diagnosis at about 2 months of gestation rather than at nearly 5 months of gestation. This procedure is the method of choice for prenatal diagnosis in the first trimester of pregnancy.

Professional Considerations

Informed consent is recommended for genetic testing.

Risks

Bleeding, hematoma, infection, intrauterine death, spontaneous abortion. Limb reduction defects may occur, possibly caused by vascular accident from decreased perfusion in distal portions of limbs or from thrombosis at the sampling site or from inadvertent amnion puncture resulting in either amniotic bands or loss of amniotic fluid, with subsequent compression and deformity. See also Amniocentesis and amniotic fluid analysis—Diagnostic. CVS involves a slightly higher fetal loss rate than amniocentesis does, with most estimates ranging from 1% to 2%.

Contraindications

Morbid obesity, retroverted uterus with intervening bowel.

Preparation

1. Arrange for a laboratory technician to be present to evaluate the sample on location.
2. Must have complete family history.
3. Provide continuous fetal heart tone monitoring.
4. See Amniocentesis and amniotic fluid analysis—Diagnostic.
5. See Obstetric ultrasonography—Diagnostic.

Procedure

1. Transabdominal CVS:
   a. The client is positioned supine.
   b. Under ultrasonic guidance, a long 20-gauge needle is inserted percutaneously through the abdomen into villous tissue.
2. Transcervical CVS:
   a. The client is placed in dorsal lithotomy position.
   b. Under ultrasonic guidance, a malleable catheter is inserted through the cervix into villous tissue.
   c. The perineum, vagina, and cervix are prepared with antiseptic solution.
   d. A sterile speculum is placed into the vagina to allow visualization of the cervix.
   e. The catheter is advanced through the cervix into the chorion frondosum under ultrasonic guidance.

Postprocedure Care

1. Suggest maternal serum alphafetoprotein (MSAFP) screening at 15-20 weeks of gestation.
2. See Amniocentesis and amniotic fluid analysis—Diagnostic.
3. See Obstetric ultrasonography—Diagnostic.

Client and Family Teaching

1. The advantage of CVS, as opposed to amniocentesis, is earlier diagnosis of genetic defects.
2. Explore the couple's expectations and review the risks and limitations of the test.
3. Refer the client with abnormal results for genetic counseling. Refer to section in this book on "Informed Consent for Genetic Testing".

Factors That Affect Results

1. Specimens not large enough invalidate the results.
2. Specimens not labeled invalidate the results.

Other Data

1. CVS is not indicated if neural tube defect is suspected.
2. The Genetic Information Nondiscrimination Act of 2008 prohibits health plans from using genetic family history or genetic test results from influencing

eligibility or premiums for health insurance. It also prohibits employers from using this information to influence decisions about hiring, terminating employment, or employment pay, promotions or privileges.

3. See also Amniocentesis and amniotic fluid analysis—Diagnostic.

Christmas Factor

See Factor IX—Blood.

Chromium—Serum

Norm. <2.1 µg/L.

Increased. Chromium toxicity, hypocholesterolemia, clients with metal or ultrahigh molecular weight polyethylene cementless total hip arthroplasty, tannery workers.

Decreased. Aging, diabetes mellitus.

Description. Chromium is a trace element normally found in the body. Chromium exists in carcinogenic form (hexavalent, Cr^{6+}) and noncarcinogenic form (trivalent, Cr^{3+}). The carcinogenic form results from industrial exposure to chromium in tanning, electroplating, steel and metal industries, photography, and the paint, dye, and explosives industries. It may cause toxicity, resulting in lung disease and respiratory tract cancer, liver and kidney impairment, dermatitis, convulsions, and coma. The noncarcinogenic form occurs naturally in soil, water, and air and is found in plants and animals, as well as almost all sources of food. Dietary chromium is thought to assist in amino acid transport, especially to the liver and heart. It may also enhance insulin activity and glucose utilization.

Professional Considerations

Consent form NOT required.

Preparation

1. Tube: Blue topped, metal free.

Procedure

1. Draw a 5-mL blood sample.

Postprocedure Care

1. Transport specimen to the laboratory for immediate spinning and separation of cells from serum.

Client and Family Teaching

1. Results are normally available within 24-48 hours.

Factors That Affect Results

1. Reject hemolyzed specimens.
2. Results are invalidated if the client has undergone a recent diagnostic test involving the injection of radioactive chromium.
3. Laboratory equipment used to measure chromium must be free of metal and stainless steel. Measurement must be performed under laminar air-flow conditions.
4. Parenteral nutrition may increase chromium levels.
5. Hemodialysis may increase chromium levels.

Other Data

1. Occupational exposure causes dermatitis, skin ulcerations, perforations of the nasal septum, asthma, and cancer of the nasal mucosa or lungs.
2. There is a loss of chromium in breast milk despite adequate dietary intake.
3. The National Academy of sciences recommends a daily intake of 50-200 µg of chromium per day for adults.
4. See also ^{51}Cr Red cell survival—Blood; Chromium—Urine.

Chromium—Urine

Norm.

Random specimen	0.0-5.0 µg/L
24-hr specimen	0.0-6.0 µg/24 hr

Increased. Aging, chromium toxicity, total hip replacement clients, tannery workers.

Decreased. Diabetes (children), pregnancy.

Description. See Chromium—Serum. This test is used to detect chromium toxicity.

Professional Considerations
Consent form NOT required.

Preparation
1. Prepare a 3-L container for chromium collection by leeching it for 48 hours in 10% nitric acid and then washing it with metal-free, distilled water.
2. Write the exact starting time of the urine collection on the laboratory requisition.

Procedure
1. If testing for occupational exposure to chromium, collect a 25-mL random urine sample at the end of the shift worked.
2. Collect a 24-hour urine specimen in an airtight, specially prepared 3-L container free of preservatives and metals.
3. Avoid contamination of the urine with stool.

Postprocedure Care
1. Compare urine quantity in the specimen container with the urinary output record for the test. If the specimen contains less urine than what was recorded as output, some of the sample may have been discarded, invalidating the test.
2. Document quantity of urine output for the collection period on the laboratory requisition.

Client and Family Teaching
1. Save all the urine voided in the 24-hour period and urinate before defecating to avoid loss of urine. If any of the urine is accidentally discarded, discard the entire specimen and restart the collection the next day.
2. Results are normally available within 24 hours.

Factors That Affect Results
1. Falsely elevated values may result from urine exposed to metal (as in collections from a metal urinal or bedpan) or contaminated with stool.
2. Laboratory equipment used to measure chromium must be free of metal and stainless steel. Measurement must be performed under laminar air-flow conditions.
3. All the urine voided for the 24-hour period must be included to avoid a falsely low result.

Other Data
1. Most laboratories currently use urine as a gross screening for toxicity. Because of the difficulty detecting small amounts of chromium in urine, serum levels are more accurate for determination of the level of toxicity.

Chromosome Analysis—Blood

Norm. A total of 46 chromosomes with 22 matched pairs plus XX for females and XY for males.

Usage. Diagnosis of chromosome abnormalities leading to Down syndrome, ring 20 syndrome (epilepsy), microphthalmia, other physical or mental retardation, and sex chromosome disorders such as Turner's syndrome or Klinefelter's syndrome; establishes sex in hypogonadism or unclear genitalia; part of the work-up for amenorrhea, infertility (male and female), frequent miscarriages, and other chromosome-related disorders and some leukemias and transitional-cell carcinoma of the bladder; used in genetic counseling for prospective parents and those with a family history of genetic disease.

Description. Chromosome analysis involves karyotyping human chromosomes from a culture of leukocytes from peripheral blood. Cell replication of the cultured leukocytes is chemically halted in metaphase, and microscopic photographs are taken of the chromosomes within the cell nucleus. The chromosome pictures are enlarged, and the chromosomes are paired, sorted, and studied for symmetry of pairs, number of chromosomes, identification of sex chromosomes, and staining patterns.

Professional Considerations
Informed consent is recommended for genetic testing.

Preparation
1. See Client and Family Teaching.

2. Preschedule this test with the laboratory.
3. Tube: Green topped.

Procedure
1. Draw a 10-mL blood sample.

Postprocedure Care
1. Write the date and time of specimen collection on the laboratory requisition.
2. Send the specimen to the laboratory immediately and refrigerate until testing. Testing must occur within 48 hours.

Client and Family Teaching
1. Fast for 3 hours and do not eat fatty foods for 12 hours before specimen collection.
2. Refer to section in this book on "Informed Consent for Genetic Testing".

Factors That Affect Results
1. Reject hemolyzed specimens or specimens received more than 24 hours after collection.

Other Data
1. Karyotyping may be completed on other tissues including tumor cells, bone marrow, amniocentesis, or buccal smear.
2. Some forms of leukemia, especially chronic myelogenous, are noted by chromosome assay of blood.
3. Chromosomal anomalies account for up to 15.7% of male infertility.
4. The Genetic Information Nondiscrimination Act of 2008 prohibits health plans from using genetic family history or genetic test results from influencing eligibility or premiums for health insurance. It also prohibits employers from using this information to influence decisions about hiring, terminating employment, or employment pay, promotions or privileges.
5. See also Banding in genetic disorders— Diagnostic.

CHS

See **Pseudocholinesterase**—Plasma.

Chymex Test for Pancreatic Function (Bentiromide Test, Chymotrypsin)—Diagnostic

Norm. Greater than 70% of the administered dose of p-aminobenzoic acid (PABA) appears in the urine of the client within 6 hours of administration.

Usage. This is a test used to evaluate pancreatic exocrine (digestive) function. It is frequently employed in the management of clients with chronic pancreatitis and may be used to determine if clients with this illness will require chronic pancreatic enzyme therapy.

Description. N-Benzoyl-L-tyrosyl-p-aminobenzoic acid (BT-PABA, bentiromide) is administered orally. The pancreatic digestive enzyme chymotrypsin cleaves this material into PABA, which is then readily absorbed across the intestinal mucosa into the systemic circulation. The PABA subsequently appears in the urine. Failure of significant amounts of PABA to appear in the urine implies reduced amounts of chymotrypsin in the intestinal tract, and the diagnosis of pancreatic insufficiency is consequently established.

Professional Considerations
Consent form NOT required.

Risks
Infection.

Contraindications
Previous history of allergic reaction to BT-PABA or PABA.
　Previous BT-PABA testing within 7 days of the test.
　The safety of this test has not been established during pregnancy.

Adverse Reactions
Central nervous system: Headache
　Respiratory: Stridor
　Gastrointestinal: Diarrhea, nausea, vomiting

Preparation
1. There are several medications and foods that interfere with the results of this test

and should be discontinued before testing (see Factors That Affect Results).
2. Pancreatic enzyme therapy can interfere with the test (creating a "false-negative" result) and should be discontinued at the discretion of the client's physician before the test.

Procedure
1. 500 mg of BT-PABA (bentiromide) is given to the client orally after an overnight fast.
2. The bentiromide is usually administered with 250 mL of water, and oral water intake is encouraged for several hours after the agent is administered.
3. All urine is collected for 6 hours after the bentiromide is given.
4. Urine volume is measured, and a sample of urine is submitted to the laboratory for PABA determination. In this manner the total amount of PABA excreted in the urine can be calculated.
5. The results of the test are determined as a percentage: the amount of PABA excreted in the urine (in milligrams) is divided by the amount of BT-PABA administered (500 mg), and this number is multiplied by 100.

Postprocedure Care
1. Complete urine output needs to be collected for 6 hours after the administration of the BT-PABA.

2. Encourage oral fluid intake.

Client and Family Teaching
1. The rationale behind the test should be discussed before the administration of the BT-PABA.
2. The client should be informed of the necessity of collecting all urine passed during the 6 hours after the administration of the BT-PABA.

Factors That Affect Results
1. Foods that interfere with urine PABA determination: prunes, cranberries (these should be eliminated from the diet for 72 hours before the test).
2. Medications that interfere with urine PABA determination: acetaminophen, chloramphenicol, certain sunscreens, local anesthetic agents, thiazide diuretics, sulfonamides.
3. Renal or hepatic insufficiency.
4. Ongoing therapy with pancreatic enzymes.

Other Data
1. An empiric trial of pancreatic enzyme therapy is occasionally done in clients with presumed pancreatic insufficiency in place of a formal BT-PABA test.
2. Other tests used to confirm the diagnosis of pancreatic exocrine insufficiency include the secretin test and the CCK-pancreozymin test.

Chymotrypsin Test
See **Chymex Test for Pancreatic Function**—Diagnostic.

Circulating Anticoagulant (CAC, Lupus Anticoagulant)—Blood

Norm. Negative. No CAC identified.

Positive. Indicates the presence of an inhibitor (CAC). There are two types of CAC: one is a specific factor inhibitor—an immunoglobulin that interferes with the function of any one clotting factor; the other is a lupus anticoagulant—an immunoglobulin that interferes with phospholipid in coagulation tests.

Description. Circulating anticoagulants (CACs) and lupus anticoagulants develop spontaneously or are acquired in association with autoimmune diseases or certain medication exposure. Clients with systemic lupus erythematosus, malignancies such as multiple myeloma, or chronic inflammatory diseases such as ulcerative colitis and rheumatoid arthritis as well as renal transplant recipients are known to develop these antibodies. CACs may also develop during complications postpartum or in clients taking chlorpromazine or similar drugs. In the laboratory they prolong the PT (prothrombin time), PTT (partial thromboplastin time), or APTT (activated partial thromboplastin time), or all of these. CACs are detected by a test called a "mixing study," in which normal plasma is added to client plasma and the PT, PTT, or APTT is repeated. Failure to correct the clotting to normal is a positive test. Additional tests are used to determine whether the CAC is a specific factor inhibitor or a lupus anticoagulant.

Professional Considerations
Consent form NOT required.

Preparation
1. Tube: Blue topped.

Procedure
1. Draw this specimen last or discard 1-2 mL of blood into a syringe or tube, leaving the needle in place.
2. Attach a second syringe or tube and draw a 5-mL blood sample into a blue topped tube.
3. Mix the specimen well by gently inverting the tube several times and transport it within 1 hour of collection.

Postprocedure Care
1. Write the collection time on the laboratory requisition.

Client and Family Teaching
1. The client must not take IV heparin for 4-8 hours, or subcutaneous heparin for 24 hours. Some other anticoagulant drugs may interfere with the test. Warfarin (Coumadin) does not interfere.

Factors That Affect Results
1. Drugs that may cause false-positive results include heparin, hirudin, and argatroban.
2. Contact of the specimen with the tissue thromboplastin may cause false-negative results. This is the reason for the double-draw procedure.
3. Reject hemolyzed, diluted, iced, or clotted specimens and specimens received more than 1 hour after collection.
4. Separate and refrigerate plasma if the test cannot be performed within 2 hours of collection.

Other Data
1. Specific factor inhibitors cause severe bleeding. Severe clinical bleeding is rare with the lupus anticoagulant unless there are other clotting abnormalities such as thrombocytopenia.
2. See also Mixing study—Plasma.

Circulating Tumor Cell Test (CCCT™, Blood Biopsy)—Blood

Norm. Negative.

Usage. May detect progression of metastatic breast cancer. Not to be used for evaluation of response to treatment.

Description. Measures the level of circulating tumor cells (CTCs) in the blood. Circulating tumor cells are extremely rare and result from epithelial shedding from the tumors of people with cancer of the breast that is in an advanced stage. This test screens for a higher than normal amount of epithelial cells in the bloodstream (Naoe, 2008), targets and removes normal cells from the sample, and then uses histologic and DNA examination on the remaining sample to pinpoint cells with cancerous morphology.

Professional Considerations
Consent form NOT required.

Preparation
1. Obtain a 20-mL syringe and CCCT test kit.

Procedure
1. Obtain a 20-mL blood sample.

Postprocedure Care
1. Package and store according to test kit instructions and send to laboratory.

Client and Family Teaching
1. There is no fasting required for this test.
2. Test results may take 2-3 weeks.

Factors that Affect Results
1. None.

Other Data
1. This test has low (less than 48%) sensitivity when used to detect disease progression.

Cisternography, CSF Flow Scan

See Cisternography, Radionuclide—Diagnostic.

Cisternography, Radionuclide (CSF Flow Studies, CSF Flow Scan)—Diagnostic

Norm. Normal cerebrospinal fluid (CSF) flow patterns at specific times after intrathecal injection of radiographic material into the lumbar area of the spinal cord.

1 hour: Basal cisterns.

3-4 hours: Radioactivity has reached the cerebral area and begun to spread to the ventricles and subarachnoid area.

24 hours: The flow of radioactivity should be complete to convexities or subarachnoid areas, without leakage or obstruction that would interfere with bilateral symmetry of flow.

48 hours: Radioactivity is primarily diffuse over the vertex but not in the brainstem area because it has been absorbed into the blood circulation. Symmetry is normal.

Usage. Brain atrophy; communicating hydrocephalus; suspected hydrocephalus related to CSF flow blockage (that is, tumor, cyst, subdural hematoma); CSF leakage (rhinorrhea); cerebrospinal fistulas; CSF leaks after spontaneous intracranial hypotension, trauma, or neurosurgery; identification of dural tear site with basal skull fracture; evaluation of the patency of a CSF shunt; and work-up of central nervous system symptoms such as personality changes, behavioral changes, and other neurologic changes.

Description. A nuclear medicine study of the brain and cerebral blood flow. Injection of a radioisotope into the subarachnoid space through a cisternal or lumbar puncture. The head is scanned at regular intervals to determine the amount of time it takes for the radioisotope to clear from the circulating CSF. Several views are taken at specific times over 24-48 hours.

Professional Considerations

Consent form IS required for the lumbar puncture, the radioactive injection, or the injection by cisternal puncture.

Risks

Same as for Lumbar Puncture—Diagnostic.

Contraindications

In elevated cerebrospinal fluid pressure; skin infection in lumbar or cisternal area.

Precautions

During pregnancy, risks of cumulative radiation exposure to the fetus from this and other previous or future imaging studies must be weighed against the benefits of the procedure. Although formal limits for client exposure are relative to this risk to benefit comparison, the United States Nuclear Regulatory Commission requires that the cumulative dose equivalent to an embryo/fetus from occupational exposure not exceed 0.5 rem (5 mSv). Radiation dosage to the fetus is proportional to the distance of the anatomy studied from the abdomen and decreases as pregnancy progresses. For pregnant clients, consult the radiologist/radiology department to obtain estimated fetal radiation exposure from this procedure.

Preparation

1. Inspect the lumbar and cisternal areas for skin infection.
2. Obtain povidone-iodine solution, 1%-2% lidocaine, a needle, a syringe, radionuclide, and a sterile lumbar puncture tray including a spinal needle.
3. Elevated CSF pressure should be ruled out before this procedure.

Procedure

1. Lumbar injection:
   a. The client is placed in a lateral position with knees drawn up and chin placed on the chest. A lumbar puncture is performed, and CSF pressure is measured. A radionuclide (indium-111, ytterbium-169, iodine-131 bound to RISA) is injected into the lumbar spine space.
   b. The client is then returned to a hospital room and usually must lie flat between studies, especially for the first series.
   c. Cisternograms or radiographic scans are completed at 4, 24, and 48 hours.
   d. The progress and flow pattern of the radiographic material is then studied for diagnostic purposes.
2. Cisternal injection:
   a. Using the lumbar puncture set, a puncture is made directly into the cisterna magna at the base of the skull. A radionuclide (indium-111, ytterbium-169,

iodine-131 bound to RISA) is injected into the cisterna magna.

b. Cisternograms are obtained in minutes, and subsequent studies are performed in 24 and 48 hours.

Postprocedure Care

1. The client should lie flat for 1-4 hours after the injection.
2. Observe for headache or neurologic changes.
3. Return the client, when scheduled, to the nuclear medicine department.

Client and Family Teaching

1. Notify the nurse or physician of any complaints of headache, dizziness, or nausea.

Factors That Affect Results

1. Movement during the scan obscures the views.

2. Improper injection may cause inadequate visualization.

Other Data

1. Cisternography is an expensive, invasive test.
2. If improper injection (rather than leak) is suspected, the study should be repeated after at least 1 week. A radiograph of the spine may be used to study a suspected leak in that area.
3. Health care professionals working in a nuclear medicine area must follow federal standards set by the Nuclear Regulatory Commission. These standards include precautions for handling the radioactive material and monitoring of potential radiation exposure.

CK and CK Isoenzymes

See **Creatine Kinase**—Serum.

Clinistix Test

See **Glucose Qualitative, Semiquantitative**—Urine.

Clinitest

See **Glucose Qualitative, Semiquantitative**—Urine.

Clonazepam—Blood

Norm. Negative.

		SI Units
Therapeutic level	10-80 µg/L	32-254 nmol/L
Panic level	≥100 µg/L	≥254 nmol/L

Panic Level Symptoms and Treatment

Symptoms. Deteriorating level of consciousness, coma.

Treatment

NOTE: Treatment choice(s) depend(s) on client's history and condition and episode history.

1. Gastric lavage is not recommended, but should be considered if within 1 hour of ingestion and if ingestion of additional lethal substance is suspected. Use warm tap water or 0.9% saline.
2. Administer activated charcoal if within 4 hours of ingestion or if symptoms are present. Repeat as necessary, as benzodiazepines undergo hepatic recirculation.
3. Monitor for central nervous system depression.
4. Protect airway. Support breathing with oxygen and mechanical ventilation, if necessary.
5. Flumazenil is not recommended for routine use in benzodiazepine overdose. Flumazenil has been used as a competitive antagonist to reverse the profound effects of benzodiazepine overdose. Use of flumazenil is contraindicated if

concomitant tricyclic antidepressants were taken or in dependence states because of risk of causing seizures from lowering of the seizure threshold and because it may precipitate symptoms of benzodiazepine withdrawal. Flumazenil may not completely reverse benzodiazepine effects. Close monitoring for re-sedation is required and repeated doses may be needed.

6. Do NOT use barbiturates.
7. Do NOT induce emesis.
8. Forced diuresis or hemodialysis will NOT remove benzodiazepines to any significant extent. No information was found on whether peritoneal dialysis will remove these drugs.

Usage. Monitoring for drug abuse; monitoring for therapeutic levels with long-term use and overdose. Treatment of convulsions or myoclonus, sedation, anxiety, hallucinogen persisting perception disorder (HPPD), labile arterial hypertension, panic disorders, unipolar depression, pedophilia, and drop episodes in Coffin-Lowry syndrome. Reduce spasticity of cerebral palsy.

Description. Clonazepam is a schedule IV benzodiazepine used for the treatment of convulsions and myoclonus. Peak levels occur within 2 hours after oral administration. The drug is metabolized in the liver and excreted by the kidneys, with a half-life of 20-40 hours. Burning mouth syndrome may occur after taking the drug.

Professional Considerations
Consent form NOT required.

Preparation
1. Tube: Red topped, red/gray topped, or gold topped.
2. MAY be drawn during hemodialysis.

Procedure
1. Collect a 5-mL blood sample.

Postprocedure Care
1. If storing, separate and freeze the serum.

Client and Family Teaching
1. If an accidental overdose occurs in clients on chronic clonazepam therapy, teach the early signs of overdose (drowsiness, ataxia, slurred speech) for which emergency department treatment must be sought in the future.
2. Refer clients with intentional overdose for crisis intervention.
3. Referrals to appropriate rehabilitation centers and therapeutic community programs should be offered to all addicted clients who may be interested.

Factors That Affect Results
1. Concomitant administration of carbamazepine, phenobarbital, phenytoin, or valproic acid may result in subtherapeutic clonazepam values.

Other Data
1. For seizures, dose adjustments are necessary after 90 days because of the development of tolerance.
2. Physical dependence can occur. Discontinuation must be accomplished by tapering off to avoid status epilepticus.
3. For the first 3 weeks of treating major depression, clonazepam with fluoxetine is superior.
4. See also Benzodiazepines—Plasma and urine.

Clorazepate Dipotassium

See **Benzodiazepines**—Plasma and Urine.

Clostridial Toxin—Serum

Norm. Negative.

Positive. Botulism (foods that are undercooked or that remain unrefrigerated, such as baked potatoes). Wound botulism from use of injected black tar heroin.

Negative. Absence of spore-forming bacterium microorganism *Clostridium botulinum*.

Botulism Symptoms and Emergency Treatment

Symptoms. Diarrhea, dizziness, double-vision, fatigue, gastrointestinal pain, headache, nausea, weakness, vomiting. Cardiac and respiratory paralysis is possible.

Treatment

NOTE: Treatment choice(s) depend(s) on client's history and condition and episode history.

1. Establish IV access.
2. Administer trivalent botulism antitoxin (Connaught Laboratories, Ltd). (Note: Anaphylaxis is possible if the antitoxin is given to clients with asthma, hay fever, horse or horse serum allergies, or past exposure to horse serum.) Follow the package insert instructions for sensitivity testing before antitoxin administration.
3. Induce vomiting with syrup of ipecac if the syrup can be given soon after ingestion of the contaminated food. (Induction of emesis is contraindicated in clients with no gag reflex or with central nervous system depression or excitation.)
4. Perform gastric lavage if emesis does not produce the contaminated food.
5. Give activated charcoal slurry.
6. Administer saline cathartic if no ileus is present.
7. Monitor for respiratory decompensation, which may occur suddenly in clients with botulism. Elective intubation is advisable for large ingestions.
8. Notify the state health department and the Centers for Disease Control and Prevention at 404-639-2206. (The after-hours medical emergency number is 404-639-2888.)

Description. Clostridia are gram-positive anaerobes of the family Bacillaceae characterized by production of exothermic spores, enzymes, and potent endotoxins. *Clostridium* species are found in soil, freshwater, and marine sediments, and some species are part of the human lower gastrointestinal tract. *C. botulinum* causes botulism, a neuroparalytic disease transmitted by the clostridial spores that survive improper cooking of food. Botulism causes acute flaccid paralysis and may lead to death if not treated with antitoxin before the onset of neurologic symptoms. Infant botulism is represented by hypotonia, feeding disruption, and a weak cry. Because of the severity of the disease and the potential for an epidemic among other clients ingesting the affected food, cases of suspected botulism must be immediately reported to the state department of health and the Centers for Disease Control and Prevention. Serum samples are used to confirm the diagnosis by identification of the toxin of *C. botulinum*.

Professional Considerations

Consent form NOT required.

Preparation

1. Vials: Aerobic and anaerobic culture vials.
2. It may be necessary for this test to be performed by an outside laboratory.

Procedure

1. Collect a 15- to 20-mL blood sample from each of two sites aseptically in the two culture vials, one for the aerobic and one for the anaerobic culture.
2. Double the amount of cultures collected for clients on whom antibiotic therapy has been instituted.

Postprocedure Care

1. Note antibiotic therapy on the laboratory requisition.

Client and Family Teaching

1. Results may not be available for several days. Empiric therapy is typically started while results are being awaited.

Factors That Affect Results

1. Antibiotic therapy may interfere with organism identification.

Other Data

1. 20-50 g of stool and the food suspected of causing botulism should also be collected and sent for testing with the serum sample. See Botulism, Diagnostic procedures—Stool.

Clostridium difficile Toxin Assay—Stool

Norm. Negative. No *C. difficile* toxin detected.

Positive. Antibiotic-related pseudomembranous enterocolitis.

Usage. Determine the presence or absence of *C. difficile* toxin A.

Description. *C. difficile* is a large, gram-positive, rod-shaped bacterium that releases two necrotizing toxins (toxin A [enterotoxin] and toxin B [cytotoxin]), causing a potentially fatal (1.5%) pseudomembranous colitis, especially in clients receiving antibiotics. *C. difficile* enterocolitis is the most common cause of diarrheal disease in hospitalized clients. Although it is part of the normal flora of the intestine, antibiotics to which it is resistant may increase the amount of *C. difficile* in the intestine. *C. difficile* enterocolitis is associated most commonly with clindamycin, ampicillin, and cephalosporin therapy but is possible with any antibiotic therapy. The test includes using enzyme immunoassay detection of antibody binding to one or more *C. difficile* toxin markers produced by the organism in the stool of a client.

Professional Considerations
Consent form NOT required.

Preparation
1. Obtain a sealed plastic feces specimen container, no preservative; a sealed sterile or nonsterile container with lid.

Procedure
1. Obtain a freshly passed fecal specimen of 25 g of solid stool or 25-50 mL of liquid stool in a sterile, tightly sealed plastic container. Normally, three sequential specimens are collected.

Postprocedure Care
1. Send the specimen to the laboratory for processing within 3-4 hours.

2. The specimen may be refrigerated for up to 24 hours before being tested.
3. Freeze the specimen if the test will not be performed within 24 hours. Transportation to an outside laboratory should be performed with the specimen stored in dry ice.

Client and Family Teaching
1. For outpatients, cohabitants should also be tested.

Factors That Affect Results
1. Exposure of the specimen to carbon dioxide may deactivate the toxins.

Other Data
1. Results generally take up to 2 days.
2. Newer and more rapid testing uses molecular methods for detection of *C. difficile*.
3. Culture is sometimes also prescribed but often recovers organisms that do not produce toxin.
4. Many normal infants and up to 21% of adults may have *C. difficile* as a transient or permanent part of their normal flora. Therefore cultures of *C. difficile* are not diagnostic.
5. *C. difficile* has been isolated in hospitals in 18% of clients (Miller et al, 2002) and from curtains, bookshelves, bedpans, and linens and accounts for 73% of pathogenic disease.
6. Infection control programs have been shown to decrease the incidence of *C. difficile* by 60%.
7. Treatment includes 10 days of oral metronidazole with vancomycin as second-line therapy (intravenous or intracolonic).

Clot Urea Solubility
See **Factor XIII**.

CMP
See **Comprehensive Metabolic Panel**—Blood.

CNH
See **Natriuretic Peptides**—Plasma.

CO

See **Carbon Monoxide**—Blood.

CO_2

See **Carbon Dioxide, Partial Pressure**—Blood; **Carbon Dioxide, Total Content**—Blood.

Coagulation Factor Assay—Blood

Norm. Factors VIII, IX, and XII are present and normal.

Usage. Detection of the type of hemophilia or other coagulation abnormalities.

Hemophilia Type	PT	PTT	Adsorbed Plasma	Aged Normal Serum
Factor III	Normal	Increase	Corrects	No change
Factor IX	Normal	Increase	No change	Corrects
Factor XI	Normal	Increase	Partial	Partial
Factor II	Normal	Increase	Corrects	Corrects

Description. A blood assay completed by special coagulation laboratories to determine the presence of a congenital or acquired blood clotting factor deficiency that may cause hemophilia or other blood coagulation disorders. The client's blood is mixed with normal serum or specially prepared plasma or serum with a known specific deficiency. The results are studied for prothrombin time (PT), partial thromboplastin time (PTT), and activated partial thromboplastin time (APTT) as well as clot solubility to urea. The pattern (see table above) of clotting, PT, PTT, and any change when cross-mixed with the special agent plasma give results that can determine the specific factor deficiency. For example, in hemophilia:

1. Test plasma adsorbed contains only factors XI and XII and so would specifically correct a client's plasma deficiency in these factors and therefore identify the problem.
2. Test plasma aged contains factors VII, IX, and XI and is known to lack factors I, V, and VIII.

Professional Considerations

Consent form NOT required.

Preparation

1. Preschedule the study with the special coagulation laboratory.
2. Tube: 2.7-mL blue topped or 4.5-mL blue topped, a control tube, and a waste tube or syringe. Also obtain a container of ice.

Procedure

1. Perform a venipuncture and withdraw 2 mL of blood into a syringe or vacuum tube. Remove the syringe or tube, leaving the needle in place. Attach a second syringe, and draw two blood samples, one in a citrated blue topped tube and the other in a control tube. The sample quantity should be 2.4 mL for a 2.7-mL tube and 4.0 mL for a 4.5-mL tube. Mix the sample gently by inverting the tube several times. Place the specimens immediately in the container of ice.

Postprocedure Care

1. Write the collection time on the laboratory requisition.
2. Refrigerate the specimen during transport, and transport it to the laboratory immediately. The test should be completed within 2 hours.
3. Observe the venipuncture site closely for any client with known coagulopathy.

Client and Family Teaching

1. The client should not have warfarin (Coumadin) therapy for 2 weeks or heparin therapy for 2 days.

Factors That Affect Results

1. Reject clotted or nonrefrigerated specimens.
2. The double-draw procedure is required to avoid contact of the blood with tissue thromboplastin, which may cause false-negative results.

3. Drugs that may cause false-negative results include bishydroxycoumarin, heparin calcium, heparin sodium, and warfarin sodium.
4. Oral contraceptives may cause abnormally high levels of factors II, VII, IX, and X.

Other Data
1. It is normal for healthy premature infants to have low (50% of normal) levels of factors II, III, IX, X, XI, and XII, even though a normal premature infant does not bleed spontaneously.

Cocaine—Blood

Norm. None detected.

		SI Units
Therapeutic range	100-500 ng/mL	330-1650 µmol/L
Panic (fatal) level	>1000 ng/mL	>3300 µmol/L

Panic Level Symptoms and Treatment
Symptoms. Short-lived CNS and sympathetic stimulation, hypertension, tachypnea, tachycardia, and mydriasis.

Treatment
NOTE: Treatment choice(s) depend(s) on client's history and condition and episode history.
1. Provide airway and cardiac support. Prolonged resuscitation is indicated if cardiac arrest occurs secondary to cocaine intoxication.
2. Induce emesis if oral ingestion. (Note: Induction of emesis is contraindicated in clients with no gag reflex or with central nervous system depression or excitation.)
3. Perform gastric lavage if oral ingestion.
4. Perform whole-bowel irrigation for ingested packs of cocaine. Administer activated charcoal into the body cavity where ingested packs are found.
5. Administer benzodiazepines for convulsions or other sympathomimetic symptoms, such as arrhythmias.
6. Do NOT use beta blockers.
7. Provide cool environment or hypothermia if the client is febrile.
8. Monitor renal function for damage from rhabdomyolysis.
9. Monitor for hypoglycemia.
10. Consider need for continuous ECG monitoring.

Usage. Determination of therapeutic cocaine levels or diagnosis of drug abuse or drug overdose.

Description. Cocaine is a schedule II central nervous system stimulant and a local anesthetic used clinically for its bronchodilator and vasoconstrictor effects, which result in increased blood pressure, respiratory rate, and heart rate. It is readily absorbed through mucous membranes, detoxified in the liver, and excreted by the kidneys, and acts for 2 hours or less. Cocaine is also a drug of abuse, and street names for it include C, coke, crack, girl, lady, happy dust, gold dust, and stardust. Cocaine administration compromises the heart's antioxidant defense system, and an overdose may lead to cardiopulmonary failure.

Professional Considerations
Consent form NOT required unless the specimen may be used for legal evidence.

Preparation
1. Tube: Green topped or lavender topped. Also obtain ice. Use of gray-top Vacutainer tube containing the cholinesterase inhibitor sodium fluoride will prevent enzymatic degradation of the blood sample.

Procedure
1. If the specimen will be used as legal evidence, have the specimen collection witnessed.
2. Draw a 5- to 10-mL blood sample and place the tube immediately on ice.

Postprocedure Care
1. If the specimen will be used as legal evidence, seal the bag and label it as legal evidence. Label the specimen with the exact time drawn, the client's name, and the specimen source. Sign the laboratory

requisition and have the witness sign it also. Laboratory personnel in receipt of the specimen must also sign the requisition and record the time of receipt on it.
2. Transport the specimen to the laboratory immediately.

Client and Family Teaching
1. For overdose, refer the client and the family for crisis intervention and psychologic support.
2. Referrals to appropriate rehabilitation centers and therapeutic community programs should be offered to all addicted clients who may be interested.
3. Cocaine can cause lung and kidney problems, heart attacks, strokes, aortic dissection, intestinal ischemia, hallucinations, feelings of suicide, and death. It is an addictive drug. When you stop using cocaine, withdrawal symptoms may include depression, lack of energy, sleep disturbances, chills, muscle aches, fast heartbeat, sweating, and chest pain.

Factors That Affect Results
1. Reject specimens not received on ice. Cocaine is rapidly hydrolyzed in blood, and iced specimens must be processed by gas chromatography within 1 hour.

Other Data
1. Because cocaine is so rapidly hydrolyzed, the blood specimen would have to be drawn just after use to show that it was positive for abuse. Therefore levels of urinary cocaine or its metabolite, benzoylecgonine, are more accurate screening methods for drug abuse.
2. The use of cocaine, even one time, can cause rhabdomyolysis, a disease that causes muscle tissue destruction.
3. Cocaine and tobacco use are associated with significant risk for spontaneous abortion.
4. Cocaine has adverse effects on fetuses (with motor development deficiencies still detectable at 2 years of age), but it has no adverse effect on the placenta.

Coccidioides Serology—Blood or CSF

Norm. IgM: negative. IgG < 1:16. Test is positive when IgM is detected or when IgG titer is greater than or equal to 1:16.

Usage. Detection of *Coccidioides* infection. Occurs primarily in desert southwest United States and can result in pericarditis or acute respiratory distress syndrome. Found in persons with HIV, occupational archeological dinosaur site workers, and donor transfer in lung transplantation.

Description. See Coccidioidomycosis skin test—Diagnostic. The *Coccidioides* serologic tests help diagnose coccidioidomycosis by detecting IgG and/or IgM antibodies. The tube precipitin test for IgM antibodies is positive 7-21 days after the start of the infection and becomes negative about 6 months later. The latex agglutination (LA) test is more sensitive than the precipitin test but produces more false-positive results than the precipitin test. The immunodiffusion test for IgG antibodies will appear positive several weeks after infection. CF test of spinal fluid is highly sensitive and specific during active infection.

Professional Considerations
Consent form NOT required.

Preparation
1. Tube: Red topped, red/gray topped, or gold topped.

Procedure
1. Draw a 4-mL blood sample.
2. An acute sample should be drawn as soon as possible after symptoms appear.
3. The convalescent sample should be drawn at least 7-14 days after the acute sample and preferably 14-21 days after the onset of symptoms.

Postprocedure Care
1. None.

Client and Family Teaching
1. Results usually take several days because the sample is normally sent to a reference laboratory.
2. Return at specified date for serial specimen collection.

Factors That Affect Results
1. Up to 10% false-positive results occur in the LA test.

Other Data
1. See also Coccidioidomycosis skin test—Diagnostic.

C

Coccidioidomycosis Skin Test—Diagnostic

Norm. Negative or no skin reaction.

Positive. Skin induration >5 mm in diameter indicates exposure to *Coccidioides* but gives no indication of duration. Associated with hypercalcemia.

Usage. Determine the exposure to fungal infections affecting the pulmonary system.

Description. *Coccidioides immitis* is a fungus found in the soil of dry climates of the southwest United States and Latin America. Spores in the dust are inhaled, causing respiratory infection that is mild and asymptomatic, or may cause acute to chronic pulmonary cavities and septic shock. A rare 1% of infected individuals develop disseminated disease or infection that is fatal. The course of the disease includes fever, malaise, and respiratory complaints, which become self-limiting as the client develops antibodies. In the disseminated form, the skin, bones, internal organs, and meninges are infected. This test is performed by injection of a *Coccidioides* antigen sample and observation for signs of an antibody reaction.

Professional Considerations
Consent form NOT required.

Preparation
1. Obtain an alcohol wipe, a syringe, a subcutaneous needle, and a *Coccidioides* antigen sample.

Procedure
1. Cleanse the volar aspect of the lower arm with an alcohol wipe and allow it to dry.

2. Inject 0.1 mL of 1:100 dilution of coccidioidin or spherulin (which is more sensitive) subcutaneously.
3. Circle the injection site with a pen or marker.

Postprocedure Care
1. Read the skin test 24 and 48 hours after the injection.

Client and Family Teaching
1. The injection causes a stinging sensation.
2. Do not wash off the marking until the test is read. Return in 24-48 hours to have the test site read.

Factors That Affect Results
1. Low dilution of the antigen preparation (that is, 1:10) may produce a cross-reaction, indicating other fungal diseases.
2. The skin test may be negative in the severe, disseminated form of the disease.

Other Data
1. Cross-reactions occur in clients with histoplasmosis.
2. The advantage of skin testing is that results are available in approximately 24-48 hours.
3. The main disadvantage is the time needed to develop antibodies.
4. Clients with facial lesions are more likely to have meningitis.
5. Fluconazole and itraconazole are effective therapies for coccidiomycosis.
6. Clients who are immunosuppressed, male, Filipino, pregnant, blood types A/B and B, and elderly appear to be at an increased risk for coccidiomycosis.

Codeine—Serum and Urine

Norm. Negative (positive cutoff 5 ng/mL).

		SI Units
Serum		
Therapeutic level	10-100 ng/mL	33-334 nmol/L
Panic level	>200 ng/mL	>668 nmol/L
Urine		
Therapeutic level	5-30 mg/L	
Panic level	31-250 mg/L	

Panic Level Symptoms and Treatment

Symptoms. CNS depression (including somnolence, convulsions, stupor, coma), ataxia, vomiting, rash and itching of the skin, respiratory depression, miosis, hypotension, and skeletal muscle flaccidity.

Treatment

NOTE: Treatment choice(s) depend(s) on client's history and condition and episode history.

1. Maintain patent airway and support breathing.
2. Administer vasopressors to support blood pressure.
3. Administer naloxone in repeated doses as needed.
4. Administer activated charcoal.
5. Administer gastric lavage.
6. Administer laxative.
7. Monitor fluid status. Administer IV fluids as needed.
8. Perform neurologic checks every hour.
9. Hemodialysis will NOT remove codeine.

Usage. Codeine therapy and codeine overdose.

Description. Codeine is a schedule II narcotic analgesic used for relief of mild to moderate pain and as an antitussive. Codeine is also found in combination with other analgesics in schedule III and IV medications. Drug effects of codeine are dose related. It is metabolized by the liver and excreted as norcodeine and conjugated morphine by the kidneys, with a half-life of 2.5-4.0 hours. Codeine can induce pancreatitis and manic psychotic episodes.

Professional Considerations

Consent form NOT required unless the specimen may be used as legal evidence.

Preparation

1. Obtain a clean urine container.
2. Tube: Red topped, red/gray topped, or gold topped.

3. The specimen MAY be drawn during hemodialysis.

Procedure

1. If the specimen may be used as legal evidence, have the specimen collection witnessed.
2. Serum: Draw a 5-mL blood specimen.
3. Urine: Collect 25 mL of urine in a clean container without preservatives. A fresh specimen may be taken from a urinary drainage bag.

Postprocedure Care

1. If the specimen is being collected for legal purposes, sign and have the witness sign the laboratory requisition. Also write the date, time, and specimen source on the requisition. Transport the specimen to the laboratory in a sealed plastic bag labeled as legal evidence. Each person handling the specimen should write the date and time he or she received the specimen on the requisition.

Client and Family Teaching

1. In the event of accidental overdose, the early signs of overdose for which to seek emergency treatment include drowsiness, ataxia, or slurred speech, or all three.
2. Refer clients with intentional overdose for crisis intervention.
3. Referrals to appropriate rehabilitation centers and therapeutic community programs should be offered to all addicted clients who may be interested.

Factors That Affect Results

1. Some metabolites may affect urine codeine levels; thus confirmatory serum codeine measurement must also be drawn.
2. Lengthened codeine half-life is associated with end-stage renal disease.

Other Data

1. Accidental overdose with codeine-containing cough medications occurs in children.

Cognitive Tests, Event-Related Potentials—Diagnostic

Norm. Normal recognition and reaction time.

Usage. Alzheimer's disease, dementia, depression, Huntington's disease, multiple sclerosis, myoclonic dystrophy, post coma unawareness, psychiatric illnesses, and other clinical or experimental situations in which cognitive function disorders are suspected.

Description. A test devised to measure perceptuomotor skills, sensory acuity, and ability to discriminate. Attention span is also tested because the client is asked to indicate it by pressing a button quickly after recognizing certain auditory or visual clues. When combined with evoked potential recordings, the test can give information about possible areas of error (such as a psychiatric disorder in which a hysterical loss of hearing shows positive brain response to sound but the client is unable to respond). Lack of expected response may be found to result from physical hearing loss rather than from psychiatric causes.

Professional Considerations
Consent form NOT required.

Preparation
1. Obtain earphones, a multichannel recorder with response button, and stimulus equipment.

Procedure
1. This test is carried out in a specialized psychophysiology laboratory.
2. The client is seated in a quiet environment in a comfortable chair.
3. After headphones are placed over the client's ears, a pattern or patterns of auditory cues are given.
4. The client must respond to the cues by pushing a button as quickly as possible to signify his or her recognition of the proper cue.

5. Visual cues consisting of patterns of light flashes are also used. A multichannel recorder notes the stimulus and response so that the time lapse as well as correctness of response can be determined.
6. In some tests, an evoked potential is also recorded and determined. One electrode (active) is placed between the vertex and the auditory meatus. Neutral electrodes are attached to the earlobes, and an evoked potential recording of the hearing test is obtained along with the above recordings.

Postprocedure Care
1. Remove the headphones.

Client and Family Teaching
1. You must cooperate if the results are to be of value. You will be asked to recognize certain demonstrated tones through earphones and respond by pressing the button provided.

Factors That Affect Results
1. Hearing loss or visual disorders impair the client's ability to respond to the auditory and visual cues.
2. The test is not helpful in clients who are unable to cooperate or comprehend the instructions.
3. Noise or other distractions in the testing environment may interfere with the client's comprehension of the testing cues.

Other Data
1. See also Brainstem auditory evoked potential—Diagnostic.

Cold Agglutinin Screen—Blood

Norm. Negative or <1:32. Titers <1:40 are positive.

Usage. This test is indicated when an antibody screen or panel is suggestive of cold autoagglutination because the cold agglutinins are interfering with the examination for irregular antibodies. It also may be performed for hemolytic anemia or as part of the work-up of painful extremities in cold weather (Raynaud's) or other suspected cold reactions, as in surgery. It is found in autoimmune hemolytic anemia, B-cell non–Hodgkin's lymphoma, chickenpox, lymphocytic leukemia, myelodysplastic syndrome,

systemic lupus erythematosus, T-cell lymphoma, and uterine sarcoma.

Description. Cold agglutinins are antibodies that are able to agglutinate (clump) type O human blood cells at cold (<20 degrees C) temperatures but not at room or higher temperatures. Cold agglutinins are present in small amounts in the circulation of many people and react at severely cold temperatures (<4 degrees C). Increased levels may follow infections. Their presence and reactivity at temperatures of 20 degrees C or below are termed "wide amplitude" cold agglutination. Positive cold agglutinins can cause agglutination or clumping of antigens, which leads to thrombosis, pain in the extremities, and hemolysis.

Professional Considerations
Consent form NOT required.

Preparation
1. Tube: Red topped, red/gray topped, or gold topped.

Procedure
1. Draw a 4-mL blood sample.

Postprocedure Care
1. The specimen is separated and then stored at 4 degrees C for 2 hours or overnight.

Client and Family Teaching
1. Results are normally available within 48 hours.

Factors That Affect Results
1. Reject hemolyzed specimens.

Other Data
1. Autoagglutination can occur in clients with positive results when exposed to cold and occurs especially in the extremities where body temperatures are normally lowest. It may also occur during surgery, especially during open-heart surgery, where the perfusate for bypass is 15-32 degrees C.
2. Cold agglutinins are not found in normal (room-temperature) blood cross-match methods.
3. This is not to be confused with Cold agglutinin titer, which is a specific test for *Mycoplasma* pneumonia. The only connection is that among other infections, *Mycoplasma* infection may cause the presence of these cold agglutinins.

Cold Agglutinin Titer—Serum

Norm. Negative or titer <32 or <1:4.

Positive. Titer >40 or >1:40 in combination with acute respiratory symptoms usually indicates *Mycoplasma* pneumoniae infection, usually *Mycoplasma* pneumonia, viral pneumonia, or primary atypical pneumonia. An agglutination reaction present even at very high titers is suggestive of *M. pneumoniae*, especially if the test is specific for anti-I antigens. Positive titers as a result of *M. pneumoniae* infection rise after about 10 days, peak at 12-25 days, and then diminish by 30 days with an acute infection. Positive titers may also indicate cirrhosis (hypertrophic, syphilitic), hemolytic anemia, Hodgkin's disease, lymphoma, mononucleosis infection, pleuropneumonia-like organism (PPLO), PNH, trypanosomiasis, and tuberculosis (febrile).

Negative. Titer <1:32 is negative for *M. pneumoniae* or related infection.

Description. Cold agglutinins are antibodies that cause clumping or agglutination of type O red blood cells at cold temperatures. The cold agglutinin titer tests for cold agglutinins at 2-8 degrees C—those antibodies that result from *M. pneumoniae* infection. A titer is the highest dilution of a serum that will demonstrate a specific antigen-antibody reaction. *M. pneumoniae* is a nonbacterial infective agent that causes a pneumonia characterized by fever and a nonproductive or nonpurulent cough.

Professional Considerations
Consent form NOT required.

Preparation
1. Tube: Red topped, red/gray topped, gold topped, or lavender topped.

Procedure
1. Draw a 4-mL blood sample.
2. Usually at least two serial samples are taken. The first is taken 1 week after the onset of illness. The second is taken 12-25 days after the onset of illness, and a third may be taken 30 days after the onset.

Postprocedure Care
1. Transport the specimen to the laboratory immediately. The blood is allowed to clot at 37 degrees C, and the serum is then separated from the cells and cooled for testing.

Client and Family Teaching
1. Results are normally available within 48 hours.

Factors That Affect Results

1. Reject hemolyzed specimens or refrigerated specimens. Refrigeration before separation of serum may cause false-negative results.
2. Antibiotic therapy may decrease antibody production.
3. False-positive results may occur in clients with malaria, congenital syphilis, peripheral vascular disease, hepatic cirrhosis, anemia, and respiratory diseases. In such cases, the titer pattern is more constant, without peaks.
4. The sample must not be allowed to clot at room temperature.

Other Data

1. Culture methods for *M. pneumoniae* are available, but the cold agglutinin titer is more reliable for diagnosis.
2. Serial titers are most helpful because the *M. pneumoniae* titers follow a specific pattern that peaks during the third to fourth week after infection.
3. Newer cold agglutinin methods that test agglutination reactions specific to major antigen types make this test much more specific. *M. pneumoniae* is related to the I-I antigen system. Anti-M or anti-P is associated with other cold agglutinin activity and diseases.

Colonoscopy—Diagnostic

Norm. The intima of the large intestine is normally orange-pink in color, with folds and smooth indentations covered with mucus. Blood vessels may be visible below the epithelial surface.

Usage. Visualization of the mucosa of the entire colon and terminal ileum. Screening for intestinal abnormalities, including diverticula, polyps, tumors, ulcerative areas, infection, inflammation, irritation, bleeding sites, or strictures. Also used to study and biopsy or remove tumors, polyps, ulcerative colitis, parasitic disease, or other causes of diarrhea.

Description. A fiberoptic endoscopy study in which the lining of the large intestine is visually examined for inflammation or other changes of the mucosal surface and for bleeding sites or strictures. The test is indicated after a positive test for fecal occult blood or after a positive screening sigmoidoscopy or double-contrast barium enema, after bleeding of the lower GI tract, and when a client experiences changing patterns of bowel function. The American Cancer Society recommends a screening colonoscopy every 10 years in adults older than age 50. See also Sigmoidoscopy—Diagnostic.

Professional Considerations

Consent form IS required.

Risks

Dysrhythmias, hemorrhage, myocardial infarction, perforation of colon, peritonitis, respiratory depression.

Contraindications

Anal bleeding (use with extreme caution), hypotension, megacolon, recent colon anastomosis, recent myocardial infarction or pulmonary embolus; retained barium from an earlier study; second or third trimester pregnancy. Sedatives are contraindicated in clients with central nervous system depression.

Preparation

1. See Client and Family Teaching.
2. A tap-water enema may be prescribed to be given just before the test and/or the client may ingest 28 tablets (42 g) of sodium phosphate or drink magnesium citrate the day before to cleanse the bowel.
3. Sedation may be prescribed, such as 2-3 mg of midazolam and 80 mg of propofol IV just before procedure.
4. Prepare suction equipment, emergency equipment, naloxone, lubricant, cytology brush, and containers of fixative for cytology specimens.
5. Record baseline vital signs.
6. Just before beginning the procedure, take a "time out" to verify the correct client, procedure, and site.

Procedure

1. The client is positioned lying on the left side with knees flexed and draped for privacy and comfort.
2. The flexible fiberoptic endoscope is inserted through the anus, and the rectum and colon are visualized. Insufflation occurs to aid in visualization. Insufflation

of CO_2 rather than air reduces abdominal pain and bowel distention after colonoscopy.

3. Specimens may be obtained for cytologic testing.

4. Photographs are taken of anomalies present.

5. Polyps may be removed with colonoscopy biopsy forceps or an electrocautery snare.

Postprocedure Care

1. Place the tissue specimens in a fixative of 10% formalin. Place the cytology specimens in 95% ethyl alcohol (ethanol). Label the specimens and send them to the laboratory immediately.

2. Observe the client and check vital signs every 15-30 minutes until fully recovered. If sedation was used, follow institutional protocol for post sedation monitoring. Typical monitoring includes continuous ECG monitoring and pulse oximetry, with continual assessments (every 5-15 minutes) of airway, vital signs, and neurologic status until the client is lying quietly awake, breathing independently, and responding appropriately to commands spoken in a normal tone.

3. After the client has fully recovered, he or she may resume a normal diet.

4. Observe for signs of colon perforation, which include abdominal pain or distention, malaise, fever, purulent rectal drainage, or lower gastrointestinal bleeding.

Client and Family Teaching

1. Follow a clear liquid diet for 48 hours before the test and resume normal diet after the test.

2. Bowel preparation is very important because it makes a significant difference in detecting abnormalities and in preventing the need for a repeat test. A laxative is usually prescribed the evening before the test, unless contraindicated. Examples are 10 ounces of magnesium citrate or 3 tablespoons of castor oil.

3. Prior to the test drink 4 liters of clear liquids, unless told not to by your physician or nurse, to minimize effects of fluid loss.

4. Make arrangements for transportation home after the procedure because driving is not permitted for 24 hours after receiving sedation.

5. Take deep, slow breaths during the procedure. The urge to defecate is normal and can be relieved with this type of breathing.

6. An increase in flatus is normal, and minor amounts of blood in the stool are expected after polyp removal.

Factors That Affect Results

1. Soapsuds enemas irritate the mucosa, increase mucus production, and hinder visibility.

2. Barium from any previous gastrointestinal work-up makes colon visualization impossible.

3. Failure to clean the lower intestine makes colon visualization impossible.

4. Strictures or other abnormalities from previous surgery, radiation, or severe, chronic inflammatory disease may interfere with passage of the colonoscope.

Other Data

1. The findings from this procedure may be useful to the surgeon during laparotomy to exclude other lesions.

2. Virtual endoscopic magnetic resonance colonography that uses three-dimensional imaging does not identify polyps smaller than 5 mm.

3. High-definition chromocolonoscopy involves spraying the colon with carmine dye and helps identify more multiple adenomas and more clients with adenoma of at least 5 mm. However, this method is seldom used during routine colonoscopy because dye application takes longer, and mean time to extubation is extended.

4. Music therapy has been shown to reduce anxiety and the need for sedation in persons undergoing colonoscopy.

5. Colonoscopy is much less expensive than CT Colonography.

Color Duplex Ultrasonography—Diagnostic

Norm. Description of normal tissues, structure, and blood flow.

Usage. Noninvasive study that is performed to assess characteristics of blood flow including alterations of normal flow (e.g., sexual dysfunction), direction of flow, and presence of flow (e.g., thrombosis of upper extremity, vertebrobasilar ischemic disease). Tissue perfusion and tumor vascularization (e.g., acute pancreatitis) can also be assessed.

Description. Color duplex refers to the fact that this test presents on the screen a simultaneous display of Doppler information and the B-mode ultrasonographic image. High-frequency sound waves are passed over the structure, and a computer analyzes the time required for the impulse to be reflected back to a transducer. The computer converts this impulse to an electrical impulse that is viewed on the screen to create a three-dimensional picture of the structure, using color as a guide. The "Doppler" effect refers to a change in frequency that occurs when the sound wave is reflected from a moving object. The computer can display this change in frequency as sound or as color changes in the pictures, or both. Different colors are used to represent flow, one color toward the transducer and another color away from the transducer. Speed of flow can be indicated by changes in the color shade.

Professional Considerations
Consent form NOT required.

Preparation
1. Obtain ultrasonic gel or paste.

Procedure
1. The client is positioned on the bed or on an examination table to allow access to the structure that is to be studied.

2. The area that is to be studied is covered with the ultrasonic gel or paste, and the transducer is slowly passed over the area. The technician may use a longitudinal or a transverse approach in an attempt to obtain the best visualization of the structure.
3. Video is obtained of the display for later review.
4. The procedure should last less than 45 minutes depending on what structures are being visualized.

Postprocedure Care
1. Remove gel or paste from the skin.
2. Return client to a comfortable position.

Client and Family Teaching
1. You will not be allowed to eat or drink during the test.
2. The test is painless and the ultrasonic waves cannot be felt.
3. You must lie as still as possible during the test.
4. The area that is being studied will be uncovered, but you will otherwise be covered.

Factors That Affect Results
1. Abdominal fat can alter the intensity of a beam "looking" at abdominal structures.
2. If the beams pass through substances such as barium, gas, or food particles, the clarity of the image can be diminished.
3. Client movement can affect the image clarity.

Color Vision Tests—Diagnostic

Norm. The client is able to identify all the colors, symbols, and patterns presented.

Usage. Screening for retinal disease or color vision deficiency (such as red-green or blue-yellow deficiency).

Description. A test using pseudoisochromatic plates with numbers or letters buried in a matrix of colored dots. Deficits can be genetic and result from one or more of the three-color cone systems, or deficits can be acquired.

Professional Considerations
Consent form NOT required.

Preparation
1. Obtain an eye patch or hand-held occluder, test kit, and pointer.

Procedure
1. One eye is occluded, and the test booklet is held approximately 14 inches (35 cm) in front of the unoccluded eye.
2. Sample plates of different patterns of primary colors with a background of a variety of colors are shown to the client, one at a time.
3. The client is asked to identify the patterns of the primary colors and to trace the patterns with a pointer.

Postprocedure Care

1. None.

Client and Family Teaching

1. Bring corrective glasses or lenses to the test.
2. There are no food or fluid restrictions.
3. The test is painless.

Factors That Affect Results

1. Conduct the test in a well-lighted area.

2. Abnormalities of the ocular media, the retina, or the optic nerve can affect results and should be ruled out if color blindness is discovered.
3. The client may be unable to cooperate and participate in the test.

Other Data

1. Color blindness may include more than one kind of spectral color.
2. Color vision is not affected by laser in situ keratomileusis (LASIX) surgery.

Colorectal Cancer Allelotyping for Chromosomes 17p and 18q (p53 or DCC Gene)—Specimen and Blood

Norm. Normal gene sequence.

Usage. Detection of mutations in tumor-suppressor genes, which are associated with approximately half of human cancers, including colorectal, breast, bladder, esophageal, liver, lung, ovarian, brain (p53), and pancreas cancers; leukemias; and male germ cell cancers (DCC).

Description. The progression of colon adenoma to invasive cancer frequently involves mutations in the p53 and DCC (deleted in colorectal cancer) genes, which are tumor-suppressor genes located on chromosomes 17p and 18q, respectively. Most attention is given to the p53 gene because it is the most common mutational event in the progression of cancer, involved in nearly half of all human cancers. p53 produces a protein that induces apoptosis in response to DNA damage, maintaining genetic stability and preventing tumor formation. Both of the alleles must be damaged in order for the mutation to be apparent. The DCC gene encodes a protein similar to an immunoglobulin, and mutations of this gene are found in several cancers. The role of both p53 and DCC in determining prognosis and treatment remains unclear, though breast cancers with p53 mutations appear to be relatively resistant to ionized radiation and seem to benefit significantly from CMF chemotherapy. The techniques used for analysis of the genes are immunohistochemical (to detect the gene product) and DNA analysis (to detect specific mutations). Analysis may be conducted on fresh, frozen, or paraffin-embedded tissue.

Professional Considerations

Consent is required for biopsy. See Biopsy, Site-specific—Specimen for risks and contraindications. Informed consent is recommended for genetic testing.

Preparation

1. Tissue specimen: Obtain solid-tissue biopsy bottle.
2. Blood: Obtain yellow topped or lavender topped tube.

Procedure

1. Obtain tissue specimen by desired procedure or draw blood and place in appropriate container. Tissue is to be frozen quickly.

Postprocedure Care

1. Apply clean, sterile dressing to biopsy site.

Client and Family Teaching

1. Results may not be available for several days.
2. Refer to section in this book on "Informed Consent for Genetic Testing".

Factors That Affect Results

1. Small specimens decrease the reliability of the results.
2. Tissue specimens must not be frozen, and blood specimens must not be clotted.

Other Data

1. The specimen must be >40% tumor.
2. Penclomedine is in clinical trials to assess its antitumor activity in colorectal carcinoma.
3. Increased risk of colorectal carcinoma is associated with variant alleles of the DNA

repair gene XRCC1 and GSTM3*B gene variant. Reduced risk of colorectal cancer is associated with phenol sulphotransferase SULTIA1*1 genotype.

4. The Genetic Information Nondiscrimination Act of 2008 prohibits health plans from using genetic family history or genetic test results from influencing eligibility or premiums for health insurance. It also prohibits employers from using this information to influence decisions about hiring, terminating employment, or employment pay, promotions or privileges.

ColoSure™ Test—Stool

Norm. Negative.

Usage. May be useful in individuals unwilling to undergo screening using methods such as fecal occult blood testing, colonoscopy, or flexible sigmoidoscopy, all of which have higher sensitivity and specificity. Not for use in individuals deemed to have an increased risk of colon cancer.

Description. Identifies altered DNA/mutation associated with colorectal cancer and with pre-cancerous adenomas. When these conditions are present, an epigenetic marker (methylated vimentin) is shed from the epithelial cells of the colon into the stool. This test requires no preparation; the sample is collected in the home, then shipped to a laboratory for analysis (Ned, Melillo, Marrone, 2011).

Professional Considerations

Informed consent is recommended for genetic testing.

Preparation

1. Test kit requires a physician prescription.
2. Obtain test kit and collection device.

Procedure

1. Place collection device into toilet.

Postprocedure Care

1. After defecation into the collection device, seal collection container and follow test kit instructions to ship the container to the testing laboratory.

Client and Family Teaching

1. Positive results are not diagnostic for colon cancer. Further diagnostic testing is necessary and may include colonoscopy or flexible sigmoidoscopy, which provides direct visualization of the colon and allows for a biopsy to be taken.
2. Refer to section in this book on "Informed Consent for Genetic Testing".

Factors That Affect Results

1. Provides 72-77% accuracy in screening for colon cancer. Less specific for colon cancer than fecal occult blood guaiac test.
2. No recommended testing interval has been determined for this test.

Other Data

1. Colon cancer is the third most common cancer in the United States.
2. The Genetic Information Nondiscrimination Act of 2008 prohibits health plans from using genetic family history or genetic test results from influencing eligibility or premiums for health insurance. It also prohibits employers from using this information to influence decisions about hiring, terminating employment, or employment pay, promotions or privileges.
3. This approved test is considered experimental by many insurance payers.
4. See also Immunochemical fecal occult blood testing; Occult blood—Stool.

Colposcopy—Diagnostic

Norm. Normal appearance of vagina and cervix. Vagina and cervix are free of lesions, and no abnormal cells or tissue are present.

Usage. Evaluation, by physician or certified nurse, of suspicious lesions or suspected cervical or vaginal cancer, evaluation of

C

abnormal cytologic characteristics of the vagina and cervix, testing for vulvar dystrophy, and screening for cervical abnormalities in women whose mothers were treated with diethylstilbestrol (DES). Collection of cervical specimen for definitive testing after abnormal Pap smear result has been obtained.

Description. The visual examination of the vagina and cervix using a lighted colposcope that magnifies the mucosal surfaces. Colposcopy helps diagnose benign and preclinical cancerous lesions of the cervix and vagina. Attachments to the colposcope include a green filter (aids in detecting abnormalities of blood vessels in the cervix), teaching arm, or video camera. If an abnormal Pap smear has been previously obtained, the colposcopy may be performed with a loop electrosurgical excision procedure (LEEP), in which a thin wire loop electrode is used to excise cervical tissue in the area of the abnormality for lesion removal and further examination.

Professional Considerations
Consent form IS required.

Risks
Bleeding, infection, mild discomfort.
Contraindications
Biopsy during colposcopy is contraindicated in the presence of anticoagulant therapy, bleeding disorders, thrombocytopenia, or heavy menses.

Preparation
1. The client should disrobe below the waist and the room should be a warm temperature.
2. Obtain a speculum, a 3% acetic acid solution, sterile cotton-tipped swabs, a colposcope, biopsy forceps, a cauterizer, a specimen cup with preservative, and sterile cotton.
3. Obtain supplies for a Pap smear, if one will be collected during the colposcopy examination.
4. Just before beginning the procedure, take a "time out" to verify the correct client, procedure, and site.

Procedure
1. The client is placed in the lithotomy position and draped for comfort and privacy.
2. The vagina and cervix are exposed with a speculum.
3. Saline may be applied to the cervix, then cervical mucus is removed with acetic acid being applied, and then Lugol's iodine can be applied to outline cervix abnormalities (abnormal epithelium does not contain glycogen and therefore will not stain).
4. The colposcope is inserted, and the walls of the vagina and cervix are visually examined for color, keratinization, lesions, blood vessel structure, inflammation, atrophy, and erosion. Suspicious areas may be biopsied, and cautery or pressure is used to control bleeding.
5. For clients with low-grade changes on a previous Pap smear, a repeat Pap smear may be taken during colposcopy.

Postprocedure Care
1. Vaginal bleeding is not abnormal. Provide a sanitary pad.

Client and Family Teaching
1. The procedure lasts about 15 to 20 minutes and may cause slight discomfort from the vaginal speculum.
2. A small amount of bleeding may occur because of the sampling of tissue.
3. Immediate complications include pain and hemorrhage and secondary hemorrhage can occur up to 14 days after.
4. Results may not be available for several days.
5. Refrain from sexual intercourse until receiving confirmation on a follow-up visit that the biopsy site has healed.

Factors That Affect Results
1. Heavy menstrual flow may interfere with adequate visualization of the cervix.

Other Data
1. Colposcopy is helpful in adding information about tumor extension.
2. Annual colposcopy provides no additional benefit compared to Papanicolaou smear for detection of cervical cancer in HIV-infected females.
3. Colposcopically directed brush cytologic testing is a safe substitute for directed biopsy in pregnant clients.

Companion

See **Glucose Monitoring Machines**—Diagnostic.

Complement, Total—Serum (CH$_{50}$)

Norm. 5-160 U/mL (75-160 kU/L, SI units), >33% of plasma CH$_{50}$ (fraction of plasma CH$_{50}$: >0.33, SI units).

Increased. Atopic dermatitis, diabetes mellitus, jaundice (obstructive), mixed connective tissue disease, myocardial infarction (acute), rheumatoid arthritis (adult, severe), thyroiditis, ulcerative colitis, and Wegener's granulomatosis.

Decreased. Allograft rejection, cirrhosis (advanced), glomerulonephritis (poststreptococcal acute, chronic), hemolytic anemia (autoimmune), hepatitis (chronic, active), hypogammaglobulinemia, kwashiorkor, lupus nephritis, malaria, multiple myeloma, rheumatic fever, serum sickness (acute), sinusitis (*Streptococcus pneumoniae, Neisseria*), subacute bacterial endocarditis (SBE), and systemic lupus erythematosus (SLE).

Usage. Evaluate and follow-up SLE client's response to therapy; screen for complement component deficiency; evaluate cases of immune complex disease, glomerulonephritis, arthritis, SBE, and cryoglobulinemia. Hypocomplementemia that accompanies some forms of renal disease may indicate immune utilization. Identification and monitoring of immune-related diseases.

Description. The complement system comprises a series of proteins that when activated serve to amplify an immune response. Activation of the complement system lends to the elaboration of potent inflammatory mediators, facilitates particle opsonization and clearance, and may result in the direct lysis of altered mammalian cells and certain bacteria. The complement system may be activated by a number of immunologic and nonimmunologic stimuli. Complement activation proceeds by either the classical or the alternative pathway (see Complement components—Serum). The test for total serum complement evaluates the integrity of the complement cascade. Total complement is depressed during the active phases of immune diseases when various individual components are significantly depressed.

Professional Considerations

Consent form NOT required.

Preparation

1. Tube: Red topped, red/gray topped, or gold topped.

Procedure

1. Draw a 4-mL blood sample.
2. Leave the specimen at room temperature to clot. Then refrigerate it at 4 degrees C for 30 minutes to 1 hour.

Postprocedure Care

1. Send the specimen to the laboratory for immediate testing.

Client and Family Teaching

1. Results are normally available within 48 hours.

Factors That Affect Results

1. Complement is heat sensitive and deteriorates rapidly. Send the specimen to the laboratory immediately.
2. Freeze the specimen at −70 degrees C if it cannot be processed immediately after 1 hour of refrigeration.

Other Data

1. Various individual components (C1-C9) may be depressed only slightly in immune disease and may not have a significant effect on the total complement level.
2. Low CH$_{50}$ levels tend to correlate with active phases of immune complex diseases such as SLE (especially if associated with nephritis and cases of glomerulonephritis).
3. Decreased complement in synovial fluid may be seen with acute arthritis. Low serum complement levels occur in some clients with severe active rheumatoid factor positive arthritis and may indicate the development of vasculitis.
4. See C1q immune complex detection—Serum; C3 complement—Serum; C3 proactivator—Serum; C4 complement—Serum; Complement components—Serum; Complement fixation—Serum.

Complement Components—Serum
Norm.

		SI Units
Classical Pathway Components		
C1	70,000-200,000 U/mL	70-200 MU/L
C1q		
Adult	14.9-22.1 mg/dL	149-221 mg/L
Maternal	9-24.8 mg/dL	90-248 mg/L
Newborn	9-20 mg/dL	90-200 mg/L
C1r		
Adult	0.025-0.10 mg/mL	0.025-0.010 g/L
C1s	0.05-0.10 g/L	0.05-0.10 mg/mL
C2	1.6-3.6 mg/dL	16-36 mg/L
C4		
Adult	10-67.5 mg/dL	100-675 mg/L
Alternative Pathway Components		
Factor D	1-5 µg/dL	1-5 mg/L
C3 Proactivator		
Adult	127-278 µg/mL	127-278 mg/L
Properdin		
Adult	10-36.5 µg/mL	10-36.5 mg/L
Cord serum	8.1-23.4 µg/mL	8.1-23.4 mg/L
Regulatory Components		
CI-INH	8-24.0 mg/dL	80-240 mg/L
C4-binding protein	18-32 mg/dL	180-320 mg/L
Factor H	40.5-71.7 mg/dL	405-717 mg/L
Factor I	0.025-0.05 mg/mL	25-50 mg/L
Anaphylatoxin inactivator	30-40 µg/mL	300-400 mg/L
S-protein	(mean) 500 µg/mL	(mean) 500 mg/L
C-3 nephritic factor	Negative	Negative
Split Products		
$C3_{desArg}$	<940 ng/mL	<940 µg/L
$C4_{desArg}$	<2.8 µg/mL	<2.8 mg/L
$C5_{desArg}$	<12 ng/mL	<12 µg/L
Bb, Ba	Negative	Negative
C4d	Trace	Trace
SC5b-9	<390 µg/mL	<390 mg/L
Terminal Pathway Components		
C3		
Adult	83-177 mg/dL	0.83-1.77 g/L
Cord serum	57-116 mg/dL	0.57-1.16 g/L
6 months	74-177 mg/dL	0.74-1.77 g/L
C5		
Adult	4.8-18.5 mg/dL	48-185 mg/L
Cord serum	3.4-6.2 mg/dL	34-62 mg/L
6 months	2.4-6.4 mg/dL	24-64 g/L
C6		
Adult	28-60 µg/mL	28-60 mg/L
Cord serum	6.9-12.7 mg/dL	69-127 mg/L

Continued

		SI Units
C7		
Adult	27-80 µg/mL	27-80 mg/L
C8		
Adult	40-106 µg/mL	40-106 mg/L
C9		
Adult	33-250 µg/mL	33-250 mg/L

Usage. Helps diagnose immune-mediated disease and genetic complement deficiency. C1q is higher in Alzheimer's disease, and C4 complement is increased in styrene occupational exposure.

Useful in acute vascular rejection, cerebral palsy, chronic renal failure, hereditary angioedema, hyperactive xenograft rejection, paroxysmal nocturnal hemoglobinuria, pemphigus vulgaris.

Description. The complement system comprises a series of proteins that, when activated, serve to amplify an immune response. Complement accounts for 10% of serum globulins. Activation of the complement system leads to the elaboration of potent inflammatory mediators, facilitates particle opsonization and clearance, and may result in the direct lysis of altered mammalian cells and foreign bacteria. The complement system may be activated by numerous immunologic and nonimmunologic stimuli. Complement activation proceeds by classical and alternative mechanisms. The components C1-C1q, C1r, C1s, C2, and C4 are activated in the classical pathway, which is stimulated when an antigen-antibody reaction occurs. Alternative pathway components—C3 proactivator, properdin, and factor D—are stimulated possibly by mechanisms other than antigen-antibody reactions. C3 and C4 levels are most often used to evaluate the integrity of the classical and alternative pathways. Levels of other individual components may be used to monitor autoimmune activity and identify a genetic deficiency of the individual component(s).

Professional Considerations
Informed consent IS recommended for genetic testing.

Preparation
1. Tube: Red topped, red/gray topped, or gold topped.

Procedure
1. Draw a 7-mL blood sample.
2. Leave the specimen at room temperature to clot. Then refrigerate at 4 degrees C for 30 minutes to 1 hour.

Postprocedure Care
1. Write the exact specimen collection time on the laboratory requisition.
2. Send the specimen to the laboratory, where testing should be performed immediately.

Client and Family Teaching
1. Results are normally available within 12 hours.
2. Refer to Appendix B: Informed Consent for Genetic Testing.

Factors That Affect Results
1. Complement is heat sensitive and deteriorates rapidly.
2. Reject hemolyzed specimens or specimens received more than 2 hours after collection.
3. Freeze the specimen at −70 degrees C if it cannot be processed immediately after 1 hour of refrigeration.

Other Data
1. Complement abnormalities in disease are commonly deficiencies rather than excesses.
2. Serial measurements are recommended.
3. The Genetic Information Nondiscrimination Act of 2008 prohibits health plans from using genetic family history or genetic test results from influencing eligibility or premiums for health insurance. It also prohibits employers from using this information to influence decisions about hiring, terminating employment, or employment pay, promotions or privileges.
4. See C1q immune complex detection—Serum; C3 complement—Serum; C3 proactivator—Serum; C4 complement—Serum; Complement fixation—Serum; Complement, Total—Serum.

Complement Fixation (Cf)—Serum

Norm. Negative test—red cell hemolysis occurs; positive test—absence of red cell hemolysis.

Positive. In the presence of antigen-antibody reactions, *Chlamydia pneumoniae*, hepatic psittacosis, Japanese encephalitis, *Mycoplasma pneumoniae*, Q fever infection, sheep or dairy farmers.

Usage. Detection of antigens, antibodies, or both, during reactions. Clinically, complement fixation is used to detect the presence of anti-DNA, immunoglobulins, and antiplatelet antibodies.

Description. CF is a two-step process based on the principle that one or more of the complement components can be fixed (used) in an antigen-antibody reaction. The test is initiated when a known amount of complement is added to the client's serum. The added complement is then fixed. The second step detects the amount of complement fixed and the proportion of antibody or antigen in the client's serum. The second step is performed when antigenic sheep red blood cells are added to the serum. The remaining unfixed complement will lyse the sheep red blood cells. Therefore lysis occurs when the complement is unfixed, an indication that the serum is deficient in either antigen or antibody. Lysis does not occur if all the complement is fixed, an indication of the presence of antigen and antibody in the serum.

Professional Considerations
Consent form NOT required.

Preparation
1. Tube: Red topped, red/gray topped, or gold topped.

Procedure
1. Draw a 4-mL blood sample.

Postprocedure Care
1. None.

Client and Family Teaching
1. Two days are required for this test because the second incubation must occur overnight.

Factors That Affect Results
1. A contaminated tube may give anticomplementary results.
2. Gonococcal vaccine may cause a false-positive gonococcal complement fixation test.
3. Tuberculosis may cause a false-positive leishmaniasis complement fixation test.
4. Brucellosis and Q fever may cause a false-positive psittacosis complement fixation test.

Other Data
1. See C1q Immune Complex Detection—Serum; C3 Complement—Serum; C3 Proactivator—Serum; C4 Complement—Serum; Complement components—Serum; Complement total—Serum.

Complete Blood Count (CBC)—Blood

Norm.

		SI Units
Hematocrit (HCT) (Whole Blood)		
Adult Females		
18-44 years	35%-45%	0.35-0.45
45-64 years	35%-47%	0.35-0.47
65-74 years	35%-47%	0.35-0.47
Pregnant		
Trimester 1	35%-46%	0.35-0.46
Trimester 2	30%-42%	0.30-0.42
Trimester 3	34%-44%	0.34-0.44
Postpartum	30%-44%	0.30-0.44

Continued

		SI Units
Adult males		
18-44 years	39%-49%	0.39-0.49
45-64 years	39%-50%	0.39-0.50
65-74 years	37%-51%	0.37-0.51
Children		
At birth	42%-68%	0.42-0.68
Cord blood	42%-60%	0.42-0.60
2 weeks	41%-65%	0.41-0.65
1 month	33%-55%	0.33-0.55
2 months	28%-42%	0.28-0.42
4 months	32%-44%	0.32-0.44
6 months	31%-41%	0.31-0.41
9 months	32%-40%	0.32-0.40
1 year	33%-41%	0.33-0.41
4 years	31%-44%	0.31-0.44
6-8 years	33%-41%	0.33-0.41
9-11 years	34%-43%	0.34-0.43
12-14 years (male)	35%-45%	0.35-0.45
12-14 years (female)	34%-44%	0.34-0.44
15-17 years (male)	37%-48%	0.37-0.48
15-17 years (female)	34%-44%	0.34-0.44

Hemoglobin (HGB)

Adult Females	12-16 g/dL	7.4-9.9 mmol/L
Pregnant		
Trimester 1	11.4-15.0 g/dL	7.1-9.3 mmol/L
Trimester 2	10.0-14.3 g/dL	6.2-8.9 mmol/L
Trimester 3	10.2-14.4 g/dL	6.3-8.9 mmol/L
Postpartum	10.4-18.0 g/dL	6.4-9.3 mmol/L
Adult Males	14.0-18.0 g/dL	8.7-11.2 mmol/L
Panic low level	<5 g/dL	<3.1 mmol/L
Panic high level	>18 g/dL	>11.2 mmol/L
Children		
At birth	15.5-24.5 g/dL	9.6-15.2 mmol/L
12-24 hours	19.0 g/dL	11.8 mmol/L
1 week	14.3-22.3 g/dL	8.9-13.8 mmol/L
2 weeks	10.7-17.3 g/dL	6.6-10.7 mmol/L
1 month to 1 year	9.9-15.5 g/dL	6.1-9.6 mmol/L
2 years	9.0-14.6 g/dL	5.6-9.0 mmol/L
4 years	9.4-15.5 g/dL	5.8-9.6 mmol/L
8-20 years	13.4 g/dL	8.3 mmol/L
Panic levels	<5 g/dL	<3.1 mmol/L
	>18 g/dL	>11.2 mmol/L

Red Blood Cells (RBCs)

Adult Females	4.0-6.2 million/μL	$4.0\text{-}6.2 \times 10^{12}$/L
Pregnant		
Trimester 1	4.0-5.0 million/μL	$4.0\text{-}5.0 \times 10^{12}$/L
Trimester 2	3.2-4.5 million/μL	$3.2\text{-}4.5 \times 10^{12}$/L
Trimester 3	3.0-4.9 million/μL	$3.0\text{-}4.9 \times 10^{12}$/L
Postpartum	3.2-5.0 million/μL	$3.2\text{-}5.0 \times 10^{12}$/L
Adult Males	4.0-6.2 million/μL	$4.0\text{-}6.2 \times 10^{12}$/L
Children		
At birth	4.1-6.1 million/μL	$4.1\text{-}6.1 \times 10^{12}$/L
1 week	5.1 million/μL	5.1×10^{12}/L

		SI Units
2 weeks	3.8-5.6 million/μL	$3.8\text{-}5.6 \times 10^{12}/L$
1 month to 1 year	3.8-5.2 million/μL	$3.8\text{-}5.2 \times 10^{12}/L$
2 years	3.6-5.5 million/μL	$3.6\text{-}5.5 \times 10^{12}/L$
4 years	4.0-5.2 million/μL	$4.0\text{-}5.2 \times 10^{12}/L$
6 years	4.7 million/μL	$4.7 \times 10^{12}/L$
8-20 years	4.8 million/μL	$4.8 \times 10^{12}/L$

Mean Cell Volume (MCV)

Adults	82-93 μm³	82-93 fL
Children		
At birth	106 μm³	106 fL
12-24 hours	105 μm³	105 fL
1 week	103 μm³	103 fL
2 weeks	90 μm³	90 fL
1 month to 1 year	82-88 μm³	82-88 fL
2 years	77 μm³	77 fL
4 years	80 μm³	80 fL
11-15 years	82 μm³	82 fL

Mean Cell Hemoglobin (MCH)

Adults	26-34 pg	1.61-2.11 fmol
Children		
At birth	38 pg	2.36 fmol
12-24 hours	38 pg	2.36 fmol
1 week	36 pg	2.23 fmol
2 weeks	33 pg	2.05 fmol
1 month to 1 year	26 pg	1.61 fmol
2 years	25 pg	1.55 fmol
4 years	26 pg	1.61 fmol
6 years	27 pg	1.67 fmol
8-20 years	28 pg	1.73 fmol

Mean Cell Hemoglobin Concentration (MCHC)

Adults	31-38%	19.2-23.58 mmol/L
Children		
At birth	36%	22.34 mmol/L
1 week	34%	21.10 mmol/L
2 weeks	33%	20.48 mmol/L
1 month to 1 year	33%-34%	20.48-21.10 mmol/L
2 years	32%	19.86 mmol/L
4 years	35%	21.72 mmol/L
6 years	34%	21.10 mmol/L
8-20 years	34%	21.10 mmol/L

White Blood Cells (WBCs)

Adult Females	4500-11,000/μL	$4.5\text{-}11.0 \times 10^9$ L
Pregnant		
Trimester 1	6600-14,100/μL	$6.6\text{-}14.1 \times 10^9$ L
Trimester 2	6900-17,100/μL	$6.9\text{-}17.1 \times 10^9$ L
Trimester 3	5900-14,700/μL	$5.9\text{-}14.7 \times 10^9$ L
Postpartum	9700-25,700/μL	$9.7\text{-}25.7 \times 10^9$ L
Adult Males	4500-11,000/μL	$4.5\text{-}11.0 \times 10^9$ L
Children		
At birth	9000-30,000/μL	$9.0\text{-}30.0 \times 10^9$ L
1 month to 1 year	6000-17,500/μL	$6.0\text{-}17.5 \times 10^9$ L
4 years	5700-16,300/μL	$5.7\text{-}16.3 \times 10^9$ L
8-20 years	4500-13,500/μL	$4.5\text{-}13.5 \times 10^9$ L

Continued

		SI Units
Differential White Blood Cells—Granulocytes		
Segmented Neutrophils (Segs)	54%-62%	0.54-0.62
Adults	3800/μL or mm³	3800 × 10⁶/L
Children		
At birth	8400/μL or mm³	8400 × 10⁶/L
12-24 hours	8870-12,100/μL or mm³	8870-12,100 × 10⁶/L
1 week	4100/μL or mm³	4100 × 10⁶/L
2 weeks	3320/μL or mm³	3320 × 10⁶/L
1 month to 1 year	2680-2750/μL or mm³	2680-2750 × 10⁶/L
2 years	2660/μL or mm³	2660 × 10⁶/L
4 years	3040/μL or mm³	3040 × 10⁶/L
6 years	3600/μL or mm³	3600 × 10⁶/L
8-20 years	3700-3800/μL or mm³	3700-3800 × 10⁶/L
Band Neutrophils (Bands)	3%-5%	0.03-0.05
Adults	620/μL or mm³	620 × 10⁶/L
Children		
At birth	2540/μL or mm³	2540 × 10⁶/L
12-24 hours	2680-3460/μL or mm³	2680-3460 × 10⁶/L
1 week	1420/μL or mm³	1420 × 10⁶/L
2 weeks	1200/μL or mm³	1200 × 10⁶/L
1 month to 1 year	990-1150/μL or mm³	990-1150 × 10⁶/L
2 years	850/μL or mm³	850 × 10⁶/L
4 years	710/μL or mm³	710 × 10⁶/L
6 years	670/μL or mm³	670 × 10⁶/L
8-20 years	620-660/μL or mm³	620-660 × 10⁶/L
Eosinophils (Eos)	1%-3%	0.01-0.03
Adults	200/μL or mm³	200 × 10⁶/L
Children		
At birth	400/μL or mm³	400 × 10⁶/L
12-24 hours	450/μL or mm³	450 × 10⁶/L
1 week	500/μL or mm³	500 × 10⁶/L
2 weeks	350/μL or mm³	350 × 10⁶/L
1 month to 1 year	300/μL or mm³	300 × 10⁶/L
2 years	280/μL or mm³	280 × 10⁶/L
4 years	250/μL or mm³	250 × 10⁶/L
6 years	230/μL or mm³	230 × 10⁶/L
8-20 years	200/μL or mm³	200 × 10⁶/L
Basophils (Basos)	<0.75%	0-0.0075
Adults	40/μL or mm³	40 × 10⁶/L
Children		
Birth to 24 hours	100/μL or mm³	100 × 10⁶/L
1 week to 6 years	50/μL or mm³	50 × 10⁶/L
8-20 years	40/μL or mm³	40 × 10⁶/L
Monocytes (Monos)	3%-7%	0.03-0.07
Adults	300/μL or mm³	300 × 10⁶/L
Children		
At birth	1050/μL or mm³	1050 × 10⁶/L
12-24 hours	1100-1200/μL or mm³	1100-1200 × 10⁶/L
1 week	1100/μL or mm³	1100 × 10⁶/L

		SI Units
2 weeks	1000/µL or mm³	1000 × 10⁶/L
1 month to 1 year	700/µL or mm³	700 × 10⁶/L
2 years	530/µL or mm³	530 × 10⁶/L
4 years	450/µL or mm³	450 × 10⁶/L
6 years	400/µL or mm³	400 × 10⁶/L
8-20 years	350-400/µL or mm³	350-400 × 10⁶/L
Lymphocytes (Lymphs)	25%-33%	0.25-0.33
Adults	2500/µL or mm³	2500 × 10⁶/L
Children		
At birth	5500/µL or mm³	5500 × 10⁶/L
12-24 hours	5800/µL or mm³	5800 × 10⁶/L
1 week	5000/µL or mm³	5000 × 10⁶/L
2 weeks	5500/µL or mm³	5500 × 10⁶/L
1 month to 1 year	6000-7000/µL or mm³	6000-7000 × 10⁶/L
2 years	6300/µL or mm³	6300 × 10⁶/L
4 years	4500/µL or mm³	4500 × 10⁶/L
6 years	3500/µL or mm³	3500 × 10⁶/L
8-20 years	2500-3300/µL or mm³	2500-3300 × 10⁶/L
Platelets (Plt)		
Adults	150,000-400,000/µL or mm³	150-400 × 10⁹/L
Panic levels	<30,000/µL or mm³	<30 × 10⁹/L
	>1,000,000/µL or mm³	>1000 × 10⁹/L
Children		
At birth	100,000-300,000/µL or mm³	100-300 × 10⁹/L
1 week	260,000/µL or mm³	260 × 10⁹/L
2 years	250,000/µL or mm³	250 × 10⁹/L
Panic levels	<20,000/µL or mm³	<20 × 10⁹/L
	>1,000,000/µL or mm³	>1000 × 10⁹/L

Increased. See individual test listings.

Decreased. See individual test listings.

Description. The complete blood count (CBC) consists of several tests that allow for the evaluation of different cellular components of the blood on a broad range of clients. The items commonly evaluated include hemoglobin, hematocrit, red blood cells, red blood cell indices, white blood cells, white blood cell differential, platelets, and microscopic examination of stained blood smears. Normal levels of the different blood components vary among different age-groups, depending on the body's needs and composition (see Norms, above). The CBC is used for physical examinations, preoperative screening, and evaluation of acute disease or symptoms of anemia or infection. Serial values are often used to track the progress of a variety of diseases and to monitor for side effects resulting from acute or chronic use of drugs that may cause blood dyscrasias. See individual test listings as follows for detailed descriptions of CBC components: Blood indices—Blood; Differential leukocyte count—Peripheral blood; Hematocrit—Blood; Hemoglobin—Blood; Platelet count—Blood; Red blood cell—Blood.

Professional Considerations
Consent form NOT required.

Preparation
1. Tube: Lavender topped.
2. Do NOT draw during dialysis.

Procedure
1. To avoid a hemodiluted sample, draw the sample from an extremity that does not have intravenous fluids infusing into it. Leaving the tourniquet in place no longer than 60 seconds, completely fill the tube with a venous blood sample. Invert and

gently rotate the tube to thoroughly mix the anticoagulant.

Postprocedure Care
1. Write the specimen collection time on the laboratory requisition.

Client and Family Teaching
1. See individual test listings.
2. Results are normally available within 4 hours.

Factors That Affect Results
1. Failure to fill the tube completely with blood causes an improper blood:anticoagulant ratio, which yields unreliable values.
2. The serum sample is stable at room temperature for 10 hours, may be refrigerated for up to 18 hours, and should not be frozen.
3. Donors in living liver donation experience significantly decreased platelet levels as long as 3 years after donation.
4. See also individual test listings.

Other Data
1. See individual test listings.

Complexed PSA

See **Prostate-Specific Antigen—Serum.**

Comprehensive Metabolic Panel (CMP)—Blood

Norm. See individual test listings: Albumin—Serum, Alkaline phosphatase, heat stable—Serum, Aspartate aminotransferase—Serum, Bicarbonate—Blood, Bilirubin—Serum, Calcium, Ioninized—Blood, Chloride—Serum, Creatinine—Serum, Glucose—Blood, Potassium—Serum, Protein, Total, Sodium, Plasma—Serum, and Urea nitrogen—Plasma or serum.

Usage. See individual test listings.

Description. The CMP is a term defined by the Centers for Medicare and Medicaid Services (CMS) in the United States to indicate a group of tests for which a bundled reimbursement is available. The panel is one of several that replace the multichannel tests, such as SMA-20. The panel is disease oriented, meaning that payment through Medicare is available only when the test is used to diagnose and monitor a disease, and payment is not available when the test is used for screening purposes in clients who have no signs and symptoms. All the tests in the panel must be carried out when a BMP is ordered.

Professional Considerations
Consent form NOT required.

Preparation
1. Tube: Red topped, red/gray topped, or gold topped.
2. Do NOT draw specimens during hemodialysis.

Procedure
1. Draw a 5-mL blood sample.

Postprocedure Care
1. None.

Client and Family Teaching
1. See individual test listings.

Factors That Affect Results
1. See individual test listings.

Other Data
1. See individual test listings.

Compression Ultrasound (CUS)—Diagnostic

Norm. Negative.

Usage. Used in conjunction with rapid ELISA D-dimer testing to assess the probability of existence of venous thrombi. Monitoring for occurrence of deep vein thrombosis in high-risk populations.

Description. Compression ultrasound (CUS) is a noninvasive diagnostic tool that has largely replaced venography (phlebography), which is the criterion standard for diagnosis of venous thrombosis. In this procedure, the transducer pressure is applied to collapse the vein being scanned. A normal vessel will collapse completely, whereas a vessel with a thrombosis will not. Although CUS poses less procedural risk than venography, it is most accurate for the detection of proximal deep vein thromboses, which occur in 85% of clients with deep vein thrombosis (DVT), and which are the source of life-threatening pulmonary emboli. However, CUS often does not identify thromboses of the calf vein(s), is unreliable in determining the patency of the pelvic veins and inferior vena cava, and is not sensitive to asymptomatic postoperative DVT. To compensate for its limitations, the CUS is often followed by a color duplex ultrasound. CUS is not indicated in nonhospitalized clients with a low clinical score for risk of DVT, if a negative D-dimer test result has been obtained. For those with moderate or higher clinical risk scores and a negative D-dimer result, the CUS is recommended. Any positive CUS confirms DVT. Michiels et al (2002) found that "the combination of a negative CUS and a negative rapid ELISA D-dimer test safely excludes DVT in clients with suspected DVT irrespective of the clinical score." Frequent involvement of both limbs suggests the use of this procedure bilaterally.

Clinical Score (Ambulatory Care Clients)	Risk of DVT	Rapid ELISA D-Dimer Test	CUS	Implications
Low	3%-10%	Negative	N/A	Negative predictive value >99% to exclude DVT
Low		Positive <1000 ng/mL	Negative	Negative predictive value >99.9% to exclude DVT
Moderate	15%-30%	Negative	Negative	Negative predictive value >99.4% to exclude DVT
Moderate	15%-30%	Positive	Negative	Probability of DVT of 3%-5% Repeat CUS recommended
High	>70%	Not recommended	Negative	Probability of DVT of 20%-30% Repeat CUS recommended

Michiels JJ, Kasbergen H, Oudega R et al: Exclusion and diagnosis of deep vein thrombosis in outpatients by sequential noninvasive tools, *Int Angiol* 21(1):9-19, 2002.

Professional Considerations
Consent form is NOT required.

Preparation
1. This test may be performed at the bedside.
2. Obtain a 3- to 7-MHz (for adults) or a 5- to 7-MHz (for children) linear transducer.

Procedure
1. Establish a baseline for comparison by evaluating the asymptomatic extremity.
2. Both noncompression and compression views are taken, beginning at the groin and proceeding distally down the common femoral vein, superficial femoral vein, and popliteal vein. Transverse views are taken both without and with augmentation at each of these vessels, followed by longitudinal views via spectral and color Doppler.
3. Repeat on the affected extremity, adding visualization of the iliac veins and inferior vena cava in the pelvis.
4. Follow with color duplex ultrasonography if further visualization of the pelvic veins and inferior vena cava is needed.

Postprocedure Care
1. Cleanse ultrasound gel off of skin.

Client and Family Teaching
1. This test is painless and noninvasive.
2. Test takes about 20 minutes to complete.
3. Radionuclide imaging may follow inconclusive tests.

Factors That Affect Results
1. CUS results may be positive for up to 6 months after an acute DVT.
2. The skill of the operator affects the accuracy of the results.

Other Data
1. The clinical score for determination of probability for DVT is a clinical model of complaints, signs, and symptoms, which has been found to be valid for estimating low, moderate, and high probability.

Computed Tomographic Percutaneous Transsplenic Portography

See **Splenoportography**—Diagnostic.

Computed Tomography of the Body (Spiral [Helical], Electron Beam [EBCT, Ultrafast], High Resolution [HRCT], 64-Slice Multidetector [MDCT])—Diagnostic

Norm. Negative. No tumor, malformations, or pathologic activity.

EBCT Norm. No coronary artery stenosis or calcification, no pulmonary embolism. EBCT has the potential to replace ventilation-perfusion scanning as the primary screening diagnostic test for pulmonary emboli. Scores range from 0-400 with a score over 100 suggesting future cardiac morbidity.

Traditional CT Usage. Determination of the extent of primary and secondary neoplasms of the neck; evaluation of bony and inflammatory abnormalities of the spine and joints, including neoplasms, fractures, dislocations, and congenital anomalies; localization of foreign bodies in the soft tissues, hypopharynx, or larynx; assessment of airway integrity after trauma; evaluation of retropharyngeal abscesses; investigation of suspected tracheal, thymic, mediastinal, and hilar masses; evaluation of problems identified on chest radiographs; staging of bronchogenic carcinoma and gastrointestinal tumors; detection of aortic aneurysm or aortic dissection; detection, localization, and characterization of lung disease; detection of mediastinal or diaphragmatic herniation; evaluation of musculoskeletal or soft-tissue trauma or neoplasms; evaluation of suspected congenital or other abnormalities of specific body organs such as the liver, gallbladder, pancreas, kidneys, adrenal gland, and spleen; identification and localization of sites of hemorrhage; assessment of the organs and structures of the peritoneal cavity and pelvis; and sometimes used to provide imaging identification and guidance for invasive procedures such as abscess drainage or amebic liver abscess, percutaneous biopsy, or aspirate for cytologic or histologic study. The newer 64-slice multidetector CT (MDCT) equipment is suitable for cardiac and coronary scanning, including perfusion scanning, e.g., CT coronary angiography and is comparable to invasive coronary angiography in low-prevalence populations, but not in higher prevalence populations. Therefore the value of CT coronary angiography is in being able to rule out coronary artery disease. MDCT has also been used in the differential diagnosis of appendicitis prior to surgery.

EBCT Usage. Used with contrast for imaging the coronary arteries and coronary artery bypass grafts; for diagnosis of aortic malformations and diseases, pulmonary emboli, and other lung diseases; and for quantifying ventricular mass and volume. Used primarily in asymptomatic clients who have risk factors for heart disease.

Spiral CT Usage. Procedure of choice for lung evaluations for cancer; greater than 90% sensitive and specific for pulmonary embolism, except when subsegmental emboli are found; superior to ultrasonography for detection of deep venous thrombosis; 100% sensitive and 98% specific for detection of aortic injury; 80%-85% sensitive for detection of metastatic liver disease; provides the most sensitivity for diagnosing kidney stone; rapid evaluation for ischemic stroke; preferred CT method for children because of reduced length of radiation exposure and reduced dose of contrast material. Spiral CT equipment often is selected as a replacement for older CT equipment; thus usage would be as described above for traditional CT.

High-Resolution CT Usage. Procedure of choice for lung evaluations for chronic infiltrative lung diseases, and for vascular evaluations, such as brain imaging for vascular malformations.

Description. *Computed tomography* (CT) is a radiographic scan that may be performed with or without contrast on virtually any portion of the body. CT is classified as a reconstructive imaging procedure because it produces a picture of the contents of a portion of the body based on the differing densities and composition of body tissues. The picture is obtained by projection of x-rays along all possible lines in the plane of the body. An x-ray detector records the intensity of the x-rays from multiple angles as it is transmitted through the tissue. A computer then reconstructs the differing intensities into pixels that appear in differing shades for differing tissues and represent an anterior-to-posterior "slice" across the plane of the body. CT is used to detect very minor differences in radiographic contrast, providing radiography that portrays boundaries between tissues that are normally indistinguishable to radiographic examination. The tissue-contrast differentiation of CT is superior to that of conventional radiography.

Electron beam CT (EBCT, Ultrafast CT) was developed specifically for evaluating the heart and other structures in the chest, such as the lungs and blood vessels. This type of CT uses an electron beam magnetically directed to take a rapid sequence of images at the speed of light, thus providing detailed information about how the heart functions throughout the cardiac cycle. Because the images can be taken so quickly, the test takes less time than a regular CT. EBCT can detect plaque and stenosis and can also detect minute amounts of calcific deposits, which can progress to coronary artery lesions.

Spiral (also called helical) CT, first available in the early 1990s, is an improvement in the CT technology that provides much improved resolution in a much shorter time than older CT imaging methods. Spiral CT enables the collection of multiple overlapping pictures taken in a continuous spiral pattern that can be fused to give a three-dimensional picture of the body. Because of the continuous nature of the imaging, less contrast material is needed, and the procedure takes only a few minutes.

High-resolution CT (HRCT) improves on traditional CT technology by providing optimized spatial resolution of body structures and better differentiation of normal from abnormal blood vessels.

The newest equipment, called *"Dual Modality Imaging"* and also known as *"3-D Body Scan,"* combines CT with functional imaging modalities such as PET or SPECT for improved imaging results. In this technique the cross-sectional CT images are fused with the metabolically differentiated PET images to produce a single three-dimensional image that provides better detection of early heart disease, cancer, and brain disorders than either modality alone. (See Dual modality imaging—Diagnostic.)

Professional Considerations

Consent form IS required if contrast material will be injected.

Risks

Allergic reaction to dye (itching, hives, rash, tight feeling in the throat, shortness of breath, bronchospasm, anaphylaxis, death); renal toxicity; hematoma or infection at the injection site for CT with contrast.

Contraindications

CT with contrast: Previous allergy to iodine, shellfish, or radiographic dye; renal insufficiency. CT is contraindicated in clients who are unable to remain motionless while lying in a supine position.

Precautions

During pregnancy, risks of cumulative radiation exposure to the fetus from these and other previous or future imaging studies must be weighed against the benefits of the procedures. Although formal limits for client exposure are relative to this risk:benefit comparison, the United States Nuclear Regulatory Commission requires that the cumulative dose equivalent to an embryo/fetus from occupational exposure not exceed 0.5 rem (5 mSv). Radiation dosage to the fetus is proportional to the distance of the anatomy studied from the abdomen and decreases as pregnancy progresses. An abdominal CT (10-slice) exposes the first trimester fetus to 2.6 rad, but the week 35 fetus to only 1.7 rad. For pregnant clients, consult the radiologist/radiology department to obtain estimated fetal radiation exposure from these procedures.

Preparation

1. For CT with contrast, see Client and Family Teaching.
2. Remove radiopaque objects such as jewelry, snaps, and electrocardiographic leads with snaps (if possible).
3. Establish intravenous access for injection of the dye and prepare emergency equipment for a possible hypersensitivity reaction.

C

4. Obtain radiographic contrast medium, if the procedure will be performed with contrast.
5. Have emergency equipment readily available if the procedure will be performed with contrast.
6. If contrast medium will be injected, just before beginning the procedure, take a "time out" to verify the correct client, procedure, and site.

Procedure

1. The client is positioned supine, with his or her head secured and resting on a headrest on a motorized handling table. For spinal studies, the lumbar spine is straightened by flexing the knees and providing a footrest.
2. The client must lie motionless as the table slowly advances through the circular opening of the scanner. The CT scanner sends a narrow beam of x-rays across the area to be imaged in a linear fashion. While a client is being scanned, the non-absorbed x-rays are detected at the same time as the beam is transmitting. This linear scan sequence is repeated at many different angles around the client's body. The data collected consist of a series of profiles that reflect the area visualized at different angles.
3. If contrast medium is to be used, it is injected intravenously at this time, and the scan is repeated. The client is observed for rash or respiratory difficulty, which may indicate reaction to the contrast medium. Reactions usually develop within 30 minutes if the client is allergic to the dye.
4. For Ultrafast and Spiral CT, the client may be asked to hold his/her breath for short periods of time. Operating in the multislice scan mode, the scanner takes several pictures as the table is advanced by a 2-mm step.

Postprocedure Care

1. Replace the electrocardiographic (ECG) leads if they were removed.
2. For CT with contrast, observe for side effects such as headache, nausea, and vomiting. Resume previous diet if no side effects have been noted.

Client and Family Teaching

1. You must lie motionless during the scan. Because this can be a frightening test, it should be described carefully to the client before he or she enters the CT room.
2. If contrast medium will be used, fast from food and fluids for 6 hours before the CT scan.
3. For Ultrafast and Spiral CT imaging, you will have to hold breath for several seconds.
4. A sensation of burning may be felt from the injection of the contrast medium.

Factors That Affect Results

1. Unavoidable internal motion of body organs such as the heart and lungs or intentional movement by the client contributes to the appearance of "tuning fork"-like streaks across the picture.
2. Radiopaque objects such as jewelry and snaps obscure visualization.
3. The literature contains differing opinions concerning findings of segmental emboli cloud when pulmonary embolus is suspected.

Other Data

1. For chest examinations, the average breast dose from EBCT is comparable to that of conventional CT scanners, despite differences in dose distribution.
2. EBCT has the potential to replace ventilation-perfusion scanning as the primary screening diagnostic test for pulmonary emboli.
3. See also Cerebral computed tomography —Diagnostic.

Computed Tomography of the Brain
See Cerebral Computed Tomography—Diagnostic.

Computed Tomography of the Heart
See Cardiac Calcium Scoring—Diagnostic.

C

Concentration Test—Urine
Norm.

		SI Units
Specific gravity	1.025-1.032	1.025-1.032
Osmolality	>800 mOsm/kg of water	>800 mmol/kg of water

Increased. Dehydration.

Decreased. Congestive heart failure, diabetes insipidus, Fanconi syndrome, hydronephrosis, hypercalcemia, hypokalemia, hypoproteinemia, nephrogenic diabetes insipidus, polycystic kidneys, pyelonephritis (chronic), and sickle cell trait. Drugs include diuretics.

Description. The urine concentration test is an evaluation of renal capacity to concentrate urine in response to fluid deprivation or to dilute the urine in response to fluid overload. Urine specific gravity and osmolality are measured after mild hypernatremia is induced by 12 hours of fluid restriction and deprivation. This test is used to detect renal impairment and evaluate renal tubular function. It is also used to differentiate deficiency of antidiuretic hormone (ADH) from renal insensitivity to ADH. In clients with normal renal function and diabetes insipidus (caused by ADH deficiency), administration of exogenous ADH causes urine osmolality to increase. In clients with renal insensitivity to ADH (nephrogenic diabetes insipidus), the exogenous ADH does not cause an increase in urine osmolality.

Professional Considerations
Consent form NOT required.

Risks
Hypotension and associated sequelae.
Contraindications
This test may be contraindicated in clients with subnormal cardiac output because of the risk of depleting plasma volume.

Preparation
1. See Client and Family Teaching.
2. Obtain baseline weight before the evening meal before the test and every 4 hours until the test is completed. Terminate the test if weight decreases more than 5% from the baseline weight or for orthostatic hypotension.
3. Obtain three 500-mL clean containers.

4. Monitor the client closely throughout the test for symptoms of severe dehydration or for surreptitious intake of fluids.

Procedure
1. Collect the entire voided urine specimens in separate, refrigerated, clean containers at 0600 (6 AM), 0800 (8 AM), and 1000 (10 AM). Record the exact time and amount of each specimen.
2. If the test is being performed to differentiate diabetes insipidus from nephrogenic diabetes insipidus, exogenous ADH (vasopressin) is administered intravenously as soon as a plateau in osmolality is reached. A final urine sample is collected, as above, in 1 hour.

Postprocedure Care
1. Resume diet and fluids.
2. Record the time and amount of each specimen collected on the laboratory requisition.
3. Refrigerate the specimens until testing.

Client and Family Teaching
1. Eat a high-protein dinner the day before the test.
2. Fluids are restricted to 200 mL the evening before the test, including the evening meal.
3. Fast from food and fluids from midnight before the test until the test is completed.
4. It is normal to feel very thirsty during the testing period, but you should not drink anything.

Factors That Affect Results
1. Failure to follow dietary and fluid restrictions will interfere with results.
2. Fluid intake over 200 mL caused by intravenous therapy invalidates the results.
3. Administration of radiographic dyes within 7 days before the test may cause increased urine osmolality.
4. Baseline glucosuria invalidates the results.

Other Data
1. None.

Condyloma Latum, Vulvar or Anal Culture for Cytology—Specimen

Norm. Negative findings.

Description. Condyloma latum is a flat, moist, papular growth that appears on the moist skin of the genital and anal areas during the secondary stages of syphilis. It is also called flat condyloma.

Professional Considerations
Consent form NOT required.

Preparation
1. Verify the collection procedure with the individual laboratory performing the test. Smears may be required to be prepared and fixed at the bedside.
2. Obtain sterile cotton swabs or Culturette, gloves, and transport medium.

Procedure
1. *Vulvar sample:* Wipe the vulva with sterile cotton or gauze. Insert a sterile, cotton-tipped swab between the vulva and leave it in place for several seconds for optimum absorption of pathogens.
2. *Anal sample:* Insert a sterile, cotton-tipped swab into the anus approximately 2 cm. Leave the swab in place several seconds for optimum absorption of pathogens. If feces are obtained, discard the swab and repeat the procedure.

Postprocedure Care
1. Place the swab in the transport medium according to the requirements of the laboratory performing the test.
2. Send the swab immediately to the laboratory.

Client and Family Teaching
1. Refer the client with positive results for follow-up care, which is necessary for prevention and early detection of sequelae.

Factors That Affect Results
1. Results are invalidated if the swab dries out before being inoculated onto culture medium or before preparation of a smear.

Other Data
1. Condyloma of the toe web is an unusual manifestation of secondary syphilis.

Conization of Cervix (Cold Knife Conization)—Diagnostic

Norm. Negative. No abnormal findings.

Usage. Follow-up study for abnormal Pap smear; atypical squamous cells of undetermined significance (ASCUS); carcinoma in situ; cervical cancer, cervical intraepithelial neoplasia (CIN); used when colposcopy, cervical cytology, and colposcopy biopsies yield inconclusive findings.

Description. Conization is a biopsy of the uterine cervix that is performed after cervical smears reveal the presence of intraepithelial neoplasias. It may be performed with dilation and curettage. The advantage that conization brings to the diagnostic process is that it provides a sample of the entire lateral margins of the transformation zone of the cervix. Cold knife conization is less expensive than laser conization and produces equally satisfactory specimens for histologic examination. The cold knife method may also be superior to the loop electrosurgical excisional procedure (LEEP) because it does not produce electrocautery artifact that interferes with examination of the cervical margins.

Professional Considerations
Consent form IS required.

Risks
Hemorrhage, infection, sepsis.
Contraindications
Anticoagulant therapy, bleeding disorders, thrombocytopenia. Sedatives are contraindicated in clients with central nervous system depression.

Preparation
1. See Client and Family Teaching.
2. Preschedule this test with the pathology laboratory. Biopsy specimens must be processed immediately.
3. Obtain Lugol's solution, a tenaculum, vasopressin, conization knife, suture material, Gelfoam or Surgicel (or electrocautery), and a sterile container.

4. Just before beginning the procedure, take a "time out" to verify the correct client, procedure, and site.

Procedure

1. This procedure can be performed under general anesthesia, though local anesthesia is less costly and the client experiences little discomfort, nausea, or vomiting.
2. The client is placed in a lithotomy position, and the cervix is painted with Lugol's solution (Schiller's test) to detect white, pale, or unstained areas, which may indicate lesions.
3. A suture may be sewn on each side of the cervix to control bleeding. The anterior lip of the cervix is lifted with a tenaculum, and vasopressin (Pitressin Synthetic) is injected into several areas to control bleeding.
4. A cone of tissue is removed from the cervical os with a cold knife (Fleming knife). Tissues that did not stain with Schiller's test are included in the cone. The specimen is transferred immediately to the laboratory in a sterile container, with or without sterile saline, according to the requirements of the laboratory performing the test.
5. Bleeding may be controlled by packing with Gelfoam or Surgicel or by cervical sutures or electrocautery.

Postprocedure Care

1. Provide sanitary pads and observe for heavy bleeding, which is abnormal.
2. Perform standard postanesthesia observations and assessments if general anesthesia or deep sedation was used.

Client and Family Teaching

1. If general anesthesia will be used, fast from food and fluids for 8 hours before the procedure.
2. A greenish-grayish discharge from the vagina caused by the presence of the Lugol's solution is normal for several days after the test.
3. Resume previous diet after the procedure.

Factors That Affect Results

1. Electrocautery should not be used because it distorts tissues and impairs diagnosis.

Other Data

1. Conization should be performed in a hospital, rather than in a physician's office.
2. Conization should be performed before dilation and curettage, which dislodges the cervical epithelium.
3. Residual dysplasia present in cold knife conization specimens is not predictive of residual dysplasia in hysterectomy specimens.
4. Residual carcinoma in situ can be present even with a negative conization margin.

Conjunctivae, Routine—Culture

Norm. No abnormal growth. Normal flora includes diphtheroids, *Staphylococcus epidermidis, Staphylococcus pyogenes, Streptococcus pneumoniae,* and *Streptococcus viridans.*

Usage. Used to establish the presence of bacterial or viral pathogens causing blepharitis, chalazion, conjunctivitis, impetigo, and stye.

Description. Conjunctivitis is an inflammation of the eye conjunctiva most commonly caused by staphylococci, nonserotypable *Streptococcus pneumoniae, Chlamydia* (causing inclusion conjunctivitis), rickettsiae, viruses, or parasites. Less commonly, the conjunctiva may be infected by *Gonococcus* and may possibly lead to blindness. Conjunctivitis may also result from allergic processes or injury to the eye. Symptoms of conjunctivitis include redness, swelling, drainage, and itching. This condition is commonly diagnosed by culture and Gram staining or Wright staining of the drainage from the lower part of the conjunctiva.

Professional Considerations

Consent form NOT required.

Preparation

1. Cleanse the skin around the eye.
2. Obtain an eye swab approved for microbiologic purposes and culture tube (Culturette).

Procedure

1. Gently but firmly wipe a sterile, cotton-tipped swab over the inflamed lower conjunctiva or inner canthus, avoiding the eyelashes.
2. Insert the swab into a Culturette tube and squeeze the ampule of medium.
3. If the specimen will be tested for *Gonococcus* (most commonly in newborns), place the swab in a Transgrow bottle, not a Culturette tube.

Postprocedure Care

1. Write the antibiotic therapy on the laboratory requisition.
2. Send the swab to the laboratory immediately.

Client and Family Teaching

1. Where inflammation is present, the swab technique may cause transient pain.

2. Wash hands after touching conjunctival area to avoid spread of infection to others.

Factors That Affect Results

1. Results are invalidated if the specimen dries out before being inoculated onto culture medium or before preparation of a slide for staining.

Other Data

1. The best results are obtained if the culture is taken before antibiotic therapy is started.
2. Candidal blepharitis is often found in immunosuppressed clients.
3. Ciprofloxacin 0.3% ophthalmic solution is effective treatment for keratitis and conjunctivitis. About 8% of conjunctivitis is resistant to ciprofloxacin.

Conjunctival Impression Cytology

See **Ocular Cytology**—Specimen.

Connecting Peptide

See **C-Peptide**—Serum.

Contraction Stress Test

See **Fetal Monitoring, External**—Diagnostic, Contraction Stress Test and Oxytocin Challenge Test.

Contrast Venography

See **Venography**—Diagnostic.

Coombs' Test, Direct (Direct Antiglobulin Test)—Serum

Norm. Negative.

Positive. Arthritis (rheumatoid), elderly clients, erythroblastosis fetalis, hemolytic anemia (autoimmune, drug induced), infection, neoplasm, renal disorders, systemic lupus erythematosus, and transfusion reaction. Drugs include (possibly as a result of IgG erythrocyte sensitization by the drugs) aminopyrine, cephalosporins, chlorpromazine, dipyrone, ethosuximide, hydralazine hydrochloride, insulin, isoniazid, levodopa, mefenamic acid, melphalan, methyldopa, methyldopate hydrochloride, oxyphenisatin, *p*-aminosalicylic acid, penicillins, phenacetin, phenytoin, phenytoin sodium, procainamide hydrochloride, quinidine gluconate, quinidine polygalacturonate, quinidine sulfate, rifampin, streptomycin sulfate, sulfonamides, tetracyclines, and Unasyn (ampicillin sodium plus sulbactam sodium).

Negative. Hemolytic anemia (nonautoimmune, non drug induced). Normal finding.

Usage. Used to show antigen-antibody reactions, differentiation of types of hemolytic anemias, testing for suspected erythroblastosis fetalis, and investigation of erythrocyte sensitization by drugs or blood transfusions.

Description. The direct Coombs' test involves adding Coombs' antihuman globulin serum to a client's washed red blood cells and observing for agglutination, which signals the presence of previously undetected IgG antibodies, complement, or immunoglobulins on the surfaces of the client's erythrocytes. The Coombs' antiglobulin contains antibodies to IgG and several complement components. The antibodies detected by the direct Coombs' test are difficult to detect any other way because they are left over from incomplete antigen-antibody reactions and, though present on the erythrocyte surfaces, remain invisible. The Coombs' antiglobulin causes completion of the antigen-antibody reaction, thus making the antibodies identifiable as they begin clumping.

Professional Considerations
Consent form NOT required.

Preparation
1. Tube: Lavender topped, red topped, red/gray topped, or gold topped.

Procedure
1. Draw a 5-mL blood sample.
2. The sample may be obtained from cord blood.

Postprocedure Care
1. Write recent transfusions and drugs on the laboratory requisition.

Client and Family Teaching
1. For positive results, the more specific direct Coombs' IgG test is indicated.

Factors That Affect Results
1. Reject hemolyzed specimens.
2. Cord blood contaminated by Wharton's jelly may yield unreliable results.
3. Cold agglutinins may cause false-positive results.
4. Drugs that may cause false-negative results in the presence of acquired hemolytic anemia include heparin calcium and heparin sodium.

Other Data
1. This test does not delineate the nature of the antibodies identified.
2. The test must be completed within 24 hours of specimen collection.
3. There is a high incidence of positive results in clients with antibodies to HIV, which indicates that this test may be helpful as a prognostic indicator for the disease course.
4. See also Antibody identification, Red cell—Blood.

Coombs' Test, Direct IgG—Serum

Norm. Negative.

Positive. Anemia (hemolytic, drug induced), autoimmune hepatitis, erythroblastosis fetalis, leukemia (chronic lymphocytic), and transfusion reaction. Drugs include (possibly as a result of IgG erythrocyte sensitization by the drugs) aminopyrine, cephalosporins, chlorpromazine, dipyrone, ethosuximide, hydralazine, hydrochloride, insulin, isoniazid, levodopa, mefenamic acid, melphalan, methyldopa, methyldopate hydrochloride, oxyphenisatin, p-aminosalicylic acid, penicillins, phenacetin, phenytoin, phenytoin sodium, procainamide hydrochloride, quinidine gluconate, quinidine polygalacturonate, quinidine sulfate, rifampin, streptomycin sulfate, sulfonamides, and tetracyclines.

Description. See Coombs' test, Direct—Serum. This test is more specific than a direct Coombs' test and is performed after a positive direct Coombs' test. The direct Coombs' IgG test mixes Coombs' antiglobulin containing only anti-IgG with the client's washed red blood cells and observes for agglutination, which signals the presence of IgG on the surface of the client's erythrocytes.

Professional Considerations
Consent form NOT required.

Preparation
1. Tube: Lavender topped.

Procedure
1. Draw a 5-mL blood sample.

Postprocedure Care
1. Write recent transfusions and drugs on the laboratory requisition.

Client and Family Teaching
1. Results are normally available within 24 hours.

Factors That Affect Results
1. Cold agglutinins may cause false-positive results.
2. False-negative results may occur in the presence of sensitized erythrocytes with less than 100-300 IgG molecules per cell.

Other Data
1. The test must be completed within 24 hours of specimen collection.

Coombs' Test, Indirect (Indirect Antiglobulin Test)—Serum

Norm. Negative.

Positive. ABO-incompatible bone marrow transplant, erythroblastosis fetalis, hemolytic anemia (drug induced), hemolytic transfusion reaction (delayed), incompatible crossmatch, maternal-fetal Rh incompatibility, and prior transfusion reaction. Drugs include levodopa, mefenamic acid, methyldopa, and methyldopate hydrochloride.

Description. This test detects unexpected circulating antibodies by exposing a client's serum to group O erythrocytes that are not affected by anti-A or anti-B antibodies but do contain other known antigens. It screens for reactions to RhDu, Kell, and Duffy antigens; pre transfusion blood screening; detection of leukocyte, platelet, or rare antibodies; and screening prenatally for fetomaternal blood incompatibility. In contrast to the direct Coombs' test, which detects antibodies already attached to erythrocytes, the indirect Coombs' test detects the presence of antibodies other than those of the ABO groups that are present in the serum. One performs the test by (1) mixing erythrocytes containing known antigens to a client's serum and allowing time for unknown antibodies in the client's serum to react with the antigens; (2) adding Coombs' antihuman globulin serum to the mixture and observing for agglutination, indicating the presence of antibodies.

Professional Considerations
Consent form NOT required.

Preparation
1. Tube: Red topped, red/gray topped, or gold topped and lavender topped.

Procedure
1. Adults: Draw a 10-mL blood sample in the red topped tube and a 5-mL blood sample in the lavender topped tube.
2. Pediatrics: Draw a 7-mL blood sample in the red topped tube and a 3-mL blood sample in the lavender topped tube.

Postprocedure Care
1. Write recent transfusions and drugs on the laboratory requisition.

Client and Family Teaching
1. Results are normally available within 24 hours.
2. If results are positive, an additional sample may be needed to perform antibody identification.

Factors That Affect Results
1. Reject hemolyzed specimens.
2. Cold agglutinins may cause false-positive results.

Other Data
1. Negative tests on pregnant women during the first 12 weeks of gestation should be repeated at 28 weeks of gestation. A positive test at 28 weeks of gestation indicates the need for antibody-identification testing.
2. This test must be completed within 48 hours of specimen collection.

Co-Oximeter Profile (Hemoglobin Profile), Arterial or Venous—Blood

Norm.

	% Hemoglobin
Carboxyhemoglobin (COHb)	Nonsmokers: <1.5%
	Smokers: <5%
	Toxic: 15%-35%
Methemoglobin (MetHb)	0.4%-1.5%
Oxyhemoglobin (O$_2$Hb, oxygen saturation)	Arterial: 94%-100%
	Venous: 60%-80%
Total hemoglobin (THb)	12%-15%
Volume % O$_2$ (%O$_2$)	15%-23%

Usage. Helps diagnose and monitor carbon monoxide poisoning. Determination of the fractional components of hemoglobin.

Description. CO-oximetry provides a breakdown of all of the components that make up the total hemoglobin values. In monitoring critically ill clients, this test can help the clinician assess the capacity for oxygenation in these clients. It can provide more accurate information than noninvasive pulse oximetry, which decreases in accuracy as hypoxemia and perfusion worsen.

Professional Considerations
Consent form NOT required.

Preparation
1. Allow time for client to relax before testing.
2. Obtain a heparinized green topped tube or lavender topped tube or a heparinized capillary tube and ice for a venous sample; or an arterial blood gas kit and ice for an arterial sample.
3. Document oxygen delivery amount and site of specimen collection on the laboratory requisition.

Procedure
1. Position client supine.
2. Venous sample: Draw at least a 0.5-mL blood sample by means of venous puncture or heelstick.
3. Arterial sample: Obtain a 1.5-mL arterial blood sample by means of arterial puncture.

Postprocedure Care
1. Place specimen immediately on ice.
2. Hold pressure over the site until bleeding stops. Assess for hematoma.

Client and Family Teaching
1. Any hematoma present will gradually reabsorb into the body over several days.

Factors That Affect Results
1. Results may not be accurate if client is also receiving methylene blue.
2. Results will be erroneous if specimen contains air bubbles.
3. Blood substitutes give less accurate or negative carboxyhemoglobin readings.

Other Data
1. See also Methemoglobin—Blood; Blood gases, Arterial—Blood; Blood gases, Venous—Blood.

Copper (Cu)—Serum

Norm.

		SI Units
Adult Females	80-155 µg/dL	12.56-24.34 µmol/L
Pregnant, 40 weeks	118-302 µg/dL	18.53-47.41 µmol/L
Adult Males	70-140 µg/dL	10.99-21.98 µmol/L
Children		
≤6 months	20-70 µg/dL	3.14-10.99 µmol/L
Infant	15-65 µg/dL	2.35-10.20 µmol/L
Child	30-150 µg/dL	4.71-23.55 µmol/L

Increased. Alzheimer's disease, anemia (aplastic, pernicious, megaloblastic of pregnancy; iron deficiency), cirrhosis (biliary), elevated C-reactive protein, glomerulonephritis, hemochromatosis, Hodgkin's disease, hyperestrogenemia, hypertension, hyperthyroidism, hypothyroidism, infection, leukemia, Löfgren's syndrome, lymphoma, myocardial infarction, occupation as worker in copper processing plant, pellagra, pregnancy, rheumatoid arthritis, sarcoidosis, systemic lupus erythematosus, and ulcerative colitis. Drugs include carbamazepine, estrogens and oral contraceptives, heroin that is homemade, phenobarbital, and phenytoin sodium.

Decreased. Burns, Down syndrome, enteral nutrition (long-term), hypoproteinemia, kwashiorkor, malabsorption, Menkes (kinky hair) syndrome, nephrosis, and Wilson's disease. Drugs include nifedipine.

Description. Copper is an essential trace element that functions in hemoglobin synthesis and activation of respiratory enzymes. Abnormally low levels cause impaired erythrocyte production and survival time and lowered catabolism by copper-containing enzymes. Copper toxicity causes jaundice, hepatic injury, headache, and vomiting and may lead to hemolytic shock. This test is most frequently used to aid diagnosis of Wilson's disease, in which serum copper levels are low, urine copper levels are high, and increased amounts of copper are deposited in body tissues.

Professional Considerations
Consent form NOT required.

Preparation
1. Preschedule this test with the laboratory.
2. Obtain a stainless-steel needle, plastic syringe, and navy blue topped tube.
3. Do NOT draw during hemodialysis or peritoneal dialysis.

Procedure
1. Draw a 10-mL blood sample in a plastic syringe, using a stainless-steel needle.
2. Transfer the sample into a navy blue–topped tube without a rubber-siliconized stopper.

Postprocedure Care
1. None.

Client and Family Teaching
1. Results are normally available within 24 hours.

Factors That Affect Results
1. The contact of serum with a rubber-siliconized stopper yields unreliable results.

Other Data
1. Serum ceruloplasmin and urine copper are usually also evaluated with this test.
2. Serial testing and copper supplementation are recommended for clients with burns.

Copper (Cu)—Urine

Norm.

		SI Units
All ages	0-60 µg/24 hours	0-0.96 µµmol/day
Wilson's disease	>100 µg/24 hours	>1.60 µmol/day

Increased. Alzheimer's disease, aminoaciduria, cirrhosis (biliary, Indian childhood), hepatitis (chronic, active), hyperceruloplasminemia, nephrotic syndrome, pellagra, proteinuria, and Wilson's disease (500-1000 mg/dL).

Description. Copper is an essential trace element that functions in hemoglobin synthesis and activation of respiratory enzymes. Abnormally low levels cause impaired erythrocyte production and survival time and lowered catabolism by copper-containing enzymes. Copper toxicity causes jaundice, hepatic injury, headache, and vomiting and may lead to hemolytic shock. This test is most frequently used to aid diagnosis of Wilson's disease, in which serum copper levels are low, urine copper levels are high, and increased amounts of copper are deposited in body tissues.

Professional Considerations
Consent form NOT required.

C

Preparation

1. Preschedule this test with the laboratory.
2. Obtain a clean polyethylene, acid-washed container, pH paper, hydrochloric (HCl) or nitric acid, and a 100-mL clean container for the aliquot.

Procedure

1. Discard the first morning urine specimen.
2. Begin to time a 24-hour urine collection.
3. Save all the urine voided for 24 hours in a room temperature, clean, 3-L, polyethylene, acid-washed container. Document the quantity of urine output during the specimen collection period. For catheterized clients, empty the urine drainage bag into the acidified collection container hourly. Include the urine voided at the end of the 24-hour period. Add HCl or nitric acid as needed to maintain pH at 2.

Postprocedure Care

1. Compare the urine quantity in the specimen container with the urinary output record for the test. If the specimen contains less urine than what was recorded as output, some of the sample may have been discarded, invalidating the test.
2. Document the urine quantity on the laboratory requisition.
3. Send a 100-mL aliquot to the lab.

Client and Family Teaching

1. Save all the urine voided in the 24-hour period and urinate before defecating to avoid loss of urine. If any urine is accidentally discarded, discard the entire specimen and restart the collection the next day.

Factors That Affect Results

1. All the urine voided for the 24-hour period must be included before the aliquot is taken to avoid a falsely low result.
2. Contact of the specimen with stool or metal invalidates results.

Other Data

1. Serum copper and serum ceruloplasmin are usually also evaluated with this test.
2. Significantly higher copper values are seen in females 15-19 years of age when compared to males.

Coproporphyrin (UCP)—Urine

Norm. Norms vary by laboratory. Consult reference range reported with results. Some reported ranges are as follows:

		SI Units
24-Hour Urine		
All	34-234 µg/24 hours	51-351 nmol/day
Adult females	1-57 µg/24 hours	1.5-86 nmol/day
Adult males	<96 µg/24 hours	<144 nmol/day
First Morning Void		
All	0.5-2.3 µg/dL	0.75-3.5 nmol/L

Increased. Acute myocardial infarction, acute poliomyelitis, anemia (hemolytic, pernicious, sideroachrestic), cirrhosis (alcoholic), coproporphyria (erythropoietic), erythroid hyperplasia, exercise, fever, hemochromatosis, hepatitis C virus, HIV, Hodgkin's disease, lead poisoning, leukemia, porphyria (congenital erythropoietic), porphyria cutanea tarda, protoporphyria (erythropoietic), thyrotoxicosis, and vitamin deficiencies. Drugs include barbiturates, chloral hydrate, chlordiazepoxide, chlorpropamide, meprobamate, and sulfonamides.

Decreased. Not clinically significant.

Description. Coproporphyrin is a compound formed during the production of the heme portion of hemoglobin. After it is metabolized, small amounts of coproporphyrin can be found in the urine of healthy individuals. Clients with one of the congenital or acquired diseases classified as the "porphyrias" secrete and excrete increased amounts of hemoglobin-precursor compounds, including coproporphyrin. This test is most frequently used with the measurement of other urine porphyrin levels to differentiate the cause and type of porphyria present.

Professional Considerations
Consent form NOT required.

Preparation
1. See Client and Family Teaching.
2. Obtain a 3-L, light-protected, clean specimen container, pH paper, sodium bicarbonate, and a 100-mL light-protected container.

Procedure
1. 24-hour urine:
   a. Discard the first morning urine specimen.
   b. Begin to time a 24-hour urine collection.
   c. Collect a 24-hour urine specimen in a refrigerated dark bottle containing 5 g of sodium carbonate. Document the quantity of urine output and keep the container tightly covered during the specimen collection period. For catheterized clients, maintain the collection bag on ice in a light-protected container and empty the bag into the refrigerated collection container hourly.
   d. Maintain the pH of the specimen between 6 and 7 by adding sodium bicarbonate as needed. Include the urine voided at the end of the 24-hour period.
   e. At the end of the collection period, mix the specimen gently and transfer a 50-mL aliquot to a light-protected container and cap tightly.
2. First morning void:
   a. Collect the entire first morning-voided urine specimen in a light-protected container.

Postprocedure Care
1. Before taking an aliquot, compare the urine quantity in the specimen container with a urinary output record for the test. If the specimen contains less urine than what was recorded as output, some of the sample may have been discarded, thus invalidating the test.
2. Send the specimen to the laboratory immediately and refrigerate it until testing.

Client and Family Teaching
1. Barbiturates, chloral hydrate, chlorpropamide, sulfonamides, meprobamate, and chlordiazepoxide will induce porphyria and should be stopped 10 days before the test.
2. Save all the urine voided in the 24-hour period and urinate before defecating to avoid loss of urine. If any urine is accidentally discarded, discard the entire specimen and restart the collection the next day.

Factors That Affect Results
1. All the urine voided for the 24-hour period must be included before the aliquot is taken to avoid a falsely low result.
2. Porphyrins decompose when exposed to light.
3. Drugs that may cause unreliable results include phenothiazines.

Other Data
1. This test is not specific for lead poisoning.
2. Uroporphyrin, protoporphyrin, delta-aminolevulinic acid (ALA), and porphobilinogen levels should also be performed.

Coronary Angiography
See Cardiac Catheterization—Diagnostic.

Coronary Artery Calcium Scoring
See Cardiac Calcium Scoring—Diagnostic.

Coronary Intravascular Ultrasonography (Coronary Sonogram, Coronary Ultrasound)—Diagnostic

Norm. Three-dimensional view of the inside of vasculature. Normal coronary vascular anatomy; absence of coronary artery narrowing or occlusion; absence of coronary artery luminal irregularities.

Usage. Provides information regarding tissue characterization, morphology, and the precise measurement of the dimensions of the coronary arteries; identification of plaque and thrombus as well as other luminal irregularities; assessment of the coronary arteries before and after coronary angioplasty; identification of the best location for the placement of arterial stents (a coil wire used to keep arteries open in clients with occluded arteries). Helps check for stent expansion after placement of intracoronary stents. Also used for the location of atherosclerotic plaque formation before removal during cardiac catheterization.

Description. An invasive ultrasound performed from a transducer within the lumen of the coronary arteries. The intravascular ultrasound uses a tiny transducer, about 1 mm in diameter, that is fed through a catheter leading to the heart from a femoral vessel. Similar to those seen in ultrasonograms and echocardiograms, ultrasound images of the inside of the arteries appear on a monitor, offering a clear picture of the inside of the vessel. The images allow visualization of tears, precise determination of the size and shape of plaque buildup or a blood clot, or evaluation of the effectiveness of an angioplasty. This procedure is extremely useful in the evaluation of left main coronary artery narrowing. It is performed with coronary catheterization and angiography. A baseline impression, depicted through tissue differentiation, can provide insight into the progression and degree of coronary artery disease. When used with other procedures, the ultrasonogram requires about 5 minutes of time to complete.

Professional Considerations

Consent form IS required. Consent for this procedure may be included with the consent for cardiac catheterization and angiography.

Risks
Prolonged bleeding, hemorrhage, cerebrovascular accident, hypotension, death.
Contraindications
No different from those for cardiac catheterization.

Preparation
1. See Cardiac catheterization—Diagnostic. No additional preparation is necessary for this procedure.

Procedure
1. An 8-French, transducer-tipped catheter is placed over a guidewire into the coronary artery. The sound beam is swept through a series of radial positions within the perimeter of a well-defined cross-sectional plane. The echo information is then converted into a "real-time" cross-sectional image of the vessel.
2. This procedure increases the length of a cardiac catheterization procedure by approximately 15 minutes and requires a larger dose of heparin.
3. Just before beginning the procedure, take a "time out" to verify the correct client, procedure, and site.

Postprocedure Care
1. Because additional heparinization is required when this procedure is added to a cardiac catheterization, the immediate postprocedure bed rest requirements may be prolonged.
2. See Cardiac catheterization—Diagnostic.

Client and Family Teaching
1. See Cardiac catheterization—Diagnostic.

Factors That Affect Results
1. None found.

Other Data
1. Complications of this procedure include the potential for lifting plaque or thrombus from the vessel lumen because the tip of the transducer actually enters the coronary artery, as well as potential complications listed under Cardiac Catheterization—Diagnostic.

Cortisol—Plasma or Serum

Norm.

		SI Units
Adult		
8-10 AM	5-28 μg/dL	138-773 nmol/L
4-6 PM	2-14 μg/dL or 1/2 morning level	55-386 nmol/L
8 PM	<50% of morning level	
Child		
8-10 AM	15-25 μg/dL	414-690 nmol/L
4-6 PM	5-10 μg/dL or 1/2 morning level	138-276 nmol/L
8 PM	<50% of morning level	

Increased. Burns, CABG (post-op), Crohn's disease, Cushing's disease, Cushing's syndrome, eclampsia, exercise, hepatic disease (severe), hyperpituitarism, hypertension, hyperthyroidism, infectious disease, obesity, osteoporosis, pancreatitis (acute), pregnancy, renal disease (severe), shock, stress (severe, heat, cold, trauma, psychologic), surgery, and virilism. Drugs include corticotropin, estrogens, oral contraceptives, yohimbine, and vasopressin.

Decreased. Addison's disease, adrenal insufficiency, adrenogenital syndrome, chromophobe adenoma, craniopharyngioma, hypoglycemia, hypophysectomy, hypopituitarism, hypothyroidism, liver disease, postpartum pituitary necrosis, rheumatoid arthritis, and Waterhouse-Friderichsen syndrome. Drugs include dexamethasone, dexamethasone acetate, and dexamethasone sodium phosphate.

Description. Cortisol is a steroidal hormone released from the adrenal cortex when stimulated by secretion of adrenocorticotropic hormone (ACTH) from the pituitary gland. Cortisol is normally secreted in a diurnal pattern, with peaks and troughs occurring during specific time periods. This test is most commonly used to aid diagnosis of Cushing's syndrome, in which multiple results compared from AM and PM reveal no diurnal variation in cortisol levels. However, plasma or serum cortisol levels are less reliable than a 24-hour urine collection for diagnosing or ruling out Cushing's syndrome.

Professional Considerations
Consent form NOT required.

Preparation
1. See Client and Family Teaching.
2. Tube: Red topped, red/gray topped, or gold topped tube for serum level; green topped or lavender topped for plasma level.

Procedure
1. Draw a 4-mL blood sample.

Postprocedure Care
1. Write the collection time on the laboratory requisition. Also note the client's status, such as "after ACTH infusion," where applicable.
2. Send the specimen to the laboratory for immediate spinning.

Client and Family Teaching
1. Fast from food and fluids for 4-8 hours before the procedure.
2. Restrict physical activity for 10-12 hours. The client should be relaxed and recumbent for 30 minutes before the test.

Factors That Affect Results
1. Reject hemolyzed or lipemic specimens.
2. Cortisol is secreted in a diurnal pattern. The highest levels occur from 5 to 10 AM, with peak levels occurring at about 8 AM.
3. Specimens collected other than in the morning should be collected before meals.
4. Collect specimens at the same time each day. Levels increase with exposure to bright light.
5. Hypoglycemic states suppress plasma cortisol response.
6. Falsely elevated results may occur from amphetamines, estrogens (within 6

weeks), ethyl alcohol (ethanol), methamphetamines, nicotine, oral contraceptives (within 6 weeks), quinacrine, and spironolactone.

7. Estrogens during pregnancy and during oral contraceptive use will falsely increase levels by increasing plasma proteins that bind with cortisol.

8. Falsely decreased results may result when there is a delay in spinning down the sample.

Other Data

1. The specimen is stable at room temperature for 1 week.

2. Extreme elevation in the morning and no variation in the evening are suggestive of carcinoma.

3. A single sleeping midnight cortisol level >50 nmol/L has 100% accuracy in the diagnosis of Cushing's syndrome, 2% more accurate than the dexamethasone suppression test alone.

Cortisol—Urine

Norm.

		SI Units
Adult	10-100 μg/day	27-276 nmol/day
Child >12 years	5-55 μg/day	14-152 nmol/day
Child <12 years	2-27 μg/day	5.5-74 nmol/day

Increased. Amenorrhea, Cushing's syndrome, hyperthyroidism, lung cancer (small cell carcinoma), pituitary tumor, pregnancy, and stress. Drugs include corticotrophin, fluticasone propionate.

Decreased. Hypothyroidism and renal glomerular dysfunction. Drugs include dexamethasone, dexamethasone acetate, dexamethasone sodium phosphate, and inhaled glucocorticoids for asthma treatment. Ingestion of grapefruit juice.

Description. Cortisol is a steroidal hormone released from the adrenal cortex when stimulated by secretion of adrenocorticotropic hormone (ACTH) from the anterior pituitary gland. Free cortisol is unconjugated cortisol filtered by the renal glomeruli into the urine. Although it comprises less than 5% of circulating cortisol, the amount filtered follows the pattern of cortisol secretion from the adrenal cortex. Because it is excreted in a diurnal pattern, a 24-hour urine sample contains the effects of both the peak and trough cortisol levels and is thus a more accurate measurement than serum levels for diagnosing or ruling out Cushing's syndrome in which continuously high levels of cortisol are secreted.

Professional Considerations

Consent form NOT required.

Preparation

1. See Client and Family Teaching.

2. Obtain a clean, 3-L urine container to which 10 g of boric acid or 20 mL of 33% acetic acid has been added.

Procedure

1. Discard the first morning urine specimen.

2. Save all the urine voided for 24 hours in a refrigerated 3-L container to which 10 g of boric acid has been added. If the specimen is more than 1 L, add 10 g of boric acid for each additional liter of urine. Include the urine voided at the end of the 24-hour period. For catheterized clients, keep the drainage bag on ice and empty urine into the collection container hourly.

3. Alternatively, obtain a room-temperature collection as described previously in a 3-L container to which 20 mL of 33% acetic acid has been added.

Postprocedure Care

1. Compare the urine quantity in the specimen container with the urinary output record for the test. If the specimen contains less urine than what was recorded as output, some of the sample may have been discarded, invalidating the test.

2. Document the quantity of urine output for the 24-hour period on the laboratory requisition.

3. The specimen should be frozen until testing occurs.

Client and Family Teaching
1. Do not take spironolactone or quinacrine for 7 days before the test.
2. Because exercise increases cortisol secretion, activity should be restricted 24 hours before the test until the collection is complete.
3. Save all the urine voided in the 24-hour period and urinate before defecating to avoid loss of urine. If any urine is accidentally discarded, discard the entire specimen and restart the collection the next day.

Factors That Affect Results
1. Stress during the test increases levels.
2. All the urine voided for the 24-hour period must be included to avoid a falsely low result.
3. Falsely elevated results may occur from amphetamines, anticonvulsants, estrogens (within 6 weeks), methamphetamines, nicotine, oral contraceptives (within 6 weeks), quinacrine, and spironolactone.

Other Data
1. Also measure creatinine concentration.

Coxsackie A or B Virus Titer—Blood

Norm. Negative. Less than a fourfold increase in titer of paired (acute and convalescent) sera.

Positive Coxsackie A. Acute febrile respiratory disease, acute flaccid paralysis, conjunctivitis (epidemic hemorrhagic), enteroviral carditis, myositis, and viral carditis.

Positive Coxsackie B. Acute febrile respiratory disease, aseptic meningitis (viral), chorioretinitis, enteroviral carditis, epidemic pleurodynia, fulminant hepatitis, hand-foot-and-mouth disease, herpangina, meningitis, myocarditis, pericarditis, pleurisy, and viral carditis.

Description. The coxsackievirus is divided into two antigenically different groups, A and B, and is of the enterovirus family. Enteroviruses are easily transmitted by the fecal-oral route and are associated with epidemics, especially in newborn nurseries. Although blood is rarely used for isolation of viruses, serologic testing may be performed to detect Coxsackie A virus or Coxsackie B virus antibodies. Twenty-three species of Coxsackie A exist. Types 1, 4, 9, 16, and 23 may infect the heart, causing pericarditis progressing to heart failure. Hand, foot and mouth disease (HFMD) is a viral infection caused by Coxsackie A virus, occurring usually in ages 10 years and younger. Coxsackie type A is also associated with a severe form of conjunctivitis and with respiratory disease. Six species of Coxsackie B exist. Types 1 to 5 may infect the heart, causing pericarditis progressing to heart failure.

These same types may cause pleurodynia, a disease of limited duration (1 week) in which the client experiences the acute onset of chest or abdominal pain along with fever and headache. Types 2 to 5 cause most cases of viral meningitis. This test involves measuring the antibody levels in both an acute and a convalescent sample of blood to detect an increase in the titer. It is a neutralization test in which diluted samples (1:2, 1:8, 1:32, 1:128, 1:512) are mixed with Coxsackie A virus or Coxsackie B virus, inoculated onto a cell culture system, and observed for antigen-antibody reactions for up to 7 days. Enterovirus antibodies respond very quickly to infection; thus the earlier the acute sample is collected, the better the chance of detecting a positive test.

Professional Considerations
Consent form NOT required.

Preparation
1. Preschedule the test with the laboratory.
2. Tube: Red topped, red/gray topped, or gold topped.

Procedure
1. Draw a 4-mL blood sample.
2. Collect an acute-phase sample promptly after symptoms appear and no more than 1 week after onset.
3. Collect the convalescent sample 2-3 days after the onset of symptoms or 2-3 weeks after the acute-phase sample.

Postprocedure Care
1. Label the specimen as either the acute sample or the convalescent sample.

2. The test should be specified as either Cox-sackie A virus titer or Coxsackie B virus titer.
3. Transport the specimen immediately to the laboratory. The sample should be clotted at room temperature, with serum and clot then separated and saved for simultaneous testing with the convalescent sample.

Client and Family Teaching

1. Results are usually available in 5 to 10 days.

Factors That Affect Results

1. Transportation of the serum to an outside laboratory may result in clot disintegration and hemolysis, thus invalidating the test.

2. After separation, samples are stable up to 6 weeks when refrigerated. Longer storage requires freezing at −20 degrees C.
3. Paired sera should be tested at the same time in the same laboratory.
4. False-negative Coxsackie A virus results may occur when the acute-phase titer is elevated as a result of past Coxsackie A virus infection.
5. False-negative Coxsackie B virus results may occur when the acute-phase titer is elevated as a result of past Coxsackie B virus infection.

Other Data

1. Other tests performed to detect Coxsackie A virus or Coxsackie B virus infection include swabs of feces and the throat.

CPA

See Color Duplex Ultrasonography—Diagnostic.

CPAP Titration Study

See Polysomnography—Diagnostic.

C-Peptide (Connecting Peptide)—Serum

Norm.

		SI Units
C-Peptide		
Adult ≤60 years	≤4.0 ng/mL	≤4.0 µg/L
Female >60 years	1.4-5.5 ng/mL	1.4-5.5 µg/L
Male >60 years	1.5-5.0 ng/mL	1.5-5.0 µg/L
Insulin:Glucose Ratio	<0.3	

Usage. Factitious (self-medication) hypoglycemia caused by exogenous insulin overdose or insulin abuse; detection of fasting hypoglycemia or insulinoma by failure to suppress C-peptide production with exogenous insulin administration; evaluation after pancreatectomy for residual islet tissue; and evaluation of insulin reserve in insulin-dependent diabetics.

Increased. Android type of obesity, cardiac dysrhythmias (prolonged QT interval), islet cell tumor, sudden death. Drugs include oral hypoglycemic agents and sulfonylureas. One study suggests that a high intake of fructose and high-glycemic foods are associated with higher C-peptide levels.

Decreased. Diabetes mellitus, pancreatic disorders in alcoholics. Drugs include rosiglitazone, troglitazone.

Description. C-peptide is an inactive amino acid residue degradation product of proinsulin. It is formed as a by-product during the endogenous conversion of proinsulin to insulin in the pancreatic beta cells and its release is unaffected by exogenous insulin administration. C-peptide levels normally correlate with insulin levels because it is released by the beta cells in amounts similar to endogenous insulin release. This test is helpful in estimating endogenous insulin levels when insulin assay is falsely elevated by insulin antibodies.

Professional Considerations
Consent form NOT required.

Preparation
1. Tube: Red topped, red/gray topped or gold topped, and gray topped, and a container of ice.

Procedure
1. Draw a 4-mL blood sample for insulin and C-peptide in a chilled, red topped tube.
2. Pack the sample for insulin in ice.
3. Draw a 4-mL blood sample for glucose in a gray topped tube.

Postprocedure Care
1. Write the collection time on the laboratory requisition.

2. Transport the specimen to the laboratory immediately.
3. The serum should be immediately separated in a chilled centrifuge and frozen in a plastic tube.

Client and Family Teaching
1. Fasting from food and fluids for 8 hours may be required before sampling.

Factors That Affect Results
1. Reject hemolyzed specimens.
2. Recent radioactive scans invalidate the results.
3. C-peptide levels do not always correlate with intrinsic insulin levels in obese clients and clients with islet cell tumors.
4. Hepatic dysfunction causes elevated levels.

Other Data
1. Perform the C-peptide measurement and insulin measurement on the same sample.
2. Pancreas graft function is attainable in clients with high preoperative C-peptide.

CPK
See **Creatine Kinase—Serum.**

CPS
See **Polysomnography—Diagnostic.**

^{51}Cr (Chromium)-Red Cell Survival—Blood

Norm.

Plasma radioactivity half-life	$\leq$2 hours
Tagged ^{51}Cr-red blood cell half-life	25-35 days
Gamma scan	Only slight spleen, liver, and bone marrow radioactivity

Increased. Thalassemia minor.

Decreased. Anemia (congenital nonspherocytic, idiopathic acquired hemolytic, megaloblastic of pregnancy, pernicious, sickle cell), distal splenorenal shunt, elliptocytosis (with hemolysis), hemoglobin C disease, hemoglobinuria (paroxysmal nocturnal), leukemia (chronic lymphatic), spherocytosis (hereditary), and uremia.

Description. Red blood cell survival time is measured by tagging a sample of the client's red blood cells (RBCs) with radioactive ^{51}Cr. Over a 4-week period, blood samples are periodically measured for radioactivity levels to determine the amount of time taken for the tagged RBCs to disappear from the circulation. Major body organs may also be scanned with a gamma camera to locate concentrations of radioactivity. The test aids in identifying the cause of anemia and sites of RBC destruction.

Professional Considerations
Consent form NOT required.

C

Preparation

1. For procedure steps 1-3, collect a sterile glass beaker containing sodium chromate.
2. For procedure steps 4-6, use green topped and lavender topped tubes.

Procedure

1. Draw a 30-mL blood sample and mix it with 100 mCi of ^{51}Cr (sodium chromate).
2. Incubate overnight.
3. Inject the mixture intravenously into the client.
4. 30 minutes later, draw a 6-mL blood sample in a lavender topped tube for measurement of baseline volumes of blood and red cells.
5. 24 hours later, draw a 6-mL blood sample in a green topped tube. Send the specimen to the laboratory for a same-day measurement of hematocrit and of ^{51}Cr with a scintillation well counter.
6. Repeat procedure 5 every 1-3 days for 4 weeks.
7. After the last sample is drawn, draw a 6-mL blood sample in a lavender topped tube for comparison measurement of blood and red cell volumes.

Postprocedure Care

1. None.

Client and Family Teaching

1. No isolation is necessary.

Factors That Affect Results

1. Conditions that decrease red blood cell volume or the proportion of tagged red cells to nontagged red cells, including blood draws, blood transfusions, chronic occult extravascular blood loss, and hemorrhage, will simulate decreased survival time.

Other Data

1. Normal tests are seen in hemoglobin C trait and sickle cell trait and elliptocytosis without hemolysis.
2. Normal red blood cell half-life is 60 days.
3. This test may also be used to predict the viability of donated red blood cells.
4. Red blood cell survival can also be measured by use of enumeration of biotinylated red blood cells, which does not expose the client to radiation.

C-Reactive Protein (CRP, High-Sensitivity CRP, HS-CRP)—Plasma or Serum

Norm.

	SI Units
Qualitative	Negative
Quantitative	
(Consult reference ranges provided with results)	
Adult	<8 µg/mL
	<0.8 mg/dL
Behring BNII assay (HS-CRP):	
Females	0.175 mg/dL
Males	0.115 mg/dL
Kamiya K-assay (HS-CRP):	
Females	0.191 mg/dL
Males	0.139 mg/dL
Cord blood	10-350 ng/mL 10-350 µg/L

AHA/CDC Risk Groups for Heart Disease

	HS-CRP
Lowest Risk	<1.0 mg/dL
Average Risk	1.0-3.0 mg/dL
Highest Risk	>3.0 mg/dL

Positive (>1:2 Titer). Active inflammatory conditions such as abscess, bronchitis, Crohn's disease, empyema, meningitis, nephritis, pancreatitis (acute), peritonitis, pharyngitis (streptococcal), pneumonia (pneumococcal), rheumatoid arthritis (acute), rheumatic fever (acute), sepsis, and urinary tract or other infections; Alzheimer's disease, ankylosing spondylitis, Castleman's tumor, gout, Graves' disease, Hodgkin's disease, Kawasaki disease, lymphoma, malignant tumor, metabolic syndrome, myocardial infarction, myxoma (of heart left atrium), necrosis, non-Hodgkin's lymphoma, postcommissurotomy syndrome, postoperatively (first week), pregnancy (after month 3), renal infarction, systemic lupus erythematosus, trauma (surgical), and tuberculosis.

Positive (if >0.3 mg/dL). Associated with increased risk of developing initial or recurrent myocardial infarction.

Usage. Monitoring of rheumatoid arthritis and rheumatic fever inflammatory processes, differentiation of Crohn's disease from ulcerative colitis, predictor of myocardial infarction (plasma levels >1.6 mg/L predict future coronary events) in women and coronary heart disease in middle-aged men, marker for existing arterial disease, detection of the presence or exacerbation of inflammatory processes (high preoperative levels indicate increased risk for postoperative infection), and monitoring response to therapy for inflammatory conditions. More reliable than ESR in evaluating inflammatory conditions. May be more useful than WBC to help diagnose serious bacterial infection in infants (Bilavsky et al, 2009).

Description. C-reactive protein (CRP) is an abnormal serum glycoprotein produced by the liver during acute inflammation. CRP is detectable within 6-10 hours after the body's inflammatory response is stimulated and may rise as high as 4000 times when the acute phase inflammatory response is peaking. Because it disappears rapidly when inflammation subsides, its detection signifies the presence of a current inflammatory process. It is the best indicator of the severity of pancreatitis when measured 48 hours after the onset of symptoms. C-reactive protein has been linked to metabolic syndrome, a group of signs that include abdominal obesity, hypertriglyceridemia, low HDL-C, hypertension, and high fasting blood glucose levels. It is now suspected that chronic inflammation as evidenced by a chronically elevated C-reactive protein level may be an additional component of the

syndrome. Its contribution is hypothesized to be regulation of the adverse lipid profile seen in metabolic syndrome. The American Heart Association and The Centers for Disease Control in 2003 jointly issued recommendations for use of CRP as a "discretionary tool" for use in evaluating clients with moderate risk of heart disease, but not for use in widespread screening for heart disease. Wakugawa et al (2006) found that elevated high-sensitivity CRP was an independent risk factor for future ischemic stroke in Japanese males, and when combined with at least one other risk factor for stroke indicates an extreme increase in the risk. C-reactive protein interacts with the complement cascade and is detected by antiserum by means of immunoassays.

Professional Considerations
Consent form NOT required.

Risks
None.

Contraindications
This test should not be done when the client has chronic inflammatory conditions, such as arthritis.

Preparation
1. Tube: Red, green, lavender, or pink topped.

Procedure
1. Draw a 4-mL blood sample.

Postprocedure Care
1. Transport the specimen to the laboratory for immediate testing. Separate plasma or serum within 1 hour.
2. Do not refrigerate the specimen. Specimen should be frozen if not tested within 24 hours after collection.

Client and Family Teaching
1. Fast from food and fluids for 4 hours before sampling.

Factors That Affect Results
1. Drugs that may cause false-positive results include oral contraceptives.
2. Drugs that may cause false-negative results as a result of suppression of inflammation include NSAIDs, steroids, and salicylates.
3. Drugs that lower C-reactive protein include NSAIDs and statins and

angiotensin-converting enzyme inhibitor plus beta-blocker use.

4. Presence of an intrauterine device may cause inflammation, which produces a positive test.
5. Overnight refrigeration of the sample may produce a false-positive result.
6. Hemolysis of specimen invalidates results.
7. Increased values may be caused by alcohol, coffee, hypertension, high protein diet, increased triglycerides or smoking.

Other Data

1. Daily measurements of C-reactive protein correlate with resolution of sepsis. A decrease in CRP by 25% or more from the previous day's level is a good indicator of resolution of sepsis, with a predictive value of 97%.
2. When C-reactive protein is positive in clients with chronic renal failure, it is predictive of future cardiovascular events and all-cause mortality.
3. Values may be normal in 35%-45% of clients with rheumatoid arthritis.

Creatine Kinase (CK)—Serum

Norm. Results are method-dependent and should be compared with the reference values of the laboratory performing the test.

		SI Units
Creatine Kinase—Total		
Adult Females	20-180 U/L	0.33-2.98 µKat/L
Ambulatory	10-70 U/L	0.17-1.16 µKat/L
≤60 years	10-55 U/L	0.17-0.92 µKat/L
>60 years	16-80 U/L	0.27-1.33 µKat/L
Adult Males	20-200 U/L	0.33-3.31 µKat/L
Ambulatory	25-90 U/L	0.42-1.50 µKat/L
<61 years	12-80 U/L	0.20-1.33 µKat/L
61-70 years	20-110 U/L	0.33-1.83 µKat/L
>70 years	22-90 U/L	0.37-1.50 µKat/L
Children		
Newborn	65-580 IU/L at 30 degrees C	1.07-9.61 µKat/L
	10-200 U/L	0.17-3.33 µKat/L
Male	0-70 IU/L at 30 degrees C	<1.16 µKat/L
Female	0-50 IU/L at 30 degrees C	<0.83 µKat/L

Total levels may be normal in acute myocardial infarction, even when the CK-MB isoenzyme is elevated. In general, total CK trends in Acute Myocardial Infarction are as follows.

Initial rise:	2-6 hours after onset of damage
Peak levels:	18-36 hours after onset of damage
Return to baseline level:	3-6 days

Creatine Kinase Isoenzymes	% of Total CK	Fraction of Total CK (SI Units)
CK_1-BB (brain)	0-3	0-0.03
CK_2-MB (heart)	0-6 or 0.3-4.9 ng/mL	0-0.06
CK_3-MM (muscle)	90-97	0.90-0.97

CK_2-MB Trends in Acute Myocardial Infarction.

Initial rise	4-8 hours after onset of damage
Peak levels	18-24 hours after onset of damage
Return to baseline level	3 days after onset of damage

Increased Total CK. Amyotrophic lateral sclerosis (values greater in limb-onset versus bulbar-onset), anoxia, atresia (biliary), bowel injury, brain tumor, burns (thermal, electrical), cancer (breast, lung, oat cell, gastrointestinal, prostatic), carbon monoxide poisoning, cardiomyopathy (cobalt-beer), carrier state (for Duchenne's muscular dystrophy), cerebrovascular accident, CNS trauma, coma (hepatic), convulsions, coughing (severe), crush syndrome, delirium tremens, dermatomyositis, ectopic pregnancy, eosinophilia-myalgia syndrome, exercise, head injury, hemodialysis, hypokalemia (severe), hypothermia, hypothyroidism, hypothyroid myopathy, infarction (bowel, cerebral, myocardial, prostate), intoxication (alcohol, salicylate), intramuscular injection (recent), labor, leptospirosis, malignant hyperthermia, meningoencephalitis, muscle spasms, muscular dystrophy (Duchenne's, limb-girdle, facioscapulohumeral), myocarditis, myoglobinuria, myopathy (from alcoholism), myotonic dystrophy, myxedema, necrosis of striated muscle, neuroleptic malignant syndrome, organ rejection (heart transplant), parturition, polymyositis, postictal state, pregnancy, prostate injury, psychosis (acute with agitation), pulmonary edema, pulmonary embolism, renal failure, renal insufficiency (chronic), Reye's syndrome, rhabdomyolysis, Rocky Mountain spotted fever, shock, skeletal muscle disorders, status epilepticus, striated muscle atrophy (acute), subarachnoid hemorrhage, surgery (bowel, cardiac, CNS, prostate), tachycardia, thyrotoxicosis, toxic shock syndrome (day 7), trauma (muscular), typhoid fever, and very muscular people. Drugs include anabolic steroids, fluvastatin, isotretinoin, and combination cerivastatin-gemfibrozil therapy.

Increased CK₁-BB (Brain). Anoxia, atresia (biliary), brain damage, cancer (breast, gastrointestinal, oat cell, prostatic, widespread malignancies), cerebrovascular accident (hemorrhage, infarction), hemodialysis, hypothermia, intestinal necrosis, labor, malignant hyperthermia, renal failure, shock, surgery (CNS), and uremia.

Increased CK₂-MB (Heart). Anoxia, burns (electrical, thermal), cancer (lung), carbon monoxide poisoning, cardiomyopathy (cobalt-beer), collagen vascular diseases, congestive heart failure (rare), coronary angiography (rare), coronary insufficiency (rare), hypothermia, hypothyroidism, malignant hyperthermia, muscular dystrophy (Duchenne's), myocardial infarction, myocarditis, myoglobinuria (severe), polymyositis, pulmonary embolism, renal insufficiency (chronic), Reye's syndrome, rhabdomyolysis, Rocky Mountain spotted fever, surgery (cardiac, valve replacement), systemic lupus erythematosus, and trauma (cardiac). Drugs include doxycycline.

Increased CK₃-MM (Muscle). Cardiac catheterization (with myocardial damage), cardioversion, coronary arteriography (with myocardial damage), hypothyroidism, intramuscular injections, muscle trauma, muscular dystrophy, myocardial infarction, psychosis (acute with agitation), Reye's syndrome, shock, surgery, and trauma (skeletal muscle).

Decreased Total CK. Addison's disease, anterior pituitary hyposecretion, connective tissue disease, hepatic disease (alcoholic), low muscle mass, metastatic neoplasia, postinfarction left ventricular remodeling (CK flux rates are decreased), and pregnancy (first half). Drugs include steroids.

Decreased CK₁-BB, CK₂-MB, CK₃-MM. Not applicable.

Description. Creatine kinase is an enzyme found in muscle and brain tissue and reflects tissue catabolism as a result of cell trauma. It catalyzes creatine-creatinine metabolism. The test is performed to detect myocardial or skeletal muscle damage or central nervous system damage, resulting in increased tissue catabolism from those areas. One can determine what type of tissue damage (tissue undergoing increased catabolism) has occurred by performing the CK isoenzyme test; this test measures the three types of isoenzymes that make up total CPK: CK₁-BB, CK₂-MB, and CK₃-MM. CK₁-BB is found mainly in brain tissue but also in smooth muscle, thyroid gland, lungs, and prostate gland. CK₂-MB is found mainly in cardiac muscle but also in the tongue, diaphragm, and skeletal muscle (scant amount). CK₃-MM is found mainly in skeletal muscle.

The isoenzyme test is usually repeated at 8- to 12-hour intervals to track trends characteristic of specific types of cell damage. Most recently, test kits have been developed to allow detection of CK_3-MM and CK_2-MB isoforms earlier than the traditional methods for CK isoenzyme detection.

Professional Considerations
Consent form NOT required.

Preparation
1. See Client and Family Teaching.
2. Tube: Red topped, red/gray topped, or gold topped.

Procedure
1. Collect a 5-mL blood sample.

Postprocedure Care
1. Send the specimen to the laboratory immediately.
2. Refrigerate the specimen if measurement will be delayed more than 2 hours. Separate the serum and freeze it if the test will not be performed within 24 hours of collection.
3. If isoenzyme measurement is desired, specify this on the laboratory requisition.

Client and Family Teaching
1. If the test is for skeletal muscle disorder evaluation, the client should avoid strenuous physical activity for 24 hours before the test.
2. Avoid ingestion of alcohol for 24 hours before the test.
3. Withhold drugs that would affect the test results (see below) for 24 hours before the test, when possible.

Factors That Affect Results
1. Necessary intramuscular (IM) injections should be given after or at least 1 hour before this test.
2. Hemolysis invalidates the results.
3. Invasive procedures and other factors that elevate CK include cardiac catheterization (with myocardial injury), cardioversion, coronary arteriography (with myocardial injury), electric shock, electrocautery, electromyography, intramuscular injections, and muscle massage (recent).
4. Drugs that may cause falsely increased CK values include aminocaproic acid, clofibrate, codeine, dexamethasone, dexamethasone acetate, dexamethasone sodium phosphate, digoxin, epsilon-aminocaproic acid, ethyl alcohol (ethanol), furosemide, glutethimide, guanethidine, halothane, heroin, imipramine, lithium carbonate, meperidine hydrochloride, morphine sulfate, phenobarbital, and succinylcholine chloride.

Other Data
1. CK is considered to be a marker for Duchenne's muscular dystrophy.
2. Evaluation of myocardial infarction should also include LDH isoenzyme measurements every 24 hours.
3. In clients suspected of acute myocardial infarction, CK-MB testing alone may reveal more information than total CK level, which may not show an elevation initially. CK-MB measurement within 9 hours of arrival provides accurate clinical assessment in 99% of cases of myocardial infarction.
4. Troponin T is superior to CK-MB for prediction of impending complications after cardiac surgical procedures.

Creatine Kinase Isoenzymes
See **Creatine Kinase**—Serum.

Creatine Phosphokinase
See **Creatine Kinase**—Serum.

Creatine—Urine

Norm.

		SI Units
Adults	<6% of urine creatinine	
Adult females	≤80 mg/24 hours	0-615 μmol/day
Pregnant	≤12% of urine creatinine	
Adult males	≤40 mg/24 hours	0-307 μmol/day
Infants	Equal to urine creatinine	
Children	≤30% of urine creatinine	

Increased. Acromegaly, Addison's disease, amyotonia congenita, burns, children (growth state), Cushing's syndrome, diabetes mellitus, disseminated lupus erythematosus, fractures, guanidinoacetate methyltransferase (GAMT) deficiency, hyperthyroidism, hypothyroidism, infections, injuries (crushing), leukemia, male eunuchoidism, muscular dystrophy, myasthenia gravis, myoglobinuria (acute paroxysmal), myopathy (alcoholic), myotonia (congenital Thomsen's disease), myotonic dystrophy, neurogenic atrophy, poliomyelitis, polymyositis, pregnancy, puerperium, starvation, X-linked mental retardation, and raw meat diet.

Decreased. Aging (fifth to ninth decade), hypothyroidism.

Description. Creatine is a compound that functions in anaerobic muscle metabolism by combining with phosphate to yield energy used in intense muscle activity for short periods of time. Normally, phosphocreatine breaks down into creatinine, which is then excreted in the urine. In some conditions, particularly muscle diseases, creatine is released in increased amounts into the bloodstream and can be measured in the urine.

Professional Considerations
Consent form NOT required.

Preparation
1. Obtain a clean 3-L, 24-hour urine container with toluene preservative.

Procedure
1. Discard the first morning urine specimen.
2. Save all the urine voided for 24 hours in a refrigerated, clean, 3-L container to which toluene preservative has been added. Include the urine voided at the end of the 24-hour period. For catheterized clients, keep the drainage bag on ice and empty urine into the refrigerated collection container hourly.

Postprocedure Care
1. Compare the urine quantity in the specimen container with the urinary output record for the test. If the specimen contains less urine than what was recorded as output, some of the sample may have been discarded, invalidating the test.
2. Document urine quantity on the laboratory requisition.
3. Send the entire specimen to the lab.

Client and Family Teaching
1. Save all the urine voided in the 24-hour period and urinate before defecating to avoid loss of urine. If any urine is accidentally discarded, discard the entire specimen and restart the collection the next day.

Factors That Affect Results
1. All the urine voided for the 24-hour period must be included to avoid a falsely low result.
2. Drugs that may cause falsely elevated results include caffeine, corticosteroids, corticotropin, cortisone acetate, desoxycorticosterone acetate, desoxycorticosterone pivalate, methyltestosterone, nitrofurantoin, nitrofurantoin sodium, phenolsulfonphthalein, and sodium benzoate.
3. Drugs that may cause falsely decreased results include anabolic steroids, androgens, and thiazide diuretics.
4. The results may be increased after 3 weeks of pregnancy.

Other Data
1. This test may be useful as a marker for testicular damage.

Creatinine—Serum

Norm.

		SI Units
Jaffe, Manual Method	0.6-1.6 mg/dL	52-142 µmol/day
Jaffe, Kinetic or Enzymatic Method		
Adults		
Females	0.5-1.1 mg/dL	44-97 µmol/L
Males	0.6-1.2 mg/dL	53-105 µmol/L
Elderly	May be lower	May be lower
Children		
Cord blood	0.6-1.2 mg/dL	53-105 µmol/L
Newborn	0.8-1.4 mg/dL	71-124 µmol/L
Infant	0.7-1.7 mg/dL	62-150 µmol/L
1 year, female	≤0.5 mg/dL	≤44 µmol/L
1 year, male	≤0.6 mg/dL	≤53 µmol/L
2-3 years, female	≤0.6 mg/dL	≤53 µmol/L
2-3 years, male	≤0.7 mg/dL	≤62 µmol/L
4-7 years, female	≤0.7 mg/dL	≤62 µmol/L
4-7 years, male	≤0.8 mg/dL	≤71 µmol/L
8-10 years, female	≤0.8 mg/dL	≤71 µmol/L
8-10 years, male	≤0.9 mg/dL	≤80 µmol/L
11-12 years, female	≤0.9 mg/dL	≤80 µmol/L
11-12 years, male	≤1.0 mg/dL	≤88 µmol/L
13-17 years, female	≤1.1 mg/dL	≤97 µmol/L
13-17 years, male	≤1.2 mg/dL	≤106 µmol/L
18-20 years, female	≤1.2 mg/dL	≤106 µmol/L
18-20 years, male	≤1.3 mg/dL	≤115 µmol/L

Increased. Values are 20%-40% higher in the late afternoon than in the morning. Acromegaly, allergic purpura, amyloidosis, analgesic abuse, azotemia (prerenal, postrenal), congenital hypoplastic kidneys, congestive heart failure, diabetes mellitus, diet (high meat content), eating disorders (dehydration, renal dysfunction), gigantism, glomerulonephritis (chronic), Goodpasture's syndrome, gout, hemoglobinuria, high dietary intake, hypothyroidism, hypovolemic shock, infants (first 2 weeks of life), intestinal obstruction, Kimmelstiel-Wilson syndrome, metal poisoning, microalbuminemia, multiple myeloma, muscle destruction, nephritis, nephropathy (hypercalcemic, hypokalemic), nephrosclerosis, pancreatitis (necrotizing), polyarteritis nodosa, polycystic disease, preeclampsia, pyelonephritis, renal artery stenosis or thrombosis, renal cortical necrosis, renal failure, renal tuberculosis, renal vein thrombosis, rheumatoid arthritis (active), scleroderma, sickle cell anemia, subacute bacterial endocarditis, systemic lupus erythematosus, testosterone therapy, toxic shock syndrome, uremia, urinary obstruction, and vomiting. Drugs include acetohexamide, acyclovir, ammonia (inhaled), amphotericin B, androgens, arginine, bleomycin-induced pulmonary toxicity, Bromsulphalein, captopril, cephalosporins (Cefoxitin, cephalexin), cimetidine, cinchophen, clofibrate, corticosteroids, diacetic acid, disopyramide phosphate, diuretics, dopamine, fenofibrate, fosinopril, fructose, gentamicin sulfate, glucose, hydralazine hydrochloride, hydroxyurea, Lipomul, lithium carbonate, losartan, mannitol, meclofenamate sodium, methicillin sodium, metoprolol tartrate, minoxidil, mithramycin, nitrofurantoin, nitrogen oxide (inhaled), propranolol, protein, pyruvate, sulfobromophthalein, sulfonamides, streptokinase, testosterone, testosterone cypionate, testosterone enanthate, testosterone propionate, triamterene, and viomycin. Herbal or natural remedies include products containing aristolochic acids (*Akebia* spp., *Aristolochia* spp.,

Asarum spp., birthwort, *Bragantia* spp., *Clematis* spp., *Cocculus* spp., *Diploclisia* spp., Dutchman's pipe, *Fang chi, Fang ji, Guang Kan-Mokutsu, Menispermum* spp., *Mokutsu, Mu tong, Sinomenium* spp., and *Stephania* spp.).

Decreased. Diabetic ketoacidosis (artifactual decrease) and muscular dystrophy. Drugs include cefoxitin sodium, cimetidine, chlorpromazine, chlorprothixene, marijuana, thiazide diuretics, and vancomycin. Herbal or natural remedies include *Cordyceps sinensis*.

Description. Creatinine is produced continuously as a nonprotein end product of anaerobic energy-producing creatine phosphate metabolism in skeletal muscle. Because it is continually and easily excreted by the renal system, increased levels indicate a slowing of the glomerular filtration rate. Creatinine is thus a very specific indicator of renal function, revealing the balance between creatinine formation and excretion. A diurnal variation in creatinine may be related to meals, with troughs occurring around 0700 (7 AM) and peaks occurring around 1900 (7 PM).

Professional Considerations
Consent form NOT required.

Preparation
1. Tube: Red topped, red/gray topped, or gold topped.
2. Do NOT draw during hemodialysis.

Procedure
1. Draw a 4-mL blood sample.

Postprocedure Care
1. Send the specimen to the laboratory promptly and refrigerate it until tested.

Client and Family Teaching
1. Avoid excessive exercise for 8 hours before the test and avoid excessive red meat intake for 24 hours before the test.

Factors That Affect Results
1. Some clients with long-standing chronic renal failure may have normal levels.
2. Drugs that may cause falsely elevated levels include amphotericin B, ascorbic acid, barbiturates, capreomycin sulfate, carbutamide, cefoxitin sodium, cephalothin sodium, chlorthalidone, clonidine, colistin sulfate, dextran, doxycycline hyclate, kanamycin, levodopa, methyldopa, methyldopate hydrochloride, nitromethane fuel inhalation, *p*-aminohippurate, phenolsulfonphthalein, and sulfobromophthalein.

Other Data
1. The specimen will remain stable for 1 week when refrigerated and for 1 month when frozen.
2. Mean creatinine values are higher in men, non-Hispanic African-Americans, and older persons and are lower in Mexican Americans.
3. Samuels et al (2011) found that 10% increases in serum creatinine levels in ICU patients coincided with higher mortality and longer ICU stays as compared to patients who had normal creatinine levels.

Creatinine—Urine

Norm.

		SI Units
Adult	14-26 mg/kg/24 hours	124-230 μmol/kg/day
Female	600-1800 mg/24 hours	5.3-16 μmol/day
Male	800-2000 mg/24 hours	7-18 μmol/day
Child	8-22 mg/kg/24 hours	71-195 μmol/kg/day

Increased. Fever, hypothyroidism, and tissue catabolism. Values are 20%-40% higher in the late afternoon than in the morning, are higher in African-Americans, and increase with age.

Decreased. Decreased renal perfusion, glomerulonephritis, cystic kidney disease,

polymyositis, pyelonephritis (chronic bilateral), and shock (hypovolemic).

Description. Creatinine is produced continuously as a nonprotein end product of anaerobic energy-producing creatine phosphate metabolism in skeletal muscle. It is continually and easily excreted by the renal system by glomerular filtration. Decreased levels of urine creatinine indicate a slowing of the glomerular filtration rate. Creatinine is thus a very specific indicator of renal function. A diurnal variation in creatinine may be related to meals, with troughs occurring around 0700 (7 AM) and peaks occurring around 1900 (7 PM). Because this test involves the collection of a 24-hour urine sample, it captures the effects of both peaks and troughs of creatinine levels.

Professional Considerations
Consent form NOT required.

Preparation
1. Obtain a clean 3-L, 24-hour urine container.

Procedure
1. Discard the first morning urine specimen.
2. Save all the urine voided for 24 hours in a refrigerated, clean, 3-L container with or without a preservative. Include the urine voided at the end of the 24-hour period. For catheterized clients, keep the drainage bag on ice and empty it into the refrigerated collection container hourly.

Postprocedure Care
1. Compare the urine quantity in the specimen container with the urinary output record for the test. If the specimen contains less urine than what was recorded as output, some of the sample may have been discarded, invalidating the test.
2. Document the quantity of urine output and the beginning and ending times of collection on the laboratory requisition.

3. Send the specimen to the laboratory immediately and refrigerate it until tested. Only prolonged storage times of 30 days at temperatures above 55 degrees C could significantly decrease levels.

Client and Family Teaching
1. Save all the urine voided in the 24-hour period and urinate before defecating to avoid loss of urine. If any urine is accidentally discarded, discard the entire specimen and restart the collection the next day.

Factors That Affect Results
1. Failure to include all the urine voided for the 24-hour period yields a falsely low result.
2. Failure to refrigerate the specimen throughout the collection period yields a falsely low result.
3. Drugs that may cause falsely elevated results include amphotericin B, ascorbic acid, barbiturates, capreomycin sulfate, carbutamide, cefoxitin sodium, cephalothin sodium, chlorthalidone, clonidine, colistin sulfate, dextran, doxycycline hyclate, kanamycin, levodopa, methyldopa, methyldopate hydrochloride, p-aminohippurate, phenolsulfonphthalein, sulfobromophthalein.
4. Drugs that may cause falsely decreased results include anabolic steroids, androgens, and thiazides.

Other Data
1. Urine creatinine is stable when refrigerated for 1 week and when frozen for 1 month.

Creatinine Clearance—Serum and Urine

Norm. Female 0.8-1.8 g/24 hours and male 1.0-2.0 g/24 hours. Corrected to 1.73 m² of body surface area.

	Adult Female		Adult Male	
		SI Units		SI Units
Age	mL/min	mL/sec	mL/min	mL/sec
≤20 years	75	1.3	80	1.3
21-30 years	90	1.5	96	1.6
31-40 years	96	1.6	102	1.7
41-50 years	102	1.7	108	1.8
51-60 years	108	1.8	114	1.9
61-70 years	114	1.9	120	2.0

Continued

	Adult Female		Adult Male	
		SI Units		SI Units
Age	mL/min	mL/sec	mL/min	mL/sec
71-80 years	120	2.0	126	2.1
81-90 years	126	2.1	132	2.2
91-100 years	132	2.2	138	2.3

	Child	
		SI Units
Age	mL/min	mL/sec
<1 year	72	1.2
1 year	45	0.8
2 years	55	0.9
3 years	60	1.0
4-5 years	71-73	1.2
6-7 years	64-67	1.1
8 years	72	1.2
9 years	83	1.4
10-11 years	89-92	1.5
12 years	109	1.8
13-14 years	86	1.4

Increased. Correlates to higher mortality risk after acute stroke. Drugs include low molecular weight heparin enoxaparin, perindopril. Herbal or natural remedies include *Cordyceps sinensis*.

Decreased. Acute coronary syndrome acute tubular necrosis, atherosclerosis (of renal artery), congestive heart failure, dehydration, elderly clients, glomerulonephritis, malignancy (bilateral renal), nephrosclerosis, obstruction (renal artery), phenacetin, polycystic kidney disease, pyelonephritis (advanced bilateral chronic), shock (cardiogenic, hypovolemic), thrombosis (renal vein), and tuberculosis (renal). Drugs include aminoglycosides, amphotericin B, captopril, cyclosporine, indomethacin, lithium, nitrendipine, and penicillins.

Description. Creatinine is produced continuously as a nonprotein end product of anaerobic energy-producing creatine metabolism in skeletal muscle. It is continually and easily excreted by the renal system by glomerular filtration. The creatinine clearance test measures both a blood sample and a urine sample to determine the rate at which creatinine is being cleared from the blood by the kidneys. Specifically, "clearance" means the amount of blood cleared of creatinine in 1 minute and is independent of urine flow rate. Decreased results occur when over 50% of renal nephrons are damaged, thus indicating impaired glomerular filtration. Creatinine clearance is thus a very specific indicator of renal function, revealing the balance between creatinine formation and excretion.

Professional Considerations
Consent form NOT required.

Preparation
1. Urine collection: Obtain clean 3-L, 24-hour urine bag or bottle(s).
2. Serum collection: Use red topped, red/gray topped, or gold topped tube(s).
3. Do NOT draw the specimen during hemodialysis.

Procedure
1. *Urine collection:*
   a. Discard the first morning urine specimen.
   b. Begin to time a 24-hour urine collection. (2-, 6-, or 12-hour urine collections can also be performed, but a 24-hour specimen is preferable although at least an 8-hour collection is recommended.)
   c. Save all the urine voided for 24 hours in a refrigerated, clean, 3-L container with or without a preservative. Include the urine voided at the end of the 24-hour period. For catheterized clients, keep the drainage bag on ice

and empty into the refrigerated collection container hourly.

2. *Serum collection:*

   a. Because the glomerular filtration rate remains stable, the serum specimen can be drawn at any time during the urine collection period. Draw a 4-mL blood sample in a red topped tube for serum creatinine.

Postprocedure Care

1. Compare the urine quantity in the specimen container with the urinary output record for the test. If the specimen contains less urine than what was recorded as output, some of the sample may have been discarded, invalidating the test.

2. Document the quantity of the urine output as well as the beginning and ending times for the 24-hour period on the laboratory requisition.

3. Send the 24-hour urine specimen to the laboratory immediately and refrigerate it until tested.

4. Urine creatinine is stable for 1 week when refrigerated and for 1 month when frozen.

Client and Family Teaching

1. Avoid strenuous exercise for 8 hours before the test.

2. For the urine test, save all the urine voided in the 24-hour period and urinate before defecating to avoid loss of urine. If any urine is accidentally discarded, discard the entire specimen and restart the collection the next day.

Factors That Affect Results

1. Failure to refrigerate the specimen throughout the collection period allows the creatinine to decompose, causing falsely low results.

2. Drugs that may cause falsely elevated results include amphotericin B, ascorbic acid, barbiturates, capreomycin sulfate, carbutamide, cefoxitin sodium, cefpirome, cephalothin sodium, chlorthalidone, clonidine, colistin sulfate, dextran, doxycycline hyclate, kanamycin, levodopa, methyldopa, methyldopate hydrochloride, *p*-aminohippurate, phenolsulfonphthalein, and sulfobromophthalein.

3. Drugs that may cause falsely decreased results include anabolic steroids, androgens, and thiazides.

Other Data

1. Elderly clients can have a normal serum creatinine level and still have renal impairment. Therefore commonly prescribed drugs usually require dose adjustments in the elderly.

2. Because this test is cumbersome to carry out, several investigational studies have evaluated alternative methods to *estimate* creatinine clearance. A meta-analysis of these studies (Wilhelm et al, 2011) found that the most accurate method for estimating creatinine clearance is using the Cockroft-Gault equation omitting body weight and actual serum creatinine level for normal sized individuals.

CRP

See C-Reactive Protein—Plasma or Serum.

Cryoglobulin

See Cryoglobulin, Qualitative—Serum.

Cryoglobulin, Qualitative—Serum

Norm. Negative.

Positive Type I Cryoglobulin. Leukemia (chronic lymphocytic), lymphoma, multiple myeloma, and Waldenström's macroglobulinemia.

Positive Type II Cryoglobulin. Lymphoma, mixed essential cryoglobulinemia, multiple myeloma, rheumatoid arthritis, and Sjögren's syndrome.

Positive Type III Cryoglobulin. Chronic infection, cytomegalovirus infection, endocarditis (infective), glomerulonephritis (poststreptococcal), hepatitis (acute viral, chronic active), infectious mononucleosis, kala-azar, leprosy, polymyalgia rheumatica, primary biliary cirrhosis, rheumatoid arthritis, scleroderma, Sjögren's syndrome, systemic lupus erythematosus, and tropical splenomegaly syndrome.

Positive Type I, II, or III. Hodgkin's disease, infection (viral), and Raynaud's disease.

Description. Cryoglobulins are abnormal serum proteins that precipitate at low laboratory temperatures and redissolve after being warmed. They cannot be identified by serum protein electrophoresis. Cryoglobulin presence in the serum causes vascular problems most commonly of the extremities and is usually associated with immunologic disease. Three types may be delineated to help differentiate the type of disease occurring. This test involves obtaining a "cryocrit" by observation for cold precipitation of cryoglobulin after at least 72 hours of storage at 4 degrees C and confirmation of the reversibility of the reaction by rewarming of the serum sample.

Professional Considerations
Consent form NOT required.

Preparation
1. See Client and Family Teaching.
2. Tube: Red topped, red/gray topped, or gold topped.

3. The syringe and red topped tube should be warmed to 37 degrees C to prevent loss of cryoglobulins.

Procedure
1. Draw a 10-mL blood sample in a tube that has been prewarmed to body temperature.

Postprocedure Care
1. Keep the specimen warm and send it to the laboratory immediately for warmed clotting at 37 degrees C.

Client and Family Teaching
1. Fast from food and fluids for 8 hours before the test.
2. Clients with positive tests should avoid exposure to cold temperatures.
3. Results may not be available for several days.

Factors That Affect Results
1. After separation of serum from the clot and subsequent serum centrifugation, refrigerate the sample for 3-7 days. Testing the sample before the end of the precipitation period may yield incorrect results.

Other Data
1. The serum should be kept under observation for 1 week to detect late-forming cryoglobulins.
2. Cryoglobulins are not to be confused with cryofibrinogen, which precipitates from plasma, rather than serum, in cold conditions.

Cryptococcal Antigen Titer, Cerebrospinal Fluid (CSF)—Specimen

Norm. Negative.

Positive. Titers of 1:8 or more indicate active meningitic *Cryptococcus neoformans* infection. Titers of 1:4 are highly suggestive of meningitic *Cryptococcus neoformans* infection.

Description. *Cryptococcus* is a yeast member of the Fungi Imperfecti group found in the soil and in contaminated bird droppings. It is believed to be transmitted to humans by inhalation from the environment. Normal host defense mechanisms prevent *Cryptococcus* from causing disease. Clients with Hodgkin's disease, sarcoidosis,

acquired immunodeficiency syndrome, or diabetes and those on corticosteroid therapy or undergoing bone marrow transplantation are more susceptible to cryptococcal infection. *Cryptococcus neoformans* is the organism that usually causes pathologic conditions in humans, with chronic meningitis being the most common manifestation. Antigen detection enables earlier diagnosis than culture. This test uses latex agglutination to detect the presence of the cryptococcal antigen in a sample of cerebrospinal fluid. The results are reported in titers, with the level of titer corresponding to the extent of infection. Serial titers may be used to monitor response to therapy.

Professional Considerations

Consent form IS required for the spinal tap. See Lumbar puncture—Diagnostic for risks and contraindications.

Preparation

1. See Lumbar puncture—Diagnostic.

Procedure

1. 5-10 mL of cerebrospinal fluid is collected through a needle inserted into the spinal canal between L3-L4 and L4-L5 or directly from the ventricles of the brain during special procedures. See Lumbar puncture—Diagnostic.

Postprocedure Care

1. See Lumbar puncture—Diagnostic.
2. Transport the specimen to the laboratory immediately.

Client and Family Teaching

1. *Cryptococcus* is not believed to be transmitted directly from person to person. Isolation of clients with positive results is unnecessary.

Factors That Affect Results

1. False-positive results may occur in clients with rheumatoid arthritis. This cross-reaction may be eliminated when the sample is treated with Pronase or the sample is boiled with disodium EDTA.
2. Several commercially available kits have demonstrated sensitivities of 93%-100% and specificities of 93%-98% for testing for cryptococcal antigen titer in cerebrospinal fluid.

Other Data

1. Amphotericin B and 5-fluocytosine (flucytosine) are used to treat cryptococcal infections.
2. A positive culture is required to confirm diagnosis of cryptococcal infections.
3. See Lumbar puncture—Diagnostic for procedural contraindications.
4. See also Cryptococcal antigen titer—Serum for further information about the disease.

Cryptococcal Antigen Titer—Serum

Norm. Negative.

Positive. Titers of 1:8 or more are indicative of active disseminated *Cryptococcus neoformans* infection; titers of 1:4 are highly suggestive of disseminated *C. neoformans* infection.

Description. *Cryptococcus* is a yeast member of the Fungi Imperfecti group found in the soil and in contaminated bird droppings. It is believed to be transmitted to humans by inhalation from the environment. Normal host defense mechanisms prevent *Cryptococcus* from causing disease. Clients with Hodgkin's disease, sarcoidosis, or acquired immunodeficiency syndrome and those on corticosteroid therapy or receiving bone marrow transplants are more susceptible to cryptococcal infection. *C. neoformans* is the genus that usually causes pathologic conditions in humans, with chronic meningitis being the most common manifestation. Other types of cryptococcal disease involve the lungs, the cutaneous tissue, the skeletal system, and a disseminated infection. Serologic antigen detection allows earlier diagnosis than culture. This test involves using latex agglutination to detect the presence of the cryptococcal antigen in a sample of serum. Detection of the cryptococcal antigen in serum usually indicates systemic cryptococcosis. Results are reported in titers, with the level of titer corresponding to the extent of infection. Serial titers may be used to monitor response to therapy.

Professional Considerations

Consent form NOT required.

Preparation

1. Tube: Red topped, red/gray topped, or gold topped.

Procedure

1. Draw a 10-mL blood sample.

Postprocedure Care

1. Transport the specimen to the laboratory immediately.

Client and Family Teaching

1. *Cryptococcus* is not thought to be transmitted directly from person to person. Isolation of the client is unnecessary.
2. Results may not be available for several days.

Factors That Affect Results

1. False-positive results may occur in clients with rheumatoid arthritis. This cross-reaction may be eliminated by treatment of the sample with Pronase or boiling of the sample with disodium EDTA.
2. There are significant differences in sensitivity among five commercially available kits that test for cryptococcal antigen in serum. Kits that pretreat the specimen with Pronase had greater specificity (97%) than kits that did not pretreat with Pronase (83%).

Other Data

1. Amphotericin B (fluconazole) and 5-fluorocytosine (flucytosine) are used to treat cryptococcal infections.
2. A positive culture is required to confirm diagnosis of cryptococcal infections.

Cryptococcus Antibody Titer—Serum

Norm. Negative.

Positive. Titers ≥1:2 are highly suggestive of cryptococcal infection. Positive IFA at titers of ≥1:16 are diagnostic for cryptococcosis.

Description. *Cryptococcus* is a yeast member of the Fungi Imperfecti group found in the soil and in contaminated bird droppings. It is believed to be transmitted to humans by inhalation from the environment. Normal host defense mechanisms prevent *Cryptococcus* from causing disease. Clients with Hodgkin's disease, sarcoidosis, acquired immunodeficiency syndrome, or diabetes mellitus and those on corticosteroid therapy are more susceptible to cryptococcal infection. *C. neoformans* is the genus that usually causes pathologic conditions in humans, with chronic meningitis being the most common manifestation. Other types of cryptococcal disease involve the lungs, the cutaneous tissue, the skeletal system, and a disseminated infection. Serologic antibody detection allows earlier diagnosis than culture. This test involves using two tests (indirect fluorescent-antibody and tube agglutination) to detect the presence of the cryptococcal antibody in a sample of serum. The results are reported as the highest dilution demonstrating agglutination when serum is combined with yeast cells.

Professional Considerations

Consent form NOT required.

Preparation

1. Tube: Red topped, red/gray topped, or gold topped.

Procedure

1. Obtain a 5-mL blood sample.

Postprocedure Care

1. None.

Client and Family Teaching

1. *Cryptococcus* is not thought to be transmitted directly from person to person. Isolation of the client is unnecessary.

Factors That Affect Results

1. False-negative results may occur in the presence of increased circulating antigens as the disease progresses. Results may then become positive as drug therapy lowers antigen levels.
2. False-positive results may occur in the presence of antibodies from past cryptococcal infections.

Other Data

1. Amphotericin B (fluconazole) and 5-fluorocytosine (flucytosine) are used to treat cryptococcal infections.
2. A positive culture is required to confirm diagnosis of cryptococcal infections.

Cryptosporidium Diagnostic Procedures—Stool

Norm. Negative.

Usage. AIDS.

Description. To detect the presence of *Cryptosporidium*, a coccidian obligate parasite that inhabits the intestinal mucosa and respiratory tracts of many animals (deer, horses, geese) and can cause diarrhea in humans. In clients with intact immune systems, cryptosporidiosis is self-limited to 2 weeks or less. In immunocompromised clients, the disease causes a severe diarrhea lasting weeks to years. In this test, *Cryptosporidium* oocysts must be distinguished from yeast cells. Iodine stains are used to differentiate yeast cells, which do stain, from *Cryptosporidium* oocysts, which do not stain. An acid-fast stain is then performed on a smear of fixed or unfixed stool to confirm the presence of *Cryptosporidium*. In a positive test, *Cryptosporidium* oocysts stain bright red, but yeast cells do not stain.

Professional Considerations

Consent form NOT required.

Preparation

1. Clarify the collection procedure with the individual laboratory that will be performing the test. Preschedule this test with the laboratory because testing must be done on a freshly collected specimen.
2. Obtain a clear container.

Procedure

1. Collect a 20-g sample of stool directly into a wide-mouthed, watertight, clean container.
2. Some laboratories require that the stool specimen be preserved immediately with a 10% formalin solution or sodium acetate-acetic acid formalin.
3. If the client is unable to defecate into the container, substitute a sheet of waxed paper and transfer the specimen into the container.
4. Repeat the collection every other day for a total of three specimens.

Postprocedure Care

1. If a fixative is used, document the consistency of the fresh sample on the laboratory requisition or include a sample of unfixed specimen in a separate container.
2. Transport the specimen to the laboratory immediately.

Client and Family Teaching

1. Contamination of the stool specimen with urine or toilet water invalidates the results.

Factors That Affect Results

1. Antimicrobial therapy causes false-negative results. The test should be repeated 5-10 days after discontinuation of antibiotic therapy.
2. Do not use polyvinyl alcohol (PVA) fixative.

Other Data

1. Handle the specimen cautiously to prevent self-contamination. *Cryptosporidium* is highly contagious.

CSF Analysis, CSF Examination

See Cerebrospinal Fluid, Glucose—Specimen; Cerebrospinal Fluid, Immunoglobulin G, Immunoglobulin G Ratios, and Immunoglobulin G Index, Immunoglobulin G Synthesis Rate—Specimen; Cerebrospinal Fluid, Routine Analysis—Specimen; Cerebrospinal Fluid, Routine, Culture and Cytology.

CSF Flow Studies

See Cisternography, Radionuclide—Diagnostic.

CST (Contraction Stress Test)

See Fetal Monitoring, External, Contraction Stress Test and Oxytocin Challenge Test—Diagnostic.

CT Coronary Angiography

See Computed Tomography of the Body—Diagnostic.

CT Scan

See Cerebral Computed Tomography—Diagnostic; Computed Tomography of the Body—Diagnostic; Tomography, Paranasal Sinuses—Diagnostic.

CT-PTSP

See Splenoportography—Diagnostic.

C-Type Natriuretic Peptide

See Natriuretic Peptides, Atrial, Pro-Brain Natriuretic Peptide, B-Type, C-Type—Plasma.

^{13}C-UBT, ^{14}C-UBT

See Urea Breath Test—Diagnostic.

Culdoscopy—Diagnostic

Norm. Normal structure and arrangement of the pelvic organs; absence of inflammatory processes, lesions, adhesions, or ectopic pregnancy; and patent fallopian tubes.

Usage. Aids in the diagnosis of endometriosis, pelvic adhesions, and pelvic abnormalities not diagnosable by palpation. Exploratory procedure for adhesions or tubal blockage causing sterility or for suspected salpingitis, ectopic pregnancy, pelvic pain, or pelvic inflammatory disease. Technique for tubal sterilization.

Description. The direct visualization of the pelvic organs through a culdoscope inserted through the cul-de-sac (rectovaginal septum) of the vagina into the pelvis. The culdoscope, or pelvic endoscope, is a surgical instrument (flexible type available) with a fiberoptic light source, lens, and light hood. Although visualization of the pelvic organs is more difficult with culdoscopy than with laparoscopy, the procedure poses less risk to the woman.

Professional Considerations
Consent form IS required.

Risks
Inadvertent amniocentesis, pain.

Contraindications
In instances of cul-de-sac mass, fixed uterine retrodisplacement, acute gynecologic infections, thickened nodular uterosacral ligaments, and in clients who are unable to maintain a knee-chest position.

Preparation
1. Pain medication may be prescribed.
2. The client should void just before the procedure and disrobe below the waist or wear a gown.
3. Obtain an antiseptic solution, a culdoscope, a cannula and a trocar, sterile water in a warmer, perineal retractor, a speculum, a tenaculum, a local anesthetic, two needles, two syringes, indigo carmine dye, a pillow, and an absorbable suture material.
4. The culdoscope is prewarmed in a sterile solution.
5. Insert an indwelling urinary catheter to prevent bladder distension from urine.
6. Just before beginning the procedure, take a "time out" to verify the correct client, procedure, and site.

Procedure
1. The client is placed face down in the knee-chest position with her thighs perpendicular to the examination table and her shoulders supported with shoulder rests.

2. A perineal retractor is inserted to expose the vaginal vault, and the area is cleansed with an antiseptic solution.
3. A speculum is inserted through the vagina to elevate the perineum, and a tenaculum is used to pull the cervix toward the symphysis pubis, thus exposing the cul-de-sac.
4. The rectovaginal septum is injected with local anesthetic in several places.
5. The trocar is inserted through a cannula and pushed through the vaginal wall at the cul-de-sac and then removed. Upon removal, pneumoperitoneum occurs, aided by the knee-chest position, as air rushes into the peritoneal cavity.
6. The culdoscope is connected to the fiber-optic light cord and inserted through the cannula into the peritoneal cavity, and the angled lens system is manipulated to methodically inspect the pelvic organs. Organs and structures inspected include the posterior uterine surface, fallopian tubes and ovaries, uterosacral ligaments, pelvic peritoneum, appendix, rectum, and sigmoid colon.
7. Dye may be injected into the uterus through the cervix, and the fallopian tubes are inspected for patency.
8. The culdoscope is removed, and the woman is assisted into a prone position with a pillow under the abdomen to force air out of the abdominal cavity. The cannula is removed, and the cul-de-sac is sutured with absorbable sutures.

Postprocedure Care
1. Notify the physician for more than a small amount of bleeding or for fever, chills, or an increase in abdominal pain.

Client and Family Teaching
1. You may experience abdominal cramping for several days after the procedure, until the air dissipates.

Factors That Affect Results
1. The value of this procedure depends on the skill of the operator.

Other Data
1. Microsurgical repair of adnexal structures is sometimes performed with culdoscopy.

Culture—Blood

See **Blood Culture—Blood; Blood Culture with Antimicrobial Removal Device—Culture.**

Culture, Cerebrospinal Fluid

See **Cerebrospinal Fluid, Routine, Culture and Cytology**—Specimen.

Culture, Routine

Norm. No growth; normal flora.

Usage. Abscess, auditory infestations, bites (animal, human), blepharitis, body cavity drainage or fluids, cervicitis, conjunctivitis, endocarditis, inflammation, otitis externa, otitis media, respiratory secretions (mostly gram-negative rods), ulcerations, urethritis, and wounds (draining, surgical traumatic, mostly *Staphylococcus aureus*).

Description. Laboratory cultures of specimens taken from various body substances are performed to isolate and identify pathogenic microorganisms causing disease. This test involves the direct microscopic inspection of a Gram-stained smear of an organism after it is grown in selected media.

Professional Considerations
Consent form NOT required.

Preparation
1. Obtain the proper specimen container for the site (see Collection Containers for Routine Cultures).
2. Label multiple collections of the same test sequentially.
3. Wear a mask to prevent inhalation of airborne microorganisms expelled with coughing while collecting tracheal or nasopharyngeal specimens.

Procedure
1. A separate specimen should be obtained for each test.

2. *Cervical culture*: Remove from the cervical os, any secretions prior to obtaining the specimen. Insert swab or brush into the endocervix to a depth of 2 cm and rotate for 30 seconds, while pressing firmly against the interior wall of the canal. Remove swab using care to avoid brushing against any tissue.

3. *Ear culture*: Insert a cotton-tipped Culturette ⅛ to ¼ inch into the external auditory canal and rotate the swab. Remove the swab without touching any other parts of the ear. Insert the swab into the Culturette tube and squeeze the end of the tube to release the contents of the medium.

4. *Eye culture*: Swab the inner canthus of the eye with a sterile cotton-tipped Culturette swab. Insert the swab into the Culturette tube and squeeze the end of the tube to release the contents of the medium.

5. *Nasal culture*: Have the client clear the nose of excess secretions and tilt back the head. Insert the cotton-tipped Culturette into the nostril until it reaches the posterior nares and swab it in a circular motion two times. Leave the swab in place for 15 seconds. Slowly remove the swab and place it in the Culturette tube. Squeeze the swab end of the tube to release the contents of the medium. Repeat this procedure using the other nostril for nares culture.

6. *Nasopharyngeal culture*: Have the client tilt back the head and open the mouth. While depressing the tongue with a tongue blade, gently swab the tonsillar area from left to right. Also swab any reddened or purulent areas. Remove the swab without touching any other parts of the mouth. Insert the swab into the Culturette tube and squeeze the end of the tube to release the contents of the medium.

7. *Semen culture*: Collect a fresh specimen in a sterile cup.

8. *Sputum culture*: A first-morning sputum specimen is recommended. Chest clapping, postural drainage, or aerosol therapy, or all three, may be helpful in mobilizing tenacious secretions just before sputum collection. Have the client cough deeply several times and expel the mucus contents mobilized into

a wide-mouthed, sterile specimen cup. Instruct the client to avoid otherwise contaminating the cup's inside or edges. Tightly cap the cup.

Collection Containers for Routine Cultures

Site	Type of Sterile Container
Ear	Cotton swab Culturette
Eye	Cotton swab Culturette
Nasal	Two cotton swab Culturettes
Nasopharyngeal	Cotton swab Culturette
Site drainage	Cotton swab Culturette
Semen	Sterile cup with lid
Sputum	Sterile cup with lid
Sputum, tracheal	Sputum trap
Wound, superficial	Cotton swab Culturette
Wound, deep	Sterile syringe

9. *Sputum, tracheal, culture*: Ventilated clients should be hyperoxygenated before starting the procedure. Place the sputum trap in-line between the suction tubing and suction catheter. Maintain the trap in an upright position. Using a sterile technique, insert the suction catheter tip into the tracheostomy, endotracheal tube, or nares and advance it into the trachea without applying suction. In 10 seconds or less, apply suction and obtain 3-5 mL of mucus for culture in the trap and remove the suction catheter. Cap the sputum trap.

10. Urethral culture: 2 hours after the last void, insert the swab or brush 1-2 cm (females) or 2-4 cm (males) and rotate in one direction for 5 seconds.

11. *Wound, superficial site drainage*: Swab the site with the cotton-tipped end of a Culturette. Avoid touching the surrounding skin with the tip. Place the swab into the Culturette tube and squeeze the swab end to release the contents of the medium. Large wounds should have several separate cultures performed from different areas of the wound.

12. *Wound, deep*: Aspirate drainage with a syringe and needle from deep inside the wound. Remove the syringe, expel the air into sterile gauze, and either cap the needle with a rubber stopper or cork or inject the contents into anaerobic

culture medium. Transport the specimen to the laboratory immediately.

Postprocedure Care

1. Label the container with the specimen collection date and time.
2. Place the specimen in a sealed plastic bag.
3. Write any recent antibiotic or antifungal therapy on the laboratory requisition.
4. Send the specimen to the laboratory immediately. Do not refrigerate it.

Client and Family Teaching

1. The specimen collection procedure is typically painless, unless pressure is placed on an area of inflammation.
2. *Sputum collection*: Deep coughs are necessary to produce sputum, rather than saliva. To produce the proper specimen, take several breaths in, without fully exhaling each, and then expel sputum with a "cascade cough."
3. Clients started on empiric therapy should continue taking drugs unless and until test results are found to be negative.
4. Results are normally available in 2-3 days.

Factors That Affect Results

1. Antibiotic or antifungal therapy initiated before the specimen is taken may produce false-negative results. Obtain the culture before starting this therapy for the most accurate identification of the causative bacteria and the best clinical results.

Other Data

1. Results for most microorganisms will not be available for 48-72 hours. Fungi and mycobacteria may take several weeks. Gram stains requested should be available within 1 hour.

2. Normal mouth flora include *Actinomyces*, anaerobic and aerobic (non–group A) streptococci, anaerobic spirochetes, Enterobacteriaceae, *Haemophilus influenzae*, *Lactobacillus*, *Pneumococcus*, *Branhamella catarrhalis*, *Bacteroides* species, *Candida* fungi, nonpathogenic *Neisseria*, *N. meningitides*, *Staphylococcus aureus*, *S. epidermidis*, *S. pyogenes*, and *Veillonella* species.
3. Normal throat flora include alpha-hemolytic and nonhemolytic streptococci, *Bacteroides*, *Candida* fungi, *Corynebacterium* species, Enterobacteriaceae, *Haemophilus influenzae*, *N. meningitides*, nonpathogenic *Neisseria*, *Pneumococcus*, *S. aureus*, and *S. pyogenes*.
4. Normal nasal flora in small amounts include *B. catarrhalis*, *C. albicans*, diphtheroids, *H. influenzae*, *Neisseria* species (except *N. gonorrhoeae* and *N. meningitides*), *S. aureus*, *S. epidermidis*, *S. pneumoniae*, and *S. pyogenes*.
5. Normal ear flora include *S. epidermidis*, *Corynebacterium*, and *S. aureus*.
6. Normal eye flora include diphtheroids, Enterobacteriaceae, *Haemophilus*, *Moraxella*, *Neisseria*, *Pneumococcus*, *Sarcina*, *Staphylococcus epidermidis*, and *S. pyogenes*.
7. Nasal cultures should generally be limited to situations where throat specimens are not easily obtained because throat cultures are usually more advantageous for diagnosing upper respiratory tract infections.
8. Time to detection closely correlates with overall response to treatment for pulmonary tuberculosis.

Culture, Skin—Specimen

Norm. Negative.

Usage. Abscesses, ache, anthrax, athlete's foot, burn infections, candidiasis, carbuncles, erysipelas, folliculitis, herpes simplex, *Microsporum audouinii* for ringworm of the scalp, *Neisseria meningitides* for meningococcemia, neutrophilic eccrine hidradenitis, *Prototheca* algae, pruritus, psoriasis, pyoderma, scrapings to collect ova or mites for scabies, *Staphylococcus aureus* or group A beta-hemolytic streptococci for impetigo, *Streptococcus pyogenes*, tinea cruris, vitiligo, warts, yaws, and other skin infections.

Description. A sample of infected lesions of the skin is incubated, and the growth patterns, bacterial cell staining, and microscopic appearance are studied for determination of the organism causing the disease process. The most common skin pathogens are *Aspergillus*, *Blastomyces*, *Candida*, *Coccidioides immitis*, *Cryptococcus*, *Enterococcus*, *Histoplasma capsulatum*, *Microsporum*,

Penicillium, Proteus, Rhizopus, Rhodotorula, Sporothrix schenckii, Staphylococcus, Strepto-coccus, and *Trichophyton* species.

Professional Considerations
Consent form NOT required.

Preparation
1. Obtain 70% alcohol, sterile water, a sterile scalpel or spatula, and a sterile petri dish or anaerobic swab culture tubes, as indicated.

Procedure
1. Cleanse the lesion site with 70% alcohol and then rinse with sterile water to eliminate the effect of alcohol on any bacteria. Allow the site to dry.
2. Scrape the edge of the lesion to obtain tissue samples or purulent drainage with a sterile scalpel or spatula. Place the sample in a sterile petri dish.
3. For an anaerobic culture, obtain purulent drainage samples from deep in the wound on a swab and carefully place them in an anaerobic culture medium.

Postprocedure Care
1. Apply a dry, sterile dressing as needed.

Client and Family Teaching
1. If started on empiric therapy, you should continue taking the prescribed drug(s) unless and until the test results are found to be negative.

Factors That Affect Results
1. Obtain specimens before starting antibiotics for the most accurate bacterial identification and best clinical outcome.
2. For burned clients, viable skin rather than eschar yields the best results.
3. Chances of inadequate sampling of the lesion can be reduced when several separate samplings of the lesion or exudate are taken.

Other Data
1. Minor normal flora of the skin include *S. aureus,* fungi of the pityriasis type, and *Staphylococcus epidermidis,* which may proliferate in clients with poor immune systems and invasive wounds.

Culture
See **Stool Culture, Routine—Stool**

Culture—Urine
See **Culture, Routine.**

Cutaneous Immunofluorescence Biopsy—Diagnostic

Norm. A descriptive, interpretive report of histologic study findings is made.

Usage. Bulbous pemphigoid, chilblain lesions, dermatitis herpetiformis, herpes gestationis, necrolytic migratory erythema, pemphigus, and porphyria cutanea tarda in scleroderma; indicated in the investigation of cutaneous forms of chronic discoid lupus erythematosus, blistering disease, and vasculitis; also used to confirm the histopathologic characteristics of skin lesions and to follow the results of treatment.

Description. A biopsy specimen of the skin is taken for direct epidermal immunofluorescent study. Direct immunofluorescence is a histologic technique whereby the skin sample is treated with fluorescein-conjugated human immunoglobulin antisera and then incubated and examined under ultraviolet radiation. Deposition of human immunoglobulins and complement components in skin tissue and lesions (indicating a disorder) is identified and differentiated by the immunofluorescent patterns demonstrated.

Professional Considerations
Consent form IS required.

Risks
Bleeding, infection.
Contraindications
May be contraindicated in bleeding disorders, anticoagulated states, and immunocompromised states.

Preparation

1. Obtain punch forceps, an antiseptic solution, gauze, and a sterile specimen container.

Procedure

1. A 4-mm punch biopsy or surgically excised specimen of involved or uninvolved skin is obtained.
2. The specimen is quick-frozen in liquid nitrogen and stored at −94 degrees F (−70 degrees C). If the specimen is to be shipped to an outside lab, it is preserved in Michel holding solution with the pH maintained between 7.0 and 7.4.
3. Just before beginning the procedure, take a "time out" to verify the correct client, procedure, and site.

Postprocedure Care

1. Apply a dry, sterile dressing to the biopsy site.

Client and Family Teaching

1. The test typically is transiently painful.
2. Place pressure over the site for 5 minutes if bleeding occurs.
3. Results may not be available for several days.

Factors That Affect Results

1. Amount of biopsy <4 mm is insufficient.
2. The reliability of the immunofluorescence technique is affected by factors such as age and site of the lesion, type of immunofluorescence, and type of immunoglobulin. For this reason, histopathologic characteristics should also be used to confirm the results.

Other Data

1. The final report may take up to 3 days.

CXR

See **Chest Radiography**—Diagnostic.

Cyanide—Blood

Norm.

		SI Units
Serum		
Nonsmoker	0.004 mg/L	0.15 μmol/L
Smoker	0.006 mg/L	0.22 μmol/L
Panic (lethal) level	>0.1 mg/L	>3.7 μmol/L
Nitroprusside therapy	0.01-0.06 mg/L	0.37-2.21 μmol/L
Whole Blood		
Nonsmoker	0.016 mg/L	0.59 μmol/L
Smoker	0.041 mg/L	1.52 μmol/L
Panic (lethal) level	>1 mg/L	>37 μmol/L
Nitroprusside therapy	0.05-0.5 mg/L	1.9-19 μmol/L

Panic Level Symptoms and Treatment

Symptoms. Headache, dizziness, abdominal pain, nausea, confusion, labored breathing, syncope, tachycardia, hypertension, convulsions, and coma before respiratory failure. Loss of consciousness, metabolic acidosis, and cardiopulmonary failure are the three most common signs of cyanide poisoning in clients who die from this problem.

Treatment

NOTE: Treatment choice(s) depend(s) on client's history and condition and episode history.

Oxygen 15 L by mask (adult) and amyl nitrate pearl inhalants (crush onto a cloth and place in front of mouth for inhalation for 15-30 seconds, remove for 15 seconds, and repeat process every 3 minutes), hydroxocobalamin 4 g in 24 hours for adults, sodium nitrate 3% (300 mg in 10 mL of sterile water given IV over 10 minutes for adult and may repeat × 1, and 0.33 mL/kg for children; if given too fast, causes hypotension), and sodium thiosulfate (12.5 g in 50 mL of sterile water under slow IV push for adult and 1.65 mg/kg as pediatric dose).

Usage. Cyanide poisoning or suicide and monitoring of cyanide levels during nitroprusside therapy.

Description. A determination of the presence of cyanide in the blood. Cyanide is a very toxic chemical that inactivates cellular respiration enzymes (cytochrome oxidase), poisoning their functional activity and causing death from asphyxia. The major cause of death from cyanide poisoning is suicide.

Professional Considerations
Consent form NOT required.

Preparation
1. Tube: Lavender topped, black topped, or green topped.

Procedure
1. Completely fill the tube with blood.

Postprocedure Care
1. If cyanide poisoning is suspected, monitor neurologic and respiratory status closely and have emergency intubation equipment and oral airway available.

Client and Family Teaching
1. Kidneys and corneas can be harvested for transplantation after the poison level falls below lethal concentrations without adverse transplantation effects.

Factors That Affect Results
1. An insufficient blood sample may cause falsely low results.

Other Data
1. Cyanide is an end product of combustion, cigarette smoke, artificial nail remover, metal, wood, plastic refineries, Laetrile, plants, grass (sorghum), and pits of peaches and apricots. Also found in acetonitrile (methyl cyanide), a common industrial organic solvent.

Cyclic Adenosine Monophosphate (cAMP, Cyclic AMP)—Serum and Urine

Norm.

		SI Units
Serum	5.6-10.9 ng/mL	17-33 nmol/L
Urine		
Total cAMP	112-188 mg/L	340-570 nmol/L
cAMP portion of creatinine	3-5 mmol/g of creatinine	
cAMP portion of glomerular filtrate	6.6-15.5 mg/L	20-47 mmol/L
cAMP nephrogenous portion of glomerular filtrate	<9.9 mg/L	<30 nmol/L

Increased. Hyperparathyroidism, malignant processes combined with hypercalcemia, manic-depressives with bipolar disorder (untreated), migraine headaches, and pseudohyperparathyroidism.

Decreased. Atopic dermatitis, chronic renal failure, hypoparathyroidism, and pseudohypoparathyroidism.

Description. Nephrogenous cyclic adenosine monophosphate (cAMP) is an enzyme that increases in production in the renal tubules in response to parathyroid hormone. cAMP influences the rate of cell protein synthesis and indirectly affects renal reabsorption of phosphate, gastrointestinal calcium absorption, and skeletal calcium mobilization. cAMP in urine is the result of renal tubular cAMP secretion and glomerulus-filtered cAMP. Thus by comparing the serum and urine levels of cAMP with the glomerular filtration rate, one can estimate the portion of cAMP secreted by the tubules. There is some evidence that it may be secreted in a diurnal pattern. In clients with hyperparathyroidism, increased levels of nephrogenous cAMP are usually found as a result of excess parathyroid hormone production. A 24-hour urine collection may reveal increased levels of cAMP as a result of excess parathyroid hormone in the system.

Professional Considerations
Consent form NOT required.

Preparation
1. See Client and Family Teaching.
2. Preschedule this test with the laboratory.
3. Tube: Red topped, red/gray topped, or gold topped for the serum sample.
4. Obtain a 3-L container with hydrochloric acid (HCl) preservative for the urine sample.
5. The client should lie recumbent throughout the urine collection.
6. For 24-hour collections, discard the first morning urine specimen and write the beginning time on the laboratory requisition.

Procedure
1. Serum collection: Draw a 5-mL blood sample.
2. Urine collection: Collect a 2- or 24-hour urine sample for cAMP and creatinine in a refrigerated 3-L container. For 24-hour collections, include the urine voided at the end of the 24-hour period. For catheterized clients, keep the drainage bag on ice and empty urine into the acidified collection container hourly.

Postprocedure Care
1. *Serum sample:*
   a. Write the specimen collection time on the laboratory requisition.
   b. Transport the specimen to the laboratory immediately for serum separation.

c. Freeze the specimen if the test cannot be performed immediately.
2. *Urine sample:*
   a. Compare the urine quantity in the specimen container with the urinary output record for the test. If the specimen contains less urine than what was recorded as output, some of the sample may have been discarded, invalidating the test.
   b. Write the ending time of collection and the total urine volume on the laboratory requisition.
   c. Send the specimen to the laboratory immediately and refrigerate it until testing.

Client and Family Teaching
1. Limit physical exertion for 4 hours before the urine test.
2. Urinate before defecating to avoid loss of urine for the urine test. If any urine is accidentally discarded, discard the entire specimen and restart the collection the next day.
3. Results may not be available for more than 24 hours.

Factors That Affect Results
1. Reject serum specimens received more than 1 hour after collection.
2. Radioactive scans within 7 days before the test invalidate the serum and urine results.
3. Impaired renal function precludes the value of this urine test because results cannot be relied on for diagnosis.
4. All the urine voided for the 24-hour period must be included to avoid a falsely low result.

Other Data
1. For differentiation of hypoparathyroidism from pseudohypoparathyroidism, see Cyclic adenosine monophosphate provocation test—Urine.

Cyclic Adenosine Monophosphate Provocation Test—Urine

Norm. Positive: a 10-20-fold increase, or 3.6-4 mmol.

Negative. Type I pseudohypoparathyroidism.

Description. A test that measures cyclic adenosine monophosphate (cAMP) response to parathyroid hormone administration.

cAMP is an enzyme that influences the rate of cell protein synthesis and indirectly affects renal reabsorption of phosphate, gastrointestinal calcium absorption, and skeletal calcium mobilization. In normal clients and those with idiopathic or postoperative hypoparathyroidism, parathyroid hormone administration causes increased renal tubular

C

production of cAMP. In clients with pseudo-hypoparathyroidism—a genetically transmitted, autosomal dominant disease resulting in tissue resistance to the effects of parathyroid hormone—the infusion fails to increase production of cAMP in the renal tubules, resulting in a negative test.

Professional Considerations
Consent form NOT required.

Risks
Allergic reaction to parathyroid hormone (itching, hives, rash, tight feeling in the throat, shortness of breath, bronchospasm, anaphylaxis, death).

Contraindications
Positive parathyroid hormone skin test. This test is contraindicated in hypercalcemia.

Precautions
Use cautiously when digitalis has been administered and in renal impairment, cardiac disease, or sarcoidosis.

Preparation
1. Preschedule this test with the laboratory.
2. Obtain 300 U of parathyroid hormone and reconstitute it with sterile water for injection, as directed on the container.
3. Obtain a needle, a syringe, and a 1-L urine collection container with hydrochloric acid (HCl) preservative.
4. Establish intravenous access with 5% dextrose in water.
5. Have emergency equipment readily available.

Procedure
1. Have the client empty the bladder.
2. Attach a new collection bag on ice for catheterized clients.
3. Administer the prescribed dose of parathyroid hormone over 15 minutes.
4. Save all the urine collected in a refrigerated, 1-L container with HCl preservative. For catheterized clients, empty the drainage bag into the collection container hourly.
5. Three hours after the completion of the infusion, mix the container gently and collect a 50- to 100-mL aliquot for cAMP measurement.

Postprocedure Care
1. Send the specimen to the laboratory immediately. Refrigerate the specimen until testing.
2. Observe the client for lethargy, anorexia, nausea, vomiting, vertigo, or abdominal cramps, which could result from the mobilization of calcium stores by parathyroid hormone administration.

Client and Family Teaching
1. You will not be permitted to drive for 24 hours after the test and should make arrangements for someone else to drive you home.

Factors That Affect Results
1. Radioactive scans within 7 days before the test invalidate the results.

Other Data
1. None.

Cyclic AMP

See Cyclic Adenosine Monophosphate—Serum and Urine.

Cystatin C—Serum

Norm. 0.5-1.0 mg/L

Usage. Helps assess renal function (Seliger, DeFilippi, 2006); evaluation and staging of chronic kidney disease. Also used to assess how well a renal allograft is functioning.

Increased. Values >1.18 mg/L predict the occurrence of CIN in patients with moderate renal insufficiency with a sensitivity of 81.8% and a specificity of 90.9% (Ishibashi et al, 2010).

Decreased. None.

Description. Cystatin C is a cellular protein involved in inhibition of proteinase, thus helping to inhibit degradation of the extracellular matrix in body tissues. It is present in many body fluids and cells, but is normally present in very low quantities in the urine. In the kidneys, cystatin C is filtered freely through the glomerular barrier into the urine, and is not reabsorbed into the tubules. For this reason, it is useful in measuring the glomerular filtration rate and is considered to be highly sensitive and specific.

Professional Considerations
Consent form NOT required.

Preparation
1. Tube: red-top or serum separator tube or green-top tube.

Procedure
1. Obtain a 2-ml blood sample.
2. Deliver to lab immediately for separation of plasma or serum.

Postprocedure Care
1. Specimen is stable for 24 hours at room temperature, 1 week refrigerated, or 3 months frozen.

Client and Family Teaching
1. Fast overnight, or for 12 hours prior to the procedure.

Factors That Affect Results
1. Values increase significantly prior to cardiac catheterization after injection of contrast materials (Malyszko, Bachorzewska-Gajawska, Poniatowski, 2009 and Kato, Sato, Yamamoto et al, 2008).
2. Values increase significantly within 8 hours of a cardiac catheterization and peak 24 hours after the procedure.

Other Data
1. The presence of cystatin C has been identified as a risk factor for peripheral arterial disease PAD), and has been shown to be a better predictor than creatinine of cardiovascular events and death (Peralta, Shlipak, Judd, 2011).
2. Levels are less affected by muscle mass, weight, age, gender, and race than are creatinine levels. Thus, considering cystatin C values, along with creatinine levels and albumin-to-creatinine ratio improves the accuracy of stratification when evaluating risk for end stage renal disease (Peralta, Shlipak, Judd, 2011). Cystatin C is also thought to be more accurate than creatinine as a marker of renal function in the elderly with reduced muscle mass from aging.

Cystic Fibrosis CFTR Mutations (Genetic Carrier Screening for Cystic Fibrosis)—Specimen

Norm. Negative

Usage. Pre-conception screening examination to detect cystic fibrosis carrier status.

Description. Cystic fibrosis (CF) is a disorder in which alterations occur in the cystic fibrosis transmembrane conductance regulator (CFTR) protein, which is critical to normal functioning of the lungs, respiratory tract, gastrointestinal tract, genitourinary tract, pancreas, liver, and sweat glands (Burns, Englund, Prince, 2009). The mutated gene occurs in highest frequency in people with northern European ancestors and those of Ashkenazi Jewish descent. CF is the second most-common condition (after sickle cell disease) that shortens the lifespan of clients with the disease. Because this is an inherited, autosomal recessive disorder, if both parents carry the altered CF gene, the chances of having a child with CF are 25%. Therefore the American Congress of Obstetricians and Gynecologists recommends that carrier screening be made available to all couples contemplating pregnancy; and they also recommend screening of all newborns for cystic fibrosis, because early diagnosis leads to improved nutritional support, which leads to improved growth and cognitive development of the child. There are over 1500 mutations of the CFTR gene. Carrier screening tests for 23 to 32 of the most common mutations. If parents test negative with this genetic carrier screening test, any children born should still be tested, because false negative results can occur. This test examines the DNA from a blood or oral mucous membrane scraping sample to detect mutations in the CFTR protein.

Professional Considerations
Informed consent IS recommended for genetic testing.

Preparation
1. Collect required questionnaire regarding client history.
2. For blood test: Tube: lavender-, pink-, or yellow topped.
3. For buccal test: 2 buccal brushes.

Procedure

1. For blood test: Collect a 5-mL blood sample.
2. For buccal test: Gently scrape the interior buccal membranes with the 2 buccal brushes.

Postprocedure Care

1. None.

Client and Family Teaching

1. Refer the client with abnormal results for genetic counseling. Refer to Appendix B, Informed Consent for Genetic Testing.
2. If the first person tested is negative for any CFTR mutation, testing of the partner is not needed.

Factors That Affect Results

1. False negative results can occur of a mutation present was not one included in the carrier screening test.

Other Data

1. The Genetic Information Nondiscrimination Act of 2008 prohibits health plans from using genetic family history or genetic test results from influencing eligibility or premiums for health insurance. It also prohibits employers from using this information to influence decisions about hiring, terminating employment, or employment pay, promotions or privileges.

Cystine, Qualitative—Urine

Norm. Negative.

Positive. Congenital cystinuria, Fanconi syndrome, Lowe syndrome, nephrolithiasis, nephrotoxicity (caused by heavy metals), pyelonephritis (acute), renal tubular acidosis, and Wilson's disease.

Description. Cystine is an amino acid normally absent or present in only low amounts in the urine. In conditions causing cystinuria >300 mg/day, smooth, waxy cystine stones form in the kidneys and may be passed into the urine. Positive qualitative results should be followed by a 24-hour collection for cystine measurement because random samples may demonstrate peaks of cystine excretion in the urine.

Professional Considerations
Consent form NOT required.

Preparation

1. Obtain a clean container.

Procedure

1. Obtain a random urine specimen of 20 mL. A fresh specimen may be taken from a urinary drainage bag.

Postprocedure Care

1. Send the specimen to the laboratory immediately.

Client and Family Teaching

1. Results are normally available within 24 hours.

Factors That Affect Results

1. Drug that may cause false-negative results include penicillamine.

Other Data

1. This test should be scheduled before an intravenous pyelogram.
2. This is not a test for cystinosis, in which the urine cystine may be normal or only slightly elevated.
3. Acalculous cystinuria does not necessarily result in urinary stone disease.

Cystography, Retrograde—Diagnostic

Norm. Normal and intact structure of the bladder and normal location of the bladder; absence of rupture, laceration, fistula, tumor, or reflux into the ureters.

Usage. Detection of anastomotic leak after surgery, bladder diverticuli, bladder tumors, calculi, clots or other foreign bodies, fistula, hematoma, pyelonephritis, and laceration or rupture of bladder, urinary tract infections, or vesicoureteral reflux. This test will often indicate irregularity of the bladder present in neurogenic bladders.

Description. Retrograde cystography is performed by filling the bladder by injection or gravity flow (by means of a syringe barrel) with opacified contrast medium and sometimes air through a catheter into the bladder. This is followed by radiographs of the pelvis and bladder with the client in several positions.

Professional Considerations
Consent form IS required.

Risks
Bleeding, infection, urinary tract obstruction. Allergic reaction to contrast medium (hives, itching, rash, tight feeling in the throat, shortness of breath, bronchospasm, anaphylaxis, death) is extremely rare. Contrast should not be used in clients who have a contrast allergy or clients who have suspected major trauma to the bladder with the possibility of venous uptake of contrast or intraperitoneal spill.

Contraindications
History of allergy to radiographic dye, iodine, or shellfish; in urethral obstruction or injury, inability to pass a urethral catheter; or during the acute phase of a urinary tract infection; pregnancy (if iodinated contrast material is used, because of radioactive iodine crossing the blood-placental barrier).

Preparation
1. Obtain a straight urinary catheter and a catheter insertion tray, 50-300 mL of radiographic dye, and a syringe.
2. The client should disrobe below the waist or wear a gown.
3. Obtain baseline vital signs.
4. Have emergency equipment readily available.
5. Just before beginning the procedure, take a "time out" to verify the correct client, procedure, and site.

Procedure
1. The client is positioned supine on the radiographic table.
2. A baseline kidney-ureter-bladder (KUB) radiograph is taken.
3. 200-300 mL (50-100 mL for infants) of radiographic dye is instilled into the bladder by a catheter inserted through the urethra. It is recommended that the contrast be instilled through gravity using the barrel of a catheter-tipped syringe.
4. After the catheter is clamped, the client is assisted to several different positions by a tilt table; the physical position changes for radiographic examination of the bladder and surrounding areas.
5. The catheter is unclamped, the bladder fluid is allowed to drain, and final radiographs are taken.

Postprocedure Care
1. Monitor vital signs every 15 minutes × 4, then every 30 minutes × 2, then hourly × 4, and then every 2 hours for 24 hours after the test only if there is gross extravasation or major trauma is identified.
2. Encourage the oral intake of fluids where not contraindicated.
3. Have the client and family members observe for signs of allergic reaction to the dye (listed under Risks) for 24 hours.
4. Observe for urinary retention or symptoms of urinary tract infection (fever; chills; tachycardia; tachypnea; abdominal, flank, or suprapubic pain; hesitancy and frequency; dysuria; and hematuria). Notify the physician of any of these signs.
5. See Client and Family Teaching.

Client and Family Teaching
1. A clear liquid diet and a cathartic the day before the test may improve the clarity of the results by minimizing intestinal gas and the amount of stool.
2. After the procedure, save all the urine voided for the next day and report chills or painful urination. Blood in the urine that lasts more than 4-6 hours is abnormal.

Factors That Affect Results
1. This test should not be performed within 1 week of a previous intestinal barium examination.
2. The clarity of the radiographic images may be diminished by the presence of excess gas or stool in the lower gastrointestinal tract.

Other Data
1. None.

Cystometry—Diagnostic

C

Norm. Normal filling pattern. Absence of residual urine; sensation of fullness at 300-500 mL; urge to void at 150-450 mL; filling bladder pressure constant until capacity reached with contraction at capacity. Normal thermal sensation when hot and cold sterile fluids are introduced into the bladder.

Usage. Evaluation of detrusor muscle function and tonicity, determination of the cause of bladder dysfunction (urinary incontinence and retention), and differentiation of the type of neurogenic bladder dysfunction.

Description. Cystometry involves assessment of bladder neuromuscular function after instillation of measured quantities of fluid or air and evaluation of the client's neurologic sensations and muscular responses. It also includes assessment of the voiding flow pattern for abnormalities. Neuromuscular dysfunction of the bladder can occur when brain or spinal cord lesions (spinal cord or brain surgery or injury; stroke) interfere with the neural pathways that transmit bladder reflexes to and from the brain or with progressive diseases (such as multiple sclerosis), congenital malformations, strokes, or postoperatively. Cystometry is most often performed in a physician's office or clinic.

Professional Considerations
Consent form IS required.

Risks
Clients with spinal cord lesions (usually with cervical lesions or a history of higher cord lesions) may exhibit autonomic dysreflexia (bradycardia, hypertension, flushing, diaphoresis, and headache) during instillation of fluid or carbon dioxide. Intravenous or oral nifedipine or propantheline bromide may help to counteract this response.

Contraindications
This procedure is contraindicated in the acute phase of urinary tract infection and in urethral obstruction.

Preparation
1. Obtain a gas cystometer, a cystometric set, a 6- or 8-French special multiple-port transducer catheter, and an irrigation solution of sterile 0.9% saline or sterile, distilled water.
2. The client should disrobe below the waist or wear a gown.
3. Just before beginning the procedure, take a "time out" to verify the correct client, procedure, and site.

Procedure
1. The client urinates into a funnel attached to a machine that plots the amount, flow, and time of voiding on a graph.
2. Residual urine volume, if any, is then measured by means of an inserted indwelling catheter.
3. As the client lies in a supine position, thermal sensation is evaluated by the client's reported sensations in response to the instillation of 30-60 mL of room temperature 0.9% sterile saline solution, followed by 30-60 mL of 29-32 degrees C, 0.9% sterile saline solution through the catheter into the bladder.
4. The fluid is then drained from the bladder.
5. The client is then placed on a special commode chair attached to a cystometrogram table or placed in the semi-upright position. The client's sensations to bladder filling are measured next after the catheter is connected to a cystometer and measured amounts of sterile fluid or carbon dioxide are instilled into the bladder. Sometimes another catheter is placed into the rectum for abdominal pressure measurement. This allows true bladder muscle (detrusor) pressure to be electronically determined (bladder pressure − abdominal pressure ≈ detrusor pressure). Needle or surface electrodes may be used to measure pelvic floor muscle activity.
6. The cystometer measures and graphically records bladder pressure and volume, along with the client's reported descriptions of sensations (such as when he or she first feels the urge to void or feels unable to go any longer without voiding) and any reported discomfort.
7. The instillation is stopped when the client feels uncomfortably full or if it is determined that there is an absence of filling sensation.
8. The air or fluid and catheter are removed, or the client may be asked to void the fluid.

9. The test may be repeated in standing or sitting positions or after the administration of bladder-tone stimulants such as bethanechol chloride.

Postprocedure Care
1. Encourage the oral intake of fluids when not contraindicated; 125 mL/hour for 24 hours is desirable.
2. Monitor fluid intake and urine output for 24 hours.
3. Observe for urinary retention, symptoms of urinary tract infection (fever; chills; tachycardia; tachypnea; abdominal, suprapubic, or flank pain; hesitancy and frequency; dysuria; and hematuria).
4. Hematuria for more than 4-6 hours is abnormal. More postprocedure discomfort may be experienced after carbon dioxide instillation than after irrigant instillation.

5. Analgesics may be prescribed for bladder spasms.

Client and Family Teaching
1. The client must lie very still during the test.
2. The client may experience bladder spasms and see blood in his or her urine after the procedure. Spasms occurring for longer than 24 hours or bloody urine for more than 4-6 hours is abnormal. Call the physician if either of these occurs.

Factors That Affect Results
1. Antihistamines may interfere with bladder function by causing relaxation.
2. Movement during the test may interfere with bladder reflexes.

Other Data
1. None.

Cystoscopy—Diagnostic

Norm. Normal structure and function of the bladder; absence of urethral strictures or abnormalities, tumors, or bladder calculi; and absence of inflammation or purulent secretions.

Usage. Diagnosis of bladder cancer (99% Stage Ta grade I), diagnosis of vesicoureteral efflux in children, evaluation and differentiation of urinary tract disorders, method for obtaining bladder and ureteral biopsy specimens, sometimes used for excision of small tumors, evaluation of hematuria and of suspected urinary tract malformation in children.

Description. Cystoscopy is the direct, transurethral visualization of the bladder and urethra with the use of a lighted, magnifying cystoscope with a variety of lenses. The cystoscope is a metal instrument with a solid obturator that is placed inside a sheath within the urethra. Flexible cystoscopy is becoming more widely used as an alternative to rigid cystoscopy. Cystoscopy is indicated after other tests (such as cystography) show abnormalities; for evaluation of symptoms such as dysuria, frequency, and incontinence; or for evaluation of hematuria. It is also used as surveillance for recurrent bladder lesions such as transitional cell carcinoma. The procedure may be performed in a hospital or office by a physician or specialist urology nurse.

Professional Considerations
Consent form IS required.

Risks
Bleeding, infection (7.8% overall and 21.7% in enterocystoplasty clients), urinary tract obstruction.
Contraindications
Acute inflammations of the urethral passage. Sedatives are contraindicated in clients with central nervous system depression.

Preparation
1. See Client and Family Teaching.
2. Obtain a cystoscopy tray, disinfectant or surgical scrub solution, a genitourinary irrigant, drapes, sterile gloves, a cystoscope with appropriate lenses, obturator and light source (today video monitoring is common and the appropriate lens connector for camera and cord connection to the video unit is recommended), filiforms and followers, and two or three sterile

specimen containers (for possible biopsy, urine for culture and sensitivity, and a urine sample for cytologic testing).

3. A sedative may be prescribed.
4. Prophylactic antibiotics do not decrease the incidence of urinary tract infection in clients with sterile urine.
5. The client should disrobe below the waist or wear a gown.
6. Obtain baseline vital signs.
7. Pad the lithotomy stirrups.
8. Have emergency equipment readily available.
9. Just before beginning the procedure, take a "time out" to verify the correct client, procedure, and site.

Procedure

1. The client is positioned in the supine position on the cystoscopic table for possible administration of general or regional anesthesia.
2. The client is then placed in the lithotomy position for external genitalia cleansing and draping and cystoscopic examination.
3. After local anesthesia (if used) is instilled into the urethra and bladder and retained for 10-20 minutes, the urethra is progressively dilated (if necessary), and a cystoscope with obturator in place is inserted through the urethra into the bladder. The cystoscope is usually placed with the obturator in place in women and under direct vision with a 0- or 30-degree lens or flexible cystoscope in men. Pain can be significantly reduced by use of 20 mL of 2% lignocaine (lidocaine) gel left in the urethra for 15 minutes.
4. Urine specimens for culture or cytologic study may be removed through the cystoscope.
5. The bladder is filled with genitourinary irrigant solution, and the lighted cystoscope is used with magnification to directly examine the interior walls, structures, and contents of the bladder and urethra.
6. The bladder is inspected for tumors, calculi, diverticula, obstructions, and other lesions. The urethra is inspected for strictures and other lesions.
7. A biopsy sample of the bladder or ureters may be taken, and tiny tumors may also be excised through the cystoscope, with bleeding controlled by electrocautery.

Postprocedure Care

1. For general anesthesia, monitor vital signs every 15 minutes × 4, then every 30 minutes × 2, and then every 2 hours × 2. Typical postanesthesia monitoring also includes continuous ECG monitoring and pulse oximetry, with continual assessments (every 5-15 minutes) of airway and neurologic status until the client is lying quietly awake, is breathing independently, and responds appropriately to commands spoken in a normal tone.
2. For local anesthesia, assist the client to a chair until strength has returned to baseline value or for at least 15-30 minutes.
3. Encourage oral intake of fluids: 125 mL/hour for 24-48 hours when not contraindicated.
4. Monitor fluid intake and urine output for 24 hours.
5. Observe for urinary retention or symptoms of urinary tract infection (fever, chills, pain [abdominal, suprapubic, or flank], tachypnea, tachycardia, hesitancy and frequency, dysuria, and hematuria). Notify the physician if any of these signs occur.
6. Observe for hematuria. Pink urine is normal initially but should clear. Frank hematuria or clotting is abnormal. Dysuria lasting more than 4-6 hours is abnormal.
7. Analgesics may be prescribed for bladder spasms, and sitz or tub baths may help decrease generalized genital area discomfort.
8. Resume diet.

Client and Family Teaching

1. Arrange for someone to drive you home if the procedure was performed using anything other than local anesthesia because you will not be permitted to drive for 24 hours after having general anesthesia. It is also suggested that someone drive you home after local anesthesia in some situations, but this is not absolutely necessary.
2. For general anesthesia, fast from food and fluids for 8 hours. For local anesthesia, consume only clear liquids for 8 hours. You may be required to take in a large amount of fluids to promote urine flow during the procedure.

3. Clients receiving local anesthesia may feel the urge to void while the cystoscope is in place.
4. After the procedure, drink 6-8 glasses of water or other fluids per day for 2 days (unless contraindicated). Watch for warning symptoms of complications (see above). Report chills, fever, dysuria, or frank blood in the urine.
5. Do not have sexual relations until the physician confirms healing.

Factors That Affect Results
1. None.

Other Data
1. Urethroscopy or retrograde pyelogram may also be combined with cystoscopy.
2. Cystoscopy may also be used as a therapeutic procedure to crush and remove calculi, perform bladder irrigation, resect tumors, or perform a transurethral resection of the prostate gland.
3. The use of intraurethral lidocaine gel has not been shown to decrease client pain during rigid cystoscopy. Anxiety has been shown to positively correlate with pain perception.

Cystourethrography, Voiding—Diagnostic

Norm. Normal formation of bladder and urethra, normal elimination of contrast medium through the urethra, and absence of retrograde movement of contrast medium into the ureters.

Usage. Detection of urinary tract congenital anomalies, vesicoureteral reflux, neurogenic abnormalities, enlarged prostate gland, urethral strictures, and bladder diverticula or polyps.

Description. Using fluoroscopy or radiography, voiding cystourethrography demonstrates the bladder filling by contrast medium instillation through a catheter into the bladder and then shows exiting of the contrast medium during voiding after removal of the catheter.

Professional Considerations
Consent form IS required.

Risks
Bleeding, hematuria, and infection. Allergic reaction to contrast (itching, hives, rash, tight feeling in the throat, shortness of breath, bronchospasm, anaphylaxis, death) is a very rare possibility, since no contrast should be absorbed into the vascular tree with this procedure.

Contraindications
Previous allergy to radiographic dye, iodine, or shellfish; in the acute phase of a urinary tract infection; urinary tract obstruction; during pregnancy (if iodinated contrast material is used, because of radioactive iodine crossing the blood-placental barrier); recent bladder surgery; and urethral obstruction, evulsion, or transection. Sedatives are contraindicated in clients with central nervous system depression.

Preparation
1. See Client and Family Teaching.
2. Obtain a balloon catheter, a contrast medium, and a syringe or tubing for instillation of the contrast medium.
3. The client should disrobe below the waist.
4. A sedative may be prescribed.
5. Have emergency equipment readily available.
6. Just before beginning the procedure, take a "time out" to verify the correct client, procedure, and site.

Procedure
1. After the client is positioned supine, a balloon catheter is inserted through the urethra into the bladder, and the balloon is inflated.
2. The bladder is filled with contrast medium by gravity or syringe instillation, and the catheter is clamped.
3. Radiographic or fluoroscopic films of the lower urinary tract are taken with the client in several positions.
4. The catheter is then removed, and the client must void in a right-sided or left-sided position with the lower leg flexed at the hip. Male testes should be shielded by lead before voiding begins.
5. Several more radiographic or fluoroscopic films of the lower urinary tract are taken during voiding.
6. If the client is unable to void, the bladder area is gently pressed to stimulate voiding.

Postprocedure Care

1. Encourage oral intake of fluids, 125 mL/hour for 24 hours when this is not contraindicated.
2. Monitor fluid intake and urine output for quantity, and monitor hematuria for 24 hours. Hematuria or dysuria that lasts more than 4-6 hours is abnormal.
3. Observe for signs of allergic reaction to the contrast (listed above) for 24 hours.
4. Observe for urinary retention or symptoms of urinary tract infection (fever, chills, pain [abdominal, suprapubic, or flank], tachypnea, tachycardia, hesitancy and frequency, dysuria, and hematuria). Notify physician for anuria present within 8 hours or for any of the above signs.
5. Analgesics may be prescribed for bladder spasms, and sitz or tub baths may help decrease generalized genital area discomfort.

Client and Family Teaching

1. A clear liquid diet and a cathartic may be prescribed the day before the exam.
2. The urge to void during the procedure is normal.
3. Drink 6-8 glasses of water or other fluids per day for 2 days (unless contraindicated). Watch for warning symptoms of complications (see above). Report chills, fever, dysuria, or frank blood in the urine.
4. In women who are breast-feeding, formula should be substituted for breast milk for 1 or more days after the procedure.

Factors That Affect Results

1. Although the clearest films result from the recumbent position, standing films are sometimes used for clients unable to void while lying down.
2. Intestinal barium studies within 1 week before the test or the presence of a large amount of gas in the lower bowel may inhibit the clarity of the films.

Other Data

1. None.

Cysts and Nipple Discharge

See Cytologic Study of Breast Cyst—Diagnostic; Cytologic Study of Nipple Discharge—Diagnostic.

Cytochemical Stain

See Leukocyte Cytochemistry—Specimen.

Cytologic Study

See Bronchial Washing—Specimen; Brushing Cytology—Specimen; Cerebrospinal Fluid, Routine, Culture and Cytology—Specimen; Cytologic Study of Breast Cyst, Effusions, Gastrointestinal Tract, Nipple Discharge, Respiratory Tract, or Urine—Diagnostic; Ocular Cytology—Specimen; Oral Cavity Cytology—Specimen.

Cytologic Study of Breast Cyst—Diagnostic

Norm. Absence of cells indicating malignancy or infection.

Usage. Determine if the breast lesion is a mass or a cyst, and determine if malignant cells are present.

Description. Breast cyst cytology is the microscopic study of the fluid or cells obtained by fine-needle aspiration. The lesion may have been detected by breast examination or mammogram. The fluid is fixed and examined by the cytologist on a microscopic slide. Any cells in the cyst fluid are studied for diagnosis of neoplasm, infective process, and, rarely, tuberculosis of the breast.

Professional Considerations

Consent form NOT required. See Needle aspiration—Diagnostic for procedure-specific risks and contraindications.

C

Preparation

1. Obtain a 21- or 23-gauge long needle, a 10-mL syringe, sterile 0.9% saline, a red- or marble topped glass tube or gold seal plastic tube, and a clean jar.
2. The client should disrobe above the waist.
3. Position the client for comfort and accessibility to the cyst and drape him or her for privacy.

Procedure

1. The aspiration site is identified. The skin is cleansed with an alcohol wipe and allowed to dry.
2. The suspect mass is immobilized by one hand while the needle is inserted with the other hand.
3. Fluid is aspirated when one draws back on the syringe.
4. A fluid drop is placed on a clean slide, and the thin edge of a second slide is used to produce a smear.
5. The slide is then fixed immediately in 95% ethyl alcohol in a clean jar.
6. If more than a minute amount of fluid has been aspirated, place the remaining fluid in a red- or marble topped tube.
7. If the specimen is minute, rinse the needle with 10 mL of sterile 0.9% saline and place the rinsed material into the tube.
8. Label the slide and the aspirate or wash with the client's name, and indicate the specimen source, noting which breast.

Postprocedure Care

1. Apply pressure to the aspiration site for a short time.
2. Write the pertinent clinical information on the laboratory requisition.
3. Send the specimens to the laboratory for immediate evaluation.

Client and Family Teaching

1. This is the diagnostic procedure of choice for breast cysts in pregnant women because there are no radiographs or anesthesia required.
2. This is a sterile procedure that takes approximately 10 minutes, with minimal discomfort.
3. Watch the area for the next 72 hours for redness, drainage, and swelling, and check for temperature >101 degrees F (>38.3 degrees C); report any of these signs to the physician or nurse.
4. Results are normally available within 48 hours.

Factors That Affect Results

1. Immediate fixation of the smear prevents drying of the sample and distortion of the findings because of contamination.
2. Some cytologists prefer specimens that were allowed to dry before being placed in the fixative. These should be specifically labeled because they are stained differently for study.
3. An insufficient sample may result when the breast lesion is not penetrated or it contains no fluid.

Other Data

1. Aspiration is an inexpensive screening procedure for evaluating breast lesions. It decreases the necessity of open surgical biopsy to determine a definitive diagnosis.
2. This test is more reliable than nipple discharge cytology for ruling out neoplasms.
3. Culture of the aspirate is usually obtained for a complete work-up.
4. There is no difference in the cytologic yield with a 21-gauge needle as compared with that of a 23-gauge needle.
5. Fine-needle aspiration is a sensitive test that must be used only in the context of other diagnostic modalities.

Cytologic Study of Effusions—Diagnostic

Norm. No tumor cells or infection.

Usage. Gout, lymphoproliferative disease, infections of or fistulas into serous cavities, metabolic arthritis, metastatic neoplasms, myeloproliferative disease, rheumatoid arthritis, rheumatoid pleuritis, systemic lupus erythematosus, and pulmonary TB.

Description. An effusion is an abnormal collection of fluid occurring most commonly in the pericardial sac, abdomen, pleural space, and synovial cavities. Effusions may be transudate caused by hydrostatic pressure differences or exudate caused by tumors or infective processes. Effusion cytology is the microscopic study of the fluid aspirate of the particular effusion and is used to differentiate the cause and type of effusion and to characterize and identify the source of infection or the tumor type.

Professional Considerations

Consent form IS required for the procedure used to obtain the specimen. See individual procedures for procedure-specific risks and contraindications.

Preparation

1. Check PT and PTT or INR. This procedure may be contraindicated in clients with coagulation defects.
2. Obtain the appropriate procedure tray, sterile gloves and drapes, povidone-iodine solution, and 1%-2% lidocaine. If a large effusion is to be drained, obtain a heparinized vacuum bottle and tubing with a clamp or stopcock.
3. Obtain baseline vital signs.
4. For a pericardiocentesis, monitor ECG continuously throughout the procedure.
5. For small or loculated effusions, an ultrasonograph- or CT-guided tap will increase the chance of obtaining a specimen.
6. Just before beginning the procedure, take a "time out" to verify the correct client, procedure, and site.

Procedure

1. Position the client appropriately for the procedure to be performed.
2. Cleanse the aspiration site and surrounding skin with povidone-iodine solution and allow it to dry.
3. Overlay the aspiration site with sterile drapes.
4. Obtain two 3- to 10-mL samples of fluid using a sterile technique by means of

arthrocentesis, pericardiocentesis, paracentesis, or thoracentesis. Place one specimen in a heparinized tube and one in a nonheparinized tube for evaluation and cytologic testing.

Postprocedure Care

1. For a thoracentesis, a postprocedure chest radiograph MUST be performed to check for a possible pneumothorax.
2. Monitor vital signs for indications of bleeding or hemodynamic changes.
3. Write the name, date, source of fluid, and symptoms on the laboratory requisition.
4. Send the specimen to the laboratory immediately. Refrigerate specimens not examined immediately.

Client and Family Teaching

1. This is a sterile procedure that takes up to 1 hour and may include moderate discomfort.
2. It is very important to stay as still as possible during the procedure to avoid injury and complications.
3. Results are normally available within 72 hours.

Factors That Affect Results

1. Results are most accurate when the specimen is examined within 1 hour of collection.

Other Data

1. This method is usually more sensitive than blind biopsy for diagnosis of pleural malignancies.
2. The addition of Ki-67 immunostaining appears more sensitive than cytomorphology alone in distinguishing benign from malignant effusions.

Cytologic Study of Gastrointestinal Tract—Diagnostic

Norm. Normal cells of the gastrointestinal tract. No tumor cells or infection.

Usage. Cytologic examination of exfoliation of the mucosa of the gastrointestinal tract to allow diagnosis of benign, precancerous, or malignant lesions of the esophagus, stomach, and duodenum. Also for amyloidosis, microscopic colitis, Crohn's disease, granulomatous inflammation, gastritis, *Helicobacter pylori*, leiomyosarcoma, lymphoma, intestinal spirochetosis, melanosis coli, Ménétrier's disease, pernicious

anemia, schistosomiasis, toxic drug effect on gastric mucosa, and Whipple's disease.

Description. Brushings or fine-needle aspirations of the mucosa of the upper gastrointestinal tract are performed during endoscopic examination. Washings of the mucosa for a specimen through a nasogastric tube may be performed when endoscopy is not available or is contraindicated or when neoplasm is clinically suspected. Brushings of the colon or rectum can be made by proctosigmoidoscopy.

Professional Considerations
Consent form NOT required for nasogastric tube method. Consent form IS required for endoscopy and sigmoidoscopy.

Risks
See individual procedures for risks and contraindications.
Contraindications
Severe gastrointestinal bleeding, varices (gastric or esophageal), and clients who are unable to cooperate.

Preparation
1. Preschedule this test with the laboratory.
2. If colon washing is to be performed, administer an oral cathartic as prescribed and collect the last bowel movement before the test to send to the laboratory with the washing specimen.
3. For collection of gastric washings for cytologic examination, obtain a nasogastric (NG) tube, a lubricant, 0.9% saline, a syringe, a 500-mL clean container, a 50% ethyl alcohol (ethanol) fixative, and dry ice.
4. For collection of endoscopic brushings for cytologic examination, obtain endoscopic equipment, a brush, glass slides labeled with the client's name, a clean container of 95% ethyl alcohol or other fixative required by the specific laboratory, and dry ice or 50% ethyl alcohol.
5. For colon washing, obtain an enema tube, 0.9% saline, a large airtight plastic container, and dry ice or 50% ethyl alcohol.
6. See Gastroscopy or gastroduodenojejunoscopy—Diagnostic; Barium enema—Diagnostic; Proctoscopy—Diagnostic; or Sigmoidoscopy—Diagnostic for other preparations, as would be appropriate for the procedure being performed.

Procedure
1. *Gastric washing:*
   a. Insert a nasogastric tube.
   b. Withdraw gastric contents with a Toomey syringe and discard.
   c. Instill 300-500 mL of 0.9% saline solution into the stomach through the NG tube.
   d. Have the client roll 360 degrees four or five times.
   e. Aspirate all the gastric contents into a clean, sealed container.
2. *Endoscopic brushings for cytology:*
   a. During endoscopy, a brushing is taken from specific lesions of the esophagus, the stomach, or the duodenal area.
   b. The brush should be rolled onto a slide to cover at least a 1.5-cm-diameter area.
   c. The slide should be immediately placed into a container of 95% ethyl alcohol (ethanol) or other required fixative.
3. *Colon washing:* Colon washing is performed just before barium enema washing.
   a. Insert the enema tubing into the colon through the rectum.
   b. Instill 100 mL of 0.9% saline solution through the tubing.
   c. Have the client roll 360 degrees several times.
   d. Drain the fluid out of the enema tubing and instill it into an airtight container.
4. *Colon or rectal brushing:*
   a. Insert the proctoscope or sigmoidoscope.
   b. Take a brushing from the lesion sites.
   c. The brush should be rolled onto a slide to cover at least a 1.5-cm-diameter area.

Postprocedure Care
1. Either pack the specimen in dry ice or preserve it with 50% ethyl alcohol.
2. Write the time and source of the specimen collection on the laboratory requisition. Each separate brushing sample should be labeled with the anatomic site of collection.
3. Transport the specimen to the cytotechnologist in the pathology laboratory immediately for fixing and microscopic examination.
4. Remove the nasogastric or enema tube.
5. Resume normal diet.
6. See Gastroscopy or gastroduodenojejunoscopy—Diagnostic; Barium enema—Diagnostic; Proctoscopy—Diagnostic; or Sigmoidoscopy—Diagnostic for other postprocedure care, as appropriate for the procedure being performed.

Client and Family Teaching
1. Eat a soft diet for the evening meal before the test.
2. Fast from food for 8-12 hours and from water for 1 hour before the procedure.

C

Factors That Affect Results

1. Washings may be performed twice. Discarding the first aspirate and sending the second aspirate for study may be more reliable, especially for gastric neoplasms.
2. Contamination of the specimen with food or barium invalidates the results.
3. Reject specimens not packed in dry ice or not received promptly after collection.
4. Reject slides that were allowed to dry before fixing or those received without fixative.
5. Reject unlabeled slides.

Other Data

1. This is not as effective a diagnostic tool as radiography or endoscopy with biopsy.
2. A negative report does not rule out malignancy.
3. Gastroscopy-guided brushings are preferable to gastric washings for cytologic study.
4. Proctosigmoidoscopic smears to investigate diarrhea should be performed with no preparation of the bowel because the exudate may be washed away, the mucosa distorted, trauma of the mucosa induced, or the evidence of disease obscured or altered.

Cytologic Study of Nipple Discharge—Diagnostic

Norm. Absence of tumor cells or infection.

Usage. Diagnosis of inflammatory disease, intraductal papilloma, mammary dysplasia with ectasia of the ducts, metastasis or suspected malignancy of the breast, and papillomatosis.

Description. Nipple discharge is considered abnormal except in lactating or pregnant women, though some discharge is caused by medication. Several nipple-discharge smears are fixed on glass slides and microscopically studied for the presence of abnormal cells indicating neoplasm or infection, and, rarely, tuberculosis of the breast. Abnormal cytology indicates increased relative risk for breast cancer.

Professional Considerations

Consent form NOT required.

Preparation

1. Explain the procedure. The client who assists should hold the fixative bottle under the breast so that the slide can be immediately placed in the fixative.
2. Obtain warmed sterile saline, 6-12 clean glass slides, 6-12 clean glass bottles of 95% ethyl alcohol (ethanol), labels, and cotton or gauze.
3. The client should disrobe above the waist.
4. Position the client so that it is convenient to obtain the specimen, and drape him or her for privacy.

Procedure

1. Vigorously cleanse the nipple and then soak it in warm saline on a cotton or gauze pad for 10-15 minutes and pat it dry.
2. Gently strip the subareolar area with a thumb and forefinger, moving toward the nipple tip. Continue until a pea-sized droplet of fluid is expressed.
3. Place the frosted side of a clean glass microscope slide on the nipple and quickly slide it across the nipple tip to obtain a smear of fluid.
4. Immediately place the slide into a small jar of 95% ethyl alcohol (ethanol) fixative.
5. Label the jar with the number of the smear and whether it was taken from the right or left breast. This is especially important when both breasts are studied.
6. Repeat steps 1 through 5 until four to six slides from each breast are obtained, if possible.

Postprocedure Care

1. Write a description of the discharge and the client's name, age, clinical symptoms, and which breast is being studied on the laboratory requisition.
2. Send the specimens to the laboratory immediately.
3. Cleanse the breast and nipple as needed.

Client and Family Teaching

1. The procedure takes about 10 minutes.
2. Results are normally available within 48 hours.
3. About 3% of breast cancers and 10% of benign lesions of the breast are associated

C

with nipple discharge. Negative cytologic results do not rule out a malignancy.

Factors That Affect Results
1. Immediate fixation of the smear prevents drying of the sample and distortion of the findings because of contamination.
2. Several (rather than one or two) slides improve results because later smears include more abnormal cells if they are present.

3. Medications that affect hormonal balance and may cause nipple discharge include chlorpromazines, digitalis, diuretics, oral contraceptives, phenothiazines, and steroids.

Other Data
1. Mammography and biopsy or aspiration are more reliable diagnostic procedures for breast malignancy than cytologic study.

Cytologic Study of Respiratory Tract—Diagnostic

Norm. Negative.

Usage. Diagnosis of respiratory neoplasms or premalignant cell changes related to chronic inflammation, inhaled toxins, tuberculosis, or asthma; diagnosis of respiratory bacterial, viral, or parasitic infections.

Description. Respiratory tract cytology is the microscopic study of the number and type of cells of the respiratory tract or sputum to detect the presence of cells abnormal for that specimen, including tumor or pretumor cells or evidence of an infective process. Any anomalies of cells are correlated to clinical data for diagnosis.

Professional Considerations
Consent form NOT required unless the sample for study is obtained by bronchoscopy.

Preparation
1. An aerosol treatment just before specimen collection may help to mobilize respiratory secretions.

Procedure
1. Three early-morning specimens are obtained.
2. Have the client rinse the mouth with water.
3. Instruct the client to inhale deeply and then exhale with a deep, expulsive cough and expectorate sputum directly into a sterile, wide-mouthed container.
4. Alternatively, bronchial secretions may be removed directly during bronchoscopy or by nasotracheal suctioning using a specimen trap.

Postprocedure Care
1. Write the client's name, the date, the specimen source, the specimen number, the

diagnosis, and the clinical symptoms on the laboratory requisition.
2. Send the specimen to the laboratory immediately.

Client and Family Teaching
1. Results are normally available within 72 hours.
2. To produce a deep sputum specimen, rather than saliva, take several deep breaths, without fully exhaling between them. When you feel as though you cannot take any more breaths, cough out forcefully and catch the sputum in the sterile cup.
3. The results may have to be confirmed by culture or biopsy.

Factors That Affect Results
1. The results are most accurate when examined within 1 hour of collection.
2. The results are invalid if the sample is saliva, rather than respiratory secretions.
3. Smoking and pharmacotherapy affect the results of the analysis.

Other Data
1. About 15% of results are false negatives.
2. Sputum cytologic findings are more likely to be negative in a client with small cell carcinoma than in one with non–small cell carcinoma of the lung.
3. Culture with or without biopsy is usually more reliable than cytologic examination for diagnosis of respiratory tract neoplasm or infection.
4. The detection of the codon-12 K-ras mutation in BALF cells aids the diagnosis of lung cancer in clients with negative cytologic findings.

Cytologic Study of Urine—Diagnostic

Norm. Normal type and amount of squamous and epithelial cells of the urinary tract and little or no cellular debris; red blood cell count ≤3; white blood cell count ≤4; no abnormal cells such as cytomegalic inclusion bodies, malignant cells, parasites, or yeasts.

Usage. Anemia (hemolytic), cerebral metachromatic leukodystrophy, cytomegalovirus infection (cytomegalic inclusion bodies), measles (cytomegalic inclusion bodies), renal hemosiderosis, screening for premalignant cell changes, transplant rejection, urinary tract infections (herpesvirus, fungi, *Schistosoma*, others), urinary tract inflammation (epithelial cells, RBCs, WBCs), and urinary tract primary or metastatic cancer (malignant cells).

Description. Urine cytology is the microscopic study of cells in urine to detect the presence of abnormal cells, including tumor or pretumor cells, or evidence of an infective process. Any abnormalities found are correlated to clinical data for a diagnosis of urinary tract neoplasm, infection, or other diseases that may affect the urine.

Professional Considerations
Consent form NOT required.

Preparation
1. Obtain a sterile container.
2. Hydrate the client ½ to 1 hour before specimen collection.

Procedure
1. Urine cytology involves centrifuging and filtering the urine, or cytocentrifuging, staining, and examining the filtered sediment.
2. For a voided specimen, have the client urinate directly into a sterile container. Tightly cover the container.
3. Catheterization may be used if it is otherwise difficult to obtain the specimen or if a high urinary tract lesion is suspected.

Postprocedure Care
1. Send the specimen to the laboratory immediately.

Client and Family Teaching
1. Discard the first morning void if collecting the sample in the morning. With the next void, urinate directly into the container and then cap it tightly.
2. Results are normally available within 48 hours.

Factors That Affect Results
1. An early-morning specimen is unsuitable because cell death occurs in the bladder overnight.
2. Recent instrumentation may cause cell injury or changes that give false-positive results.
3. Hypotonic solutions used as washing during cystourethroscopy procedures may alter the results by directly affecting cell structure and appearance.
4. Chemotherapeutic agents such as cyclophosphamide may alter the results.

Other Data
1. A voided specimen is preferred except when specific study of high urinary tract areas is needed. Urine from each ureter may be studied and compared.
2. Cytomegalovirus (CMV) can be diagnosed by urine cytologic examination. Several specimens are recommended because cytomegalovirus is not shed continuously. The presence of CMV in the urine may indicate CMV disease or an asymptomatic reactivation of CMV disease. The herbs *Geum japonicum*, *Syzygium aromaticum*, and *Terminalia chebula* have demonstrated anti-murine CMV activity in mice.

Cytology

See **Cytologic Study**—Specimen and **Cytologic Study of Urine**—Diagnostic.

Cytomegalic Inclusion Disease, Cytology—Urine

Norm. Negative for inclusion body cells.

Positive. Cytomegalovirus infections of a disseminated type.

Description. Cytomegalovirus is a member of the herpesvirus family and causes cytomegalic inclusion disease, a generalized infection in infants and small children caused by intrauterine, natal, or postnatal exposure to infected secretions (blood, cervical secretions, urine, saliva, breast milk, or semen). The mode of transmission to immunocompromised clients is unknown. Cytomegalic inclusion disease symptoms may range from none in healthy-appearing children to generalized symptoms of a severe infection; the disease is characterized by the presence of intranuclear or intracellular inclusion bodies in the kidney that are excreted in the urine. The disease may also affect the salivary glands, lung, liver, pancreas, and brain, where inclusion bodies may also be found. Severe symptoms may be fatal.

Professional Considerations

Consent form NOT required.

Preparation

1. Obtain a clean-catch urine kit.
2. Hydrate the client for $\frac{1}{2}$ to 1 hour.
3. The specimen should be obtained at least 3 hours after the last void, but should not be the first morning void.

Procedure

1. Urine cytology involves centrifuging and filtering the urine, or cytocentrifuging, staining, and examining the filtered sediment.
2. The clean-catch urine technique must be used to decrease the risk of specimen contamination. See clean-catch collection instructions in the test Body fluid, Routine—Culture.
3. A fresh specimen may be taken from a clean urinary drainage bag.

Postprocedure Care

1. Send the specimen to the laboratory immediately.

Client and Family Teaching

1. Provide collection instructions (above) if the client will be obtaining the specimen independently.
2. This test is one of the most reliable and rapid methods for diagnosing cytomegalovirus infection. Several specimens are recommended because cytomegalovirus is not shed continuously.

Factors That Affect Results

1. Specimens should be tested within 6 hours.

Other Data

1. Cytomegalic inclusion bodies are often found in clients with cancer undergoing chemotherapy and in transplant clients receiving immunosuppressive drugs.
2. Inclusion bodies may also be found in smears and brushings from other sources, such as bronchoalveolar lavage fluid and biopsy specimens of cytomegalovirus-infected tissues.
3. Positive urine culture with the occurrence of CMV retinitis signifies CMV retinitis in the contralateral eye of clients with unilateral disease.
4. The herbs *Geum japonicum, Syzygium aromaticum,* and *Terminalia chebula* have demonstrated anti-murine CMV activity in mice.

Cytomegalovirus Antibody—Serum

Norm. Negative.

IgM	<1:8
IgH	<1:8 for those exposed
IgG	<1:16 for those exposed

Positive. A fourfold increase in the antibody titer between the acute and convalescent specimens or IgM >1:8 in a single specimen indicates a primary cytomegalovirus infective process. Cytomegalovirus (CMV) infections include congenital CMV, spontaneous CMV mononucleosis (heterophil-negative mononucleosis), posttransfusion CMV mononucleosis, and CMV in immunosuppressed clients. Disseminated infections may cause CMV retinitis, esophagitis, hepatitis, and ileocolitis. Positive in aphthous stomatitis, lichen planus, Ménière's disease, pulmonary fibrosis, and scleroderma.

Description. Cytomegalovirus is a herpesvirus. The virus is present in a large segment of the population early in life without causing apparent disease. Serologic prevalence studies show that 60%-90% of U.S. adults, depending on socioeconomic level, and very old people are positive for antibodies to CMV. Because the presence of disease is unusual, host factors predisposing to the disease should be investigated when the disease is manifested. CMV mononucleosis usually occurs in older adults, compared to Epstein-Barr mononucleosis, and presents with a lower incidence of pharyngitis and lymphadenopathy. Congenital CMV may cause a variety of developmental abnormalities and neurologic deficits in the infant or young child. In the immunosuppressed client, pulmonary or systemic infections may occur. Clients receiving tissue transplants (liver, heart, lung, kidney, and bone) are also at high risk for manifested infections. CMV immune status should be performed on all organ transplant candidates before surgery. Blood for transfusion to seronegative transplant clients and all premature neonates should be from donors without CMV antibodies.

Professional Considerations
Consent form NOT required.

Preparation
1. Tube: Red topped, red/gray topped, or gold topped.

Procedure
1. Draw a 3-mL blood sample. Label the tube as the acute sample.

2. 10-14 days later, repeat the test and label the tube as the convalescent sample.

Postprocedure Care
1. Results are normally available within 72 hours.

Client and Family Teaching
1. It is important to return in 10 days to 2 weeks for follow-up sampling to determine if the infection is clearing up.
2. Acyclovir, ganciclovir, and foscarnet are used for treatment of cytomegalovirus infections.

Factors That Affect Results
1. False-positive low titer results may occur in clients exposed to the Epstein-Barr virus, but a high titer confirms CMV. May also be falsely positive in those with rheumatoid factor in their serum.

Other Data
1. The titer is not valid for the study of infants under 6 months of age because they may have maternal antibodies present in their serum.
2. In a CMV-positive client, CMV may be cultured from urine. The presence of the virus in the urine may indicate CMV disease or an asymptomatic reactivation of CMV. The finding of a positive CMV blood culture has a much higher correlation with the presence of CMV disease.
3. CMV antibody titers are of little value in determining the presence of CMV infection in immunocompromised clients because of the high incidence of CMV seropositive clients in the general public. Viral isolation is necessary for diagnosis.
4. The herbs Geum *japonicum*, *Syzygium aromaticum*, and *Terminalia chebula* have demonstrated anti-murine CMV activity in mice.

Cytoplasmic Neutrophil Antibodies
See Antineutrophil Cytoplasmic Antibody Screen—Serum.

D & C
See Dilation and Curettage—Diagnostic.

DCP
See Des-gamma-carboxy Prothrombin (DCP)—Serum

D-Dimer Test (Fibrin Degradation Fragment)—Blood

Norm. <0.4 µg/mL.

Positive. Indicates in vivo fibrinolytic activity. Value >4 µg/mL indicates possible DVT in clients with a moderate DVT risk and a normal compression ultrasound. Value >120 µg/L (plus plasmin-antiplasmin complex >5.25 nmol/L) was predictive of a 2.5 times the average risk of a future MI in males and females >65 years in a study by Cushman et al (1999). Similar findings of more than 2 times the risk for ischemic heart disease when D-dimer is elevated were published in 2004 by Lowe et al and in 2005 by Smith et al.

Usage. Diagnostic criterion for acute thrombosis (including arterial, coronary, and deep vein) and of pulmonary thromboembolism and disseminated intravascular coagulation. Also used to help monitor defibrination therapy, fibrinolysis (primary and secondary), malignancy (ovarian), postoperative fibrinolytic therapy, pregnancy (especially postpartum period), preeclampsia, rheumatoid arthritis (juvenile), sickle cell anemia vasoocclusive crisis, surgery, and unstable angina. May help identify clients at high risk for stroke progression.

Description. An assay used to measure the amount of clot breakdown products specific for cross-linked fragments (D-dimer) derived from fibrin. A positive test indicates that thrombus formation is occurring. The test can be performed on whole blood without the removal or interference of fibrinogen. It does not distinguish lysis of physiologic and pathologic thrombi but distinguishes between fibrinogenolysis and fibrinolysis. The test has a 93% sensitivity for large emboli and a 50% sensitivity for smaller subsegmental emboli. A negative D-dimer test in the presence of a normal compression sound has a negative predictive value of 99%.

Professional Considerations
Consent form NOT required.

Preparation
1. Tube: Blue topped if other coagulation tests are being drawn at the same time.

Procedure
1. Completely fill a blue topped tube.
2. The specimen is stable for 8 hours at room temperature or for 6 months at 20 degrees C.

Postprocedure Care
1. Assess the client for other signs of thrombosis, emboli, or venoocclusive disease.

Client and Family Teaching
1. Results are normally available within 48 hours.

Factors That Affect Results
1. D-Dimer levels increase with increasing levels of tumor marker CA 125 in ovarian cancer, with increasing titers of rheumatoid factors, after electrical cardioversion, and with letrozole therapy in advanced breast cancer.
2. False positive results may occur when rheumatoid factor is present or after surgery or traumatic injury.

Other Data
1. May be of use in venoocclusive disease associated with sequelae of bone marrow transplantation in oncology.
2. A normal D-dimer value excludes pulmonary embolus in 30% of clients.
3. A negative D-dimer result does not rule out the possibility of a pulmonary embolism. False-negative D-dimers are not uncommon for pulmonary emboli.
4. Should be included as follow-up for clients having repaired aortic dissections.

Dehydroepiandrosterone Sulfate (DHEA-S)—Serum and Urine, 24-Hour

Norm.

Serum

Adult female	0.5-2.8 µg/mL
	or 200-800 ng/dL

Continued

		SI Units
Premenopausal	60-340 µg/dL	1.6-8.9 µmol/L
	or 820-3380 ng/mL	
Postmenopausal	<130 µg/dL	
	or 100-610 ng/mL	
Pregnant (term)	230-1170 ng/mL	
Adult male	130-550 µg/dL	3.4-14.4 µmol/L
	or 270-1400 ng/dL	
Prepubertal male	2000-3350 ng/mL	
Newborn	1670-3640 ng/mL	
Child	100-600 ng/dL	
Urine		
Female	0.2-1.8 mg/day	0.7-6.2 µmol/day
Male	0.2-2 mg/day	0.7-6.9 µmol/day

Increased. Acute stress, Addison's disease, adrenal cortex adenoma and carcinoma, Cushing's disease, ectopic ACTH-producing tumors, female acne and hirsutism, hyperthyroidism, oligomenorrhea in female athletes, polycystic ovarian syndrome (increased, but less than 800 µg/dL, less than 20.8 mmol/L SI units), Stein-Leventhal syndrome, and virilizing congenital adrenal hyperplasia.

Decreased. Adrenal insufficiency (primary and secondary), chronic fatigue syndrome, Crohn's disease, diabetes mellitus under poor blood glucose control, low libido, ulcerative colitis. Low levels in amniotic fluid indicate anencephaly in the fetus. Drugs include carbamazepine, dexamethasone, phenytoin.

Description. Dehydroepiandrosterone sulfate (DHEA-S) is the most abundant steroid in the circulation. It arises primarily from the adrenal cortex and is converted to testosterone. Although not androgenic itself, it is a specific and stable marker of adrenal androgen production. Levels are normally elevated in neonates and then decrease considerably until 7 years of age. At puberty, increased levels of DHEA-S from the adrenals result in axillary and pubic hair growth, preceding gonadal androgen secretion.

Professional Considerations
Consent form NOT required.

Preparation
1. *Blood test*: Tube: red topped, red/gray topped, gold topped, or green topped.

2. *Urine test*: Obtain a 3-L, 24-hour urine jug without preservative.

Procedure
1. *Blood test*: Obtain a 4-mL blood sample.
2. *Urine test*:
   a. Discard the first morning-urine specimen.
   b. Save all the urine voided for 24 hours. Include the urine voided at the end of the 24-hour period. For catheterized clients, keep the drainage bag on ice and empty urine into the collection container hourly.

Postprocedure Care
1. Freeze the serum specimen if it is not tested within 1 hour.
2. *Urine*:
   a. Compare the urine quantity in the specimen container with the urinary output record for the test. If the specimen contains less urine than what was recorded as output, some urine may have been discarded, thus invalidating the test.
   b. Document the quantity of urine output for the collection period on the laboratory requisition.
   c. It is best to send the entire specimen to the laboratory so that it can be measured and mixed well before being tested.

Client and Family Teaching
1. Avoid radionuclide scans for 24 hours before this test.
2. Urine: Save all the urine voided in the 24-hour period and urinate before defecating to avoid loss of urine. If any urine

is accidentally discarded, discard the entire specimen and restart the collection the next day.

3. Results are normally available within 24 hours.

Factors That Affect Results

1. Radionuclides administered in the last 24 hours may increase DHEA-S levels.
2. Phenytoin and carbamazepine cause DHEA-S levels to decrease.
3. Medications, including amlodipine and manidipine, improve insulin resistance and increase DHEA and DHEA-S levels.
4. Changes in DHEA-S serum concentrations may occur with antidepressant medication.

Other Data

1. For those who exercise strenuously, such as marathon runners, DHEA-S levels will be elevated at the completion of the exercise period and for up to 36 hours after.
2. Levels decline with age in men and women. Individuals differ in the amount of DHEA-S secreted and, for unknown reasons, DHEA-S levels positively correlate with longevity. Low levels also decrease the development of atherosclerosis.
3. Women with levels >70 mg/dL have successful labor inductions.
4. A significant positive correlation exists between bone mineral density and serum DHEA-S levels in postmenopausal women.

Densitometry

See **Bone Densitometry**—Diagnostic.

Denver Developmental Screening Test (DDST), Denver II—Diagnostic

Norm. Age-appropriate tasks should be demonstrated for each area tested in children between 1 month and 6 years of age.

Usage. The Denver Developmental Screening Test (DDST) tests children in the following areas: gross and fine motor development, language skills, and personal-social skills. Norms for each chronologic age are provided. Although not diagnostic by itself, this frequently used test can identify children (such as those with HIV, hypoxic-ischemic encephalopathy, or blindness) who have global problems or problems in one specific area. This test can also be used to track children over time.

Description. The DDST is a skills test that was revised in 1990 as the Denver II to include 125 items. These easily administered items were picked to prevent any bias against gender, ethnicity, maternal education, or place of residence. Most skills are objectively visualized by the tester, but caregiver verbal reports are adequate to pass some of them.

Professional Considerations
Consent form NOT required.

Preparation

1. Provide a quiet room with all the equipment needed for the test:
   a. Denver Development Screening forms available in pads of 100 sheets from Denver Development Materials.
   b. Denver Development Screening kit, which includes a ball, bell, and other objects needed to perform test.

Procedure

1. Determine the chronologic age of child (see manual for explanation of age adjustment for preterm birth) and draw age line on scoring sheet.
2. Begin testing child with items in approximation but to the left of the age line. This establishes confidence. See manual for directions on repeating test items and giving instructions to child.
3. Continue testing along age line and then to the right of the age line until child fails items in each of the four categories.

Postprocedure Care

1. Explain results to parent or caregiver. Show adult the scoring sheet.

Client and Family Teaching

1. The test usually takes less than 1 hour and helps identify potential developmental problems in the child.
2. A parent or person familiar to the child will be asked to stay with the child during the screening.
3. Results are completely available within 48 hours.

Factors That Affect Results

1. Environmental distractions interfere with validity of the results.

2. Testing by untrained clients. Screening should be performed only by clients who have successfully completed a written and an observational proficiency test.

Other Data

1. The Denver examination is less reliable for children less than 30 months of age and more than $4\frac{1}{2}$ years of age. For younger children, use the Revised Denver Prescreening Developmental Questionnaire (R-PDQ).

11-Deoxycortisol (Compound S, 11-DOC) Test—Diagnostic

Norm. Clients >3 months: 0-0.8 µg/dL.

Usage. Basal levels aid in diagnosis of adrenal carcinoma and congenital adrenal hyperplasia; used to measure response when metyrapone is given to diagnose adrenal insufficiency and Cushing's disease. Low levels found in amyloidosis and posttraumatic stress disorder (PTSD). High levels found in adrenocortical tumors.

Description. Blood test used to determine a specific metabolic block in the synthesis of cortisol. Cortisol is synthesized by two successive hydroxylations of 17-alpha-hydroxyprogesterone. The first results in 11-deoxycortisol, which is then catalyzed by 11-beta-hydroxylase to yield cortisol. This test is used with the metyrapone test to allow diagnosis of primary and secondary adrenal insufficiency. Metyrapone blocks the conversion of 11-deoxycortisol to cortisol, which then stimulates the adrenals to produce more 11-deoxycortisol. A blood level of 11-deoxycortisol that is not elevated after metyrapone administration indicates the presence of adrenal insufficiency.

Professional Considerations

Consent form NOT required.

Preparation

1. Tube: Green topped.

Procedure

1. Obtain a 7-mL blood sample.

Postprocedure Care

1. Deliver the specimen to the laboratory immediately. Separate and freeze the plasma.

Client and Family Teaching

1. Results are normally available within 48 hours.

Factors That Affect Results

1. Results are increased if the client is taking any glucocorticoids, such as hydrocortisone, dexamethasone, or prednisone.

Other Data

1. 11-Deoxycortisol has no glucocorticoid activity.
2. See also Metyrapone test—Serum.

Des-Gamma-Carboxy Prothrombin (DCP)—Serum

Norm. 0.0-7.4 ng/mL.

DCP-positive result indicates that the features of HCC are more aggressive than DCC-negative HCC.

Usage. Detection of hepatocellular carcinoma (HCC) (Fujikawa, Shiraha, Yamamoto, 2009); determination of aggressiveness of HCC; differentiation of HCC from non-malignant hepatic disease. Used in conjunction with alpha-fetoprotein (AFP), des-gamma-carboxy prothrombin can increase the sensitivity and specificity for diagnosing HCC. Less useful than AFP in detecting HCC in early stages. More reliable than AFP for determining the aggressiveness and invasiveness of HCC.

Increased. Hepatocellular carcinoma, vitamin K deficiency. Drugs include

D

Warfarin and any drugs that impair or inhibit vitamin K production.

Description. Des-gamma-carboxy pro-thrombin (DCP) is an abnormally functioning protein produced by the liver when either a deficiency of vitamin K is present, or when the client has an aggressive form of hepatocellular carcinoma. This enzyme-linked immunoassay test may or may not be used in conjunction with tissue testing for DCP.

Professional Considerations
Consent form NOT required.

Preparation
1. Tube: Red topped or serum separator tube.

Procedure
1. Collect a 3-mL blood sample.

Postprocedure Care
1. Allow blood sample to clot for 30 minutes before centrifuging.
2. Store sample at 2-8 degrees centigrade for up to 1 week until testing.

Client and Family Teaching
1. Tissue samples may also be tested. When DCP is also present in HCC cancer tissue, a poorer prognosis is expected.

Factors That Affect Results
1. Decreasing levels of DCP are seen when treatment for hepatocellular carcinoma is effective.

Other Data
1. Specificity is 91% for hepatocellular carcinoma.

Desipramine

See **Tricyclic Antidepressants**—Plasma or Serum.

DEXA

See **Bone Densitometry**—Diagnostic.

Dexamethasone Suppression Test—Diagnostic

Norm. 24-hour urine values should be <50% baseline values.

Plasma cortisol	<5 μg/dL
Urine-free cortisol	<25 μg/24 hours
Urine for 17-OHCS	4 μg/24 hours

Positive. High levels of serum cortisol and 17-OHCS are present after dexamethasone is administered. Occurs in adrenal hyperplasia, adrenal incidentalomas, adrenal tumors, aldosteronism (primary), bulimia nervosa, chronic fatigue syndrome, chronic renal failure, Cushing's disease, depression, oat cell cancer of the lung, and schizophrenics with suicide attempts.

Description. Screening test for Cushing's disease and for depression. The test can be performed after administration of a low or high dose of dexamethasone or as an overnight test with a morning blood draw.

Dexamethasone is a potent synthetic glucocorticoid that is used to test the integrity of the hypothalamic-pituitary-adrenal axis. When given to normal clients, it decreases the production of cortisol and other adrenal steroids through the usual feedback systems. In clients with Cushing's disease or depression, there is no suppression of ACTH. The low test dose is for screening. If results are positive, a high-dose test is given to determine the cause of Cushing's disease. If there is suppression with the high-dose test, it indicates a pituitary origin of the excess cortisol. If there is no suppression, it indicates an adrenal or ectopic tumor.

Professional Considerations
Consent form NOT required.

Preparation
1. Obtain a 3-L plastic container.
2. Tube: Green topped, red topped, red/gray topped, or gold topped.

3. Baseline values for plasma cortisol, urine-free cortisol, and urine 17-OHCS should be known.

Procedure

1. Obtain a 5-mL blood sample for plasma cortisol level.
2. Overnight test consists of administering 1 mg of dexamethasone orally at 1100 (11 AM) followed by venipuncture for cortisol level the next day at 0800 (8 AM).
3. The low-dose test includes a baseline measurement of urine-free cortisol or 17-OHCS followed by oral dexamethasone 0.5 mg every 6 hours for 2 days followed by a 24-hour urine for free cortisol or 17-OHCS collected on day 2.
4. The high-dose test includes a baseline measure of urine-free cortisol or 17-OHCS followed by oral dexamethasone 2 mg every 6 hours for 2 days followed by a 24-hour urine for urine-free cortisol or 17-OHCS collected on day 2.

Postprocedure Care

1. Send the blood sample to the laboratory within 30 minutes for serum separation and freezing.

Client and Family Teaching

1. Oral dexamethasone will be given at a specific time the evening before the blood sampling. The blood and urine samples will be collected at specific times the next day.
2. *Urine*: Save all the urine voided in the 24-hour period and urinate before defecating to avoid loss of urine. If any urine is accidentally discarded, notify the physician immediately because the test results will be invalid.

Factors That Affect Results

1. Failure to ingest oral dexamethasone or a radioactive scan performed within the previous 24 hours will elevate the results. For depressed clients, methylene blue is added to the dexamethasone tablets, and urinary excretion of the dye is monitored to indicate that the drug was ingested.
2. False-positive results occur with acute illnesses, alcoholism, anorexia nervosa, dehydration, preclinical Cushing's syndrome (PCS), severe depression, diabetes (unstable), electroconvulsive therapy after treatment day 1, fever, high stress, malnutrition, nausea, obesity, pregnancy, and temporal lobe disease. Drugs include aspirin (drug overdose), barbiturates, carbamazepine, estrogens, glutethimide, meprobamate methaqualone, methyprylon, oral contraceptives, phenytoin, reserpine, rifampin, spironolactone, stilbestrol, and tetracycline.
3. False-negative results occur with Addison's disease, hypopituitarism, and in clients who metabolize dexamethasone at an abnormally slow rate. Drugs include benzodiazepines (high dose), corticosteroids, and cyproheptadine.
4. Using 1 mg of dexamethasone results in lower sensitivity in Japanese and Asian people with major depressive episodes when compared to Caucasians. Low-dose 0.5 mg DST is better in Japanese and Asian clients.

Other Data

1. Levels in some clients with Cushing's disease may be suppressed by 50%, but these clients can be identified by the metyrapone test.
2. As a screening test for depression, it is 90% specific and 45% sensitive.
3. Female survivors of sexual abuse have significantly suppressed plasma cortisol in response to dexamethasone.
4. See also Metyrapone test—Serum.

DHEA

See **Dehydroepiandrosterone Sulfate**—Serum and Urine, 24-Hour.

Dialyzable Calcium

See **Calcium, Ionized**—Blood.

Diascan

See **Glucose Monitoring Machines**—Diagnostic.

Diazepam—Serum

Norm. Negative.

		SI Units
Diazepam		
Therapeutic range	0.2-1.0 µg/mL	0.70-3.51 µmol/L
Panic level	>5.0 µg/mL	>17.55 µmol/L
Lethal level	720 µg/mL	
Nordiazepam		
Therapeutic range	0.06-1.80 µg/mL	
Toxic level	>2.50 µg/mL	

Panic Level Symptoms and Treatment

Symptoms. Ataxia, cyanosis, coma, convulsions, diminished reflexes, mental confusion, respiratory depression, somnolence, slurred speech, vertigo.

Treatment

NOTE: Treatment choice(s) depend(s) on client's history and condition and episode history.

1. Gastric lavage is not recommended, but should be considered if within 1 hour of ingestion and if ingestion of additional lethal substance is suspected. Use warm tap water or 0.9% saline.
2. Administer activated charcoal if within 4 hours of ingestion or if symptoms are present. Repeat as necessary, because benzodiazepines undergo hepatic recirculation.
3. Monitor for central nervous system depression.
4. Protect airway. Support breathing with oxygen and mechanical ventilation, if necessary.
5. Flumazenil is not recommended for routine use in benzodiazepine overdose. Flumazenil has been used as a competitive antagonist to reverse the profound effects of benzodiazepine overdose. Use of flumazenil is contraindicated if concomitant tricyclic antidepressants were taken or in dependence states because of the risk of causing seizures from lowering the seizure threshold and because it may precipitate symptoms of benzodiazepine withdrawal.
6. Flumazenil may not completely reverse benzodiazepine effects. Close monitoring for re-sedation is required and repeated doses may be needed.
7. Do NOT use barbiturates.
8. Do NOT induce emesis.
9. Forced diuresis or hemodialysis will NOT remove benzodiazepines to any significant extent. No information was found on whether peritoneal dialysis will remove these drugs.

Increased. Drug abuse, overdose, and suicide.

Description. Diazepam is a benzodiazepine derivative that acts on the limbic and subcortical levels of the central nervous system, producing sedation, skeletal muscle relaxation, and anticonvulsant effects. Absorbed from the gastrointestinal tract, metabolized by the liver, and excreted in the urine and stool, peak plasma concentration is 1-2 hours, half-life is 21-46 hours, and steady-state levels occur in 5-10 days.

Professional Considerations

Consent form NOT required unless sample is being collected as legal evidence.

Preparation

1. Tube: Red topped, red/gray topped, or gold topped.
2. MAY be drawn during hemodialysis.

Procedure

1. Have the specimen collection witnessed if being collected for legal evidence.
2. Obtain a 5-mL blood sample.

3. For a therapeutic dose evaluation, draw the sample 2 hours after oral ingestion of diazepam.

Postprocedure Care

1. For specimens collected for legal evidence, write the client's name, date, exact time of collection, and specimen source on the lab requisition. Sign and have the witness sign the lab requisition.
2. Transport the specimen to the laboratory immediately in a sealed plastic bag marked as legal evidence. All persons handling the specimen should sign and mark the time of receipt on the laboratory requisition.
3. Observe for side effects of ataxia, drowsiness, lethargy, nausea, nystagmus, tinnitus, and vertigo, which often subside after continued therapy.

Client and Family Teaching

1. Discuss the need for psychologic intervention with the family and the client if panic or lethal doses have been determined. Refer for crisis intervention for intentional overdose.

2. Referrals to appropriate rehabilitation centers and therapeutic community programs should be offered to all addicted clients who may be interested.
3. Expect intensive care unit placement for severe overdose.
4. Death is rare in overdose when diazepam is taken alone.

Factors That Affect Results

1. Naltrexone (opiate antagonist) delays the peak level of diazepam by 1 hour.
2. Proton pump inhibitor (PPI) medications have metabolic interactions with diazepam.

Other Data

1. Heavier sedation occurs in persons with liver disease.
2. Long-term use may deplete the body of trace elements: zinc, iron, and copper.
3. Lorazepam is the first-line therapy in preference to diazepam in adults with convulsive status epilepticus.
4. See also Benzodiazepines—Plasma and urine.

Diethylpropion

See Amphetamines—Blood.

Differential Leukocyte Count (Diff)—Peripheral Blood

Norm.

		SI Units
White Blood Cells (WBCs)		
Adult Females	4500-11,000/μL	4.5-11.0 × 10⁹/L
Pregnant		
Trimester 1	6600-14,000/μL	6.6-14.1 × 10⁹/L
Trimester 2	6900-17,100/μL	6.9-17.1 × 10⁹/L
Trimester 3	5900-14,700/μL	5.9-14.7 × 10⁹/L
Postpartum	9700-25,700/μL	9.7-25.7 × 10⁹/L
Adult Males	4500-11,000/μL	4.5-11.0 × 10⁹/L
Children		
Newborn	9000-30,000/μL	9.0-30.0 × 10⁹/L
3 months	5700-18,000/μL	5.7-18.0 × 10⁹/L
1 year	6000-17,500/μL	6.0-17.5 × 10⁹/L
3 years	5700-16,300/μL	5.7-16.3 × 10⁹/L
10 years	4500-13,500/μL	4.5-13.5 × 10⁹/L

		SI Units

Differential White Blood Cells Granulocytes

Segmented Neutrophils (Segs) | 40%-75% | 0.40-0.75
Adults | 3800/μL | 3800 × 10⁶/L
Children | |
Birth | 8400/μL | 8400 × 10⁶/L
12 hours | 12,100/μL | 12,100 × 10⁶/L
24 hours | 8870/μL | 8870 × 10⁶/L
1 week | 4100/μL | 4100 × 10⁶/L
2 weeks | 3320/μL | 3320 × 10⁶/L
1-2 months | 2750/μL | 2750 × 10⁶/L
4 months | 2730/μL | 2730 × 10⁶/L
6 months | 2710/μL | 2710 × 10⁶/L
8 months | 2680/μL | 2680 × 10⁶/L
10 months | 2600/μL | 2600 × 10⁶/L
12 months | 2680/μL | 2680 × 10⁶/L
2 years | 2660/μL | 2660 × 10⁶/L
4 years | 3040/μL | 3040 × 10⁶/L
6 years | 3600/μL | 3600 × 10⁶/L
8-14 years | 3700/μL | 3700 × 10⁶/L
16-20 years | 3800/μL | 3800 × 10⁶/L

Band Neutrophils (Bands) | |
Proportion | 0%-10% | 0.00-0.10
Adults | 620/μL | 620 × 10⁶/L
Children | |
Birth | 2540/μL | 2540 × 10⁶/L
12 hours | 3460/μL | 3460 × 10⁶/L
24 hours | 2680/μL | 2680 × 10⁶/L
1 week | 1420/μL | 1420 × 10⁶/L
2 weeks | 1200/μL | 1200 × 10⁶/L
1 month | 1150/μL | 1150 × 10⁶/L
2 months | 1100/μL | 1100 × 10⁶/L
4-10 months | 1000/μL | 1000 × 10⁶/L
12 months | 990/μL | 990 × 10⁶/L
2 years | 850/μL | 850 × 10⁶/L
4 years | 710/μL | 710 × 10⁶/L
6 years | 670/μL | 670 × 10⁶/L
8 years | 660/μL | 660 × 10⁶/L
10 years | 645/μL | 645 × 10⁶/L
12-14 years | 640/μL | 640 × 10⁶/L
16-20 years | 620/μL | 620 × 10⁶/L

Eosinophils (Eos) | |
Proportion | 0%-5% | 0.00-0.05
Adults | 200/μL | 200 × 10⁶/L
Children | |
Birth | 400/μL | 400 × 10⁶/L
12-24 hours | 450/μL | 450 × 10⁶/L
1 week | 500/μL | 500 × 10⁶/L
2 weeks | 350/μL | 350 × 10⁶/L
1 month-1 year | 300/μL | 300 × 10⁶/L
2 years | 80/μL | 280 × 10⁶/L
4 years | 250/μL | 250 × 10⁶/L
6 years | 230/μL | 230 × 10⁶/L
8-20 years | 200/μL | 200 × 10⁶/L

Continued

		SI Units
Basophils (Basos)		
Proportion	0%-1%	0-0.01
Adults	40/μL	40×10^6/L
Children		
Birth-24 hours	100/μL	100×10^6/L
1 week-8 years	50/μL	50×10^6/L
10-20 years	40/μL	40×10^6/L
Monocytes (Monos)		
Proportion	2%-14%	0.02%-0.14%
Adults	300/μL	300×10^6/L
Children		
Birth	1050/μL	1050×10^6/L
12 hours	1200/μL	1200×10^6/L
24 hours-1 week	1100/μL	1100×10^6/L
2 weeks	1000/μL	1000×10^6/L
1 month	700/μL	700×10^6/L
2 months	650/μL	650×10^6/L
4 months	600/μL	600×10^6/L
6-8 months	580/μL	580×10^6/L
10-12 months	550/μL	550×10^6/L
2 years	530/μL	530×10^6/L
4 years	450/μL	450×10^6/L
6 years	400/μL	400×10^6/L
8-12 years	350/μL	350×10^6/L
14 years	380/μL	380×10^6/L
16-18 years	400/μL	400×10^6/L
20 years	380/μL	380×10^6/L
Lymphocytes (Lymphs)		
Proportion	25%-40%	0.25-0.40
Adults	2500/μL	2500×10^6/L
Children		
Birth-12 hours	5500/μL	5500×10^6/L
24 hours	5800/μL	5800×10^6/L
1 week	5000/μL	5000×10^6/L
2 weeks	5500/μL	5500×10^6/L
1 month	6000/μL	6000×10^6/L
2 months	6300/μL	6300×10^6/L
4 months	6800/μL	6800×10^6/L
6 months	7300/μL	7300×10^6/L
8 months	7600/μL	7600×10^6/L
10 months	7500/μL	7500×10^6/L
12 months	7000/μL	7000×10^6/L
2 years	6300/μL	6300×10^6/L
4 years	4500/μL	4500×10^6/L
6 years	3500/μL	3500×10^6/L
8 years	3300/μL	3300×10^6/L
10 years	3100/μL	3100×10^6/L
12 years	3000/μL	3000×10^6/L
14 years	2900/μL	2900×10^6/L
16 years	2800/μL	2800×10^6/L
18 years	2700/μL	2700×10^6/L
20 years	2500/μL	2500×10^6/L

Increased White Blood Cell Count. Abscess, actinomycosis, amebiasis, Andersen's disease, anemia (acquired hemolytic), anorexia, anoxia, anthrax, appendicitis, bacterial infections, blastomycosis, bronchitis, burns, chickenpox, cholecystitis (acute), choledocholithiasis, cholera, cirrhosis (with necrosis), colon cancer, convulsive seizures, Crohn's disease, croup, Cushing's syndrome, cytomegalovirus, dengue fever, diphtheria, dissecting aortic aneurysm, diverticulitis, diverticulosis, dysproteinemia, eclampsia, electrical injury, emotional stress, empyema (acute subdural), endocarditis, Epstein-Barr virus, erythroblastosis fetalis, exercise, exposure to ultraviolet radiation, fascioliasis, fatty liver, fever of undetermined origin, G6PD deficiency, gangrene, glomerulonephritis (poststreptococcal), gout (acute), halothane toxicity, heart transplant rejection, hemorrhage, hepatitis (alcoholic), hepatoma, hookworm, Hodgkin's disease, idiopathic myelofibrosis, infection (bacterial, parasitic), infectious mononucleosis, intestinal obstruction, ketoacidosis, lactic acidosis, legionnaires' disease, leukemia, leukocytosis, lymphoma, meningitis, menstruation, myocardial infarction, myocarditis, pancreatitis, paroxysmal tachycardia, peritonitis, pneumomediastinum, pneumonia, poisoning (arthropods, chemicals, metals, venom), polycythemia vera, postoperative surgical stress, pregnancy, preleukemia, pylephlebitis, rat-bite fever, red blood cell hemolysis, retroperitoneal fibrosis, rheumatic fever, rubeola, sepsis, shock, smallpox, stress, strongyloidiasis, suppurative cholangitis, systemic lupus erythematosus, tonsillitis, toxic shock syndrome, transfusion reaction, trauma, trichuriasis, tuberculosis, tularemia, tumor necrosis, ulcers, ultraviolet radiation, uremia, yellow fever, visceral larva migrans, Wegener's granulomatosis, and Weil's disease. Drugs include allopurinol, anesthetics, atropine sulfate, barbiturates, diethylcarbamazine, epinephrine bitartrate, epinephrine borate, epinephrine hydrochloride, erythromycin, steroids, streptomycin sulfate, and sulfonamides. Herbs or natural remedies that increase granulocyte colony-stimulating factor (GCSF) include Japanese *sho-saiko-to* (TJ-9, *xiao chaihu tang*, Minor *Bupleurum* Combination), and those that increase lymphocyte counts include *Viscum album* (European mistletoe; Plenosol, viscumin and viscotoxin) and *Echinacea purpurea* (purple coneflower; echinacin).

Increased Neutrophils. Acute infections, allergies, anemia, anoxia, anxiety, appendicitis, asthma, burns, cancer, chickenpox, cholecystitis, cholera, colitis, Cushing's syndrome, dermatitis, diabetic acidosis, Di Guglielmo's disease, diphtheria, diverticulitis, diverticulosis, eclampsia, electroconvulsive therapy treatment, emphysema, empyema, endocarditis, fear, G6PD deficiency, gangrene, gout, hemorrhage, inflammation, ketoacidosis, labor and delivery, leukemia, leukocytosis, lymphoma, meningitis (purulent), myocardial infarction, osteomyelitis, otitis media, pancreatitis, panic, peritonitis, pernicious anemia, pneumonia, poisoning (carbon monoxide, lead, mercury, arsenic, turpentine), polycythemia vera, postoperative surgical stress, pulmonary infarction, pyelonephritis, pyemia, rheumatic fever, rheumatoid arthritis, salpingitis, scarlet fever, septicemia, smallpox, smoking, thyroiditis, tonsillitis, transfusion reaction, typhus, and uremia. Drugs include acetylcholine, benzene, blood stored for more than 2 days at room temperature, carbon monoxide, casein, chlorpropamide, corticosteroids, corticotropin, digitalis, epinephrine, ethylene glycol, heparin, histamine, insect venoms, lead, lithium, mercury, potassium chloride, and turpentine.

Increased Bands. Pharyngitis.

Increased Segs. Pernicious anemia.

Increased Eosinophils. Addison's disease, allergies, asthma, atheroembolic renal disease, brucellosis, cancer (bone, brain, ovary, testes), chorea, coccidioidomycosis, dermatitis, diverticulitis, diverticulosis, eczema, gangrene, hay fever, Hodgkin's disease, leprosy, leukemia (chronic granulocytic), leukocytosis, Löffler's syndrome, malaria, metastatic carcinoma, parasitic infections, pemphigus, pernicious anemia, phlebitis, polycythemia vera, pruritus caused by jaundice, psoriasis, radiation therapy, rheumatoid arthritis, rhinitis, sarcoidosis, scarlet fever, sickle cell anemia, Sjögren's syndrome, splenectomy, thrombophlebitis, tuberculosis, and ulcerative colitis. Drugs include allopurinol, antibiotics (associated with allergic reactions), aminosalicylic acid, anticonvulsants, blood stored for more than 2 days at room temperature, cephalosporins, chlorpropamide, digitalis, heparin, imipramine, methotrexate, nitrofurantoin, penicillin, phenothiazine, procainamide, procarbazine, propranolol, quinidine, streptomycin, sulfonamides, and tetracycline.

Increased Basophils. Allergic reaction to foods/drugs/inhalants, chickenpox, chronic myelogenous erythroderma, Heinz body anemia, Hodgkin's disease, hypothyroidism, irradiation, leukemia, leukocytosis, myelofibrosis, myxedema, nephrosis, periarteritis nodosa, polycythemia vera, serum sickness, sinusitis, smallpox, splenectomy, ulcerative colitis, and urticaria. Drugs include antithyroids, desipramine, and estrogens.

Increased Lymphocytes. Brucellosis, cytomegalovirus, diverticulitis, diverticulosis, endocarditis, hepatitis, Hurler's syndrome, infectious mononucleosis, leukocytosis, lymphocytic leukemia, pertussis, syphilis, toxoplasmosis, and xerostomia. Drugs include aspirin, blood stored for more than 2 days at room temperature, carbon disulfate poisoning, haloperidol, lead intoxication, levodopa, phenytoin, and tetrahydrochloride poisoning.

Increased Monocytes. Brucellosis, carbon disulfide poisoning, Epstein-Barr virus, Hodgkin's disease, leukemia (AML, CML), leukocytosis, multiple myeloma, phosphorus poisoning, rheumatoid arthritis, salmonellosis, sarcoidosis, syphilis, systemic lupus erythematosus, tetrahydrochloride poisoning, tuberculosis, and ulcerative colitis. Drugs include haloperidol and methsuximide.

Decreased White Blood Cell Count. Agranulocytosis, acquired immune deficiency syndrome (AIDS), alcoholism, amyloidosis, anaphylactic shock, anemia (aplastic, pernicious), anorexia nervosa, anthrax, arsenic poisoning, brucellosis, cachexia, chemical toxicity, chemotherapy, cirrhosis, Colorado tick fever, dengue fever, disseminated lupus erythematosus, Felty's syndrome, Gaucher disease, heavy chain disease, hepatitis (infectious, viral), Hodgkin's disease, hypersplenism, hypothermia, idiopathic myelofibrosis, infection (severe bacterial, viral), influenza, legionnaires' disease, leishmaniasis, leukemia (some forms), leukopenia, lymphoma, measles, mononucleosis, myxedema,

paratyphoid fever, pharyngitis, *Pneumocystis* pneumonia, preleukemia, protein therapy, psittacosis, Q fever, radiation therapy, renal trauma, rheumatic fever, rubella, sepsis neonatorum, shock, Sjögren's syndrome, stiffman syndrome, stomatitis, strongyloidiasis, toxoplasmosis, tuberculosis, tularemia, and typhoid fever. Drugs include acetaminophen, aminoglutethimide, aminopyrine, antibiotics, antineoplastics, antithyroids, arsenicals, aurothioglucose, bismuth, chloramphenicol, chloroquine phosphate, diazepam, diethylcarbamazine, ethotoin, furosemide, immunosuppressives, meprobamate, methyldopa, methyldopate hydrochloride, methsuximide, phenothiazines, phenylbutazone, phenytoin, phenytoin sodium, primidone, procainamide hydrochloride, quinacrine hydrochloride, quinine sulfate, sulfonamides, and vitamin A.

Decreased Neutrophils. Acromegaly, Addison's disease, agranulocytosis, anaphylactic shock, anorexia nervosa, aplastic anemia, brucellosis, cachexia, carcinoma, Chédiak-Higashi syndrome, chemotherapy, cirrhosis, Colorado tick fever, dengue fever, Felty's syndrome, folic acid deficiency, Gaucher disease, hypersplenism, hypopituitarism, hypothyroidism, infections, infectious hepatitis, infectious mononucleosis, influenza, iron deficiency anemia, kala-azar, malaria, measles, mumps, myelofibrosis, myeloma, paratyphoid fever, paroxysmal nocturnal hemoglobinuria, pernicious anemia, pneumonia, psittacosis, radiation therapy, Rocky Mountain spotted fever, rubella, rubeola, sarcoma, septicemia, thyrotoxicosis, tularemia, typhoid fever, vitamin B_{12} deficiency, and yellow fever. Drugs include alcohol, aminophylline, aminopyrine, ampicillin, antipyrine, arsenic, aspirin, barbiturates, carbimazole, cephalothin, chemotherapeutic agents, chloramphenicol, chlorpromazine, chlorpropamide, cinchophen, DDT, diazepam, dinitrophenol, diuretics, electroconvulsive therapy treatment, gold salts, imipramine, indomethacin, isoniazid, mephenytoin, 6-mercaptopurine, methaphenolene hydrochloride, methicillin, *p*-aminobenzoic acid, penicillin, phenacetin, phenylbutazone, phenylhydrazine, phenytoin, procainamide, quinine, rauwolfia, streptomycin, sulfonamides, tolbutamide, tripelennamine hydrochloride, and urethan.

Decreased Eosinophils. Acromegaly, anemia (aplastic), coccidioidomycosis, congestive heart failure, Cushing's syndrome, disseminated lupus erythematosus, eclampsia, fascioliasis, Goodpasture's syndrome, hypersplenism, infections, infectious mononucleosis, schistosomiasis, and stress. Drugs include adrenocorticotropic hormone, corticotropin, epinephrine, glucocorticoids, methysergide, niacin, niacinamide, procainamide, and thyroxine.

Decreased Basophils. Acute infection, anaphylaxis, Cushing's syndrome, hyperthyroidism, ovulation, pregnancy, radiation therapy, thyrotoxicosis, and stress. Drugs include chemotherapy, corticosteroids, corticotropin, procainamide, and thiotepa.

Decreased Lymphocytes. Aplastic anemia, Cushing's syndrome, Hodgkin's disease, immunoglobulin deficiencies, leukemia (chronic granulocytic, monocytic), lymphosarcoma, renal failure, systemic lupus erythematosus, thymic hypoplasia in children, and uremia. Drugs include asparaginase, chlorambucil, cortisone, epinephrine, glucocorticoids, lithium compounds, mechlorethamine, niacin, nitrogen mustard, and radiation therapy to the lymphatics.

Decreased Monocytes. Aplastic anemia and hairy-cell leukemia. Drugs include blood stored for more than 2 days at room temperature.

Description. The differential white blood cell count (Diff) provides an assessment of each leukocyte distribution on two stained glass slides of peripheral blood. One hundred white blood cells are identified and then classified (differentiated) according to their morphology. A relative percentage of each type of cell is then determined and reported. White blood cells (leukocytes) function in the body's immune defense system. Three main types of white blood cells exist: granulocytes, monocytes, and lymphocytes; they are identified and counted by microscopic examination of stained blood films. Granulocytes, manufactured by bone marrow, are subdivided into neutrophils, eosinophils, and basophils and function in bacterial phagocytosis. Neutrophils are further subclassified as either segmented or band neutrophils. Segmented neutrophils (Segs) are more mature and have two to five lobes, which increase (shift to the right) during pathologic conditions. Band neutrophils (Bands) are less mature and increase in number (shift to the left) during conditions causing increased white blood cell (WBC) production. Eosinophils are leukocytes that contain course round granules. Eosinophils become active in the later stages of inflammation. These cells act as phagocytes and are active in allergic reactions and parasitic infections. Eosinophils are under the influence of the adrenal cortex. Monocytes are manufactured by bone marrow and function both in antigen recognition and in phagocytosis of cellular debris. Lymphocytes formed by the lymphatic system function in humoral and cell-mediated immune responses to foreign antigens.

Professional Considerations
Consent form NOT required.

Preparation
1. Tube: Lavender topped glass or lavender sealed plastic.
2. Screen client for the use of herbal preparations or natural remedies such as Japanese *sho-saiko-to* (TJ-9, *xiao chaihu tang*, Minor *Bupleurum* Combination); those that increase lymphocyte counts include *Viscum album* (European mistletoe; Plenosol, viscumin, and viscotoxin) and *Echinacea purpurea* (purple coneflower, echinacin).

Procedure
1. Draw a 3.5-mL blood sample.
2. Do not leave tourniquet in place longer than 60 seconds.

Postprocedure Care
1. Apply pressure at the site of the venipuncture because bleeding may occur because of disease entity.
2. Record the collection time because counts vary according to time of day.

Client and Family Teaching
1. Results are normally available within 24 hours.

Factors That Affect Results
1. In leukemia, cryofibrinogenemia, and cryoglobulinemia, WBC results performed on an electronic cell counter are unreliable. The counts must be performed manually.

2. The most accurate leukocyte counts are obtained from capillary punctures. For EDTA-anticoagulated blood (lavender topped tube), the most accurate counts are obtained within 4 hours of specimen collection.

3. The serum sample is stable at room temperature for 10 hours and refrigerated for 18 hours and should not be frozen.

4. Leukocyte differential relative values reported as percentages should be converted to absolute values by multiplication of the percentage by the total WBC count before interpretation.

Other Data

1. "Shift to the left" means that there are an increased number of immature neutrophils in the peripheral blood. Neutrophils are usually illustrated from left (young cells) to right (mature cells) in the differential. A low total WBC count with a left shift indicates a recovery from bone marrow depression or an infection of such intensity that the demand for neutrophils in the tissue is greater than the capacity of the bone marrow to release them in the circulation. A high total WBC count with a left shift indicates an increased release of neutrophils by the bone marrow in response to an overwhelming infection or inflammation.

2. "Shift to the right" means cells have more than the usual number of nuclear segments. This is found in liver disease, Down syndrome, or megaloblastic and pernicious anemia.

3. The eosinophil count may be used with the Thorn test to evaluate adrenocortical stimulation.

4. An automated WBC count may not reveal the "shifts."

5. Differential leukocyte counts do not differ in clients with or without chronic graft-versus-host disease after allogeneic bone marrow transplant.

Diffusing Capacity for Carbon Monoxide (DL$_{CO}$, Transfer Factor)—Diagnostic

Norm. The predicted values are based on prediction equations calculated according to gender, age, height, weight, and hemoglobin level. Results are considered abnormal if they are less than 80% of the predicted values. The average normal for resting subjects by the single-breath and steady-state methods is 25 mL/min/mm Hg.

Usage. Identify and monitor the course of parenchymal lung disease processes and pulmonary hypertension in scleroderma; monitor for pulmonary drug toxicity; distinguish chronic bronchitis (normal DL$_{CO}$) from emphysema (low DL$_{CO}$); distinguish interstitial fibrosis from pleural fibrosis.

Increased. Alveolar hemorrhage, asthma, polycythemia. Diseases or conditions associated with increased pulmonary blood flow such as left-to-right shunts, tachycardia, and exercise. Medications include inhaled budesonide corticosteroid.

Decreased. Acute myocardial infarction, alveolar fibrosis (associated with sarcoidosis, asbestosis, berylliosis, ex-smokers with asthma and COPD, pneumoconiosis in coal miners, idiopathic pulmonary fibrosis, O$_2$ toxicity, or silicosis), asbestosis, bone marrow transplant following total body irradiation, bronchiolitis obliterans with organizing pneumonia, diseases associated with anemia (such as chronic renal failure), histiocytosis X, lung resection, metal fume fever, mitral stenosis, mixed connective tissue diseases (dermatomyositis, inflammatory bowel disease, polymyositis, rheumatoid arthritis, Wegener's granulomatosis), obstructive lung diseases (emphysema, cystic fibrosis), parenchymal loss or replacement, pneumonia, posture of upright position, primary pulmonary hypertension, pulmonary edema, pulmonary emboli, restrictive lung disease, space-occupying lesions, systemic disease with pulmonary involvement (progressive systemic sclerosis, scleroderma, systemic lupus erythematosus). Drugs include amiodarone and bleomycin affecting the alveolocapillary membrane, marijuana smoking, acute and chronic ethyl alcohol ingestion, freebasing cocaine, cigarette smoking.

Description. Carbon monoxide (CO) is a gas that is readily taken from the alveolus and bound to hemoglobin (Hb) in pulmonary capillary blood. The diffusing capacity rate of the lung provides a measure of the lung's gas-exchange mechanism. It assesses the amount of functioning pulmonary capillary bed in contact with functioning alveoli. Therefore it can provide useful information on gas-exchange properties of the lung. Thus transport or flow or uptake of carbon monoxide is a unique way to noninvasively determine the ability of the alveolar capillary membrane to transport oxygen into the blood. It is reported in cubic centimeters (of CO) per minute per millimeters of Hg or millimoles (of CO) per minute per kilopascals at 0 degrees C, 760 mm Hg, dry (i.e., STPD). There are several methods for determining the DL$_{CO}$. The two most commonly used in the clinical setting are the steady-state technique and the single-breath technique.

Comparison of Steady-State and Single-Breath Methods for Determination of DL$_{CO}$

Steady State	Single Breath
Generally easier for the subject to perform because no special breathing maneuvers are required.	Far less susceptible to development of CO back-pressure and to effects of V/Q abnormalities.
Adaptable to use during exercise and other applications where breath holding is not feasible.	Tends to be more reproducible. Generally yields higher values (than steady-state methods) in a given subject.

Professional Considerations
Consent form NOT required.

Preparation
1. Assess medication record for recent analgesic that may depress respiratory function.
2. Bronchodilators and intermittent positive-pressure breathing therapy may be withheld before the tests.
3. The client should wear loose-fitting and comfortable clothing the day of the test.
4. Document the client's age, gender, height, and weight on the test requisition.
5. Dentures should not be removed.
6. See Client and Family Teaching.

Procedure
1. The equipment used for this test consists of a sample pump and bag, a calibrated spirometer of test gas, and both a helium analyzer and a carbon monoxide analyzer.
2. The client is positioned sitting upright with feet on the floor.
3. A nose clip is applied to ensure consistent air flow through the mouth.
4. *Single-breath maneuver:*
   a. The client exhales completely, rapidly inhales from the spirometer to reach maximum capacity, and then holds his or her breath for 10 seconds.
   b. Upon exhalation, 0.5-1.0 liter of exhaled air is collected and analyzed for helium and carbon monoxide.
   c. The test is repeated after 4 minutes.
   d. Note: Variations of this test have been published, with a second method measuring DL$_{CO}$ on inhalation, breath holding, and exhalation. A third method is designed for clients who cannot hold their breath for 10 seconds or achieve an adequate flow rate and is based on a slow, submaximal breath and requires different equipment.
5. *Steady-state method:*
   a. The client is instructed to breathe in and out through the mouthpiece while exercise is done or other maneuvers are carried out; measurements are taken.

Postprocedure Care
1. Resume all medications including bronchodilators and intermittent positive-pressure breathing therapy.
2. Test results are normally available within 30 minutes.

Client and Family Teaching
1. Teach proper breathing technique for the test.
2. The procedure takes approximately 20 minutes.

3. Refrain from smoking or eating a heavy meal for 3-4 hours before the test.
4. Refrain from drinking alcohol for 24 hours before the test.

Factors That Affect Results

1. Reasonable airway mechanics, lung volumes, and client cooperation are required for accurate measurements.
2. An inadequate seal around the mouthpiece invalidates the results.
3. A supine body position increases DL_{CO}.
4. Exercise increases diffusing capacity.
5. Gastric distention, hypoxia, narcotics, sedatives, and pregnancy may alter the results.
6. Bronchodilators administered before the tests may obscure true pulmonary function.
7. Results are adjusted for high or low hemoglobin (Hb) levels using the following equation:

$$\text{Corrected } DL_{CO} = \text{Actual } DL_{CO} \times 10.2 + \text{Observed Hb (g/dL)}/1.7 + \text{Observed Hb (g/dL)}$$

8. Single-breath method results are invalidated and reported with anecdotal notation for any of the following reasons:
   a. Inspired vital capacity (VC) <90% of highest historical VC.
   b. Client is unable to hold breath at least 9 seconds or holds longer than 11 seconds.
   c. Client inspires too slowly (such as longer than 2.5-4 seconds).
9. Females have lower diffusing capacity for carbon monoxide relative to body size.

Other Data

1. Diffusion capacity for carbon monoxide is routinely performed in a pulmonary function laboratory.
2. Proper interpretation of results needs to account for inherent assumptions regarding CO distribution and timing procedures.
3. The abbreviation for the single-breath method is $DL_{CO}{}^{SB}$.
4. A DL_{CO} value of at least 70% predicts low post-pneumonectomy complications.
5. Decreasing DL_{CO} is an excellent predictor of subsequent development of isolated PHT as a late stage complication in limited cutaneous scleroderma.

Diffusion-Weighted Imaging

See **Magnetic Resonance Imaging**—Diagnostic.

Digital Mammography

See **Mammography**—Diagnostic.

Digital Subtraction Angiography (DSA) and Transvenous Digital Subtraction—Diagnostic

Norm. Normal carotid arteries, vertebral arteries, abdominal aorta and branches, renal arteries, and peripheral vessels.

Usage. Aneurysms, aortic valvular stenosis, arterial occlusion, bypass surgery (postoperative), carotid stenosis, dural sinus thrombosis, hepatocellular carcinoma, jugular tumors, nutcracker renal phenomenon, pheochromocytoma, pulmonary emboli, thoracic outlet syndrome, and ulcerative plaques.

Description. A noninvasive computer imaging procedure that allows examination of the arteries in the body after an IV injection of contrast medium. Images of the cardiac region are subtracted from images obtained after contrast medium injection as the dense images of soft tissue and bone are removed by the computer. There is less discomfort and risk of complications than with an arteriogram, but visualization of the arteries is less precise, and visualization of stenotic lesions in sequential branches may not occur.

Professional Considerations
Consent form IS required.

Risks
Allergic reaction to dye (itching, hives, rash, tight feeling in the throat, shortness of breath, bronchospasm, anaphylaxis, death), aphasia, hemiplegia, hemorrhage, infection, paresthesia, renal toxicity from contrast medium, thromboemboli.

Contraindications
Recent myocardial infarction, severe renal failure, previous allergy to dye, iodine, or shellfish; during pregnancy (because of radioactive iodine crossing the blood-placental barrier).

Preparation
1. Assess for normal renal function.
2. Have emergency equipment readily available.
3. Glycogen may be administered intravenously to reduce motion artifacts by stopping peristalsis.
4. Record baseline vital signs.
5. Just before beginning the procedure, take a "time out" to verify the correct client, procedure, and site.

Procedure
1. A local anesthetic is given over the basilic or cephalic veins in the antecubital area.
2. Venous catheterization is performed and iodine contrast medium is injected at a rate of 14 mL/second.
3. Radiographic images are taken of arteries made visible by the contrast medium.

Postprocedure Care
1. Monitor vital signs every 15 minutes until stable.
2. Observe the puncture site of catheterization for infection, hemorrhage, and hematoma.
3. Force fluids after the procedure to help flush the contrast medium through the kidneys. A liter of IV fluid may be given as a precautionary measure to clients having an increased risk of developing renal toxicity from the contrast medium, such as the elderly, and clients with dehydration, diabetes, or multiple myeloma.
4. Monitor renal function (BUN and creatinine) for 2 days after the procedure in all clients to be sure the levels remain normal. If the levels become abnormally elevated, indicating nephrotoxicity, continuous IV fluids should be given until the levels return to normal limits. An adverse reaction to IV contrast medium should be noted in a prominent place on the chart and the client informed that he or she should not receive a contrast medium in the future.
5. If the study is necessary in a client with renal insufficiency, a newer, less nephrotoxic agent should be used, even though it is more expensive, and the client should be well hydrated.

Client and Family Teaching
1. You must remain still during the procedure.
2. The procedure takes approximately 45 minutes.
3. In women who are breast-feeding, formula should be substituted for breast milk for 1 or more days after the procedure.

Factors That Affect Results
1. Small amounts of motion by the individual including swallowing and respirations obscure results.
2. Intracardiac or intra-arterial injection of contrast medium can also obscure results.

Other Data
1. The femoral vein may also be used for catheterization.
2. Flat panel detectors represent the most suitable substitute for digital subtraction angiography.

Dilation and Curettage (D & C)—Diagnostic

Norm. No abnormal cells.

Usage. Acquired and congenital cervical stenosis, cancer, diagnosis and treatment of abnormal uterine bleeding, dysmenorrhea, insertion of an IUD, insertion of a radium device for treatment of cancer, pedunculated leiomyomas, preceding a hysterography or hysteroscopy, and uterine polyps.

Description. A widening of the cervical canal with a dilator and then a scraping of the uterine canal with a curette. The test is performed for diagnostic purposes less frequently than in the past because other modalities, such as endometrial biopsy, hysteroscopy, and pelvic ultrasonography, have become available for use. D & C is usually performed therapeutically after an incomplete abortion or miscarriage.

Professional Considerations
Consent form IS required.

Risks
The primary complication is perforation of the uterus. If a perforation occurs and the client is stable, a laparoscopy can be performed to evaluate the perforation. If a perforation is suspected during a suction curettage, a laparoscopy must be performed to continue the procedure to be sure that bowel is not aspirated into the uterus. If the client becomes unstable, emergency surgery is necessary. Arthralgias, though uncommon, can be painful side effects.

Contraindications
Clients with coagulopathies or active vaginal infections.

Preparation
1. Ascertain any drug allergies.
2. Perineal shave may be preferred.
3. The client should void before the procedure.
4. An enema may be prescribed before the procedure.
5. An intravenous line may be initiated.
6. Obtain containers of 10% formalin solution for tissue specimens.
7. Measure and document baseline vital signs.
8. Just before beginning the procedure, take a "time out" to verify the correct client, procedure, and site.

Procedure
1. Regional or general anesthesia (thiopental-isoflurane most cost-effective) is initiated.
2. The cervical canal is dilated with a dilator, and the uterine canal is scraped with a curette.
3. Tissue specimens are placed in containers of 10% formalin and sent to the

laboratory for analysis. If an infection is suspected, part of the specimen should be placed in a sterile container without fixative and sent to the laboratory for culture and sensitivity.

Postprocedure Care
1. Assess vital signs every 15 minutes until stable and then every hour × 4 after general anesthesia. Additional monitoring after general anesthesia typically includes continuous ECG monitoring and pulse oximetry, with continual assessments (every 5-15 minutes) of airway, vital signs, and neurologic status until the client is lying quietly awake, is breathing independently, and responds appropriately to commands spoken in a normal tone.
2. After regional anesthesia, assess vital signs when the procedure is completed and continue to monitor if unstable.
3. Assess the perineal pad for color and amount of drainage.
4. Assess for postanesthesia sensation.
5. Assess and medicate for cramping.
6. Dexamethasone 8 mg IV is an effective antiemetic for preventing postoperative nausea and vomiting 0-24 hours after propofol-based anesthesia after D & C.

Client and Family Teaching
1. The procedure takes approximately 45 minutes.
2. The procedure is accompanied by cramping similar to menstrual cramps. Medications will be given to keep this tolerable.
3. Call the physician for signs of infection: temperature higher than 101 degrees F (38.3 degrees C), pelvic or vaginal pain, purulent vaginal drainage, or excessive bleeding.

Factors That Affect Results
1. None found.

Other Data
1. Hysteroscopy does not improve the sensitivity of D & C in detecting hyperplasia or endometrial carcinoma but is superior in detecting focal lesions of the uterine cavity in postmenopausal bleeding.

Dinitrophenylhydrazine (DNPH) Test—Diagnostic

Norm. Normal amino acid screen.

Usage. Biotinidase deficiency, cystinuria, fructose-1,6-diphosphatase deficiency, Hartnup's homocystinuria disease, ketosis, lactic acidosis, maple syrup urine disease, oasthouse urine disease, PKU, seizures, tyrosinemia, tyrosinosis, and unexplained mental retardation.

Description. Metabolic screening test to detect inherited disorders in the metabolism of branched-chain amino acids.

Professional Considerations
Consent form NOT required.

Preparation
1. Obtain a clean specimen container.

Procedure
1. Obtain a 15-mL random urine specimen.

Postprocedure Care
1. Keep the urine sample refrigerated or frozen.

Client and Family Teaching
1. Results are normally available within 72 hours.

Factors That Affect Results
1. Radiopaque contrast dye may increase the results.
2. Falsely elevated results occur if valproic acid, penicillin derivatives, or benzoic acid preservatives have been ingested within 3 days of the urine collection.

Other Data
1. A 24-hour urine sample may also be obtained.
2. Peritoneal dialysis may be used to clear amino acids from the body.
3. One of the branched-chain amino acids produces a metabolite that causes the urine to smell like maple syrup.
4. The test can also be performed on a newborn heelstick blood spot as part of the neonatal screening for metabolic disorders.

Dipyridamole-Thallium Scan

See **Heart Scan**—Diagnostic.

Direct Antiglobulin Test

See **Coombs' Test, Direct**—Serum.

Discovery Imaging

See **Dual Modality Imaging**—Diagnostic.

Disopyramide Phosphate—Serum

Norm.

	Trough
Therapeutic	2-5 μg/mL
Panic level	>7 μg/mL

Panic Level Symptoms and Treatment
Symptoms. Prolonged Q-T interval and ventricular tachycardia, heart failure, hypotension.

Treatment

NOTE: Treatment choice(s) depend(s) on client's history and condition and episode history.

1. Stop medication.
2. Monitor ECG for R-on-T phenomenon.
3. Support airway, breathing, and blood pressure.
4. Hemodialysis WILL remove disopyramide. No information was found on the effect of peritoneal dialysis on disopyramide levels.

Usage. Monitoring for therapeutic dosage during disopyramide phosphate.

Description. A quinidine-like type 1a anti-dysrhythmic agent used to treat atrial and ventricular dysrhythmias. It depresses myocardial responsiveness, slows automaticity, and raises the cardiac tissue threshold, prolonging the effective refractory period. It also prolongs cardiac conduction. Disopyramide is metabolized by the liver, with a half-life of 4-10 hours. Up to 80% is excreted in the urine. Steady-state levels are reached after 25-30 hours. Overdose treatment includes catecholamine infusion and gastric lavage to restore blood pressure followed by percutaneous cardiopulmonary support. Known to produce cardiac arrhythmias in clients receiving macrolide antibiotics (erythromycin, clarithromycin) simultaneously with disopyramide, hypoglycemia in clients who have type 2 diabetes mellitus, neuropathy, and pneumonitis.

Professional Considerations

Consent form NOT required.

Preparation

1. Note the time the last dose was taken.
2. Note on the laboratory requisition if the client is taking phenytoin because this may cause decreased levels of disopyramide phosphate.
3. Obtain a siliconized red topped or gold-sealed tube.
4. Do NOT draw this specimen during hemodialysis.

Procedure

1. Draw a 4-mL TROUGH blood sample.
2. Draw a peak sample 2-3 hours after the oral dose.
3. Draw a trough sample just before the next dose.

4. Obtain serial measurements at the same time each day.

Postprocedure Care

1. Assess the results before administration of the next dose.

Client and Family Teaching

1. The next dose of medication is dependent on these test results.
2. Explain the need and timing of the peak and trough blood samples.
3. Refer clients with intentional overdose for crisis intervention.

Factors That Affect Results

1. Results are elevated in renal and hepatic dysfunction and with drug use of azithromycin.
2. Blood levels are difficult to monitor because the levels of free (unbound) disopyramide change considerably over a dosing interval.
3. Metabolism increases with concomitant treatment with phenobarbital, phenytoin, and rifampin.
4. Interaction of disopyramide with propranolol includes bradycardia and arrhythmia in chick embryos.

Other Data

1. Other trade names include DSP, Napamide, Norpace, and Rythmodan.
2. Metabolite has an anticholinergic effect, causing dry mouth, urinary retention, constipation, blurred vision, exacerbation of glaucoma, and dryness of bronchial secretions.
3. Use with caution with myasthenia gravis because it may precipitate a crisis.
4. Do not use with clients in heart failure or shock.
5. More than 6 mg/mL may be needed to suppress ventricular dysrhythmias.
6. Enhances the effect of warfarin and oral antihyperglycemics. Does not affect digoxin and digitoxin levels.
7. Improves myocardial oxygen supply-demand balance in clients with hypertrophic obstructive cardiomyopathy (HOCM) and controls hypotension and bradycardia in neurocardiogenic syncope.
8. Cibenzoline has comparable efficacy to disopyramide for the prevention of recurrence of atrial tachyarrhythmia and is better tolerated.

DNA Ploidy (Stem Line DNA Analysis)—Specimen

Positive. Aneuploid, polyploid.

Negative. Diploid.

Usage. Determining prognosis in bladder cancer (squamous), breast cancer, hepatocellular carcinoma (HCC), laryngeal squamous-cell carcinoma, and ovarian cancer.

Description. Malignant cells demonstrate greater proliferation than normal cells and tend to have disordered cellular division whereby aneuploid DNA is present in individual cells. This abnormality increases with the degree of malignancy. Clinical studies indicate that the proportion of proliferating cells in a breast tumor biopsy specimen and the degree of aneuploidy have prognostic significance for breast cancer. Longer disease-free periods after treatment tend to occur in individuals whose tumor has lower degrees of proliferation and fewer aneuploid cells.

Professional Considerations

A consent form IS required for the biopsy used to obtain the specimen.

Preparation

1. Obtain a sterile formalin specimen container.
2. The specimen may be obtained by needle or surgical biopsy.

Procedure

1. Place the tissue specimen in a sterile formalin specimen container.

Postprocedure Care

1. Send the specimen to pathology as soon as possible.

Client and Family Teaching

1. DNA ploidy is only one means of measuring the degree of malignancy and prognosis of breast cancer. Other prognostic factors include status of axillary nodes, presence of estrogen and progesterone receptors, tumor size and extension into chest wall or skin, and distant metastasis.
2. Use a mild analgesic for biopsy site pain.

Factors That Affect Results

1. An inadequate sample size may yield false-negative results.

Other Data

1. DNA ploidy analysis may offer additional prognostic information in individuals with prostatic adenocarcinoma, lymphoma, bladder carcinoma, renal cell carcinoma, malignant melanoma, and head and neck cancers.
2. Most early-stage prostate cancers are diploid. Aneuploidy is associated with hormone resistance. Aneuploidy and tetraploidy are associated with advanced prostate cancer.
3. Relatively few cells are needed to perform DNA ploidy flow cytometry. Therefore tumors and response to treatment can be monitored for changes in the DNA content of the cells by serial needle biopsy.

DNPH

See Dinitrophenylhydrazine Test—Diagnostic.

Doppler Ultrasonographic, Transcranial

See Doppler Ultrasonographic Flow Studies—Diagnostic.

Doppler Ultrasonographic Flow Studies, Transcranial

See Doppler Ultrasonographic Flow Studies—Diagnostic.

D

Doppler Ultrasonographic Flow Studies (Includes Carotid Doppler, Carotid Artery Echography, Carotid Artery Ultrasonography, Duplex Ultrasonography, Transcranial Doppler Ultrasonography)—Diagnostic

Norm. Normal intracranial arterial flow velocity. Normal carotid artery anatomy or unimpeded blood flow of that portion of the circulation evaluated.

Usage. *Transcranial Doppler ultrasonography* is used to evaluate blood flow through the cerebral arteries. Diagnostic in intracranial aneurysms, arteriovenous malformations, and moyamoya syndrome. Allows assessment of blood supply in intracranial neoplasms. Used intraoperatively to monitor velocity in the middle portion of the cerebral artery during carotid endarterectomy. Used in the evaluation of collateral circulation stenosis, vasoconstriction as a result of insult, and cerebral dynamics after head injury and in establishing brain death in adults. Used to predict the risk of stroke in children with sickle cell anemia. *Carotid Doppler ultrasonography, carotid artery ultrasonography,* and *carotid artery echography* are used for detection or preoperative evaluation of atherosclerotic carotid artery disease and cerebrovascular disease. *Duplex ultrasonography* is used for evaluation of conditions such as renal artery stenosis and deep vein thrombosis, and postoperatively for evaluating carotid endarterectomy and cardiac function. When evaluating for deep vein thrombosis (DVT), the flow of the vessel is studied as the vessel is compressed. If the vessel cannot be completely compressed to eliminate flow, the test is very sensitive and specific for DVT in a symptomatic client.

Description. A noninvasive, hand-held mechanical ultrasonograph that uses a low-frequency (2-2.5 MHz) sector transducer through temporal, orbital, and suboccipital acoustic windows of the skull. Constant-frequency ultrasonic waves are transmitted into the vessel of interest by a transducer in the form of either fixed-wave or pulsed signals. Using the color and power technique of the Doppler signal instead of the frequency shift, it records the anatomy, flow direction, and mean blood flow velocity in real-time imaging. Doppler ultrasonography can display very small quantitative and qualitative volumes, allowing great morphologic detail. Inferences about the presence of obstruction to blood flow can be made with this procedure. When this technique is combined with a static image of the vessel provided by B-mode imaging ultrasonography, the procedure is referred to as "duplex Doppler ultrasonography." When a color image is generated by changes in blood flow, the term "color Doppler" is applied.

Professional Considerations

Consent form is NOT required.

Preparation

1. Although portable ultrasonographic equipment is available, this test is frequently performed within the radiology suite.
2. Occasionally clients are required to fast before abdominal ultrasonographic procedures. No other pretest preparation or medication is required.
3. Remove any restrictive clothing to allow access to the portion of the client's body to be studied.
4. The client is usually positioned recumbent with a small pillow supporting the head.
5. See Client and Family Teaching.

Procedure

1. The test is generally performed in a darkened room either by a radiology technician or by a radiologist who is seated at the bedside.
2. Acoustic jelly is applied to the skin on the area over the part of the circulatory system of interest.
3. The ultrasound transducer is applied to the skin, and acoustic jelly and ultrasonographic recordings are made. The procedure is painless and usually brief (minutes).
4. Ultrasonic waves are released from the transducer and reflected back to it. An image is then generated within the ultrasound apparatus where it is displayed on a viewing screen. The sound waves used during the test are not audible to the client.
5. For transcranial Doppler ultrasonography, a time-averaged mean blood

flow velocity of >200 cm/second is indicative of cerebral ischemia. Stenosis >60% diameter reduction is reported immediately.

Postprocedure Care

1. Wipe ultrasonic gel from the client's body.
2. Although preliminary results of the procedure may be available in the radiology suite, the client should be informed that a physician interpretation is required before the test results are available.

Client and Family Teaching

1. The test takes approximately 60 minutes, can be performed at the bedside, and is painless and safe.
2. Results are usually available in 24 hours.
3. Vascular (carotid) surgery may occur because of the test results, and this will require special educational and emotional support for the client and family.

Factors That Affect Results

1. The accuracy of this test is highly dependent on the skill of the operator (technician or radiologist) and the interpreter of the results.
2. The body habitus of the client and the technical condition of the equipment may affect the test results.
3. Accurate transmission and reflection of ultrasonographic signals can be affected by the presence of calcium (bone or calcification deposits) or gas overlying the vessel of interest, and condition may preclude the achievement of accurate results.
4. Intramural calcification may inhibit sound penetration, leading to false-positive results.

5. Flow velocity is age dependent and decreases continuously from early childhood to adulthood.
6. Detection of small aneurysms is limited by insonation angles and spatial resolution.
7. Transcranial procedure:
   a. ICP, blood pressure and volume, hematocrit, and subarachnoid hemorrhage affect flow velocity in transcranial Doppler scanning.
   b. False-negative exams of vasospasm are associated with chronic high blood pressure, increased intracranial pressure, severe spasm of the carotid siphon, and distal vasospasm.
   c. Use of tobacco and caffeine can affect the results.
   d. In clients with occlusive cerebrovascular disease, false-positive and false-negative results have been reported when one is evaluating for cross flow through the anterior and posterior communicating arteries.

Other Data

1. In previous years carotid endarterectomy was almost always preceded by carotid arteriography; however, the high diagnostic accuracy of carotid ultrasonography (when performed by experienced operators) has eliminated this requirement in many cases.
2. Most accurate for diagnosis of proximal DVT but less reliable in isolated calf vein thrombi.
3. See also Ankle-brachial index—Diagnostic.

Doppler Ultrasonographic Flow Studies

See Doppler Ultrasonographic Flow Studies—Diagnostic.

Doxepin

See Tricyclic Antidepressants—Plasma or Serum.

Drug Screen

See Toxicology, Drug Screen—Blood or Urine.

D

Dual Energy X-Ray Absorptiometry

See **Bone Densitometry**—Diagnostic.

Dual Modality Imaging (3-D Body Scan, PET/CT, SPECT/CT, Biograph, Discovery VH Hawkeye, Discovery VI Positrace, Discovery LS, Gemini)—Diagnostic

Norm. Findings are interpreted by a radiologist specializing in the types of imaging used.

Usage. Cancer staging via precise localization of tumor-targeted radiopharmaceuticals; monitoring response to radioimmunotherapy. More accurate assessment of myocardial perfusion than other single-mode studies. Planning for and evaluating success of radiation therapy.

Description. Dual modality imaging combines different types of imaging techniques to simultaneously evaluate functional structure and metabolic physiology. Traditional single-mode structural imaging includes ultrafast computed tomography (CT) and magnetic resonance imaging (MRI). Traditional functional imaging that evaluates the physiology occurring in tissues includes positive emission tomography (PET) and single-photon emission computed tomography (SPECT). Dual-mode imaging combines one of the structural imaging techniques with one of the functional imaging techniques, and data are acquired by one machine containing both the x-ray component and the radionuclide detector during only one procedure. After both sets of images are acquired, computer software then merges the data and fuses the images to give results that are more sensitive and specific than a single procedure alone, and that overcomes many limitations of each single procedure. In addition, simultaneous imaging can provide improved attenuation correction and anatomic mapping and overcome issues with the body being positioned differently for tests taken at two separate times. In the 3-D Body Scan, cross-sectional CT images are fused with the metabolically differentiated PET images to produce a single three-dimensional image that provides better detection of early heart disease, cancer, and brain disorders than either modality alone.

Professional Considerations

Consent form IS required.

Risks

See risks described for each separate mode of imaging to be combined with the specific equipment listed under Preparation, 1.

Contraindications

See contraindications described for each separate mode of imaging to be combined with the equipment listed under Preparation, 1.

Precautions

See contraindications described for each separate mode of imaging to be combined with the equipment listed under Preparation, 1.

Preparation

1. See separate preparation information, depending on the modalities combined in the dual-mode imaging equipment:
   a. Magnetic resonance imaging—Diagnostic.
   b. Positron emission tomography—Diagnostic.
   c. Single-photon emission computed tomography, Brain—Diagnostic.
   d. Computed tomography of the body—Diagnostic.
2. Document clinical indications on the test requisition. This helps guide the interpreter to provide the most relevant test interpretation, and it also is essential for many types of procedure reimbursement.
3. Just before beginning the procedure, take a "time out" to verify the correct client, procedure, and site.

Procedure

1. The client is positioned supine on the scanning table. See procedure for individual led listing.

Postprocedure Care

1. Assess the venous access site for infiltration.

Client and Family Teaching

1. You will have to hold breath for several seconds.
2. It is important to lie still for the test.
3. A sensation of burning may be felt from the injection of the contrast.

Factors That Affect Results

1. See individual tests as described under Preparation, 1. Factors that affect the

results for all tests are considerably reduced by the dual-mode imaging technique.

Other Data

1. GE Medical Systems manufactures the Discovery VH Hawkeye, Discovery VI Positrace, and Discovery LS Imaging Systems. Siemens Medical manufactures the Biography imaging system. Phillips Medical Systems manufactures the Gemini imaging system.

D-Xylose Absorption Test (Xylose Tolerance Test)—Diagnostic

Norm.

Time after Ingestion	Serum D-Xylose Level	SI Units
Adults		
Fasting	0 mg/dL	0 mmol/L
After ingesting 25 g		
1-Hour sample	21-57 mg/dL	1.40-3.80 mmol/L
2-Hour sample	32-58 mg/dL	2.13-3.87 mmol/L
3-Hour sample	19-42 mg/dL	1.27-2.80 mmol/L
4-Hour sample	11-29 mg/dL	0.74-1.93 mmol/L
5-Hour sample	6-48 mg/dL	0.40-3.21 mmol/L
After ingesting 5 g		
2-Hour sample	20-60 mg/dL	1.33-4.00 mmol/L
Children >10 years	Serum D-Xylose Level 1 Hour after Ingestion	
Fasting	0 mg/dL	0 mmol/L
<6 months of age (after	15-58 mg/dL	1.00-3.87 mmol/L ingesting 0.5 g/kg)
6 months-16 years (after	20-58 mg/dL	1.33-3.87 mmol/L ingesting 0.5 g/kg)

Urine	Grams of D-Xylose Excreted in Urine During 5 Hours after Ingestion	Fraction of Xylose Excreted in Urine
Adults		
Age 17-64 after ingesting 25 g	4-10 g	16%-40%
Age 17-64 after ingesting 5 g	1.2-2.0 g	20%-40%
≥65 after ingesting 25 g	3.5-10 g	14%-40%
≥65 after ingesting 5 g	1.2-2.0 g	20%-40%
Children	n/a, because dose varies by weight	16%-40% excreted in 5 hours

Increased. Disaccharidase deficiencies, Hodgkin's disease, malabsorption, status post gastrectomy, radiation side effects of small intestine, and scleroderma.

Decreased. Amyloidosis, ascariasis, blind loop syndrome, celiac disease, Crohn's disease, cystic fibrosis, diarrhea, immunoglobulin deficiency, massive bacterial

overgrowth in small bowel, pancreatitis, pellagra, postoperatively (after bowel resection), radiation enteritis, short bowel syndrome, tropical sprue, Whipple's disease, and any other jejunal mucosal disease.

Description. D-Xylose is a pentose (carbohydrate) that is not metabolized by the body and is normally absorbed by the proximal portion of the small bowel and excreted unchanged by the kidney into the urine. The test is used to distinguish malabsorption from maldigestion because it helps evaluate the efficiency of mucosal absorption efficiency. In clients with normal renal function, results indicate whether the absorptive abilities of the mucosa are impaired. In clients with malabsorption, both serum and urine values would be lower than the norms. Urine D-xylose is measured along with serum D-xylose to provide information related to renal retention. In clients with renal problems, the urine collection is not done.

Professional Considerations

Consent form NOT required.

Preparation

1. See Client and Family Teaching.
2. Obtain a large brown urine container and three red topped, marble topped, or gold topped tubes.
3. Assess renal function laboratory data (BUN, creatinine).

Procedure

1. At 0800 (8 AM), instruct the client to void and discard the sample.
2. Draw a fasting blood sample of 4 mL and write on the tube the date and time collected and "fasting sample."
3. D-Xylose dose:
   a. Adults: Give 25 g of D-xylose dissolved in 250 mL of water by mouth.
   b. Children: Give 0.5 g of D-xylose per kilogram of body weight, up to 25 g.
   c. For clients unable to take 25 g, a 5-g dose may be used.
4. Follow with 250 mL of water orally.
5. No further fluids or food should be given until the test is completed.
6. Collect all the urine voided for 5 hours after ingestion of D-xylose in a refrigerated container.
7. *Adults*: Draw a 5-mL blood specimen for D-xylose levels 60 and 120 minutes after ingestion of D-xylose. Some tests may also include 3-hour, 4-hour, and 5-hour collections. Label the tube with the date and time collected as well as the number of hours since ingestion (e.g., "1 hour sample").

8. *Children*: Draw a 5-mL blood specimen for D-xylose levels 60 minutes after ingestion of D-xylose. Include the date and time collected and label as the 1-hour sample.
9. Document on the laboratory requisition the total dose of D-xylose administered and the total volume of urine collected.

Postprocedure Care

1. Resume fluids and diet as prescribed.

Client and Family Teaching

1. Adults must fast for 8 hours and children for 4 hours before drinking prescribed D-xylose.
2. Do not eat foods containing pentoses: fruits, jams, jellies, and pastries.
3. You will not be able to smoke during the test.
4. You will need to rest quietly during the test. The D-xylose commonly causes mild diarrhea.
5. The test involves specifically timed specimens.
6. The test takes several hours. Bring reading material or other diversions to the test.

Factors That Affect Results

1. Failure to collect all urine voided during the testing time will produce a falsely low result.
2. Drugs that will increase absorption in the intestines include aspirin, atropine, and indomethacin. Other drugs that interfere with the test results include colchicine, digitalis, MAO inhibitors, nalidixic acid, neomycin, opium alkaloids, and phenelzine.
3. Poor renal function will decrease urinary output, and vomiting will decrease the amount of D-xylose consumed or absorbed.
4. The urine amount of D-xylose may be decreased by dehydration, delayed gastric emptying, renal insufficiency, reduced circulation, third spacing of fluid (such as in pregnancy and ascites), and hypothyroidism, but these will not affect the serum levels.
5. Massive bacterial overgrowth in the small bowel may decrease the amount of D-xylose available for absorption by the

small bowel and therefore decrease the serum and urine levels.

Other Data

1. Because an abnormal D-xylose test is suggestive of small bowel mucosal

disease, a biopsy should be performed as the next step.

2. Radioactive isotope 14C-xylose breath test is an alternative test for the diagnosis of celiac disease.

Duplex Ultrasonography

See Doppler Ultrasonic Flow Studies—Diagnostic.

Ear, Routine—Culture

See Culture, Routine.

Eastern Equine Encephalitis Virus Titer—Specimen

Norm. Titer <1:10.

Positive. A fourfold increase in titer between acute and convalescent specimens supports the diagnosis of eastern equine encephalitis.

Negative. Normal finding or bacterial infection.

Description. Eastern equine encephalitis is an inflammation of the brain caused by an arbovirus that attacks the central nervous system. The mode of transmission to humans is through the bite of a mosquito of the genus *Culex*. High risk when in contact with deciduous wetlands.

Professional Considerations
Consent form NOT required.

Preparation

1. Tube: Red topped, red/gray topped, or gold topped.
2. Assess for fever and symptoms of meningitis and meningoencephalitis, including convulsions, abnormal reflexes, extremity rigidity, and bulging of the fontanelle in infants. In children, assess for headache, drowsiness lasting 2-3 days, nausea, and vomiting. In adults, assess for frontal

headache, photophobia, nausea, and vomiting.

Procedure

1. Draw a 4-mL blood sample.

Postprocedure Care

1. Send the specimen to the laboratory immediately.
2. Draw a convalescent sample 14 days later.

Client and Family Teaching

1. The convalescent sample will be drawn in 2 weeks to see if the treatment is working.
2. The mortality in the United States is 65%-75%. Survivors often have significant neurologic disabilities.

Factors That Affect Results

1. Failure to collect a convalescent sample will result in the inability to show a rising of antibody titer between the acute and convalescent phases of the disease.

Other Data

1. Common hosts include mosquitoes, birds, ducks, fowl, and horses.
2. MRI is a sensitive test to identify early radiographic signs including involvement of the basal ganglia and thalamus.

EBCT

See Computed Tomography of the Body—Diagnostic.

ECG

See Electrocardiography—Diagnostic.

E

Echinococcosis Serologic Test—Blood

Norm. IHA 1:2-1:64.

Usage. Echinococcosis.

Description. Echinococcosis is a tapeworm infection common among clients in contact with sheep or cattle. Any member of the dog family may serve as a definitive host for the adult tapeworm. Dogs are infected by feeding on the offal of domestic animals or on animal parts at butchering time. Children are at a high risk of ingesting eggs excreted by dogs because of their close contact with their pet dogs. Humans are the intermediate host. The eggs become blood borne and form cysts in the liver and other parts of the body such as the heart, lungs, and bone. It may take 5-20 years for a cyst to grow large enough to cause symptoms. Common in persons associated with goats or sheep or who live in Turkey or in Muslim communities of southern Israel. In addition, there is a high seroprevalence in Castilla y León in Spain.

Professional Considerations
Consent form NOT required.

Preparation
1. Tube: Red topped, red/gray topped, or gold topped.
2. Obtain recent history for possible animal contact.

Procedure
1. Draw a 4-mL blood sample.

Postprocedure Care
1. Surgical resection of the cyst is the treatment of choice.
2. Aspiration of the cyst contents should not be attempted for a diagnosis because of the danger of rupture and leakage of the contents. This could cause an acute allergic reaction, anaphylactic shock, or dissemination of the infection.

Client and Family Teaching
1. Results are normally available within 72 hours.
2. Treatment with benzimidazole compounds (mebendazole, albendazole) may take years or decades.

Factors That Affect Results
1. False-positive results may occur in clients with a history of cirrhosis, collagen disease, systemic lupus erythematosus, or schistosomiasis.

Other Data
1. Positive titers occur in 35%-50% of cases with hydatid lung cysts and in 85% with hydatid liver cysts.
2. Removal of the cyst does not dramatically lower the antibody titer. It may persist for years.

Echocardiography (Echo, Heart Sonogram, Heart Ultrasonogram)—Diagnostic

Norm. No abnormalities.

Usage. Atrial septal defect, aortic stenosis or regurgitation, atrial tumors, bradycardia, cardiac tamponade, cardiomyopathy, congenital heart disease, effusion (pericardial), embolization of artery, endocarditis, idiopathic hypertrophic subaortic stenosis, lymphoma metastasis, Marfan syndrome, mitral regurgitation or stenosis, mitral valve prolapse, myocardial infarction post evaluation for wall-motion abnormalities, myocarditis, panic disorder, patent ductus arteriosus, pericarditis, subacute bacterial endocarditis (SBE), transposition of the great arteries, tricuspid atresia, ventricular septal defect, and other cardiac defects.

Description. Echocardiography is a noninvasive, acoustic imaging procedure that determines the size, shape, position, thickness, and movements of the heart valves, walls, and chambers during each cardiac cycle. It records the echoes created by the deflection of short pulses of an ultrasonic beam off the cardiac structures onto an oscilloscope. The time required for the ultrasonic beam to be reflected back to the transducer from differing densities of tissue is converted by a computer to an electrical impulse displayed on an oscilloscopic screen to create a two-dimensional picture of the heart in different projections. The resolution of the oscilloscope recording obtained is determined by the frequency of the beam.

Lower frequencies penetrate further but provide less resolution than higher frequencies. Echocardiography can also be performed transesophageally (TEE) with the transmitter inserted into the esophagus similar to an endoscope. This gives a clearer view of the valves and endocardium, especially in the presence of obesity or severe chronic obstructive pulmonary disease (COPD).

Professional Considerations
Consent form NOT required.

Preparation
1. The client should disrobe above the waist or wear a gown.

Procedure
1. With the client in a supine or recumbent position, conductive gel is placed over the third and fourth intercostal spaces to the left of the sternum.
2. A transducer is angled directly over the intercostal spaces or beneath the xiphoid process to direct ultrasonic waves that are displayed on the oscilloscopic machine and printed in the M (motion) mode on a recorder.
3. The client may also be placed on the left side to obtain a different view of the heart and may occasionally be asked to perform certain maneuvers or to inhale amyl nitrite (a gas with a slightly sweet odor) to record changes in heart function.
4. For a transesophageal echocardiogram, the throat is anesthetized with spray, and the transducer is passed orally into the esophagus. (See Transesophageal ultrasonography—Diagnostic for more information.)

Postprocedure Care
1. Remove the conductive gel from the skin.
2. For a transesophageal echocardiogram, oral fluids must be held until the local anesthetic is no longer in effect and the gag reflex has returned.

Client and Family Teaching
1. The procedure takes 30-60 minutes, can be performed at the bedside, and is painless.
2. Remain as still as possible.
3. Results are normally available within 24 hours.

Factors That Affect Results
1. Thick chests, COPD, obesity, chest wall abnormalities or scar tissue, or dressings may alter the display of ultrasonic waves on the recorder.
2. Pulmonary hypertension reduces the accuracy of Doppler measurements of pulmonary artery systolic pressure.
3. Better resolution can be obtained for children than for adults because their thinner, less dense chest wall enables use of a higher-frequency, shorter-wavelength sound.
4. Improper placement of the transducer.

Other Data
1. Very sensitive test in detecting pericardial effusion.
2. Side effects of amyl nitrite, which has a short duration of action, are dizziness, flushing, and tachycardia.
3. See also Stress test, Pharmacologic—Diagnostic; Transesophageal uiltrasonography—Diagnostic.

Echoencephalography

See Brain Ultrasonography—Diagnostic.

Echography/Echogram

See Abdominal Aorta Ultrasonography—Diagnostic; Brain Ultrasonography—Diagnostic; Breast Ultrasonography—Diagnostic; Echocardiograph—Diagnostic; Eye and Orbit Ultrasonography—Diagnostic; Gallbladder and Biliary System Ultrasonography—Diagnostic; Gynecologic Ultrasonography—Diagnostic; Kidney Ultrasonography—Diagnostic; Liver Ultrasonography—Diagnostic; Obstetric Ultrasonography—Diagnostic; Pancreas Ultrasonography—Diagnostic; Prostate Ultrasonography—Diagnostic; Spleen Ultrasonography—Diagnostic; Thyroid Ultrasonography—Diagnostic; Transesophageal Ultrasonography—Diagnostic; or Urinary Bladder Ultrasonography—Diagnostic.

Ecstasy

See **Amphetamines**—Blood.

EEG

See **Electroencephalography**—Diagnostic.

EGD

See **Esophagogastroduodenoscopy**—Diagnostic.

EKG

See **Electrocardiography**—Diagnostic.

EKG, Signal-Averaged

See **Signal-Averaged Electrocardiography**—Diagnostic.

Electrocardiography (ECG, EKG)—Diagnostic

Norm. Normal sinus rhythm, no dysrhythmias.

Usage. Anesthesia, angina pectoris, anxiety, atrial septal defect, beriberi, bradycardia, carbon monoxide poisoning, chest pain, coarctation of the aorta, congestive heart failure, eating disorders (bradycardia, low-voltage changes, prolonged QTc interval, inverted T waves, depressed ST segments), effusion (pericardial), emergency monitoring, endocarditis, heart murmur, ischemia, myocardial infarction (MI), pacemaker function, palpitations, panic disorder, patent ductus arteriosus, pericarditis, preoperative evaluation, pulmonic stenosis, respiratory distress, surgery, syncope, tetralogy of Fallot, transposition of the great arteries, tricuspid atresia, ventricular hypertrophy, ventricular septal defect, and yellow fever.

Description. Recording of the heart's electrical current using electrodes from 12 different leads: bipolar limb leads I, II, III; augmented limb leads aVR, aVL, aVF; and precordial chest leads V_1-V_6. The heart's electrical activity takes three forms on the ECG: the P wave, which signifies atrial depolarization; the QRS complex, which signifies ventricular depolarization; and the T wave, which signifies ventricular repolarization. This test identifies conduction abnormalities and dysrhythmias, monitors recovery from MI, and helps evaluate the effectiveness of cardiac medications. Single-lead tracings monitor the presence and type of electrical conduction during cardiac emergencies and during insertion of a temporary transvenous pacemaker.

Professional Considerations
Consent form NOT required.

Preparation
1. The client should disrobe above the waist.
2. Cleanse the skin where the electrodes will be placed by rubbing it lightly with an alcohol wipe and then scraping gently with the edge of an electrode.
3. Check the paper supply.

Procedure
1. Single-channel recording:
   a. The client is positioned supine.
   b. Five electrodes are placed over clean fleshy skin with the conductor ends pointing upward. Electrodes are positioned on the right arm, the left arm, the right leg, and the left leg; the lead is sequentially repositioned for

E

6-second recording at locations V_1-V_6 on the chest.

c. The machine is turned on, and the recording is begun.

d. In nonautomatic machines, turn the lead selector to lead l and run it for 6 seconds for each lead from I through aVF. Then turn the lead selector to neutral and determine the proper placement for leads V_1-V_6 before recording. The position of V_1 is at the fourth intercostal space, right sternal border. V_2 is at the fourth intercostal space, left sternal border. V_3 is midway between V_2 and V_4. V_4 is at the left midclavicular line at the fifth intercostal space. V_5 follows V_4 in a straight line over the fifth intercostal space to the anterior axillary line, and V_6 follows V_5 in a straight line over the fifth intercostal space to the left midaxillary line.

e. The procedure takes 15 minutes.

f. During emergencies, three electrodes can be placed for monitoring: the white lead on the right upper chest, the black lead on the left upper chest, and the red lead on the lower left lateral chest.

2. *Simultaneous 12-channel recording:*

a. The client is positioned supine.

b. The limb leads are connected to electrodes, and each is attached to a limb.

c. Leads V_1-V_6 are connected to electrodes and attached to the chest wall in the locations described under procedure 1.

d. The machine is activated, and a simultaneous recording of all 12 channels is printed automatically by the electrocardiograph machine.

e. The procedure takes 5-10 minutes.

Postprocedure Care

1. Label the ECG with client's name, room number, date, time, and episodes of chest pain during the procedure.

2. Remove the electrodes and cleanse the skin of any residual conductive gel.

Client and Family Teaching

1. You should not move or talk during the procedure.

Factors That Affect Results

1. Body movement, poor skin cleansing, or improper electrode placement produces an artifact, which may necessitate repeating the test.

2. The results should be interpreted in comparison with prior electrocardiograms, if available.

Other Data

1. MI produces three changes on the ECG: elevated ST indicates formation of ischemia, and then the T wave flattens and becomes inverted with an enlarged Q wave appearing, which indicates necrosis.

2. See also Holter monitor—Diagnostic; Signal-averaged electrocardiography—Diagnostic.

3. The abbreviation "EKG" is often spoken and written instead of the more proper "ECG" to decrease confusion with "EEG" (electroencephalogram).

Electroencephalography (EEG)—Diagnostic

Norm. Normal electrical brain activity as recorded by the EEG instrument.

Usage. Used as a diagnostic tool in the diagnosis of Alzheimer's disease (declining D alpha values), attention-deficit/hyperactivity disorder (ADHD), different central nervous system disorders including tumors, infections, and various encephalopathic states. Special use involves the characterization of various types of seizure disorders and also the determination of the anatomic locus of seizure activity within the brain (the "seizure focus"). The EEG is also of value in the determination of central nervous system death ("brain death"). It is occasionally helpful in establishing the diagnosis of various neurosensory disorders when used in its applied forms (the recording of "visual evoked" and "auditory evoked potentials").

Description. Using a special cap, electroconductive gel, and electrodes, an EEG recording of the electrical potentials of the cerebral cortex of the brain is taken and subsequently analyzed to determine the presence or absence of various waveform activities.

Professional Considerations

Consent form NOT required.

Preparation

1. See Client and Family Teaching.
2. Although portable EEG equipment is available, the test is generally conducted in an EEG lab by a neurologist or an EEG technician.
3. Sedative drugs and prolonged fasting (hypoglycemia) can influence the test and should be avoided if possible.

Procedure

1. The client is placed in a recumbent position in a darkened room.
2. A cap with numerous plastic electrode locators is placed on the client's head, and the openings in the electrode locators are filled with electroconductive gel.
3. Electrodes are inserted through the locators into proximity with the client's scalp. (It is not necessary to shave or puncture the scalp to accomplish this step.)
4. EEG recordings are made in the supine position. The client may be asked to perform various physical maneuvers during the test; occasionally recordings are made during sleep.

Postprocedure Care

1. Electrodes and EEG cap are removed and the gel is wiped from the scalp.

Client and Family Teaching

1. Pretest orientation with a description of the method used to attach the electrodes is important.
2. Shaving of the scalp hair is not necessary for this test.
3. Hair should be free of products such as gel or hair spray, which could interfere with conductivity to the electrodes.

4. It is important to lie still throughout the test.
5. If the EEG is used as an adjunct in the determination of brain death, a detailed description of the test and the rationale behind its use in this setting should be given to the family.
6. The procedure may take up to 2 hours.

Factors That Affect Results

1. Hypoglycemia (prolonged fasting) may decrease response time, leading to an abnormal pattern.
2. Certain sedative drugs can affect the EEG pattern.
3. Caffeine causes significant reduction of total EEG power at fronto-parieto-occipital central electrode positions of both hemispheres when subjects have their eyes open.
4. Oily hair or hair spray interferes with the recording because it reduces conductivity to the electrodes.
5. Sleep, motor activity on the part of the client, muscle tension, and various external sensory stimuli may interfere with the waveform patterns and prolong the test.

Other Data

1. Prolonged (semiambulatory) EEG recordings may be valuable in the management of certain clients with epilepsy.
2. The EEG may be used as an evaluation tool in the management of anesthesia and sedation.
3. A single negative EEG finding should not rule out a seizure disorder. Serial or repeated EEG tracings are necessary.
4. See also Visual evoked potential—Diagnostic.

Electrolytes Panel (EP)—Blood

Norm. See individual test listings: Bicarbonate—Blood, Carbon dioxide total count—Blood, Chloride—Serum, Potassium—Plasma or serum, and Sodium, Plasma—Serum or urine.

Usage. See individual test listings.

Description. The Electrolytes Panel is a term defined by the Centers for Medicare and Medicaid Services (CMS) in the United States to indicate a group of tests for which

a bundled reimbursement is available. The panel is one of several that replace the multichannel tests, such as SMA-6. The panel is disease oriented, meaning that payment through Medicare is available only when the test is used to diagnose and monitor a disease and payment is not available when the test is used for screening purposes in clients who have no signs and symptoms. All the tests in the panel must be carried out when a basic metabolic panel (BMP) is ordered.

Professional Considerations

Consent form NOT required.

Preparation

1. Tube: Red topped, red/gray topped, or gold topped.
2. Do NOT draw specimens during hemodialysis.

Procedure

1. Draw a 5-mL blood sample.

Postprocedure Care

1. None.

Client and Family Teaching

1. See individual test listings.

Factors That Affect Results

1. See individual test listings.

Other Data

1. See individual test listings.

Electrolytes—Plasma or Serum

See also Anion Gap—Blood; Carbon Dioxide—Blood; Chloride—Serum; Potassium—Plasma or Serum; Sodium, Plasma—Serum or Urine.

Norm.

		SI Units
Anion Gap	7-17 mEq/L	7-17 mmol/L
Carbon Dioxide, Total Content		
Adults	22-30 mEq/L or 38-50 mm Hg	22-30 mmol/L
Panic levels	<15 mEq/L or >50 mEq/L	<15 mmol/L >50 mmol/L
Neonates-2 years	32-44 mm Hg	
Children >2 years	22-26 mEq/L	22-26 mmol/L
Chloride		
Children and adults	97-107 mEq/L	97-107 mmol/L
Premature infants	95-110 mEq/L	95-110 mmol/L
Full-term infants	96-106 mEq/L	96-106 mmol/L
Panic levels	<80 mEq/L or >115 mEq/L	<80 mmol/L or >115 mmol/L
Potassium		
Adults	3.5-5.3 mEq/L	3.5-5.3 mmol/L
Premature Infants		
Cord blood	5.0-10.2 mEq/L	5.0-10.2 mmol/L
2 days	3.0-6.0 mEq/L	3.0-6.0 mmol/L
Full-Term Newborn		
Cord blood	5.6-12.0 mEq/L	5.6-12.0 mmol/L
Newborn	3.7-5.0 mEq/L	3.7-5.0 mmol/L
Infants	4.1-5.3 mEq/L	4.1-5.3 mmol/L
Children	3.4-4.7 mEq/L	3.4-4.7 mmol/L
Panic Levels		
Adults	<2.5 mEq/L or >6.6 mEq/L	<2.5 mmol/L or >6.6 mmol/L
Newborn	<2.5 mEq/L or >8.1 mEq/L	<2.5 mmol/L or >8.1 mmol/L
Sodium		
Adults	136-145 mEq/L	136-145 mmol/L
Umbilical cord	116-166 mEq/L	116-166 mmol/L
Infants	139-146 mEq/L	139-146 mmol/L
Children	138-145 mEq/L	138-145 mmol/L

Usage. Evaluate the four electrolytes at once and compare their relative values. Evaluate acid-base balance and determine the anion gap [$Na+ - (Cl^- + HCO_3^-)$]. Serum sodium levels <133 mEq/L seen in cerebral salt wasting syndrome.

Description. The electrolyte panel is a series of tests performed on one tube of blood. The tests commonly included are Anion gap—Blood; Carbon dioxide total count—Blood; Chloride—Serum; Potassium—Plasma or serum; and Sodium, Plasma—Serum or urine. See individual test listings for further description.

Professional Considerations
Consent form NOT required.

Preparation
1. Tube: Red topped, red/gray topped, or gold topped.
2. Do not allow the client to clench-unclench the hand before blood drawing.
3. Do NOT draw specimens during hemodialysis.

Procedure
1. Collect the specimen without a tourniquet or quickly after tourniquet application, to prevent stasis.
2. Using a 20-gauge or larger needle, draw a 5-mL blood sample.
3. Do not aspirate strongly or push plunger into the vacuum tube too forcefully.

Postprocedure Care
1. Write the collection time on the laboratory requisition.
2. Transport the specimen to the laboratory within 15 minutes.

Client and Family Teaching
1. Do NOT clench-unclench the fist before blood drawing.
2. Results are normally available within 24 hours.

Factors That Affect Results
1. Hemolysis of the specimen abnormally elevates the potassium level and invalidates results.
2. Hypoalbuminemia lowers anion gap.
Adjustment of anion gap (with albumin concentrations in g/L) = Observed anion gap + 0.25 × [(Normal albumin)(Observed albumin)]
If the albumin is given in g/dL, the factor is 2.50.

Other Data
1. Cognitive status assessed by the Mini-Mental Examination correlates to serum sodium and serum chloride levels in the elderly.
2. See individual test listings.

Electrolytes—Urine

See also Chloride—Urine; Potassium—Urine; Sodium, Plasma—Serum or Urine.

Norm.

		SI Units
Chloride		
Adults	110-250 mEq/24 hours or 9 g/L	110-250 mmol/day
Children	15-115 mEq/L	15-115 mmol/L
Potassium		
Adults (intake dependent)	25-123 mEq/24 hours	25-123 mmol/day
Children	17-57 mEq/24 hours	17-57 mmol/day
Sodium		
Adults	75-200 mEq/24 hours	75-200 mmol/day
Children		
Newborn 6-10 years	14-40 mEq/24 hours	14-40 mmol/day
Females	20-69 mEq/24 hours	20-69 mmol/day
Males 10-14 years	41-115 mEq/24 hours	41-115 mmol/day
Females	48-168 mEq/24 hours	48-168 mmol/day
Males	63-177 mEq/24 hours	63-177 mmol/day

Usage. Evaluate renal function and fluid volume status by noting the amount of each electrolyte excreted and determine the anion gap $[(Na^+ + K^+) - Cl^-]$. A ratio of urine sodium to urine chloride of >1.16 identifies 51.6% of persons with bulimia nervosa.

Description. Urine electrolyte testing involves a series of tests performed on a sample of urine. The urine specimen may be random or a timed 12-hour or 24-hour urine. Tests commonly included are Chloride—Urine; Potassium—Urine; and Sodium, Plasma—Serum or urine. See individual test listings for further description.

Professional Considerations
Consent form NOT required.

Preparation
1. Obtain a specimen container, a 3-L container without preservatives, or a pediatric urine collection device or bag and tape, depending on whether the sample is to be a random sample or a 24-hour urine collection.
2. Write the beginning time of the collection on the laboratory requisition and the specimen container.
3. Note the diuretic or glucocorticoid therapy on the laboratory requisition.

Procedure
1. Obtain a random fresh urine specimen from a void or a urinary catheter drainage bag.
2. For a 24-hour specimen, discard the first morning urine specimen.
3. Save all the urine voided for 24 hours in a refrigerated, clean, 3-L container without preservatives. Document the quantity of the urine output during the specimen collection period. Include urine voided at the end of the 24-hour period. For catheterized clients, keep the drainage bag on ice and empty the urine into the collection container hourly.
4. Pediatric or infant specimen collection:
   a. Place the child in a supine position with the knees flexed and the hips externally rotated and abducted.
   b. Cleanse, rinse, and thoroughly dry the perineal area.
   c. To prevent the child from removing the collection device or bag, a diaper may be placed over the genital area.
   d. *Females:* Tape the pediatric collection device or bag to the perineum. Starting at the area between the anus and vagina, apply the device or bag in an anterior direction.
   e. *Males:* Place the pediatric collection device or bag over the penis and scrotum and tape it to the perineal area.
   f. Empty the collection device or bag into the refrigerated collection container hourly.

Postprocedure Care
1. For a 24-hour specimen, compare the urine quantity in the specimen container with the urinary output record for the test. If the specimen contains less urine than what was recorded as output, some of the sample may have been discarded, invalidating the test.
2. Document the quantity of urine and the collection ending time on the laboratory requisition.
3. Send the specimen to the laboratory and refrigerate it.
4. See also individual test listings.

Client and Family Teaching
1. Save all the urine voided in the 24-hour period and urinate before defecating to avoid loss of urine. Avoid contaminating the urine with toilet tissue or stool. If any urine is accidentally discarded, discard the entire specimen and restart the collection the next day.

Factors That Affect Results
1. All the urine voided for the 24-hour period must be included in the 24-hour specimen to avoid a falsely low result.
2. For spot urine testing, potassium levels are higher at night than in the morning, and sodium levels are higher in the morning than at night.
3. See also individual test listings.

Other Data
1. Urine osmolality is often requested at the same time as urine electrolytes.
2. See also individual test listings.

E

Electromyelography

See **Electromyography and Nerve Conduction Studies**—Diagnostic.

Electromyography (EMG) and Nerve Conduction Studies (Electromyelogram)—Diagnostic

Norm. Electromyelogram: no electrical activity at rest. A variety of abnormal electrical patterns produced by diseased muscles at rest and during activity exist and may allow diagnosis of specific myopathy. Nerve conduction studies: normal nerve conduction varies depending on the nerve studied but is in the range 40-70 m/sec.

Usage. Nerve conduction studies combined with electromyography can provide useful clues to the existence of neuromuscular disease, primary myopathy, and neuropathic states. Specific disease states that are diagnosed with these techniques include carpal tunnel syndrome, myasthenia gravis, various forms of myositis, Guillain-Barré syndrome, and the myopathies. Electromyography of the pelvic floor muscles may be conducted as part of urodynamics testing.

Description. *Electromyogram*: One or more needles are inserted into the muscle to be studied. Electrodes are also attached to the skin. Recordings are made at rest after an interval has elapsed subsequent to the needle insertion. Recordings are repeated during a period of voluntary muscle contraction by the client.
Nerve conduction study: Electroconductive gel is applied over the nerve to be studied. Electrodes are attached to the nerve to be studied, and an electric current is applied so that velocity measurements can be made. This process can be performed for both motor and sensory nerves.

Professional Considerations
Consent form IS required.

Risks
Bleeding, interference with pacemaker function, infection at the site of needle insertion.

Contraindications
History of bleeding disorder or chronic anticoagulation therapy, pacemaker.

Preparation
1. Client will bathe or shower the day of the test.
2. Avoid skin cosmetic products.
3. The physician ordering the tests may ask the client to avoid tobacco and caffeine for several hours before the procedures.
4. Fasting before the tests is not necessary.
5. Just before beginning the procedure, take a "time out" to verify the correct client, procedure, and site.

Procedure
1. *Electromyography*: Most procedures are performed with the client either in the sitting or in the supine position. Electrodes are inserted into the muscle of interest and recordings are made at rest and during voluntary contraction of the muscle. For pelvic floor EMG, a combination of needles or copper wires will be inserted into the pelvic floor periurethral muscles and small patches may also be applied to the anal mucosa. The test takes from 30 minutes to an hour to complete.
2. *Nerve conduction study*: A conductive gel is applied to the skin over the nerve of interest, and electrodes are attached at either end of the segment to be studied. An electric current is applied to the nerve segment, and the conduction velocity is measured.

Postprocedure Care
1. The conductive gel is cleaned from the skin.
2. Hospitalized clients may require transport from the testing location back to their rooms.
3. Local application of ice or a cold pack may alleviate postprocedure pain associated with EMG needle placement.

Client and Family Teaching
1. The needles used in the EMG procedure are disposable, and the risk of infection is consequently minimal.

2. Pain may occur during and after insertion of the EMG needles. This is generally minor, and a local anesthetic is not usually given. Minor discomfort may be associated with the nerve conduction procedure.

Factors That Affect Results

1. Cooperation of the client.
2. Drugs that affect neuromuscular conduction.
3. Artifacts can occur when there are electrical potentials in the environment, which can be generated by microwave ovens, other electrical devices, room lighting, and high voltage fluoroscopic generators.

Performing the test in a lead-lined room can prevent such artifacts. Technical artifacts related to placement of the electrodes and physical artifacts related to client movement are also possible.

Other Data

1. These techniques may be helpful in the early detection of subclinical diabetic neuropathy.
2. Portable equipment is available and can be used in the performance of these procedures.
3. This application has primarily been used in the workplace to screen large numbers of workers for carpal tunnel syndrome.

Electromyography (EMG)

See Electromyography and Nerve Conduction Studies—Diagnostic.

Electron Beam CT

See Computed Tomography of the Body—Diagnostic.

Electron Microscopy (Cardiomyopathy, Nerve Tissue, Small Bowel Mucosa)—Diagnostic

Norm. No abnormality or disease noted.

Usage. Doxorubicin HCl (Adriamycin) cardiotoxicity, cardiomyopathy, Hand-Schüller-Christian disease, liver disease, neuropathy, renal disease, tumors, and Whipple's disease.

Description. An examination of a thin section of tissue for microscopic evaluation. Used to define tumor classification when light microscopy is insufficient. Environmental scanning electron microscope allows wet insulating samples to be imaged without specimen preparation.

Professional Considerations

Consent form NOT required for this test.

Preparation

1. Prepare for the surgical excision.
2. Obtain a sterile container filled with 0.9% saline.

Procedure

1. Obtain a fresh unfixed tissue specimen and place it into a container of 0.9% saline.

Postprocedure Care

1. Deliver the specimen to the laboratory immediately so that the proper fixative can be applied.

Client and Family Teaching

1. Results are normally available within 72 hours.

Factors That Affect Results

1. Specimens should NOT be placed into formalin.

Other Data

1. Useful in diagnosing or differentiating leukemia or lymphoma, sarcoma, and endocrine and brain tumors.
2. This is an expensive and time-consuming procedure.

Electronic Crossmatch

See Type-and-Crossmatch—Blood.

Electronystagmography (Eye Movement, ENG) Test—Diagnostic

Norm. Normal eye movement free of nystagmus.

Usage. Brain lesion, dizziness (not valuable in community-derived sample of dizzy elderly subjects >65 years old), falls in elderly >65 years of age (best fall indicator is ocular motor battery), unilateral hearing loss, neurotoxicity related to antiepileptic drugs, nystagmus, tinnitus, and vertigo.

Description. Technique for recording eye movements allowing exact quantification of physiologic and pathologic nystagmus. The test picks up subtle spontaneous nystagmus and also helps differentiate peripheral from central nystagmus. The battery of tests includes visual ocular control, the search for pathologic nystagmus with fixation and with eyes open in darkness, and measurement of induced physiologic nystagmus (caloric and rotational). The test can be helpful in identifying a vestibular lesion and localizing it within the peripheral and central pathways. It also provides serial tracings to compare a client's pattern over time.

Professional Considerations

Consent form NOT required.

Risks

Water caloric test: perforation of the eardrum.

Contraindications

In clients with pacemakers or with a perforated eardrum.

Preparation

1. None.

Procedure

1. Small electrodes are taped to the skin on either side of each eye.
2. Tests include calibration, gaze nystagmus, pendulum tracking, optokinetics, positional tests, and water caloric test.
   a. *Calibration test*: The client holds head straight and fixed and follows with the eyes a stylus, from the right side to the middle and then to the left side.
   b. *Gaze nystagmus test*: The client must close his or her eyes and perform an arithmetic task for 30 seconds while eye motion is recorded. Then eye motion is recorded with the eyes open and fixed looking straight ahead.
   c. *Pendulum tracking*: A 20-second eye motion recording is made as the client looks straight ahead and follows a pendulum with the eyes. This is followed by a 30-second recording of eye motion as the client stares straight ahead with the eyes closed.
   d. *Optokinetics test*: Two 30-second recordings of eye motion are made as the client stares straight ahead and then follows a target across the visual field from right to left and then from left to right.
   e. *Positional tests*: A 5-second baseline recording of eye motion is obtained, followed by a recording of eye motion as the client follows the following nine commands:
      i. "With head erect and eyes forward, turn your head quickly to the right."
      ii. "With head erect and eyes forward, turn your head quickly to the left."
      iii. "Sit erect with eyes closed and quickly lie flat on your back with your eyes still closed."
      iv. "Sit up quickly from the lying position with your eyes closed."
      v. "Lie on your back with your eyes closed and quickly turn your body and head to the right."
      vi. "Lie on your back with your eyes closed and turn your body and head to the left."
      vii. "Sit erect with your eyes forward and closed and lay your head back quickly so that it hangs over the back of the chair."
      viii. "Quickly pick up your head from over the back of the chair to the erect position."
      ix. "Quickly put your head back to the right so that it hangs over the back right side of the headrest on

the chair and then repeat this by putting your head to the left so that it hangs over the back left side of the headrest on the chair."

f. *Water caloric test*: The client is positioned at a 30-degree head-of-bed elevation with the eyes closed. Water is instilled directly into the ear canal so that it hits the tympanic membrane, while eye motion is simultaneously recorded. This is followed by a 60-second recording with the eyes open and a final recording with the eyes closed until nystagmus disappears or for 3 minutes.

Postprocedure Care
1. Remove electrodes.
2. Assess for dizziness, nausea, or weakness.

Client and Family Teaching
1. The test takes less than 1 hour.
2. The client must be cooperative and able to follow commands to ensure the accuracy of the test results.

Factors That Affect Results
1. CNS stimulants will increase eye movement, and depressants will decrease eye movement.
2. Poor eyesight.
3. Loose electrodes.
4. Requires considerable cooperation on the part of the client and skill on the part of the operator in conducting and interpreting the test.

Other Data
1. Results are reported as normal, borderline, or abnormal.

Electrophysiologic Study (EPS)—Diagnostic

Norm. Negative for ability to induce dysrhythmias. Normal cardiac conduction system mapping. No reentrant pathways identified.

Usage. To document the anatomy and physiologic substrates of episodic dysrhythmias by reproducing them so that the mechanism can be identified. Helps diagnose cardiac conduction defects, circuit reentry, ectopic foci, syncope of unexplained cause, tachydysrhythmias, and ventricular preexcitation syndromes; evaluates the effectiveness of antidysrhythmic medications or ablation; helps determine proper choice of a pacemaker; maps the cardiac conduction system before ablation; determines the need for an implanted defibrillator to prevent sudden cardiac death; and records intracardiac electrocardiograms.

Description. Electrophysiologic study involves the introduction of an electrode catheter under fluoroscopy through a peripheral vein or artery and into the cardiac chambers or sinuses and the performance of programmed electrical stimulation of the heart. Clients who may require EPS include survivors of sudden cardiac death, those with syncope with other than cardiac causes ruled out, and clients with dysrhythmias. Clients who usually require repeat EPS are those who have undergone antidysrhythmic therapy or catheter ablation since the last study. EPS is usually performed in a special laboratory or operating room by a cardiologist, with a specially trained registered nurse and a technician in attendance, certified in ACLS (Advanced Cardiac Life Support).

Professional Considerations
Consent form IS required.

Risks
Arterial injury (rare), cardiac perforation or rupture, cerebrovascular accident, death, fatal dysrhythmias, hemorrhage (rare), infection, insertion-site hematoma, major venous thrombosis, myocardial infarction, pericardial effusion, pulmonary embolus.
Contraindications
Bleeding disorders, thrombocytopenia. Sedatives are contraindicated in clients with central nervous system depression.

Preparation
1. Antidysrhythmic drugs are usually discontinued for several days before the test, when tolerated, for initial EPS. For evaluation of effectiveness of antidysrhythmic therapy, drug levels should reach a steady state before EPS. This may take several days or even a few weeks for drugs such as amiodarone.

2. The client should fast from food overnight and from fluids for 4 hours before the test.
3. Establish intravenous access.
4. If left ventricular stimulation that requires an arterial EPS route is planned, preheparinization may be prescribed.
5. Have emergency cart and defibrillator or cardioverter readily available.
6. A sedative may be prescribed.
7. Obtain baseline vital signs. Monitor vital signs and level of consciousness continuously throughout the procedure. Observe respiratory status closely throughout the procedure, especially if a sedative is administered.
8. Just before beginning the procedure, take a "time out" to verify the correct client, procedure, and site.

Procedure

1. The client is positioned on the procedure table, and the peripheral pulses distal to the insertion site are marked. The location and baseline quality of the pulses are documented.
2. A baseline electrocardiogram is obtained. The leads are left in place for continuous cardiac monitoring.
3. The insertion site is cleansed with povidone-iodine solution, allowed to dry, and draped.
4. An introducer (sheath, Cordis) catheter is introduced, using the Seldinger technique, through a femoral, brachial, subclavian, or jugular vein. An arterial approach is used for stimulation of the left ventricle. A size 5F, 6F, or 7F electrode catheter is advanced under fluoroscopy to the heart.
5. Intracardiac electrocardiograms are recorded.
6. After proper catheter position is verified, the following or any combination may be performed, depending on the purpose of the study (an amnestic such as midazolam may be administered before induction of dysrhythmias):
   a. Mapping of the electrical system and pathways, with characterization of the electrical properties of the cardiac conduction system.
   b. Measurement of conduction times, refractory periods, and recovery times of different portions of the heart.
   c. Pacing of the atria may be performed, and extra stimuli may be added at specific intervals, to evaluate whether they can stimulate dysrhythmias.
   d. Attempts to induce dysrhythmias by delivery of a small electrical charge to specific locations of the chamber walls.
   e. Overdrive pacing.
   f. Antidysrhythmic drug effectiveness may be evaluated by administration of the drug to terminate stimulated dysrhythmias.
7. Induced dysrhythmias that are poorly tolerated (that is, cause hypotension, loss of consciousness) may be terminated by overdrive pacing, cardioversion, or defibrillation.
8. The catheter is removed, and pressure is applied to the site for 10 minutes, or at least until 10 minutes after bleeding stops. A pressure dressing is placed over the site.

Postprocedure Care

1. Assess and document the following every 15 minutes × 4, then every 30 minutes × 4, then hourly × 4, and then every 4 hours until 24 hours after the procedure:
   a. Vital signs.
   b. Insertion site for bleeding or hematoma.
   c. Color, motion, temperature, sensation, and the presence and quality of pulses in the extremity distal to the insertion site as compared to baseline value, and those for the opposite extremity. Notify the physician of any changes from baseline assessment.
2. If deep sedation was used, follow institutional protocol for post sedation monitoring. Typical monitoring includes continuous ECG monitoring and pulse oximetry, with continual assessments (every 5-15 minutes) of airway, vital signs, and neurologic status until the client is lying quietly awake, is breathing independently, and responds appropriately to commands spoken in a normal tone.
3. For bleeding at insertion site, apply firm pressure for 10 minutes. If bleeding continues after 10 minutes, continue holding pressure, and notify physician.
4. A sandbag may be placed over the insertion site for several hours.

5. Maintain continuous electrocardiographic monitoring and observe for dysrhythmias for at least 24 hours.
6. Resume diet.
7. If antidysrhythmic drugs were administered during EPS or begun after EPS, observe cardiac monitor pattern for their effect.

Client and Family Teaching
1. Fast from food from midnight the night before the procedure. Fluids may be taken up to 4 hours before the test, but no caffeine is permitted.
2. The procedure takes up to 8 hours.
3. Because this procedure can be frightening, good explanations are necessary. Inform the client of the following information: you will have to lie as motionless as possible on your back, and feelings of flushing, anxiousness, dizziness, and palpitations are common during EPS. EPS will cause abnormal heart rhythms, and the doctors, nurses, and technicians are skilled at quickly treating these rhythms. The procedure may take 1-8 hours. After EPS, you must lie with the extremity distal to the insertion site motionless for

several (usually 8) hours, and a sandbag may be in place over the site. Vital signs, the insertion site, and affected extremity circulation will be checked frequently after EPS.

Factors That Affect Results
1. Antidysrhythmic drugs that are not completely cleared from the body before initial EPS may result in a falsely normal study.

Other Data
1. Subsequent treatment based on EPS findings may include antidysrhythmic drugs, ablation, implantation of an implantable cardioverter defibrillator (ICD), implantation of a rapid atrial pacemaker (overdrive pacing), combinations of the above, or other techniques.
2. African-Americans have significantly lower rates of utilization of EPS and ICD procedures and higher subsequent death rates (Alexander et al, 2002).
3. EPS can elicit latent atrial flutter or tachycardia in clients with refractory atrial fibrillation.
4. See also His bundle electrography—Diagnostic.

EMG
See **Electromyography and Nerve Conduction Studies**—Diagnostic.

Endometrium, Anaerobic—Culture

Norm. No growth of anaerobic bacteria.

Positive. Actinomycosis, endometriosis, and pelvic inflammatory disease.

Description. The endometrium is the interior uterine mucosal layer formed of epithelium. This is the uterine layer that proliferates and sheds in response to hormonal effects throughout the menstrual cycle. Because the uterus is an anaerobic environment, anaerobic endometrial infections may cause symptoms of severe abdominal pain and bloating, menstrual irregularities, and infertility problems. Endometrial culture is performed when any of the above is suspected.

Professional Considerations
Consent form NOT required.

Preparation
1. Obtain disinfectant, a sterile syringe, a vaginal speculum, and an anaerobic transport tube.

Procedure
1. Place the client in the dorsal lithotomy position with feet in the stirrups and drape her for comfort and privacy.
2. Insert the vaginal speculum and disinfect the cervix; then, using a sterile syringe, aspirate material through the cervical os.
3. Expel air bubbles from the syringe and place the collected material into the anaerobic tube.

Postprocedure Care
1. Provide a sanitary pad for the client for minor bleeding.

2. Transport the specimen to the laboratory within 30 minutes.
3. Include the site of the specimen and list any recent antibiotic therapy on the laboratory requisition.

Client and Family Teaching

1. A feeling of pelvic cramping similar to a strong menstrual cramp is normally felt during insertion of the aspiration tube through the cervix. Prostaglandin inhibitors, such as ibuprofen or naproxen sodium, will lessen the discomfort and may be taken before or after the procedure, or at both times.
2. Minor spotting on a sanitary pad is normal during the 24 hours after the procedure.

3. Notify the physician for excessive bleeding or purulent drainage, increasing pelvic pain, or temperature >101 degrees F (38.3 degrees C).
4. Take showers, rather than tub baths, for 3-4 days.
5. Do not have sexual relations for 7 days after the procedure.
6. Results are normally available within 72 hours.

Factors That Affect Results

1. Do not refrigerate the sample(s).

Other Data

1. This test is not optimal for fungus culture.
2. Actinomycosis may be associated with endometritis and pelvic inflammatory disease from use of IUD contraception.

Endomysial Antibody (EMYA)—Serum

Norm. No endomysial antibody detected.

Usage. Noninvasive measure for screening and diagnosis of celiac sprue and duodenal villous atrophy (78% sensitivity). May be used with jejunal biopsy, a definitive diagnostic standard.

Description. Indirect immunofluorescent test that measures endomysial antibodies that react against the endomysial component of smooth muscle in the duodenum and jejunum. With a positive endomysial antibody titer, there is a suggested association between celiac disease and sclerosing cholangitis, primary biliary cirrhosis, autoimmune connective tissue disease, insulin-dependent diabetes mellitus, or inflammatory bowel disease. It has approximately 80% sensitivity and 95% specificity in untreated clients.

Professional Considerations
Consent form NOT required.

Preparation

1. Tube: Red topped or red/gray topped.

Procedure

1. *Adults:* Draw a 4-mL blood sample.
2. *Children*: Draw a 2-mL blood sample.

Postprocedure Care

1. None.

Client and Family Teaching

1. Test results will be available in a few days.
2. Dietary therapy with removal of all foods containing wheat, rye, and barley gluten.

Factors That Affect Results

1. Current or recent cigarette smoking associated with EMA-negative status.

Other Data

1. The serum is stable for 7 days if refrigerated and 1 year if frozen.
2. Celiac Sprue Association telephone: 877-272-4272; website: http://www.csaceliacs.info (USA).

Endoscopic Retrograde Cholangiopancreatography (ERCP)—Diagnostic

Norm. Patent bile ducts, duodenal papilla, pancreatic ducts, and gallbladder.

Usage. Determine the cause of cirrhosis, evaluate jaundice, obtain tissue samples

from the pancreatobiliary tree, and diagnose cholangitis, pancreatic cancer, pancreatitis, pancreatic cysts, pancreatic ductal lesions, pancreas divisum, and papillary stenosis. After the ERCP, by endoscopy, cysts can be drained, stones can be removed from the common bile duct, and stents can be placed across biliary or pancreatic strictures.

Description. Endoscopic retrograde cholangiopancreatography (ERCP) is the radiographic viewing of the hepatobiliary tree and pancreatic ducts through an endoscope using contrast medium injected through the ampulla of Vater. ERCP is used for detection of common bile duct stones when the probability for this condition is high. A newer test—endoscopic ultrasound (EUS)—is also used for detection of stones in the common bile duct. EUS is less risky because it does not involve exposure to radiation. See Endoscopic ultrasonography—Diagnostic.

Professional Considerations
Consent form IS required.

Risks
Cholangitis, dysrhythmias, hemorrhage, pancreatitis, perforation of intestine, peritonitis, sphincter of Oddi dysfunction.

Contraindications
Anticoagulant therapy, bleeding disorders, renal insufficiency, thrombocytopenia. Sedatives are contraindicated in clients with central nervous system depression.

Precautions
During pregnancy, risks of cumulative radiation exposure to the fetus from this and other previous or future imaging studies must be weighed against the benefits of the procedure. Although formal limits for client exposure are relative to this risk/benefit comparison, the United States Nuclear Regulatory Commission requires that the cumulative dose equivalent to an embryo/fetus from occupational exposure not exceed 0.5 rem (5 mSv). Radiation dosage to the fetus is proportional to the distance of the anatomy studied from the abdomen and decreases as pregnancy progresses. For pregnant clients, consult the radiologist/radiology department to obtain estimated fetal radiation exposure from this procedure.

Preparation
1. A kidney-ureter-bladder (KUB) flat-plate radiograph of the abdomen is taken to determine the absence of barium.
2. See Client and Family Teaching.
3. Obtain a topical anesthetic, sedative, and endoscope.

4. Establish intravenous access.
5. Antibiotic prophylaxis before ERCP results in fewer cases of cholangitis in clients with obstructive jaundice.
6. Just before beginning the procedure, take a "time out" to verify the correct client, procedure, and site.

Procedure
1. A topical anesthetic is applied to the oropharyngeal area.
2. Sedatives are given intravenously.
3. The client is placed in the left lateral position.
4. The endoscope is inserted through the esophagus to the stomach and then into the duodenum.
5. The client is then placed in the prone position, the papilla is cannulated with a catheter, and contrast dye is injected into the pancreatic or bile ductal system.
6. Several radiographs are taken, and then biopsy specimens may be taken if desired.

Postprocedure Care
1. The client should have nothing by mouth until the gag reflex returns.
2. If deep sedation was used, follow institutional protocol for post sedation monitoring. Typical monitoring includes continuous ECG monitoring and pulse oximetry, with continual assessments (every 5-15 minutes) of airway, vital signs, and neurologic status until the client is lying quietly awake, is breathing independently, and responds appropriately to commands spoken in a normal tone.
3. Assess for the complications of urinary retention and intra-abdominal hematoma.
4. Transient rise in serum liver enzymes is common up to 24 hours after ERCP.

Client and Family Teaching
1. Fast from food and fluids for 12 hours before and after the procedure until the gag reflex returns.
2. The procedure takes approximately 1 hour.

Factors That Affect Results
1. Retained barium can obstruct viewing.

Other Data
1. Up to 95% of the pancreatic duct and 85% of the biliary duct can be visualized by an experienced physician.

2. Useful in differentiating surgical from medical jaundice.
3. Therapeutic ERCP has a significantly higher complication rate (4.6%) and higher death rate (0.5%) when compared to diagnostic ERCP.
4. Magnetic resonance cholangiopancreatography (MRCP) may make diagnostic ERCP obsolete and is more effective in the evaluation of intrahepatic stones. ERCP is not well-suited for intrahepatic stones because of the frequency of biliary strictures and the angulation of the ducts. ERCP is, however, more sensitive in detecting common bile duct stones than is computed tomography cholangiography.
5. For detection of pancreatobiliary malignant obstruction, MRCP, ERCP, and EUS provide similar diagnostic results.
6. Factors that may indicate the presence of gallstones include clinical jaundice or elevated bilirubin, liver function tests, and common bile duct dilation (identified via ultrasound).

Endoscopic Ultrasonography (EUS)—Diagnostic

Norm. Requires interpretation. Lipomas image as bright and echogenic. Tumors are usually dark and hypoechogenic, often with irregular borders.

Usage. Gastrointestinal (GI) cancer staging; imaging of lymph node metastasis from the GI tract to help determine TNM staging; screening for cancer in clients with Barrett's esophagus; screening for recurrence of GI cancer of all types. Provides guidance for fine-needle aspiration biopsies of the abdominal organs and lymph nodes. EUS-guided FNA may help diagnose lung masses adjacent to the esophagus. More sensitive than upper GI endoscopy for diagnosing varices. Evaluation for the presence of stones in the common bile duct. More accurate than any other tests for detection of pancreatic cancer. Simple tool to assess and diagnose aberrant right subclavian artery (ARSA). Some therapeutic uses are also being investigated.

Description. One of the newest uses for ultrasonography involves taking ultrasound images from within the GI tract. EUS improves diagnostic accuracy by reducing artifacts that occur from anatomic structures and gas when imaging from the exterior of the body. Because the ultrasound probe is much closer to the area being examined, higher frequency ultrasound can be used, which normally is not an option when imaging from greater distances. Higher frequencies can provide clearer images of smaller areas and better detail of the layers of the GI tract, which are often the site where cancer begins.

Professional Considerations
Consent form IS required.

Risks
Vasovagal bradycardia and drug-induced tachycardia are likely dysrhythmias; esophageal perforation; bleeding; transient hypoxemia; oversedation.
Contraindications
Esophageal obstructions, stenosis, fistula, or dysphagia; history of radiation therapy to the esophagus or surrounding area (mediastinum); acute penetrating chest injuries. Neonates and young children are not candidates because of the unavailability of specially sized scopes. Sedatives are contraindicated in clients with central nervous system depression and in clients who cannot tolerate lying flat.

Preparation
1. See Client and Family Teaching.
2. Document clinical indications on the test requisition. This helps guide the interpreter to provide the most relevant test interpretation.
3. Start an IV infusion at KVO (keep vein open) rate for administration of sedation or emergency medications.
4. Remove dentures and eyeglasses. Have the client void before the procedure.
5. Obtain local anesthetic spray.
6. A drying agent is typically given to reduce secretions (that is, glycopyrrolate 0.1-0.2 mg IV). Some clients require a small IV dose of an antianxiety agent (such as midazolam or diazepam). Prophylactic

E

antibiotics are usually given if the client has a prosthetic valve.

7. Just before beginning the procedure, take a "time out" to verify the correct client, procedure, and site.

Procedure

1. The client is monitored continuously: heart rate and rhythm by cardiac monitor, blood pressure by noninvasive monitor, and O_2 by pulse oximetry.

2. Position the client in the left lateral decubitus position.

3. Topical anesthesia per physician preference is used to numb the throat and suppress the gag reflex. This may be repeated several times during the procedure.

4. The client should be awake enough to follow commands, but drowsy. This procedure may also be performed on a fully anesthetized or intubated client.

5. The client is asked to open the mouth and flex the neck forward in a chin-to-chest position.

6. The lidocaine-lubricated probe is inserted, and the client is asked to swallow.

7. A small flexible tube equipped with an ultrasonic probe and camera at the tip is inserted through the mouth or rectum and advanced into the GI tract. Ultrasonic images are taken at points appropriate to the clinical indications for the procedure.

8. The nurse remains with the client to monitor respiratory status, vital signs, and cardiac rhythm and to assess the need for further sedation or suctioning.

Postprocedure Care

1. Continue assessment of respiratory status. If deep sedation was used, follow institutional protocol for post sedation monitoring. Typical monitoring includes continuous ECG monitoring and pulse oximetry with continual assessments (every 5-15 minutes) of airway, vital signs, and neurologic status until client

reaches level 3, 2, or 1 on the Ramsay Sedation scale.

2. Once the gag reflex has returned, the client can resume fluids. Full diet is not recommended until 3 hours after procedure.

Client and Family Teaching

1. This procedure involves having a narrow, flexible tube inserted through your mouth and esophagus into your stomach and small intestine and having an ultrasound picture taken from inside the body.

2. Fast for 6-8 hours before the test. Medications may be taken with a small amount of water as directed by the physician. You will have to remove your dentures and eyeglasses, but you should keep your hearing aid on so that you can hear the physician's instructions.

3. You will be given a sedative for the procedure. You should arrange for someone to drive you home because you may be drowsy after the procedure and will not be permitted to drive.

4. Do not eat or drink for 4-6 hours before the procedure. Take any prescription medications with a small sip of water.

5. Bowel preps may be ordered for lower EUS.

6. The test takes about 45 minutes.

7. The tongue and throat may feel swollen after the topical anesthetic; the mouth and lips will feel sticky and dry if a drying agent is used. Do not eat or drink after the procedure until the numbness is gone.

8. Home instructions: Promptly report persistent sore throat, dysphagia, stiff neck, and epigastric, substernal, or abdominal pain that worsens with breathing or movement.

Factors That Affect Results

1. None found.

Other Data

1. None found.

ENFD

See **Epidermal Nerve Fiber Density Test**—Specimen.

Entamoeba histolytica, Serologic Test—Blood

Norm. Negative, IHA titer <1:128, CF titer <1:8.

Positive. Diarrhea (inflammatory or HIV related), dysentery, liver abscess, lung abscess, perianal ulcers, perineal ulcers, salpingitis. A fourfold rise in titer supports the diagnosis of *Entamoeba* infection.

Negative. Bacterial infection of the intestines.

Description. *Entamoeba histolytica* is a protozoon that causes intestinal disease transmitted in infected food and water by flies and by direct contact, causing acute diarrhea. Abscesses may form on the liver (75% found in right lobe), lungs, and brain, causing death. Prevalence in the United States is lowest in winter (22%-27%) and highest between July and October (36%-43%). This test cannot distinguish between amoebic liver abscess and intestinal amebiasis.

Professional Considerations
Consent form NOT required.

Preparation
1. See Client and Family Teaching.
2. Tube: Red topped, red/gray topped, or gold topped.

Procedure
1. Draw a 4-mL blood sample.

Postprocedure Care
1. Resume previous diet.
2. Draw convalescent sample 14-21 days after acute sample.

Client and Family Teaching
1. Fast from food and fluids from midnight until after the test has been completed.
2. *Entamoeba histolytica* amebiasis is treated with metronidazole 750 mg TID for 10 days (for extraintestinal form), paromomycin 30 mg/kg in 3 divided doses for 7 days, or diloxanide 500 mg TID for 10 days (for intraluminal and extraintestinal trophozoites), except during pregnancy.
3. Return in 2-3 weeks to have a follow-up sample drawn. This will help determine whether the infection is responding to treatment.

Factors That Affect Results
1. Ulcerative colitis may cause false-positive results.

Other Data
1. 99% of serologic test results are positive 1 week after infection and may remain positive for as long as 2 years after curative therapy.
2. *Entamoeba histolytica* amebiasis is a reportable disease in most areas.

EOS

See **Differential Leukocyte Count—Peripheral Blood.**

Eosinophil Count

See **Differential Leukocyte Count—Peripheral Blood.**

EP

See **Protoporphyrin, Free Erythrocyte—Blood; Electrolytes Panel—Blood.**

Ephedrine

See **Amphetamines—Blood.**

Epidermal Nerve Fiber Density Test (ENFD)—Specimen

Norm. *Thigh:* 21.1±10.4 per millimeter (mean±SD); 60% higher than calf specimen
Calf: 13.8±6.7 per millimeter at the distal part of the leg

Values at or below the fifth percentile of reported norms are considered abnormal and diagnostic for small diameter nerve fiber neuropathy (McArthur, Stocks, Hauer et al, 1998).

	Fibers/Millimeter Length of Epidermis		
	Abnormal, Positive for SDNF Neuropathy	Low-Normal Range (Suspicious for Early or Mild Neuropathy)	Lower Limit of Normal
Thigh	Less than 6.8	6.8 to 8	6.8
Calf	Less than 5.4	5.4-5.7	5.4
Foot	Less than 3.1	3.1-4.5	3.1

Usage. A highly sensitive and specific test that helps detect small fiber neuropathy (SFN) of the sensory nerves when tests such as electromyography, nerve conduction studies, quantitative sensory testing, or laser-evoked potentials are negative. Also used to assess progression of this condition and response to treatment.

Description. Small diameter nerve fiber (SDNF) neuropathy is characterized by damage to the small nerve fibers located in the internal organs, skin, and nerves of the periphery of the body. When the unmyelinated and thin-myelinated small sensory nerve fibers are damaged, the symptoms that result include numbness, paresthesias, hypersensitivity to touch, and even small amounts of pressure, such as that of clothing on the skin, can cause pain. Routine evaluation for neuropathy includes electromyelogram (EMG) testing; however, this type of testing only measures large nerves. When an EMG test is negative, a tissue biopsy can be used to count the number of small fiber nerves to measure the density of sensory nerves that are small-fiber nerve tissue. This test is often used in conjunction with the sweat gland nerve fiber density test (SGNFD), which measures small nerve fiber density of autonomic nerve fibers, which can also be affected in small fiber neuropathy (Devigli, Tugnoli, Penza et al, 2008).

Professional Considerations
Consent form IS required.

Preparation
1. Obtain test kit. Place cool pack in freezer for return shipping.
2. Obtain 2% lidocaine, 1mL syringe, test kit vials containing Zamboni's fixative and dry sterile dressing, sterile scissors, and chemocautery solution.
3. See Client and Family Teaching.

Procedure
1. Cleanse the biopsy site with an alcohol swab.
2. Inject approximately 0.5 mL of 2% lidocaine with epinephrine in a 1-cm circle or "V" pattern around the site.
3. Obtain biopsy of the thigh, calf, or foot using a 3mm punch to a depth of 2 mm. Specific locations recommended are those where an established norm is known:
   a. *Thigh:* at the pubis level, 20 cm distal to the iliac spine
   b. *Calf:* lateral side, 10 cm above the lateral malleolus
   c. *Foot:* dorsum, above the extensor digitorum brevis muscle.
4. Remove the sample without damaging the epithelium by pushing down on the epithelium next to the sample, then attaching forceps to the dermal side and lifting the sample, then cutting the base to detach the specimen.
5. Split sample into two vials and label with location of the biopsy site.
6. Leave in fixative overnight. Pour off fixative, then rinse with buffer solution × 2. Fill vial with cryoprotectant, then place inside a cool pack and mail to the testing lab.
7. The count includes separating the sample into 5 subsets, then counting the number of epidermal fibers that cross the basement membrane.

Postprocedure Care
1. Apply an aluminum-based chemocautery to the site. Apply pressure dressing to site.

2. Remove pressure, apply triple-antibiotic, then apply a dry sterile dressing.

Client and Family Teaching

1. The test is performed in a physician's office and takes about 15 minutes.
2. Expect bruising and mild aching at site for up to 24 hours. Leave the original dressing in place and keep the site dry for 1-2 days to minimize the risk of infection and bleeding. If bleeding occurs, apply firm pressure to site for 10 minutes. Once the dressing is removed, you will be able to shower normally and allow the site to get wet.
3. Although a highly sensitive test, normal results do not rule out the presence of neuropathy.
4. Results will be available within 2 weeks.

Factors That Affect Results

1. Sensitivity for detecting small fiber neuropathy is 88.4%. Specificity is 95%-97%.
2. Location of the biopsy affects results. The more distal the site, the lower the normal results.

Other Data

1. Small fiber neuropathy can be caused by a variety of conditions, including alcoholism, amyloidosis, diabetes (most common cause) (Lauria, Devigli, 2007), Fabry disease, inflammatory bowel disease, lupus, Lyme disease, malnutrition/nutritional deficiency, and Sjögren's syndrome.
2. See also Sweat gland nerve fiber density test—Specimen.

Epinephrine—Blood

See Catecholamines—Plasma.

EPS

See Electrophysiologic Study—Diagnostic.

Epstein-Barr Virus (EBV), Serology—Blood

Norm. Negative; no virus found.

Increased. Autoimmune thyroiditis, breast carcinoma, Burkitt's lymphoma, dysplasia, Epstein-Barr virus, gastric adenocarcinoma, head and neck tumors, HIV, Hodgkin's disease, hyperplasia, infectious hepatitis, infectious mononucleosis, lung carcinoma, lymphocytic leukemia, lymphoepithelioma, nasopharyngeal carcinoma, non-Hodgkin's lymphoma, post-transplant lymphoproliferative disorders in lung transplant, prostatic intraepithelial cancer, sarcoidosis, and systemic lupus erythematosus.

Description. Epstein-Barr virus is a B-lymphocyte human herpesvirus that is the causative agent of infectious mononucleosis. The mode of transmission is through direct contact with the saliva of an infected client. Signs and symptoms, after a 4- to 8-week incubation period, include malaise, anorexia, chills, fever, cervical lymphadenopathy, pharyngitis, splenomegaly, hepatitis, and peripheral atypical lymphocytosis. An Epstein-Barr virus panel includes four antibody levels: IgM VCA (viral capsid antigen), IgG VCA, EA (early antigen), and EBNA (Epstein-Barr nuclear antigen). The pattern of reactivity is helpful in distinguishing recent primary infection, reactivated infection, or remote inactive infection. Individual laboratories will give their reference range with the test results.

Professional Considerations

Consent form NOT required.

Preparation

1. Tube: Red topped, red/gray topped, or gold topped.
2. Write the date of the onset of illness on the laboratory requisition.

Procedure

1. Draw a 3-mL blood sample.

Postprocedure Care

1. Refrigerate the serum after separation.

Client and Family Teaching

1. Results are normally available within 72 hours.

Factors That Affect Results

1. Cytomegalovirus in clients who have had organ transplants will cause a positive result for EBV serology.
2. Posttransfusion reactions of blood and blood products will cause a temporary increase in EBV serologic features.
3. False-positive results occur in clients with collagen vascular disease such as rheumatoid arthritis, leukemia, lymphoma, or HIV.

Other Data

1. Up to 20% of people are negative for heterophil antibodies (see Monospot screen—Blood) with infectious mononucleosis.
2. In the presence of clinical findings of infectious mononucleosis with negative heterophil and specific viral antibody tests, primary cytomegalovirus infection should be considered.
3. Antibody titers for EBV are needed only if there is a question of a false-positive result on the Monistat rapid slide test for EBV.
4. Many people with chronic fatigue syndrome present with high antibody titers for EBV, but these are probably unrelated to the disease process.
5. IgG avidity assay is a supplementary test that distinguishes between acute and past infections better than the lysate immunoblot banding test.
6. EBV-associated lymphoproliferative disease is a life-threatening complication following hematopoietic stem cell transplantation. May be prevented with pre-emptive therapy with rituximab.
7. See also Monospot screen—Blood.

ERCP

See Endoscopic Retrograde Cholangiopancreatography—Diagnostic.

Ergonovine Maleate Test—Diagnostic

Usage. Aids in the diagnosis of coronary spasm during coronary arteriography, echocardiography, and electrophysiologic studies in clients with variant angina and no major occlusions of the coronary arteries.

Description. Ergonovine maleate (Ergotrate) stimulates contractions of vascular smooth muscle. It is administered during the cardiac procedure to produce and evaluate the effects of the resulting coronary artery spasm. The IV initial phase half-life is 1-5 minutes. The terminal phase half-life is 0.5-2.0 hours. This drug is no longer commercially available in the United States.

Professional Considerations
Consent form IS required.

Risks

Adverse drug effects may occur with ergonovine: nausea and vomiting, dizziness, headache, tinnitus, diaphoresis, palpitations, transient chest pain, dyspnea, thrombophlebitis, hematuria, water intoxication, nasal congestion, diarrhea, and allergic phenomena, including shock. Ergonovine-induced hypertension has been accompanied by headaches, severe dysrhythmias, seizures, and cerebrovascular accidents. Hypotension has also been reported. See also individual procedures for procedure-specific risks.

Contraindications or Precautions
Previous allergy to ergot, hypertension, pregnancy, toxemia, untreated hypocalcemia. Use ergonovine with extreme caution in the presence of renal or hepatic dysfunction, coronary artery disease, peripheral vascular disease, or sepsis. See also individual procedures for procedure-specific contraindications.

Preparation

1. See the listing for the procedure that is being performed.

Procedure

1. 0.1-0.4 mg of ergonovine maleate is given slowly intravenously with dilution.

Postprocedure Care

1. See the specific procedure for postprocedure care.
2. Observe for adverse drug effects (listed under Risks).

Client and Family Teaching

1. Inform the client about the approximate time length of the procedure that will be used with ergonovine administration.

Factors That Affect Results

1. None found.

Other Data

1. Hypertension may occur if the client is given the IV dose too rapidly or without dilution or if ergonovine is used along with a regional anesthetic or vasoconstrictor.
2. This drug is also used to stimulate contractions of the uterus to prevent and treat postpartum and postabortion hemorrhage caused by uterine atony.
3. Ergonovine test is not necessary for diagnosis of coronary artery spasm if client's exercise test or thallium perfusion scan is negative. Use of 123I-MIBG SPECT scan is feasible under these circumstances.

Erythrocyte

See Red Blood Cell—Blood.

Erythrocyte Protoporphyrin (EP)

See Protoporphyrin, Free Erythrocyte—Blood.

Erythrocyte Sedimentation Rate

See Sedimentation Rate, Erythrocyte—Blood.

Erythropoietin (EPO)—Serum

Norm. 7-36 milli-immunochemical units/mL.

Increased. Absolute erythrocytosis, acute lymphocytic leukemia, aplastic anemia, cerebellar hemangioblastomas, chronic obstructive pulmonary disease, hepatoma, high altitudes, hypoxia, kidney transplant rejection, myelodysplastic syndromes, nephrectomy, nephroblastoma, pheochromocytoma, pregnancy, renal cancer, renal cysts, and sickle cell anemia (thrombotic events). Drugs include hydroxyurea treatment in sickle cell disease.

Decreased. Acute neuropsychiatric porphyrias, autoimmune diseases, cancer, Hodgkin's disease, polycythemia rubra vera, and renal failure (chronic). Hemoperfusion with polymyxin B–immobilized fiber (PMX-F). EPO declines with repeated chemotherapy and in lead toxicity if blood values of lead are >32 mg/dL.

Description. Erythropoietin is a glycoprotein produced in the peritubular cells in the renal cortex of the kidney. It is released in response to renal hypoxia and stimulates the formation and development of erythrocytes in the bone marrow.

In healthy persons there is an inverse correlation between serum EPO and hematocrit: an exponential increase in EPO levels occurs as hematocrit decreases.

Professional Considerations

Consent form NOT required.

Preparation

1. Tube: Red topped, red/gray topped, or gold topped.

Procedure

1. Draw a 5-mL blood sample.

Postprocedure Care

1. Note on the laboratory requisition the amount of oxygen delivery because oxygen influences erythrocyte function.

Client and Family Teaching

1. The results are normally available within 24 hours.

Factors That Affect Results

1. Morning values are higher than afternoon values because of the diurnal rhythm of secretion.
2. Blood donation increases serum values.

Other Data

1. Useful in differentiating primary from secondary polycythemia.
2. May not reliably detect ectopic erythropoietin-like substances, and so neoplasia cannot be excluded.
3. Can be used as a measure of oxygenation in critically ill clients.

Esophageal Acidity Test (Tuttle Test)—Diagnostic

Norm.

Esophageal pH	>5.0
Esophageal reflux pH	≤5.0

Usage. Helps diagnose gastroesophageal reflux.

Description. A test that evaluates the integrity of the esophageal sphincter by measuring the pH of gastric and esophageal contents using a pH electrode attached to an esophageal catheter introduced through the mouth and esophagus. This test may be performed' with esophageal manometry.

Professional Considerations

Consent form IS required.

Risks

Aspiration and chemical bronchitis, vasovagal response.

Contraindications

Clients at high risk for poor tolerance of a vasovagal reaction (i.e., clients with known cardiac instability).

Preparation

1. See Client and Family Teaching.
2. Verify that the client has fasted.
3. Obtain a gastric catheter with a pH electrode, and 300 mL of 0.1% N hydrochloric acid (HCl).
4. Establish intravenous access. Have 0.9% saline and atropine on hand for use in the event a vasovagal response occurs.
5. The client should void just before the test.
6. Just before beginning the procedure, take a "time out" to verify the correct client, procedure, and site.

Procedure

1. Place the client in a high-Fowler's position.
2. Assess for vasovagal reaction, dysrhythmia, cyanosis, or coughing during the procedure.
3. Introduce the catheter with a pH electrode through the mouth to the back of the throat. Instruct the client to swallow, perform the Valsalva maneuver, or lift the legs to stimulate reflux to catheter level, and then determine the pH.
4. If the pH is normal, pass the catheter into the stomach, instill 300 mL of 0.1% N HCl over 3 minutes, and repeat step 2.

Postprocedure Care

1. Assess vital signs every 30 minutes × 2. Extend assessments as needed if the client was treated for a vasovagal reaction during the procedure.

Client and Family Teaching

1. Fast from midnight before the test and avoid smoking for 24 hours before the test.
2. Do not drink alcohol for 24 hours before the test.
3. The physician may want you to stop taking adrenergic blockers, antacids, anticholinergics, cimetidine, cholinergics, corticosteroids, and reserpine for 24 hours before the test. Check with your doctor before stopping any of your medicine.
4. You must swallow a catheter with a small electrode attached, which will measure the amount of acid in your esophagus and stomach. After the measurements are taken, the electrode will be slowly pulled out of your stomach.
5. The test takes 30 minutes or less.
6. The results are immediately available.

Factors That Affect Results

1. Antacids, anticholinergics, and cimetidine may decrease pH. Adrenergic blockers, cholinergics, corticosteroids, ethyl alcohol (ethanol), and reserpine may increase pH.

Other Data

1. None.

Esophageal Manometry—Diagnostic

E

Norm.

Esophageal pressures	Equal bilaterally
Motility	Smooth peristalsis proximally to distally
Spasm	None
Proportion of propulsive waves	56% median
Proportion of simultaneous waves	10%

Usage. Assessment and diagnosis of achalasia, dysphagia, esophageal reflux, spasm, motility abnormalities, and hiatal hernia.

Description. In esophageal manometry, a multilumen esophageal catheter is introduced through the mouth and oropharynx into the esophagus, and pressures along the esophagus are measured as the client performs a series of swallowing maneuvers. The test helps identify locations of abnormal contractions and peristalsis in the esophagus as well as areas of increased pressure that would indicate esophageal spasm and achalasia. The test may be performed with the esophageal acidity (Tuttle) test and the acid perfusion (Bernstein) test. It has been used extensively in the research setting in the study of esophageal motility disorders and is less commonly used in the clinical setting.

Professional Considerations

Consent form IS required.

Risks

Vasovagal reaction, dysrhythmia, cyanosis, or coughing.

Contraindications

Clients at high risk for poor tolerance of a vasovagal reaction (that is, clients with known cardiac instability).

Preparation

1. Verify that the client has fasted.
2. The client should void just before the test.
3. Obtain a gastric catheter, a swallowing sensor, water, and a syringe.
4. Just before beginning the procedure, take a "time out" to verify the correct client, procedure, and site.

Procedure

1. Place the client in a high-Fowler's position.
2. Introduce the catheter through the mouth to the back of the throat. Instruct the client to swallow the catheter several times until it has passed into the esophagus to the proper level.
3. Reposition the client in a supine position.
4. Attach the swallowing sensor to the client's neck.
5. The client is then asked to swallow small amounts of water injected into the mouth with a syringe, and the esophageal pressures are measured. This is followed by several dry swallows with corresponding pressure measurements.

Postprocedure Care

1. Assess vital signs every 30 minutes × 2. Extend assessments as needed if the client was treated for a vasovagal reaction during the procedure.
2. Observe for cholinergic side effects: bradycardia, diaphoresis, dizziness, flushing, muscle cramping, nausea, urinary urgency, and vomiting.

Client and Family Teaching

1. Fast from midnight before the test and avoid smoking for 24 hours before the test.
2. Do not drink alcohol or take any of these drugs within 2 days before the test: bethanechol, diltiazem or other calcium channel blockers, chlordiazepoxide, cimetidine, Donnatal, erythromycin, famotidine, Inderal or other beta blockers, lansoprazole, Levsin, metoclopramide, L-hyoscyamine, nitroglycerin or other nitrates, nizatidine, omeprazole, or ranitidine.
3. Arrange for transportation home because you will not be allowed to drive for 12-24 hours after receiving edrophonium chloride.
4. You must swallow a catheter with a small electrode attached. You will then be asked

to swallow several times, first with small amounts of water injected into the mouth and then without water. The catheter and neck sensor will measure the pressures in the esophagus as you swallow. After the measurements are taken, the catheter will be slowly pulled out of the stomach.

5. The test takes 30 minutes or less.

6. Irritation of nose and throat are common problems for up to 8 hours post procedure.

Factors That Affect Results
1. None.

Other Data
1. See also Esophageal acidity test—Diagnostic.

Esophageal Radiography—Diagnostic

Norm. Normal size and normal peristalsis.

Usage. Achalasia, esophageal varices, esophagitis, locating a foreign body, gastrointestinal (GI) bleeding, guidance for balloon dilatation of stricture, head and neck cancer, impaction, hiatal hernia, polyps.

Description. A radiographic and fluoroscopic examination of the esophagus for patency, structure, and motility. When examined with the stomach, duodenum, and upper jejunum, this test is known as an upper GI series.

Professional Considerations
Consent form IS required.

Risks
This procedure carries minimal risks.
Contraindications
Dysphagia, ileus.
Precautions
During pregnancy, risks of cumulative radiation exposure to the fetus from this and other previous or future imaging studies must be weighed against the benefits of the procedure. Although formal limits for client exposure are relative to this risk:benefit comparison, the United States Nuclear Regulatory Commission requires that the cumulative dose equivalent to an embryo/fetus from occupational exposure not exceed 0.5 rem (5 mSv). Radiation dosage to the fetus is proportional to the distance of the anatomy studied from the abdomen and decreases as pregnancy progresses. For pregnant clients, consult the radiologist/radiology department to obtain estimated fetal radiation exposure from this procedure.

Preparation
1. Verify that the client has fasted.

2. Just before beginning the procedure, take a "time out" to verify the correct client, procedure, and site.

Procedure
1. A plain radiograph of the esophagus is taken in the supine position.
2. Barium sulfate, approximately 400 mL, is then swallowed with the client in a standing position in front of the fluoroscope, and radiographs are again taken.
3. Follow-up radiographs at 24 hours may be performed.
4. The procedure takes 45 minutes.

Postprocedure Care
1. Resume diet.
2. Observe for passage of barium in the stool for 2-3 days.
3. A laxative may be needed to evacuate barium.
4. Encourage the oral intake of fluids to help prevent barium impaction.

Client and Family Teaching
1. Fast from food and fluids from midnight the day of the test.
2. Drink 4-6 glasses of water per day (unless contraindicated) for 2-3 days after the test to promote barium excretion. Barium stools will look grayish white. Notify health care provider if unable to pass barium in stool within 3 days.
3. Results are normally available within 24 hours.

Factors That Affect Results
1. Retained barium from a previous examination interferes with the quality of the radiographic images.

Other Data
1. Esophageal varices are difficult to identify and are usually a sign of liver cirrhosis.
2. Barium comes in flavors but is still described as unpleasant to swallow.

Esophagogastroduodenoscopy (EGD)—Diagnostic

Norm. Normal upper gastrointestinal tract (that is, esophageal mucosa is smooth and pink, with visible submucosal blood vessels; stomach mucosa is composed of continuous, deeper red rugal folds; duodenal lining is covered with villi). All surfaces are free of ulcers, varices, bleeding, and lesions.

Usage. Biopsy, cancer, dysphagia, esophagitis, gastric ulcers, hiatal hernia, Mallory-Weiss tear, odynophagia (painful swallowing), postoperative examination of the gastrointestinal (GI) tract, and upper GI bleeding.

Description. Visualization of the esophagus, stomach, and upper duodenum with a fiberoptic scope that has a lighted mirror lens on the end. EGD is less sensitive than endoscopic ultrasound for detection of varices of the esophagus and stomach. See Endoscopic ultrasonography—Diagnostic.

Professional Considerations

Consent form IS required.

Risks

Gastrointestinal perforation and hemorrhage, aspiration, infection, respiratory arrest, death.

Contraindications

Zenker's diverticulum or large aortic aneurysm. Sedatives are contraindicated in clients with central nervous system depression.

Precautions

During pregnancy, risks of cumulative radiation exposure to the fetus from this and other previous or future imaging studies must be weighed against the benefits of the procedure. Although formal limits for client exposure are relative to this risk:benefit comparison, the United States Nuclear Regulatory Commission requires that the cumulative dose equivalent to an embryo/fetus from occupational exposure not exceed 0.5 rem (5 mSv). Radiation dosage to the fetus is proportional to the distance of the anatomy studied from the abdomen and decreases as pregnancy progresses. For pregnant clients, consult the radiologist/radiology department to obtain estimated fetal radiation exposure from this procedure.

Preparation

1. Verify that the client has fasted.
2. The client should urinate and attempt to defecate before the procedure to increase comfort.
3. The client should remove dentures, partial plates, and jewelry.
4. Assess for allergies to anesthetics.
5. Establish intravenous access.
6. Obtain specimen containers (one with 95% ethyl alcohol and the other with 10% formaldehyde), an endoscope, and an intravenous sedative.
7. Measure and record heart rate, blood pressure, and respiratory rate.
8. Attach electrodes for continuous ECG monitoring and initiate continuous-pulse oximetry measurement.
9. Atropine may be prescribed to dry secretions before the test.
10. Infusion of erythromycin before EGD reduces the need for second-look endoscopy in clients with upper GI bleeding.
11. Just before beginning the procedure, take a "time out" to verify the correct client, procedure, and site.

Procedure

1. A topical, bitter-tasting anesthetic is applied to the throat and a mouth guard inserted if the client has teeth.
2. Intravenous sedation is given.
3. The endoscope is inserted into the esophagus and slowly advanced to the duodenum.
4. Air is instilled to distend any area to aid in visualization.
5. Biopsy specimens or photos may be taken.

Postprocedure Care

1. If deep sedation was used for the procedure, follow institutional protocol for post sedation monitoring. Typical monitoring includes continuous ECG monitoring and pulse oximetry, with continual assessments (every 5-15 minutes) of airway, vital signs, and neurologic status until the client is lying quietly awake, is breathing independently, and responds appropriately to commands spoken in a normal tone.

2. Resume previous diet after the gag reflex returns and sedation has worn off, usually 2 hours after the procedure.
3. Observe for signs of perforation: pain, fever, dyspnea, tachycardia, cyanosis, and pleural effusion.

Client and Family Teaching
1. Ambulatory clients should arrange for transportation home because they will not be allowed to drive for 12 hours after the procedure.
2. Fast from food and fluids for 8 hours before the test.
3. You may receive medication to dry secretions during the test, and this will cause a dry mouth. Sedation may also be used to cause a relaxed state, which may or may not result in sleeping through the test. After a local anesthetic is sprayed into the back of the throat, you will be positioned lying on the side, and the flexible scope will be inserted through the mouth. Suction will remove any draining saliva. Pressure may be felt as the scope advances through the esophagus into the stomach. Feelings of bloating but not pain are common.
4. The procedure lasts about 40 minutes.
5. Results are normally available within 24 hours.
6. Complications in elderly include arrhythmia, elevated blood pressure >50 mm Hg, increased pulse rate, and decreased oxygen saturation.

Factors That Affect Results
1. If the client moves excessively during the procedure, the risk of perforation is increased.

Other Data
1. Emergency EGD diagnostic accuracy is 80%-85%.

ESR
See **Sedimentation Rate, Erythrocyte**—Blood.

Esterase Stain—Diagnostic

Norm. Descriptive interpretation by hematologist.

Usage. Granulocytic sarcoma, leukemia.

Description. Stain of bone marrow to distinguish normal and leukemic cells of neutrophils, monocytes, and their precursors.

Professional Considerations
Consent form NOT required.

Preparation
1. Obtain glass slides, a lancet, a capillary tube, and a bone marrow tray.

Procedure
1. Obtain a bone marrow specimen and a fingerstick collection for peripheral blood smear.

Postprocedure Care
1. Assess the bone marrow aspiration site for bleeding or hematoma.
2. The client must lie flat for 1-2 hours after the procedure.
3. Send the specimen slides to the laboratory immediately.

Client and Family Teaching
1. Bone marrow aspiration is very painful but only for a brief moment.
2. Results are normally available within 24 hours.

Factors That Affect Results
1. Poor bone marrow sample will decrease the amount or quality of the cells, leading to inaccurate interpretation.

Other Data
1. Staining of fresh specimens enhances assessment.
2. See also Bone marrow aspiration analysis—Specimen for professional considerations related to the bone marrow aspiration procedure.

Estradiol—Serum

Norm.

		SI Units
Menstruating Females		
Midfollicular	24-114 pg/mL	87-420 pmol/L
Midluteal	80-273 pg/mL	295-1005 pmol/L
Periovulatory	62-534 pg/mL	228-1965 pmol/L
Postmenopausal Females	20-88 pg/mL	57-323 pmol/L
Females Taking Oral Contraceptives	12-50 pg/mL	44-184 pmol/L
Adult Males	20-75 pg/mL	74-276 pmol/L
Prepubertal Males	2-8 pg/mL	11-29 pmol/L

Increased. Adrenal tumors, breast cancer risk, cirrhosis, gynecomastia in males, hyperthyroidism, in vitro fertilization success of ovulation induction and pregnancy (fourth day of gonadotropin therapy), Klinefelter's syndrome, liver tumors, ovarian neoplasm, polycystic ovary syndrome.

Decreased. Amenorrhea, eating disorders, hypopituitarism, infertility, menopause, osteoporosis, ovarian hypofunction, pituitary disease, and polycystic ovary syndrome.

Description. Estradiol is an estrogenic hormone secreted by the ovary and by the placenta that acts on the mucosa of the uterus to stimulate endometrial growth in preparation for the progestational stage. Other actions include follicle-stimulating hormone (FSH) suppression and luteinizing hormone (LH) stimulation. Estradiol levels help evaluate ovarian function, menstrual abnormalities, feminization disorders, and estrogen-producing tumors. Estradiol production diminishes or stops during menopause. Ozcakir et al (2002) found that the estradiol level at the time of intrauterine insemination did not seem to affect the pregnancy rate in nonandrologic and non-peritubal factor infertility.

Professional Considerations

Consent form NOT required.

Preparation

1. Tube: Red topped, red/gray topped, or gold topped.

Procedure

1. Draw a 3-mL blood sample.

Postprocedure Care

1. Write the collection time and the client's sex and present menstrual cycle phase on the laboratory requisition.
2. Transport the specimen to the laboratory immediately for spinning and freezing within 1 hour.

Client and Family Teaching

1. Results are normally available within 24 hours.

Factors That Affect Results

1. Reject the specimen if the client has had a radioactive scan within 7 days.
2. Highest levels occur 1 day before the LH surge and again after corpus luteum formation.
3. Drugs that may falsely elevate results include ampicillin, cortisone (large doses), diethylstilbestrol, hydrochlorothiazide, meprobamates, phenazopyridine, prochlorperazine, and tetracyclines.
4. An herb that may falsely elevate results is cascara sagrada (*Rhamnus purshiana*).

Other Data

1. The specimen is stable at room temperature for 1 week, in a frost-free refrigerator for 1 year, and in a nondefrosting freezer for 3 years.
2. This test should not be used to evaluate fetal well-being because it does not measure estriol.

Estradiol Receptor and Progesterone Receptor in Breast Cancer—Diagnostic

Norm.

		SI Units
Negative	<6 fmol/mg cytosol protein	<6 nmol/kg cytosol protein
Borderline	6-10 fmol/mg cytosol protein	6-10 nmol/kg cytosol protein
Positive	>10 fmol/mg cytosol protein	>10 nmol/kg cytosol protein

Usage. Used to predict response to hormonal therapy in clients with breast cancer.

Description. Estrogen receptors and progesterone receptors are intracellular proteins that specifically bind estrogens and progesterones. The establishment of receptor status in clients with breast cancer is crucial because the receptors are the most predictive factor for the response to hormonal therapies for primary and metastatic breast cancer. They are the only tumor markers recommended for routine clinical use in breast cancer by the Tumor Marker Panel of the American Society of Clinical Oncology. Clients whose tumors express the estrogen and progesterone receptors respond more often and have longer disease-free periods and overall survival rates when treated with hormonal therapy. Although receptor status is important in determining which clients are likely to benefit from endocrine therapy, estrogen and progesterone receptor status is only a weak predictor of long-term relapse and mortalities and is not to be used alone to assign a client to a particular prognostic grouping. It should be noted that breast cancers that are initially hormone dependent might progress to a hormone-independent form, despite the continued expression of the receptor. This may limit the long-term usefulness of the hormonal therapies. Historically these receptors were measured by means of biochemical assays, but there are now highly specific monoclonal antibodies and immunohistochemical techniques available to assess estrogen and progesterone receptor status. When receptor status is determined using biochemical assays, sampling error may occur if the sample does not contain enough tumor, if there is significant desmoplastic response, or if there is a delay in the processing of the specimen. A value of less than 3 fmol/mg is considered negative when measured by the biochemical assay. Using the immunocytochemical assay, which measures the concentration of receptors by staining them with monoclonal antibodies, avoids sampling error. An additional advantage to the monoclonal assay is the ability to assay formalin-fixed, paraffin-embedded tissue. Most labs have chosen 10%-20% positive cells as the cutoff for receptor positivity, though recent studies have suggested that clients whose tumors contain as few as 1% weakly positive cells have significantly improved disease-free periods and overall survival when treated with hormonal therapy. Clients with a negative receptor status have at most an 8% chance of response to hormonal therapy.

Professional Considerations

Consent form IS required for biopsy. See Biopsy, Site-specific—Specimen for procedure-specific risks and contraindications.

Preparation

1. *Biochemical assay or frozen-tissue immunoassay*: Obtain a 60-mg solid tumor biopsy bottle (fluorescent pink), a waxed cardboard container or plastic tube without fixative, and a needle biopsy tray.
2. *Immunohistochemistry on paraffin block*: Obtain a biopsy bottle containing 10% formalin and a biopsy tray. Use of fixatives other than 10% formalin may not yield satisfactory results.

Procedure

1. Local anesthetic is not used because it may destroy receptors and lead to a false-negative result.
2. 0.5-1.0 mg of solid tumor tissue is removed, with care taken to remove excess fat and blood, both of which may lead to false-positive results.

3. *Biochemical assay or frozen-tissue immunoassay*: The tissue is immediately cut into small pieces and assayed. If the assay is unable to be performed immediately, the tissue should be frozen on dry ice, in a cryostat, or in liquid nitrogen within 20 minutes of collection. The specimen will be rejected if thawed or formalin fixed. The specimen should not be placed in foil, gauze, or fixative.

4. *Immunohistochemistry on paraffin block*: Tissue is placed in 10% formalin for not longer than 48 hours, preferably 12-24 hours. A paraffin block is then made on which an immunoassay to measure concentration of receptors may be performed.

Postprocedure Care

1. Apply a dry, sterile dressing to the biopsy site.
2. Mild analgesics may be used for postprocedure pain.
3. Depending on where the assay is performed, results may not be available for several days.

Client and Family Teaching

1. A small sample of breast tissue will be removed with a hollow needle. The breast will not be numbed with an anesthetic because this can cause false-negative results, and so there will be discomfort for a short time. The procedure takes a few minutes and leaves no scar.
2. Use mild analgesia for postprocedure pain if needed.
3. Results may not be available for several days.

Factors That Affect Results

1. Specimens not frozen within 20 minutes will falsely decrease results.
2. Antiestrogen preparations taken within the last 2 months may cause a negative estradiol receptor response.

Other Data

1. 50%-70% of breast cancers are positive.
2. Women with ER-negative breast cancer have an increased risk of a second ER-negative tumor, as compared to women with ER-positive breast cancer.

Estriol, Serum—24-Hour Urine

Norm.

	Total Estriol	SI Units
Serum		

A diurnal pattern is present, with the highest levels occurring in the mid to late afternoon.

Weeks of Pregnancy		
30-32	31-330 ng/mL	108-1145 nmol/L
34-36	45-350 ng/mL	156-902 nmol/L
36-38	48-570 ng/mL	167-1978 nmol/L
40	95-460 ng/mL	330-1596 nmol/L
Urine		
Week 30 of pregnancy	6-18 mg/24 hours	21-62 µmol/24 hours
Week 35 of pregnancy	9-28 mg/24 hours	31-97 µmol/24 hours
Week 40 of pregnancy	13-42 mg/24 hours	45-146 µmol/24 hours
Females, nonpregnant	0-54 mg/24 hours	0-188 µmol/24 hours
Males	0.3-2.4 mg/24 hours	1.0-8.2 µmol/24 hours
Children	0.3-2.4 mg/24 hours	1.0-8.2 µmol/24 hours
Panic level	4 ng/mL or 40% below the average of two prior values	

Increased. Feminizing tumors, true precocious puberty, liver cirrhosis, and multiple pregnancy. Drugs include oxytocin.

Decreased. Abortion, anemia, anencephaly, choriocarcinoma, diabetes mellitus, erythroblastosis fetalis, fetal adrenal aplasia,

E

fetal Down syndrome, fetal encephalopathy, fetal growth retardation, gynecomastia, hemoglobinopathy, hepatic disease, hydatidiform mole, intrauterine death, menopause, neural tube defects, postmaturity, preeclampsia, Rh immunization, and Smith-Lemli-Opitz syndrome. Drugs include betamethasone, corticosteroids (large doses), dexamethasone, diuretics, estrogens, glutethimide, mandelamine, meprobamate, penicillins, phenazopyridine, phenolphthalein, probenecid, and senna (*Cassia* species). Herbs or natural remedies include cascara sagrada (*Rhamnus purshiana*).

Description. Estriol is an estrogen synthesized in the placenta by a fetal hormone. Serum estriol levels are used to evaluate fetal and placental function for abnormalities such as growth retardation and fetal death. Low serum estriol has been associated with increased risk for X-linked ichthyosis. Estriol levels must be evaluated in consideration of the number of weeks of gestation because levels vary during pregnancy. Because serum levels fluctuate throughout the day, serial levels over time are used to evaluate the status of the fetus and the placenta.

Professional Considerations
Consent form NOT required.

Preparation
1. Tube: Red topped, red/gray topped, or gold topped.
2. Obtain a clean, 3-L container without preservative.

Procedure
1. *Serum test*: Draw a 5-mL blood sample.
2. *Urine test*:
   a. Discard the first morning urine specimen.

b. Begin to time a 24-hour urine collection.
c. Save all the urine voided for 24 hours in a clean 3-L container. Document the quantity of urine output during the specimen collection period. Include the urine voided at the end of the 24-hour period.

Postprocedure Care
1. Mix the 24-hour urine specimen gently and obtain a 100-mL aliquot to send to the laboratory.

Client and Family Teaching
1. Discard the first specimen of the morning, and then save all the urine voided in a 24-hour period; urinate before defecation to avoid loss of urine. If any urine is accidentally discarded, discard the entire specimen and restart the collection the next day.
2. Results are normally available within 24 hours after completion of the urine collection.
3. Refer pregnant clients with low serum estriol levels for genetic counseling.

Factors That Affect Results
1. Draw serum levels at the same time of the day for each sample.
2. Reject the specimen if the client has had a radioactive scan within 48 hours.
3. Levels are higher in Asian and African-American women compared to Hispanic and Caucasian women.

Other Data
1. Single values are not as meaningful as a trend in a series of measurements.
2. Reduction of estradiol by decreasing dietary fat intake by 12% decreases the risk for breast cancer in women.

Estrogen Receptor Assay
See **Estradiol Receptor and Progesterone Receptor in Breast Cancer**—Diagnostic.

Estrogens, Nonpregnant
See **Estrogens**—Serum and 24-Hour Urine.

E

Estrogens—Serum and 24-Hour Urine

Norm.

	Total Estrogens	SI Units
Serum	**pg/mL**	**ng/L**
Premenopausal females	60-400	60-400
Postmenopausal females	<130	<130
Males	10-130	10-130
Children	<25	<25
24-Hour Urine	**g/g Creatinine**	**mg/mol Creatinine**
Adult Females		
Follicular phase	7-65	0.79-7.35
Midcycle peak	32-104	3.62-11.75
Luteal phase	8-135	0.90-15.26
Adult Males	4-23	0.45-2.60

Increased in Serum. Amenorrhea, corpus luteum cyst, feminizing tumors, fibrocystic disease, hypogonadism in males, and Stein-Leventhal syndrome. Drugs include chlortetracycline, estrogens, levodopa, oral contraceptives, phenothiazines, tetracyclines, and vitamins. Herbs or natural remedies include cascara sagrada (*Rhamnus purshiana*).

Increased in Urine. Adrenocortical tumor, HIV-positive males, ovarian or testicular tumors, and virilization. Drugs include acetazolamide (in pregnant women), cascara, chlortetracycline, clomiphene, corticotropin, hydrochlorothiazide (in pregnant women), levodopa, phenothiazines, testosterone, tetracyclines, and vitamins.

Decreased in Serum. Amenorrhea, anorexia nervosa, dysmenorrhea, infertility, menopause, menorrhagia, menstruation, metrorrhagia, osteoporosis, psychogenic stress, and Turner's syndrome. Drugs include acetazolamide, glucose, hydrochlorothiazide, phenothiazines, tetracyclines, and vitamins. Herbs or natural remedies include cascara sagrada (*Rhamnus purshiana*).

Decreased in Urine. Amenorrhea, breast cancer risk factor, menopause, ovarian dysfunction, and Simmonds' disease. Drugs include acetazolamide, glucose, hydrochlorothiazide, phenothiazines, senna, tetracyclines, and vitamins. Herbs or natural remedies include cascara sagrada (*Rhamnus purshiana*).

Description. Estrogen is a hormone produced in the ovaries, testes, placenta, and adrenals that influences the development and maintenance of the female sex organs. Estrogen levels in females fluctuate in predictable amounts throughout the menstrual cycle, with the highest amounts produced during ovulation and the levels greatly decreasing during the latter phase of the cycle. Decreasing estrogen and rising progesterone levels signal the body that pregnancy has not occurred and leads to sloughing of the uterine lining. Serum and urine tests may be performed independently.

Professional Considerations
Consent form NOT required.

Preparation
1. Tube: Red topped, red/gray topped, or gold topped. Also obtain ice.
2. Obtain urine collection bottle containing 10 mL of glacial acetic acid or boric acid.
3. Screen client for the use of herbal preparations or natural remedies such as ginseng.

Procedure
1. Serum: Draw a 1.5-mL blood sample. Place the specimen on ice.
2. Discard the first morning void, and then collect all the urine voided in a refrigerated, 24-hour urine bottle containing glacial acetic acid. For catheterized clients, keep the drainage bag on ice and empty the bag into a refrigerated collection container hourly.

Postprocedure Care
1. Write the client's age, sex, and current menstrual cycle phase on the laboratory

requisition. For urine samples, document the quantity of urine output and the ending time for the 24-hour collection on the laboratory requisition.
2. Place the blood or urine specimen on ice. Deliver to the laboratory within 30 minutes after the collection has been completed.

Client and Family Teaching
1. Discard the first specimen of the morning, and then save all the urine voided in a 24-hour period; urinate before defecation to avoid loss of urine. If any urine is accidentally discarded, discard the entire specimen and restart the collection the next day.
2. Results are normally available within 48 hours.

Factors That Affect Results
1. Reject the specimen if the client has received a radioactive scan within the last 48 hours.
2. An incomplete urine specimen may cause falsely decreased results.
3. Herbs and natural remedies with additive effects to estrogens include ginseng.

Other Data
1. Do NOT use this test in pregnant females or to assess fetal well-being because it does not measure estriol.
2. Risk for coronary artery disease is decreased by exposure to estrogen.
3. Ingestion of alcohol by postmenopausal women who are on estrogen replacement therapy may increase their risk for breast cancer.

Ethanol

See **Alcohol**—Blood; **Toxicology, Volatiles Group by GLC**—Blood or Urine.

Ethchlorvynol—Blood

Norm. Negative.

		SI Units
Therapeutic level	5-10 μg/mL	35-70 μmol/L
Toxic level	>20 μg/mL	>138 μmmol/L
Panic level	>25 μg/mL	>175 μmol/L

Panic Level Symptoms and Treatment
Symptoms. Nausea, vomiting, hypotension, bradycardia, respiratory depression, hypothermia, coma.

Treatment
NOTE: Treatment choice(s) depend(s) on client's history and condition and episode history.
1. Monitor for noncardiogenic pulmonary edema.
2. Protect airway and support breathing.
3. Perform gastric lavage with warm tap water or normal saline if the client is treated soon after ingestion.
4. Give activated charcoal.
5. Seizure precautions: use phenobarbital or diazepam or restart ethchlorvynol, and then taper off drug if convulsions occur.
6. Administer resin or charcoal hemoperfusion if comatose.
7. Note: Hemodialysis and peritoneal dialysis will NOT remove ethchlorvynol from the bloodstream.
8. Provide cardiovascular and respiratory support of symptoms.

Usage. Drug abuse and overdose.

Description. A nonbarbiturate sedative-hypnotic drug that is absorbed through the gastrointestinal tract and metabolized in the liver, with a half-life of up to 20 hours. Duration of action is 5 hours.

Professional Considerations
Consent form NOT required.

Preparation
1. Tube: Red topped or red/gray topped.
2. Do NOT use alcohol wipe at venipuncture site.

3. The specimen MAY be drawn during hemodialysis.

Procedure

1. Cleanse the site with povidone-iodine solution, and then draw a 5-mL blood sample.

Postprocedure Care

1. Monitor cardiovascular, respiratory, and neurologic status for symptoms of overdose and provide support as needed.

Client and Family Teaching

1. For accidental overdose, teach client and family about proper dosing and side effects as well as interactions of the drug with alcohol and the signs for which medical attention must be sought.
2. For intentional overdose, refer the client and family for psychiatric counseling and crisis intervention.
3. Referrals to appropriate rehabilitation centers and therapeutic community programs should be offered to all addicted clients who may be interested.

4. If activated charcoal was given for elevated levels, the client should drink 4-6 glasses of water each day for 2 days to prevent constipation. The activated charcoal will cause stools to be black for a few days.

Factors That Affect Results

1. Peak blood levels occur 1.0-1.5 hours after ingestion.
2. The refrigerated specimen remains stable at 0-6 degrees C for several days.

Other Data

1. Sedative effects are potentiated by alcohol.
2. Ethchlorvynol interacts with monoamine oxidase (MAO) inhibitors, tricyclic antidepressants, alcohol, barbiturates, central nervous system depressants, and oral anticoagulants. Transient delirium has been reported when used concurrently with amitriptyline.
3. Intravenous use may precipitate pleural effusion.

Ethosuximide—Blood

Norm. Negative.

	Trough	SI Units
Therapeutic level	40-110 μg/mL	280-780 μmol/L
Panic level	>200 μg /mL	>1420 μmol/L

Overdose Symptoms and Treatment

Symptoms. Nausea, vomiting, lethargy.

Treatment

NOTE: Treatment choice(s) depend(s) on client's history and condition and episode history.

1. Give activated charcoal slurry.
2. Administer saline cathartic unless client has an ileus.
3. Give sorbitol cathartic.
4. Perform gastric lavage if soon after ingestion.
5. Protect airway and support breathing.
6. Administer neurologic checks every hour.
7. Forced diuresis is not helpful.
8. Hemodialysis WILL remove ethosuximide.

Increased. Drug abuse and overdose.

Decreased. Absence of ethosuximide use and convulsions during ethosuximide use.

Description. Anticonvulsant used in the treatment of petit mal seizures and is the first choice drug for treatment of epileptic negative myoclonus. Depresses motor cortex and elevates central nervous system threshold to stimuli. Absorbed from the gastrointestinal (GI) tract. Half-life of 40-60 hours in adults and 30-50 hours in children. Metabolized by the liver and excreted slowly in the urine. Steady-state levels are reached after 8-12 days in adults and 6-10 days in children.

Professional Considerations

Consent form NOT required.

Preparation

1. Tube: Green topped, red/gray topped, or gold topped.
2. Do NOT draw during hemodialysis.

Procedure

1. Draw a 4-mL TROUGH blood sample.
2. Obtain serial measurements at the same time each day.

Postprocedure Care

1. Monitor for overdose symptoms and provide support as needed.

Client and Family Teaching

1. Results are normally available within 24 hours.
2. Seek medical attention if early warning signs of drug overdose are noted: fatigue, drowsiness, confusion, difficulty waking up, slurred speech, unsteady gait.
3. If activated charcoal was given for elevated levels, the client should drink 4-6 glasses of water each day for 2 days to prevent constipation. The activated charcoal will cause stools to be black for a few days.
4. Refer clients with overdose for crisis intervention.
5. Referrals to appropriate rehabilitation centers and therapeutic community programs should be offered to all addicted clients who may be interested.

Factors That Affect Results

1. Peak levels occur 2-4 hours after dose.

Other Data

1. Adverse effects include gastric disturbances, lymphadenopathy, psychiatric disorders, and a lupus-like syndrome.
2. Neurotoxic interaction with valproate is possible.
3. Hypersensitivity to succinimides may cause adverse reactions, including pancytopenia, dizziness, myopia, vaginal bleeding, urticaria, swelling of tongue, and hirsutism.
4. Research, using rats, shows that estrogen increases EEG episodes of seizures.

Ethyl Alcohol

See Alcohol—Blood; Toxicology, Volatiles Group by GLC—Blood or Urine.

Ethylene Glycol—Serum and Urine

Norm. Serum and urine: negative.

		SI Units
Serum panic level	>2 mEq/L	>2 mmol/L
Serum lethal level	>30 mEq/L	>30 mmol/L

Poisoning Symptoms and Treatment

Symptoms

1. Within the first hour, the client appears drunk, followed by coma with convulsions.
2. During the first 12 hours, hypertension and an elevation in leukocytes occur.
3. Within 12-24 hours, cardiopulmonary failure, acute renal failure, and metabolic acidosis (with increased anion gap and osmolal gap) occur. Other symptoms include abdominal pain and tetany.

Treatment

NOTE: Treatment choice(s) depend(s) on client's history and condition and episode history.

1. Hemodialysis is the treatment of choice. Both hemodialysis and peritoneal dialysis WILL remove ethylene glycol.
2. Fomepizole has been found to be effective as an antidote to ethylene glycol and can eliminate the need for dialysis, except in clients with renal problems or levels >50 mg/dL. Administer IV loading dose of 15 mg/kg followed by maintenance dose of 10 mg/kg every 12 hours × 4, followed by 15 mg/kg every 12 hours to reach therapeutic fomepizole level >8.6 mg/mL. Continue until ethylene glycol concentrations are undetectable. Dosing frequency must be increased if dialysis is also used.

    Monitor for hyperventilation secondary to acidemia.

Usage. Evaluation for ethylene glycol poisoning; monitoring response to treatment for ethylene glycol poisoning.

Description. Ethylene glycol is a compound contained in antifreeze and other automotive products that, when ingested and metabolized, causes toxicity to the body. After ingestion, oxalic acid is excreted by the kidneys, causing oxalate crystals in the urine, acidosis, tetany, and renal failure. The minimum lethal dose is approximately 100 mL, but any amount ingested may produce toxic symptoms. Half-life is 3 hours without treatment, 2.5 hours with dialysis, and 17 hours with concomitant orally administered ethyl alcohol.

Professional Considerations
Consent form NOT required.

Preparation
1. Serum: Tube: gray topped, red/gray topped, or gold topped.
2. Do NOT draw during hemodialysis.
3. Urine: Obtain a clean specimen container.

Procedure
1. Serum: Draw a 4-mL blood sample.
2. Urine: Obtain a random urine sample in a clean container.

Postprocedure Care
1. Store the blood or urine sample at 4 degrees C.
2. Observe for seizures or coma, and assess for renal failure.

Client and Family Teaching
1. Explain the possible side effects of ethylene glycol ingestion (described above) and that the client will require intensive care monitoring for up to 48 hours or longer.

Factors That Affect Results
1. An uncooperative client may require catheterization to obtain a urine specimen.
2. Ethylene glycol is rapidly metabolized; therefore levels may not be obtainable. In this case, examination of urine under a Wood's lamp may reveal oxalate crystals characteristic of the metabolism of ethylene glycol.

Other Data
1. Ethyl glycol can also be detected in gastric secretions.
2. Highest known concentration that a person survived is 1889 mg/dL.

ETOH

See Alcohol—Blood; Toxicology, Volatiles Group by GLC—Blood or Urine.

Euglobulin Clot Lysis—Blood

Norm. Lysis in 1.5-4 hours.

Panic level: 100% lysis in 1 hour.

Panic Level Symptoms and Treatment
Symptoms. Bleeding from wounds, phlebotomy sites, or intracerebrally, or all three.

Treatment
NOTE: Treatment choice(s) depend(s) on client's history and condition and episode history.
1. Discontinue any drugs (listed below) contributing to shortened lysis time.
2. Place the client on bleeding precautions.
3. Monitor neurologic status for signs of intracerebral bleeding.

Usage. Urokinase and streptokinase monitoring.

Increased or Longer Lysis Time. Diabetes mellitus type 2 in women, dialysis (hemodialysis, continuous ambulatory peritoneal), polycystic ovary syndrome.

Decreased or Shortened Lysis Time. Disseminated intravascular coagulation (DIC), fibrinolysis, hemorrhage, pancreatic or pulmonary surgery, and pyrogen reactions. Drugs include asparaginase, clofibrate, dextran, epinephrine, misoprostol, streptokinase, and urokinase.

Description. Euglobulin clot lysis provides a measure of fibrinogen activity by measuring plasminogen and plasminogen activator, which are proteins important in preventing fibrin clot formation.

Professional Considerations
Consent form NOT required.

Preparation
1. Tube: 2.7-mL blue topped tube or 4.5-mL blue topped tube, a control tube, and a waste tube or syringe. Also obtain a container of ice.
2. Schedule the test with the laboratory before drawing blood because the sample must be centrifuged within 30 minutes of obtaining the specimen.

Procedure
1. Avoid taking the sample from an extremity into which intravenous fluids are infusing.
2. Withdraw 2 mL of blood into a syringe or vacuum tube. Remove the syringe or tube, leaving the needle in place. Attach a second syringe, and draw two blood samples, one in a citrated blue topped tube and the other in a control tube. The sample quantity should be 2.4 mL for a 2.7-mL tube and 4.0 mL for a 4.5-mL tube. Place the specimens immediately into a container of ice.

Postprocedure Care
1. Deliver specimens to the laboratory for processing within 30 minutes.

Client and Family Teaching
1. Avoid strenuous physical activity for 1 hour before sampling.

Factors That Affect Results
1. Aminocaproic acid (Amicar) neutralizes urokinase and streptokinase.
2. Lysis time may be shortened in clients who have exercised within the last hour.
3. Venipuncture that is rough, including pumping the fist or massaging the vein, may shorten lysis time.

Other Data
1. Heparin does not affect results.

EUS
See Endoscopic Ultrasonography—Diagnostic.

Exactech
See Glucose Monitoring Machines—Diagnostic.

Excretion Fraction of Filtered Sodium—Blood and Urine

Norm. 1-2 excretion fraction (F).

Increased. Acute tubular necrosis, renal failure, uremia, and urinary obstruction. Drugs include diuretics.

Decreased. Azotemia, glomerulonephritis, and hepatorenal syndrome.

Description. A sensitive and specific test for acute tubular necrosis that requires assays of both urine and serum sodium and creatinine levels. The excretion fraction is calculated by the following equation:

Excretion fraction (F) =
[(Urine sodium/Plasma sodium) ×
(Plasma creatinine/Urine creatinine)] × 100

Professional Considerations
Consent form NOT required.

Preparation
1. Tube: Red topped, red/gray topped, or gold topped. Also obtain a urine cup.
2. List diuretics on the laboratory requisition.

Procedure
1. Obtain a 10-mL random urine specimen.
2. Draw a 7-mL blood sample.

Postprocedure Care
1. Send specimens to the laboratory within 2 hours.

Client and Family Teaching
1. Results are normally available within 12 hours.

Factors That Affect Results
1. See individual tests (Sodium, Plasma—Serum or urine; Creatinine—Serum; Creatinine—Urine).

Other Data
1. Timed specimens are not required.

Excretory Urography

See Intravenous Pyelography—Diagnostic.

Exercise Stress Test

See Stress/Exercise Test—Diagnostic.

Exophthalmometry Test—Diagnostic

Norm. 12-20 mm. Eyes differ by less than 3 mm.

Usage. Cellulitis, enophthalmos, exophthalmos, periostitis, retinoblastoma, thyroid disease, tumors of the eye, and xanthomatosis.

Description. Measures the amount of forward protrusion of the eye by means of an exophthalmometer. The exophthalmometer is a horizontal, calibrated bar with movable 45-degree mirrors on both sides.

Professional Considerations
Consent form NOT required.

Preparation
1. If previous examination results are available, calibrate the bar to the baseline reading.

Procedure
1. Position client upright, facing the examiner, with eyes on the same level.
2. Hold the horizontal bar of the exophthalmometer in front of the client's eyes and parallel to the floor.
3. Move the two concave carriers against the lateral orbital margins and record the reading.
4. Measure each eye separately.
5. Have the client fixate his or her right eye on your left eye. Using the locked inclined mirrors, superimpose the apex of the right cornea on the scale, and record the reading.
6. Repeat the procedure with the client's left eye fixated on the examiner's right eye and record the reading.

Postprocedure Care
1. For abnormal results, refer to a specialist.

Client and Family Teaching
1. The test is painless.

Factors That Affect Results
1. Failure to set calibrated bar at baseline value.

Other Data
1. Use of steroids may contribute to exophthalmos.

Extractable Nuclear Antigen (ENA Complex)

See Anti-RNP Test—Diagnostic; Anti-Sm Test—Diagnostic.

Eye and Orbit Ultrasonography (Eye and Orbit Echograms, Eye and Orbit Sonograms)—Diagnostic

Norm. Negative for foreign body, cyst, inflammation, tumor, retinal detachment, or optic nerve atrophy. Orbit is of proper size, shape, and concavity.

Usage. Alternative to direct ophthalmoscopic visualization of the interior of the eye when cataract, fundal opacity, or vitreous hemorrhage is present; detection of intraocular foreign body or tumor; detection of retrobulbar optic nerve, optic nerve atrophy, or optic nerve tumor; differentiation of intraocular melanoma; eye measurement before lens implant; and evaluation of fundal abnormalities, intactness of retina, and the vitreous humor.

Description. Evaluation of the eye and orbit by the creation of an oscilloscopic picture from the echoes of high-frequency sound waves passing over the eye and eyelid (acoustic imaging). The time required for the ultrasonic beam to be reflected back to the transducer from differing densities of tissue is converted by a computer to an electrical impulse displayed on an oscilloscopic screen to create both a linear waveform and a two-dimensional dot-pattern picture of the structures. The B-scan mode is used to evaluate the optic disc, and the A-scan mode is used to evaluate optic nerve disease. Water immersion of the eye may also be used with the eye ultrasonogram to enhance images of the anterior part of the globe. The immersion of the transducer in water lifts it away from the eye, while still preventing air from obscuring the image. The transducer provides the best picture when it is at least 5-8 mm away from the structures being imaged. A newer method, ultrasound biomicroscopy, is able to provide even better images of the relationship of the structures of the anterior globe of the eye than conventional immersion ultrasonography.

Professional Considerations
Consent form NOT required.

Preparation
1. A sedative or general anesthetic may be used for children being evaluated for retinoblastoma or other purposes. The child should fast from food and fluids for 4 hours if general anesthesia will be used.
2. Remove metal objects such as eyeglasses or jewelry from the client's head and neck.
3. Obtain anesthetic eyedrops and conductive gel. If water immersion is to be performed, obtain an ocular drape and 0.9% sterile saline.

Procedure
1. The client is positioned supine in bed or on a procedure table.
2. After anesthetic eyedrops are administered, a transducer coated with conductive gel is slowly passed over a clear, methylcellulose eye form applied to the eye to form an airtight seal. The resulting waveform provides eye measurements and helps delineate the presence of abnormal tissue or structure.
3. The eye cup is removed and the eyelid closed. The gel-coated transducer is then slowly passed over the eyelid. A two-dimensional image of the eye and orbit is displayed on the oscilloscope.
4. Water immersion (sometimes performed):
   a. A waterproof drape is fastened around the orbit.
   b. After anesthetic drops are instilled, the eyelid is retracted, and the eye is flooded with warm, sterile 0.9% saline.
   c. The transducer is immersed into the water and moved slowly across the eye.
   d. The client may be asked to move the eye in specific directions.
   e. The water is then drained and the drape removed.
5. The procedure takes less than 30 minutes. Permanent photographs of the oscilloscopic recordings are made.

Postprocedure Care
1. Remove conductive gel from the eyelid(s) after the anesthetic effects have worn off (to prevent corneal damage).
2. If general anesthesia was administered, monitor vital signs every 15 minutes × 4, then every 30 minutes × 2, and then hourly × 4. Additional monitoring typically includes continuous ECG monitoring and pulse oximetry, with continual assessments (every 5-15 minutes) of airway, vital signs, and neurologic status until the client is lying quietly awake, is

breathing independently, and responds appropriately to commands spoken in a normal tone.

Client and Family Teaching

1. The procedure is noninvasive, painless, and poses no risk; it is important for you to relax the eyelid during the procedure.
2. You may hear an echo that sounds like repetitious humming or a musical note as the eye structures reflect the ultrasonic beam.
3. Avoid rubbing your eyes until the anesthetic effects have worn off (about $\frac{1}{2}$ hour). Infants or small children may need to be restrained during this time.

Factors That Affect Results

1. None found.

Other Data

1. None found.

Eye Culture and Sensitivity

See Conjunctivae, Routine—Culture.

Factor, Fitzgerald (High-Molecular-Weight Kininogen)—Plasma

Norm. Activated partial thromboplastin time (APTT) normal or 25-35 seconds (ellagic acid $[C_{14}H_6O_8]$ activation products) or 30-45 seconds (diatomaceous earth activation products) after mixing the sample with plasma known to be deficient for the Fitzgerald factor.

Increased. Congenital deficiency of the Fitzgerald factor, factor XI (sometimes), factor XII deficiency (sometimes), and high-molecular-weight kininogen deficiency. Drugs include bishydroxycoumarin, heparin calcium, heparin sodium, and warfarin sodium.

Decreased. Not applicable.

Description. Fitzgerald factor deficiency is a rare, autosomal recessive trait affecting the intrinsic pathway of coagulation that results in an abnormal APTT and coagulation time without other factor deficiencies. Fitzgerald factor interferes with plasminogen activation, immune pathway activation, and generation of the vasoactive polypeptide bradykinin. The client is asymptomatic for bleeding.

Professional Considerations

Consent form NOT required.

Preparation

1. Preschedule this test with the laboratory.
2. Tube: 2.7- or 4.5-mL blue topped. Also obtain ice.

Procedure

1. Withdraw 2 mL of blood into a syringe or vacuum tube. Remove the syringe or tube, leaving the needle in place. Attach a second syringe, and draw a 2.4-mL sample in a 2.7-mL tube or a 4.0-mL sample in a 4.5-mL tube. Place the specimens immediately in a container of ice.
2. Gently tilt the tube five or six times to mix.

Postprocedure Care

1. Place the specimen on ice immediately.
2. Write the collection time on the laboratory requisition.
3. Transport the specimen to the laboratory immediately, discard the ice, and refrigerate the specimen. The sample should be centrifuged and refrigerated within 1 hour of collection. Freeze the plasma if the test will not be performed within 24 hours of specimen collection.

Client and Family Teaching

1. The client should not have warfarin therapy for 2 weeks or heparin therapy for 2 days before the test.
2. Results are normally available within 24 hours.

Factors That Affect Results

1. Failure to discard the first 1-2 mL of blood may result in specimen contamination with tissue thromboplastin.

2. Reject hemolyzed or clotted specimens, specimens not completely mixed, tubes partially filled with blood, specimens diluted or contaminated with heparin, specimens not placed on ice, or specimens received more than 1 hour after collection.

Other Data

1. Compare results to prior PTT and APTT.
2. See Activated partial thromboplastin substitution test—Diagnostic; Activated partial thromboplastin time and partial thromboplastin time—Plasma.

Factor, Fletcher (Prekallikrein)—Plasma

Norm. Activated partial thromboplastin time (APTT) normal or 30-45 seconds (diatomaceous earth activator) after mixing the sample with plasma known to be deficient for the Fletcher factor.

Increased. Fletcher factor deficiency, hepatic disease, prekallikrein deficiency, and uremia. Drugs include bishydroxycoumarin, heparin sodium, heparin calcium, and warfarin sodium.

Decreased. Not applicable.

Description. Rare condition of prolonged APTT and prekallikrein deficiency. The APTT shortens only after prolonged contact activation. The deficiency is believed to be inherited as an autosomal recessive trait in which the client is asymptomatic for bleeding. Fletcher factor is believed to function as a necessary component in the activation of factors XI and XII. To detect a deficient Fletcher factor, an APTT test is conducted on the sample and then repeated with a diatomaceous earth activator and lengthened incubation time from 3 to 10 minutes. The deficiency is suggested if the second APTT test is corrected.

Professional Considerations

Consent form NOT required.

Preparation

1. Preschedule this test with the laboratory.
2. Tube: 2.7-mL or 4.5-mL blue topped. Also obtain ice.

Procedure

1. Withdraw 2 mL of blood into a syringe or vacuum tube. Remove the syringe or tube, leaving the needle in place. Attach a second syringe, and draw a 2.4-mL sample in a 2.7-mL tube or a 4.0-mL sample in a 4.5-mL tube. Place the specimens immediately in a container of ice.
2. Gently tilt the tube five or six times to mix.

Postprocedure Care

1. Place the specimen on ice immediately.
2. Write the collection time on the laboratory requisition.
3. Transport the specimen to the laboratory immediately, discard the ice, and refrigerate the specimen. The sample should be centrifuged and refrigerated within 1 hour of collection. Freeze the plasma if the test will not be performed within 24 hours of collection.

Client and Family Teaching

1. The client should not have warfarin therapy for 2 weeks or heparin therapy for 2 days before the test.
2. Results are normally available within 24 hours.

Factors That Affect Results

1. Failure to discard the first 1-2 mL of blood may result in specimen contamination with tissue thromboplastin.
2. Reject hemolyzed or clotted specimens, specimens not completely mixed, tubes partially filled with blood, specimens not received on ice, specimens diluted or contaminated with heparin, or specimens received more than 1 hour after collection.
3. Ellagic acid activation products should not be used for this test.

Other Data

1. Compare results to prior PT and APTT.
2. See Activated partial thromboplastin substitution test—Diagnostic; Activated partial thromboplastin time and partial thromboplastin time—Plasma.

Factor I

See Fibrinogen—Plasma.

Factor II (Prothrombin)

See Prothrombin Time and International Normalized Ratio—Blood.

Factor V (Labile Factor, Proaccelerin, Ac-Globulin)—Blood

Norm. 50%-150% of normal (control sample) activity. Half-life is 12-36 hours.

Increased. Not applicable.

Decreased. Alpha-globulin deficiency, disseminated intravascular coagulation, factor V deficiency, factor V inhibitors (circulating), fibrinogenolysis, HELLP syndrome, hepatic disease, labile factor deficiency, leukemia (acute), parahemophilia, postoperatively, proaccelerin deficiency, and radioactive phosphorus therapy. Drugs include anisindione, bishydroxycoumarin, carbimazole, dicumarol, phenprocoumon, and warfarin sodium.

Description. Factor V is a vitamin K–dependent glycoprotein synthesized in the liver. It is part of the prothrombin-converting complex that functions in the extrinsic pathway of blood clotting. Specifically it is a cofactor that accelerates the conversion of prothrombin to thrombin. Factor V deficiency is an inherited, autosomal recessive condition that occurs with equal frequency in men and women. The symptoms can be mild to severe and include bruising easily, frequent nosebleeds, menorrhagia, and prolonged bleeding after traumatic episodes, including operative and dental procedures. One performs the test by first performing a prothrombin time (PT) on the client's plasma. A factor V–deficient plasma substrate is then mixed with the client's plasma, and the degree of correction in the PT is determined and compared to the degree of correction obtained by normal plasma. The *Factor V Leiden mutation,* newly identified in the 1990s, is a molecular defect in factor V, which makes it resistant to anticoagulant activation by protein C. The Leiden mutation is identified by performing an activated protein C resistance test and confirming an abnormal result with DNA evaluation for the Leiden mutation.

Professional Considerations
Consent form NOT required.

Preparation
1. Preschedule this test with the laboratory.
2. Tube: 2.7- or 4.5-mL blue topped. Also obtain ice.

Procedure
1. Withdraw 2 mL of blood into a syringe or vacuum tube. Remove the syringe or tube, leaving the needle in place. Attach a second syringe, and draw a 2.4-mL sample in a 2.7-mL tube or a 4.0-mL sample in a 4.5-mL tube. Place the specimens immediately in a container of ice.
2. Gently tilt the tube five or six times to mix.

Postprocedure Care
1. Place the specimen on ice immediately.
2. For clients with coagulopathy, hold pressure over the sampling site for at least 5 minutes and observe the site closely for development of a hematoma.
3. Write the collection time on the laboratory requisition.
4. Take the iced specimen to the laboratory immediately because factor V is labile in drawn blood samples.

Client and Family Teaching
1. The client should not have warfarin therapy for 2 weeks or heparin therapy for 2 days before the test.
2. Results are normally available within 24 hours.
3. Seek medical attention for signs of bleeding (that is, hematoma, bleeding of gums, wounds, petechiae, confusion, changing level of consciousness).

Factors That Affect Results

1. Failure to discard the first 1-2 mL of blood may result in specimen contamination with tissue thromboplastin.
2. Reject hemolyzed or clotted specimens, specimens not completely mixed, tubes partially filled with blood, specimens not on ice, specimens diluted or contaminated with heparin, or specimens received more than 2 hours after collection.
3. Some drugs that may cause shortened prothrombin time include meprobamate, barbiturates, ethchlorvynol, glutethimide, oral contraceptives, and vitamin K.
4. Some drugs that may cause prolonged prothrombin time include antibiotics, chloral hydrate, hydroxyzine hydrochloride, hydroxyzine pamoate, iothiouracil, methylthiouracil, phenylbutazone, phenyramidol, phosphorus (toxicity), propylthiouracil, salicylates, sulfonamides, tolbutamide, and vitamin A.

Other Data

1. The coagulation factor Roman numerals identify order of discovery rather than their order in the stages of clot formation.
2. Platelet transfusion is a common treatment.
3. See Activated partial thromboplastin substitution test—Diagnostic; Activated partial thromboplastin time and partial thromboplastin time—Plasma.

Factor VII (Stable Factor, Proconvertin, Autoprothrombin I)—Blood

Norm. 50%-150% of normal (control sample) activity. Half-life is 6 hours.

Increased. Pregnancy (late) and thromboembolism, uremia. Drugs include oral contraceptives.

Decreased. Factor VII deficiency, hemorrhagic disease of the newborn, hepatic carcinoma, hepatitis, jaundice (obstructive), kwashiorkor, menstrual cycle, proconvertin autoprothrombin I deficiency, stable factor deficiency, and vitamin K deficiency. Drugs include anisindione, bishydroxycoumarin, dicumarol (dicoumarin), metformin, phenprocoumon, and warfarin sodium. Diet including olive oil.

Description. Factor VII is a vitamin K–dependent beta globulin synthesized in the liver. It is activated in the extrinsic pathway during blood clotting and in turn activates tissue thromboplastins, with excess amounts of factor VII present in serum and plasma when clotting is completed. Both forms of the rare factor VII deficiency are autosomal recessive and affect both males and females. Bleeding symptoms may be severe, including cerebral hemorrhage. One performs the test by first determining the prothrombin time (PT) of the client's plasma. A factor VII–deficient plasma substrate is then mixed with the client's plasma, and the degree of correction in the PT is determined and compared to the degree of correction obtained by normal plasma.

Professional Considerations

Consent form NOT required.

Preparation

1. Preschedule this test with the laboratory.
2. Tube: 2.7-mL or 4.5-mL blue topped.

Procedure

1. Withdraw 2 mL of blood into a syringe or vacuum tube. Remove the syringe or tube, leaving the needle in place. Attach a second syringe, and draw a 2.4-mL sample in a 2.7-mL tube or a 4.0-mL sample in a 4.5-mL tube. Place the specimen immediately in a container of ice.
2. Gently tilt the tube five or six times to mix.

Postprocedure Care

1. For clients with coagulopathy, hold pressure over the sampling site for at least 5 minutes and observe the site closely for development of a hematoma.
2. Write the collection time on the laboratory requisition.
3. Transport the specimen to the laboratory immediately. Centrifuge and leave the specimens at room temperature.

Client and Family Teaching

1. The client should not have coumarin therapy for 2 weeks before the test.
2. Results are normally available within 24 hours.
3. Seek medical attention for signs of bleeding (that is, hematoma, bleeding of gums,

wounds, petechiae, confusion, changing level of consciousness).

Factors That Affect Results
1. Failure to discard the first 1-2 mL of blood may result in specimen contamination with tissue thromboplastin.
2. Reject hemolyzed or clotted specimens, specimens not completely mixed, tubes partially filled with blood, specimens not refrigerated, or specimens received more than 2 hours after collection.
3. Cold temperatures activate factor VII. Do not refrigerate or freeze the plasma.
4. Drugs that may cause shortened PT include barbiturates, ethchlorvynol, glutethimide (Dorimide), meprobamate, oral contraceptives, and vitamin K.

5. Some drugs that may cause prolonged prothrombin time include antibiotics, chloral hydrate, hydroxyzine hydrochloride, hydroxyzine pamoate, iothiouracil, methylthiouracil, phenylbutazone, phosphorus (toxicity), propylthiouracil, salicylates, tolbutamide, and vitamin A.

Other Data
1. After separation of plasma, factor VII is stable for 4 days at 25-37 degrees C.
2. The coagulation factor Roman numerals identify order of discovery rather than their order in the stages of clot formation.
3. See Prothrombin time and international normalized ratio—Blood.

Factor VIII (Antihemophilia Factor, AHF)—Blood

Norm. 50%-150% of normal (control sample) activity.

Mild deficiency	5%-25%
Moderately severe deficiency	1%-5%
Severe deficiency	<1%
von Willebrand's disease	1%-50%
Plasma level	Approximately 100 mg/L

Increased. Coronary artery disease, exercise, hyperthyroidism, hypoglycemia, macroglobulinemia, myocardial infarction (factor VIII antigen), pregnancy, and surgery. Drugs include oral contraceptives and sudden discontinuance of bishydroxycoumarin and warfarin sodium.

Decreased. Disseminated intravascular coagulation, factor VIII inhibitor (from childbirth, multiple myeloma, neoplasms, penicillin allergy, rheumatoid arthritis, or systemic lupus erythematosus), fibrinolysis, hemophilia A, and von Willebrand's disease.

Description. Factor VIII is a glycoprotein believed to be made up of two components that are easily dissociated. One component contains von Willebrand factor (vWf), newly recognized as the initiator of platelet adhesion in combination with collagen and glycoprotein Ib. The second component contains factor VIII Ag, a protein antigen, and factor VIII (measured by this test), which refers to the coagulant activity. Factor VIII is the antihemophilia (A) factor essential for thromboplastin generation in stage I of the intrinsic coagulation pathway. Factor VIII deficiency is usually transmitted as a sex-linked, recessive condition. One performs this test by first determining the partial thromboplastin time (PTT) of the client's plasma. A factor VIII–deficient plasma substrate is then mixed with the client's plasma, and the degree of correction in the PTT is determined and compared to the degree of correction obtained by normal plasma.

Professional Considerations
Consent form NOT required.

Preparation
1. Preschedule this test with the laboratory.
2. Tube: 2.7- or 4.5-mL blue topped. Also obtain ice.

Procedure
1. Withdraw 2 mL of blood into a syringe or vacuum tube. Remove the syringe or tube, leaving the needle in place. Attach a second syringe, and draw a 2.4-mL sample in a 2.7-mL tube or a 4.0-mL sample in a 4.5-mL tube. Place the specimen immediately in a container of ice.
2. Gently tilt the tube five or six times to mix.

Postprocedure Care

1. For clients with coagulopathy, hold pressure over the sampling site for at least 5 minutes and observe site closely for development of a hematoma.
2. Transport the specimen to the laboratory immediately, discard the ice, and refrigerate the specimen. The sample should be centrifuged and refrigerated within 1 hour. Freeze the plasma if the test will not be performed within 24 hours of collection.

Client and Family Teaching

1. The client should not have warfarin therapy for 2 weeks or heparin therapy for 2 days before the test.
2. Results are normally available within 24 hours.

Factors That Affect Results

1. Failure to discard the first 1-2 mL of blood may result in specimen contamination with tissue thromboplastin.

2. Reject hemolyzed or clotted specimens, specimens not completely mixed, tubes partially filled with blood, specimens not on ice, or specimens received more than 1 hour after collection.

Other Data

1. The coagulation factor Roman numerals identify order of discovery rather than their order in the stages of clot formation.
2. There is currently less-than-optimal standardization of this test.
3. Previous terminology used for factor VIII includes factor VIIIC, AHG, and AHF.
4. Factor VIII is stable in polyvinylchloride bags for continuous infusion by ambulatory mini pump.
5. See also Activated partial thromboplastin substitution test—Diagnostic; Activated partial thromboplastin time and partial thromboplastin time—Plasma.

Factor VIII R:Ag

See von Willebrand Factor Antigen—Blood.

Factor IX (Christmas Factor, Hemophilic Factor B, Plasma Thromboplastin Component, PTC)—Blood

Norm. 50%-150% of normal (control sample) activity. Plasma level about 4 mg/L. Half-life is 20 hours.

Increased. Drugs include hormone replacement therapy.

Decreased. Hemophilia B (Christmas disease), hepatic disease, nephrotic syndrome, and vitamin K deficiency. Drugs include anisindione, bishydroxycoumarin, dicumarol (dicoumarin), heparin calcium, heparin sodium, phenprocoumon, and warfarin sodium.

Description. Factor IX is a vitamin K–dependent beta globulin essential in stage I of the intrinsic coagulation system as an influence on the amount of thromboplastin available. It is deficient in the inherited, sex-linked disease of hemophilia B, with bleeding symptoms similar to hemophilia A but usually milder. Factor IX deficiency may also be acquired in severe hepatic dysfunction.

One performs the test by first determining the partial thromboplastin time (PTT) of the client's plasma. A factor IX–deficient plasma substrate is then mixed with the client's plasma, and the degree of correction in the PTT is determined and compared to the degree of correction obtained by normal plasma.

Professional Considerations

Consent form NOT required.

Preparation

1. Preschedule this test with the laboratory.
2. Tube: 2.7- or 4.5-mL blue topped. Also obtain ice.

Procedure

1. Withdraw 2 mL of blood into a syringe or vacuum tube. Remove the syringe or tube, leaving the needle in place. Attach a second syringe, and draw a 2.4-mL sample in a 2.7-mL tube or a 4.0-mL sample in a 4.5-mL tube.

F

2. Gently tilt the tube five or six times to mix.

Postprocedure Care
1. Place the specimen on ice immediately.
2. For clients with coagulopathy, hold pressure over the sampling site for at least 5 minutes and observe the site closely for development of a hematoma.
3. Write the collection time on the laboratory requisition.
4. Transport the specimen to the laboratory immediately. The specimen should be centrifuged and refrigerated within 2 hours, where it will remain stable for several weeks.

Client and Family Teaching
1. The client should not have coumarin therapy for 2 weeks or heparin therapy for 2 days before the test.
2. Results are normally available within 24 hours.
3. Seek medical attention for signs of bleeding (that is, hematoma, bleeding of gums, wounds, petechiae, confusion, changing level of consciousness).

Factors That Affect Results
1. Reject hemolyzed or clotted specimens, specimens not completely mixed, tubes partially filled with blood, specimens not refrigerated, specimens diluted or contaminated with heparin, or specimens received more than 2 hours after collection.
2. Failure to discard the first 1-2 mL of blood may result in specimen contamination with tissue thromboplastin.

Other Data
1. The coagulation factor Roman numerals identify order of discovery rather than their order in the stages of clot formation.
2. Treatment with factor IX can result in anaphylaxis and nephrotic syndrome.
3. See also Activated partial thromboplastin substitution test—Diagnostic; Activated partial thromboplastin time and partial thromboplastin time—Plasma.

Factor X (Stuart-Prower Factor)—Blood

Norm. 50%-150% of normal (control sample) activity. Plasma level about 12 mg/L. Half-life is 30-50 hours.

Increased. Normal pregnancy. Drugs include oral contraceptives.

Decreased. Factor X deficiency, hepatic disease, and vitamin K deficiency. Drugs include anisindione, bishydroxycoumarin, dicumarol (dicoumarin), phenprocoumon, and warfarin sodium.

Description. A vitamin K–dependent proenzyme alpha globulin active in both the intrinsic and extrinsic coagulation pathways. Factor X deficiency can be inherited and also acquired in severe hepatic dysfunction and causes usually mild bleeding and prolonged prothrombin time (PT) and activated partial thromboplastin time (APTT). One performs the test by first determining the PT of the client's plasma. A factor X–deficient plasma substrate is then mixed with the client's plasma, and the degree of correction in the PT is determined and compared to the degree of correction obtained by normal plasma.

Professional Considerations
Consent form NOT required.

Preparation
1. Preschedule this test with the laboratory.
2. Tube: 2.7- or 4.5-mL blue topped.

Procedure
1. Withdraw 2 mL of blood into a syringe or vacuum tube. Remove the syringe or tube, leaving the needle in place. Attach a second syringe, and draw a 2.4-mL sample in a 2.7-mL tube or a 4.0-mL sample in a 4.5-mL tube.
2. Gently tilt the tube five or six times to mix. Place the specimen immediately in a container of ice.

Postprocedure Care
1. For clients with coagulopathy, hold pressure over the sampling site for at least 5 minutes and observe the site closely for development of a hematoma.
2. Transport the specimen to the laboratory immediately. The specimens should be left at room temperature, with the stopper in place until tested within 24 hours.

F

Client and Family Teaching

1. The client should not have coumarin therapy for 2 weeks or heparin therapy for 2 days before the test.
2. Results are normally available within 24 hours.
3. Seek medical attention for signs of bleeding (that is, hematoma, bleeding of gums, wounds, petechiae, confusion, changing level of consciousness).

Factors That Affect Results

1. Failure to discard the first 1-2 mL of blood may result in specimen contamination with tissue thromboplastin.
2. Reject hemolyzed or clotted specimens, specimens not completely mixed, tubes partially filled with blood, specimens diluted or contaminated with heparin, or specimens received more than 2 hours after collection.

3. Some drugs that may cause shortened prothrombin time include barbiturates, ethchlorvynol, glutethimide, meprobamate, oral contraceptives, and vitamin K.
4. Some drugs that may cause prolonged prothrombin time include antibiotics, chloral hydrate, hydroxyzine hydrochloride, hydroxyzine pamoate, iothiouracil, methylthiouracil, phenylbutazone, phosphorus (toxicity), propylthiouracil, salicylates, tolbutamide, and vitamin A.

Other Data

1. The coagulation factor Roman numerals identify order of discovery rather than their order in the stages of clot formation.
2. See Activated partial thromboplastin time and partial thromboplastin time—Plasma.

Factor XI (Plasma Thromboplastin Antecedent, PTA)—Blood

Norm. 65%-135% of normal (control sample) activity. Plasma level about 7 mg/dL. Half-life is 40-80 hours.

Increased. Not applicable.

Decreased. Congenital heart disease, factor XI deficiency (common in Ashkenazi Jews), hepatic disease, newborns (transient), pregnancy, and vitamin K deficiency. Drugs include anisindione, bishydroxycoumarin, dicumarol (dicoumarin), heparin calcium, heparin sodium, phenprocoumon, and warfarin sodium.

Description. Factor XI is a beta globulin active in stage I of the intrinsic coagulation pathway and missing, defective, or deficient in hemophilia C, an inherited, autosomal recessive deficiency that occurs in both sexes and causes prolonged coagulation evidenced by mild bleeding after surgical procedures. One performs the test by first determining the partial thromboplastin time (PTT) of the client's plasma. A factor XI–deficient plasma substrate is then mixed with the client's plasma, and the degree of correction in the PTT is determined and compared to the degree of correction obtained by normal plasma.

Professional Considerations
Consent form NOT required.

Preparation

1. Preschedule this test with the laboratory.
2. Tube: 2.7- or 4.5-mL blue topped. Also obtain ice.

Procedure

1. Withdraw 2 mL of blood into a syringe or vacuum tube. Remove the syringe or tube, leaving the needle in place. Attach a second syringe, and draw a 2.4-mL sample in a 2.7-mL tube or a 4.0-mL sample in a 4.5-mL tube.
2. Gently tilt the tube five or six times to mix.

Postprocedure Care

1. Place the specimen on ice immediately.
2. For clients with coagulopathy, hold pressure over the sampling site for at least 5 minutes and observe the site closely for development of a hematoma.
3. Write the collection time on the laboratory requisition.
4. Transport the specimen to the laboratory immediately, discard the ice, and refrigerate the specimens. The sample should be centrifuged and refrigerated within 2 hours.

Client and Family Teaching

1. The client should not have warfarin therapy for 2 weeks or heparin therapy for 2 days before the test.
2. Results are normally available within 24 hours.
3. Seek medical attention for signs of bleeding (that is, hematoma, bleeding of gums, wounds, petechiae, confusion, changing level of consciousness).

Factors That Affect Results

1. Failure to discard the first 1-2 mL of blood may result in specimen contamination with tissue thromboplastin.
2. Reject hemolyzed or clotted specimens, specimens not completely mixed, tubes partially filled with blood, specimens not refrigerated, specimens diluted or contaminated with heparin, or specimens received more than 2 hours after collection.
3. The test for factor XI deficiency must be performed on a freshly collected specimen.
4. Freezing the specimen may falsely elevate results.

Other Data

1. The coagulation factor Roman numerals identify order of discovery rather than their order in the stages of clot formation.
2. Factor XI concentrate use is associated with the development of venous thromboembolic disease.
3. See also Activated partial thromboplastin substitution test—Diagnostic; Activated partial thromboplastin time and partial thromboplastin time—Plasma.

Factor XII (Hageman Factor)—Blood

Norm. 50%-150% of normal (control sample) activity. Plasma level: 23-47 mg/mL. Half-life is 52-60 hours.

Increased. After alcohol intake or exercise, high risk for coronary heart disease.

Decreased. Factor XII deficiency, nephrotic syndrome, and pregnancy. Diet including olive oil or sunflower oil.

Description. Factor XII is a beta globulin or gamma globulin enzyme, the active form of which initiates the intrinsic coagulation pathway. Its deficiency is inherited as an autosomal recessive defect with bleeding symptoms usually absent and causes a prolonged partial thromboplastin time (PTT). One performs the test by first determining the PTT of the client's plasma. A factor XII–deficient plasma substrate is then mixed with the client's plasma, and the degree of correction in the PTT is determined and compared to the degree of correction obtained by normal plasma.

Professional Considerations

Consent form NOT required.

Preparation

1. Preschedule this test with the laboratory.
2. Tube: 2.7- or 4.5-mL blue topped. Also obtain ice.

Procedure

1. Withdraw 2 mL of blood into a syringe or vacuum tube. Remove the syringe or tube, leaving the needle in place. Attach a second syringe, and draw a 2.4-mL sample in a 2.7-mL tube or a 4.0-mL sample in a 4.5-mL tube.
2. Gently tilt the tube five or six times to mix.

Postprocedure Care

1. Place the specimen on ice immediately.
2. For clients with coagulopathy, hold pressure over the sampling site for at least 5 minutes and observe the site closely for development of a hematoma.
3. Write the collection time on the laboratory requisition.
4. Transport the specimen to the laboratory immediately, discard the ice, and refrigerate the specimen. The sample should be centrifuged and refrigerated within 2 hours. Freeze the plasma if the test will not be performed within 24 hours of collection.

Client and Family Teaching

1. The client should not have warfarin therapy for 2 weeks or heparin therapy for 2 days before the test.

2. Results are normally available within 24 hours.
3. Seek medical attention for signs of bleeding (that is, hematoma, bleeding of gums, wounds, petechiae, confusion, changing level of consciousness).

Factors That Affect Results

1. Failure to discard the first 1-2 mL of blood may result in specimen contamination with tissue thromboplastin.
2. Reject hemolyzed or clotted specimens, specimens not completely mixed, tubes partially filled with blood, specimens not refrigerated, specimens diluted or contaminated with heparin, or specimens received more than 2 hours after collection.

Other Data

1. The coagulation factor Roman numerals identify order of discovery rather than their order in the stages of clot formation.
2. See also Activated partial thromboplastin substitution test—Diagnostic; Activated partial thromboplastin time and partial thromboplastin time—Plasma.

Factor XIII (Fibrin-Stabilizing Factor, Clot Urea Solubility)—Blood

Norm. Clot is insoluble in 5 M urea for at least 24 hours. Half-life of factor XIII is 100 hours.

Increased. Factor XIII is more often increased than decreased in most clients.

Decreased. Agammaglobulinemia, Crohn's disease, factor XIII deficiency, hepatic disease, hyperfibrinogenemia, lead poisoning, malaria (*Plasmodium falciparum*), multiple myeloma, postoperatively, and ulcerative colitis.

Description. Factor XIII is an alpha globulin that, in its active form, stabilizes fibrin clots. Its deficiency is a rare, inherited, autosomal recessive condition that may result in symptoms ranging from abnormal bleeding from cuts and bleeding in joints to cerebral hemorrhage and infant death from umbilical cord hemorrhage. One performs the test by adding calcium chloride to the sample and clotting the mixture at 37 degrees C for $\frac{1}{2}$ hour, and then placing the clot in 5 M urea and observing hourly for clot dissolution. Clots from clients with factor XIII deficiency will dissolve within 1-3 hours.

Professional Considerations

Consent form NOT required.

Preparation

1. Tube: 2.7- or 4.5-mL blue topped. Also obtain ice.

Procedure

1. Withdraw 2 mL of blood into a syringe or vacuum tube. Remove the syringe or tube, leaving the needle in place. Attach a second syringe, and draw a 2.4-mL sample

in a 2.7-mL tube or a 4.0-mL sample in a 4.5-mL tube. Place the specimens immediately in a container of ice.
2. Gently tilt the tube five or six times to mix.

Postprocedure Care

1. Place the specimens on ice immediately.
2. For clients with coagulopathy, hold pressure over the sampling site for at least 5 minutes and observe the site closely for development of a hematoma.
3. Write the collection time on the laboratory requisition.
4. Transport the specimens to the laboratory immediately, discard the ice, and refrigerate the specimens.

Client and Family Teaching

1. The client should not have warfarin therapy for 2 weeks or heparin therapy for 2 days before the test.
2. Results are normally available within 24 hours.
3. Seek medical attention for signs of bleeding (that is, hematoma, bleeding of gums, wounds, petechiae, confusion, changing level of consciousness).

Factors That Affect Results

1. Reject hemolyzed or clotted specimens, specimens not completely mixed, tubes partially filled with blood, specimens not refrigerated, specimens diluted or contaminated with heparin, or specimens received more than 2 hours after collection.
2. The presence of only 1% of normal levels of factor XIII is enough to provoke a normal test result.

F

Other Data

1. The coagulation factor Roman numerals identify order of discovery rather than their order in the stages of clot formation.
2. Factor XIII is used as a treatment for scleroderma and status post coronary surgery to decrease bleeding and reduce the need for blood transfusions. It is a useful supplementation (5000 U initially, followed by 20 IU/kg body weight three times a day for up to 3 weeks) in the treatment of acute graft-versus-host disease of the bowel post stem cell transplantation. Used to prevent development of leakage syndrome and myocardial edema in children undergoing surgery for congenital heart conditions.

FAMILION® Test—Blood

Norm. Negative

Usage. Used to confirm diagnosis when the diagnosis of long QT syndrome is inconclusive; and to risk stratify individuals with known long QT syndrome (Goldenberg, Moss, Bradley, 2008). May also be used to identify asymptomatic family members who may be at risk for long QT syndrome, and allow for prophylactic treatment.

Description. The cardiac conduction abnormality of long QT syndrome is estimated to occur as a result of an inherited/genetic disorder 75% of the time (Moss, Shimizu, Wilde, 2007). Long QT syndrome occurs when ventricular repolarization is longer than normal, causing a long QT interval on the ECG, placing the patient at risk for *R on T phenomenon* in which the next depolarization occurs before the ventricles are completely repolarized. This leads to ventricular tachycardia and fibrillation. Clients with long QT syndrome are at increased risk for sudden cardiac death. Conditions in which there are disruptions in the flow of ions across the cardiac membrane during depolarization and repolarization are called *channelopathies*. This test analyzes the gene sequence and variants of the 5 major cardiac ion channel genes that affect the flow of cardiac ions, and risk stratifies any variant findings as follows:

Class	Risk of Harmful Sequelae
I	Definitely or probably deleterious
II	Possibly deleterious
III	Unlikely/not expected to be deleterious
IV	Not deleterious

In addition to a physical exam and history, electrocardiographic testing, and traditional scoring systems, the risk stratification results of this genetic test can help guide decision-making about the range of treatment options for long QT syndrome.

Professional Considerations

Informed consent is recommended for genetic testing.

Preparation

1. Complete patient history questionnaire.
2. Tubes: 2 Lavender topped EDTA.

Procedure

1. Collect two 10-mL blood samples.

Postprocedure Care

1. None.

Client and Family Teaching

1. Refer the client with abnormal results for genetic counseling. Refer to Appendix B, "Informed Consent for Genetic Testing".

Factors That Affect Results

1. Sensitivity of this test is 99%, but specificity is not known.

Other Data

1. The Genetic Information Nondiscrimination Act of 2008 prohibits health plans from using genetic family history or genetic test results from influencing eligibility or premiums for health insurance. It also prohibits employers from using this information to influence decisions about hiring, terminating employment, or employment pay, promotions, or privileges.
2. The FAMILION® test is offered by Genaissance Pharmaceutical of New Haven, Connecticut.
3. This test is also marketed for use identifying Brugada syndrome, short QT syndrome, and catecholaminergic polymorphic ventricular tachycardia (CPVT), but cannot provide risk stratification.

F

Fast MRI
See Magnetic Resonance Imaging—Diagnostic.

Fasting Blood Sugar
See Glucose—Blood.

Fat, Semiquantitative—Stool

Norm.

Neutral fat	<50 globules/HPF
Fatty acids	<100 globules/HPF

Increased. Amyloidosis, beta-lipoprotein deficiency, bile salt deficiency, blind loop syndrome, celiac disease, cystic fibrosis, diarrhea, diverticulosis, enteritis, hepatobiliary disease, hypogammaglobulinemia, increased peristalsis, ingestion of castor oil or mineral oil, intestinal fistula, lymphangiectasis, lymphoma, pancreatic disease (cancer, chronic pancreatitis, enzyme deficiency, mucoviscidosis), postoperatively (bowel resection), sprue, Whipple's disease, and Zollinger-Ellison syndrome.

Decreased. Persons fed medium-chain-triglyceride-enriched formula.

Description. Fecal fat is measured to aid diagnosis of conditions causing poor absorption of dietary fat, resulting in steatorrhea.

Professional Considerations
Consent form NOT required.

Preparation
1. Obtain a clean plastic specimen container and a clean toilet-seat urine collection container.
2. The client is to ingest 60 g of fat a day for 3-6 days.
3. Avoid use of suppositories, oily lubricants, or mineral oil in the perianal or genital areas for 3 days before and during specimen collection.

Procedure
1. Collect 20 mL of stool in a clean glass or plastic container.

Postprocedure Care
1. Cleanse the anal area.

Client and Family Teaching
1. Explain the need to avoid use of rectal, vaginal, or genital-area oils, lubricants, or suppositories for 3 days before the test. The client should urinate before defecating and then defecate sample into the urine collection container and transfer the stool sample to the specimen container with a wooden spatula.
2. Results may take several days.

Factors That Affect Results
1. Send fresh random stool samples to the laboratory within 2 hours.

Other Data
1. Bedtime laxatives may be needed for constipated clients.
2. Some malabsorption syndromes such as tropical sprue may not show increased fecal fat.

FDP
See Fibrinogen Breakdown Products—Blood.

Febrile Agglutinins—Serum

Norm. Negative, or less than a fourfold rise in titer between acute and convalescent samples or a titer less than 1:40.

Normal Dilutions.

	Negative	Suggestive Of Disease* with Single Serum Titer of
Salmonella antibody	<1:80	
Brucella antibody	<1:80	>1:160
Francisella antibody	<1:40	>1:80
Rickettsia antibody	<1:40	

*When accompanied by clinical symptoms.

Usage. Suspected infection with *Brucella*, *Francisella* (tularemia), *Proteus*, *Rickettsia* (Rocky Mountain spotted fever, typhus), *Salmonella* (paratyphoid, salmonellosis, and typhoid). Chronic granulomatous disease.

Description. Febrile agglutination tests are performed to identify the cause of febrile illnesses. Bacterial antibodies to the above organisms will agglutinate in vitro if present in the serum in sufficient concentrations to indicate current or past infection. In this test, the sample containing suspected antigens is mixed with a client's serum and observed for an agglutination reaction. The sample is heated and observed for clumping and unclumping. A sample that clumps upon warming and unclumps upon cooling is considered a positive test. A positive reaction is followed by serial dilutions of serum and retesting. The results are expressed as the highest titer showing agglutination. Agglutination at a titer greater than 1:40 indicates the presence of antibodies to any of the above four organisms. Agglutination at a titer greater than 1:80 indicates the presence of antibodies to the *Brucella* or *Salmonella* organisms.

Professional Considerations

Consent form NOT required.

Preparation

1. Tube: Red topped, red/gray topped, or gold topped. Cool the tube in the refrigerator or on ice before specimen collection.

Procedure

1. Draw a 10-mL blood sample and label it as the acute sample. Repeat the test every 3-5 days. Draw the final sample in 10-14 days and label it as the convalescent sample.

Postprocedure Care

1. Send the specimens to the laboratory immediately.

Client and Family Teaching

1. Two samples must be taken about 2 weeks apart to identify a trend in levels that can pinpoint the cause of the fever. The client may be treated empirically before the second sample is taken.

Factors That Affect Results

1. Reject hemolyzed specimens.
2. Chronic exposure to or vaccination against the above-mentioned organisms may cause high titers.
3. Immunosuppressed clients may be infected but have low or negative titers.
4. Antibiotic therapy causes low initial titers.
5. *Brucella* antigen skin tests may elevate titers.
6. Many cross-reactions are possible.

Other Data

1. Results are given as the highest dilution in which a positive reaction with the antigen occurs.
2. A blood culture for the above organisms should be performed concurrently.
3. Failure rate is 22% when tularemia is being treated with streptomycin antibiotic. Retreatment with ciprofloxacin is recommended followed by ofloxacin if needed.
4. Oculoglandular tularemia is an uncommon conjunctivitis caused by a tick or insect bite and is most common in the state of Arkansas.
5. See also Brucellosis agglutinins—Blood; Rocky Mountain spotted fever serology—Serum; or Tularemia agglutinins—Serum.

Fecal Fat, Quantitative, 72-Hour—Stool

Norm.

Adult, 60 g of fat/day diet	2-6 g/24 hours, or <20% of total solids, or 7-21 mmol/day
Adult, fat-free diet	<4 g/day
Breast-fed infant	<1 g/day
Child up to 6 years old	<2 g/day

Increased. Amyloidosis, beta-lipoprotein deficiency, bile salt deficiency, blind loop syndrome, celiac disease, Crohn's disease, cystic fibrosis, diarrhea, diverticulosis, enteritis, Graves' disease, hepatobiliary disease, hypogammaglobulinemia, increased peristalsis, ingestion of castor oil or mineral oil, intestinal fistula, lymphangiectasis, lymphoma, pancreatic disease (cancer, chronic pancreatitis, enzyme deficiency, mucoviscidosis), postoperatively (bowel resection), sprue (celiac), Whipple's disease, and Zollinger-Ellison syndrome. Drugs include lanreotide and orlistat (Xenical). Dietary intake of >40 g of olestra per day increased levels to those of steatorrhea clients.

Description. Fecal fat is measured to aid diagnosis of conditions causing poor absorption of dietary fat resulting in steatorrhea. The value of this test is that the amount of dietary fat intake is known and used in evaluation of the results.

Professional Considerations
Consent form NOT required.

Preparation
1. Obtain 500-mL clean plastic containers, dry ice, and a clean toilet-seat urine collection container.

Procedure
1. Collect all stools, using a urine collection container in the toilet, on the fourth, fifth, and sixth days of the specified diet and place the stools in the clean plastic containers.
2. Keep the specimen containers refrigerated during the collection period.

Postprocedure Care
1. Freeze the specimens on dry ice if the testing will not be performed within 24 hours.
2. Record the date and time of each specimen collected.

Client and Family Teaching
1. The client is to ingest 50-150 g of fat per day for 3-6 days.
2. Avoid suppositories, oily lubricants, or mineral oil in the perianal or genital areas for 3 days before and during collection.
3. Avoid contaminating the stool with urine or toilet paper.
4. Results may take several days.

Factors That Affect Results
1. Reject specimens submitted in improper containers such as cartons, coffee cans, or plastic bags.
2. False-negative results are most commonly caused by failure to collect all stools.
3. False-positive results are caused by dietary ingestion of olestra found in some potato chips.

Other Data
1. Bedtime laxatives may be needed for constipated clients.
2. Some clients with malabsorption syndromes such as tropical sprue may not show increased fecal fat excretion.

Fecal Immunochemical Testing

See Immunochemical Fecal Occult Blood Testing—Stool

Fecal Leukocytes, Stool—Diagnostic

Norm. No leukocytes present.

Usage. Determine the type of diarrhea, invasive or noninvasive, to the mucosa of the colon. If no fecal leukocytes are present in the stool specimen, an antidiarrheal medication can be given. If fecal leukocytes are present, an antidiarrheal medication should not be given. The results of this test will be readily available, whereas a culture will take several days.

Description. The presence of fecal leukocytes in the stool indicates that the cause of the diarrhea is an organism such as Shiga toxin–producing *E. coli* or a process that is breaking the mucosal barrier of the colon, such as *Salmonella, Shigella, Amoeba, Campylobacter, Helicobacter,* or *Yersinia* infections, Crohn's disease, and chronic inflammatory bowel disease. Fecal leukocytes are usually not present in infectious processes that do not invade the mucosa, such as "viral enteritis," toxin-mediated diarrhea, or infections with noninvasive *E. coli*. The absence of blood and fecal leukocytes usually means that the diarrhea process is transient and can be treated symptomatically. *Clostridium difficile* may or may not be associated with leukocytes in the stool (fecal leukocyte stain is 14% sensitive and 90% specific); therefore if it is suspected, a stool culture should be sent and no antidiarrheal agent given until the results are confirmed as negative.

Professional Considerations
Consent form is NOT required.

Preparation
1. Obtain a stool specimen container.

Procedure
1. Instruct the client to collect a stool sample, or use a bedpan so that the sample can be obtained.
2. Send the specimen to the laboratory.

Postprocedure Care
1. Keep the rectal area as clean and as dry as possible to prevent skin breakdown.
2. If diarrhea is frequent, encourage fluids and check serum electrolytes for abnormalities.

Client and Family Teaching
1. Avoid contaminating the stool with toilet tissue or urine.
2. Results are normally available within 48 hours.

Factors That Affect Results
1. None.

Other Data
1. Stool cultures should be obtained from all clients with fecal leukocytes to differentiate acute infection from inflammatory bowel syndrome. In the absence of fecal leukocytes, stool cultures are usually negative.

Fenfluramine

See **Amphetamines**—Blood.

Ferric Chloride Test—Diagnostic

Norm. No color change when the diagnostic reagent (ferric chloride) is added to the urine.

Usage. Of value in the diagnosis of epidemic dropsy and certain drug intoxications (salicylates and phenothiazines), and in the diagnosis of several inborn errors of amino acid metabolism (phenylketonuria, maple syrup urine disease, and alkaptonuria). Also occasionally used to detect melanin in the urine.

Description. A spot urine sample is obtained. Ferric chloride solution is added to the urine sample, and characteristic color changes occur depending on the pathologic condition present (that is, purple with salicylates, purple-pink with phenothiazines, gray with melanin, for example).

Condition	Color Change in Urine
Alcoholism	Red or red-brown
Alkaptonuria	Blue or green, fades quickly
Diabetes	Red or red-brown
Drug ingestion	
Acetophenetidines	Red
Aminosalicylic acid	Red-brown
Antipyrines	Red
Cyanates	Red
Phenol derivative	Violet
Phenothiazines	Purple-pink
Salicylates	Stable purple
Histidinemia	Green or blue-green

Condition	Color Change in Urine
Maple syrup urine disease	Blue
Phenylketonuria	Blue or blue-green, fades to yellow
Starvation	Red or red-brown
Tyrosinosis	Green, fades in seconds
Other products	
Alpha-Ketobutyric acid	Purple, fades to red-brown
Bilirubin	Blue-green
o-Hydroxyphenyl-acetic acid	Mauve
o-Hydroxyphenyl-pyruvic acid	Red
Pyruvic acid	Deep gold-yellow or green
Xanthurenic acid	Deep green, later brown

Professional Considerations
Consent form NOT required.

Preparation
1. Several drugs can influence the test and cause a color change when the ferric chloride reagent is added to the urine. These include salicylates (aspirin and related drugs) and phenothiazine-related compounds. These should be avoided if possible before the test.
2. Fasting is not required before the test, and no other pretest preparation is necessary.

Procedure
1. Urine is collected from the client into a clean container and submitted to the diagnostic laboratory for analysis.
2. In the laboratory ferric chloride is added to the urine sample, and the technician waits for a color change to occur.

Postprocedure Care
1. No special postprocedure care of the client is required.

Client and Family Teaching
1. The client and appropriate family members should be oriented as to the rationale behind the test before it is performed.
2. Several of the conditions diagnosed with this test represent inborn errors of metabolism.
3. Genetic counseling may be indicated once the diagnosis of these disorders is established.

Factors That Affect Results
1. Preparation and storage of the ferric chloride reagent.
2. Ingestion of certain drugs (salicylates and phenothiazines) may cause a color change when the ferric chloride is added to the urine sample.

Other Data
1. The ferric chloride test is rather insensitive because it relies on a gross (qualitative) color change observed by a technician. Other more sensitive tests (including chromatography) may be helpful in the diagnosis of several of the disorders listed above.

Ferritin—Serum
Norm.

		SI Units
Adult Females		
≤40 years	7-282 ng/mL	7-282 µg/L
>40 years	12-263 ng/mL	12-263 µg/L
Adult Males	6-323 ng/mL	16-323 µg/L
Children		
Newborn	25-200 ng/mL	25-200 µg/L
1 month	200-600 ng/mL	200-600 µg/L
2-5 months	50-200 ng/mL	50-200 µg/L
6 months	7-140 ng/mL	7-140 µg/L
1-15 years	7-140 ng/mL	7-140 µg/L

Iron Toxicity: Serial measurements over 1000 µg/L.

Increased. Carcinoma (generalized, hepatic), cirrhosis, hemochromatosis (idiopathic), hepatic disease (acute, chronic), hepatic necrosis, hepatitis, hepatoma, Hodgkin's disease, hyperthyroidism, inflammation (chronic), iron intake (excessive dietary or by blood transfusion), jaundice (obstructive), leukemia, multiple myeloma, polycythemia, renal disease (chronic), respiratory infection (upper) with fever, rheumatoid arthritis, siderosis, and tissue trauma. Transfusion-related: Anemia (chronic, hemolytic, megaloblastic, pernicious, sideroblastic), myelodysplastic syndrome, Sickle cell disease, thalassemia (major, minor). Drugs include alcohol (wine ethanol), ascorbic acid (women only), iron, and hormonal contraceptives.

Decreased. Acid peptic disease, adenoma of GI tract, anemia (iron deficiency), colon cancer, hemodialysis, IgG-positive people, inflammatory bowel disease, pregnancy, rigorous athletic training, and surgery (gastrointestinal).

Description. An iron-storing protein manufactured in the liver, spleen, bone marrow, tumor cells, and sites of inflammation. Evaluation of ferritin levels is most often performed in the differential diagnosis of several types of anemia. Serum ferritin has been found to be more specific and sensitive and specific than serum transferrin receptor for differentiating iron-deficiency anemia from anemia of chronic disease in elderly clients with anemia. However, in infants, serum ferritin is less accurate in identifying iron deficiency than is serum transferrin receptor and the serum transferrin receptor:serum ferritin ratio.

Professional Considerations

Consent form NOT required.

Preparation

1. Tube: Red topped, red/gray topped, or gold topped.

Procedure

1. Draw a 4-mL blood sample.

Postprocedure Care

1. Centrifuge and freeze samples.

Client and Family Teaching

1. Results may not be available for several days.

Factors That Affect Results

1. Reject specimens if the client had a radioactive scan within 48 hours before specimen collection.
2. Deruisseau et al (2004) found that serum ferritin levels were lowered in college-age males who weight-trained.

Other Data

1. Hemolyzed samples are acceptable.
2. Ferritin <50 ng/mL is predictive of a serious GI tract pathologic condition.
3. Goel et al (2003) found that a serum ferritin (SF) "concentration of >40 micro g/dL and a rise in SF concentration with increasing gestation should alert the clinician regarding the possibility of preterm delivery."
4. Elevated ferritin levels a few hours after cerebral vascular accident (CVA) and weeks after the CVA are predictive of a poor prognosis.
5. Risk of iron toxicity increases as the number of lifetime transfusions approaches the 10 to 20 range or cumulative transfusions of packed red blood cells equating to 120mL/kg.

Fetal Fibronectin (fFN, Oncofetal Fibronectin)—Specimen

Norm. >0.050 µg/mL

Usage. Assay indicated for use in clients with higher than average risk for preterm delivery. Findings are evaluated in conjunction with other clinical information as an aid to rapidly assess the risk of preterm delivery in symptomatic and asymptomatic pregnant women between 24 and 34 weeks of completed gestation. This test provides an advantage over other assessments of risk for preterm delivery, such as digital examination and measurement of contraction frequency, because it is less subjective, and thus can prevent unnecessary activity restrictions and medications to slow delivery.

Description. Qualitative test for the detection of fetal fibronectin (fFN) in cervicovaginal secretions. fFN can be detected in cervicovaginal secretions of women throughout pregnancy by use of a monoclonal antibody–based immunoassay. fFN is elevated in cervicovaginal secretions during the first 24 weeks of pregnancy but diminishes between 24 and 34 weeks in normal pregnancies. The significance of its presence in the vagina during the first 24 weeks of pregnancy is not understood. However, it may simply reflect the normal growth of the extra villous trophoblast population and the placenta. Detection of fFN in cervicovaginal secretions between 24 and 34 completed weeks of gestation is reported to be associated with preterm delivery in symptomatic and asymptomatic pregnant women. Ninety-nine percent of pregnant women with signs and symptoms of preterm delivery who test negatively for fFN do not deliver within the next 14 days. A positive fFN result is the single best predictor of impending delivery. However, there is a high false-positive rate as up to 40% of those with positive results experience full-term deliveries.

Professional Considerations
Consent form NOT required.

Contraindications
Symptomatic women with one or more of the following conditions: advanced cervical dilatation (>3 cm), rupture of amniotic membranes, cervical cerclage, moderate or gross vaginal bleeding; OR asymptomatic women with one or more of the following conditions: multiple gestations, cervical cerclage, placenta previa (partial or complete), sexual intercourse in the preceding 24 hours. Test is also contraindicated when the pregnancy is less than 22 weeks of gestation.

Preparation
1. See Client and Family Teaching.
2. Obtain a polyester-fiber (Dacron) swab, sterile gloves, speculum.
3. The client should disrobe below the waist.
4. Position the client recumbent on a gynecologic examination table in the lithotomy position and drape for comfort and privacy.

Procedure
1. NOTE: Specimen must be obtained before digital examination.
2. Cervicovaginal swab: Collection from *symptomatic* women:
   a. Insert a sterile speculum into the vagina. You should collect the specimen from the posterior fornix of the vagina during a sterile speculum examination by slightly rotating the Dacron swab for approximately 10 seconds to absorb the cervicovaginal secretions. Remove swab and immerse Dacron tip into buffered collection tube. Break the swab shaft even with the top of the tube. Align the shaft of the swab with the hole inside the tube cap and push the cap down tightly to seal the tube.
3. Cervicovaginal swab: Collection from *asymptomatic* women:
   a. Insert a sterile speculum into the vagina. You should collect the specimen from either the posterior fornix of the vagina or the ectocervical region of the external cervical os during a sterile speculum examination by slightly rotating the Dacron swab for approximately 10 seconds to absorb the cervicovaginal secretions. Remove swab and immerse Dacron tip into buffered collection tube. Break the swab shaft even with the top of the tube. Align the shaft of the swab with the hole inside the tube cap, and push the cap down tightly to seal the tube.

Postprocedure Care
1. Write the client's age, the reason for the study, and calculated gestational weeks on the lab requisition.
2. Document any signs or symptoms of preterm delivery in the client's record.
3. Send specimen to the laboratory immediately.

Client and Family Teaching
1. It is customary practice for the physician to discuss with the client the purpose of the procedure and risks associated with the procedure. Arrangements for discussing the results of the test should be made by the client's physician.

Factors That Affect Results

1. A positive fetal fibronectin result may be observed for clients who have experienced cervical disruption caused by but not limited to events such as sexual intercourse, digital cervical examination, or vaginal probe ultrasonography.
2. Care must be taken not to contaminate the swab or cervicovaginal secretions with lubricants, soaps, or disinfectants (such as K-Y Jelly, povidone-iodine solution [Betadine], hexachlorophene). Lubricants or creams may physically interfere with absorption of the specimen onto the swab. Soaps or disinfectants may interfere with the antibody-antigen reaction.
3. Cotton swabs absorb the fetal fibronectin and are not acceptable for this assay.
4. Results obtained from pregnant women who have had intercourse within the previous 24 hours before collection are difficult to interpret.
5. Test interference from the following components has not been ruled out: douches, white blood cells, bacteria, and bilirubin.
6. Results should be interpreted with caution when a specimen is obtained from a client with unconfirmed gestational age.
7. Rupture of membranes should be ruled out before the assay is performed, since fFN is found in both amniotic fluid and the fetal membranes.

Other Data

1. Other research studies in fFN testing have been done in the field of embryo and trophoblast implantation.
2. "Oncofetal" fibronectin was the name given to the molecule by researchers Matsuura and Hakomori (1985) who discovered the FDC-6 antibody; they originally demonstrated the antibody's capability of binding to tumor cells and tissues. The company marketing the "fetal" fibronectin test (which uses the FDC-6 antibody), dropped the "onco" portion of the test name to avoid raising concern that the test or reasons for use has any association with cancer.

Fetal Hemoglobin (HbF)—Blood

Norm.

Adults	0-2% of total hemoglobin
Children	
Newborn	60%-90% of total hemoglobin
1-5 months	<75% of total hemoglobin
6-12 months	<5% of total hemoglobin
1-20 years	<2% of total hemoglobin

Increased. Anemia (aplastic, megaloblastic, nonhereditary refractory normoblastic, pernicious, refractory, sickle cell, spherocytic), anorexia nervosa, bone marrow metastasis, bulimia nervosa, diabetes, Down syndrome, erythroleukemia, hereditary persistence of fetal hemoglobin, hyperthyroidism, hypothyroidism, infants (small for gestational age, chronic intrauterine anoxia, developmental abnormalities), leukemia, lymphoma, macroglobulinemia, multiple myeloma, myelofibrosis, paroxysmal nocturnal hemoglobinuria, post cord blood stem cell transplant, pregnancy (fetal blood leakage into mother's blood), spherocytosis, sudden infant death syndrome (SIDS), thalassemia (beta major, minor), thyrotoxicosis, trisomy 13-15, D trisomy, and trisomy 21. Drugs include anticonvulsants.

Decreased. Multiple chromosome abnormality (C/D translocation).

Description. HbF, the hemoglobin present during fetal development, contains a polypeptide globin chain that is different from that in adult hemoglobin. It composes most of the hemoglobin of a newborn's red blood cells. Over the first 6 months of life, most of the fetal hemoglobin is replaced by adult hemoglobin, though a small portion of HbF may persist throughout the life span. This test is most often used to differentiate thalassemia and other hemoglobinopathies in which abnormalities may be found in the polypeptide globin chains.

Professional Considerations

Consent form NOT required.

Preparation

1. Tube: Lavender topped or green topped.

Procedure

1. Draw a 2-mL blood sample.

Postprocedure Care

1. None.

Client and Family Teaching

1. Results may take several days.

Factors That Affect Results

1. Reject specimens older than 4 days at room temperature.

Other Data

1. Sample is stable at room temperature for 4 days.

Fetal Hemoglobin Stain

See **Betke-Kleihauer Stain**—Diagnostic.

Fetal Monitoring, External—Diagnostic

Norm. Fetal heart rate (FHR) and variability normal.

FHR	120-160 bpm
FHR variability	5-25 bpm

Usage. Monitoring FHR and uterine contractions, evaluation of fetal effects of stressed and nonstressed situations, assessment of the need for internal fetal monitoring, and monitoring of fetal well-being during the oxytocin challenge test.

Description. A noninvasive test in which an electronic transducer is placed on the pregnant abdomen to amplify the FHR while a cardiotachometer records FHR and pressure sensors record uterine contractions. External fetal monitors record fluctuations in the baseline FHR and detect variability between beats. This test is able to detect FHR accelerations and decelerations in response to uterine contractions.

Professional Considerations

Consent form NOT required.

Preparation

1. Obtain a fetal heart monitor and an electroconductive gel.
2. Cleanse the transducer and transducer connections.

Procedure

1. The client is placed in a semi-Fowler's or left lateral position with the abdomen exposed.
2. The transducer is coated with electroconductive gel and strapped over the abdominal area with the most distinct fetal heart tones. For active labor, this is the fundus.
3. The alarm limits for FHR are set, and test recordings are started to ensure that the system is functioning properly.
4. For active labor, baseline FHR is recorded and calculated over a 10-minute period and then monitored continuously as labor progresses. The recording is evaluated for abnormalities in FHR and FHR response to contractions, drugs, or maternal position.
5. Transducer location may need adjustment in response to fetal movement in utero.

Postprocedure Care

1. Weekly external fetal monitoring is indicated for diabetes, hypertension, fetal growth retardation, and pregnancy over 42 weeks of gestation.

Client and Family Teaching

1. For antepartal testing, the client should eat a full meal just before the test.
2. The test poses no risk of harm to the client or the fetus.

Factors That Affect Results

1. Maternal position may cause fetal distress. The left side-lying position best promotes oxygen delivery to the fetus.
2. Maternal obesity may interfere with the adequacy of recordings.
3. Artifact may result from poor transducer connections, or dried electroconductive gel on the transducer.

Other Data

1. Events that cause changes in the FHR recordings during active labor are handwritten on the graphic recording. These include maternal movement, administration of drugs, and procedures.

Fetal Monitoring, External, Contraction Stress Test (CST) and Oxytocin Challenge Test (OCT)—Diagnostic

Norm. Fetal heart rate (FHR) and variability normal.

FHR	110-160 bpm
FHR variability	5 bpm: minimal variability
	6-25 bpm: moderate variability
	greater than 25 bpm: pronounced variability

Usage. To stimulate labor, to evaluate fetal responses to contractions. CST/OCT administered as a result of nonreactive non–stress test (NST). CST is one measure used to evaluate the quality of placental perfusion and fetal well-being. This test is usually conducted after 32 weeks of gestation.

Description. A noninvasive procedure in which the fetus is electronically monitored and uterine contractions are stimulated. A regular contraction pattern is achieved for the purpose of evaluating fetal responses and making predictions regarding fetal outcome to labor.

Interpretation of CST/OCT

Negative = No decelerations during entire procedure; long-term viability (LTV) is present. Uterine contractions have no adverse effect on fetus (deceleration). Is predictive of continued fetal well-being for 7 days.

Positive = At least half of contractions obtained are accompanied by late decelerations. Prognosis is poor in the presence of decreased LTV. Vigorous management is indicated.

Equivocal = Test needs to be repeated within 24 hours.

Hyperstimulation = >4 contractions in 10 minutes, or contractions lasting longer than 90 seconds, or <60 seconds between contractions.

Suspicious = Late decelerations present in less than half of contractions. LTV usually present.

Unsatisfactory = Quality of tracing too poor to provide accurate interpretation.

Professional Considerations

Consent form is NOT required, but maternal permission should be obtained. Client needs to be informed that the effect of oxytocin may induce labor.

Contraindications

Preterm labor, placenta previa.

Preparation

1. Complete a 20-minute monitor strip for a baseline FHR and uterine activity. Observe fetal movement and changes in FHR.
2. Test must be conducted in an intrapartal unit in the event of nonreassuring outcomes that require immediate interventions.

Procedure

1. For exogenous oxytocin release by oxytocin (Pitocin) infusion, begin an intravenous infusion of lactated Ringer's, dextrose with saline, or normal saline. Add oxytocin piggyback IV infusion at 0.5 milliunit (mU)/minute. Test period conducted until client achieves three uterine contractions, each lasting 40 seconds, within a 10-minute period. Increase oxytocin rate per protocol until contraction pattern is achieved.
2. For endogenous oxytocin release, see Client and Family Teaching.

Postprocedure Care

1. Continue to observe and document fetal patterns and changes in uterine activity. Watch for uterine hyperstimulation.
2. Discontinue oxytocin; monitor client's blood pressure and pulse rate until contractions have subsided.

Client and Family Teaching

1. For endogenous oxytocin release by nipple stimulation, instruct client to brush or massage a nipple until contractions begin, or for 10 minutes. If there are no contractions after 10 minutes, ask client to brush or massage other nipple.

Factors That Affect Results

1. CST/OCT has a <2% false-negative rate and a >50% false-positive rate.

Other Data

1. CST/OCT is more sensitive to fetal oxygen reserves than is NST.

2. In the presence of variable decelerations, regardless of the outcome of the test, amniotic fluid infusion may be indicated.

Fetal Monitoring, External, Non–Stress Testing (NST)—Diagnostic

Norm. Reactive: Fetal heart rate (FHR) and variability normal.

FHR	110-160 bpm
FHR variability	
Minimal	5 bpm
Moderate	6-25 bpm
Pronounced	greater than 25 bpm

Usage. Monitoring FHR and uterine patterns under normal, nonstressful circumstances during late pregnancy (third trimester). This test is able to detect FHR accelerations as associated with fetal movement. In the presence of uterine contractions, decelerations may be observed.

Description. A noninvasive test in which an electronic transducer is placed on the pregnant abdomen to amplify the FHR while a cardiotachometer records FHR and a pressure sensor (tocodynamometer) records any uterine contractions. A baseline FHR is determined, fetal movements are recorded, and any change in FHR associated with the fetus's own movement is evaluated. A result classified as "reactive" indicates that blood and oxygen flow to the fetus is adequate and correlates with fetal survival.

Interpretation of NST

Reactive = At least 2 accelerations of greater than 15 beats above baseline during 20 minutes.

Nonreactive = None of the reactive criteria met; long-term variability minimal.

Unsatisfactory = Unable to obtain adequate tracing; fetal patterns are borderline for criteria. Reschedule testing as indicated by condition.

Professional Considerations

Consent form NOT required. Client agreement is recommended.

Preparation

1. Obtain a fetal heart monitor and an electroconductive gel.
2. Cleanse the transducer, tocodynamometer, and monitor connections with alcohol pads.

Procedure

1. The client is instructed to empty her bladder and then is placed in a left lateral or semi-Fowler's position (with left hip roll) with the abdomen exposed. Use Leopold's maneuvers to determine fetal outline. Palpate fetal spine and locate occiput. The most distinct fetal heart tones are obtained over area of the fetal shoulders (usually lower left or lower right quadrant).
2. The transducer is coated with electroconductive gel and strapped over the location of fetal heart tone.
3. The alarm limits for FHR are set, and a baseline heart rate over a 2-minute period is determined.
4. Assess uterine fundus to locate area where contractions are best palpated and not affected by fetal position. Strap tocodynamometer over this area.
5. Client is monitored for a minimum of 30 minutes. During this time, monitor will electronically record any fetal movements, including kicking. If monitor does not have this capacity, client will be asked to press a button each time a movement is felt in order to record activity.
6. Fetus should exhibit accelerations during a 20-minute period. Acceleration is defined as an increase of 15 bpm over fetal baseline rate, lasting 15 seconds.

Postprocedure Care

1. Weekly external fetal monitoring is indicated for diabetes, hypertension, fetal growth retardation, and pregnancy >42 weeks of gestation.
2. In the event of a nonreactive result, client will be scheduled for a contraction stress test (CST)/oxytocin challenge test (OCT).

Client and Family Teaching

1. For antepartal testing, the client should eat a full meal just before the test.
2. The test poses no risk or harm to the client or the fetus.

Factors That Affect Results

1. False-positive result associated with inadequate testing time, maternal hypotension, and maternal medications.

2. False-negative result associated with improper placement of monitoring devices.

Other Data
1. None.

Fetal Monitoring, Internal—Diagnostic

Norm. Fetal heart rate (FHR) and variability normal.

FHR	110-160 bpm
FHR variability	
Minimal	5 bpm
Moderate	6-25 bpm
Pronounced	<25 bpm

Maternal Contractions and Intrauterine Pressure During Labor

Prelabor	<3 contractions over 10 minutes
	25-40 mm Hg contraction pressure
First stage	<6 contractions over 10 minutes
	8-12 mm Hg baseline pressure
	30-40 mm Hg contraction pressure
Second stage	1 contraction about every 2 minutes
	10-20 mm Hg baseline pressure
	50-80 mm Hg contraction pressure

Usage. Monitoring of beat-to-beat variability of FHR and rate and pressure monitoring of uterine contractions during labor. Often used as an adjunct to external fetal monitoring. More accurate than external fetal monitoring, especially in cases of maternal obesity. Internal monitoring is less affected by fetal or maternal movement than external monitoring.

Description. During this invasive monitoring procedure, a sterile fetal scalp electrode and a uterine catheter are inserted through the vaginal canal for the purpose of FHR and uterine-contraction measurements during labor after 3-cm cervical dilatation and rupture of membranes. Internal monitoring is recommended over external monitoring for a better assessment of the effects of labor on the fetus and to provide interpretation of quality of contraction pattern.

Professional Considerations
Consent form IS required.

Risks
Maternal uterine perforation; intrauterine infection; and fetal scalp infection, abscess, or hematoma.
Contraindications
Active genital herpes.
Precaution
Test should be performed only when the fetal presenting part is the head.

Preparation
1. Obtain an antiseptic solution, sterile gloves, a fetal scalp electrode and guide, a pressure catheter for intrauterine contraction monitoring, a catheter guide, a transducer, a fetal heart monitor, and a topical antibiotic.
2. Ascertain that membranes are ruptured and that the presenting part is the fetal head.

Procedure
1. The client is placed in a dorsal lithotomy position.
2. The perineal area is cleansed with antiseptic solution.
3. A sterile vaginal examination is performed to measure cervical dilatation and identify a fetal scalp location over bone for electrode placement.
4. The electrode is guided through the vaginal canal and cervical os and gently screwed into place on the fetal scalp.
5. The electrode wires are connected to the fetal monitor. Correct placement and functioning of the system are verified when a FHR signal is demonstrated by the fetal monitor.
6. The pressure-sensitive catheter for monitoring uterine contractions is then guided into place, through the cervix, a shallow distance to the uterus. The distal end is connected to a pressure transducer for continuous monitoring of intrauterine pressure. The monitor is calibrated to zero for a uterine pressure baseline value.
7. Continue monitoring FHR and contraction pattern as with external monitoring.

8. Just before beginning the procedure, take a "time out" to verify the correct client, procedure, and site.

Postprocedure Care
1. Cleanse the fetal scalp electrode site with antiseptic at the time of delivery.
2. Document observed laceration(s) of the baby's scalp.

Client and Family Teaching
1. Explain procedure to client. Internal fetal monitoring poses risks (listed above) but provides much better assessment of how well the fetus is tolerating the labor process than external fetal monitoring does.

Factors That Affect Results
1. Drugs that affect the sympathetic and parasympathetic nervous systems may influence FHR.
2. The maternal position may cause fetal distress. The left side-lying position best promotes oxygen delivery to the fetus.

Other Data
1. The internal scalp electrode may be inserted and removed by a registered nurse who has received specialized preparation in this skill or by a physician. The intrauterine pressure catheter may be inserted only by a physician.

Fetoscopy—Diagnostic

Norm. Normal fetal development. Absence of neural tube defects.

Usage. Diagnosis of malformation of the fetus. Detection of neural tube defect. Blood samples may be obtained to test for sickle cell anemia and hemophilia.

Description. Fetoscopy is an endoscopic procedure that allows direct examination of the fetus by means of the fetoscope.

Professional Considerations
Consent form IS required.

Risks
Abortion or premature labor; amnionitis (antibiotics may be given prophylactically to prevent this complication).

Contraindications
Anteriorly placed placenta, bleeding disorder, hypertensive crisis, incompetent cervix, history of spontaneous abortion or premature labor.

Preparation
1. To prevent excessive fetal activity during the procedure, the mother may be given meperidine (Demerol), which crosses the placenta and quiets the fetus.
2. Obtain a local anesthetic and a fetoscopy tray.

3. Just before beginning the procedure, take a "time out" to verify the correct client, procedure, and site.

Procedure
1. The abdominal wall of the mother is anesthetized with a local anesthetic.
2. An ultrasound examination is then used to locate the fetus and placenta.
3. A small incision is made in the abdominal wall, and the fetoscope is inserted through the abdominal wall into the amniotic cavity. The fetus is visualized for obvious malformations, such as neural tube defects.

Postprocedure Care
1. Apply a dry, sterile dressing to the fetoscopy site.

Client and Family Teaching
1. This procedure poses risks (listed above).
2. A local anesthetic will be used to prevent pain. The client will feel pressure as the fetoscope is inserted.
3. The test takes about 40 minutes.

Factors That Affect Results
1. Excessive movement of the mother may obscure results.

Other Data
1. None.

Fetus Examination After Death

See **Autopsy**—Diagnostic.

FFDM

See **Mammography**—Diagnostic.

Fibrin Breakdown Products

See **Fibrinogen Breakdown Products**—Blood.

Fibrin Degradation Fragment

See **D-Dimer**—Blood.

Fibrin Degradation Products

See **Fibrinogen Breakdown Products**—Blood.

Fibrin Split Products, Protamine Sulfate Test—Blood

Norm. Negative test.

Positive Test. Deep vein thrombosis, disseminated intravascular coagulation (DIC), infarcts, Kasabach-Merritt syndrome, postoperative blood vessel clots, and pulmonary embolism.

Description. Protamine sulfate added to the blood sample helps differentiate between conditions producing secondary fibrinolysin (positive test) and conditions producing primary fibrinolysin (negative test). It is primarily used as a screening test for DIC, which produces secondary fibrinolysin.

Professional Considerations
Consent form NOT required.

Preparation
1. Tube: Blue topped.
2. Perform this test before implementing heparin therapy.

Procedure
1. Draw a 3-mL blood sample.

Postprocedure Care
1. For clients with coagulopathy, hold pressure over the sampling site for at least 5 minutes and observe the site closely for development of a hematoma.
2. Write the collection time on the laboratory requisition.
3. Do NOT shake the tube or place it on ice.
4. Transport the specimen to the laboratory immediately for incubation.

Client and Family Teaching
1. Results are normally available within 2 hours.
2. Seek medical attention for signs of bleeding (that is, hematoma, bleeding of gums, wounds, petechiae, confusion, changing level of consciousness).

Factors That Affect Results
1. Reject hemolyzed specimens or specimens received more than 2 hours after collection.
2. Drugs that may produce a false-positive result include heparin calcium and heparin sodium.

Other Data
1. Assess for signs of shock from bleeding: tachycardia, hypotension, and clammy cold skin.

Fibrin Stabilizing Factor

See **Factor XIII**—Blood.

Fibrinogen (Factor I)—Plasma

Norm. Quantitative is 200-400 mg/dL (2.0-4.0 g/L, SI units).

Lower values can occur in newborns.

Increased. Arthritis (rheumatoid), familial paroxysmal peritonitis (familial Mediterranean fever, periodic disease), hepatitis, infection (acute), and menstruation.

Decreased. Abortion (septic, missed), anemia (acquired hemolytic), burns (severe), carcinoma (prostate, lung, metastasis), circulating fibrinogen inhibitors, cirrhosis, coagulation factor deficiency, congenital fibrinogen disorders (afibrinogenemia, hypofibrinogenemia, dysfibrinogenemia), cryoglobulinemia, disseminated intravascular coagulation (DIC), eclampsia, embolism (amniotic fluid, fat, meconium), leukemia, lymphoma, macroglobulinemia, multiple myeloma, septicemia, shock, snakebite, thrombotic thrombocytopenic purpura, transfusion reaction, and trauma. Drugs include asparaginase, bezafibrate, perindopril, phenobarbital drug poisoning, streptokinase, ticlopidine, and urokinase. Elevation slows or stops with the administration of glycoprotein IIB/IIIA inhibitors.

Description. Fibrinogen (factor I) is a heat-stable, complex polypeptide that converts to the insoluble polymer of fibrin after thrombin enzymatic action and combines with platelets to clot the blood. Synthesized in the liver, fibrinogen increases in diseases associated with tissue damage or inflammation. There is some evidence that it may be useful as a predictor of arteriosclerotic disease. One performs this test by adding thrombin to the client's plasma and measuring the amount of time taken for clotting to occur at standard dilutions. The amount of fibrin is then calculated based on the thrombin clotting time.

Professional Considerations

Consent form NOT required.

Preparation

1. Tube: 2.7- or 4.5-mL blue topped.

Procedure

1. Withdraw 2 mL of blood into a syringe or vacuum tube. Remove the syringe or tube, leaving the needle in place. Attach a second syringe and draw two blood samples, one in a citrated blue topped tube and the other in a control tube. The sample quantity should be 2.4 mL for a 2.7-mL tube and 4.0 mL for a 4.5-mL tube. Draw a 5-mL blood sample in a sodium citrate–anticoagulated blue topped tube.

Postprocedure Care

1. For clients with coagulopathy, hold pressure over sampling site for at least 5 minutes and observe site closely for development of a hematoma.
2. Transport the specimens to the laboratory immediately for spinning. The specimens are then stable for 3 days when refrigerated.

Client and Family Teaching

1. Seek medical attention for signs of bleeding (that is, hematoma, bleeding of gums, wounds, petechiae, confusion, changing level of consciousness).

Factors That Affect Results

1. Reject hemolyzed specimens or tubes partially filled with blood.

Other Data

1. Active bleeding or administration of a blood transfusion within 1 month before the test invalidates results.
2. Normally a prothrombin time and an activated partial thromboplastin time can also be performed on this specimen.
3. See also Activated partial thromboplastin time and thromboplastin time—Plasma.

Fibrinogen Breakdown Products (Fibrin Degradation Products, FDP)—Blood

Norm. 2-10 µg/mL. Panic range: >40 µg/mL.

Increased. Abruptio placentae, aneurysm, blood transfusion reaction, brain damage, burns, carcinomatosis, cirrhosis (alcoholic), congenital heart disease, deep vein thrombosis, disseminated intravascular coagulation, internal bleeding (newborns), intrauterine death, myocardial infarction, organ rejection (renal transplant), parturition, post cesarean birth, preeclampsia, pregnancy (third trimester), pulmonary embolism, pulmonary infarction, renal disease, respiratory distress (newborns), rheumatoid arthritis, sepsis, shock, squamous cell carcinoma of the oral cavity, subdural hematoma, sunstroke, surgical complications, and tissue damage (extensive). Drugs include barbiturates (large doses causing coma), megestrol acetate (high-dose), oral contraceptives containing desogestrel (DSG), streptokinase, and urokinase.

Decreased. Not clinically significant.

Description. Seven split products result from splitting fibrin or fibrinogen as a result of attack by plasmin during dissolution of fibrin clots. These split products, labeled A, B, C, D, E, X, and Y, indicate recent clotting activity. Greatly increased amounts interfere with hemostatic plug formation and indicate abnormal amounts of fibrinolysis. Levels >40 mg/mL are highly suggestive of disseminated intravascular coagulation.

Professional Considerations
Consent form NOT required.

Preparation
1. Tube: 2.7- or 4.5-mL blue topped. Also obtain ice.

Procedure
1. Withdraw 2 mL of blood into a syringe or vacuum tube. Remove the syringe or tube, leaving the needle in place. Attach a second syringe, and draw a 2.4-mL sample in a 2.7-mL tube or a 4.0-mL sample in a 4.5-mL tube. Place the specimens immediately in a container of ice.
2. Gently tilt the tube until a clot forms.

Postprocedure Care
1. For clients with coagulopathy, hold pressure over the sampling site for at least 5 minutes and observe the site closely for development of a hematoma.
2. Place the specimens on ice.

Client and Family Teaching
1. Results are normally available within 4 hours.
2. Seek medical attention for signs of bleeding (that is, hematoma, bleeding of gums, wounds, petechiae, confusion, changing level of consciousness).

Factors That Affect Results
1. Reject specimens of nonclotted blood.
2. Reject specimens if the tube is mixed vigorously.
3. If heparin is to be administered, do so after this specimen is drawn.

Other Data
1. This test does not distinguish between conditions producing primary fibrinolysin activity and those producing secondary fibrinolysin activity.

Fibrinoligase

See Factor XIII—Blood.

Fibrinopeptide A (FPA)—Blood

Norm. 0.6-1.9 mg/mL

Increased. Cellulitis, disseminated intravascular coagulation, infection, leukemia, systemic lupus erythematosus.

Decreased. Elevation slows or stops with the administration of glycoprotein IIB/IIIA inhibitors.

Description. A peptide involved in thrombus formation after vascular endothelial damage occurs and a platelet plug develops. Fibrinopeptides A and B split off from fibrinogen that is circulating in the blood and form soluble fibrin monomer complexes, which become the base on which a fibrin clot builds. The presence of increased fibrinopeptide A indicates that coagulation is occurring.

Professional Considerations
Consent form NOT required.

Preparation
1. Tube: 2.7- or 4.5-mL blue topped.

Procedure
1. Withdraw 2 mL of blood into a syringe or vacuum tube. Remove the syringe or tube, leaving the needle in place. Attach a second syringe, and draw two blood samples, one in a citrated blue topped tube and the other in a control tube. The sample quantity should be 2.4 mL for a 2.7-mL tube and 4.0 mL for a 4.5-mL tube. Draw a 5-mL blood sample in a sodium citrate–anticoagulated blue topped tube.

Postprocedure Care
1. For clients with coagulopathy, hold pressure over sampling site for at least 5 minutes and observe site closely for development of a hematoma.
2. Transport the specimens to the laboratory immediately for spinning. The specimens are then stable for 3 days when refrigerated.

Client and Family Teaching
1. Seek medical attention for signs of bleeding (that is, hematoma, bleeding of gums, wounds, petechiae, confusion, changing level of consciousness).

Factors That Affect Results
1. Reject hemolyzed specimens or tubes partially filled with blood.

Other Data
1. See also Soluble fibrin monomer complex—Serum.

Fibroblast Skin Culture

Norm. Requires interpretation.

Usage. Gardner's syndrome, hereditary tyrosinemia (type 1), Hurler's syndrome, Marfan syndrome, and mucopolysaccharidosis.

Description. Fibroblasts, large stellate spindle-shaped connective tissue cells, are common in developing or repairing tissues, where they are associated with protein and collagen synthesis. The test is used to help identify gene coding for genetic diseases through cytogenetic study.

Professional Considerations
Consent form IS required.

Risks
Bleeding, infection.
Contraindications
None.

Preparation
1. Obtain povidone-iodine solution, a sterile needle, a knife, and a sterile container.
2. See Biopsy, Site-specific—Specimen.

Procedure
1. Cleanse the site to be biopsied with povidone-iodine solution and allow it to dry.
2. Raise the skin with a sterile needle.
3. Excise a 2-gram skin snip just below the needle with the knife.
4. Place the skin snip in a sterile container.

Postprocedure Care
1. Send the skin biopsy without fixative to the laboratory.

Client and Family Teaching
1. The test involves taking a tiny sample of skin for testing, Pain is minimal enough that a local anesthetic is often not needed.

Factors That Affect Results
1. None.

Other Data
1. A scleral punch may also be used for the biopsy.

Fine-Needle Aspiration Biopsy

See **Needle Aspiration**—Diagnostic.

FISH Test

See **Fluorescence In Situ Hybridization**—Urine

FIT Test

See Immunochemical Fecal Occult Blood Testing—Stool

Five Prime Nucleotidase

See 5′-Nucleotidase—Serum.

Flat-Plate Radiography of Abdomen (Kidney-Ureter-Bladder, KUB, Scout Film)—Diagnostic

Norm. Normal-sized kidneys as judged by radiopaque renal outlines, no abdominal calcifications, no abdominal free air, no evidence of intramural bowel gas, no evidence of bowel distention to indicate possible obstruction or ileus, no rib or pelvic fractures, no evidence of nephrolithiasis or cholelithiasis.

Usage. A screening abdominal radiograph used to rule out acute abdominal disease processes to include colonic perforation, obstruction, or ileus. Occasionally helpful in the diagnosis of cholelithiasis and nephrolithiasis. At times helpful in establishing the diagnosis of chronic pancreatitis (in this disorder abdominal calcifications can be seen occasionally on KUB film).

Description. A plain abdominal film exposed from anterior to posterior (AP) with the client in the supine position. The lower portion of the radiograph displays the superior portion of the symphysis pubis, and the superior portion of the film shows the upper margins of the renal shadows.

Professional Considerations
Consent form NOT required.

Precautions
During pregnancy, risks of cumulative radiation exposure to the fetus from this and other previous or future imaging studies must be weighed against the benefits of the procedure. Although formal limits for client exposure are relative to this risk:benefit comparison, the United States Nuclear Regulatory Commission requires that the cumulative dose equivalent to an embryo/fetus from occupational exposure not exceed 0.5 rem (5 mSv). Radiation dosage to the fetus is proportional to the distance of the anatomy studied from the abdomen and decreases as pregnancy progresses. For pregnant clients, consult the radiologist/radiology department to obtain estimated fetal radiation exposure from this procedure.

Preparation
1. The radiograph may be taken either in the x-ray department or in the client's room with portable equipment.
2. No special preparation of the client is necessary before the radiography.

Procedure
1. The client is placed in the supine position.
2. Radiographic shields are placed over the gonadal areas.
3. The client is asked to expire and hold his or her breath. The film is exposed at the end of expiration.

Postprocedure Care
1. No special postprocedure care is required. The client may require transport back to his or her nursing care unit if the film is done in the radiology department.

Client and Family Teaching
1. The risk of malignancy from plain abdominal radiographic procedures is minimal.
2. Radiographic damage to the gonads is prohibited by abdominal shielding of these areas during the radiographic procedure.

Factors That Affect Results

1. Respiration artifact (the client breathing during exposure of the radiograph).
2. Inappropriate positioning of the radiograph cassette leading to abdominal areas missed when the film is exposed.
3. Underexposure or overexposure of the film.

Other Data

1. The KUB is considered to be a screening procedure. More powerful diagnostic radiologic procedures (computed tomography, magnetic resonance imaging scans, barium studies) may be required to establish the diagnosis.

Flecainide—Plasma or Serum

Norm. Negative.

		SI Units
Therapeutic trough	0.2-1.0 μg/mL	0.5-2.4 μmol/L
Panic level	>1.0 μg/mL	>2.4 μmol/L

Overdose Symptoms and Treatment

Symptoms. Overdose will produce effects that are extensions of pharmacologic effects. AV nodal escape rhythms and prolongation of QRS and QT intervals. ECG abnormalities associated with overdose have included bradycardia, atrioventricular block, regular ventricular tachycardia with a right bundle branch that progressed to polymorphous tachycardia, substantial prolongation of the P-R and Q-T intervals, widened P waves. Sudden death may occur.

Treatment

NOTE: Treatment choice(s) depend(s) on client's history and condition and episode history.

1. Provide symptomatic and supportive care with ECG, blood pressure, and respiratory monitoring.
2. There is no specific antidote.
3. Hemodialysis will NOT remove flecainide.

Increased. Hepatic or renal dysfunction. Drugs include amiodarone, cimetidine, and propranolol.

Decreased. Drugs include phenobarbital and rifampin.

Description. Flecainide is a class 1C antidysrhythmic used for ventricular dysrhythmias and reducing atrial defibrillation threshold in clients treated with low-energy internal atrial cardioversion. It is metabolized and excreted by the liver and kidneys, with a half-life of 20 hours and steady-state levels reached by 3-5 days after therapy is started. Safe to take during pregnancy.

Professional Considerations

Consent form NOT required.

Preparation

1. If the client is also taking propranolol or quinidine, indicate this on the laboratory requisition.
2. Tube: Red topped, red/gray topped, gold topped, or green topped.
3. MAY be drawn during hemodialysis.

Procedure

1. Draw the blood sample just before the next scheduled dose.
2. Draw a 2-mL blood sample.

Postprocedure Care

1. Send the specimen to the laboratory promptly. Plasma or serum must be separated within 2 hours.

Client and Family Teaching

1. Results are normally available within 24 hours.
2. Refer clients with intentional overdose for crisis intervention.

Factors That Affect Results

1. Propranolol and quinidine cause unreliable results when the spectrofluorometric method is used.
2. Refer clients with intentional overdose for crisis intervention.

Other Data

1. Plasma levels >1.2 mg/mL in clients with renal dysfunction are associated with serious side effects and sudden death.
2. Administration in persons with implanted AAIR pacemaker because of sick sinus syndrome can cause failure of pacing.
3. Can cause diffuse infiltrative lung disease. Treatment includes discontinuation of flecainide and prednisone treatment.
4. Interaction of flecainide with topical timolol maleate and verapamil includes bradycardia.
5. Changes in serum concentration of flecainide (pilsicainide and pirmenol) can be estimated from changes in the duration of f-QRS on signal-averaged ECG, and periodic monitoring of the ECG may help reduce blood samples that monitor drug concentrations.

Fletcher Factor

See **Factor, Fletcher—Plasma**.

Flexible Sigmoidoscopy

See **Sigmoidoscopy—Diagnostic**.

Flucytosine—Serum

Norm.

		SI Units
Therapeutic level	25-100 μg/mL	195-775 μmol/L
Panic level	>125 μg/mL	>970 μmol/L

Panic Level Symptoms and Treatment

Symptoms. Panic levels correlate poorly with clinical symptoms. May have adverse effects on renal, hepatic, and hematopoietic systems and include acute cerebellopathy.

Treatment

NOTE: Treatment choice(s) depend(s) on client's history and condition and episode history.

1. Flucytosine can be eliminated by hemodialysis (50%), peritoneal dialysis, and, in part, hemofiltration.

Usage. Monitoring for therapeutic and toxic levels of the drug.

Description. An orally effective systemic antifungal drug that is a secondary agent often used with amphotericin B for treating serious, deep-seated mycotic infections caused by *Candida* and *Cryptococcus* species. Is less effective but less toxic than amphotericin B. Ancobon is well absorbed and well distributed throughout the body, and the majority is excreted unchanged by the kidneys. Half-life is 3-6 hours.

Professional Considerations

Consent form NOT required.

Preparation

1. Tube: Red topped, red/gray topped, or gold or green topped.
2. Do NOT draw during hemodialysis.

Procedure

1. Draw a 5-mL blood sample 2 hours after oral administration for peak levels and immediately before oral administration for trough levels.

Postprocedure Care

1. None.

Client and Family Teaching

1. Inform the client or the family of the rationale for the test.
2. Results are normally available in 24 hours.
3. Refer clients with intentional overdose for crisis intervention.

Factors That Affect Results

1. Ancobon half-life may increase up to 200 hours in clients with renal failure.

Other Data

1. There is a 57% failure rate when flucytosine is used alone for treatment.

2. There is a 68% clinical response for treatment of cryptococcal meningitis in persons with AIDS using amphotericin B and flucytosine.

3. Flucytosine can be combined with both amphotericin B and fluconazole.

Fluorescein Angiography (Eye Fundus)—Diagnostic

Norm. No leakage of dye from blood vessels of the retina during any of the following phases.

Filling Stage. Begins 12-15 seconds after dye injection; noted when retinal vessels begin filling with dye.

Choroidal Flush. The retina fluoresces and appears evenly mottled throughout the capillaries.

Arterial Stage. Noted when arteries begin to fill with dye.

Arteriovenous Stage. Noted when arteries have filled with dye and veins begin to fill with dye.

Venous Stage. The arteries have emptied, and the veins have become filled and then emptied.

Late Stage. $\frac{1}{2}$ to 1 hour after injection, the dye has circulated throughout the body, and recirculation of the retinal vessels can be seen.

Usage. Evaluation of retinopathy, tumors, retinal circulation abnormalities (occlusion, stenosis, dilatation, aneurysm, arteriovenous shunt), or papilledema. Identification of leakage and retinal thickening for subsequent laser treatment.

Description. A radiographic examination of the retinal vasculature after rapid injection of fluorescein dye. Fluorescein angiography provides rapid and direct acquisition of sequential images of the vasculature and the ability to manipulate the fluorescein images with the computer. For example, the processor can adjust for fluorescein leakage into the vitreous, cataracts, or cloudy corneas. It also provides the ability to display fluorescein images and color fundus images for comparison during laser treatment. The rapidly available images are also used to help explain the disease process to the client being examined.

Professional Considerations

Consent form IS required.

Risks

Allergic reaction (itching, hives, rash, tight feeling in the throat, shortness of breath, bronchospasm, anaphylaxis, death), or seizure reaction to sodium fluorescein.

Contraindications

Previous allergy to sodium fluorescein; clients who are unable to keep their eyes open for the test.

Precautions

During pregnancy, risks of cumulative radiation exposure to the fetus from this and other previous or future imaging studies must be weighed against the benefits of the procedure. Although formal limits for client exposure are relative to this risk:benefit comparison, the United States Nuclear Regulatory Commission requires that the cumulative dose equivalent to an embryo/fetus from occupational exposure not exceed 0.5 rem (5 mSv). Radiation dosage to the fetus is proportional to the distance of the anatomy studied from the abdomen and decreases as pregnancy progresses. For pregnant clients, consult the radiologist/radiology department to obtain estimated fetal radiation exposure from this procedure.

Preparation

1. Obtain mydriatic eyedrops and 5% or 10% sodium fluorescein.

2. Administer mydriatic eyedrops as prescribed 15-30 minutes before the test.

3. Insert a heparin lock intravenously.

4. Have emergency equipment, including diazepam or phenytoin, available in case of allergic or seizure reaction.

5. Just before beginning the procedure, take a "time out" to verify the correct client, procedure, and site.

Procedure

1. Dilating eyedrops are administered.
2. The client's chin and forehead rest against the fundus camera, and one arm is extended to the side.
3. The client is instructed to open the eyes very wide, close the mouth, and look forward. The client can blink normally.
4. Baseline fundus photographs are taken.
5. Fluorescein dye is injected quickly and may cause facial flushing or nausea.
6. Photographs of the fundus of the eye are taken every second for 25-45 seconds. Late-phase photographs are taken 30 minutes later, if needed.

Postprocedure Care

1. Discontinue the heparin lock.

Client and Family Teaching

1. Clients with glaucoma should omit mydriatic eyedrops the day of the test.
2. Do not drive for at least 2 hours after the test.
3. Protective eyewear may be necessary for at least 2 hours after the test if the environment is bright or sunny.
4. Yellow discoloration of the skin and urine is normally present for up to 2 days.

Factors That Affect Results

1. Cataracts may interfere with fundal view.

Other Data

1. None.

Fluorescein Meniscus Test

See **Schirmer Tearing Eye Test**—Diagnostic.

Fluorescence In Situ Hybridization (FISH, UroVysion™ FISH) Test—Urine

Norm. Negative: Specimen has less than 4 cells with gains for 2 or more chromosomes or less than 12 cells with homozygous loss of both copies of 9p21.

Positive: Specimen has at least 4 cells with gains for 2 or more chromosomes or at least 12 cells with homozygous loss of both copies of 9p21.

Usage. Detection and surveillance of primary and secondary bladder adenocarcinoma to monitor for recurrence (Asali, 2007). Used for clients with hematuria where bladder cancer is suspected. Not for use in evaluating routine hematuria, unless other risk factors for bladder cancer are present. Used in conjunction with cystoscopy.

Description. Fluorescence in situ hybridization is a genetic test that detects anomalies in the urine such as aneuploidy for chromosomes 3, 7, 17, and loss of the 9p21 locus, and can also detect deletion, duplication, or amplification of specific genes. This highly sensitive and specific analysis of the DNA sequence in bladder cells present in the urine offers advantages over conventional urine cytology, which often produces false-positive results.

Professional Considerations

Consent form NOT required.

Preparation

1. Supplies: a clean urine specimen container and 50% ethanol.

Procedure

1. Obtain at least a 35-mL sample of urine in a clean container. The FDA approved type of sample is voided urine; however, testing is often done on urine that is voided, catheterized, stomal, or washing from bladder, ureter, or kidney. Any excess urine over 60 mL may be submitted in a second tube.
2. Add an equal volume of 50% ethanol containing 2% polyethylene glycol (Carbowax preservative).

Postprocedure Care

1. Refrigerate for up to 3 days after mixing with preservative, if not shipped immediately to the testing lab. Store and transport at 2 to 8 degrees Centigrade.

Client and Family Teaching

1. A positive result may indicate the need for further testing to determine the source of the cancer.

2. Test results will be available within 2 weeks.

Factors That Affect Results

1. False positive results may occur in non-urothelial bladder carcinoma, or in clients who have a history of prostate or endometrial cancer, or who have received chemotherapy; therefore test should not be used for diagnosis.
2. Results are invalidated if the urine contains high amounts of bacteria, granulocytes, or if crystalluria or hematuria is present.
3. At least 50 bladder cells must be present in the urine sample to perform FISH testing.

Other Data

1. FISH testing takes longer and costs more, but is more sensitive (over 90% sensitivity and specificity) than conventional cytology (10%-25% sensitivity).
2. This test is available from Abbott Molecular.

Fluorescent Rabies Antibody (FRA)—Specimen

Norm. Negative. Requires interpretation.

Positive. Rabies.

Description. The rabies rhabdovirus causes an acute viral infection of the central nervous system of a variety of animals characterized by neurotropic ribonucleic acid (RNA) viral presence in the saliva, urine, feces, brain, and spinal cord. This virus is occasionally transmitted to humans by an infected skunk, squirrel, cat, bat, dog, or other animal, and is 99% fatal if symptoms appear before treatment is instituted. The serum of a human bitten by a rabid animal is examined by immunofluorescence to detect a significant serum antibody rise. This test can be used for antemortem diagnosis in clients who have never received rabies vaccine or passive antibody.

Professional Considerations

Consent form NOT required.

Preparation

1. Tube: Red topped, red/gray topped, or gold topped

Procedure

1. Draw a 7-mL human blood sample and send it to the laboratory along with animal brain. (See Animals and rabies, Negri bodies, Brain tissue—Specimen.)

Postprocedure Care

1. None.

Client and Family Teaching

1. Results are normally available in 24 hours.
2. Both preexposure and postexposure prophylaxis is available against rabies.

Factors That Affect Results

1. None.

Other Data

1. Animal survival for 10 days makes rabies unlikely.
2. Rabies is a reportable disease in most areas, as are animal bites.
3. Rabies can also be detected by reverse transcriptase-PCR method using saliva, CSF, and skin biopsy samples from the client.

Fluorescent Treponemal Antibody–Absorbed Double-Stain (FTA-Abs DS) Test—Serum

Norm. Nonreactive.

Usage. Serologic confirmation of syphilis when nontreponemal tests are positive.

Description. Syphilis is a complex, sexually transmitted disease characterized by a wide range of symptoms that imitate other diseases and is caused by the organism *Treponema pallidum*. This test provides the most sensitive detection of treponemal antibodies for syphilis in all stages. It differentiates biologic false-positive results from true syphilis-positive results and can help diagnose syphilis when definite clinical signs are present but other tests are negative. This test is positive in the treponemal diseases of bejel, pinta, syphilis, and yaws. Before testing, the serum is treated to remove antibodies that could cause false-positive results. The technique involves using fluorescence microscopy with special filters that decrease the amount of natural fluorescence from the background of the specimen. Fluorescein-conjugated antibodies to IgG are added as a counterstain to the stained specimen, and the treponemes are identified as they fluoresce in combination with the antibodies.

Professional Considerations
Consent form NOT required.

Preparation
1. Tube: Red topped, red/gray topped, or gold topped.

Procedure
1. Draw a 3-mL blood sample.

Postprocedure Care
1. None.

Client and Family Teaching
1. Results are normally available in 24 hours.
2. If testing positive:
   a. Notify all sexual contacts from the last 90 days (if early stage) to be tested for syphilis.
   b. Syphilis can be cured with antibiotics. These may worsen the symptoms for the first 24 hours.
   c. Do not have sex for 2 months and until after repeat testing has confirmed that the syphilis is cured. Use condoms after that for 2 years. Return for repeat testing every 3-4 months for the next 2 years to make sure the disease is cured.
   d. Do not become pregnant for 2 years because syphilis can be transmitted to the fetus.
   e. If left untreated, syphilis can damage many body organs, including the brain, over several years.

Factors That Affect Results
1. Reject hemolyzed specimens or chylous serum samples.
2. False-positive results may be caused by antinuclear antibodies, drug abuse, elevated or abnormal globulins, pregnancy, or systemic lupus erythematosus (beaded pattern).

Other Data
1. This test may remain positive indefinitely for clients previously infected with syphilis. Thus it is not useful for monitoring clinical response to treatment for syphilis.
2. Borderline results necessitate repeating the test.
3. Prenatal universal screening may no longer be justified economically unless a there is a high incidence of seroprevalence of syphilis in the client's geographic region.

Fluoroscopy—Diagnostic

Norm. Requires interpretation. Usually there is symmetric, synchronous pulmonary and diaphragmatic motion. Diaphragmatic excursion = 2-4 cm. Absence of calcification in the coronary arteries.

Usage. Assessment of diaphragmatic function; localization of lung mass for percutaneous biopsy, mediastinal mass, pleural effusion, pleural lesion, and pulmonary disease; screening tool for detection of coronary artery disease; infrequent applications of fluoroscopy other than that of the chest include gastrointestinal imaging, venography, myelography, and genitourinary fluoroscopy.

Description. A radiographic examination of pulmonary motion using a fluoroscopic screen containing calcium tungstate crystals, which fluoresce when struck by x-rays. When the x-ray passes through the body, dense areas allow less radiation to pass through onto the fluoroscopic screen than do less dense areas. The resulting pattern of light and dark areas aids in the diagnosis of pathophysiologic conditions. Fluoroscopy can reveal subtle nodular or parenchymal calcifications and coronary artery calcifications better than regular radiographs. The test takes about 5 minutes and includes less than 1 minute of x-ray exposure.

Professional Considerations
Consent form IS required.

Risks
Radiation exposure, radiodermatitis, infection.

Contraindications
Pregnancy and during breast-feeding.

Precautions

During pregnancy, risks of cumulative radiation exposure to the fetus from this and other previous or future imaging studies must be weighed against the benefits of the procedure. Although formal limits for client exposure are relative to this risk:benefit comparison, the United States Nuclear Regulatory Commission requires that the cumulative dose equivalent to an embryo/fetus from occupational exposure not exceed 0.5 rem (5 mSv). Radiation dosage to the fetus is proportional to the distance of the anatomy studied from the abdomen and decreases as pregnancy progresses. For pregnant clients, consult the radiologist/radiology department to obtain estimated fetal radiation exposure from this procedure.

Preparation

1. The client should remove all upper body clothing, jewelry, and metal items.
2. Just before beginning the procedure, take a "time out" to verify the correct client, procedure, and site.

Procedure

1. The client stands with the chest between the x-ray tube and the fluoroscopic screen.
2. Remove electrocardiographic monitoring leads and patches containing metal snaps and safety pins. Move invasive lines out of the fluoroscopic field if possible.
3. Wear a lead apron if remaining in the room.
4. Proceed with fluoroscopy. The client turns in different projections for the procedure.

Postprocedure Care

1. None.

Client and Family Teaching

1. Inform the client or family of the rationale for the test.
2. The client must remove all jewelry or metal objects from the trunk of the body.
3. The client must not be pregnant.
4. Results will be available after examination of the procedure results by a radiologist.
5. In women who are breast-feeding, formula should be substituted for breast milk for 1 or more days after the procedure.

Factors That Affect Results

1. Metallic objects may interfere with the quality of films obtained by fluoroscopy.

Other Data

1. A videotape of the film may be made for later examination.
2. Fluoroscopy delivers more radiation than a chest radiograph does.

Fluoxetine

See **Selective Serotonin Reuptake Inhibitors—Blood.**

Fluphenazine

See **Phenothiazines.**

Flurazepam—Serum

Norm. Negative.

	Therapeutic Ranges	SI Units
Hydroxyethyl-flurazepam metabolite	0-4 ng/mL	0-9 nmol/L
n-Desalkylflurazepam metabolite	10-140 ng/mL	21-300 nmol/L
Flurazepam panic level	>2000 ng/mL	>4300 nmol/ L

Panic Level Symptoms and Treatment

Symptoms. Dizziness, somnolence, impaired coordination, slurred speech, confusion, coma, and diminished reflexes. Hypotension, respiratory depression, and apnea may occur if the dose has been large.

Treatment

NOTE: Treatment choice(s) depend(s) on client's history and condition and episode history.

1. Gastric lavage is not recommended, but should be considered if within 1 hour of ingestion and if ingestion of additional lethal substance is suspected. Use warm tap water or 0.9% saline.
2. Administer activated charcoal if within 4 hours of ingestion or if symptoms are present. Repeat as necessary, because benzodiazepines undergo hepatic recirculation.
3. Monitor for central nervous system depression.
4. Protect airway. Support breathing with oxygen and mechanical ventilation, if necessary.
5. Flumazenil is not recommended for routine use in benzodiazepine overdose. Flumazenil has been used as a competitive antagonist to reverse the profound effects of benzodiazepine overdose. Use of flumazenil is contraindicated if concomitant tricyclic antidepressants were taken or in dependence states because of the risk of causing seizures from lowering of the seizure threshold and because it may precipitate symptoms of benzodiazepine withdrawal. Flumazenil may not completely reverse benzodiazepine effects. Close monitoring for resedation is required and repeated doses may be needed.
6. Do NOT use barbiturates.
7. Do NOT induce emesis.
8. Forced diuresis or hemodialysis will NOT remove benzodiazepines to any significant extent. No information was found on whether peritoneal dialysis will remove these drugs.

Positive. Drug abuse, overdose, and seizures.

Negative. Absence of drug in serum.

Description. Flurazepam is a schedule IV, long-acting benzodiazepine anxiolytic and hypnotic used for the treatment of insomnia and irregular sleeping habits. Flurazepam depresses the central nervous system and relaxes the skeletal muscles. It is absorbed from the gastrointestinal tract within 1 hour, metabolized by the liver, and excreted via the kidneys, with a half-life of up to 100 hours.

Professional Considerations

Consent form NOT required.

Preparation

1. Tube: Red topped, red/gray topped, or gold topped.
2. MAY be drawn during hemodialysis.

Procedure

1. Draw a 5-mL blood sample.

Postprocedure Care

1. None.

Client and Family Teaching

1. Inform the client or family of the rationale for the test.
2. Results are normally available within 24 hours.
3. If activated charcoal was given for elevated levels, the client should drink 4-6 glasses of water each day for 2 days to prevent constipation. The activated charcoal will also cause stools to be black for a few days.
4. Refer clients with intentional overdose for crisis intervention.
5. Referrals to appropriate rehabilitation centers and therapeutic community programs should be offered to all addicted clients who may be interested.

Factors That Affect Results

1. Stable at room temperature with considerable breakdown at 240 days.

Other Data

1. See also Benzodiazepines—Plasma and urine.

Flurazepam Hydrochloride

See Benzodiazepines—Plasma and Urine.

FMR1 Testing for Fragile X Associated Disorders—Blood

Norm.

	(cytosine-guanine-guanine) Repeat Range
Normal	≤54 repeats
Premutation carrier	55 to 200 repeats
Full mutation	≥200 repeats

Usage. Indications for this DNA test include males over age 50 presenting with new tremor or ataxia, females experiencing infertility related to ovarian failure at a premature age.

Description. Fragile X-associated tremor/ataxia syndrome (FXTAS) is a fairly common disorder displayed in older men in which a premutation or excessive repeat patterns occurs in the fragile X gene. This premutation in males leads to Parkinson-like symptoms of ataxia and progressive tremor, and is also accompanied by deterioration in executive cognitive function. The greater the number of excess repeat patterns, the greater the chance that more severe symptoms will develop. 20%-30% of males who carry this premutation develop FXTAS; females who carry the premutation are at risk for ovarian dysfunction. A third fragile-X associated disorder, which involves a full mutation in the FMR1 gene, is fragile X syndrome (American College of Obstetricians and Gynecologists Committee on Genetics, 2010), which causes mental retardation.

Professional Considerations

Informed consent IS recommended for genetic testing.

Preparation

1. Have client complete fragile X-associated disorders questionnaire.

2. Tube: Lavender topped or yellow topped.

Procedure

1. Collect a 10-mL whole blood sample.

Postprocedure Care

1. Store sample at room temperature and test within 48 hours of collection.

Client and Family Teaching

1. Test results will be available within 2 weeks.
2. Genetic counseling is recommended for family members of clients testing positive for the FMR1 premutation (Hagerman, Hagerman, 2004). Males pass on the permutation to all female offspring. Premutations tend to expand in the offspring of carriers, and pose the risk of full mutation.
3. Refer to Appendix B, "Informed Consent for Genetic Testing".

Other Data

1. This polymerase chain reaction test is more accurate than the Southern blot test.
2. FXTAS was not known as a diagnosis until 2001.
3. Treatment for FXTAS is symptomatic (Fragile X Clinical Research Consortium, 2012).
4. The Genetic Information Nondiscrimination Act of 2008 prohibits health plans from using genetic family history or genetic test results from influencing eligibility or premiums for health insurance. It also prohibits employers from using this information to influence decisions about hiring, terminating employment, or employment pay, promotions, or privileges.

FMRI

See **Magnetic Resonance Imaging**—Diagnostic.

FMT

See **Schirmer Tearing Eye Test**—Diagnostic.

Foam Stability Index—Amniotic Fluid

Norm. Fetal lung maturity indicated by ≥0.47.

Fetal lung immaturity indicated by ≤0.46.

Usage. Foam stability index (FSI) of amniotic fluid uncontaminated by blood or meconium provides a direct measure of fetal lung maturity by determining the amount of surfactant in amniotic fluid and thus helps determine the risk for respiratory distress syndrome (RDS) or hyaline membrane disease. The test helps the clinician decide whether to delay delivery of the fetus. The test is commonly done before repeat cesarean delivery when gestational age is uncertain and for other indications including medical or obstetric conditions such as severe maternal hypertension, renal disease, or preterm labor. Results indicating immaturity of the fetal lungs may lead to delay of delivery through use of tocolytics to suppress preterm labor or postponement of elective delivery.

Description. Pulmonary surfactant is measured in the amniotic fluid by noting the ability of the fluid to form a stable surface film that can support a ring of foam around a test tube. Proteins, bile acids, and salts of free fatty acids also will form a stable foam; these are removed from the foam by adding ethanol, which competes with these substances for a position in the surface foam. A fixed volume of amniotic fluid is mixed with a solution of 95% ethanol in increasing volumes. The largest fraction of ethanol in which the amniotic fluid is capable of supporting a ring of bubbles 360 degrees around the tube is recorded; this fraction is the FSI.

Professional Considerations

Consent form IS required for the amniocentesis. See Amniocentesis and amniotic fluid analysis—Diagnostic routine analysis.

Preparation

1. See Amniocentesis and amniotic fluid analysis—Diagnostic routine analysis.

Procedure

1. See Amniocentesis and amniotic fluid analysis—Diagnostic routine analysis.

Postprocedure Care

1. See Amniocentesis and amniotic fluid analysis—Diagnostic routine analysis.

Client and Family Teaching

1. This test evaluates fetal lung maturity but is only sensitive in 86% of cases.
2. Test results are quickly available.

Factors That Affect Results

1. Amniotic fluid must be obtained via amniocentesis; fluid from vaginal pool not acceptable.
2. Fluid must be collected in clean, untreated tubes.
3. Amniotic fluid contaminated with blood or meconium gives a false lung maturity result.
4. Amniotic fluid must be tested immediately or refrigerated at 4 degrees C.
5. Test must be performed with fluid between 20 degrees and 25 degrees C.

Other Data

1. This test has up to a 50% false-maturity and false-immaturity result.
2. Test results are interpreted as "mature" versus "immature" when there is actually a continuum of maturity
3. Artificial surfactant and antenatal corticosteroids have decreased RDS mortality and thus have lessened the need for fetal maturity testing. However, the American College of Obstetrics and Gynecology recommends pulmonary maturity testing for all planned elective deliveries at less than 39 weeks of amenorrhea.
4. An older, unstandardized form of this test was called the Shake Test.

Foley Catheter Tip—Culture

See **Foreign Body, Routine**—Culture.

Folic Acid, Red Blood Cells—Blood

Norm. Folate present in packed cells (ng/mL).

		SI Units
Adults		
≤60 years	95-503 ng/mL	215-1132 nmol/L
>60 years	150-450 ng/mL	340-1020 nmol/L

Increased. Folic acid supplements, myelodysplastic syndrome.

Decreased. Alcoholism, anemia (pure vitamin B_{12} deficiency, hemolytic megaloblastic, pernicious, sickle cell), blind loop syndrome, celiac disease, coronary artery disease, Crohn's disease, dermatitis herpetiformis, diet (inadequate intake), folate coenzyme dysfunction, hepatic disease, lactation (without increased dietary folate), leukopenia, hemodialysis, hyperthyroidism, iron and folate deficiency, leukemia (acute myelomonocytic), malabsorption syndromes, malignancy, malnutrition, mania, myeloproliferative disease, myelosclerosis, neoplastic diseases, pregnancy (without increased dietary folate), renal failure, sprue (tropical, nontropical), thrombocytopenia, and vitamin B_{12} deficiency. Drugs include aminopterin, anticoagulants (chronic), anticonvulsants, chloroquine hydrochloride, chloroquine phosphate, ethyl alcohol (ethanol), glutethimide, hydroxychloroquine sulfate, isoniazid, methotrexate, oral contraceptives (long-term), phenobarbital, phenytoin, primaquine phosphate, pyrimethamine, quinacrine hydrochloride, quinine sulfate, smoking cigarettes, and sulfonamides.

Description. Folic acid (folate) is a vitamin and amino acid needed for normal functioning of red and white blood cells. It is formed by bacteria in the intestines, stored in the liver, and found in foods such as eggs, milk, leafy vegetables, yeast, liver, and fruits. Folate is absorbed in the jejunum and functions in the metabolism of amino acids and nucleotides, affecting all tissues that undergo a large amount of cell multiplication. Folate deficiency causes megaloblastic anemia and eventually leukopenia and thrombocytopenia. Folic acid is believed to play a role in birth defects such as spina bifida, anencephaly, and orofacial clefts. Symptoms of deficiency take about 3 months to appear and can be caused by inadequate intake, increased body demand,

or folate antagonism by drugs. Red blood cells contain more folate than the serum does, and this measurement of folic acid is less sensitive to recent dietary intake of folic acid than the serum folic acid test is.

Professional Considerations
Consent form NOT required.

Preparation
1. Tube: Red topped, red/gray topped, or gold topped, and lavender topped; ascorbic acid.

Procedure
1. Draw a 5-mL blood sample in a red topped tube.
2. Draw a 5-mL blood sample in a lavender topped tube.
3. Prepare a hemolysate by adding 0.5 mL of EDTA blood to 4.5 mL of ascorbic acid and freeze immediately.

Postprocedure Care
1. Protect the specimen from light by inserting it into a paper bag.

Client and Family Teaching
1. Results are normally available within 24 hours.

Factors That Affect Results
1. Reject specimens if the client had a radioactive scan within 48 hours before specimen collection.
2. Bacterial contamination of the specimen may invalidate the results.
3. A standard multivitamin increases RBC folate levels in clients on hemodialysis.

Other Data
1. The same specimen from step 1 under Procedure may be used for serum folic acid level.
2. The recommended dietary intake of folate is 400 mg/day.
3. RBC folate level is higher in Caucasian men and women compared to African-American men and women or Mexican-American men and women, respectively.

Folic Acid (Vitamin B₉)—Serum

Norm.

		SI Units
Adults		
≤60 years	1.8-9 ng/mL	4.1-20.4 nmol/L
>60 years	1.2-12 ng/mL	4.1-27.2 nmol/L

Increased. Folic acid supplements.

Decreased. Alcoholism, Alzheimer's disease, anemia (pure vitamin B_{12} deficiency, hemolytic, megaloblastic, pernicious, sickle cell), bacterial overgrowth, blind loop syndrome, celiac disease, Crohn's disease, dermatitis herpetiformis, diet (inadequate intake), folate coenzyme dysfunction, hemolytic processes or conditions, hepatic disease, lactation (without increased dietary folate), leukopenia, hemodialysis, hyperthyroidism, insufficient dietary intake, iron and folate deficiency, jejunal diseases, leukemia (acute myelomonocytic), malabsorption syndromes, malignancy, malnutrition, myeloproliferative disease, myelosclerosis, neoplastic diseases, pregnancy (without increased dietary folate), renal failure, short bowel syndrome, sprue (tropical, nontropical), stroke, thrombocytopenia, and vitamin B_{12} deficiency. Drugs include alcohol, aminopterin, anticoagulants (chronic), anticonvulsants, chloroquine hydrochloride, chloroquine phosphate, ethyl alcohol, glutethimide, hydroxychloroquine sulfate, isoniazid, methotrexate, oral contraceptives (long-term), phenobarbital, phenytoin, primaquine primidone, phosphate, pyrimethamine, quinacrine hydrochloride, quinine sulfate, sulfonamides, and triamterene.

Description. Folic acid (folate) is a vitamin and amino acid needed for normal functioning of red and white blood cells. It is formed by bacteria in the intestines, stored in the liver, and found in foods such as eggs, milk, leafy vegetables, yeast, liver, and fruits. Folate is absorbed in the jejunum and functions in the metabolism of amino acids and nucleotides, affecting all the tissues that undergo a large amount of cell multiplication. Folate deficiency causes megaloblastic anemia and eventually leukopenia and thrombocytopenia. Folic acid is believed to play a role in birth defects such as spina bifida, anencephaly, and orofacial clefts as well as reducing cardiovascular morbidity and mortality. Symptoms of deficiency take about 3 months to appear and can be caused by inadequate intake, increased body demand, or folate antagonism by drugs. Serum contains less folate than the red blood cells do. This measurement of folic acid is more sensitive than the red blood cell folic acid test to recent dietary intake of folic acid.

Professional Considerations
Consent form NOT required.

Preparation
1. Tube: Red topped, red/gray topped, or gold topped.
2. See Client and Family Teaching.

Procedure
1. Draw a 4-mL blood sample before any injections of vitamin B_{12}.

Postprocedure Care
1. Protect the specimen from light by inserting it into a paper bag.
2. Transport the specimen to the laboratory and refrigerate the serum until tested.
3. If the specimen will not be tested within 24 hours, the serum should be frozen at −10 degrees C and protected from light.

Client and Family Teaching
1. Do not eat food 8 hours before sampling. Water is permitted.
2. Results are normally available within 24 hours.

Factors That Affect Results
1. Reject hemolyzed specimens and samples not frozen or not protected from light.
2. Hemolysis falsely elevates results.
3. Drugs that are folate antagonists, such as methotrexate and pentamidine, and cigarette smoking, antacids, anticonvulsants, and NSAIDs may induce a deficiency state.
4. Levels may decrease in clients taking oral contraceptives.

Other Data
1. The same specimen may be used for one portion of the red blood cell folic acid level test.
2. Levels fall below normal 21-28 days after deficiency begins.
3. Most women still receive less folate than the 0.4 mg/day recommended. Women of childbearing age need 400 mg/day intake of folic acid.
4. Folic acid supplements reduce methotrexate gastrointestinal side effects in clients with rheumatoid arthritis.
5. In the United States, since 1998, flour is enriched with folic acid to help prevent birth defects and decrease coronary artery disease.

Follicle-Stimulating Hormone (FSH, Follitropin)—Serum

Norm. Normal ranges will vary among laboratories and are dependent on which international system of measurement is used.

		SI Units
Adult Females		
LH:FSH Ratio	<3:1	<3:1
Premenopausal	3-8 mIU/mL	3-8 IU/L
Follicular phase	3.85-8.78 mIU/mL	3.85-8.78 IU/L
Midcycle peak	4.54-22.51	4.54-22.51 IU/L
Luteal phase	1.79-5.12 mIU/mL	1.79-5.12 IU/L
Pregnant	Low to undetectable	
Menopausal	16.74-113.59 mIU/mL	16.74-113.59 IU/L
Postmenopausal	16.74-113.59 mIU/mL	16.74-113.59 IU/L
Adult Males	1.27-19.26 mIU/mL	1.27-19.26 IU/L
Children, Prepubertal	0.5-3.7 mIU/mL	0.5-3.7 IU/L

Increased. Acromegaly (early), amenorrhea (primary), anorchism, castration, endometrial ablation, gonadal failure, hyperpituitarism, hypogonadism, hypothalamic tumor, hysterectomy, Klinefelter's syndrome, male climacteric, menopause, menstruation, orchidectomy, ovarian failure, pituitary tumors, precocious puberty, premature menopause, seminiferous tubule failure, seminoma, Stein-Leventhal syndrome (polycystic ovary syndrome), testicular agenesis, testicular destruction (caused by radiation or mumps orchitis), testicular failure, testicular feminization syndrome (complete), and Turner's syndrome (primary hypogonadism). Drugs include excessive cigarette smoking.

Decreased. Adrenal hyperplasia, amenorrhea (secondary), anorexia nervosa, anovulatory menstrual cycle, delayed puberty, hypogonadotropism, hypophysectomy, hypothalamic dysfunction, neoplasm (adrenal, ovarian, testicular), panhypopituitarism, and prepubertal child. Drugs include chlorpromazine, estrogens, oral contraceptives, progesterone, and testosterone.

Description. When released from the anterior pituitary gland, follicle-stimulating hormone (FSH) in women promotes maturation of the ovarian follicle, which produces estrogen. As levels of estrogen rise, luteinizing hormones are produced. Together, FSH and luteinizing hormone induce ovulation. In men, FSH produces spermatogenesis and luteinizing hormone stimulates the secretion of androgens. This test aids in the differential diagnosis of hypogonadism, infertility, menstrual disorders, and precocious puberty.

Professional Considerations
Consent form NOT required.

Preparation
1. Tube: Red topped, red/gray topped, or gold topped or lavender topped.

Procedure
1. Draw a 4-mL blood sample between 6 and 7 AM.

Postprocedure Care
1. Write the beginning date of the female's last menstruation on the laboratory requisition.
2. Send the specimen to the laboratory immediately for separation and freezing of serum.

Client and Family Teaching
1. Results are normally available within 24 hours.
2. Repeating the test is often required to ensure an accurate diagnosis.

Factors That Affect Results
1. Reject hemolyzed specimens or if the client had a radioactive scan within 48 hours.
2. Radionuclides cause a falsely decreased FSH level.
3. Values should be compared with the norms for the laboratory performing the test.

Other Data
1. Several daily specimens are recommended because of episodic release of FSH from the pituitary gland.

Follicle-Stimulating Hormone (FSH, Follitropin)—Urine

Norm.

		SI Units
Adult Females	3-12 IU/24 hours	3-12 IU/day
Follicular phase	2-15 IU/24 hours	2-15 IU/day
Midcycle peak	8-60 IU/24 hours	8-60 IU/day
Luteal phase	2-10 IU/24 hours	2-10 IU/day
Menopausal	35-100 IU/24 hours	35-100 IU/day
Adult Males	2-18 IU/24 hours	>2-18 IU/day
>61 years	>2-18 IU/24 hours	
Female Children		
Neonate-12 months	<1.4 IU/24 hours	<1.4 IU/day
12 months-8 years	<4.0 IU/24 hours	<4.0 IU/day
9-10 years	1-4 IU/24 hours	1-4 IU/day
11-12 years	1-8 IU/24 hours	1-8 IU/day
13-14 years	1-10 IU/24 hours	1-10 IU/day
Male Children		
Neonate-12 months	<1.4 IU/24 hours	<1.4 IU/day
12 months-8 years	<4.5 IU/24 hours	<4.5 IU/day
9-10 years	1-5 IU/24 hours	1-5 IU/day
11-12 years	1.5-5 IU/24 hours	1.5-5 IU/day
13-14 years	2-12 IU/24 hours	2-12 IU/day

Increased. Acromegaly (early), amenorrhea (primary), anorchism, castration, eating disorders, gonadal failure, hyperpituitarism, hypogonadism, hypothalamic tumor, hysterectomy, Klinefelter's syndrome, male climacteric, menopause, menstruation, orchiectomy, ovarian failure, pituitary tumors, precocious puberty, premature menopause, seminiferous tubule failure, seminoma, Stein-Leventhal syndrome (polycystic ovary syndrome), testicular agenesis, testicular destruction (caused by radiation or mumps orchitis), testicular failure, testicular feminization syndrome (complete), and Turner's syndrome (primary hypogonadism).

Decreased. Adrenal hyperplasia, amenorrhea (secondary), anorexia nervosa, anovulatory menstrual cycle, delayed puberty, hypogonadotropism, hypophysectomy, hypothalamic dysfunction, nonconceptive cycles, neoplasm (adrenal, ovarian, testicular), panhypopituitarism, and prepubertal child. Drugs include chlorpromazine, estrogens, oral contraceptives, progesterone, and testosterone.

Description. When released from the anterior pituitary gland, follicle-stimulating hormone (FSH) in women promotes maturation of the ovarian follicle, which produces estrogen. As levels of estrogen rise, luteinizing hormones are produced. Together, FSH and luteinizing hormone induce ovulation. In men, FSH produces spermatogenesis, and luteinizing hormone stimulates the secretion of androgens. Urine FSH levels are more useful than serum levels because a 24-hour collection will reflect both the peaks and lows of the episodic FSH secretion. This urine test aids in the differential diagnosis of hypogonadism, infertility, menstrual disorders, and precocious puberty.

Professional Considerations
Consent form NOT required.

Preparation
1. Obtain a 3-L container with boric acid additive.
2. Write the beginning time of the collection on the laboratory requisition.

Procedure
1. Discard the first morning urine specimen.
2. Collect all the urine voided in a 24-hour period in a refrigerated, 3-L container to which 10 g of boric acid has been added. Document the quantity of urine output during the collection period. Include the

urine voided at the end of the 24-hour period. For catheterized clients, keep the drainage bag on ice and empty urine into the collection container hourly.

Postprocedure Care

1. Write the total amount of urine in the 24-hour sample on the laboratory requisition.
2. Gently mix the container and send a 50-mL aliquot to the lab.
3. Best storage is at 4 degrees C without any additive.

Client and Family Teaching

1. Save all the urine voided in the 24-hour period and urinate before defecating to avoid loss of urine. If any urine is accidentally discarded, discard the entire specimen and restart the collection the next day.
2. Results are normally available within 24 hours.
3. The test should be repeated to ensure an appropriate diagnosis.

Factors That Affect Results

1. Radionuclides cause a falsely decreased FSH level.

Other Data

1. Several 24-hour urine specimens are recommended because of episodic release of FSH from the pituitary gland.

Follitropin

See Follicle-Stimulating Hormone—Serum.

Follitropin

See Follicle-Stimulating Hormone—Urine.

Foreign Body, Routine—Culture

Norm. No growth.

Usage. Aids diagnosis of infection caused by invasive lines, catheters, and other foreign bodies. Part of the work-up for suspected septic processes in clients on hyperalimentation or with other invasive lines. Determination of sensitivity of line-sepsis microorganisms to antibacterial therapy.

Description. Includes the culturing of heart valves, dialysis catheters, Swan-Ganz or other central line tip, and intrauterine devices. Test also includes culture of indwelling urinary catheters. Nosocomial urinary tract infections associated with the presence of indwelling urinary catheters account for up to 40% of urinary tract infections.

Professional Considerations

Consent form NOT required.

Preparation

1. Obtain povidone-iodine solution, a sterile container or a red topped tube, and sterile gloves.
2. For urinary catheter tip culture, obtain sterile scissors, a 20-mL syringe, and a sterile specimen cup or red topped tube.

Procedure

1. *Invasive lines:*
   a. Remove the line site dressing.
   b. Cleanse the line insertion site and surrounding skin with povidone-iodine and allow to dry.
   c. Remove the invasive line, taking care not to contaminate the distal portion with skin or other objects.
   d. Insert the tip (distal end) into a sterile, red topped tube or sterile container. Cut the distal 1.5-inch tip with sterile scissors, allowing the tip to drop into the container.
2. *Indwelling urinary catheter:*
   a. Using a syringe, remove the water that is inside the balloon of the catheter.
   b. Remove the catheter, using sterile gloves and being careful not to contaminate the tip.

c. While holding the tip over or inside a sterile container, cut off at least 1 inch with sterile scissors and allow the tip to fall into the container.

d. Close the container.

Postprocedure Care

1. Write the type of catheter and the removal site on the requisition.
2. Write the collection time on the laboratory requisition.
3. Transport the specimen to the laboratory within 1 hour.
4. Do not refrigerate or incubate the specimen.

Client and Family Teaching

1. Specimen collection is usually painless.
2. Incubation of the culture may take 24-48 hours.

Factors That Affect Results

1. Reject specimens if received more than 2 hours after collection.
2. Contamination of the urinary catheter specimen with the external genital area may obscure the validity of the results. This is a frequent occurrence in the collection of the tip.

Other Data

1. Irritation of the urethra is minimized by total deflation of the balloon, which holds from 5 to 30 mL of sterile water.
2. Most ingested foreign bodies are found within 24 hours and are common in Southeast Asia and Singapore as otolaryngologic emergencies. Few require culture.

FPA

See Fibrinopeptide A—Blood.

FRA

See Fluorescent Rabies Antibody—Specimen.

Fractional Excretion of Sodium in Urine

See Renal Indices—Diagnostic.

Fractional Urine

See Urinalysis, Fractional—Urine.

Free Calcium

See Calcium, Ionized—Blood.

Free Metanephrines

See Metanephrines, Total, 24-Hour Urine, and Free—Plasma.

Free PSA

See Prostate-Specific Antigen—Serum.

Frozen Tissue Section—Diagnostic

Norm. Interpreted by pathologist.

Usage. Rapid diagnosis on biopsied tissue while surgery is in progress.

Description. The rapid freezing and slicing of tissue for pathologic examination and interpretation. Using frozen tissue section samples as a basis for diagnosis, though NOT 100% accurate, has consistently proved to be a highly accurate method for rapid diagnosis. This method may also be used for fluorescent microscopy and for identification of fats and enzymes undetectable by other methods.

Professional Considerations
Consent form IS required for the procedure used to obtain the specimen. See Biopsy, Site-specific—Specimen for procedure-specific risks and contraindications.

Preparation
1. Preoperative teaching involving the type of procedure required for the sampling to proceed.
2. See Client and Family Teaching.

Procedure
1. Place the moistened, fixed or unfixed tissue on a freezing microtome table.
2. Allow carbon dioxide to enter the table through the side perforations.
3. Freeze the tissue and slice it into thin sections by means of the cryostat.
4. Attach the frozen section to a glass slide.
5. Stain the nucleus of the cells with a hematoxylin dye.
6. Stain the cytoplasm of the cells with eosin dye.
7. Examine the slide microscopically and interpret.

Postprocedure Care
1. See individual procedure listings.

Client and Family Teaching
1. Preparation for the procedure is necessary.
2. Fast from food and fluids for 12 hours before the procedure.
3. Call the physician for signs of infection at the procedure site: increasing pain, redness, swelling, purulent drainage, or for temperature >101 degrees F (>38.2 degrees C).
4. Supply information on possible support groups available for the diagnosis.

Factors That Affect Results
1. Poor tissue sample.

Other Data
1. Microscopic examination is often able to confirm a diagnosis of a specific lesion.
2. Frozen sections have been reported as false-positive and false-negative results. A fresh section is best for accuracy.

Fructosamine (Glycated Serum Protein, GSP)—Serum

Norm. Normal ranges vary according to method.

Adult		
Nondiabetic	1.5-2.7 mmol/L	
Diabetic	>2.0-5.0 mmol/L	
Child	5% below adult levels	

Usage. Evaluate diabetic control, reflecting glucose concentrations over a shorter time period (2-3 weeks) than that represented by glycated hemoglobin (hemoglobin A_{1c}) (4-8 weeks). Can be used as an index of longer-term control than glucose levels especially in diabetic clients with abnormal hemoglobin, in clients with gestational diabetes, and in children with type 1 diabetes.

Description. Fructose is a carbohydrate found in fruit and honey and a product of sucrose hydrolysis. Used for monitoring diabetic control, especially when changes in diabetic treatment are sought within weeks, instead of months as per the Hgb A_{1c} test.

Professional Considerations
Consent form is NOT required.

Preparation
1. Tube: Red topped, red/gray topped, or gold topped.
2. See Client and Family Teaching.

Procedure
1. Draw a 5-mL blood sample.

Postprocedure Care
1. None.

Client and Family Teaching
1. Abstain from food and drink 12 hours before the test.
2. Results are normally available within 24 hours.

Factors That Affect Results
1. Albumin levels <3.0 g/dL may falsely lower fructosamine concentrations.

Other Data
1. Hemoglobin, ascorbic acid, and ceruloplasmin inhibit fructosamine generation.
2. Fructosamine >285 mmol/L associated with 4.3-fold increase in cardiovascular mortality.
3. Risk of colorectal adenoma increases with level of fructosamine.

Fructose Challenge Test—Diagnostic

Norm. Lack of significant change in serum glucose, phosphorus, and magnesium concentrations after intravenous fructose administration. Lack of a decrease in serum glucose level after an oral fructose load. Normal plasma fructose level is <10 mg/dL or <6 mmol/L (SI units).

Usage. The intravenous fructose challenge test and an oral fructose challenge test are used in the evaluation of several inherited disorders of fructose metabolism including essential fructosuria, hereditary fructose intolerance, and fructose-1,6-diphosphatase deficiency, and to aid in the diagnosis of steatohepatitis.

Description. Fructose disorders all are inherited as autosomal recessive traits. Essential fructosuria is a clinically benign disorder. Fructose-1,6-diphosphatase deficiency is a clinically severe and often terminal illness in the newborn that is frequently diagnosed by clinical clues that do not involve fructose-loading tests. Hereditary fructose intolerance is a disorder, seen in children as well as adults, that is caused by a deficiency of fructose-1-phosphate aldolase. This condition, characterized by an aversion to sweet foods, may be diagnosed by use of the intravenous fructose challenge test. In this test, a weight-based dose of intravenous fructose is administered intravenously, and serial blood and urine samples are obtained.

Professional Considerations
Consent form IS required.

Risks
Profound hypoglycemia is likely to occur in clients with hereditary fructose intolerance.

Contraindications
Known fructose intolerance. Ancillary medical conditions in which hypoglycemia would impose unacceptable risk to the client (certain forms of cardiac and neurologic disease).

Preparation
1. See Client and Family Teaching.
2. Insert an indwelling intravenous catheter for the administration of fructose, for obtaining blood samples, and if the emergent administration of intravenous glucose is needed.
3. Insert an indwelling urinary catheter if urine samples will be measured.
4. Obtain 10 red topped, red/gray topped, or gold topped tubes.
5. Obtain blood glucose monitoring machine and associated supplies.
6. Obtain parenteral glucose solution ($D_{50}W$).
7. Have emergency equipment readily available.
8. Just before beginning the procedure, take a "time out" to verify the correct client, procedure, and site.

Procedure
1. The client is positioned recumbent.
2. Draw a 7-mL baseline blood sample for serum glucose, fructose, potassium, phosphorus, magnesium, and urate determination.
3. If urine testing will be included, collect a 2-hour baseline urine sample for urate, phosphorus, lactate, alanine, magnesium, and fructose determination.
4. Administer 200 mg/kg (body weight) of 20% fructose solution intravenously over

a 1-minute period for children or over a 2-minute period for adults.

5. Repeat step 2 above, drawing the blood sample immediately after the injection and then at 5, 10, 15, 20, 30, 45, 60, 90, and 120 minutes after the fructose infusion.

6. Urine measurements of fructose, lactate, alanine, magnesium, and phosphorus are occasionally performed during the fructose challenge test.

7. Serum glucose is monitored frequently during the test with cutaneous blood glucose monitoring.

Postprocedure Care

1. Write beginning and ending times of each urine collection on the laboratory requisition.

2. Perform cutaneous blood glucose measurement frequently and observe closely for signs of hypoglycemia for several hours after the test.

3. Discontinue urinary catheter.

4. Discontinue intravenous catheter once it is determined that hypoglycemia is no longer a risk.

Client and Family Teaching

1. Consume a diet free of fructose and sucrose during the 3 weeks before the test.

2. This test is needed to help diagnose hereditary fructose intolerance. This is a condition in which modifying your diet to reduce fructose in your food can improve your prognosis.

3. This test may cause you to feel hypoglycemic. If this occurs, it will be quickly treated.

Factors That Affect Results

1. Accurately timed and labeled serum and urine samples are essential.

2. Abnormally low fructose levels may result if the urine specimen is not tested when it is still fresh.

3. Timed studies of this type are often best performed in special diagnostic areas where the personnel are familiar with the diagnostic procedure.

Other Data

1. Hereditary fructose intolerance is associated with hypoglycemia after intravenous fructose administration. Other phenomena observed in these clients during the test include a rise in serum magnesium and uric acid levels, a fall in serum phosphorus level, and a decrease in urine phosphorus excretion after the fructose administration.

2. Infants fed with a sucrose-containing formula that is hydrolyzed to fructose will exhibit more severe symptoms than breast-fed infants, who are usually asymptomatic, because lactose is not catabolized by the fructose enzyme.

3. Liver biopsy specimens examined for metabolites of fructose may also be used for diagnosis of hereditary fructose intolerance.

4. Treatment for hereditary fructose intolerance is a fructose-free and sucrose-free diet.

FSH

See Follicle-Stimulating Hormone—Serum.

FSH

See Follicle-Stimulating Hormone—Urine.

FSH:LH Ratio

See Follicle-Stimulating Hormone—Serum; Luteinizing Hormone—Blood.

FT$_4$

See Thyroid Test: Thyroxine Free—Serum.

FTA-Abs

See Fluorescent Treponemal Antibody-absorbed Double-stain Test—Serum.

Full Field Digital Mammography

See Mammography—Diagnostic.

Functional MRI

See Magnetic Resonance Imaging—Diagnostic.

Fungal Antibody Screen—Blood

Norm. Negative.

Usage. Rapid detection of antifungal antibodies. Monitoring effectiveness of therapy for fungal infections.

Description. Fungi are slow-growing, eukaryotic organisms that can grow on living and nonliving organic materials and are subdivided into yeasts and molds. Only a few fungi species infect humans. Normal host defense mechanisms limit the damage they cause superficially. Viral serologic testing for fungal antibodies aids in the diagnosis of aspergillosis, blastomycosis, coccidioidomycosis, *Cryptococcus* antigen, fungal infections, histoplasmosis, and *Sporothrix* antibodies. Antibodies to fungi may be found soon after infection and increase as the infection progresses. Diagnosis of a fungal infection is confirmed when the convalescent sample demonstrates a rise in titer from the acute sample.

Professional Considerations

Consent form NOT required.

Preparation

1. Tube: Red topped, red/gray topped, or gold topped.
2. See Client and Family Teaching.

Procedure

1. Draw a 10-mL blood sample.
2. Acute and convalescent samples are required. Obtain the acute sample as soon as possible after onset. Draw the convalescent sample in 1-2 weeks.

Postprocedure Care

1. Send the specimen to the laboratory for immediate separation and freezing of the serum.

Client and Family Teaching

1. Fast for 12 hours before the test.
2. A repeat specimen is required in 1-2 weeks.
3. The treatment will usually be started prophylactically.

Factors That Affect Results

1. Reject hemolyzed specimens, tubes partially filled with blood, or specimens received more than 2 hours after collection.
2. Recent fungal antigen skin tests may cause falsely high results.
3. Blastomycosis and histoplasmosis antigens may cross-react to cause falsely high results. Cystic fibrosis may cause false-positive results for coccidioidomycosis.
4. False-negative results may be caused by immunosuppression from mycoses.

Other Data

1. Factors that predispose clients to fungal infections by lowering the normal host defense mechanisms include administration of broad-spectrum antibiotics, invasive lines, poor nutritional status, parenteral nutrition, surgery, trauma, long-term use of steroids, and chemotherapy for cancer treatment. Other significant risk factors are age more than 60 years and staying in an intensive care unit.

Fungus, Cerebrospinal Fluid

See **Cerebrospinal Fluid, Routine**—Culture and Cytology.

FV Leiden

See **Factor V**—Blood.

FXTAS Testing

See **FMR1 Testing for Fragile X Associated Disorders**—Blood

G6PD

See **Glucose-6-phosphate Dehydrogenase, Quantitative**—Blood.

Galactokinase—Blood

Norm.

Adults	12.1-39.7 mU/g Hb
Children	
2-18 years	11.0-53.6 mU/g Hb
<2 years	11.0-150.0 mU/g Hb
Infants	3-4 times adult values

Increased. Not clinically significant.

Decreased. Galactokinase deficiency, galactosemia, and juvenile cataracts.

Description. Galactokinase is an enzyme that functions in the metabolism of galactose to glucose in the liver, a deficiency of which may result in galactosemia. Galactokinase deficiency is one of three forms of galactosemia, an autosomal recessively transmitted inborn error of metabolism located on chromosome 9p13 and characterized by the inability to convert galactose into glucose with mutations found in the GALK1 gene. This form of galactosemia results in the appearance of infantile or childhood cataracts and long-term complications of speech disorders, mental retardation, ataxia, and (in females) hypergonadotropic hypogonadism.

Professional Considerations
Consent form NOT required.

Preparation
1. Preschedule this test with the laboratory.
2. Tube: Green topped, and a container of ice.

Procedure
1. Draw a 5-mL blood sample.

Postprocedure Care
1. Place the specimen on ice immediately.
2. Write the collection time on the laboratory requisition.
3. Send the specimen to the laboratory within 2 hours. Keep the specimen on ice until tested.

Client and Family Teaching
1. Results are normally available within 24 hours.
2. Diet counseling is strongly recommended if the test is positive.
3. Stress the importance of follow-up examination.
4. Refer clients with positive results for genetic counseling.

Factors That Affect Results
1. Reject specimens that were not placed on ice or were not received in the laboratory within 2 hours after collection.

Other Data
1. Homozygotes have a form of galactosemia with cataracts but without mental retardation or liver disease.

G

G

Galactose-1-Phosphate—Blood

Norm. <1 mg% of galactose-1-phosphate per 100 mL of lysed packed red blood cells. 18.5-28.5 U/g hemoglobin.

Increased. Transferase deficiency (classical) galactosemia.

Decreased. Idiopathic presenile cataracts.

Description. Galactose-1-phosphate is a metabolite that results after the action of galactokinase on galactose. It is found in red blood cells, subsequently converted to glucose-1-phosphate by galactose-1-phosphate uridyltransferase, and used for energy by the body. In clients with galactosemia who are ingesting milk and milk products, the level of galactose-1-phosphate rises and may become toxic. This test is used to monitor the dietary compliance of clients with galactosemia.

Professional Considerations
Consent form NOT required.

Preparation
1. Preschedule this test with the laboratory.
2. Tube: Green topped.

Procedure
1. Draw a 2-mL blood sample and gently invert the tube three times.

Postprocedure Care
1. Write the collection time on the laboratory requisition.
2. Refrigerate specimens until tested.

Client and Family Teaching
1. Results are normally available within 24 hours.
2. If results are positive, the client and family will require diet counseling regarding a galactose-free diet.
3. Galactose toxicity may cause failure to thrive, liver dysfunction, mental retardation, and vomiting or diarrhea.

Factors That Affect Results
1. Reject specimens received in the laboratory more than 3 hours after collection.

Other Data
1. Evaluation for hypergalactosemia should include hepatic ultrasonography.

Galactose-1-Phosphate Uridyltransferase, Erythrocyte—Blood

Norm.

		SI Units
Adult	5.9-9.5 μmol/hr/mL	98-158 U/L
Heterozygote	2.0-4.8 μmol/hr/mL	33-80 U/L
Homozygote	0.0 μmol/hr/mL	0.0 U/L
Other norms		
Normal	18-28 U/g Hb	
Possible carrier state	5-18.5 U/g Hb	

Increased. Not applicable.

Decreased. Galactose-1-phosphate uridyltransferase deficiency and transferase-deficiency (classical) galactosemia.

Description. Galactose-1-phosphate uridyltransferase is an enzyme active in the metabolism of galactose to glucose in the liver. It catalyzes the conversion of galactose-1-phosphate into glucose-1-phosphate. Deficiency of galactose-1-phosphate uridyltransferase is the most common cause of galactosemia. In this test, measurements of this enzyme are performed on the hemolysate of washed erythrocytes.

Professional Considerations
Consent form NOT required.

Preparation
1. Tube: Green topped, and a container of ice.

Procedure
1. Draw a 2-mL blood sample and then gently invert the tube three times.

Postprocedure Care
1. Place the specimen immediately on ice.

Client and Family Teaching

1. If the results are positive, the client and family will require diet counseling regarding a galactose-free diet.

Factors That Affect Results

1. Reject the specimen if it contains recently transfused blood to avoid a possible false-negative result.

2. Reject hemolyzed specimens or specimens not received on ice.

Other Data

1. Treat galactosemia with a lactose-free diet.
2. See also Galactose-1-phosphate uridyltransferase, Qualitative—Blood.

Galactose-1-Phosphate Uridyltransferase, Qualitative—Blood

Norm. Negative.

Positive. Transferase-deficiency (classical) galactosemia.

Description. A qualitative screen for galactosemia and differential diagnosis of milk intolerance in the newborn. This enzyme catalyzes the conversion of galactose-1-phosphate into glucose-1-phosphate in the liver. Galactosemia is an autosomal recessively transmitted inborn error of metabolism characterized by the inability to convert galactose into glucose. This causes deposits of galactose-1-phosphate in body tissues, resulting in vomiting, diarrhea, failure to thrive, liver dysfunction, splenomegaly, and cataracts in the infant. Symptoms appear a few days after a milk diet is started. Deficiency of galactose-1-phosphate uridyltransferase is the most common form of galactosemia. Early detection of galactosemia enables institution of a lactose-free diet and avoidance of complications of galactose toxicity. The test involves examining specially treated filter paper with a drop of dried blood under fluorescent lights after timed exposure to ultraviolet radiation. In a negative test (enzyme present), the blood fluoresces. In a positive test (enzyme absent), the blood will not fluoresce.

Professional Considerations

Consent form NOT required.

Preparation

1. Preschedule this test with the laboratory.
2. Write the client's birth date on the laboratory requisition.
3. Obtain galactosemia-screening filter paper.

Procedure

1. Obtain three drops of blood from an infant heelstick on the lateral curvature of the heel.
2. Place each drop in a circle on galactosemia-screening filter paper and allow to dry.
3. Heparinized blood may also be used (green topped tube).

Postprocedure Care

1. Apply a dressing to the heelstick site.
2. Label the filter paper with the client's name and identification.
3. Store the specimen at room temperature. Protect it from heat if it is transferred to an outside laboratory.

Client and Family Teaching

1. Results are normally available within 24 hours.
2. If results are positive, the family will require diet counseling regarding a galactose-free diet.

Factors That Affect Results

1. This test should be performed during the first 3 days after the infant is born.
2. False-negative results may occur up to 3 months after blood transfusion if the Beutler-Baluda screening method is used.

Other Data

1. Treat galactosemia with a lactose-free diet.
2. Blood testing is considered more reliable than urine testing in screening for galactosemia.
3. Positive results should be confirmed with a quantitative galactose-1-phosphate uridyltransferase measurement.

Galactose, Screening Test for Galactosemia—Urine

Norm. <10 mg/dL. Galactostix has a lower limit of sensitivity of 100 mg/dL.

Increased. Galactokinase deficiency, galactose-1-phosphate uridyltransferase deficiency, and galactosemia.

Description. A urine screen for galactosemia and differential diagnosis of milk intolerance in the newborn after a positive Benedict's or Clinitest result and a negative glucose oxidase test for glucose. Urine galactose measurements are performed by chromatography.

Professional Considerations
Consent form NOT required.

Preparation
1. Obtain a clean container with a lid, pediatric urine collection device, and tape.

Procedure
1. Obtain at least a 10-mL random urine specimen in a clean container.
2. Place the infant supine, with the knees flexed and the hips externally rotated and abducted.
3. Cleanse, rinse, and thoroughly dry the perineal area.
4. To prevent the child from removing the collection device, a diaper may be placed over the genital area.
5. *Females*: Tape the pediatric collection device to the perineum. Starting at the area between the anus and vagina, apply the device in an anterior direction.
6. *Males*: Place the pediatric collection device over the penis and scrotum and tape it to the perineal area.

Postprocedure Care
1. Send the specimens to the laboratory and refrigerate them if not tested immediately.

Client and Family Teaching
1. If the results are positive, the family will require diet counseling regarding a galactose-free diet.
2. Results are normally available within 24 hours.

Factors That Affect Results
1. None found.

Other Data
1. Blood testing is more reliable than urine testing in screening for galactosemia.
2. Positive results should be confirmed with a quantitative galactose-1-phosphate uridyltransferase measurement.
3. See also Galactose-1-phosphate uridyltransferase, Qualitative—Blood.

Gallbladder and Biliary System Ultrasonography—Diagnostic

Norm.

Gallbladder	
Appearance	Sonolucent; free of sludge or stones
Location	Anterior to the right kidney, lateral to the pancreas and duodenum
Shape	Circular on transverse scans
	Pear shaped on longitudinal scans
	7-10 cm long and 2-3 cm wide with a capacity of 30-50 mL
Walls	Sharply defined and smooth, 1-2 mm thick
Cystic Duct	
Appearance	Not sonolucent because of lumen; Heister's valves visible
Shape	Serpentine
Common Bile Duct	
Shape	Linear; internal diameter <6 mm
Hepatic Duct	
Lumen	Internal diameter <4 mm

Usage. Diagnosis of cholelithiasis and cholecystitis and differential diagnosis of the cause of jaundice (obstructive versus nonobstructive). Useful in adults with hereditary spherocytosis and those with Gilbert syndrome.

Description. Evaluation of the gallbladder, cystic duct, and common bile duct by the creation of an oscilloscopic picture from the echoes of high-frequency sound waves passing over these areas. The time required for the ultrasonic beam to be reflected back to the transducer from differing densities of tissue is converted by a computer to an electrical impulse displayed on an oscilloscopic screen to create a three-dimensional picture of the gallbladder and biliary duct system. This noninvasive test has replaced oral cholecystography for evaluation of the biliary system. The presence of sludge causes low-level echoes in the interior of the gallbladder. Acute cholecystitis causes the walls to appear thickened and sonolucent because of edema. Cholelithiasis is demonstrated by a dilated interior, with shadows present. Biliary tree gas causes shadows. Polyps appear as sharply defined masses, whereas carcinoma appears as a poorly defined mass. In obstructive jaundice, dilatation of the gallbladder and biliary duct system is detected.

Professional Considerations

Consent form NOT required.

Risks

If sincalide is given: infection.

Contraindications

Administration of sincalide is contraindicated in pregnancy and in children.

Preparation

1. See Client and Family Teaching.
2. Some scans may require intravenous access.

Procedure

1. The client is positioned supine and instructed to hold his or her breath during the scans.
2. A lubricated transducer is passed slowly over the right upper quadrant of the abdomen with transverse scans (moving from the midline to the right side) taken

every 1 cm from the xiphoid process to the right subcostal area.
3. As the gallbladder borders are identified, they are marked on the client's skin.
4. Longitudinal and oblique scans are then taken every 5 mm between the marked borders of the gallbladder.
5. The client is then turned to a steep, left lateral decubitus position, and the scan is repeated from the right costal margin.
6. The client may then be positioned upright to observe for movement of suspected stones away from the walls of the gallbladder or cystic duct.
7. If contractility of the gallbladder is to be evaluated, intravenous sincalide may be injected or a fatty meal may be ingested, and the scan is repeated in 30 minutes.
8. Photographs are taken of the oscilloscopic display.

Postprocedure Care

1. Remove the lubricant from the skin.
2. Resume previous diet.

Client and Family Teaching

1. Consume a diet free of fat the day before the test.
2. Fast for 8-12 hours before the ultrasonography, but drink plenty of fluids.
3. It is important to lie as motionless as possible during the ultrasonography.

Factors That Affect Results

1. Gallstones appear as shadows when well mixed with bile, but if the gallbladder is full of stones, shadows are difficult to detect.
2. Sincalide may cause nausea. Movement during nausea may interfere with results.
3. Dehydration interferes with adequate contrast between organs and body fluids.
4. Very small stones (<1-2 mm) in the gallbladder must be differentiated from polyps by repositioning of the client. The stones will move downward with gravity, whereas polyps will remain stable.
5. The more abdominal fat present, the greater is the attenuation (reduction in sound wave amplitude and intensity), which interferes with the clarity of the picture.

Other Data

1. Gallbladder cancer cannot usually be diagnosed by sonography.

G

Gallbladder Scan

See **Hepatobiliary Scan**—Diagnostic.

Gallium Scan

See **Gallium Scan of Bone, Brain, Breast, or Liver**—Diagnostic.

Gallium Scan of Bone—Diagnostic

Norm. Normal patterns of bone gallium uptake as interpreted by a nuclear medicine physician.

Usage. Detection of osteomyelitis, joint infections, and metastatic bone neoplasms (Wilms' tumor) or Hodgkin's disease.

Description. Nuclear medicine scan using gallium-67 citrate to localize inflammatory lesions of the bone, bone marrow, and cartilage. Although the bones normally absorb the gallium-67 citrate, abnormal areas of inflammation or tumors appear as areas of increased uptake of the radiopharmaceutical.

Professional Considerations

Consent form IS required.

Risks

Allergic reaction to the radiopharmaceutical (itching, hives, rash, tight feeling in the throat, shortness of breath, bronchospasm, anaphylaxis, death), infection.

Contraindications

Previous allergic reaction to the same radiopharmaceutical. This test is usually contraindicated during pregnancy and breast-feeding.

Preparation

1. Inject the client with a gallium-67 citrate radiopharmaceutical intravenously 48-72 hours before the test. Exception: For the detection of acute inflammatory lesions, scan at 6-24 hours and then again at 48-72 hours.
2. If the pelvis is to be scanned, the bladder should be emptied completely just before the procedure.
3. See Client and Family Teaching.
4. Just before beginning the procedure, take a "time out" to verify the correct client, procedure, and site.

Procedure

1. The client is positioned under the gamma (Anger) camera or a scintillation camera.
2. Serial images are obtained anteriorly and posteriorly while an uptake probe and detector head measure the radiation emissions.
3. The client must lie motionless throughout the scan.

Postprocedure Care

1. See Client and Family Teaching.

Client and Family Teaching

1. Increase oral intake of fluids, where not contraindicated, beginning 24 hours before the scan.
2. The scan takes 30-60 minutes and is painless.
3. The camera will make clicking noises during the scan.
4. It is important to lie motionless during the scan.
5. Drink 6-8 glasses of water and other fluids each day for 2 days after the test (unless contraindicated).
6. Results are normally available 24 hours after the completion of the scan.

Factors That Affect Results

1. Lesions <1-2 cm in size will not be detectable with a gallium scan.
2. False-positive results may be obtained in the presence of leukopenia.

Other Data

1. Gallium is excreted by the kidney and colon in 24-48 hours.
2. This test does not distinguish between benign and malignant lesions.
3. Health care professionals working in a nuclear medicine area must follow federal standards set by the Nuclear Regulatory Commission. These standards include precautions for handling the radioactive material and monitoring of potential radiation exposure.

Gallium Scan of Brain—Diagnostic

Norm. Normal pattern of brain-tissue gallium uptake as interpreted by a nuclear medicine physician.

Usage. Screening and localizing intracranial neoplasms, identification of cerebrovascular accident or tumor recurrence after surgical excision, and differentiation of localized inflammations of central nervous system (abscesses).

Description. A nuclear medicine scan in which radiopharmaceutical gallium-67 or gallium-68 is injected intravenously and a scintillation camera is used to obtain photographs of the meninges and brain soft tissue 24-48 hours later. The gallium is transported to the brain tissue via cerebrospinal fluid and plasma, where it binds to the transferrin receptor sites of soft-tissue cells of neutrophilic lactoferrin. Tumors and inflammatory lesions frequently contain large concentrations of these two proteins. A positive scan will have distinct patterns of gallium uptake that differ from normal tissue uptake. For example, neoplasms will appear as dense areas with increased gallium uptake, whereas inflammatory lesions (most frequently abscesses) appear on the scan as well-localized areas of increased gallium uptake that are encapsulated. Finally, cerebral hemorrhages will differ from normal gallium uptake, appearing as irregular, diffuse areas of uptake. This is attributable to the vascular occlusion and tissue damage associated with cerebrovascular accidents.

Professional Considerations

Consent form IS required.

Risks

Allergic reaction to the radiopharmaceutical (itching, hives, rash, tight feeling in the throat, shortness of breath, bronchospasm, anaphylaxis, death), infection.

Contraindications

Previous allergic reaction to the same radiopharmaceutical. This test is usually contraindicated during pregnancy and breast-feeding.

Preparation

1. The client is injected intravenously with radiopharmaceutical gallium-67 or gallium-68 from 6 to 48 hours before the scan.

2. See Client and Family Teaching.
3. Just before beginning the procedure, take a "time out" to verify the correct client, procedure, and site.

Procedure

1. The client is positioned under the scintillation camera, and serial images are obtained from anterior, posterior, lateral, and, occasionally, vertex views.
2. The client must lie motionless throughout the scan.

Postprocedure Care

1. See Client and Family Teaching.

Client and Family Teaching

1. Increase oral intake of fluids, where not contraindicated, beginning 24 hours before the scan.
2. The scan takes 30-60 minutes and is painless.
3. The camera may touch the body and will make a clicking noise during the scan.
4. It is important to lie motionless during the scan.
5. Drink 6-8 glasses of water and other fluids each day for 2 days after the test (unless contraindicated).
6. Results are normally available 24 hours after the completion of the scan.

Factors That Affect Results

1. Lesions <1-2 cm in size may not be detectable with a gallium scan.
2. Lesions located at the base of the brain, such as pituitary adenomas, may be difficult to detect because of the increased vascularity of the area and the difficulty in positioning the camera for clear images.
3. False-positive results may be obtained in the presence of leukopenia.
4. Pediatric neoplasms will most frequently appear intrafrontally, whereas adult neoplasms will most often be located supratentorially.

Other Data

1. Gallium is excreted by the kidney and colon in 24-48 hours.
2. Gallium scanning does not differentiate malignant from benign tumors.
3. Health care professionals working in a nuclear medicine area must follow federal standards set by the Nuclear Regulatory

G

Commission. These standards include precautions for handling the radioactive material and monitoring of potential radiation exposure.

Gallium Scan of Breast—Diagnostic

Norm. Normal pattern of breast gallium uptake as interpreted by a nuclear medicine physician.

Usage. Detection and location of tumor or inflammatory lesions of the breast, evaluation of lymphomas, and identification of recurrent tumors after chemotherapy or radiation therapy.

Description. Nuclear medicine scan using gallium-67 citrate to localize neoplasms and inflammatory lesions of the breast tissues and lymph nodes. It is believed that the gallium binds to the transferrin and lactoferrin circulating in plasma and soft tissue. Tumors and lesions containing neutrophils also have large concentrations of these two beta globulins, causing the gallium clearance to be slower than that in normal tissue. Therefore these abnormalities appear on the scan as abnormally large concentrations of gallium uptake.

Professional Considerations
Consent form IS required.

Risks
Allergic reaction to the radiopharmaceutical (itching, hives, rash, tight feeling in the throat, shortness of breath, bronchospasm, anaphylaxis, death), infection.

Contraindications
Previous allergic reaction to the same radiopharmaceutical. This test is usually contraindicated during pregnancy and breast-feeding.

Preparation
1. The client is injected with a gallium-67 citrate radiopharmaceutical intravenously 48-72 hours before the scan.
2. See Client and Family Teaching.
3. Just before beginning the procedure, take a "time out" to verify the correct client, procedure, and site.

Procedure
1. The client is positioned either erect or recumbent under a gamma (Anger) camera or rectilinear scanner in the nuclear medicine department.
2. Serial images are obtained anteriorly and posteriorly, and occasional lateral views may be required.
3. The client must lie motionless during the scan.

Postprocedure Care
1. See Client and Family Teaching.

Client and Family Teaching
1. Increase intake of fluids, where not contraindicated, beginning 24 hours before the scan.
2. The camera will make clicking noises during the scan.
3. It is important to lie motionless during the scan.
4. Drink 6-8 glasses of water and other fluids per day for 2 days after the scan.

Factors That Affect Results
1. Breast tissue has an increased affinity for gallium uptake during pregnancy, lactation, and menarche. These conditions may produce a false-positive result.
2. Drugs that may cause false-positive results include oral contraceptives.
3. Lesions <1-2 cm in size may not be detectable with a gallium scan.

Other Data
1. Gallium is excreted by the kidney and colon in 24-48 hours.
2. Gallium scanning does not differentiate malignant from benign tumors.
3. The scan takes 30-60 minutes to perform.
4. Health care professionals working in a nuclear medicine area must follow federal standards set by the Nuclear Regulatory Commission. These standards include precautions for handling the radioactive material and monitoring of potential radiation exposure.

Gallium Scan of Liver—Diagnostic

Norm. Symmetric patterns of liver gallium uptake. Requires interpretation.

Usage. Detection of hepatomas, abscesses, biopsy sites, and alcoholic cirrhoses and evaluation of recurrent lymphomas or tumors after chemotherapy and radiation therapy.

Description. Nuclear medicine scan of the liver using gallium-67 citrate radiopharmaceutical. Normal liver tissue will absorb gallium in a symmetric fashion. Abscesses appear as a "rim sign," heavily concentrated areas of gallium uptake surrounding a cold center. The cold center is an area where no inflammation exists. Abscesses are rich with lactoferrin in the neutrophils, and gallium appears to bind to the lactoferrin, making the abscess visible. Tumors appear as heavily concentrated areas of gallium with normal symmetric gallium uptake in the surrounding liver tissue.

Professional Considerations
Consent form IS required.

Risks
Allergic reaction to the radiopharmaceutical (itching, hives, rash, tight feeling in the throat, shortness of breath, bronchospasm, anaphylaxis, death), infection.

Contraindications
Previous allergic reaction to the same radiopharmaceutical. This test is usually contraindicated during pregnancy and breast-feeding.

Preparation
1. The client is injected with a gallium-67 citrate radiopharmaceutical intravenously 48-72 hours before the scan.
2. See Client and Family Teaching.
3. Just before beginning the procedure, take a "time out" to verify the correct client, procedure, and site.

Procedure
1. The client is positioned either erect or recumbent under a gamma (Anger) camera or rectilinear scanner in the nuclear medicine department.
2. Serial images are obtained anteriorly and posteriorly, and occasionally lateral views may be required.
3. The client must lie motionless during the scan.

Postprocedure Care
1. See Client and Family Teaching.

Client and Family Teaching
1. Increase oral intake of fluids, where not contraindicated, 24 hours before the scan.
2. A clear-liquid diet may be prescribed for the day before the test.
3. Cleansing enemas may be prescribed the morning before the test.
4. The camera will make clicking noises during the scan.
5. The scan takes 30-60 minutes to perform.
6. Drink 6-8 glasses of water and other fluids per day for 2 days (where not contraindicated) after the scan.

Factors That Affect Results
1. Normal hepatic gallium uptake may obscure the detection of abnormal para-aortic nodes in Hodgkin's disease, resulting in a false-negative scan.
2. Localization of neutrophils labeled with gallium into fresh operative sites and inflamed peritoneum limits this test's usefulness in clients who have recently undergone surgery.

Other Data
1. Gallium is excreted by the kidney and colon in 24-48 hours.
2. Gallium scanning does not differentiate malignant from benign tumors.
3. Health care professionals working in a nuclear medicine area must follow federal standards set by the Nuclear Regulatory Commission. These standards include precautions for handling the radioactive material and monitoring of potential radiation exposure.

Gamma Globulin (IgG, Quantitative IgG)—Plasma

Norm.

		SI Units
Adults	550-1750 mg/dL or 0.5-1.4 g/dL	5.5-17.5 g/L
Children		
Pediatric cord blood	660-1800 mg/dL	6.6-18 g/L
Newborn	831-1231 mg/dL	8.3-12.3 g/L
1-3 months	311-549 mg/dL	3.1-5.5 g/L
4-6 months	241-613 mg/dL	2.4-6.1 g/L
7-12 months	442-880 mg/dL	4.4-8.8 g/L
13-24 months	553-971 mg/dL	5.5-9.7 g/L
2-3 years	709-1075 mg/dL	7.1-10.8 g/L
3-5 years	701-1257 mg/dL	7.0-12.6 g/L
6-8 years	667-1179 mg/dL	6.7-11.8 g/L
9-11 years	889-1359 mg/dL	8.9-13.6 g/L
12-16 years	822-1170 mg/dL	8.2-11.7 g/L

Increased. AIDS, chronic granulomatous infections, cystic fibrosis of the pancreas, hepatitis (chronic), hyperimmunization, infection, juvenile rheumatoid arthritis, Laënnec's cirrhosis, multiple myeloma (IgG myeloma), myxoma of left atrium of heart, nonimmune chronic idiopathic neutropenia in adults, pulmonary tuberculosis, serum protein monoclonal gammopathy, Sjögren's syndrome, and systemic lupus erythematosus. Drugs include aminophenazone, anticonvulsants, asparaginase, ethotoin, hydralazine hydrochloride, mephenytoin, methadone, oral contraceptives, phenylbutazone, phenytoin, and phenytoin sodium prompt.

Decreased. Agammaglobulinemia, heavy chain disease, IgA myeloma, leukemia (chronic lymphocytic), lymphoid aplasia, macroglobulinemia, nephrotic syndrome, and type I dysgammaglobulinemia. Drugs include cancer chemotherapeutic agents, dextrans, methylprednisolone, methylprednisolone acetate, methylprednisolone sodium succinate, and phenytoin.

Description. Protein IgG is the major immunoglobulin of blood that possesses antibody activity against viruses, some bacteria, and toxins. It is the only immunoglobulin that crosses the placenta. Used to evaluate humoral immunity, monitor therapy in IgA G myeloma, and evaluate clients, especially those with a propensity to infections.

Professional Considerations
Consent form NOT required.

Preparation
1. See Client and Family Teaching.
2. Tube: Red topped, red/gray topped, or gold topped.

Procedure
1. Draw a 5-mL blood sample.

Postprocedure Care
1. Note vaccinations, immunizations, or toxoid administration within the previous 6 months on the laboratory requisition.
2. Note administration of blood products within the previous 6 weeks on the laboratory requisition.
3. Send the specimen to the laboratory immediately.

Client and Family Teaching
1. Do not eat or drink, except for water, for 12 hours before sampling.
2. Results are normally available within 24 hours.

Factors That Affect Results
1. Vaccination, immunization, and toxoid administration within 6 months before the test may affect results.
2. Receipt of blood products within 6 weeks before the test may affect results.
3. Drug or radiation treatment for cancer may cause decreased results.

Other Data
1. Electrophoresis is a more precise measurement for gamma globulins.

Gamma-Glutamyltransferase—Blood

See Gamma-Glutamyltranspeptidase—Blood.

Gamma-Glutamyltranspeptidase (GGTP, Gamma-Glutamyltransferase)—Blood

Norm.

Adult females	4-25 U
	8-50 mU/mL
	3.5-13 IU/L
	3-33 U/L at 37°C
Adult males	7-40 U
	12-89 mU/mL
	4-23 IU/L
	9-69 U/L at 37°C
Children	
Cord blood	190-270 U/L at 37°C
Premature infants	<140 U/L at 37°C
1-3 days	56-233 U/L at 37°C
4-21 days	0-130 U/L at 37°C
3-12 weeks	4-120 U/L at 37°C
3-6 months	
female	5-35 U/L at 37°C
male	5-65 U/L at 37°C
>6 months	15-85 IU/L at 37°C
female	5-55 IU/L at 37°C
male	
1-15 years	0-23 U/L at 37°C

Usage. Evaluation of progression of liver disease and hepatic metastasis, screening for alcoholism, and as legal evidence in rape. A marker related to oxidative stress. A marker of insulin resistance when non-alcoholic fatty liver disease or obesity is present.

Increased. Acetaminophen toxicity, alcoholism, alpha$_1$-antitrypsin deficiency, biliary atresia, cholecystitis (caused by biliary obstruction), cholestasis (intrahepatic), cirrhosis (biliary, Laënnec's), congestive heart failure, fatty liver, hepatic carcinoma (metastatic), hepatitis (acute, chronic), home parenteral nutrition associated cholestasis, jaundice (obstructive), Kawasaki disease, lipoid nephrosis, liver disease, metabolic syndrome, mononucleosis-like syndrome (MLS), myocardial infarction, obesity (extreme), pancreatic carcinoma, pancreatitis (acute), primary biliary cirrhosis, renal carcinoma, and systemic lupus erythematosus. Drugs include alcohol, glutethimide, high-dose 5-FU arterial infusion chemotherapy, methaqualone, phenobarbital, phenytoin, phenytoin sodium, and rosiglitazone. Increased meat consumption and low fruit consumption.

Decreased. Improving cardiovascular risk factors.

Description. GGTP is a biliary excretory enzyme that assists in the transfer of amino acids and peptides across cellular membranes. It is found in the liver, kidneys, pancreas, brain, heart, salivary glands, and prostate gland. Progression of carcinoma is associated with increasing levels, and regression of carcinoma is associated with decreasing GGTP levels.

Professional Considerations
Consent form NOT required.

Preparation
1. See Client and Family Teaching.
2. Tube: Red topped, red/gray topped, or green topped.

Procedure
1. Draw a 4-mL blood sample.

Postprocedure Care
1. The specimen may be frozen.

Client and Family Teaching
1. Fast, except for drinking water, for 8 hours and refrain from drinking alcohol for 24 hours before the test.

Factors That Affect Results
1. Reject hemolyzed specimens.
2. Elevation may occur with phenytoin or phenobarbital therapy; one of the alternative tests—leucine aminopeptidase (LAP) or 5′-nucleotides—is preferable.
3. High meat consumption will elevate results.
4. Echinacea taken for 8 weeks or longer may cause hepatotoxicity.

Other Data
1. The stability of specimens is as follows: room temperature, 5 days; refrigerated, 7 days; frozen −4 degrees F (−20 degrees C), 90 days.

2. GGTP is more accurate than alkaline phosphatase for hepatic disease because it is unaffected by abnormalities of skeletal muscles.

Gamma-Hydroxybutyric Acid (GHB, Gamma-Hydroxybutyrate, Liquid Ecstasy)—Blood or Urine or Human Hair

Norm. Negative for blood or urine, <8.4 ng/mg/scalp hair.

Possible Outcome in Average-Sized Adults	Ingestion Amount	Plasma or Serum Level	Urine Level
Euphoria	100 mg		1100 mg/L
Coma	4 g (just under 1 teaspoon)	>2.5 mmol/L	
Death possible	10 g		

Overdose Symptoms and Treatment

Clients who receive supportive treatment commonly regain consciousness spontaneously up to 5 hours after ingestion of GHB. Left untreated, GHB overdose of >10 g can lead to death.

Symptoms

Agitation or aggression (more common in daily users)

Amnesia occurs in 13% of users.

Ataxia

Cardiovascular depression (such as bradycardia)

Central nervous system depression (somnolence progressing to coma) occurs in 66%. Coma can occur when a 2- to 4-g dose (about ½ to 1 teaspoon) is ingested in an adult of average size.

Emesis is possible.

Hypothermia often occurs when another substance is co-ingested.

Nystagmus

Respiratory depression, respiratory acidosis

Hypotension

Hypothermia

Emergence phenomenon as the client regains consciousness may include agitation, myoclonus, confusion, and combativeness.

Treatment

NOTE: Treatment choice(s) depend(s) on client's history and condition and episode history.

1. Perform frequent neurologic checks.
2. Follow aspiration precautions.
3. Provide airway support, including oxygen and rapid-sequence intubation and mechanical ventilation as needed.
4. Provide continuous cardiac monitoring. Use atropine, neostigmine, or physostigmine if symptomatic bradycardia is present or worsening.
5. Establish intravenous access.
6. Stimulate client frequently.
7. Consider what treatment is needed for possible co-ingested substances.
8. Most clients who recover have no further symptoms and can be discharged after being observed for 6 hours.
9. Naloxone, flumazenil, and anticonvulsants all have been shown NOT to reduce GHB levels or symptoms in humans.
10. Withdrawal symptoms of visual hallucinations, tachycardia, tremor, nystagmus, and diaphoresis have been successfully treated with administration of benzodiazepines and phenobarbital (Schneir et al, 2001).

Usage. Determining drugs of abuse used in clients with overdose symptoms or central nervous system depression where the cause is unknown. Postmortem values are the following: cardiac blood, 55-409 mg/L; femoral blood, 17-44 mg/L; vitreous humor, 3.9-20 mg/L.

Description. GHB is a drug used legally outside of the United States as a sedative adjunct to anesthesia, in treating alcohol-withdrawal syndrome, and in treating narcolepsy. It is also sold and used worldwide as an illegal "street drug" and has been used for weight loss or muscle production and in date rape. In the human body, GHB is a naturally occurring derivative of GABA and is believed to have an inhibitory role in neurotransmission and to help regulate sleep cycles, temperature regulation, and glucose metabolism. When large doses are ingested, GHB causes a feeling of euphoria accompanied by central nervous system depression progressing to coma. GHB levels may indicate ingestion of either GHB or its precursor drug gamma-butyrolactone (GBL). GHB is water soluble and rapidly metabolized, having an onset of 15-30 minutes orally and 2-15 minutes IV, duration of 3 hours, and a half-life of 27 minutes. The drug is excreted rapidly in urine in <10 hours. It is metabolized to succinic acid and carbon dioxide, with the majority of GHB leaving the body in expired carbon dioxide. GBL has a longer half-life because of its solubility in lipids and thus may have a longer duration of action. Although GHB is regulated by law, GBL is not and is sold in over-the-counter body-building supplements. In this test, a sample of blood or urine is tested using gas chromatography–mass spectrometry methods.

Professional Considerations

Consent form IS usually required because specimens may be used as legal evidence.

Preparation

1. Tube: Red topped, green topped, or blue topped.
2. Obtain clean specimen container for urine collection.
3. Obtain a container of ice.

Procedure

1. Obtain a 3-mL blood sample or a ≥7-mL random or straight-catheterized urine specimen. Place sample immediately on ice.

Postprocedure Care

1. Write the client's name, the date, exact time of collection, and specimen source on the laboratory requisition. Sign, and have the witness sign, the laboratory requisition.
2. Transport the specimen to the laboratory immediately in a sealed plastic bag marked as legal evidence. All clients handling the specimen should sign and mark the time of receipt on the laboratory requisition.
3. Freeze specimen if sent off-site for testing.

Client and Family Teaching

1. Refer client and family or significant others for follow-up counseling and/or crisis intervention services. Offer drug abuse recovery resources as appropriate.
2. Survivors of sexual assault should be referred to appropriate crisis-counseling agencies as well as for gynecologic follow-up examination.
3. Because clients with overdose often are unaware of the dangers of GHB, educate client about this.

Factors That Affect Results

1. At 12 hours after ingestion, GHB can no longer be detected in urine.

Other Data

1. People who ingest GHB recreationally are often found to have taken more than one toxic substance.
2. High use reported in body builders, gay persons, and HIV-positive persons.
3. Many states have enacted laws reclassifying GHB as a controlled substance.
4. In the United States, report GHB cases to the Drug Enforcement Administration in Washington, DC, 877-801-7974, for blood values >5 mg/mL and urine values >10 mg/mL.
5. Blood concentrations <30 mg/L and urine concentrations <20 mg/L may represent only endogenous GHB production.
6. Production of GHB increases with time after death in postmortem liver.

Gas Ventilation Lung Scan—Diagnostic

Norm. Radioactive gas is distributed equally in both lungs with normal "wash-in" and "wash-out" phases.

Usage. Used with a lung perfusion scan to diagnose, identify, and evaluate regions of lung tissue that are not ventilated during respirations. Some conditions in which this may occur include pulmonary embolism, chronic obstructive pulmonary disease, and parenchymal disease (bronchogenic carcinoma).

Description. A nuclear medicine scan in which the client inhales air mixed with radiolabeled gas (xenon-133) through a mask. A gamma (Anger) camera images the gas distribution of the posterior lung fields through three phases: phase 1 is the "wash-in" phase in which the buildup of radioactive gas occurs. In phase 2, equilibrium occurs. Phase 3 is the "wash-out" phase, in which the gas is removed from the lungs. Decreased areas of ventilation will appear lighter with longer than normal wash-out phases.

Professional Considerations

Consent form NOT required.

Risks

Dizziness, fetal damage.

Contraindications

In clients who are unable to follow directions.

Precautions

During pregnancy, risks of cumulative radiation exposure to the fetus from this and other previous or future imaging studies must be weighed against the benefits of the procedure. Although formal limits for client exposure are relative to this risk:benefit comparison, the United States Nuclear Regulatory Commission requires that the cumulative dose equivalent to an embryo/fetus from occupational exposure not exceed 0.5 rem (5 mSv). Radiation dosage to the fetus is proportional to the distance of the anatomy studied from the abdomen and decreases as pregnancy progresses. For pregnant clients, consult the radiologist/radiology department to obtain estimated fetal radiation exposure from this procedure.

Preparation

1. Obtain baseline vital signs and continue to monitor vital signs every 10-15 minutes.
2. Remove jewelry and metal objects.

Procedure

1. The client is positioned erect or supine throughout the scan.
2. The client inhales a mixture of air and radioactive xenon-133 gas through a mask and holds his or her breath for 20 seconds. For mechanically ventilated clients, krypton-85 gas should be substituted for xenon-133.
3. The client's chest is scanned with a gamma camera as he or she exhales.

Postprocedure Care

1. None.

Client and Family Teaching

1. The test is painless and takes about 15-30 minutes.
2. Results are normally available after interpretation by a radiologist.

Factors That Affect Results

1. An improperly fitting or loose seal on the ventilation mask interferes with the proper mixing of air and gas and allows radioactive gas to contaminate the surrounding air.

Other Data

1. None.

Gastric Acid Analysis Test (Peptavlon Stimulation Test)—Diagnostic

Norm. Within normal limits.

Basal (Prestimulation) Acid Output (BAO) Is the Gastric Acid Secreted without Stimulation		SI Units
Adult Female		
Normal	1-4 mEq/hour	1-4 mmol/hour
Duodenal ulcer	3-8 mEq/hour	3-8 mmol/hour
Gastric carcinoma	0-3 mEq/hour	0-3 mmol/hour
Gastric ulcer	1-3 mEq/hour	1-3 mmol/hour
Atrophic gastritis	0 mEq/hour	0 mmol/hour
Pernicious anemia	0 mEq/hour	0 mmol/hour
Zollinger-Ellison syndrome	>20 mEq/hour	>20 mmol/hour

Basal (Prestimulation) Acid Output (BAO) Is the Gastric Acid Secreted without Stimulation		SI Units
Adult Male		
Normal	2-5 mEq/hour	2-5 mmol/hour
Duodenal ulcer	5-10 mEq/hour	5-10 mmol/hour
Gastric carcinoma	0-3 mEq/ hour	0-3 mmol/hour
Gastric ulcer	1-5 mEq/hour	1-5 mmol/hour
Atrophic gastritis	0 mEq/hour	0 mmol/hour
Pernicious anemia	0 mEq/hour	0 mmol/hour
Zollinger-Ellison syndrome	>20 mEq/hour	>20 mmol/hour
Maximum (Stimulated) Acid Output (MAO) Is the Gastric Acid Output After Stimulation (Sum of Four 15-Minute Specimens)		
Adult Female		
Normal	7-15 mEq/hour	7-15 mmol/hour
Duodenal ulcer	10-20 mEq/hour	10-20 mmol/hour
Gastric carcinoma	0-5 mEq/hour	0-5 mmol/hour
Gastric ulcer	5-15 mEq/hour	5-15 mmol/hour
Atrophic gastritis	0 mEq/hour	0 mmol/hour
Pernicious anemia	0 mEq/hour	0 mmol/hour
Zollinger-Ellison syndrome	35-60 mEq/hour	35-60 mmol/hour
Adult Male		
Normal	5-26 mEq/hour	5-26 mmol/hour
Duodenal ulcer	15-35 mEq/hour	15-35 mmol/hour
Gastric carcinoma	0-20 mEq/hour	0-20 mmol/hour
Gastric ulcer	10-20 mEq/hour	10-20 mmol/hour
Atrophic gastritis	0 mEq/hour	0 mmol/hour
Pernicious anemia	0 mEq/hour	0 mmol/hour
Zollinger-Ellison syndrome	35-60 mEq/hour	35-60 mmol/hour
BAO:MAO Ratio		
Normal	1:2.5-1:5.0	0.3-0.6
Gastric ulcer/gastric carcinoma		20%
Gastric ulcer/duodenal ulcer		20%-40%
Duodenal ulcer/Zollinger-Ellison syndrome		40%-60%
Zollinger-Ellison syndrome		>60%
Peak Acid Output (PAO) Is 2 × Total Values of the Two Highest 15-Minute MAO Samples; BAO:PAO Ratio		
Adult Female		0.23
Adult Male		0.29

Usage. Diagnosing and evaluating atrophic gastritis, duodenal ulcer, gastric carcinoma, gastric ulcer, Ménétrier's disease, pernicious anemia, postoperative stomal ulcer, and Zollinger-Ellison syndrome.

Increased. Duodenal ulcer, gastric ulcers in some cases, *Helicobacter pylori* infection, obesity, peptic ulcer disease, pyloric ulcer, and Zollinger-Ellison syndrome. Drugs include adrenergic blockers, alcohol, alseroxylon, caffeine, calcium salts, cholinergics, cigarette smoking, corticosteroids, deserpidine, ethyl alcohol (ethanol), NSAIDs, rescinnamine, and reserpine.

Decreased. Achlorhydria, anemia (pernicious), gastric atrophy, gastric neoplasm, gastric ulcer, and gastritis. Drugs include antacids, anticholinergics, beta-blocking agents, cimetidine, famotidine, lansoprazole, nizatidine, ranitidine hydrochloride, and tricyclic antidepressants.

Description. Gastric acid consists of hydrochloric acid (HCl), electrolytes, and mucus and is colorless and very acidic, with a pH of <2.5. It is normally secreted by the parietal cells of the stomach in response to the presence of gastrin during the gastric phase of digestion. In the presence of tumors, ulcerative disease, or pernicious anemia, the rate of gastric acid secretion can be accelerated or diminished. The Peptavlon (pentagastrin) stimulation test involves a 1-hour aspiration of stomach secretions. A basal and four 15-minute collections are made after subcutaneous injection of Peptavlon. Peptavlon normally stimulates gastric acid secretion within 10 minutes, with peaks occurring at approximately 30 minutes. By measuring the rate and volume of gastric acid secretion in response to Peptavlon, one can evaluate gastric function. Pernicious anemia and atrophic gastritis result in hyposecretion of gastric acid. Hypersecretion and the rate of secretion can indicate location and type of ulcerative disease, Zollinger-Ellison syndrome, and the need for surgical intervention.

Professional Considerations
Consent form NOT required.

Preparation
1. See Client and Family Teaching.
2. Obtain a Levin tube, lubricant, eight clean plastic containers without preservative, a Toomey syringe, suction equipment, a marker or grease pencil, and Peptavlon (pentagastrin).
3. Prepare the suction apparatus and tubing.

Procedure
1. Position the client sitting or lying on the left side.
2. Insert a Levin tube with a radiopaque tip through the client's nose or mouth into the stomach. Position the Levin tube tip in the lumen below the stomach fundus and confirm the placement by radiography or fluoroscopy.
3. Reposition the client to a sitting position and wait at least 10 minutes before proceeding further.
4. Apply low continuous suction to the Levin tube. At 15 and 30 minutes, withdraw two specimens with a Toomey syringe and discard the aspirate.
5. Begin continuous aspiration of gastric contents, using the syringe, for a total of 60 minutes. Collect the aspirate into the collection containers (labeled 1, 2, 3, 4), using a new collection container every 15 minutes until the basal acid output collection is complete.
6. Administer Peptavlon 6 mg/kg of body weight subcutaneously and begin post stimulation collections, as in the previous step, immediately. The poststimulation collection should continue for 1 hour. Observe for hypersensitivity reaction.

Postprocedure Care
1. Send all 8 containers identified as basal or post stimulation to the laboratory for analysis.
2. Remove the Levin tube.
3. Refrigerate the specimens if testing will be delayed more than 4 hours.
4. Resume previous diet.
5. Observe for nausea and vomiting.

Client and Family Teaching
1. Fast from food after the evening meal the day before testing and from water for 1 hour before the test.
2. Do not smoke or chew gum, and avoid stressful situations for 4 hours before the test.
3. The test involves the insertion of a tube through the nose into the stomach and periodic removal of the stomach contents with a syringe through the tube. The test may cause symptoms of indigestion because a drug that stimulates gastric acid secretion is given. Mild, temporary discomfort may be experienced during the tube insertion.
4. The test takes more than 3 hours. Bring reading material or other diversional activity.

Factors That Affect Results
1. Histamine antagonists or anticholinergics and antacids should be discontinued 72 and 12 hours before the test. If, however, the objective is to test the effectiveness of a histamine antagonist on acid secretions, the drugs should be continued, and the basal output of gastric acid should be performed 1 hour after administration of a morning dose.
2. Stimuli that may increase gastric acid production include smoking, the sight or odor of food, or stimuli that cause the client to become angry, fearful, or depressed.

Other Data
1. Peptavlon use in children is not indicated.

2. The test must be used with caution in conditions of esophageal varices, esophageal diverticula, esophageal stenosis, malignant neoplasm of the esophagus, aortic aneurysm, gastric hemorrhage, and congestive heart failure.

Gastric Acid Secretion Test (Gastric Acid Stimulation Test)—Diagnostic

Norm. Within normal limits.

Basal (Prestimulation) Acid Output (BAO) Is the Gastric Acid Secreted without Stimulation		SI Units
Adult Female		
Normal	1-4 mEq/hour	1-4 mmol/hour
Duodenal ulcer	3-8 mEq/hour	3-8 mmol/hour
Gastric carcinoma	0-3 mEq/hour	0-3 mmol/hour
Gastric ulcer	1-3 mEq/hour	1-3 mmol/hour
Atrophic gastritis	0 mEq/hour	0 mmol/hour
Pernicious anemia	0 mEq/hour	0 mmol/hour
Zollinger-Ellison syndrome	>20 mEq/hour	>20 mmol/hour
Adult Male		
Normal	2-5 mEq/hour	2-5 mmol/hour
Duodenal ulcer	5-10 mEq/hour	5-10 mmol/hour
Gastric carcinoma	0-3 mEq/hour	0-3 mmol/hour
Gastric ulcer	1-5 mEq/hour	1-5 mmol/hour
Atrophic gastritis	0 mEq/hour	0 mmol/hour
Pernicious anemia	0 mEq/hour	0 mmol/hour
Zollinger-Ellison syndrome	>20 mEq/hour	>20 mmol/hour
Maximum (Stimulated) Acid Output (MAO) Is the Gastric Acid Output after Stimulation (Sum of Four 15-Minute Specimens)		
Adult Female		
Normal	7-15 mEq/hour	7-15 mmol/hour
Duodenal ulcer	10-20 mEq/hour	10-20 mmol/hour
Gastric carcinoma	0-5 mEq/hour	0-5 mmol/hour
Gastric ulcer	5-15 mEq/hour	5-15 mmol/hour
Atrophic gastritis	0 mEq/hour	0 mmol/hour
Pernicious anemia	0 mEq/hour	0 mmol/hour
Zollinger-Ellison syndrome	35-60 mEq/hour	35-60 mmol/hour
Adult Male		
Normal	5-26 mEq/hour	5-26 mmol/hour
Duodenal ulcer	15-35 mEq/hour	15-35 mmol/hour
Gastric carcinoma	0-20 mEq/hour	0-20 mmol/hour
Gastric ulcer	10-20 mEq/hour	10-20 mmol/hour
Atrophic gastritis	0 mEq/hour	0 mmol/hour
Pernicious anemia	0 mEq/hour	0 mmol/hour
Zollinger-Ellison syndrome	35-60 mEq/hour	35-60 mmol/hour
BAO:MAO Ratio		
Normal	1:2.5-1:5	0.3-0.6
Gastric ulcer/gastric carcinoma		20%
Gastric ulcer/duodenal ulcer		20%-40%
Duodenal ulcer/Zollinger-Ellison syndrome		40%-60%
Zollinger-Ellison syndrome		>60%
Peak Acid Output (PAO) Is 2 × Total Values of the Two Highest 15-Minute MAO Samples; BAO:PAO Ratio		
Adult Female		0.23
Adult Male		0.29

G

Usage. Diagnosis and evaluation of duodenal ulcer, gastric carcinoma, gastric ulcer, pernicious anemia, postoperative stomal ulcer, and Zollinger-Ellison syndrome.

Increased. Duodenal ulcer, gastric ulcers in some cases, peptic ulcer disease, pyloric ulcer, and Zollinger-Ellison syndrome. Drugs include adrenergic blockers, alseroxylon, caffeine, calcium salts, cholinergics, corticosteroids, deserpidine, ethyl alcohol (ethanol), rescinnamine, and reserpine.

Decreased. Achlorhydria, anemia (pernicious), Crohn's disease, gastric atrophy, gastric neoplasm, gastric ulcer, and gastritis. Nasojejunal feeding tubes in mechanically ventilated clients. Drugs include antacids, anticholinergics, beta-blocking agents, cimetidine, famotidine, nizatidine, ranitidine hydrochloride, and tricyclic antidepressants.

Description. Gastric acid is secreted by the parietal cells of the stomach in response to neurologic and hormonal stimulation. Gastric acid is secreted during the gastric phase of digestion and aids in the breakdown of proteins and in the absorption of vitamin B_{12}, folic acid, and iron. It consists of hydrochloric acid (HCl), electrolytes, enzymes, and mucus. It is colorless and very acidic, with a pH of <2.5. In the presence of tumors, ulcerative disease, or pernicious anemia, the rate of gastric acid secretion by the parietal cells can be altered. A diagnostic gastric acid stimulation test involves aspirating and collecting basal and maximal acid outputs. Histalog (betazole, a histamine analog) or histamine diphosphate is injected intramuscularly to stimulate gastric acid secretion. By measurement of the rate and volume of gastric acid, gastric function can be evaluated.

Professional Considerations
Consent form NOT required.

Risks
Allergic reaction to injection (itching, hives, rash, tight feeling in the throat, shortness of breath, bronchospasm, anaphylaxis, death).
Contraindications
Positive skin test. Use of histamine diphosphate is contraindicated for clients who have a history of asthma, paroxysmal hypertension, urticaria, or other allergic conditions. Histalog (betazole hydrochloride) has a lower incidence of side effects than histamine diphosphate.

Preparation
1. Perform a skin test to determine hypersensitivity by injecting 0.1 mL of Histalog or histamine diphosphate subcutaneously. Wait 30 minutes for a reaction to occur. If the wheal exceeds 10 mm in diameter, do not perform the stimulation portion of this test.
2. Obtain a Levin tube, lubricant, 8-12 clean plastic containers without preservative, a Toomey syringe, suction equipment, a marker or grease pencil, and histamine diphosphate or Histalog.
3. Prepare suction apparatus and tubing.
4. See Client and Family Teaching.

Procedure
1. Position the client sitting or lying on the left side.
2. Insert a Levin tube with a radiopaque tip through the client's nose or mouth into the stomach. Position the tube tip in the lumen below the stomach fundus and confirm the placement by radiography or fluoroscopy.
3. Reposition the client to a sitting position and wait at least 10 minutes before proceeding further.
4. Apply low continuous suction to the Levin tube. At 15 and 30 minutes, withdraw two specimens with a Toomey syringe and discard the aspirate.
5. Begin continuous aspiration of the gastric contents, using the syringe, for a total of 60 minutes. Collect the aspirate into the collection containers (labeled 1, 2, 3, 4), using a new collection container every 15 minutes until basal acid output collection is complete.
6. Administer Histalog (betazole hydrochloride) 0.5 mg/kg of body weight, or histamine diphosphate 0.1 mg/kg of body weight, intramuscularly, and begin poststimulation collections, as in the preceding step, immediately. Observe for hypersensitivity reaction.
7. Poststimulation collection should continue for 1 hour (four specimens) if histamine diphosphate was used, or for 2 hours (eight specimens) if Histalog was used.

G

Postprocedure Care

1. Send all 8-12 containers, identified as basal or post stimulation, to the laboratory.
2. Remove the Levin tube.
3. Resume previous diet.
4. Observe for nausea and vomiting.

Client and Family Teaching

1. Fast from food for 12 hours and from water for 1 hour before the procedure.
2. Do not smoke or chew gum, and avoid stressful situations for 4 hours before the test.
3. The test involves the insertion of a tube through the nose into the stomach and periodic removal of the stomach contents with a syringe through the tube. The test may cause symptoms of indigestion because a drug that stimulates gastric acid secretion is given. Mild, temporary discomfort may be experienced during tube insertion. Lidocaine jelly may be used as lubricant to decrease discomfort of tube insertion.

4. The test takes more than 2 hours.
5. Results are normally available within 24 hours.

Factors That Affect Results

1. Histamine antagonists or anticholinergics and antacids should be discontinued 72 and 12 hours, respectively, before the test. If, however, the objective is to test the effectiveness of a histamine antagonist on acid secretions, the drugs should be continued, and the basal output of gastric acid should be performed 1 hour after administration of a morning dose.
2. Stimuli that may increase gastric acid production include smoking, the sight or odor of food, or stimuli that cause the client to become angry, fearful, or depressed.
3. Peak acid output after Histalog may not occur until the second hour after administration.

Other Data

1. None.

Gastric Analysis—Specimen

Norm.

Bile	Absent or minimal
Mucus	Appears evenly mixed
Blood	Absent or scant
Fasting acidity	2.5 mEq/L
Quantity produced	62 mL/hour
pH	1.0-2.5

Usage. Anemia (pernicious), stomach pain and burning, ulcers, and Zollinger-Ellison syndrome. Can also determine the presence of *Helicobacter pylori*.

Description. This test analyzes the contents of the stomach for acidity, appearance, and volume.

Professional Considerations

Consent form NOT required.

Risks

Complications of nasogastric tube insertion include bleeding, dysrhythmias, esophageal perforation, laryngospasm, and decreased mean pO_2.

Contraindications

Esophageal varices.

Preparation

1. The client should fast for 12 hours.
2. The client should not smoke tobacco or chew gum for 6 hours.
3. Obtain a nasogastric tube, a lubricant, a Toomey syringe, and a clean container.

Procedure

1. Pass a nasogastric tube into the stomach.
2. Aspirate all gastric contents into a clean container.
3. Remove the nasogastric tube.

Postprocedure Care

1. Refrigerate the sample if not tested within 4 hours.

Client and Family Teaching

1. Fast for 12 hours, and do not chew gum or smoke cigarettes for 6 hours before the test.
2. The test involves the insertion of a tube through the nose into the stomach and removal, with a syringe, of the gastric contents through the tube. The insertion may be uncomfortable and may cause a pressure like feeling or may cause you to gag and cough. You will be asked to take

sips of water and swallow to make the tube insertion easier. Removal of the stomach contents causes no pain.

3. Further tests may be indicated, based on the results of this analysis.

Factors That Affect Results

1. Stimuli that may increase gastric acid production include chewing gum, smoking, the sight or odor of food, or stimuli that cause the client to become angry, fearful, or depressed.

2. Drugs that may increase gastric acid production include adrenergic blockers, caffeine, calcium salts, cholinergics, corticosteroids, ethyl alcohol (ethanol), and reserpine.

3. Drugs that may decrease gastric acid production include antacids, anticholinergics, beta-blocking agents, cimetidine, famotidine, nizatidine, ranitidine hydrochloride, and tricyclic antidepressants.

4. Use of Hemoccult slides, as opposed to Gastroccult slides, may lead to a false-negative result if the pH of the gastric secretion is <4.

Other Data

1. Small amounts of bile may be present because of gagging during insertion of the nasogastric tube.

2. Scant amounts of blood may be present because of trauma during insertion of the nasogastric tube.

Gastric Analysis, Basal Nocturnal Acid Output—Diagnostic

Norm

Basal Acid Output (BAO)		SI Units
Adult Female		
Normal	1-4 mEq/hour	1-4 mmol/hour
Duodenal ulcer	3-8 mEq/hour	3-8 mmol/hour
Gastric carcinoma	0-3 mEq/hour	0-3 mmol/hour
Gastric ulcer	1-3 mEq/hour	1-3 mmol/hour
Atrophic gastritis	0 mEq/hour	0 mmol/hour
Pernicious anemia	0 mEq/hour	0 mmol/hour
Zollinger-Ellison syndrome	>20 mEq/hour	>20 mmol/hour
Adult Male		
Normal	2-5 mEq/hour	2-5 mmol/hour
Duodenal ulcer	5-10 mEq/hour	5-10 mmol/hour
Gastric carcinoma	0-3 mEq/hour	0-3 mmol/hour
Gastric ulcer	1-5 mEq/hour	1-5 mmol/hour
Atrophic gastritis	0 mEq/hour	0 mmol/hour
Pernicious anemia	0 mEq/hour	0 mmol/hour
Zollinger-Ellison syndrome	>20 mEq/hour	>20 mmol/hour

Usage. Aids diagnosis of pernicious anemia, duodenal or stomal ulcer, Ménétrier's disease, and Zollinger-Ellison syndrome.

Increased. Duodenal ulcer, gastric ulcers in some cases, peptic ulcer disease, pyloric ulcer, and Zollinger-Ellison syndrome. Drugs include adrenergic blockers, alseroxylon, caffeine, calcium salts, cholinergics, corticosteroids, deserpidine, ethyl alcohol (ethanol), rauwolfia, rescinnamine, and reserpine.

Decreased. Achlorhydria, anemia (pernicious), gastric atrophy, gastric neoplasm, gastric ulcer, and gastritis. Drugs include antacids, anticholinergics, beta-blocking agents, cimetidine, famotidine, nizatidine, ranitidine hydrochloride, and tricyclic antidepressants.

Description. Basal nocturnal acid output is the rate of secretion of acid by the stomach when the client is calm and resting, after a 12-hour fast, and at least 24 hours after the last dose of medications that increase or decrease gastric acid. It is measured in millimoles of titratable acidity per hour.

Professional Considerations
Consent form NOT required.

Risks

Complications of nasogastric tube insertion include bleeding, dysrhythmias, esophageal perforation, laryngospasm, and decreased mean pO_2.

Contraindications

In clients with esophageal varices, evaluate risk versus benefit in severely thrombocytopenic clients at risk for hemorrhage.

Preparation

1. See Client and Family Teaching.
2. Obtain a Levin tube, a lubricant, four clean plastic containers without preservative, a Toomey syringe, suction equipment, and a marker or grease pencil.
3. Prepare the suction apparatus and tubing.

Procedure

1. Position the client sitting or lying on the left side.
2. Insert a Levin tube with a radiopaque tip through the client's nose or mouth into the stomach. Position the tube tip in the lumen below the stomach fundus and confirm the placement by radiography or fluoroscopy.
3. Reposition to a sitting position. Wait at least 10 minutes before proceeding further.
4. Apply low, continuous suction to the Levin tube. At 15 and 30 minutes, withdraw two specimens with a Toomey syringe and discard the aspirate.
5. Begin continuous aspiration of gastric contents using the syringe, for a total of 60 minutes. Collect the aspirate into the collection containers (labeled 1, 2, 3, 4), using a new collection container every 15 minutes until basal acid output collection is complete.

Postprocedure Care

1. Send all four sequentially labeled containers to the laboratory.
2. The specimens should be refrigerated if not tested within 4 hours.
3. Remove the nasogastric tube.
4. Resume previous diet.

Client and Family Teaching

1. Fast for 12 hours, and do not chew gum or smoke cigarettes during the 6 hours before the test.
2. The test takes about 2 hours. Bring reading material or other diversions.
3. The test involves the insertion of a tube through the nose into the stomach and removal, with a syringe, of the gastric contents through the tube. The insertion may be uncomfortable and may cause a pressurelike feeling or cause you to gag and cough. You will be asked to take sips of water and swallow to make the tube insertion easier. Removal of the stomach contents causes no pain.

Factors That Affect Results

1. Reject specimens if contaminated with bile.
2. Stimuli that may increase gastric acid production include smoking, the sight or odor of food, or stimuli that cause anger, fear, or depression.
3. The amount of gastric acid increases as body weight increases.

Other Data

1. This test is sometimes followed by stimulation of gastric acid production with pentagastrin or histamine. See also Gastric acid analysis test—Diagnostic; Gastric acid secretion test—Diagnostic.

Gastric Aspirate, Routine—Culture

Norm. Negative. No growth.

Usage. Aids in the diagnosis pulmonary as well as gastrointestinal infections. One gastric aspirate in children <6 years old provides 50% yield of *Mycobacterium tuberculosis*.

Positive. Growth of microorganisms may be secondary to carcinoma or to puncture of the stomach with concomitant peritonitis or intra-abdominal abscess.

Description. One performs this test by withdrawing a small sample of gastric aspirate through a nasogastric tube and culturing the sample for the growth of microorganisms.

Professional Considerations
Consent form NOT required.

Risks
Complications of nasogastric tube insertion include bleeding, dysrhythmias, esophageal perforation, laryngospasm, and decreased mean pO_2.

Contraindications
Esophageal varices.

Preparation
1. Obtain a nasogastric tube, a lubricant, a sterile syringe, and a sterile specimen tube.

Procedure
1. Pass a nasogastric tube into the stomach.
2. Using a sterile syringe, aspirate a minimum of 2 mL of gastric contents into the sterile tube.
3. Remove the nasogastric tube.

Postprocedure Care
1. Write the collection time on the laboratory requisition.
2. Send the sample to the laboratory within 30 minutes.

Client and Family Teaching
1. The test involves the insertion of a tube through the nose into the stomach and removal, with a syringe, of the gastric contents through the tube. The insertion may be uncomfortable and may cause a pressure-like feeling or cause you to gag and cough. You will be asked to take sips of water and swallow to make the tube insertion easier. Removal of the stomach contents causes no pain.
2. Do not swallow sputum just before or during the procedure. Suction will be provided to help remove sputum from the back of the mouth.
3. Results are normally available within 48 hours.

Factors That Affect Results
1. Reject specimens received more than 30 minutes after collection.

Other Data
1. The esophagus and stomach are the two usually sterile areas of the gastrointestinal tract.
2. Clients who are unable to expectorate sputum may swallow it, thus contaminating their gastric aspirate.

Gastric Cytology—Specimen

See Cytologic Study of Gastrointestinal Tract—Diagnostic.

Gastric pH—Specimen

Norm. 1.0-2.5.

Increased. Duodenal ulcer, evaluation after vagotomy, marginal ulcer, peptic ulcer disease, and Zollinger-Ellison syndrome. Drugs include esomeprazole, omeprazole, rabeprazole, ranitidine, and tramadol.

Decreased. Achlorhydria, hypochlorhydria, and pernicious anemia.

Description. Gastric pH expresses hydrogen ion concentration of the gastric contents. It is a reflection of the amount of hydrochloric acid (HCl) produced by the parietal cells of the stomach in response to gastrin stimulation.

Professional Considerations
Consent form NOT required.

Risks
Complications of nasogastric tube insertion include bleeding, dysrhythmias, esophageal perforation, laryngospasm, and decreased mean pO_2.

Contraindications
Esophageal varices.

Preparation
1. Obtain a nasogastric tube, a lubricant, a syringe, a clean container, and a pH Test-Tape.
2. See Client and Family Teaching.

Procedure
1. Pass a nasogastric tube into the stomach.
2. Aspirate a minimum of 2 mL of gastric contents into the clean container.

3. Dip the pH Test-Tape into the specimen and compare the color change with that on the Test-Tape container.
4. Remove the nasogastric tube.

Postprocedure Care

1. None.

Client and Family Teaching

1. Do not eat for 8 hours before the test. Do not smoke cigarettes or chew gum for 4 hours before the test. Avoid stressful situations during the 4 hours immediately before the test.
2. The test involves the insertion of a tube through the nose into the stomach and removal, with a syringe, of the gastric contents through the tube. The insertion may be uncomfortable and may cause a pressure-like feeling or cause you to gag and cough. You will be asked to take sips of water and swallow to make the tube insertion easier.

Factors That Affect Results

1. Stimuli that may increase gastric acid production include smoking, the sight or odor of food, or stimuli that cause anger, fear, or depression.
2. Postprandial time with acidic pH in stomach is significantly increased in clients with chronic pancreatitis.

Other Data

1. Gastric carcinoma is associated with decreased acidity.

Gastrin—Serum

Norm.

		SI Units
Fasting		
≤60 years	<100 pg/mL	<47.7 pmol/L
	or <200 pg/mL	<95.4 pmol/L
>60 years		
Upper 15% of population	100-800 pg/mL	47.7-381.6 pmol/L
Postprandial	95-250 pg/mL	45.3-119.2 pmol/L
Zollinger-Ellison syndrome	≤60,000 pg/mL	≤28,620 pmol/L
	Often 100-500 pg/mL	Often 47.7-238.3 pmol/L

Increased. Achlorhydria, anemia (pernicious), atrophic gastritis, carcinoma (of the body of the stomach), Crohn's disease, duodenal ulcer, elderly clients, gastric ulcer, G-cell hyperplasia (antrum of the stomach), *H. pylori* infection, hypercalcemia (chronic), hyperparathyroidism, hypochlorhydria, pancreatic neuroendocrine tumor, peptic ulcer disease (with Zollinger-Ellison syndrome), pyloric obstruction with gastric distention, renal disease (chronic, end-stage), sarcoidosis, short-bowel syndrome, status post vagotomy, uremia, and Zollinger-Ellison syndrome. Drugs include acetylcholine chloride, calcium carbonate, calcium chloride, cholinergics, insulin, lansoprazole, and proton pump inhibitors.

Decreased. Drugs include anticholinergics and tricyclic antidepressants.

Description. Gastrin is a hormone secreted by the G-cells of the antrum of the stomach and by the pancreatic islets of Langerhans. Its secretion is stimulated by alkalinity, by distention of the stomach antrum, by vagal stimulation (such as chewing, tasting, or smelling), and by the presence of peptides, amino acids, alcohol, or calcium in the stomach. Its secretion is inhibited by gastric acidity by a negative-feedback system. Gastrin is absorbed into the blood and returned to the stomach, where it stimulates the secretion of gastric acid under the mediation of histamine. Other effects of gastrin include increased gastrointestinal motility and stimulation of insulin, pepsin, and intrinsic factor secretion. Catabolism of gastrin occurs in the kidneys. Serum gastrin measurement is accomplished by radioimmunoassay.

Professional Considerations

Consent form NOT required.

Preparation

1. See Client and Family Teaching.
2. Tube: Red topped, red/gray topped, or gold topped.

G

Procedure

1. Draw a 2-mL blood sample.

Postprocedure Care

1. Write the collection time on the laboratory requisition.

Client and Family Teaching

1. Fast from food for 12 hours and from alcohol for 24 hours before the test.
2. Do not chew gum or smoke cigarettes for 4 hours before the test.
3. Results are normally available within 24 hours.

Factors That Affect Results

1. Reject hemolyzed specimens, specimens drawn in anticoagulated tubes, or specimens not received in the laboratory within 30 minutes after collection.
2. Reject grossly lipemic samples, which may yield falsely elevated serum gastrin values as determined by radioimmunoassay.

3. Food, especially high-protein food, causes an increase in gastrin secretion.
4. Hypoglycemia caused by insulin increases gastrin secretion.
5. Drugs that may indirectly cause increased gastrin secretion in response to drug suppression of gastric acidity include antacids, beta-blocking agents, cimetidine, famotidine, nizatidine, and ranitidine hydrochloride.
6. Drugs that may indirectly cause depressed gastrin secretion in response to drug-stimulated increased gastric acidity include adrenergic blockers, alseroxylon, caffeine, calcium salts, corticosteroids, deserpidine, ethyl alcohol (ethanol), rauwolfia, rescinnamine, and reserpine.

Other Data

1. 15%-26% of clients with Zollinger-Ellison syndrome have Wermer's syndrome: hyperparathyroidism, islet cell tumors, pituitary tumors, Cushing's syndrome, and hyperthyroidism.

Gastrointestinal Cancer Antigen

See Ca 19-9—Blood.

Gastroscopy or Gastroduodenojejunoscopy (GJD)—Diagnostic

Norm. Cardiac and pyloric sphincters are intact. Rugal folds of the stomach are continuous. No blood or lesions are detected. Blood vessels are not visible.

Usage. Detection of gastric cancer, gastric ulcer, gastritis, hiatal hernia, and Mallory-Weiss tears; investigation of unexplained weight loss or dysphagia; and to obtain brushings of gastric mucosa to help determine infectious states such as *Helicobacter pylori* infection.

Description. Gastroscopy involves the insertion through the esophagus of a lighted flexible fiberoptic endoscope into the stomach and upper portion of the small intestine, with concurrent visual examination of the mucosal lining for active bleeding sites, varices, ulcers or perforations, lesions, or tears. The procedure takes approximately 30 minutes. Gastroduodenojejunoscopy involves advancing the instrument further into the small intestine to evaluate the

integrity of the jejunum as well as any structural or obstructive abnormalities.

Professional Considerations

Consent form IS required.

Risks

Gastrointestinal perforation and hemorrhage, peritonitis, aspiration, respiratory arrest, death.

Contraindications

Thrombocytopenia. Sedatives are contraindicated in clients with central nervous system depression.

Preparation

1. See Client and Family Teaching.
2. Dentures should be removed.
3. A sedative may be prescribed.
4. Obtain baseline vital signs.
5. Follow facility policy and procedure for clients receiving conscious sedation.
6. Obtain a blood pressure cuff, lidocaine spray, a suction machine and tubing, an

endoscope, pulse oximetry, and a gastroscopy cart. A cardiac monitor may be required with some clients.

7. Just before beginning the procedure, take a "time out" to verify the correct client, procedure, and site.

Procedure

1. A blood pressure cuff is left in place on the client's arm, and vital signs along with pulse oximetry are monitored on an individual basis throughout the procedure.
2. The mouth and oropharynx are anesthetized locally.
3. Oral secretions are suctioned or allowed to drain out as they accumulate.
4. The client is placed in a left lateral position with the head tilted forward.
5. As the endoscope is advanced into the esophagus, the head is slowly tilted back.
6. The esophagus and cardiac sphincter are examined as the endoscope is advanced. The endoscope is rotated clockwise as it is advanced into the stomach and the stomach lining, and the cardiac and pyloric sphincters are examined. The scope is advanced through the pylorus into the duodenal bulb and beyond the bulb apex into the second portion of the pH duodenum. Advancement can continue into the jejunum as well. Photographs of suspicious areas and biopsy specimens or brushings may also be taken. Sclerotherapy is commonly performed during this procedure if active bleeding is noted. Polypectomies are also common. The endoscope is slowly withdrawn.

Postprocedure Care

1. Fasting is required until the gag reflex returns.
2. Continue assessment of respiratory status. If deep sedation was used, follow institutional protocol for postsedation monitoring. Typical monitoring includes continuous ECG monitoring and pulse oximetry, with continual assessments (every 5-15 minutes) of airway, vital signs, and neurologic status until the client is lying quietly awake, is breathing independently, and responds to commands spoken in a normal tone.

3. Observe for symptoms of complications, which may include hypotension; pallor; tachycardia (from bleeding); shoulder, neck, back, or abdominal pain (from perforation); or tachypnea and rales caused by pulmonary edema after thoracic perforation.
4. Use of topical and injected local anesthetics has been associated with methemoglobinemia in rare instances. Consider this condition in clients exhibiting signs and symptoms of hypoxia refractory to oxygen therapy.

Client and Family Teaching

1. Fast from food and fluids for 8-12 hours before the procedure.
2. Arrange for someone else to drive you home because clients receiving sedation should not drive until 24 hours later.
3. It is important to swallow when asked as the endoscope is being inserted through the mouth and advanced into the stomach.

Factors That Affect Results

1. The client must be able to swallow.

Other Data

1. This test is to be performed with caution in clients with perforated ulcer, aortic aneurysm, recent bleeding esophageal varices, or Zenker's diverticulum.
2. Complications of this procedure include esophageal, thoracic, gastric, or diaphragmatic perforation.

Gemini Imaging

See Dual Modality Imaging—Diagnostic.

GeneOhm™ *C. diff* Assay

See *C. difficile* Amplified Probe—Stool.

Genital, Bacillus *Haemophilus ducreyi*—Culture

Norm. No growth

Usage. Distinguishes genital chancroid from other genital ulcerations such as syphilis, herpes genitalis, lymphogranuloma venereum, granuloma inguinale, and traumatic ulcer.

Description. The causative agent of the chancroid genital ulcer, *Haemophilus ducreyi* is a nonmotile, gram-negative bacillus transmitted by direct sexual contact. It is more common in warm climates than in cold climates and is contagious until completely healed. Genital ulceration increases the risk of transmission of HIV infections.

Professional Considerations
Consent form NOT required.

Preparation
1. Obtain one or more of the following culture media: agar supplemented with IsoVitaleX™, agar with CVA enrichment, agar with vancomycin (3 mg/L).

Procedure
1. Cleanse the ulcer and the area surrounding it with three culture kit towelettes.

Cleanse the ulcer from front to back, and discard each towelette after one pass from front to back.
2. Swab the base of the ulcer with a sterile cotton swab, and transfer the culture directly onto one or more culture media.

Postprocedure Care
1. Transport the culture to the laboratory immediately.

Client and Family Teaching
1. Describe the procedure if the client is to collect the specimen independently.
2. Results are normally available in 48 hours.

Factors That Affect Results
1. For successful growth, inoculation of the culture medium must be performed immediately.
2. The isolation rate is improved when more than one type of medium is used.

Other Data
1. If the results are negative, the test should be repeated because of common difficulty in growing *H. ducreyi*.

Genital, *Candida albicans*—Culture

Norm. No growth of *Candida*. Normal flora present.

Usage. Candidiasis (moniliasis), urethritis, and vulvovaginitis.

Description. *Candida albicans* is a fungus that is often part of the normal human skin flora but may also be transmitted sexually. It may cause infections of the skin, nails, and mucous membranes and may also cause a disseminated infection in debilitated individuals. Predisposing factors for *C. albicans* infections include diabetes mellitus, infection with human immunodeficiency virus, general debilitation, and broad-spectrum antibiotic therapy. *C. albicans* is a common cause of vaginitis in females.

Professional Considerations
Consent form NOT required.

Preparation
1. Obtain three or four towelettes, a Culturette or sterile cotton swab, and a red topped tube.

Procedure
1. Collect the specimen by cleansing the vulva and peritoneal area with three or four culture kit or microbiologic towelettes. Cleanse the area from front to back and discard each towelette after one pass from front to back. Alternatively, swab the urethral orifice, vulva, or vagina with a sterile cotton swab and place it into a sterile tube.

Postprocedure Care
1. Document the specimen source and site, the symptoms, recent antibiotic therapy, and the collection time on the laboratory requisition.
2. Send the specimen to the laboratory within 2 hours.

Client and Family Teaching
1. Results are normally available within 24-48 hours.
2. *C. albicans* infection is curable with oral and topical medication. The medication

must be continued for the full course of treatment to cure the infection.

3. Future prevention for *C. albicans* infection should include avoidance of nylon pantyhose and underwear and, if the client is diabetic, maintenance of normal blood glucose levels.

4. Do not have sexual relations until your physician confirms that the infection is gone.

5. Do not use feminine hygiene sprays or douche during the treatment.

Factors That Affect Results

1. Results may be negative if antibiotic therapy was started before specimen collection.

2. Results are invalidated if the specimen is refrigerated.

Other Data

1. At least 48 hours are required for results.

2. Consider testing for sexually transmitted diseases because *Candida* colonization has been associated with *Trichomonas vaginalis*.

Genital, *Neisseria gonorrhoeae*—Culture

Norm. All sites negative for *Neisseria gonorrhoeae*.

Vaginal culture	Normal flora
Vulvar culture	Normal flora
Urethral culture	Normal flora
Prostatic fluid culture	No growth
Endocervical culture	No growth

Usage. Cervicitis, dysuria, endometritis, epididymitis, gonorrhea, menstrual irregularities, pelvic inflammatory disease, pelvic peritonitis, perihepatitis, proctitis, prostatitis, salpingitis, urethral stricture, urethritis, vaginitis, and vulvovaginitis.

Description. *N. gonorrhoeae* is a pyogenic, gram-negative, oxidase-positive coccus that is an obligate parasite of humans. It is the causative organism of the sexually transmitted infection gonorrhea. *N. gonorrhoeae* inhabits the mucous membranes of the genital tract and may also be found in the oral mucosa of clients who engage in oral sex and in the rectum of clients who engage in anal sex. Symptoms include dysuria, purulent urethral discharge, proctitis, and pharyngitis. Females are often asymptomatic. Left untreated, gonorrhea leads to skin lesions, arthritis, meningitis, and reproductive problems. *N. gonorrhoeae* is most often found in the urethra of males and the cervix and perineum of females.

Professional Considerations

Consent form NOT required.

Preparation

1. Wait 1 hour after urination to collect urethral specimens.

2. Obtain three or four towelettes, a Culturette or cotton swab, and culture media (Transgrow, Jembec, or Thayer-Martin).

Procedure

1. Collect the specimen with a Culturette swab and either place it in a Culturette tube and then squeeze the tube tip to release the ampule of medium or inoculate the specimen directly onto culture media.

2. A rectal culture may also be collected for suspected gonorrheal proctitis by insertion of a sterile Culturette swab into the rectum. The swab should be held in place for 15 seconds and then removed and placed into the Culturette tube.

Postprocedure Care

1. Write the specimen source and site, time of collection, sex, age, symptoms, and recent antibiotic therapy on the laboratory requisition.

2. Transport the specimen to the laboratory within 1 hour. If it was inoculated directly onto Thayer-Martin medium, transport the specimen to the laboratory immediately and insert it into a carbon dioxide incubator.

Client and Family Teaching

1. Review the specimen collection procedure with the client.

2. Results are normally available within 48 hours.

3. Gonorrhea infection is treatable with antibiotics. Resistance to quinolone and

penicillin antibiotics is at high levels in Asia, Pacific Islands, and California.
4. If the results are positive, provide the client with the appropriate information on sexually transmitted diseases.
   a. Notify all sexual partners from the last 90 days to be tested for gonorrhea infection.
   b. Do not have sexual relations until your physician confirms that the infection is gone.
5. Do not use feminine hygiene sprays or douche during the treatment.
6. Wear underpants and pantyhose that have a cotton lining in the crotch.
7. Take showers instead of tub baths until the infection is gone.

Factors That Affect Results
1. Reject specimens received more than 30 minutes after collection.
2. Do not refrigerate samples. *N. gonorrhoeae* is easily destroyed by cold.

Other Data
1. The sensitivity pattern of *N. gonorrhoeae* is ceftriaxone 100%, azithromycin 100%, tetracycline 65.7%, penicillin 40%, and ciprofloxacin 5.7%.
2. Cipro resistance is seen in South Africa.

Gentamicin—Blood

Norm.

		SI Units
Peak therapeutic level	6-10 µg/mL	12-20 µmol/L
Peak panic level	>12 µg/mL	>24 µmol/L
Trough therapeutic level	<2 µg/mL	<4 µmol/L
Trough panic level	>2 µg/mL	>4 µmol/L

Overdose Symptoms and Treatment
Both sustained peak levels and trough levels that are high can be toxic.
Symptoms. Loss of hearing, acute tubular necrosis.

Treatment
NOTE: Treatment choice(s) depend(s) on client's history and condition and episode history.
   Both hemodialysis and peritoneal dialysis WILL remove gentamicin.

Usage. Evaluation of appropriateness of dosing during gentamicin therapy.

Description. Gentamicin is an aminoglycoside antibiotic effective against gram-positive and gram-negative bacteria, including *Pseudomonas aeruginosa, Klebsiella, Proteus, Escherichia*, and *Serratia*. It is excreted by the kidney, with accumulation in renal tubular cells. The half-life is 2-3 hours, with steady-state levels reached in 10-15 hours in clients with normal renal function. Gentamicin has a narrow range of therapeutic value. Thus it is important to monitor gentamicin levels throughout therapy, beginning from the time it reaches a steady state. In clients with baseline renal impairment, monitoring should be initiated sooner than recommended in this procedure. Gentamycin causes calcium and magnesium renal wasting in adults.

Professional Considerations
Consent form NOT required.

Preparation
1. Tube: Red topped, red/gray topped.
2. Write any recent antibiotic therapy on the laboratory requisition.
3. Do NOT draw during hemodialysis.

Procedure
1. For every 8-hour gentamicin administration, levels should be measured after dose number 5. For every 12-hour dosing, levels should be measured after dose number 3.
2. Draw a 4-mL blood sample. Draw a trough specimen just before the gentamicin dose. Draw a peak specimen 30 minutes to 3 hours after completion of the intravenous dose or 15-60 minutes after completion of the intramuscular dose.

G

Postprocedure Care

1. Label the tube and laboratory requisition with the specimen collection time and indicate whether it is a peak or trough specimen.
2. Send the specimen promptly to the laboratory. The sample should be spun within 1 hour, with the serum then frozen or refrigerated until testing.

Client and Family Teaching

1. The test helps determine whether the antibiotic is being given at the safe and effective dose.
2. The trough level is drawn before the antibiotic dose, and the peak level is drawn after the dose.
3. Results are normally available within 24 hours.

Factors That Affect Results

1. Increased results may be attributable to gentamicin nephrotoxicity.
2. Serum separator gel tubes can absorb serum gentamicin and falsely decrease obtained levels.

Other Data

1. Daily creatinine and beta$_2$-microglobulin levels should be monitored during gentamicin therapy.
2. Gentamicin nephrotoxicity is more likely to occur when other nephrotoxic drugs are administered during gentamicin therapy.
3. Neonates receiving gentamicin should have their hearing assessed before starting therapy and then every day until therapy is completed. Hearing testing should be performed on adults if possible before starting therapy. If the client can cooperate, Weber, Rinne, and whisper testing can be done at the bedside or clinic to assess and monitor hearing status. Notify client to report tinnitus, vertigo, or hearing loss immediately to the prescribing clinician or nurse. Intake and output should be monitored closely throughout gentamicin therapy.
4. Controlled mechanical ventilation has been shown to decrease levels of gentamicin.

GGTP—Blood

See **Gamma-Glutamyltranspeptidase**—Blood.

GHB

See **Gamma-Hydroxybutyric Acid**—Blood or Urine or Human Hair.

Ghrelin—Plasma

Norm. 77.52-98.06 pg/mL;
22.94-29.03 fmol/mL (SI units).

Increased.* Bulimia nervosa, weight loss. (Exception: Ghrelin levels do not increase when weight is reduced in people who have had gastric bypass surgery.)

Decreased.* Obesity, Short bowel syndrome, status post gastric bypass. Drugs include growth hormone.

Description. Ghrelin is a growth hormone–releasing peptide found in the stomach and

*Note: Increased and Decreased sections above summarize findings from research. Since Ghrelin has been discovered only recently, many studies have not yet been replicated.

in many other organs and tissues throughout the body. This peptide's function in the stomach is best understood, but its function throughout the rest of the body is still being studied. Ghrelin levels have been shown to increase before meals, causing an increase in glucose level, which increases the appetite. Ghrelin also stimulates the release of insulin from the islet cells of the pancreas. Ghrelin levels decrease after meals, possibly in response to increased plasma glucose. In those on weight-reduction diets, Ghrelin baseline levels have been found to increase (Cummings et al, 2002). This effect indicates a potential role of Ghrelin in weight regain experienced by many dieters. Other effects of Ghrelin include stimulating the release of adrenocorticotropic hormone, epinephrine, and glucose.

Professional Considerations
Consent form NOT required.

Preparation
1. Tube: 2.7- or 4.5-mL blue topped tube.

Procedure
1. Withdraw 2 mL of blood into a syringe or vacuum tube. Remove the syringe or tube, leaving the needle in place. Attach a second syringe, and draw two blood samples, one in a citrated blue topped tube and the other in a control tube. The sample quantity should be 2.4 mL for a 2.7-mL tube and 4.0 mL for a 4.5-mL tube. Draw a 5-mL blood sample in a sodium citrate–anticoagulated blue topped tube.

Postprocedure Care
1. Transport the specimens to the laboratory immediately for spinning and refrigeration.

Client and Family Teaching
1. Results may not be available for at least 3 days.

Factors That Affect Results
1. Reject hemolyzed specimens or tubes partially filled with blood.
2. Use of heparin anticoagulant can cause falsely high values.

Other Data
1. Ghrelin is being studied for possible vasodilatory effects.

GICA
See **Ca 19-9**—Blood.

Gilchrist's Skin Test
See **Blastomycosis Skin Test**—Diagnostic.

Globulin—Plasma

Norm.

		SI Units
Total		2.5 g of protein
Alpha$_1$	0.1-0.4 g/dL	1%-5% of total
Alpha$_2$	0.4-1.0 g/dL	4.6%-14% of total
Beta	0.5-1.5 g/dL	7.3%-15% of total
Gamma	0.5-1.7 g/dL	8%-21% of total

Increased Alpha$_1$ Globulin. Burns, carcinomatosis, focal episodes as a result of tumors, chemical injury, dehydration, diabetes mellitus, glomerulonephritis, Hodgkin's disease, inflammation (acute), lymphoma, necrosis, pregnancy, trauma, and ulcerative colitis. Drugs include estrogens.

Increased Alpha$_2$ Globulin. Acute infection, adrenal insufficiency, allergies, asthma, burns (haptoglobin, ceruloplasmin), carcinomatosis, chemical injury (haptoglobin, ceruloplasmin), Cushing's syndrome, dehydration, diabetes mellitus (advanced), focal episodes as a result of tumors (haptoglobin, ceruloplasmin), Hodgkin's disease, hypernephroma, hyperparathyroidism, hyperthyroidism, hypoalbuminemia, infarction (haptoglobin, ceruloplasmin), inflammation (haptoglobin, ceruloplasmin), leukemia (myelogenous), lymphoma, myxedema, necrosis (haptoglobin, ceruloplasmin), nephrosis, nephrotic syndrome, peritonitis (familial paroxysmal), pregnancy, rheumatic fever, rheumatoid arthritis, sarcoidosis, severe acute respiratory syndrome (SARS), systemic lupus erythematosus, trauma (haptoglobin, ceruloplasmin), and ulcerative colitis. Drugs include adrenocorticosteroids (haptoglobin) and estrogens (ceruloplasmin).

Increased Beta Globulin. Biliary cirrhosis, carcinoma (complement), chickenpox, chronic iron deficiency anemia (transferrin), cirrhosis, Cushing's disease (complement), dehydration, diabetes mellitus, dysproteinemia (familial, idiopathic), hepatitis (viral), hypercholesterolemia, hyperparathyroidism, hypothyroidism, macroglobulinemia, malignant hypertension (complement), nephrosis, nephrotic syndrome, nonfasting specimen, pregnancy (transferrin), obstructive jaundice, polyarteritis nodosa (complement), and sarcoidosis.

Increased Gamma Globulin. Amyloidosis, aortic arch syndrome, bacterial endocarditis, carcinoma, chickenpox, Crohn's disease, chronic inflammations, chronic lymphocytic leukemia, cirrhosis, congestive heart failure, cryoglobulinemia, cystic fibrosis, dehydration, Hashimoto's disease, hepatitis (viral), Hodgkin's disease, hypergammaglobulinemia, infection, leukemia (myelocytic, monocytic, myelogenous), liver disease, lymphogranuloma venereum, macroglobulinemia, malignant lymphoma, myasthenia gravis, multiple myeloma, myxedema, myxoma of left heart atrium, obstructive jaundice, polymyositis, retroperitoneal fibrosis, rheumatic fever, rheumatoid arthritis, sarcoidosis, systemic lupus erythematosus, temporal arteritis, tertiary syphilis, toxoplasmosis, trichinosis, tuberculosis, visceral larva migrans, and Waldenström's macroglobulinemia.

Decreased Alpha$_1$ Globulin. Alpha$_1$-antitrypsin deficiency, hepatitis (viral), malabsorption, nephrotic syndrome, scleroderma, and starvation.

Decreased Alpha$_2$ Globulin. Hepatitis (viral), liver disease (haptoglobin), malabsorption, malnutrition (ceruloplasmin), megaloblastic anemia (haptoglobin), nephrotic syndrome (ceruloplasmin), protein-losing enteropathy (ceruloplasmin), red blood cell hemolysis (haptoglobin), scleroderma, starvation, and Wilson's disease (ceruloplasmin). Drugs include estrogens (haptoglobin).

Decreased Beta Globulin. Atransferrinemia (transferrin), autoimmune disease, malabsorption, protein malnutrition (transferrin), scleroderma, starvation, steatorrhea, systemic lupus erythematosus, and ulcerative colitis.

Decreased Gamma Globulin. Allergies, amyloidosis, asthma, Bruton's disease, Cushing's syndrome, heavy chain disease, hyperglycinemia, hypogammaglobulinemia, leukemia (lymphocytic), lymphoma, malabsorption, nephrosis, nephrotic syndrome,

malabsorption, protein-losing enteropathy, scleroderma, starvation, steatorrhea, thymic tumor, and ulcerative colitis.

Description. Globulins are plasma proteins formed mainly in the liver, but also in the lymphatic and reticuloendothelial systems. There are three types of proteins in the family of globulins: alpha, beta, and gamma. Alpha$_1$ globulin comprises alpha$_1$-antitrypsin, alpha$_1$-acid glycoprotein, alpha-fetoprotein, cortisol-binding protein, and thyroxine-binding globulin. Alpha$_2$ globulin comprises haptoglobin, alpha$_2$-macroglobulin, and ceruloplasmin. Beta globulin comprises transferrin, beta-lipoprotein, and complement components. Gamma globulin comprises IgG, IgA, IgM, IgD, and IgE antibodies. Functions served by the globulins include buffers in acid-base balance; transporters of constituents of blood such as lipids, vitamins, hormones, iron, copper, and enzymes; and antibody activity.

Professional Considerations
Consent form NOT required.

Preparation
1. See Client and Family Teaching.
2. Tube: Red topped, red/gray topped, or gold topped.
3. Do NOT draw specimen during hemodialysis.

Procedure
1. Draw a 7-mL blood sample.

Postprocedure Care
1. Vaccinations and immunizations within the previous 6 months should be noted on the laboratory requisition.
2. Blood product administration or antitoxin administration within the previous 6 weeks should be noted on the laboratory requisition.

Client and Family Teaching
1. Fast for 8 hours before the test.

Factors That Affect Results
1. Reject hemolyzed specimens.

Other Data
1. The globulin level may be estimated by subtraction of albumin from total protein.

G

Glomerular Basement Membrane Antibody—Serum

Norm. Negative.

Positive. Antiglomerular basement membrane disease including glomerulonephritis (crescentic) and Goodpasture's syndrome. Positive in systemic vasculitis presenting as pulmonary-renal syndrome.

Description. Antibodies specific for the glomerular basement membrane (GBM) bind to specific antigens, causing an immune response leading to various anti-GBM diseases. This test identifies the presence of circulating GBM antibodies and is positive in 87% of clients with anti-GBM–associated Goodpasture's syndrome and 60% of clients with anti-GBM–associated glomerulonephritis. Goodpasture's syndrome is a rare disease characterized by necrotizing glomerulonephritis and hemorrhagic pneumonitis, which may result in renal failure and death.

Professional Considerations

Consent form NOT required.

Preparation

1. See Client and Family Teaching.
2. Tube: Red topped, red/gray topped, or gold topped.

Procedure

1. Draw a 4-mL blood sample.

Postprocedure Care

1. Transport the specimen to the laboratory immediately.
2. Freeze the serum if the test is not run immediately.

Client and Family Teaching

1. Fast (except for water) for 8 hours before the test.

Factors That Affect Results

1. Antibiotic administration may produce a false-negative result.
2. Up to 20% of results may be false negatives.

Other Data

1. In addition to a specimen of blood, a kidney or lung biopsy may also be evaluated for the presence of the antibody.

Glucagon—Plasma

Norm. Norms vary by laboratory.

		SI Units
Big glucagon	34-192 pg/mL	34-192 ng/L
Proglucagon	<28 pg/mL	<28 ng/L
Glucagon	2-60 pg/mL	2-60 ng/L
Small glucagon	8-54 pg/mL	8-54 ng/L
Adult	20-100 pg/mL	20-100 ng/L
Cord blood	0-215 pg/mL	0-215 ng/L
Newborn–3 days	0-1750 pg/mL	0-1750 ng/L
4 days–14 years	0-148 pg/mL	0-148 ng/L

Increased. Acromegaly, burns, cirrhosis, Cushing's syndrome, diabetes mellitus (average 1525 ± 578 pg/mL [1525 ± 578 ng/L]), diabetic ketoacidosis, familial hyperglucagonemia, glucagonoma (levels >900 pg/mL [900 ng/L, SI units]), HIV, hyperosmolality, hypoglycemia, Japanese encephalitis, luteal phase of menstrual cycle, necrotizing dermatitis, pancreatic islet cell lesion, pancreatitis (acute, severe), pheochromocytoma, postoperatively, renal failure (average 500-580 pg/mL, 500-580 ng/L), stress, trauma, and uremia. Drugs include amino acids, cholecystokinin-pancreozymin, danazol, fructose infusion, gastrin, glucocorticoids, insulin, nifedipine, and sympathomimetic amines. Diet high in fat or carbohydrates.

Decreased. Cystic fibrosis, hypoglycemia (related to chronic pancreatitis), idiopathic glucagon deficiency, insulinoma, neoplastic replacement of pancreas, pancreatitis (chronic), and status post pancreatectomy.

Drugs include atenolol, pindolol, propranolol, secretin, and stevioside. Treatments include acupuncture.

Description. Glucagon is a peptide hormone manufactured in and secreted by the alpha-cells of the pancreatic islets of Langerhans. Hypoglycemia, beta-adrenergics, and amino acids stimulate the secretion of glucagon, whereas increasing insulin levels inhibit its secretion. Glucagon increases blood glucose concentration by increasing the breakdown of glycogen to glucose and stimulates activity of phosphorylase, the enzyme that initiates the first step in gluconeogenesis. This test is most often used as an aid in the diagnosis of glucagonoma, an alpha islet–cell neoplasm occurring most often in females after menopause, and hypoglycemia caused by chronic pancreatitis or idiopathic glucagon deficiency.

Professional Considerations
Consent form NOT required.

Preparation
1. See Client and Family Teaching.
2. Tube: Lavender topped, and ice.

Procedure
1. Draw a 10-mL blood specimen into a chilled tube.
2. Place the specimen immediately on ice.

Postprocedure Care
1. Send the specimen to the laboratory immediately.
2. Current administration of insulin or catecholamines, or both, should be noted on the laboratory requisition.

Client and Family Teaching
1. Fast for 10-12 hours before the test.
2. Because exercise and stress elevate plasma glucagon levels, the client should be relaxed and recumbent for 30 minutes before the test.

Factors That Affect Results
1. Results are invalidated if the client had a radioactive scan within 48 hours.
2. Reject hemolyzed specimens.
3. Prolonged fasting, stress, or current use of insulin or catecholamines may elevate glucagon levels.

Other Data
1. Because of the influence on glucagon secretion, serum insulin and glucose levels should also be measured.
2. This test should not be performed for poorly controlled diabetic clients.
3. Stimulation or suppression tests may be needed to confirm a diagnosis of idiopathic glucagon deficiency or hypoglycemia caused by chronic pancreatitis.

Gluco Chek
See Glucose Monitoring Machines—Diagnostic.

Glucometer
See Glucose Monitoring Machines—Diagnostic.

Glucoscan
See Glucose Monitoring Machines—Diagnostic.

Glucose—Blood
Norm. Dependent on time and content of last meal. In normal clients, glucose levels return to the fasting level (given in these norms) within 2 hours after the last meal.

		SI Units
Whole Blood		
Adults	60-89 mg/dL	3.3-4.9 mmol/L
>60 years	68-98 mg/dL	3.8-5.4 mmol/L
Children		
Cord blood	38-82 mg/dL	2.1-4.6 mmol/L
Premature infant	17-51 mg/dL	0.9-2.8 mmol/L
Neonate	25-51 mg/dL	1.4-2.8 mmol/L
Newborn to 24 hours	34-51 mg/dL	1.9-2.8 mmol/L
Newborn >24 hours	42-68 mg/dL	2.3-3.8 mmol/L
Child	51-85 mg/dL	2.8-4.7 mmol/L
Serum		
Adults	65-100 mg/dL	3.6-5.5 mmol/L
>60 years	80-115 mg/dL	4.4-6.4 mmol/L
Children		
Cord blood	45-96 mg/dL	2.5-5.3 mmol/L
Premature infants	20-60 mg/dL	1.1-3.3 mmol/L
Neonates	30-60 mg/dL	1.7-3.3 mmol/L
Newborn to 24 hours	40-60 mg/dL	2.2-3.3 mmol/L
Newborn >24 hours	50-80 mg/dL	2.8-4.4 mmol/L
Child	60-100 mg/dL	3.3-5.5 mmol/L

NOTE: Whole-blood glucose values are about 15% less than serum glucose values because of greater dilution.

Panic Levels		
Adults	<40 mg/dL	<2.2 mmol/L
	or >700 mg/dL	or >38.6 mmol/L
Neonates	<30 mg/dL	<1.6 mmol/L
	or >300 mg/dL	>16.0 mmol/L

Diagnostic for Diabetes		
Fasting plasma glucose	At least 126 mg/dL	At least 7.0 mmol/L
2-hour post-prandial plasma glucose	At least 200 mg/dL	At least 11.1 mmol/L

Diagnostic for Gestational Diabetes		
Fasting plasma glucose during pregnancy	At least 92 mg/dL	At least 5.1 mmol/L

Screening for Pre-diabetes		
Fasting plasma glucose	100 to 125 mg/dL	5.5 to 6.9 mmol/L
2-hour post-prandial plasma glucose	140 to 199 mg/dL	7.8 to 11.0 mmol/L

Panic Level Symptoms and Treatment—Increased

Symptoms. Abdominal pain, fatigue, muscle cramps, nausea, polyuria, thirst, and vomiting.

Treatment

NOTE: Treatment choice(s) depend(s) on client's history and condition and episode history.

1. Administer subcutaneous or intravenous injection of insulin per sliding scale. Intravenous insulin is typically administered by continuous infusion for panic levels accompanied by reduced level of consciousness. Hourly adjustments are based on subsequent blood glucose measurements.
2. Perform hourly neurologic checks.
3. Monitor hourly intake and output.

4. Monitor for hypokalemia as side effect of treatment.

Panic Level Symptoms and Treatment—Decreased

Symptoms. Confusion, headache, hunger, irritability, nervousness, restlessness, sweating, and weakness.

Treatment

NOTE: Treatment choice(s) depend(s) on client's history and condition and episode history.

1. Administer oral form of glucose followed by oral ingestion of carbohydrates. For neonates or unconscious clients, give IV glucose or IV/IM glucagon.

Increased. Acromegaly, anesthesia, burns, carbon monoxide poisoning, cerebrovascular accident, convulsions, Cushing's disease, Cushing's syndrome, cystic fibrosis, diabetes mellitus, eclampsia, encephalitis, erectile dysfunction, gigantism, hemochromatosis, hemorrhage, hyperosmolar hyperglycemic nonketotic coma (HHNK), hyperadrenalism, hyperpituitarism, hypertension, hyperthyroidism, hypervitaminosis A (chronic), infections, injury, malnutrition (chronic), meningitis, myocardial infarction, obesity, pancreatic carcinoma, pancreatic insufficiency, pancreatitis (chronic), pheochromocytoma, pituitary adenoma, pregnancy, shock, subarachnoid hemorrhage, stress, trauma, and Wernicke's encephalopathy. Drugs include anabolic steroids, androgens, arginine, ascorbic acid, asparaginase, aspirin, atenolol, baclofen, benzodiazepines, bisacodyl (prolonged use), chlorpromazine, chlorthalidone, cimetidine, clonidine, corticosteroids, corticotropin, dextran, dextrothyroxine, diazoxide, disopyramide phosphate, epinephrine, epinephrine bitartrate, epinephrine borate, epinephrine hydrochloride, estrogens, ethacrynic acid, furosemide, glucose infusions, haloperidol, heparin calcium, heparin sodium, hydralazine hydrochloride, hydrochlorothiazide, imipramine, indomethacin, isoniazid, isoproterenol hydrochloride, levodopa, levothyroxine sodium/T_4, lithium carbonate, magnesium hydroxide (prolonged high doses), meperidine, mercaptopurine, methimazole, methyldopa, methyldopate (hydrochloride), metronidazole, nalidixic acid, niacin, nicotine, nicotinic acid, oral contraceptives, oxazepam, p-aminosalicylic acid, phenolphthalein, phenytoin, phenytoin sodium, progestins, promethazine hydrochloride, propranolol (in diabetic clients), propylthiouracil, protease inhibitors, reserpine, rifampin, risperidone, ritodrine hydrochloride, sildenafil, terbutaline sulfate, tetracyclines, thiazides/thiazide diuretics, thyroglobulin, thyroid medications, tolbutamide (SMA methodology), and triamterene. In addition, intensive dose statin therapy has been associated with an increased incidence of new-onset diabetes.

Decreased. Addison's disease, adrenal medulla unresponsiveness, alcoholism, carcinoma (adrenal gland, stomach, fibrosarcoma), cirrhosis, cretinism, diabetes mellitus (early), dumping syndrome, exercise, fever, Forbes' disease (type III glycogen deposition disease), fructose intolerance, galactosemia, glucagon deficiency, hepatic phosphorylase deficiency (type VI glycogen storage disease), hepatitis, hyperinsulinemia, hypopituitarism, hypothermia, hypothyroidism, infant of diabetic mother, insulin overdose (factitious hypoglycemia), insulinoma, kwashiorkor, leucine sensitivity, malnutrition, maple syrup urine disease, muscle phosphofructokinase deficiency (type VII glycogen storage disease), myxedema, pancreatic islet cell tumor, pancreatitis, postoperatively (after gastrectomy or gastroenterostomy), postprandial hypoglycemia, Reye's syndrome, Simmonds' disease, vomiting, von Gierke's disease (type I glycogen storage disease), Waterhouse-Friderichsen syndrome, and Zetterstrom syndrome. Drugs include acetaminophen, allopurinol, amphetamines, aspirin, atenolol, beta-adrenergic blockers, caffeine, cerivastatin, chlorpropamide, clofibrate, edetate disodium, ethyl alcohol (ethanol), gatifloxacin, guanethidine sulfate, isoniazid, insulin, isocarboxazid, marijuana, nitrazepam, oral hypoglycemic agents, p-aminosalicylic acid, pargyline hydrochloride, phenacetin, phenazopyridine, phenelzine sulfate, phenformin, propranolol (in diabetics), tetracyclines, theophylline, and tranylcypromine sulfate. Herbs or natural remedies include *zhi mu* ("know-mother," *Anemarrhena asphodeloides*, an herb) and *shi gao* ("stone-plaster," calcium sulfate, gypsum) taken in combination; *xuan shen* ("black ginseng," *Scrophularia ningpoensis*, figwort) and *cang zhu* ("green-*shu*/*zhu* herb," *Atractylodes lancea*, var. ovata) taken in combination; *shan yao* ("mountain-medicine," *Dioscorea batatas*, potato yam) and *huang qi* ("yellow-old 60," *Astragalus reflexistipulus*, or *A. hoantchy*, yellow vetch) taken in combination; and karela (*Momordica charantia*, balsam apple) taken in combination with chlorpropamide. Herbs or natural remedies include teas (decoctions, infusions) containing chromium, karela, ginseng, guar gum, *meshasringi* (*Gymnema sylvestre*, *mesha shringi*, Indian milkweed vine), *methi* (fenugreek leaves), syzygium cumini (jambul), tundika (*Coccinia indica*).

Description. Glucose is a monosaccharide found naturally occurring in fruits. It is also formed from the digestion of carbohydrates and the conversion of glycogen by the liver and is the body's main source of cellular energy. Glucose is essential for brain and erythrocyte function. Excess glucose is stored as glycogen in the liver and muscle cells. Hormones influencing glucose metabolism include insulin, glucagon, thyroxine, somatostatin, cortisol, and epinephrine. Fasting glucose levels are used to help diagnose diabetes mellitus and hypoglycemia. A randomly timed test for glucose is usually performed for routine screening and nonspecific evaluation of carbohydrate metabolism. The American Diabetes Association criteria for diagnosis of diabetes mellitus include a fasting plasma glucose level of >126 mg/dL (7 mmol/L).

Professional Considerations
Consent form NOT required.

Preparation
1. See Client and Family Teaching.
2. Tube: Red topped, red/gray topped, or gold topped or gray topped.
3. Observe for signs of hypoglycemia (weakness, slurred speech, confusion, somnolence, pallor, palpitations, convulsions) in fasting clients.
4. Screen client for the use of herbal preparations or natural remedies such as chromium, karela, ginseng, guar gum, meshasringi, methi, and tundika.

Procedure
1. Draw a 4-mL blood sample.

Postprocedure Care
1. Send the sample to the laboratory for immediate spinning. If transport is delayed, refrigerate the sample.
2. The time of the client's last pretest meal, the sample collection time, and the time of the last pretest insulin or oral hypoglycemic agent (if applicable) should be noted on the laboratory requisition.

Client and Family Teaching
1. Fast (except for water) for 8-12 hours before collection for fasting specimen.
2. Withhold morning insulin or oral hypoglycemic agent until after fasting blood sample has been drawn.
3. Refer newly diagnosed diabetic clients for diabetic teaching and long-term medical follow-up care.
4. Resume diet after the fasting specimen has been drawn.
5. Watch for signs of hypoglycemia and hyperglycemia. Teach appropriate intervention.

Factors That Affect Results
1. Reject specimens received more than 1 hour after collection to prevent falsely low results.
2. Falsely decreased glucose values may occur when the glucose oxidase/peroxidase procedure is used or if the client has recently taken acetaminophen or oxycodone.

Other Data
1. Spun samples are stable for 8 hours.
2. In a client with diabetes, the blood specimen should be drawn before insulin treatment or administration of oral hypoglycemic drugs.
3. Factitious hypoglycemia by unprescribed or excessive use of sulfonylureas is biochemically indistinguishable from insulinoma. Factitious hypoglycemia has also been reported by unprescribed and intentionally excessive use of insulin.
4. Revised American Diabetes Association 2012 guidelines for the diagnosis of diabetes call for a diagnosis of diabetes when fasting plasma blood glucose is 126 mg/dL or higher and for a diagnosis of prediabetes when the level is 100-125 mg/dL.

Glucose, 2-Hour Postprandial—Serum

Norm.

		SI Units
Newborn to 50 years	65-140 mg/dL	3.6-7.7 mmol/L
50-60 years	65-150 mg/dL	3.6-8.3 mmol/L
>60 years	65-160 mg/dL	3.6-8.8 mmol/L
American Diabetes Association diagnosis of diabetes (after 75-g glucose load)	>200 mg/dL	>11 mmol/L

Usage. Screening for diabetes mellitus and assessing control of hyperglycemia.

Increased. Acromegaly, anoxia, anxiety, brain tumor, cirrhosis, convulsive disorders, Cushing's disease, Cushing's syndrome, diabetes mellitus, dumping syndrome (after gastrectomy), hepatic disease (chronic), hyperlipoproteinemia, hyperthyroidism, infarction (myocardial, cerebral), lipoproteinemias, malnutrition, malignancy, nephrotic syndrome, pancreatitis, pheochromocytoma, preeclampsia, pregnancy, sepsis, and stress (physical, emotional). Drugs include those discussed under Glucose—Blood.

Decreased. Addison's disease, adrenal insufficiency, anterior pituitary insufficiency, congenital adrenal hyperplasia, hepatic insufficiency, hyperinsulinism, hypoglycemia, hypopituitarism, hypothyroidism, insulinoma, islet cell adenoma, malabsorption syndrome, myxedema, steatorrhea, and von Gierke's disease. Drugs include those discussed under Glucose—Blood.

Description. The 2-hour postprandial glucose test is the measurement of serum glucose level 2 hours from the beginning of a meal containing a specific amount of carbohydrate. In normal clients, glucose should return to fasting levels within 2 hours after the ingestion of the test meal.

Professional Considerations

Consent form NOT required.

Preparation

1. See Client and Family Teaching.
2. Tube: Gray topped, and test meal.

Procedure

1. Draw a 5-mL blood sample 2 hours after beginning ingestion of the designated test meal.

Postprocedure Care

1. Refrigerate specimens not sent to the laboratory within 1 hour.

Client and Family Teaching

1. Eat a high-carbohydrate (200-300 g) diet for 3 days before the test.
2. Fast (except for water) for 8-12 hours and abstain from alcohol for 36 hours before the test.
3. When possible, drugs affecting the results should be stopped 3-21 days before the test.
4. Insulin and oral hypoglycemic agents should be withheld the morning of the test.
5. Eat a meal containing 75-100 g of carbohydrate within 20 minutes during the testing period.
6. Avoid strenuous activity, caffeine, and nicotine after the meal until the sample is drawn.

Factors That Affect Results

1. Falsely increased values may occur with strenuous activity, inhalation of nicotine, ingestion of caffeine during the test, and in 10% of healthy older adults without a pathologic process.
2. Falsely decreased glucose values may occur with acetaminophen and oxycodone when the glucose oxidase/peroxidase procedure is used.
3. Stresses caused by acute illness, infection, pregnancy, or surgery invalidate the results.

Other Data

1. An abnormally elevated test indicates the need for a glucose tolerance test.

G

Glucose, Cerebrospinal Fluid

See **Cerebrospinal Fluid, Glucose**—Specimen.

Glucose, Qualitative, Semiquantitative—Urine

Norm. Negative.

Five-Drop Method		Two-Drop Method	
Negative	Blue-green	Negative	Blue-green
0.25%	Green	Trace	Dark green
0.5%	Olive-green	0.5%	Green
0.75%	Brown-green	1%	Olive-green
1%	Gold	2%	Brown-green
2%	Orange	3%	Gold
		>5%	Orange

Positive. Adrenal disorders, central nervous system disease, diabetes mellitus, eclampsia, Fanconi syndrome, glomerulonephritis, glucose administration, heavy-metal poisoning, hepatic disease, hyperalimentation, infections, nephrosis, pregnancy, presence of reducing substances and sugars other than glucose in the urine (copper-reduction method only), thyroid disorders, total parenteral nutrition, and toxic renal tubular disease. Drugs include ammonium chloride, asparaginase, carbamazepine, corticosteroids, dextrothyroxine sodium, indomethacin, isoniazid, lithium carbonate, nicotinic acid, phenothiazines, and thiazide diuretics.

Negative. Negative results occur with Clinistix when sugars other than glucose are present in the urine.

Description. A random urine specimen is tested either by copper reduction (Clinitest) or by the enzymatic glucose oxidase method (Clinistix) for the presence of glucose. Semiquantitative determination includes reagent strips called R-strip and T-strip.

Clinitest is a copper-reduction tablet test used to detect melituria and to detect and monitor urine glucose and non-glucose carbohydrate levels. Urine glucose levels up to 2% may be measured with the five-drop method, and up to 5% may be measured with the two-drop method. Copper-reduction methods are helpful when the test purpose is to detect both glucose and non-glucose carbohydrates present in the urine, as in metabolic disease or parenteral nutrition administration.

Clinistix test is a qualitative dipstick method of urine glucose testing that involves an oxidation reaction between urine, impregnated enzymes, and a chromogen, resulting in a color change proportional to the amount of glucose present in the urine. Clinistix is classified as a glucose oxidase method of urine glucose testing. The advantage of glucose oxidase methods over copper-reduction tests is that this method is specific for glucose and unaffected by other carbohydrates and reducing substances.

Professional Considerations
Consent form NOT required.

Preparation
1. Clinitest:
   a. Obtain a 50-mL clean plastic container, a test tube, a dropper, and urine test tablets.
   b. Dark blue tablets should be discarded. Use only fresh tablets, which are light blue and flecked with dark blue.
   c. Avoid touching the tablets. To avoid burns, wash the affected area quickly if skin contact occurs.
   d. A fresh-voided, postprandial specimen is recommended.
2. Clinistix test:
   a. For a Clinistix test, obtain a 50-mL clean plastic container and urine test strips.
   b. Keep the Clinistix bottle tightly capped. Open the bottle to quickly remove a reagent strip and then recap it before performing test.

c. Light exposure and moisture speed the degradation of Clinistix. Inspect the strip before use, even if the contents of bottle have not expired. If the strip is darkened, discard it and the bottle from which it was taken.

Procedure

1. Have the client completely empty the bladder and then drink at least 8 ounces of fluid; 30 minutes later, have the client void at least 20 mL of urine into a clean plastic container. A fresh specimen may be taken from a urinary drainage bag. Refrigerate the specimen if it is not tested promptly.
2. Clinitest:
   a. Five-drop method: Add 5 drops of urine to a clean test tube and rinse the dropper with water. Then add 10 drops of water to a test tube.
   b. Add one Clinitest tablet to this mixture.
   c. Recap the Clinitest jar tightly.
   d. Observe the color changes during the boiling phase. Be careful because the tube is hot!
   e. Glucose concentration >2 g/dL causes a rapid color change to orange during the boiling phase. If this occurs, the test should be repeated as described previously, using 2 drops instead of 5 drops of urine and comparing results to the Clinitest color chart for the two-drop test.
   f. 15 seconds after the boiling stops, agitate the test tube and immediately compare the mixture color to the Clinitest color chart. Record the results as shown in the table above.
3. Clinistix test:
   a. Dip the Clinistix reagent strip into the urine, making sure to completely immerse the test pad for 2 seconds.
   b. While removing the strip, slide the pad side against the edge of the container.
   c. Exactly 30 seconds after removal of the strip from the urine, compare the color of the test pad to the colors on the bottle.
   d. Record the results as negative, light, medium, or dark.

Postprocedure Care

1. Discard the specimen and the reagent strip, if used. Rinse the test tube, if used, with water.

Client and Family Teaching

1. New diabetic clients must learn home glucose testing, which may be with or without a machine.
2. Do not contaminate the urine specimen with stool or toilet tissue.
3. For home monitoring, provide the written instructions and a flow sheet so that the client can record the test results.
4. Watch for signs of hyperglycemia and hypoglycemia (see Glucose—Blood for symptoms and treatment).

Factors That Affect Results

1. Failure to perform the test on a fresh or refrigerated specimen invalidates the results.
2. Copper-reduction method (Clinitest):
   a. The color charts for the two-drop and five-drop methods are different and must be used with the appropriate test.
   b. Failure to protect tablets from moisture can result in false findings and possibly an explosion.
   c. Use of discolored or dark blue tablets invalidates the results.
   d. The presence of radiographic contrast medium in the urine may cause false-negative results.
   e. Reducing substances that cause a false-positive test include aminosalicylic acid, ampicillin, ampicillin sodium, ascorbic acid, camphor, cephalosporins, chloral hydrate, chloramphenicol, chloroform, creatinine, formaldehyde, fructose, galactose, glucosamine, glucuronic acid, homogentisic acid, isoniazid, ketones, levodopa, maltose, menthol, metolazone, nitrofurantoin, nitrofurantoin sodium, penicillin G benzathine, penicillin G potassium, pentose, phenol, salicylates, streptomycin sulfate, tetracyclines, turpentine, and uric acid.
3. Glucose oxidase method (Clinistix):
   a. Clinistix strips must be compared with the color chart on the bottle from which they were taken.
   b. Use of darkened strips or those exposed to prolonged moisture or air invalidates the results.
   c. Drugs that may cause false-negative results with Clinistix include ascorbic

acid, levodopa, methyldopa, methyldopate hydrochloride, phenazopyridine, and salicylates.

Other Data

1. If the client is receiving ascorbic acid, hydrochlorides, levodopa, peroxides, phenazopyridine, or salicylates, use Clinitest tablets.

2. Other available glucose oxidase urine testing strips include Diastix, n-Multistix, and Tes-Tape.

3. These tests are now used less frequently to monitor urine glucose levels in clients with diabetes because of the availability of more precise techniques for blood glucose self-monitoring and blood testing for hemoglobin A_{1c}.

Glucose, Quantitative, 24-Hour—Urine

Norm. ≤ 100 mg/24 hours (≤ 5.6 mmol/day, SI units).

Increased. Adrenal disorders, central nervous system disease, diabetes mellitus, eclampsia, Fanconi syndrome, glomerulonephritis, glucose administration, heavy-metal poisoning, hepatic disease, hyperalimentation, infections, nephrosis, pregnancy, thyroid disorders, and toxic renal tubular disease. Drugs include ammonium chloride, asparaginase, carbamazepine, corticosteroids, dextrothyroxine sodium, indomethacin, isoniazid, lithium carbonate, nicotinic acid, phenothiazines, and thiazide diuretics.

Description. A quantitative measurement of urine glucose may detect glucose spillage into the urine that occurs intermittently and thus may not be detected by random urine glucose measurement. The enzymatic glucose oxidase method is used to detect the presence and amount of glucose. However, the test is performed in the laboratory on an aliquot of a 24-hour urine collection, and the results are reported as numeric values.

Professional Considerations
Consent form NOT required.

Preparation

1. Obtain a 3-L, 24-hour urine collection bottle containing toluene preservative.
2. For pediatric collections, also obtain a pediatric urine-collection device and tape.
3. Write the beginning time of collection on the laboratory requisition.

Procedure

1. Adult collection:
   a. Discard the first morning urine specimen.
   b. Save all the urine voided for 24 hours in a refrigerated, clean, 3-L container to which toluene preservative has been added. For catheterized clients, keep the drainage bag on ice and empty the urine into the refrigerated collection container hourly.
   c. Document the quantity of urine output during the collection period. Include the urine voided at the end of the 24-hour period.
2. Pediatric collection:
   a. Place the child in a supine position with the knees flexed and the hips externally rotated and abducted.
   b. Cleanse, rinse, and thoroughly dry the perineal area.
   c. To prevent the child from removing the collection device, a diaper may be placed over the genital area.
   d. *Females:* Tape the pediatric collection device to the perineum. Starting at the area between the anus and vagina, apply the device in the anterior direction.
   e. *Males:* Place the pediatric collection device over the penis and scrotum and tape it to the perineal area.
   f. After each void, empty the collection device into a refrigerated, 3-L container to which toluene preservative has been added.

Postprocedure Care

1. Refrigerate the specimen until it is tested.
2. Compare the urine quantity in the specimen container with the urinary output record for the test. If the specimen contains less urine than what was recorded as output, some of the sample may have been discarded, invalidating the test.
3. Document the quantity of urine output and the ending time on the laboratory requisition.

4. Send the specimen to the laboratory for measurement.

Client and Family Teaching

1. Save all the urine voided in the 24-hour period and urinate before defecating to avoid loss of urine. If any urine is accidentally discarded, discard the entire specimen and restart the collection the next day.

Factors That Affect Results

1. All the urine voided for the 24-hour period must be included to avoid a falsely low result.
2. Drugs that may cause false-negative results with Clinistix include ascorbic acid, levodopa, methyldopa, methyldopate hydrochloride, phenazopyridine, and salicylates.
3. Failure to refrigerate the specimen throughout the collection period decreases accuracy of the results because of bacterial growth.

Other Data

1. This test aids in the regulation of diet and medication in clients with diabetes mellitus.
2. Because of the problem with incomplete urine collections, laboratories sometimes check the creatinine present in the urine to validate that the sample represents a full 24 hours.

Glucose, Semiquantitative—Urine

See Glucose, Qualitative, Semiquantitative—Urine.

Glucose Alert—Diagnostic

See Glucose Monitoring Machines—Diagnostic.

Glucose Monitoring Machines—Diagnostic

Norm. Whole-blood glucose values are about 15% less than serum glucose values as a result of greater dilution.

Whole Blood		SI Units
Adults	60-89 mg/dL	3.3-4.9 mmol/L
>60 years	68-98 mg/dL	3.8-5.4 mmol/L
Children		
Cord blood	38-82 mg/dL	2.1-4.6 mmol/L
Premature infant	17-51 mg/dL	0.9-2.8 mmol/L
Neonate	25-51 mg/dL	1.4-2.8 mmol/L
Newborn to 24 hours	34-51 mg/dL	1.9-2.8 mmol/L
Newborn >24 hours	42-68 mg/dL	2.3-3.8 mmol/L
Child	51-85 mg/dL	2.8-4.7 mmol/L

Usage. Chronic glucose monitoring for diabetes mellitus, monitoring for hypoglycemia in newborn, and bedside whole-blood glucose analysis.

Description. Blood glucose monitoring is generally considered to be more reliable for diabetic glucose monitoring than urine glucose levels. This is particularly true for clients with an abnormally low renal threshold for glucose reabsorption after glomerular filtration. The term "glucose monitoring machines" encompasses a variety of reflectance meters (including voice-activated machines) that can be used to quickly quantitate whole-blood glucose levels. In general, the technique involves blood to be dropped onto a reagent strip so the blood is absorbed up into the strip, inserting the strip into the reflectance meter, and then following the manufacturer's recommended steps for processing. The result is generally obtained within 3 to 10 seconds and has been estimated to cost as little as one twentieth of a "stat" laboratory glucose measurement. Home meters need to be verified at regular intervals, as one third of readings deviated significantly in one study (Henry et al, 2001).

Professional Considerations
Consent form NOT required.

Preparation
1. Verify that the client's hematocrit level is within the range for which the specific brand of machine is designed to be accurate. If the hematocrit is outside the required range, perform the glucose blood test instead of this test.
2. Verify that the machine has been calibrated within the time requirements specified by the manufacturer.
3. Obtain an alcohol wipe, a 2.5-mm lancet (or a needle and a syringe), a reagent strip, a cotton ball, a reflectance meter, sterile gauze, and a capillary tube if heelstick blood will be used.
4. Read the instructions for the specific reflectance meter to be used.

Procedure
1. Fingerstick capillary method:
   a. Cleanse the lateral aspect of the pad of the finger with an alcohol wipe and allow the area to dry.
   b. Using a 2.5-mm lancet, puncture the lateral aspect of the pad of the finger. Wipe the first drop of blood away with sterile gauze.
   c. Holding the puncture site dependent, allow a second, large drop of blood to accumulate and drop onto the reagent strip, making sure there is enough blood to completely cover the pad of the reagent strip. The pad of the finger may be very gently and repeatedly pressed to encourage blood flow, but avoid milking the finger.
   d. Follow directions for the specific reflectance meter being used.
2. Heelstick capillary method:
   a. Prewarming the heel is not necessary.
   b. Avoid puncturing over previous puncture sites or puncturing the posterior curvature of the heel.
   c. Cleanse an area on the medial or lateral plantar surface of the heel with 70% alcohol and allow the area to dry.
   d. Using a 2.5-mm lancet, puncture the heel until a free flow of blood is obtained. Wipe the first drop of blood away with sterile gauze.
   e. Holding the puncture site dependent, allow a second, large drop of blood to accumulate and drop onto the reagent strip, making sure that there is enough blood to completely cover the pad of the reagent strip. Avoid milking the heel.
   f. Follow the directions for the specific reflectance meter being used.
3. Venous method:
   a. Obtain a 4-mL venous blood sample in a syringe or green topped tube.
   b. Completely cover the pad of the reagent strip with a drop of the blood specimen.
   c. Follow the directions for the specific reflectance meter being used.

Postprocedure Care
1. Hold pressure to the site until the bleeding stops. Leave puncture sites open to the air to heal.

Client and Family Teaching
1. Teach the newly diagnosed client with diabetes how to perform a fingerstick and use a reflectance meter.
2. Watch for signs of hyperglycemia and hypoglycemia (see Glucose—Blood for symptoms and treatment).
3. Bring a home reflectance meter to office appointments with the physician so that technique and machine calibration may be assessed.

Factors That Affect Results
1. After the skin is cleansed with alcohol, the skin must be allowed to dry completely before the puncture is performed.
2. Failure to follow timing instructions exactly as recommended by the manufacturer may cause inaccurate results.
3. The most accurate and reliable results are obtained when the reflectance meter is calibrated according to the schedule recommended by the manufacturer.
4. For glucose levels >400 mL/dL, accuracy of Chemstrip bG and the Accu-Chek reflectance meter has been shown to improve when a 4-mL specimen of

heparinized blood is diluted with 2 mL of 0.9% saline and the corresponding result is multiplied by 3 to correct for dilution.

5. Vigorous milking of the heel or finger may cause falsely low results because of dilution of the specimen with interstitial fluid.

6. Many conditions and drugs affect glucose levels (see Glucose—Blood for symptoms and treatment).

Other Data

1. In normal clients, blood glucose levels return to fasting levels within 2 hours postprandially.

2. Glucose monitoring machine: competency of the operator may be evaluated by assessment of results of control solutions.

3. Incidence of significant error ranges from 6%-76%.

Glucose Tolerance Test (GTT, OGTT)—Blood

Norm. (Serum Levels)

Intravenous GTT		SI Units
Fasting	70-105 mg/dL	3.9-5.8 mmol/L
5 minutes	300-400 mg/dL	16.5-22.0 mmol/L
30 minutes	180-200 mg/dL	9.9-11.0 mmol/L
1 hour	160-180 mg/dL	8.8-9.9 mmol/L
2 hours	≤140 mg/dL	≤7.7 mmol/L
≥3 hours	70-105 mg/dL	3.9-5.8 mmol/L
Oral GTT		
Fasting	70-105 mg/dL	3.9-5.8 mmol/L
30 minutes	150-160 mg/dL	8.3-8.8 mmol/L
1 hour	160-170 mg/dL	8.8-9.4 mmol/L
1.5 hours	145-155 mg/dL	8.0-8.5 mmol/L
2 hours	≤120 mg/dL	≤6.6 mmol/L
3 hours	70-105 mg/dL	3.9-5.8 mmol/L

Usage. Evaluation of clients with symptoms of diabetic complications but with fasting glucose levels <140 mg/dL and screening during pregnancy for gestational diabetes (a single fasting value of at least 5.1 mmol/L or 92 mg/dL, 1-hour cut-off of at least 9.99 mmol/L or 180 mg/dL or 2-hour cut-off of at least 5.1 mmol/L 92 mg/dL). The American Diabetes Association (ADA) lowered the threshold to diagnose diabetes to 126 mg/dL or 7.0 mmol/L for a fasting plasma glucose level or 2-hour OGTT cut-off of at least 200 mg/dL or 11.1 mmol/L and advised that the oral glucose tolerance test not be used in routine practice. The ADA recommended in 2011 that the Hb A_{1c} test be used for diagnosis of diabetes. The World Health Organization recommends retaining the OGTT for persons with a fasting glucose level of >6.1 mmol/L. Also used in combination with growth hormone measurement when acromegaly is suspected, in which case there will be a lack of growth hormone to the glucose load.

Increased Results (Decreased Glucose Tolerance). Acromegaly, aldosteronism (primary), central nervous system lesions, Cushing's syndrome, cystic fibrosis, diabetes mellitus, Forbes' disease (type III glycogen deposition disease, debrancher deficiency, limit dextrinosis), gigantism, hemochromatosis, hepatic damage (severe), hyperlipidemia (types III, IV, V), hyperthyroidism, Louis-Bar's syndrome, myocardial infarction, neoplasm, pancreatic tumor (islet cell), pancreatitis (chronic), pheochromocytoma, pregnancy, uremia, and von Gierke's disease (type I glycogen storage disease, glucose-6-phosphatase deficiency). Drugs include anabolic steroids, androgens, arginine, ascorbic acid, asparaginase, aspirin, baclofen, benzodiazepines, bisacodyl (prolonged use), chlorpromazine, chlorthalidone, cimetidine, clonidine, corticosteroids, corticotropin, dextran, dextrothyroxine, diazoxide, disopyramide phosphate, epinephrine, epinephrine bitartrate, epinephrine borate, epinephrine hydrochloride, estrogens, ethacrynic acid, furosemide, glucose infusions, haloperidol, heparin calcium, heparin sodium, hydralazine hydrochloride, imipramine, indomethacin, isoniazid, isoproterenol hydrochloride, levodopa, levothyroxine sodium, lithium carbonate, magnesium hydroxide (prolonged high doses), mercaptopurine, methimazole, methyldopa, methyldopate hydrochloride), nalidixic acid, nicotine, nicotinic acid, oral contraceptives, oxazepam, p-aminosalicylic acid, phenolphthalein, phenytoin, phenytoin sodium, progestins, promethazine hydrochloride, propranolol (in diabetic clients), propylthiouracil, reserpine, ritodrine hydrochloride, terbutaline sulfate, tetracyclines, thiazides, thyroglobulin, thyroid, tolbutamide (SMA methodology), and triamterene.

Decreased Results (Increased Glucose Tolerance). Addison's disease (oral GTT only), celiac disease (oral GTT only), hepatic disease, hypoglycemia, hypoparathyroidism (oral GTT only), hypothyroidism (oral GTT only), islet cell adenoma, malabsorption (oral GTT only), narcotic addiction, pancreatic islet cell hyperplasia, and sprue (oral GTT only). Drugs include allopurinol, amphetamines, beta-adrenergic blockers, caffeine, chlorpropamide, clofibrate, edetate disodium, ethyl alcohol (ethanol), guanethidine sulfate, insulin, isocarboxazid, isoniazid, marijuana, nitrazepam, oral hypoglycemic agents, p-aminosalicylic acid, pargyline hydrochloride, phenacetin, phenazopyridine, phenelzine sulfate, phenformin, propranolol (in diabetic clients), and tranylcypromine sulfate.

Description. Glucose is a monosaccharide formed from the digestion of carbohydrates and the conversion of glycogen by the liver and is the body's main source of cellular energy. The glucose tolerance test is most commonly used to aid in the diagnosis of diabetes mellitus. If blood glucose levels peak at higher than normal levels at 1 and 2 hours (after injection or ingestion of glucose) and are slower than normal to return to fasting levels, diabetes mellitus is confirmed.

Professional Considerations
Consent form NOT required.

Preparation
1. See Client and Family Teaching.
2. Tubes: Gray topped × 6-7.

3. Label each tube as shown in the table below (See Procedure 4).

Procedure
1. Begin the test between 7 and 9 AM.
2. Draw a 1-4-mL venous blood sample.
3. Intravenous GTT: Inject a standardized intravenous solution of 0.5 g/kg of body weight of 50% glucose, or 50 mL of 50% glucose intravenously over 4 minutes.
4. Oral GTT: Adults should completely ingest a solution containing 75-100 g of glucose within 5 minutes.

Tube Number	Intravenous GTT	Oral GTT
1	Fasting	Fasting
2	5 minutes	30 minutes
3	30 minutes	1 hour
4	1 hour	1.5 hours
5	2 hours	2 hours
6	3 hours	3 hours
7	4 hours	4 hours

For children, the dosages are as follows:
  <18 months: 2.5 g/kg
  18 months-3 years: 2.0 g/kg
  3 years-12 years: 1.75 g/kg
  >12 years: 1.25 g/kg (100-g limit)
5. Repeat step 2 at the following precise time intervals after infusion or ingestion of glucose is started.
6. If evaluating for postprandial hypoglycemia, draw an additional sample at 4 hours.

Postprocedure Care
1. Current administration of medications known to affect the test results should be noted on the laboratory requisition.
2. Send blood samples to the laboratory immediately or refrigerate them.

Client and Family Teaching
1. Eat a high-carbohydrate (200-300 g) diet for 3 days before testing.
2. Avoid alcohol, coffee, and smoking for 36 hours before testing.
3. Fast (except for water) for 10-16 hours.
4. When possible, drugs affecting results should be stopped 3-21 days before the test.

5. Insulin and oral hypoglycemic agents should be withheld the morning of the test.
6. Avoid strenuous exercise for 8 hours before and after the test.
7. Because the test requires multiple blood samples, suggest bringing a book or other quiet diversion to the test because it usually requires a minimum of 3 hours.
8. Alert the client to the symptoms of hypoglycemia and instruct the client to report these symptoms immediately.

Factors That Affect Results

1. No eating, smoking, or exercise is permitted during the testing period. Caffeine interferes with the accuracy of the results.
2. Water may be given to help ease the collection of urine specimens.
3. Failure to adhere to a high-carbohydrate diet for 3 days before the test may produce abnormally increased results.
4. Stresses caused by acute illness, pregnancy, or surgery invalidate the results.
5. Slight increases are normal in clients more than 50 years of age (up to 1 mg/dL per year for ages more than 50 years).
6. When the glucose oxidase/peroxidase procedure is used, falsely decreased glucose values may occur when the client has recently taken acetaminophen or oxycodone.

Other Data

1. This test usually takes 3-5 hours.
2. 10 mL of urine for glucose measurement may also be collected at the same time as the blood samples.
3. The intravenous glucose tolerance testing method is recommended for clients who may have impaired or erratic intestinal absorption of glucose.
4. The oral glucose tolerance test has been shown to be unreliable for use in the evaluation of reactive hypoglycemia.
5. In a client with non–insulin-dependent diabetes (type 2), fasting serum glucose levels may be within normal range, but insufficient secretion of insulin after ingestion of carbohydrates causes serum glucose to increase sharply and return to normal slowly.
6. If a client develops severe hypoglycemia during the test, draw a blood sample, record the time on the laboratory requisition, and discontinue the test. Have the client ingest an oral form of glucose or administer intravenous glucose according to the physician's orders.
7. A 2-hour glucose level is better than a fasting level alone in identifying older adults at increased risk of major incident cardiovascular events (Smith et al, 2002).
8. A 2-hour glucose ≥11.1 mmol/L increases risk for preterm delivery.

Glucose-6-Phosphate Dehydrogenase (G6PD, G-6-PD), Quantitative—Blood

Norm. Norms vary according to the test method used:
140-280 U/billion cells

125-280 U/dL packed red blood cells
8.6-18.6 U/g hemoglobin
4.5-10.8 U/g hemoglobin

Zinkham Method (30 degrees C)		SI Units
Newborn	7.8-14.4 U/g Hb	0.50-0.93 U/mol Hb
	226-418 U/1012 Ercs*	0.23-0.42 U/L Ercs
	2.65-4.90 U/mL Ercs	2.65-4.90 kU/L Ercs
Adult	5.5-9.3 U/g Hb	0.35-0.60 U/mol Hb
	160-270 U/1012 Ercs	0.16-0.27 U/L Ercs
	1.87-3.16 U/mL Ercs	1.87-3.16 kU/L Ercs

*Ercs, Electronic counters.

Increased. Anemia (pernicious, megaloblastic), hepatic coma, hyperthyroidism, leptospirosis, myocardial infarction, and Werlhof's disease (idiopathic thrombocytopenic purpura).

Decreased. Anemia (congenital nonspherocytic hemolytic), congenital G6PD deficiency, favism, and nonimmunologic hemolytic disease of the newborn. Drugs include cefoperazone/sulbactam, gentamicin sulfate, netilmicin sulfate, and tocopherol acetate. Herbicide 4-chlorophenoxyacetic acid (4-CPA).

Description. Glucose-6-phosphate dehydrogenase (G6PD) is an enzyme normally present in the erythrocytes. This enzyme is part of the pentose phosphate pathway that metabolizes glucose and functions to protect cells from damage by oxidizing agents. This test measures G6PD levels in red blood cells, thereby detecting deficiencies of this enzyme. G6PD deficiency is a sex-linked genetic disorder found mostly in males that results in hyperbilirubinemia, jaundice, and hemolysis of erythrocytes, producing anemia after the receipt of certain drugs. Drugs that may precipitate hemolytic episodes in affected individuals include acetanilide, acetylphenylhydrazine, antipyrine, ascorbic acid, aspirin, chloramphenicol, nalidixic acid, naphthalene, nitrofuran, nitrofurantoin, pentaquine, phenacetin, phenylhydrazine, primaquine, probenecid, quinacrine, quinidine, quinine, sulfonamides, and vitamin K. Other precipitants include diabetic acidosis, fava bean ingestion, infections (viral, bacterial), and septicemia.

Professional Considerations
Consent form NOT required.

Preparation
1. Tube: Lavender topped, blue topped, or green topped.

Procedure
1. Draw a 3-mL blood sample.
2. Invert the tube gently several times to mix the sample.

3. Handle the sample gently to prevent hemolysis.

Postprocedure Care
1. Recent blood transfusion or current or recent ingestion of antimalarials, aspirin, fava beans, nitrofurantoin, phenacetin, sulfonamides, or vitamin K should be noted on the laboratory requisition.

Client and Family Teaching
1. Refer the client with elevated levels for long-term medical follow-up care.
2. Clients testing positive should receive thorough disease teaching, including which drugs place the client at risk for a hemolytic episode.
3. Refer clients testing positive for genetic counseling.

Factors That Affect Results
1. Reject hemolyzed specimens to avoid false-negative results.
2. False-negative results may occur after a blood transfusion or a hemolytic episode.

Other Data
1. Several methods are available to test for G6PD deficiency. The method used by the particular laboratory determines the type of blood tube used.
2. G6PD deficiency is demonstrated most frequently in African-Americans, Greeks, Sardinians, and Sephardic Jews. Incidence is 2.1% in Iran.

Glucose-6-Phosphate Dehydrogenase (G6PD, G-6-PD) Screen—Blood

Norm. Enzyme activity detected.

Increased. Not applicable.

Decreased. Anemia (congenital nonspherocytic hemolytic), congenital G6PD deficiency, favism, and nonimmunologic hemolytic disease of the newborn.

Description. G6PD is an enzyme normally present in erythrocytes. This enzyme is part of the pentose phosphate pathway that metabolizes glucose and functions to protect cells from damage by oxidizing agents. This test measures G6PD levels in red blood cells, thereby detecting deficiencies of this enzyme. G6PD deficiency is a sex-linked genetic disorder, found mostly in 6% of males and 1% in females of African, Mediterranean, and Far East populations, that results in hemolysis of erythrocytes, producing anemia after the receipt of certain drugs and contractile dysfunctions of the heart. Drugs that may precipitate hemolytic episodes in affected individuals include acetanilide, acetylphenylhydrazine, antipyrine, ascorbic acid, aspirin, butyl nitrite inhalation, chloramphenicol, metformin, nalidixic acid, naphthalene, nitrofuran, nitrofurantoin, pentaquine, phenacetin, phenylhydrazine, primaquine, probenecid, quinacrine, quinidine, quinine, sulfonamides, topical henna, and vitamin K. Other precipitants include diabetic acidosis, fava bean ingestion, infections (viral, bacterial), lead poisoning and septicemia.

Professional Considerations
Consent form NOT required.

Preparation
1. Tube: Lavender topped.

Procedure
1. Draw a 2-mL blood sample.
2. Invert the tube gently several times to mix the sample.
3. Handle the sample gently to prevent hemolysis.

Postprocedure Care
1. Recent blood transfusion or current or recent ingestion of antimalarials, aspirin, fava beans, nitrofurantoin, phenacetin, sulfonamides, or vitamin K should be noted on the laboratory requisition.

Client and Family Teaching
1. Results are normally available within 24 hours.
2. Clients testing positive should receive thorough disease teaching, including which drugs place the client at risk for a hemolytic episode.
3. Refer clients testing positive for genetic counseling.

Factors That Affect Results
1. Reject hemolyzed specimens to avoid false-negative results.
2. False-negative results may occur after a blood transfusion or a hemolytic episode.

Other Data
1. G6PD deficiency is demonstrated most frequently in African-Americans, Greeks, Sardinians, and Sephardic Jews and people from the United Arab Emirates.

Glutethimide—Blood

Norm.

		SI Units
Therapeutic	2-6 µg/mL	9-28 µmol/L
Toxic level	>20 µg/mL	>92 µmol/L
Panic level	>30 µg/mL	>135 µmol/L

Overdose Symptoms and Treatment
Symptoms. Central nervous system depression, cerebral edema, hypotension, paralysis, respiratory depression, spasticity, and tachycardia. Death may occur at doses >30 mg/mL.

Treatment
NOTE: Treatment choice(s) depend(s) on client's history and condition and episode history.
1. Administer gastric lavage of water and castor oil in a 1:1 mix because glutethimide is soluble in lipids.
2. Hemodialysis will NOT but hemoperfusion WILL remove glutethimide.

Usage.
Glutethimide abuse and glutethimide overdose.

Description.
Glutethimide is a schedule III, piperidine-derivative, nonbarbiturate sedative-hypnotic with actions similar to barbiturates used for temporary insomnia, preoperative sedation, and during stage 1 of labor. It is primarily stored in fat tissue, hydroxylized in the liver, and excreted primarily by the kidneys, with a biphasic half-life of 5-22 hours.

Professional Considerations
Consent form NOT required.

Preparation
1. Tube: Red topped, red/gray topped, or gold topped, black topped, or lavender topped.
2. MAY be drawn during hemodialysis.

Procedure
1. Draw a 7-mL blood sample.

Postprocedure Care
1. Observe closely for symptoms of overdose. This includes continuous ECG and airway monitoring, frequent neurologic

G

checks, and vital sign measurement every 15-60 minutes.

Client and Family Teaching

1. Be alert for symptoms of overdose (see Postprocedure Care) and seek medical attention if they occur.
2. Refer clients with intentional overdose for crisis intervention.
3. Referrals to appropriate rehabilitation centers and therapeutic community programs should be offered to all addicted clients who may be interested.

Factors That Affect Results

1. Serial measurements for glutethimide are recommended because of the variable release of the drug from adipose tissue.

Other Data

1. Death rate is highest in glutethimide intoxication in suicidal poisonings.

Glycated Hemoglobin

See Glycosylated Hemoglobin—Blood

Glycated Serum Protein

See Fructosamine—Serum.

Glycosylated Hemoglobin (GHb, Glycohemoglobin, (Glycated hemoglobin, Hb A$_{1a}$, Hb A$_{1b}$, Hb A$_{1c}$)—Blood

Norm.

	Percentage of Total Hb
Total of Hb A$_{1a}$, Hb A$_{1b}$, and Hb A$_{1c}$	5.5-8.8
Diabetes under control	7.5-11.4
Diabetes less well controlled	11.5-15
Diabetes out of control	greater than 15
Ketoacidosis	14.3-20
High-performance liquid chromatography	
Hb A$_{1a}$	1.8
Hb A$_{1b}$	0.8
Hb A$_{1c}$	1.0-5.6
Increased risk of developing diabetes mellitus	5.7-6.4
Diagnostic of diabetes	Greater than 6.5

Usage. Screening for and diagnosing diabetes mellitus; ongoing monitoring status of glucose control in clients with diabetes. Targets set by clinicians may vary, based on individual characteristics due to the variability of instances of hypoglycemia. Target Hgb A$_{1c}$ in clients over age 60 is generally less than 8.0% and at less than 6.0% in this age group, there is increased risk for mortality (Huang et al, 2011).

The American Diabetes Association (2011) recommendations for screening children for diabetes mellitus include screening every 3 years beginning at age 10 or at start of puberty if earlier, if any of the following apply:

• There is type 2 diabetes in first- or second-degree relative or the mother had gestational diabetes during the child's fetal development

• Child is Native American, African American, Latino, Asian American, Pacific Islander)

• Symptoms or conditions indicative of possible insulin resistance are present: (acanthosis nigricans, hypertension, dyslipidemia, PCOS, or small-for-gestational-age birth weight)

Increased. Diabetes mellitus, glycosuria, hyperglycemia, hypothyroidism, and polycystic ovary syndrome.

Decreased. See Factors That Affect Results, #3.

Description. Glycosylated hemoglobin is blood glucose bound to hemoglobin (Hb) and includes forms Hb A_{1a}, Hb A_{1b}, and Hb A_{1c}. Hb A_{1c} is bound covalently to the terminal acid of the beta chain and is gradually glycosylated throughout the 120-day red blood cell life span, and forms the largest portion of the three glycosylated Hb fractions. The amount of glycosylated hemoglobin found and stored in erythrocytes depends on the amount of glucose available. Glycosylated hemoglobin measurements exclude short-term fluctuations in glucose. Hb A_{1c} is a reflection of how well blood glucose levels have been controlled for up to the previous 4 months. Hyperglycemia in diabetic clients is usually the cause of an increase in Hb A_{1c}.

Professional Considerations
Consent form NOT required.

Preparation
1. Tube: Lavender topped, green topped, or gray topped.

Procedure
1. Draw a 5-mL blood sample.
2. Invert the tube gently several times to mix the sample.

Postprocedure Care
1. Send the specimen to the laboratory for prompt spinning.

Client and Family Teaching
1. The test evaluates the effectiveness of diabetes therapy over a period of several months, and so more samples will be needed in the future.
2. The client should maintain his or her prescribed medication or diet regimen between physician visits.

3. An Hb A_{1c} <7% is the target for diabetic clients.

Factors That Affect Results
1. Reject hemolyzed specimens.
2. Falsely increased values may be attributable to fetal-maternal transfusion, hemodialysis, hereditary persistence of fetal hemoglobin, neonates, and pregnancy. Testing for persistent diabetes after delivery in women with recent gestational diabetes is unreliable because iron stores are low and hemoglobin levels are undergoing reassimilation.
3. Falsely decreased values may be attributed to anemia (hemolytic, pernicious, sickle cell), chronic loss of blood, effects of splenectomy, hemoglobin F (fetal hemoglobin) accounting for more than 10% of total hemoglobin, renal failure (chronic), and thalassemias or drug use of monoclonal antibodies.
4. For diagnosing pre-diabetes in adolescents, fasting plasma glucose may be a better indicator, because sensitivity of Hb A_{1c} is less for adolescents (sensitivity 5.0%) than for adults (23.1%) (Lee, Wu, Tarini et al, 2011).
5. Racial differences in Hb A_{1c} include higher levels in blacks than white clients, given the same fasting plasma glucose level.

Other Data
1. Glycosylated hemoglobin cannot be used to monitor control of diabetic clients with chronic renal failure because levels are significantly lower as a result of shortened erythrocyte survival.
2. In type 2 diabetes, repaglinide/metformin combination is better than nateglinide/metformin for glycemic control, and glimepiride neutralizes weight effect.
3. Paynter et al (2011) found that adding Hb A_{1c} to cardiovascular risk assessment models improved the predictive ability of the models.
4. Point of care Hb A_{1c} tests are not appropriate for diagnosing diabetes.

Gonorrhoeae Culture

See **Genital,** *Neisseria gonorrhoeae*—Culture.

Gram Stain—Diagnostic

Norm.

Body fluid, drainage, or wound	Interpretation required
Urine	No organisms detected

Usage. Diagnostic. Anthrax meningitis (CSF), bacterial vaginosis, Barrett's esophagus, cough (sputum sample), effusion (abdominal or pleural), empyema, gonorrhea, impetigo, infections from catheters, *Legionella*, pulmonary nocardiosis, tuberculosis, and wounds.

Sputum. Cough (productive), fever, infections, and pneumonia.

Urine. Cystitis and urethritis.

Description. Gram staining divides bacteria into two groups according to their staining properties: gram negative and gram positive. The staining involves placing drops of crystal violet dye onto the specimen sample, washing off the violet stain, and flooding the smear with an iodine solution followed by a 95% ethyl alcohol (ethanol) solution. Gram-positive cells remain blue, and gram-negative cells are decolorized by the alcohol. The specimen is then stained with a red dye called "safranin O," which colors the gram-positive cells red and leaves the gram-negative cells appearing purple. The cell wall structure is the basis of the Gram reaction. Gram staining of specimens aids in decision-making for early, broad-spectrum antibiotic therapy. Gram stain is 67.9% sensitive for detection of bacteria in blood cultures.

Professional Considerations

Consent form NOT required.

Preparation

1. *Diagnostic:* Obtain a sterile container or swab.
2. *Sputum:* Obtain a sterile sputum container or suction tubing, suction source, and sputum trap.
3. *Urine:* Obtain a sterile container and clean-catch urine specimen collection kit, or a straight catheter or a syringe and needle if the specimen will be collected from an indwelling catheter.
4. See Client and Family Teaching.

Procedure

1. *Diagnostic:*
   a. Obtain the specimen using a sterile technique and a sterile container or swab.
   b. Avoid contamination of the sample with surrounding tissue.
2. *Sputum:*
   a. Collect an early-morning sputum sample into a sterile sputum container.
   b. Specimens are of best quality when obtained by direct suctioning into a sputum trap.
   c. For expelled specimens, have the client sit up, take two or three deep breaths without fully exhaling each breath, and then cough expulsively to mobilize the sputum from the respiratory tract directly into the sterile specimen container.
3. The clean-catch urine technique must be used to decrease the risk of specimen contamination. See clean-catch collection instructions in the test Body fluid, Routine—Culture.

Postprocedure Care

1. Write the specimen source, the diagnosis, and recent antibiotic therapy on the laboratory requisition.
2. Place the specimen in the refrigerator if not delivered to the microbiology area immediately after collection.

Client and Family Teaching

1. *Sputum:* Cough the specimen directly into the container and avoid holding the sputum in the mouth. Deep coughs are necessary to produce sputum, rather than saliva. To produce the proper specimen, take several breaths in, without fully exhaling each, and then expel sputum with a "cascade cough."
2. *Urine:* See clean-catch collection instructions in the test Body fluid, Routine—Culture.

Factors That Affect Results

1. Epithelial cells will appear in the specimen if it is contaminated with mucosal surfaces.
2. Saliva contamination of sputum specimens invalidates the results.

Other Data

1. Gram staining is not useful for identifying species of bacteria but can be suggestive of certain broad species.
2. A culture and sensitivity study of the specimen should also be performed to confirm the diagnosis and proper choice of antibiotic.

3. Compared to Gram stain of vaginal secretions, the cervical Papanicolaou smear has fair sensitivity (55%) and excellent positive predictive value (96%) in the diagnosis of bacterial vaginosis.

Granulocyte

See **Differential Leukocyte Count**—Peripheral Blood.

Growth Hormone (Somatotropin, GH) and Growth Hormone–Releasing Hormone (GHRH)—Blood

Norm.

Growth Hormone		SI Units
Adults, Female	<10 ng/mL	<440 pmol/L
>60 years	1-14 ng/mL	44-616 pmol/L
Adults, Male	≤5 ng/mL	≤220 pmol/L
>60 years	0.4-10 ng/mL	18-440 pmol/L
Children		
Cord blood	10-50 ng/mL	440-2200 pmol/L
Newborn	15-40 ng/mL	660-1760 pmol/L
Child	<20 ng/mL	<880 pmol/L
Growth Hormone–Releasing Hormone		
All ages	<100 ng/L	

Increased GH. Acromegaly, anorexia nervosa, deep sleep states, diabetic adolescents, gigantism, hypoglycemia, hyperpituitarism, infants, starvation, and surgery. Drugs include arginine, beta-adrenergic blockers, estrogens, gamma-butyryl lactone (GBL), gamma-hydroxybutyrate (GHB) (which can increase levels up to 40 ng/mL), glucagon, levodopa, and oral contraceptives. Herbs or natural remedies include St. John's wort (*Hypericum perforatum and calycinum*), which contains hypericin, Qi-training.

Increased GHRH. Acromegaly because of ectopic secretion of GHRH.

Decreased GH. Acute lymphoblastic leukemia, chronic atrophic gastritis, congenital growth hormone deficiency, congenital pituitary hypoplasia, dwarfism, failure to thrive, growth hormone deficiency, Hallermann-Streiff syndrome, hyperglycemia, hypothalamic degeneration, hypopituitarism, lesion (pituitary or hypothalamus), and pituitary fibrosis or calcification. Drugs include corticosteroids, phenothiazines, and selective serotonin reuptake inhibitors (SSRI). Urban pollutants.

Description. Growth hormone (GH) is a polypeptide anterior pituitary hormone essential for body growth. GH synthesis and release are controlled by the hypothalamus through growth hormone–releasing factor (GHRF) and growth hormone release–inhibiting hormone (GHRIH). GH stimulates the production of RNA and protein synthesis and mobilizes fatty acids and insulin. It is influenced by several drugs as well as exercise and stress.

Professional Considerations
Consent form NOT required.

Preparation
1. See Client and Family Teaching.
2. Tube: Red topped, red/gray topped, or gold topped.

G

3. Have the client recline for 30 minutes before sampling.
4. Screen client for the use of herbal preparations or natural remedies such as St. John's wort.

Procedure
1. Draw a 4-mL blood sample.

Postprocedure Care
1. Write the collection time and client's recent activity (sleeping, eating, resting, walking) on the laboratory requisition.
2. Current administration of corticosteroids or phenothiazines should be noted on the laboratory requisition.
3. Transport the specimen to the laboratory immediately. The serum should be separated into a plastic container and frozen until testing.

Client and Family Teaching
1. Fast and limit physical activity for 10-12 hours before the test.

2. A second blood sample may have to be drawn the next day for comparison to the first sample.

Factors That Affect Results
1. Reject specimens if the client had a radioactive scan within the previous 48 hours.
2. Growth hormone in serum samples is unstable at room temperature.
3. False-negative GHRH results are possible if ectopic secretion occurs directly into the hypophyseal-portal system.

Other Data
1. Serial measurements are recommended because of the episodic release of growth hormone.
2. This test may be performed as part of a GH-stimulation test, using arginine, glucose, glucagon, levodopa, insulin-induced hypoglycemia, or other methods.

GSP

See Fructosamine—Serum.

Guthrie Test for Phenylketonuria—Diagnostic

Norm. Negative or <3 mg/dL.

Usage. Neonatal screening for phenylketonuria (PKU).

Description. The Guthrie test is a bacterial inhibition assay in which elevated levels of phenylalanine cause growth of the bacterium *Bacillus subtilis* around the blood sample. If growth occurs around the bacterium, the diagnosis of PKU is suggested; further blood testing is needed to confirm the diagnosis.

Phenylketonuria is an autosomal recessive inherited disorder with a frequency of 1 in 10,000 live births. This condition is caused by a deficiency of the enzyme phenylalanine hydroxylase, which leads to an accumulation of phenylalanine and deficiency of tyrosine in the blood. Resultant symptoms include neurologic conditions such as mental retardation, microcephaly, seizures, and hyperactivity, as well as eczema, growth retardation, and a musty odor. If treatment with a restricted phenylalanine diet is begun early,

these symptoms can be minimized and even prevented.

PKU testing is performed in the newborn period on a metabolic screening filter paper. Although states vary in the panel of conditions they test, all states test for PKU.

Professional Considerations
Consent form NOT required.

Preparation
1. Obtain supplies: 2.0-2.5 lancet, alcohol wipe, gauze pads, gloves, and blood collection form (filter paper) with completed information.

Procedure
1. Warm heel for 3-5 minutes with warm, wet cloth or heel warmer with foot lowered below the heart to increase blood flow.
2. Clean heel with alcohol wipe and dry with sterile gauze.
3. Puncture the lateral third of the plantar surface of the heel. Wipe first drop of blood away with gauze pad and, when

another large drop of blood collects, lightly touch the filter paper, making sure to fill the designated circle completely. Fill in all circles on the filter paper in the same manner.

Postprocedure Care

1. Place pressure on the heel for 1-2 minutes, and then cover with sterile gauze or a bandage.
2. Allow the form to dry on a flat surface for a minimum of 4 hours and mail to the laboratory within 24 hours.

Client and Family Teaching

1. Inform parents that the sample is sent to the state laboratory and that they will be informed of an abnormal result within 2 weeks.
2. When positive results are found, call the family immediately, repeat the test, and institute a low-phenylalanine diet with consultations to a nutritionist and geneticist.

Factors That Affect Results

1. Method of sample collection: Samples must be carefully collected. The heel should not be squeezed excessively, blood spots on the filter paper should not be touched, the sample should be air-dried, and the sample should not be applied with a capillary tube.
2. Factors that produce false-negative results:
   a. *Protein intake:* Child must have had 24 hours of protein feedings (either breast milk or formula) in order for the test to be valid.
   b. *Antibiotic use:* Test should be repeated if child had been taking antibiotics when the sample was collected.
3. Factors that produce false-positive results: goat milk intake, total parenteral nutrition, severe illness, layering of blood on test paper.

Other Data

1. Test should be performed, if possible, before a transfusion.
2. Each circle on the filter paper needs to be completely filled.
3. If the baby is <48 hours old at the time of collection, a repeat sample should be obtained within the first week of life.

Gynecologic Ultrasonography (Gynecologic Echogram, Gynecologic Sonogram, Pelvic Sonogram, Pelvic Ultrasound)—Diagnostic

Norm. Normal size, shape, and position of pelvic structures (uterus, ovaries, fallopian tubes); negative for cyst, foreign body, stones, or tumor.

Usage. Evaluation of the size, shape, and position of bladder, ovaries, vagina, and uterus; detection of pelvic cyst, ectopic pregnancy, endometrial abnormalities, foreign body (such as intrauterine device), hydatidiform mole, stones, or masses; differentiation of solid from liquid masses; infertility work-up (monitoring the ovarian follicle or screening for uterine cavity abnormalities); monitoring of pelvic tumor response to therapy; and transvaginal sonography have an added advantage of providing information regarding the cervical and uterine vascular supplies.

Description. Gynecologic ultrasonography (ultrasound) is the evaluation of the pelvic structures by the creation of an oscilloscopic picture from the echoes of high-frequency sound waves passing over the pelvic area (acoustic imaging). The time required for the ultrasonic beam to be reflected back to the transducer from differing densities of tissue is converted by a computer to an electrical impulse displayed on an oscilloscopic screen to create a three-dimensional picture of the pelvic contents. Both transabdominal and transvaginal methods may be used. Traditional transabdominal methods are more helpful for the evaluation of large cysts and fibroids, whereas the newer, transvaginal method is more specific for ruling out ectopic pregnancy or evaluating endometrial abnormalities. Transvaginal methods have also been shown to provide better depictions of the fine structures and individual organs of the pelvic cavity and are better tolerated by the subject because a full bladder is not required. Gynecologic ultrasonography may be used as an adjunct to the pelvic bimanual examination in women who are at risk for ovarian cancer.

Professional Considerations
Consent form NOT required.

Preparation
1. This test should be performed before intestinal barium tests or after the barium is cleared from the system.
2. The client should disrobe below the waist or wear a gown.
3. Obtain ultrasonic gel.
4. See Client and Family Teaching.

Procedure
1. *Transabdominal method*
   a. The client is positioned supine in bed or on a procedure table.
   b. The pelvic area is covered with ultrasonic gel, and a lubricated transducer is passed slowly and firmly over the lower abdomen at a variety of angles and at 1- to 2-cm intervals.
   c. The client may be repositioned to a right or slight left decubitus position so that better pictures of the ovaries or the adnexal area may be obtained.
   d. A water enema may be administered if more specific evaluation of the adnexal area is required.
   e. Photographs are taken of the oscilloscopic pictures.
   f. The procedure takes less than 30 minutes.
2. *Transvaginal method*
   a. The client is positioned in the dorsal lithotomy position or on a conventional examination table, with a pillow supporting the hips.
   b. A sterile, nonreservoir condom containing ultrasonic gel is placed over the transducer, and air bubbles are worked out of it. The condom is then coated with a sterile lubricant.
   c. The client or the examiner may insert the transducer into the vagina until it touches the posterior or anterior walls.
   d. The transducer is rotated 90 degrees against the vaginal vault to obtain sagittal and coronal scans of the uterus.

The probe is pulled back 2-3 cm to examine the cervix. Using identified landmarks, the ovaries and fallopian tubes are pictured. All possible angles are scanned. The client may be repositioned slightly to facilitate imaging.

Postprocedure Care
1. Remove the lubricant from the skin.
2. Allow the client to void.
3. Disinfect the transducer probe by soaking in glutaraldehyde solution for 10 minutes.

Client and Family Teaching
1. The procedure is painless and carries no risks.
2. If transabdominal ultrasonography is to be performed, drink 1 quart of water during the hour before the test, and refrain from voiding during this time. The full bladder provides an acoustic window for imaging.
3. If transvaginal ultrasonography is to be performed, fast from fluids for 4 hours before the procedure, and void just before the procedure.

Factors That Affect Results
1. Dehydration interferes with adequate contrast between organs and body fluids.
2. Intestinal barium or gas obscures results by preventing proper transmission and deflection of the high-frequency sound waves. This problem is particularly pronounced with pelvic ultrasonography as the result of the proximity of the large bowel.
3. The more abdominal fat present, the greater is the attenuation (reduction in sound wave amplitude and intensity), which interferes with the clarity of the transabdominal picture.
4. Transvaginal techniques are not adequate for very large masses.

Other Data
1. Further studies may include tomography or other radiographic imaging.

Hageman Factor
See **Factor XII**—Blood.

Haloperidol—Serum

Norm. Negative.

Therapeutic level	3-20 µg/L
Panic level	>25 µg/L

Panic Level Symptoms and Treatment

Symptoms. Hypotension, sedation with respiratory depression severe enough to cause a shocklike state, severe extrapyramidal neuromuscular reactions (dystonia, hyperreflexia, and oculogyric crises), and rhabdomyolysis with hypertonia as part of neuroleptic malignant syndrome (NMS).

Treatment

NOTE: Treatment choice(s) depend(s) on client's history and condition and episode history.

1. Ipecac may be used to induce vomiting, with due regard for haloperidol's antiemetic properties and aspiration hazards. Induction of vomiting is contraindicated in clients with no gag reflex or with central nervous system depression or excitation. Gastric lavage may also be used, followed by activated charcoal and saline cathartics. Intravenous diphenhydramine (Benadryl) can be used to treat extrapyramidal symptoms.
2. Hemodialysis and peritoneal dialysis will NOT remove haloperidol.

Usage. Periodic monitoring for therapeutic levels in clients receiving haloperidol. Screening for haloperidol toxicity or overdose.

Description. Haloperidol is a butyrophenone that acts as an antipsychotic, sedative, and antiemetic. It depresses the central nervous system, directly acts on the chemoreceptor trigger zone (CTZ), and inhibits catecholamines. This drug is used in agitation, schizophrenia, and the manic phase of manic-depressive psychosis and to manage vocal utterances in Gilles de la Tourette's syndrome. It is absorbed in the gastrointestinal tract, concentrated in the liver, and excreted in the urine and in bile. Has been known to induce torsades de pointes.

Professional Considerations

Consent form NOT required.

Preparation

1. Tube: Red topped, red/gray topped, or gold topped.

2. May require assistance if the client is uncooperative.
3. MAY be drawn during hemodialysis.

Procedure

1. Obtain a 3-mL blood sample.

Postprocedure Care

1. Refrigerate the specimen.

Client and Family Teaching

1. For periodic monitoring, it is not necessary to restrict food or fluids.
2. If activated charcoal was given for elevated levels, the client should drink 4-6 glasses of water each day for 2 days to prevent constipation. The activated charcoal will also cause stools to be black for a few days.
3. Refer clients with intentional overdose for crisis intervention.
4. Referrals to appropriate rehabilitation centers and therapeutic community programs should be offered to all clients who may be interested.

Factors That Affect Results

1. Therapeutic norms are not well established; laboratory values vary among clients on equal doses.
2. Significant lowering of serum haloperidol level occurs with the coadministration of carbamazepine and/or barbiturates.
3. Increased levels can occur in clients using the drug fluoxetine and in smokers with a 2D6*10 homozygous genotype.

Other Data

1. For consistency, collect the specimen at least 12 hours after the last dose (trough level).
2. Extrapyramidal effects occur frequently during the first few days and are dose related although they can occur even with small doses.
3. Diphenhydramine may interfere with some methods used to measure haloperidol.
4. Haloperidol can cause cardiac arrhythmias, including Q-T interval lengthening, amplification of hypokalemia and hypomagnesemia, and in overdose may cause myocarditis.
5. Fatty liver increases susceptibility to adverse effects.
6. Endovascular cooling has been successful in treating neuroleptic malignant syndrome.

Ham's Test (Acidified Serum Test Acid Hemolysin Test)—Blood

Norm. Negative, <5% lysis.

Usage. Paroxysmal nocturnal hemoglobinuria (PNH) or the PNH abnormality.

Description. For Ham's test, a blood sample is taken from the client, mixed with his or her own serum and with a sample of serum from an ABO-compatible donor, acidified, and examined for lysis. The presence of lysis in the client's own serum is definitive in the diagnosis of PNH. This rare condition, in which hemoglobin is found in the urine during and after sleep, is believed to be related to red blood cell hypersensitivity to higher levels of carbon dioxide and a resulting decrease in the plasma pH, though the cause of this disease is unknown.

Professional Considerations
Consent form NOT required.

Preparation
1. Tube: Red topped AND lavender topped.

Procedure
1. Draw a 3-mL blood sample in each tube.

Postprocedure Care
1. Defibrinate the sample immediately.

Client and Family Teaching
1. Results are normally available within 24 hours.

Factors That Affect Results
1. Hemolysis of the specimen invalidates results.
2. Transfusion of red blood cells within the last 3 weeks may cause false-negative results.
3. False-positive results may occur in dyserythropoietic anemia, spherocytosis, aplastic anemia, and leukemia.

Other Data
1. PNH has been a candidate for myeloproliferative disease occurring in 55%-65% of cases of myeloid metaplasia and primary myelofibrosis.
2. The paroxysmal nocturnal hemoglobinuria (PNH) gel test can replace Ham's test for screening.
3. 40% positive Hams test for PNH associated with CD59 or CD55 erythrocyte deficiency.

Haptoglobin (Hp)—Serum

Norm.

		SI Units
Adult	26-237 mg/dL	0.5-2.37 g/L; 260-2370 mg/L
Newborn	5-48 mg/dL	0.05-4.8 g/L; 50-480 mg/L

Usage. Serves as an index of hemolysis, investigates hemolytic transfusion reactions, identifies suspected ahaptoglobinemia, serves as serum tumor marker for glioblastoma, breast, pancreatic and hepatocellular cancers and helps establish proof of paternity.

Increase. Abscess, acute rheumatic disease, arterial disease, Behçet disease, biliary obstruction, burns, hematologic toxicities in persons receiving gemcitabine, infection, inflammation, malaria, malignancies, myasthenia gravis, myocardial infarction, peptic ulcer, pneumonia, pregnancy tissue necrosis, tuberculosis, and ulcerative colitis. Drugs include anabolic steroids, corticosteroids, and oral contraceptives.

Decrease. Ahaptoglobinemia, artificial heart valve implantation, G6PD deficiency, hemolysis (intravascular or extravascular), hemolytic anemia, liver disease, malarial infestation, megaloblastic anemia, mononucleosis (infectious), sickle cell anemia, systemic lupus erythematosus (SLE), thalassemia, tissue hemorrhage, and transfusion reaction (hemolytic). Drugs include dapsone, estrogens, methyldopa, and tamoxifen.

Description. Haptoglobin is an alpha$_2$ globulin that combines with hemoglobin that has been released as the result of red blood cell destruction. Its primary function is to preserve the body's iron stores from being excreted in the urine. Haptoglobin can be depleted rapidly by any condition that destroys red blood cells.

Professional Considerations
Consent form NOT required.

Preparation
1. Tube: Red topped, red/gray topped, or gold topped.

Procedure
1. Draw a 4-mL blood sample.

Postprocedure Care
1. Report abnormal vital signs on the laboratory requisition.
2. Deliver the specimen to the laboratory immediately, taking care not to shake it.

Client and Family Teaching
1. Results may not be available for several days.
2. Call the physician if noting symptoms of hemolysis, which include back pain, chills, distended neck veins, fever, flushing, hypotension, tachycardia, and tachypnea.

Factors That Affect Results
1. Hemolysis of the specimen invalidates results.
2. Specimen contact with peroxidase or other oxidants may falsely elevate the result.

Other Data
1. Do not consider this test alone for diagnosis.
2. Haptoglobin levels rise to normal by 4 months of age.
3. In about 1% of the population (4% of African-Americans), haptoglobin is permanently absent (congenital ahaptoglobinemia).
4. Negative correlation between umbilical cord haptoglobin during delivery and bilirubin value on 5th day making haptoglobin a predictor of neonatal jaundice.

Hawkeye Imaging
See Dual Modality Imaging—Diagnostic.

Hb
See Glycosylated Hemoglobin—Blood.

HBDH
See Hydroxybutyrate Dehydrogenase—Blood.

---

hCFHrp
See BTA test for Bladder Cancer—Diagnostic.

---

hCG
See Human Chorionic Gonadotropin, Beta Subunit—Serum, or Pregnancy Test, Routine, Serum and Qualitative—Urine.

HCO$_3^-$
See Bicarbonate—Blood.

Hct
See Hematocrit—Blood.

H

Hcy

See **Homocysteine**—Plasma or Urine.

HcySU

See **Homocysteine**—Plasma or Urine.

HDL, HDL-C

See **High-Density Lipoprotein Cholesterol**—Blood.

HE4

See **Human Epididymis Protein 4**—Blood.

Head-Up Tilt Table Test

See **Tilt Table Test**—Diagnostic.

Hearing Test for Loudness, Recruitment

See **Audiometry Test**—Diagnostic.

Heart Scan—Diagnostic

Norm. Electron Beam CT (EBCT): No evidence of coronary artery stenosis or calcification. Scores range from 0-400 with a score over 100 suggesting future cardiac morbidity.

Technetium-99m Stannous Pyrophosphate (Radiolabeled PYP). No evidence of myocardial ischemia.

Thallium-201. No evidence of myocardial ischemia or infarction.

Multigated Blood Pool Study (MUGA). Normal (55%-65%) ejection fraction, symmetric contraction of the left ventricle.

Nitroglycerin MUGA. Normal (55%-65%) ejection fraction, symmetric contraction of the left ventricle.

Sestamibi or Sestamibi-dipyridamole Exercise Testing and Scan. No evidence of diminished perfusion, ischemia, or infarction.

Usage. Aneurysm, angina, cardiomegaly, coronary artery disease, myocardial infarction, and presurgical evaluation.

Dipyridamole Injection. Replaces the treadmill portion of the test for clients with chronic lung disease, peripheral vascular disease, impaired mobility, medication therapy that prevents demonstration of maximal exercise effort (calcium-channel blockers, beta-adrenergic blockers), or post–myocardial infarction risk stratification.

Description. Heart scan encompasses any of several noninvasive scans that involve radiopharmaceutical injection.

The *electron beam CT (EBCT)* scan detects and quantifies the degree of calcified atherosclerotic plaques in any coronary artery. Radiation exposure is minimal (FDA states <50 rad per organ/tissue) at 0.8 rad to chest and 2.5 rad to abdomen.

The *PYP scan* is used to determine the occurrence, extent, and prognosis of myocardial infarction. Technetium-99m stannous pyrophosphate is believed to combine with the calcium in damaged myocardial cells, forming a spot on the scan. Such spots appear within 12 hours of infarction, are most prominent 48-72 hours after an infarction, and disappear within 1 week. A spot that does not disappear indicates continued myocardial damage.

The *thallium-201 scan* is used to show myocardial perfusion, location, and extent of acute or chronic myocardial infarction or coronary artery disease; also shows effectiveness of angioplasty, angina therapy, or grafted coronary arteries. An analog of potassium, this radionuclide is absorbed into healthy tissue while avoiding damaged tissue, forming spots on the scan. Ischemic areas (which eventually absorb isotope) can be differentiated from infracted areas (which never absorb isotope) by repeating the scan within 5 minutes. May be performed under stress. Thallium scans are often combined with dipyridamole administration (described below) because this causes greater thallium uptake and improved quality of images and accuracy of diagnoses. The combination is used for clients who are unable to perform exercise treadmill or bicycle testing in conjunction with their scan.

The *MUGA scan* is used to assess the function of the left ventricle and show myocardial wall abnormalities. Once the isotope is injected, the heart appears as a map with all four chambers, and the great vessels are visualized simultaneously. A series of images are taken during systole (low isotope in left ventricle) and diastole (high isotope in left ventricle). These can be shown like a movie or superimposed to show the left ventricular function, and the ejection fraction can be calculated. May be performed under stress.

The *nitroglycerin scan* is an additional feature of the MUGA scan. Another series of images is taken to evaluate the effectiveness of sublingual nitroglycerin administration. May be performed under stress.

The *sestamibi exercise testing and scan* is used to evaluate cardiac perfusion before and after a treadmill exercise test. The injected radiopharmaceutical ^{99m}Tc-pertechnetate (sestamibi) is taken up by ischemic or infarcted cardiac cells that did not improve in perfusion with exercise and is seen as a "hot spot" in nuclear imaging.

The *sestamibi-dipyridamole stress test and scan* is used in clients who cannot walk on a treadmill or pedal a bicycle because of physical mobility limitations. Dipyridamole is an antiplatelet drug used in nuclear medicine

for its coronary artery vasodilatory action. It causes increased endogenous adenosine levels, which causes an effect on the perfusion of the heart muscle similar to that of an exercise test. For this test, the cardiac perfusion is compared in scans taken before and after the tracer and dipyridamole injections. Because the areas that vasodilate can draw blood flow from less perfused areas, the test can cause ischemia and infarction. Thus this test carries specific risks related to the radiopharmaceutical administered and requires a cardiologist to be present in many institutions.

The *single-photon emission computed tomography (SPECT) scan* is a newer nuclear medicine procedure in which the radiopharmaceutical technetium-99m hexamethyl propylene amine oxime is injected intravenously. This substance decomposes and remains for several hours in the heart and other tissues, where it can be detected with the SPECT camera. The camera sends images to a computer that can reproduce visual images, or "slices," of the heart along several planes. An advantage of SPECT imaging over older nuclear medicine scans is that it can produce clear, more accurate images.

Professional Considerations
Consent form IS required.

Risks
Persantine (dipyridamole): chest pain (angina), ECG changes, and ischemia, including infarction, bronchospasm, nausea, vomiting, hypotension, headache, dyspnea, facial flushing. Radiopharmaceutical or radiolabeled albumin: allergic reaction (itching, hives, rash, tight feeling in the throat, shortness of breath, bronchospasm, anaphylaxis, death).

Treadmill testing: cardiac ischemia, including myocardial infarction, dysrhythmias, hypotension, hypertension, dizziness.
Contraindications
Clients who are unable to lie motionless for the scan; women who are breast-feeding; previous allergic reaction to radiopharmaceutical or radiolabeled albumin if use is planned.

Dipyridamole. Previous allergy to dipyridamole; unstable cardiac status; allergy to aminophylline (which is used as an antidote to adverse effects of dipyridamole); aminophylline or pentoxifylline taken within the last 48 hours; severe asthma or bronchospasm.

Relative Contraindications, Dipyridamole. Congestive heart failure, status post heart transplantation, bilateral carotid artery disease, days 1-3 after acute myocardial infarction.

Treadmill Testing. Active unstable angina, recent significant changes in ECG, alcohol intoxication, uncontrolled dysrhythmias, chest pain, acute infection, cardiac inflammation (myocarditis, pericarditis), acute congestive heart failure, coronary insufficiency syndrome, digitalis toxicity, heart blocks (2°, 3°), thrombophlebitis, recent pulmonary embolism, inability to walk on a treadmill or pedal a bicycle.

Precautions

During pregnancy, risks of cumulative radiation exposure to the fetus from imaging studies must be weighed against the benefits of the procedure. Although formal limits for client exposure are relative to this risk:benefit comparison, the United States Nuclear Regulatory Commission requires that the cumulative dose equivalent to an embryo/fetus from occupational exposure not exceed 0.5 rem (5 mSv). Radiation dosage to the fetus is proportional to the distance of the anatomy studied from the abdomen and decreases as pregnancy progresses. For pregnant clients, consult the radiologist/radiology department to obtain estimated fetal radiation exposure from any of these procedures.

Preparation

1. Assess for history of hypersensitivity to radioactive dyes.
2. Have emergency equipment readily available. This includes aminophylline to counteract the side effects of dipyridamole if the dipyridamole test is to be performed.
3. For scans conducted with stress testing, obtain a baseline 12-lead ECG.
4. See Client and Family Teaching.
5. Just before beginning the procedure, take a "time out" to verify the correct client, procedure, and site.

Procedure

1. *Electron beam CT (EBCT) scan*: No IV access required. Position supine on scanner table. Three electrodes are placed on the inferior-anterior chest. An ECG tracing is obtained. Then the client's arms are placed over head and the client holds breath while the scanner passes above body from the shoulders to the hips. Then one image taken during each heart beat as confirmed by ECG tracing. Total time for test is 30 minutes.
2. *PYP*: Technetium-99m stannous pyrophosphate (20 mCi) is injected 2-3 hours before the test. Images are taken from different angles, with a total of 30-60 minutes being used for imaging.
3. *Thallium-201*: Resting imaging takes place within the first few hours of cardiac symptoms. The radionuclide is injected, and scanning begins within 5 minutes. For stress scanning, an intravenous line is started, and a blood pressure cuff and ECG leads are attached. After 15 minutes on a treadmill or bicycle, the client is injected with radioactive thallium; 15 minutes later, imaging occurs for 1 hour, with a repeat scan performed within the next 24 hours. The thallium-201 dose is 1.5-3 mCi.
4. *Thallium-dipyridamole*: ECG and blood pressure are monitored continuously throughout this scan. After the resting image is taken and the radionuclide is injected, dipyridamole is injected intravenously over 4 minutes. Some clients may be asked to perform mild exercise, which improves blood flow through the coronary arteries, increases uptake of the thallium, and reduces the side effects of the dipyridamole. Thallium is then injected about 4 minutes later, when peak coronary blood flow is expected, and the final scan is taken. Aminophylline may be infused prophylactically or in response to adverse side effects of the dipyridamole. The client may then return for redistribution imaging in about 4 hours.
5. *MUGA*: 15-20 mCi of ^{99m}Tc-pertechnetate is tagged to serum albumin or red blood cells; 1 minute after injection, imaging begins. The client should be in a supine position though the client may be asked to exercise. The procedure takes 1 hour.

6. *Nitroglycerin*: A cardiologist assesses a baseline MUGA scan, injects nitroglycerin, takes another scan, and repeats this procedure until blood pressure reaches desired level.

7. *Sestamibi exercise testing and scan*: After a 12-lead ECG machine is attached to chest electrodes, the nuclear medicine technician injects the tracer and completes a resting scan, which lasts approximately 30 minutes. The ECG and blood pressure are then measured continuously as the client completes the exercise portion of the test on a treadmill. Heart rate, blood pressure, and ECG are recorded every 1-2 minutes during each 3-minute stage. If vital signs and ECG have remained stable, the nuclear medicine technician then injects additional tracer 1 minute before the client comes off the treadmill. The final scan of another 30 minutes is then completed.

8. *Sestamibi-dipyridamole stress test and scan*: After a 12-lead ECG machine is attached to chest electrodes, the nuclear medicine technician injects the tracer and completes a resting scan, which lasts approximately 30 minutes. The client is instructed to perform isometric hand grips until dipyridamole injection to help prevent the drug's side effects. The ECG and blood pressure are then monitored continuously as a dose of dipyridamole is injected over 4 minutes. 2-7 minutes later, the nuclear medicine technician injects the sestamibi tracer. The side effects of Persantine may include chest pain, dysrhythmias, nausea, vomiting, bronchospasm, headache, flushing, or dizziness and hypotension. The side effects may be treated with intravenous aminophylline, which acts as an adenosine receptor agonist. 30 minutes after the tracer injection, the final scan is completed.

9. *Single-photon emission computed tomography (SPECT) scan*: The client is transported to the nuclear medicine department, positioned supine on the scanning table, and left to rest quietly for approximately 10 minutes. A radiopharmaceutical is injected intravenously and allowed to circulate. The SPECT scan is then taken while the client lies motionless.

Postprocedure Care

1. Monitor the pulse, blood pressure, and respirations every 15 minutes × 2.

2. For scans that involved stress testing or administration of dipyridamole, the client is monitored until vital signs or ECG patterns, or both, return to baseline values.

Client and Family Teaching

1. Do not take drugs or drink caffeine-containing beverages for 6 hours before testing (24 hours for the SPECT scan).

2. Some tests take several hours. Bring reading material or other diversional activity.

3. *PYP, thallium-201, dipyridamole*: Fast for 4 hours before the test.

4. *Dipyridamole*: Do not take drugs containing aminophylline for 48 hours before the test.

5. *Thallium-201, MUGA, nitroglycerin*: Report fatigue, pain, or shortness of breath immediately, particularly if stress (exercise) is used.

6. You may be asked to move into different positions during the scan.

7. Drink plenty of fluids for 24 hours after the procedure.

8. For positive results reduce modifiable risk factors: smoking cessation, dietary modification, maintain healthy BP and cholesterol levels.

Factors That Affect Results

1. Digitalis and quinidine alter contractility. Notation should be made on the chart.

2. Bundle branch block, left ventricular hypertrophy, or hypokalemia.

3. Thallium-201 scans may produce false-negative results in clients with single-vessel disease.

4. MUGA does not give positive results for 24 hours after myocardial infarction (MI), and so it cannot be used to diagnose acute MI.

5. Radionuclides or radioactive tracers with long half-lives from recent scans will interfere with the quality of the images.

Other Data

1. The larger the perfusion defect, the poorer the prognosis.

2. Abnormalities of the heart scan may indicate the need for further studies or cardiac catheterization.

3. Health care professionals working in a nuclear medicine area should wear a film badge at waist level (the level closest to the client).
4. Technetium half-life is 6 hours. Thallium half-life is 73 hours.
5. Health care professionals working in a nuclear medicine area must follow federal standards set by the Nuclear Regulatory Commission. These standards include precautions for handling the radioactive material and monitoring of potential radiation exposure.
6. The MUGA scan is used to monitor cardiac function in clients receiving cardiotoxic antineoplastic chemotherapy.
7. See also Stress/exercise test—Diagnostic; Stress test, Pharmacologic—Diagnostic.

Heart Shunt Scan—Diagnostic

Norm. Normal pulmonary transit time and chamber-filling sequence.

Usage. Determines improper shunting of blood in heart disorders, especially in children.

Description. The heart shunt scan is an angiography study used to examine the transit of a bolus of technetium-99m into the jugular vein. Images are taken to follow the bolus on its journey through the heart chambers to visualize any abnormal shunting of blood between chambers.

Professional Considerations
Consent form IS required.

Risks
Infection.
Contraindications
During pregnancy or breast-feeding.

Preparation
1. Have emergency equipment readily available.

Procedure
1. With the client positioned in a 20-degree Fowler's position, radionuclide is injected into the external jugular vein.
2. Scanning is performed for approximately 45 minutes.

Postprocedure Care
1. Assess the venipuncture site for bleeding, hematoma.
2. Observe the client carefully for up to 60 minutes after the study for a possible (anaphylactic) reaction to the radionuclide.
3. Wear rubber gloves when discarding urine that is voided up to 24 hours after the procedure. Wash the gloved hands with soap and water before removing the gloves. Wash the ungloved hands after the gloves have been removed.

Client and Family Teaching
1. Meticulously wash the hands with soap and water after each void for 24 hours.

Factors That Affect Results
1. None.

Other Data
1. This test is specific for left-to-right shunt and right-to-left shunt.
2. Health care professionals working in a nuclear medicine area should wear a film badge at waist level (the level closest to the client).
3. Health care professionals working in a nuclear medicine area must follow federal standards set by the Nuclear Regulatory Commission. These standards include precautions for handling the radioactive material and monitoring of potential radiation exposure.
4. Technetium half-life is 6 hours.

Heart Sonogram

See Echocardiography—Diagnostic.

Heart Ultrasound

See Echocardiography—Diagnostic.

Heavy Metals—Blood and 24-Hour Urine

Norm.

Blood		SI Units
Antimony	0.052 ± 0.019 µg/dL	4.35 ±1.6 nmol/L
Arsenic	2-23 µg/L	0.03-0.31 µmol/L
Chronic poisoning	100-500 µg/L	1.33-6.65 µmol/L
Acute poisoning	600-9300 µg/L	7.98-124 µmol/L
Bismuth	0.1-3.5 µg/L	0.5-16.7 nmol/L
Cadmium	0.4 µg/L	
Smokers	0.6-3.9 µg/L	5.3-34.7 nmol/L
Nonsmokers	0.3-1.2 µg/L	2.7-10.7 nmol/L
Toxic	100-3000 µg/L	0.9-26.7 µmol/L
Cobalt	0.11-0.45 µg/L	1.9-7.6 nmol/L
Copper		
Infants	20-70 µg/dL	3.1-11 µmol/L
Child, 6 years	90-190 µg/dL	14.1-29.8 µmol/L
Child, 12 years	80-160 µg/dL	12.6-25.1 µmol/L
Adult male	70-140 µg/dL	11.0-22.0 µmol/L
Adult female	80-155 µg/dL	12.6-24.3 µmol/L
Pregnant	118-302 µg/dL	18.5-47.4 µmol/L
Lead		
Child	<25 µg/dL	<1.21 µmol/L
Adult	<40 µg/dL	<1.93 µmol/L
Industry exposure	<65.4 µg/dL	<2.90 µmol/L
Toxic concentration	≥100 µg/dL	≥4.83 µmol/L
Toxic concentration in children	≥25 µg/dL	≥1.21 µmol/L
Mercury	0-10 µg/mL blood	<50 nmol/L blood
Selenium	58-234 µg/L	0.74-2.97 µmol/L
Thallium	<0.5 µg/dL	<24.5 nmol/L
Toxic concentration	10-800 µg/dL	0.5-39.1 µmol/L
Zinc	70-150 µg/dL	10.7-23 µmol/L

24-Hour Urine		SI Units
Antimony	<10 µg/L	<82.1 µmol/L
Toxic concentration	≥10 µg/L	≥82.1 µmol/L
Arsenic	5-50 µg/L random sample; 8.55 µg/g creatinine; <100 µg/L in 24-h sample	0.067-0.665 µmol/L
Chronic poisoning	50-5000 µg/L	0.67-66.5 µmol/L
Acute poisoning	1000-20,000 µg/L	13.3-266 mmol/L
Bismuth	0.3-4.6 µg/L	1.4-22 nmol/L
Cadmium	0.5-4.7 µg/L	4.4-41.8 nmol/L
Industrial exposure	10-580 µg/L	0.09-5.16 µmol/L
Cobalt	1-2 µg/L	17-34 nmol/L
Copper	2-80 µg/L	0.03-1.26 µmol/L
Lead	<80 µg/L; 0.63 mug/g creatinine	<0.39 µmol/L
Industrial exposure	<120 µg/L	<0.58 µmol/L
Mercury		
Adult	<50 µg/L 24 hours	<0.05 µmol/L
Toxic concentration	>50 µg/24 hours	>0.25 µmol/L
Platinum	<0.01 µg/L	<0.01 µmol/L
Selenium	7-160 µg/L	0.09-2.03 µmol/L
Toxic concentration	>400 µg/L	>5.08 µmol/L

Continued

24-Hour Urine		SI Units
Thallium	<2 μg/L; <20 μg/L with occupational exposure; hair <15 ng/gram	<9.8 nmol/L
Toxic concentration	1-20 μg/L	4.9-97.8 μmol/L
Zinc	150-1200 μg/L	2.3-18.4 μmol/L
Toxic concentration	>1200 μg/L	>18.4 μmol/L

Toxic or Poisoning Symptoms and Treatment

Symptoms

Antimony: Vomiting.

Arsenic: Gastric pain, vomiting, profuse diarrhea, confusion, convulsions, hypotension, heart failure, pulmonary edema, shock, ventricular dysrhythmias, coma, and death in acute poisoning; and diarrhea, scaling and bronze pigmentation of skin called "raindrops in the dust", hair loss, anemia, liver disease, Mees lines (transverse white striae on fingernails), metallic taste and peripheral neuropathy (2-8 weeks post exposure) in chronic poisoning.

Bismuth: Weakness, decreased appetite, fever, halitosis, black gum line, rheumatic-type pain, and renal damage.

Cadmium: Pneumonia, pulmonary edema, and cardiovascular collapse from inhalation; violent gastrointestinal symptoms from acute ingestion; and osteomalacia and renal dysfunction from chronic ingestion.

Cobalt: Thyroid gland hyperplasia, giant cell pneumonitis, hypersensitivity pneumonitis, pulmonary fibrosis, bronchiolitis obliterans, cardiomyopathy, nerve damage, and myxedema.

Copper: Nausea, vomiting, headache, diarrhea, abdominal pain, Wilson's disease, Indian childhood cirrhosis, noncaseating granuloma, pulmonary fibrosis.

Lead: Initial anorexia, severe abdominal pain, vomiting, peripheral neuropathy, irritability, and apathy. Also anemia, constipation, hepatotoxicity, pancreatitis, saturnine gout, hypertension, sperm abnormalities. In BLLs between 40-70 μg/dL symptoms similar to depression, 80-150 μg/dL memory problems, insomnia, personality changes, and over 150 μg/dL encephalopathy, seizure, coma, papilledema.

Mercury: Acute = chills, GI upset, poor appetite, dry mouth, constriction of bilateral visual fields, paresthesia, weakness, cough, dyspnea, ARDS. Chronic = fatigue, headache, loss of memory, apathy, emotional instability, Swift-Feer disease (usually seen in infants/children = autonomic hypertension, tachycardia, dermatologic pruritus, rash, oral ulcers and musculoskeletal changes including weakness and loss of tone), paresthesia, ataxia, deafness, dysarthria, visual deterioration, dysphagia, coma, and death.

Nickel: Contact dermatitis, irritability of gastrointestinal and respiratory systems, diffuse interstitial pneumonitis, and cerebral edema with severe poisoning. Little data to support carcinogenic potential. Treatment: sodium diethyldithiocarbamate (investigational chelating agent).

Selenium: Garlic smell in breath and urine, metallic taste, headaches, nausea, vomiting, pneumonia, and pulmonary edema.

Thallium: Early sign is painful peripheral neuropathy in feet/legs often misdiagnosed as Guillain-Barré. Alopecia begins 5-14 days after exposure. Ataxia, pulmonary edema, vomiting, constipation, restlessness, delirium, and coma. Antidote is Prussian blue (Radiogardase®).

Vanadium: Rhinitis, wheezing, nasal hemorrhage, conjunctivitis, cough, sore throat, and chest pain.

Zinc: Cough, chest discomfort, tachycardia, hypertension, gastrointestinal irritation, nausea, vomiting, diarrhea, and metallic taste in mouth.

Treatment

NOTE: Treatment choice(s) depend(s) on client's history and condition and episode history.

Antidotes for heavy-metal poisoning include BAL (British anti-Lewisite, dimercaprol), deferoxamine, dimercaprol, and EDTA. Heavy metals respond to hemodialysis or hemoperfusion in varying degrees (poor to well). FDA approved antidote for cesium is Prussian blue (Radiogardase®).

Usage. Screening for heavy-metal toxicity from overexposure, ingestion, or occupational exposure. Disorders for individual metals found under test listings for individual metals. Drugs that may further increase some values include carbamazepine, estrogens, oral contraceptives, penicillamine, phenobarbital, phenytoin, and sodium salts.

Description. Heavy metals include antimony, arsenic, bismuth, cadmium, cobalt, copper, lead, mercury, nickel, selenium, thallium, vanadium, and zinc.

Antimony exposure occurs in cigarette smokers, miners, smelters, and ore-refinery workers.

Arsenic is found naturally in food (seafood, rice, mushrooms, poultry) and the environment as well as in pesticides. Increased values found in immigrant farm workers and electronic, metal, glass, and ceramic workers. Treatment is by chelating agents BAL 3-4 mg/kg IM q 4-12 hours or DMSA 10mg/kg orally every 8 hours × 5 days then every 12 hours as needed.

Bismuth exposure occurs in workers in cosmetic, disinfectant, and pigment industries. It may also occur as a result of treatment for syphilis.

Cadmium accumulates in the lungs, liver, and kidneys by exposure to food, water, air, and cigarette smoke. Increased urine levels found in persons working/living near waste recycling centers. Levels increase with age.

Cobalt, a component of vitamin B_{12}, is found in most foods. It is also used to treat some resistant anemias and some radiosensitive malignancies. Occupational exposure occurs with glass and ceramic pigmentation, electroplating, chemical and petroleum industries, grinding and sharpening of hard metal tools, and animal-feed manufacturing.

Copper is a trace element found in normal diets. It is one of the few heavy metals that are potentially harmful at low levels as well as at toxic levels. Toxic levels may be caused by Buerger disease, the use of copper IUDs, ingestion of contaminated substances, electroplating, metal reclamation, roasting, crushing, smelting, and fungicide exposure. The biliary tract is the primary route of elimination. Gastrointestinal symptoms occur around whole blood levels near 3 mg of Cu per liter. Treatment is by chelating agents ($CaNa_2$-EDTA, BAL) or fungicide exposure.

Lead is absorbed into the body by the ingestion of lead-containing paint or after industrial exposure such as in occupation of battery plant, metal welder, painter, construction worker, lead miner, firing range worker, glass blower, ship builder (bone lead levels are higher in men in blue-collar occupations) or fragments of lead shot in game birds. Increased in Buerger disease, ingestion of "moonshine" alcohol, second hand cigarette smoke ingestion and in immigrant farm workers. Exposure adversely affects a child's academic achievement and reduces cognitive abilities and increases sterility in exposed adults. CDC states no level of lead in children can be specified as safe. Treatment includes chelation therapy (oral DMSA or parenteral Calcium EDTA).

Mercury is found in fungicides (antifungals in paints), industrial processes, cosmetics, explosives, dyes, pigments, preservative in some vaccines and contact lens solutions, and fish (living in polluted water). It can also be ingested in the form of mercury salts. High mercury levels have been noted among dental workers, persons with amalgam fillings, and persons with acute atopic eczema. High values are a risk factor for ischemic heart disease. After acute exposure blood samples are reliable for 2-3 days. Treatment of choice is DMSA, dialysis may also be needed.

Nickel is ubiquitous in soil, water, and many foods. Nickel does not accumulate in humans, and acute toxicity is usually related to exposure to nickel carbonyl. Current data are insufficient to indicate risk of carcinogenesis from nickel exposure.

Selenium is a metal used for the activity of human glutathione peroxidase. Exposure occurs as a result of the manufacture of glass, paints, dyes, electronic equipment, fungicides, rubber, and semiconductors. Decreased in Buerger disease.

Thallium is present in cosmetics, pesticides, and some medications. It is absorbed through intact skin and mucous membranes.

Vanadium is a corrosion-resistant metal that does not occur in nature. The primary source of exposure is from the diet. Occupational exposure occurs during boiler-cleaning operations as a result of the generation of vanadium oxide dust. The kidneys are the primary route of excretion. Toxicity overall is low.

Zinc is a trace metal important for cellular growth and metabolism. Toxicity can occur from industrial exposure and consumption of acidic food or beverages from galvanized containers. Decreased in Buerger disease.

Professional Considerations
Consent form NOT required.

Preparation
1. *Blood:*
   a. Tube: Metal-free tube containing EDTA anticoagulant.
   b. Do NOT draw specimens during hemodialysis.
2. *24-hour urine:*
   a. Obtain a 3-L, plastic, acid-washed collection container. Use a plastic bedpan or urinal for voided specimens.
   b. Write the beginning date and the time of collection on the container and the laboratory requisition.

Procedure
1. *Blood:* Draw a 10-mL blood sample.
2. *24-hour urine:* Save all the urine in a 3-L plastic, acid-washed container for 24 hours.

Postprocedure Care
1. Do NOT spin blood.
2. *24-hour urine:* Record the total volume and the ending time of collection on the specimen container and label the container with the client information.
3. Refrigerate the specimen(s).

Client and Family Teaching
1. *24-hour urine:* Save all the urine voided for the next 24 hours and urinate before defecating to avoid contaminating the urine specimen with stool. If any urine is accidentally discarded, discard the entire specimen and restart the collection the next day.

Factors That Affect Results
1. A diet high in heavy metals may elevate results.
2. Occupational exposure may elevate results.
3. A recent seafood diet may cause increased arsenic values.

4. A diurnal variation exists such that the highest copper levels are found in the morning.
5. Copper levels are 8%-12% higher in African-Americans.
6. Drugs that may further increase some values include dimercaprol, loop diuretics (intravenous), naproxen, penicillamine, sodium chloride, and thiazide diuretics.

Other Data
1. Make sure the specimen for the 24-hour urine is not voided into a metal bedpan or urinal.
2. Urine is the preferred specimen for arsenic if symptoms are present or in acute exposure. Blood testing is reliable within 10 days after acute arsenic poisoning, but urine results are detectable for weeks.
3. Supplemental vanadyl sulfate, used by some athletes to enhance weight training, can increase vanadium levels.
4. Many asymptomatic occupationally exposed workers have elevated vanadium levels.
5. Except for lead and cadmium, evidence is lacking on toxicity levels.
6. In the absence of acute toxicity, serial testing is usually more informative when applied in context with physical examination and knowledge of exposure history.
7. Blood lead levels have been correlated with higher levels of serum total cholesterol and high-density lipoprotein.
8. Increased intake of ascorbic acid has been shown to decrease blood lead levels.
9. Genetic linkages: Lead—Chromosome 3; Cadmium—2, 18, 20, X; Mercury—5; Selenium—4, 8; Zinc—2.
10. American College of Medical Toxicology states that post-challenge urinary metal testing has not been scientifically validated, has no demonstrated benefit, and may be harmful when applied in assessment and treatment of patients with metal poisoning.
11. See also Arsenic—Blood, hair, nails or urine; Cadmium—Serum and 24-hour urine; Copper—Serum; Copper—Urine; Lead—Blood and urine; Mercury—Blood and urine; Thallium—Serum or 24-hour urine; Zinc—Blood.

Heinz Body Stain—Diagnostic

Norm. Negative.

Positive. G6PD deficiency, Heinz body anemia, hemolytic anemia, homozygous beta-thalassemia, and after splenectomy. Drugs include acetanilid, aminosalicylic acid, analgesics, aniline, antipyretics, chlorates, hydroxylamine, naphthalene, nitrobenzene, phenol derivatives, phenothiazines, phenylhydrazine, phenylsemicarbazide, pyridine, resorcin, salicylazosulfidine, sodium sulfoxone, sulfapyridine, sulfones, tolbutamide, and large doses of vitamin K.

Negative. No Heinz body identified.

Description. Heinz bodies are small, irregular particles of denatured hemoglobin within mature red blood cells. These appear when stained with methyl violet or cresyl blue but not under Wright-stained preparations. The presence of Heinz bodies in a stained specimen indicates an abnormal hemoglobin structure.

Professional Considerations
Consent form NOT required.

Preparation
1. Tube: Lavender topped.
2. Contact the laboratory to arrange for testing.

Procedure
1. Draw a 3.5-mL blood sample.
2. Invert the tube gently several times to adequately mix the sample and the anticoagulant.

Postprocedure Care
1. Refrigerate the specimen.
2. Current administration of antimalarials, furazolidone, nitrofurantoin, phenacetin, procarbazine, or sulfonamides should be noted on the laboratory requisition.

Client and Family Teaching
1. Results are normally available within 24-48 hours.

Factors That Affect Results
1. Hemolysis or clotting of the specimen invalidates the results.
2. Antimalarials, dapsone, furazolidone (in infants), nitrofurantoin, phenacetin, phenylhydrazine, procarbazine, resorcin, and sulfonamides can cause false-positive results.

Other Data
1. Heinz bodies per cell vary from 1 to 20.
2. G6PD deficiency often affects Dutch, German, or French individuals.

Helical CT

See **Computed Tomography of the Body**—Diagnostic.

Helicobacter pylori Antigen Test—Stool

Norm. Negative for the presence of *H. pylori* antigens.

Usage. Provides earlier evaluation than the urea breath test of the success of treatment for *H. pylori* infection.

Description. See Urea breath test—Diagnostic. The *H. pylori* stool antigen test is one of the newest tests developed to evaluate for the persistence of bacteria and detects the *H. pylori* antigen that is shed in the stool of clients with active *H. pylori* infection. A positive test as early as 7 days after the completion of treatment indicates that the treatment was not successful. This test's early usefulness is as sensitive and specific as the urea breath test, which should not be performed for at least 4-6 weeks after treatment, for evaluation of treatment success. Prevalence in asymptomatic Japanese is 37.5%. Cytotoxin-associated gene (cagA) detected in 50%-60% fecal specimens.

Professional Considerations
Consent form NOT required.

Preparation
1. Obtain a clean container.

Procedure
1. Obtain a small sample of stool in a clean, dry container.

2. The stool is smeared on a Microplate coated with *H. pylori* antibodies and incubated, and the resulting color change is compared to a chart. The greater the degree of color change, the greater the amount of *H. pylori* antigen in the stool sample.

Postprocedure Care
1. None.

Client and Family Teaching
1. Do not take omeprazole, lansoprazole, or pantoprazole within 14 days before the test.
2. Do not take bismuth mixtures (e.g., Pepto-Bismol) within 1 month before the test.
3. Test results are normally available in about 3 hours.
4. Intake of yogurt, containing *Lactobacillus acidophilus* and *Bifidobacterium lactis*, twice a day for 6 weeks suppresses *H. pylori* infection.
5. Active *H. pylori* are shed by vomitus also.

Factors That Affect Results
1. Recent intake of bismuth-containing compounds (Pepto-Bismol) or lansoprazole may cause false-negative results.
2. Sensitivity is 93.1%. Specificity is 94.6%. This is comparable to other test methods such as those listed below.

Other Data
1. See also *Campylobacter*-like-organism test—Specimen; *Helicobacter pylori* quick office serology, Serum and titer—Blood; and Urea breath test—Diagnostic.
2. HpSA ImmunoCard STAT is an accurate test for *H. pylori* infection, but has a low sensitivity in children.
3. Sensitivity and specificity of stool-PCR is 62.5% and 92.3%.
4. Detection of alkyl hydroperoxidase reductase protein (AhpC) antigen by immunoblotting in stool is useful non-invasive method for accurate diagnosis of *H. pylori* in adolescents and children.

Helicobacter pylori Quick Office Serology, Serum and Titer—Blood

Norm. Negative.

Usage. Duodenal ulcers, gastric cancer, gastric ulcers, gastritis (chronic), lymphoma (stomach), and peptic ulcers.

Description. *H. pylori* are heterogeneous S- or C-shaped, gram-negative bacilli with a smooth outer coat and two to four unipolar flagella. The virulence of these organisms varies geographically. They were first detected in the stomachs of clients with gastritis around 1990 and have now been shown to be the major cause of active chronic gastritis. In addition, the evidence that *H. pylori* play a major role in the pathophysiology of duodenal and peptic ulcers and possibly gastric ulcers is compelling. An association between *H. pylori* and gastric cancer and lymphoma of the stomach may also exist. There is no known natural reservoir for *H. pylori* in the environment, but it is believed that these organisms are spread by the fecal-oral or oral-oral route and include vomitus as a mode of transmission. The Quick Office Serology test may be performed in the physician's office in 20 minutes on serum, providing a yes-or-no answer to the presence of IgA and IgG antibodies to *H. pylori*. Laboratory-based serology tests are more specific than office-based tests in that they quantitate antibody levels, providing titers so that antibody levels can be monitored after therapy. An elevated antibody level indicates active or recent infection. Because antibodies remain in the blood long after the infection is eradicated, this test cannot evaluate response to treatment. Instead, the urea breath test should be used to confirm eradication after treatment (see Urea breath test—Diagnostic).

Professional Considerations
Consent form NOT required.

Preparation
1. Tube: Red topped, red/gray topped, or gold topped.

Procedure
1. Draw a 3-mL blood sample.

Postprocedure Care
1. If shipping the sample to an off-site laboratory, keep the specimen cool with frozen coolant from April through

October and with refrigerated coolant from November through March.

Client and Family Teaching

1. Because serologic tests may remain positive for many months after successful treatment for *H. pylori*, other tests are also recommended for evaluating progress (endoscopy or breath test).
2. Intake of yogurt, containing *Lactobacillus acidophilus* and *Bifidobacterium lactis*, twice a day for 6 weeks suppresses *H. pylori* infection.

Factors That Affect Results

1. Serologic testing alone is associated with high false-positive rates because of past infection without active disease.

Other Data

1. These tests require 1 mL of serum.
2. *H. pylori* affects about 20% of clients younger than 40 years and 50% of those older than 60 years. *H. pylori* is uncommon in young children
3. Associated genes include sabA (91.3%), cagA (65%), vacA (97.5%), iceA (97.5%), babA2 (48.8%).
4. More than 90% of duodenal ulcers are caused by *H. pylori*.
5. Noninvasive ^{13}C-labeled urea breath test is useful for initial assessment.
6. The A2142G and A2143G mutations in the 235 rRNA gene are associated with clarithromycin resistance.
7. See also *Campylobacter*-like-organism test—Specimen.

HELLP (Hemolysis, Elevated Liver Enzymes, Low Platelets) Syndrome Panel—Serum

Norm. Blood pressure within normal limits or below 160/110 mm Hg. Complete blood count (CBC) and liver enzymes within normal limits.

Usage. Laboratory studies of blood values and liver enzymes will confirm diagnosis of syndrome. Tests repeated daily or every 8-12 hours in severe cases. Serves as a foundation for client care.

Description. Pregnancy-related syndrome associated with severe cases of pregnancy-induced hypertension (PIH)/preeclampsia, affects 60% primigravidas, occurs overall in 4%-12% of clients with increased risk in twin pregnancies, and most often presents in 28-32 weeks of pregnancy. Overall incidence 0.17%-0.85% of all births or 1:400 pregnant women. Pathophysiologic cause of syndrome is unknown. Persistent hypertension results in a decrease in intrinsic vasodilators (prostacyclin and nitric oxide) and increased production of vasopressors such as thromboxane. A chain of events leads to widespread vasospasms, acute renal failure, pulmonary edema, ascites, pleural effusion, ARDS, DIC, and/or multiple-organ damage. Postpartum hemorrhage occurs frequently when platelet count <40,000/μL.

Hepatic dysfunction caused by vasospasms affects:

- Metabolism of free fatty acids → increased plasma levels of fatty acids → aberrations in membranes of red blood cells (RBCs).
- Liver function, namely, AST (formerly SGOT), ALT (formerly SGPT), LDH.
- Endothelial integrity, platelet adherence, fibrin deposits. Increased sensitivity to angiotensin II, associated with PIH, heightens effect of angiotensin II on cells, causing them to contract. Increased prostacyclin (vasodilator and aggregation inhibitor) contributes to platelet "stickiness."

Laboratory values associated with HELLP syndrome:

ALT (SGPT) >50 U/L
AST (SGOT) >72 U/L
Bilirubin >1.2 mg/dL
BUN >10 mg/dL
Cr >2 mg/dL
Hct <32%
Hgb <10 mg/dL
LDH >350 IU/L
Plasma fibrinogen <300 mg/dL
PLT <100,000/mm^3
PT/PTT prolonged
Uric acid >10 mg/dL

Signs or symptoms associated with HELLP syndrome:

Blood pressure: 160/110 mm Hg or systolic >30 mm Hg or diastolic >15 mm Hg over baseline value

Dependent edema that progresses to non-dependent edema of upper arms, upper legs, abdomen, face, and neck

Epigastric pain, right upper abdominal quadrant tenderness

Hemolytic anemia: fatigue, pallor, dyspnea

Jaundice

Proteinuria: +4

Pulmonary edema

Professional Considerations

Consent form NOT required.

Preparation

1. Tube: Red topped, red/gray topped, or gold topped for liver function tests.
2. Do NOT draw during hemodialysis.
3. Lavender topped tube for platelets.
4. Obtain intravenous access for possible blood product infusion(s).
5. Obtain baseline vital signs.

Procedure

1. Draw a 4-mL blood sample.
2. Management with fresh-frozen plasma and packed RBCs. Avoid platelet transfusion because platelet consumption will occur.
3. Monitor vital signs frequently.

Postprocedure Care

1. Specimen may be refrigerated but not frozen.
2. For clients with HELLP syndrome, the critical period is 24 hours postpartum. During this time, the client's condition often worsens before improvement is seen.

Client and Family Teaching

1. Results available within an hour.

2. Clients with HELLP syndrome usually deliver by cesarean section and need to receive therapeutic blood components.
3. Mother is very ill and her condition will be of concern for at least 48 hours after delivery.
4. Preeclampsia subjective complaints include malaise, epigastric pain, nausea, vomiting, headache, and visual disturbances.
5. Condition of the baby will depend on gestational age at time of delivery, effects of uteroplacental insufficiency (associated with PIH), and maternal hemorrhage before delivery.

Factors That Affect Results

1. Delivery of fetus will correct preeclampsia. HELLP syndrome is complicated by disseminated intravascular coagulation (DIC) and potential liver rupture.
2. Hemolysis affects serum laboratory results for liver function.

Other Data

1. Usually develops between 20 and 37 weeks of gestation. Maternal mortality can be as high as 60%.
2. CT and MRI play a complementary role to sonography in diagnosis.
3. Severe folate deficiency may mimic HELLP syndrome.
4. Treatment may include recombinant activated factor VII given IV at dose 90 microg/kg twice and/or dexamethasone or methylprednisolone (125-250 mg IV 3-4 times per day). In grave cases use of IV urapidil or hydralazine followed by oral nifedipine or metoprolol is used.
5. Increased plasma protein 13 (PP13) in serum of mothers in third trimester indicates pre-eclampsia or HELLP.

Hemagglutination Treponemal Test for Syphilis (HATTS)—Serum

Norm. Titer <1:160.

Usage. Serologic confirmation of syphilis when nontreponemal antibody tests are positive.

Description. Syphilis is a complex, sexually transmitted disease characterized by a wide range of symptoms that imitate other diseases and is caused by the organism *Treponema pallidum*. In this test, the client's serum is heat-treated and mixed with *T. pallidum*–sensitized turkey red blood cells, incubated, and compared with a control. A positive result occurs when agglutination occurs in the test sample but not in the control. Positive results will occur in treponemal diseases of bejel, pinta, syphilis, and yaws.

Professional Considerations

Consent form NOT required.

Preparation

1. See Client and Family Teaching.
2. Tube: Red topped, red/gray topped, or gold topped.

Procedure
1. Draw a 7-mL blood sample.

Postprocedure Care
1. Send the specimen to the laboratory and refrigerate it until it is tested.
2. All cases of syphilis should be reported to the Centers for Disease Control and Prevention in Atlanta, Georgia, at: 404-639-2206.
3. Sexual contacts should be notified in the event of positive results.

Client and Family Teaching
1. Fast overnight before the test.
2. Refer clients with elevated titers for medical management, which is necessary to slow or prevent the sequelae of syphilis.
3. If testing positive:
   a. Notify all sexual contacts from the last 90 days (if in the early stage) to be tested for syphilis.
   b. Syphilis can be cured with antibiotics. These may worsen the symptoms for the first 24 hours.
   c. Do not have sex for 2 months and until after repeat testing has confirmed that the syphilis is cured. Use condoms after that for 2 years. Return for repeat testing every 3-4 months for the next 2 years to make sure the disease is cured.
   d. Do not become pregnant for 2 years because syphilis can be transmitted to the fetus.

e. If left untreated, syphilis can damage many body organs, including the brain, over several years. Neurosyphilis (late stage) is very difficult to treat with currently available regimens.

Factors That Affect Results
1. False-positive results may be attributable to hepatitis, infectious mononucleosis, leprosy, rheumatoid arthritis, or systemic lupus erythematosus.
2. False-negative results may occur in clients with AIDS. Treponemal antigen tests demonstrate greater accuracy in detecting late-stage infection in clients with HIV.

Other Data
1. This test may remain positive indefinitely for clients previously infected with syphilis. Thus it is not useful for monitoring clinical response to treatment for syphilis.
2. Benzathine penicillin G is the drug of choice to treat syphilis. Severe disease or immunosuppressed clients may require intravenous therapy. Consider doxycycline, ceftriaxone, or tetracycline with PCN allergy. Oral therapy with 2.0 grams of azithromycin is an alternative therapy.
3. Serial quantitative cardiolipin antigen testing is used for monitoring treatment response.
4. False-positive results have been reported in IV drug users infected with HIV and hepatitis B virus.

Hematocrit (Hct)—Blood
Norm.

		SI Units
Females		
Adult	37%-47%	0.37-0.47
Pregnant	30%-46%	0.30-0.46
Adult Males	40%-54%	0.40-0.54
Cord blood	42%-60%	0.42-0.60
Children		
Neonates	40%-68%	0.40-0.68
3 months	29%-54%	0.29-0.54
1-2 years	35%-44%	0.35-0.44
6-10 years	31%-45%	0.31-0.45
Panic Levels	<15% or >60%	<0.15 or >0.60

Panic Level Symptoms and Treatment—Increased

NOTE: Treatment choice(s) depend(s) on client's history and condition and episode history.

Cause	Symptoms	Possible Treatments
Hemoconcentration	Decreased pulse pressure and volume, decreased skin turgor, decreased venous filling, dry mucous membranes, low central venous pressure, orthostatic hypotension, tachycardia, thirst, and weakness	Administer IV fluids. Monitor hematocrit. Stop or reduce dose of diuretics if they are contributors to condition.
True polycythemia overtransfusion	Extremity pain and redness, facial flushing, irritability, anasarca decreasing QRS voltage with severe fluid overload	Administer IV fluids. Monitor hematocrit. Observe for signs of thrombosis. Perform bloodletting by venipuncture (phlebotomy).
Hemodilution	Rales, anxiety, edema, hypertension, jugular venous distention, restlessness, and shortness of breath	Administer diuretics. Restrict sodium. Restrict fluids. Monitor hematocrit and intake and output. Administer oxygen.
Blood loss	Hypotension, bleeding, hypoxia	Identify and treat cause of bleeding. Give isotonic fluids. Perform blood transfusion. Administer omeprazole (if blood loss is caused by bleeding esophageal varices). Protect airways; administer oxygen as needed.

Increased. Addison's disease, blood doping (autologous transfusion to improve athletic performance), burns (severe), dehydration (severe), diabetes mellitus, diarrhea, eclampsia, erythrocytosis, hemoconcentration, hemorrhage, pancreatitis (acute), polycythemia, shock, and tetralogy of Fallot. Any condition that increases red blood cells (RBCs).

Decreased. Anemia, bone marrow hyperplasia, burns (severe), cardiac decompensation, cirrhosis, congestive heart failure, cystic fibrosis, fatty liver, fluid overload, hemolytic reactions to chemicals or drugs or prosthetics, hemorrhage, hydremia of pregnancy, hyperthyroidism, hypothyroidism, idiopathic steatorrhea, intestinal obstruction (late), leukemia, overhydration, pancreatitis (hemorrhagic), pneumonia, and pregnancy. Also, conditions that decrease RBCs. Drugs include acetaminophen, acetohexamide, aminosalicylic acid, amphotericin, antimony potassium tartrate, antineoplastic agents, antibiotics, atabrine hydrochloride, chloramphenicol, chloroquine hydrochloride or phosphate, doxapram hydrochloride, ethosuximide, ethotoin, furazolidone, haloperidol, hydralazine hydrochloride, indomethacin, isocarboxazid, isoniazid, mefenamic acid, mephenytoin, mercurial diuretics, metaxalone, methaqualone, methsuximide, methyldopa, methyldopate hydrochloride, nitrates, nitrofurantoin, novobiocin sodium, oleandomycin, oxyphenbutazone, paramethadione, pargyline hydrochloride, penicillins, phenacemide, phenelzine sulfate, phenobarbital, phensuximide, phenylbutazone, phenytoin sodium, phytonadione, primidone, radioactive agents, rifampin, spectinomycin hydrochloride, sulfonamides, tetracyclines, thiazide diuretics, thiocyanates, thiosemicarbazones, tolazamide, tolbutamide, tranylcypromine sulfate, trimethadione, tripelennamine hydrochloride, troleandomycin, valproic acid, vegetarian diet, vitamin A, and zidovudine (AZT).

Description. Hematocrit is the percentage of red blood cells in a volume of whole blood.

Professional Considerations

Consent form NOT required.

Preparation

1. Tube: Lavender topped or heparinized capillary tube with a red band on the anticoagulant end.
2. Do NOT draw during hemodialysis.

Procedure

1. Draw a 3.5-mL blood sample from an extremity that does not have intravenous fluids infusing into it to avoid hemodiluted samples. Do not leave the tourniquet in place for longer than 1 minute during collection.
2. For a capillary puncture (fingers, toes, heels), establish a free flow of blood to minimize dilution with tissue fluid. Fill the capillary tube from the red-banded end to about two-thirds capacity and seal this end with clay.
3. For a central venous access device, temporarily stop all fluids infusing through ports, prepare injection port with povidone-iodine solution or alcohol, using only 10-mL syringes flush with 10 mL of 0.9% NaCl, and immediately withdraw 10 mL of discard blood. Withdraw required blood volume with new syringes and transfer specimen to appropriate tubes. Flush port with 10 mL of 0.9% NaCl. (Refer to your facility's policy and procedure manual or obtain related current standards from Intravenous Nursing Society, Oncology Nursing Society, or North American Vascular Access Network.) Flush solutions and discard volumes may vary by client population and published guidelines.

Postprocedure Care

1. Invert the tube gently 10 times to mix.
2. Refrigerate the sample after 10 hours. Do not freeze it.

Client and Family Teaching

1. Results are normally available within less than 24 hours.

Factors That Affect Results

1. Hemolysis of the specimen invalidates results.
2. Results are elevated with dehydration or leukocytosis over 100 x 10^9/L.
3. False elevations occur with glucose × 400 mg/dL.
4. Obtain the specimen before bath, shower, or massage because these can cause a temporary rise in the value.
5. High altitude may increase the value.
6. Level may measure as normal, even in the condition of blood loss, because of compensatory mechanisms and/or overlying conditions such as dehydration.

Other Data

1. The hematocrit value is approximately three times the value of the hemoglobin.
2. Hematocrit does not detect iron deficiency in infants, but ferritin level will for those 9-18 months of age.
3. Consider hemoglobin levels with pulse oximetry—if hemoglobin is low and oxygen saturation is 100%, oxygenation could be clinically and significantly inadequate.
4. Clients older than 64 years with a hematocrit less than 39% should be treated routinely using preoperative storage of autologous blood.

Hemoccult

See **Occult Blood**—Stool.

Hemoglobin (Hb, Hgb)

Norm.

		SI Units
Females	12-16 g/dL	7.45-9.90 mmol/L
Pregnant	10-15 g/dL	6.3-9.9 mmol/L
Males	13.6-18.0 g/dL	8.44-11.17 mmol/L

Continued

		SI Units
Children		
Neonates	14-27 g/dL	8.69-16.76 mmol/L
3 months	10-17 g/dL	6.21-10.55 mmol/L
1-2 years	9-15 g/dL	5.58-9.31 mmol/L
6-10 years	11-16 g/dL	6.82-9.92 mmol/L
Panic Levels	<5 g/dL	<3.10 mmol/L
	>20 g/dL	>12.41 mmol/L

Panic Level Symptoms and Treatment—Increased. See Hematocrit—Blood.
Panic Level Symptoms and Treatment—Decreased. See Hematocrit—Blood.

Increased. Burns (severe), congestive heart failure, chronic obstructive pulmonary disease (COPD), dehydration, diabetic retinopathy, diarrhea, erythrocytosis, hemorrhage, hemoconcentration, high altitudes, intestinal obstruction (late), polycythemia vera, snorers, and thrombotic thrombocytopenic purpura. Also conditions that increase red blood cells (RBCs). Drugs include gentamicin, methyldopa, and pentoxifylline.

Decreased. Andersen's disease, anemia (iron deficiency), carcinomatosis, cirrhosis, cystic fibrosis, deoxygenated blood (2% decrease), diabetes mellitus type I (predicts mortality), fat emboli, fatty liver, fluid retention, hemolysis, hemolytic reaction to chemicals or drugs or prosthetics, hemorrhage, Hodgkin's disease, hydremia of pregnancy, hyperthyroidism, hypervitaminosis A, hypothyroidism, idiopathic steatorrhea, intravenous overload, leukemia, lymphoma, otitis media, platelet apheresis, pregnancy, renal cortical necrosis, sarcoidosis, severe hemorrhage, systemic lupus erythematosus, tetralogy of Fallot, and transfusion of incompatible blood. Also, conditions that decrease RBCs or hemoglobin (organophosphate insecticides). Drugs include antibiotics, antineoplastic agents, Apresoline (hydralazine HCl with hydrochlorothiazide), aspirin, hydantoin derivatives, indomethacin, linezolid, losartan, monoamine oxidase inhibitors, primaquine, rifampin, sulfonamides, tridione, and zidovudine (AZT); vegetarian diet.

Description. Hemoglobin is the oxygen-carrying pigment of the RBCs. It is composed of amino acids that form a single protein called "globin" and a compound called "heme." Heme contains iron atoms and the red pigment porphyrin. Each erythrocyte contains approximately 300 million molecules of hemoglobin.

Professional Considerations
Consent form NOT required.

Preparation
1. Tube: Lavender topped or heparinized capillary tube with a red band on the anticoagulant end.
2. Do NOT draw specimen during hemodialysis.

Procedure
1. Draw a 3.5-mL blood sample from an extremity that does not have intravenous fluids infusing into it. Do not leave the tourniquet in place for longer than 1 minute during collection.
2. For capillary puncture (fingers, toes, heels), establish a free flow of blood to minimize dilution with tissue fluid. Fill the capillary tube from the red-banded end to about two-thirds capacity and seal this end with clay.
3. Central venous catheter (see Hematocrit—Blood).

Postprocedure Care
1. Invert the tube gently 10 times to mix it.
2. The specimen is stable at room temperature for 10 hours; then refrigerate it for up to 18 hours total.

Client and Family Teaching
1. Results are normally available within less than 24 hours.

Factors That Affect Results
1. Hemolysis of the specimen invalidates the results.
2. Results are falsely elevated by lipemic samples and leukocytosis >30 × 10⁹/L.
3. Obtain the specimen before bath, shower, or massage because these can cause a temporary increase in the value.

4. High altitude may increase the value.
5. The mean hemoglobin level in African-Americans is 0.4-1.0 g/dL lower than that in Caucasians after the first decade of life.
6. During exercise, arterial hemoglobin saturation falls.

Other Data

1. The hemoglobin value is approximately one third the value of the hematocrit.
2. Recent animal studies of hemoglobin have indicated that it may play a role in blood pressure regulation by carrying and releasing "super–nitric oxide," a form of gas that causes relaxation of muscle cells in peripheral blood vessels.
3. Dialysis patients have increased mortality if hematocrit is low or high and EPO use with Hct >13g/dl may increase mortality in those with ESRD or CKD.
4. After ischemic stroke, Hct >50 independent predictor of mortality in women.
5. One unit of blood (300 mL) transfused will change the Hct between 0.7% and 3.1%.

Hemoglobin A₁ₐ

See Glycosylated Hemoglobin—Blood.

Hemoglobin A₁ᵦ

See Glycosylated Hemoglobin—Blood.

Hemoglobin A₁ᵪ

See Glycosylated Hemoglobin—Blood.

Hemoglobin A₂—Blood

Norm.

		SI Units (Mass Fraction)
Cord blood	0%-1.8%	0-0.018
Birth to 6 months	0-3.5%	0-0.035
>6 months	1.5%-3.5%	0.015-0.035
Beta-thalassemia		
Trait	3.7%-6.5%	0.037-0.065
Sickle cell trait	1.7%-4.5%	0.017-0.045

Increased. Anemia (megaloblastic) and beta-thalassemia (homozygous). Blacksmith occupation.

Decreased. Anemia (iron deficiency, microcytic, sideroblastic), alpha-thalassemia, beta-thalassemia, erythroleukemia, gene mutation 0/00, hemoglobin A₂-Monreale mutation, and hemoglobin H disease.

Description. Hemoglobin A₂ is a normally present hemoglobin component constituting 2%-3% of the normally present hemoglobin. Found in 2%-3% of Mauritanian populations and 1.5% worldwide population are carriers of β-thalassemia. This test is used to help differentiate hemoglobin abnormalities. Classic phenotype of heterozygous β-thalassemia is increased Hb A₂, RBC, and decreased MCV and MCH.

Professional Considerations
Consent form NOT required.

Preparation
1. Tube: Lavender topped.

Procedure
1. Draw a 2-mL blood sample, without hemolysis.

Postprocedure Care

1. Invert the tube gently 10 times to mix.

Client and Family Teaching

1. Results are normally available within 24-48 hours.

Factors That Affect Results

1. Hemolysis or clotting of the specimen invalidates the results.
2. Clients with both beta-thalassemia and iron deficiency may demonstrate normal

Hb A_2 levels and may need to be retested after taking iron supplements.
3. In clients who have received recent blood transfusions, the results may be unreliable.

Other Data

1. Hb A_2 cannot be measured in the presence of HbC, HbE, or HbO.
2. 52 genotypes have been observed in thalassemia.

Hemoglobin Electrophoresis—Blood

Norm.

		SI Units (Hb Fraction)
Hemoglobin A	>95%	>0.95
Infants	10%-30%	0.10-0.30
Hemoglobin A_2	1.5%-3.5%	0.01-0.04
Hemoglobin F	<2%	<0.02
Neonates	70%-80%	0.70-0.80
1 month	70%	0.70
2 months	50%	0.50
3 months	25%	0.25
6 months-1 year	3%	0.03
Hemoglobin C	Absent	
Hemoglobin D	Absent	
Hemoglobin E	Absent	
Hemoglobin H	Absent	
Hemoglobin S	Absent	

Usage. Congenital dyserythropoietic anemia, Heinz-body anemia, hemoglobin C disease (trait=45%, disease >90%), hemolytic anemia (HbD and HbE), microcytic anemia, sickle cell anemia (HbS: trait = 20%-40%, disease = 80%-100%), and thalassemia minor (HbH).

Description. A screening procedure in which the hemoglobin molecules migrate in solution in response to electrical currents such that the different components and their percentages can be determined. Common in people of the Aegean region of Turkey.

Hemoglobins A, A_2, and F are types of hemoglobin that are found normally in the body.

Hemoglobin C causes red blood cells to sickle at times because of osmotic fragility. It occurs in 2%-3% of the African-American population.

Hemoglobins D and E rarely occur by themselves though the anemias are without

symptoms. When either occurs in combination with sickle cell anemia or thalassemia, the disease takes a more serious form.

Hemoglobin H is known to develop many inclusion bodies within the red blood cell, resulting in a damaged cell membrane and premature cell death (40 days). It also disrupts transport of oxygen to tissues by binding with rather than releasing the oxygen.

Hemoglobin S is the most common of the abnormal hemoglobin traits, occurring in 10% of the African-American population. Its presence results in a sickling distortion of the red blood cells in response to reduced oxygen levels.

Professional Considerations

Consent form NOT required.

Preparation

1. Tube: Lavender topped.

Procedure
1. Draw a 2.5-mL blood sample.

Postprocedure Care
1. Deliver the specimen to the laboratory immediately because abnormal hemoglobins are unstable.
2. Recent (within the past 4 months) blood transfusion(s) should be noted on the laboratory requisition.

Client and Family Teaching
1. The client should wear a medical identification tag if chronic anemia is present.
2. If the sickle cell trait or the disease is present, offer genetic counseling.

Factors That Affect Results
1. Red blood cell transfusion within the previous 4 months may mask or reduce the presence of abnormal hemoglobins.
2. Hemoglobins A_2, C, and S may be decreased in iron deficiency.
3. False-negative tests occur in hemoglobin S with clients with polycythemia or in those less than 3 months of age.

Other Data
1. More than 350 variants of Hb have been recognized.
2. Changes in the proportion of normal types of hemoglobin may imply a hemolytic disease.

Hemoglobin (Free), Plasma and Qualitative—Urine

Norm.
Urine. Negative.

Blood		SI Units
Normal	<3 mg/dL	<0.47 µmol/L
Hemoglobinemia	>10 mg/dL	>1.55 µmol/L
Intravascular hemolysis	>30 mg/dL	>4.65 µmol/L
Hemoglobinuria occurs at	>150 mg/dL	>23.25 µmol/L
Cherry-red plasma occurs at	>200 mg/dL	>31 µmol/L

Increased in Plasma. Autoimmune hemolytic anemia, burns, cold hemagglutinins, disseminated intravascular coagulation, falciparum malaria, intravascular hemolysis, leptospirosis, lupus erythematosus, paroxysmal nocturnal hemoglobinuria, septicemia, sickle cell anemia, thrombosis, transfusion reaction, and traumatic hemolysis. Drugs include analgesics, antimalarials, cinchona alkaloids, nitrofurantoins, sulfonamides, and sulfones. Clients receiving fluid substitute of hydroxyethylstarch (HES).

Positive in Urine. Autoimmune hemolytic anemia, blackwater fever, bladder irrigation, burns, *Clostridium perfringens* infection, disseminated intravascular coagulation, hemolytic anemia, kidney infarctions, malaria, paroxysmal nocturnal hemoglobinuria, poisonings, pregnancy, transfusion reaction, and transurethral prostatectomy. Drugs include arsenic, bacitracin, ciprofloxacin, coumadin, cyclophosphamide, fenoprofen, gold salts, indomethacin, mebendazole, nitrofurantoin, phenacetin, phenothiazines, phenylbutazone, polymyxin B, quinine, and suprofen.

Description. Free hemoglobin is hemoglobin that escapes from erythrocytes during intravascular hemolysis. A small amount of hemoglobin is normally present, but it is increased in the bloodstream and urine after massive hemolysis.

Professional Considerations
Consent form NOT required.

Preparation
1. Tube: Red topped, red/gray topped, or gold topped, and green topped for plasma sample.
2. Obtain a sterile plastic specimen container for the urine sample.
3. If the female client is menstruating, reschedule the urine test.

Procedure
1. *Plasma*: Do NOT draw from an extremity with intravenous solution infusing. Draw the blood sample using an 18-gauge needle with an attached infusion tubing as follows:

a. Gently place the tourniquet around the upper arm. Follow this with venipuncture of the antecubital vein with as little trauma as possible.

b. Release the tourniquet and clamp the tubing as soon as flashback occurs.

c. Collect 3 mL of blood in the red topped tube. Remove the top from the green topped tube, and collect 5 mL of blood. Replace the top of the heparinized green topped tube.

d. Clamp the tubing, withdraw the needle, and apply pressure to the venipuncture site.

2. *Urine:* Obtain a 20-mL random urine specimen in a sterile plastic container.

Postprocedure Care

1. *Plasma:* Send the specimen to the laboratory immediately. The plasma must be separated from the cells within 1-2 hours.

2. *Urine:*

a. Do not shake the specimen.

b. Dip a commercial dipstick in the urine and match the stick with a color block or chart, or send the stick to the laboratory immediately.

c. Refrigerate the specimen if the test is not performed within 1 hour.

Client and Family Teaching

1. Urinate before defecating and avoid contaminating the urine with toilet tissue.

Factors That Affect Results

1. Hemolysis of blood specimens invalidates the results. The specimen-collection procedure is critical because any damage to red blood cells can produce falsely elevated results.

2. False-positive urine results may occur if the specimen is contaminated with menstrual blood.

3. Ascorbic acid (or medications containing ascorbic acid as a preservative, such as antibiotics) may cause false-negative urine tests by inhibiting reagent activity.

4. Bromides, copper, iodides, and oxidizing agents cause false-positive urine tests.

Other Data

1. If plasma hemoglobin levels are increased, encourage periods of rest to preserve usable hemoglobin.

2. Free hemoglobin can often be detected in the urine when red blood cells cannot because they lyse in strongly alkaline or dilute urine.

3. The urine test is often part of a routine analysis.

Hemoglobin Profile

See CO-oximeter Profile, Arterial or Venous—Blood.

Hemoglobin S

See Hemoglobin Electrophoresis—Blood; Sickle Cell Test—Blood.

Hemoglobin, Unstable, Heat-Labile Test—Blood

Norm. <5% (<0.05 factor, SI units).

Increased. Heinz body anemia and iron deficiency anemia.

Description. Unstable hemoglobin is a type of hemoglobin, normally absent, that precipitates faster than normal hemoglobin. After precipitation, unstable hemoglobin forms Heinz bodies, inclusions attached to erythrocyte membranes that increase the fragility of the red blood cell and lead to hemolysis. In Heinz body and iron deficiency anemia, a small percentage of hemoglobin becomes denatured when subjected to acid and heated to 50 degrees C.

Professional Considerations
Consent form NOT required.

Preparation

1. Tubes: Two lavender topped.

Procedure

1. Draw a 3.5-mL blood sample in each of both tubes.

Postprocedure Care

1. Invert the tube 10 times gently to mix the specimen.

Client and Family Teaching

1. Results are normally available within 24 hours.

Factors That Affect Results

1. Reject specimens received more than 3 hours after collection.

Other Data

1. The test should be run with a normal control.

Hemoglobin, Unstable, Isopropanol Precipitation Test—Blood

Norm. Negative. No precipitation at 40 minutes.

Positive. Heinz body anemia and slight opacity at 10 minutes in the presence of hemoglobin H. The abnormal chain of Hb Mont Saint-Aignan is a variant associated with hemolytic anemia. Autosomal dominant Hemoglobin Pitie-Salpetriere identified in Japanese persons.

Description. Unstable hemoglobin is a type of hemoglobin, normally absent, that precipitates faster than normal hemoglobin. After precipitation, unstable hemoglobin forms Heinz bodies, inclusions attached to erythrocyte membranes that increase the fragility of the red blood cell and lead to hemolysis. Unstable hemoglobin is detectable when subjected to isopropanol.

Professional Considerations
Consent form NOT required.

Preparation

1. Inform the laboratory of the time the specimen will be arriving.
2. Tube: Lavender topped.

Procedure

1. Draw a 2-mL blood sample.

Postprocedure Care

1. Invert the sample gently 10 times to mix.
2. Send the specimen to the laboratory immediately because the test must be run with fresh blood.

Client and Family Teaching

1. Results are normally available within 24 hours.

Factors That Affect Results

1. The presence of hemoglobin F may cause a false-positive result.

Other Data

1. More sensitive than heat denaturization.

Hemophilic Factor B

See Factor IX—Blood.

Hepatic Function Panel (HFP)—Blood

Norm. See individual test listings: Alanine Aminotransferase—Serum, Albumin—Serum, urine, and 24-hour urine, Alkaline phosphatase—Serum, Aspartate aminotransferase—Serum, and Bilirubin—Serum.

Usage. See individual test listings.

Description. The HFP is a term defined by The Centers for Medicare and Medicaid Services (CMS) in the United States to indicate a group of tests for which a bundled reimbursement is available. The panel is disease-oriented, meaning that payment through Medicare is available only when the test is used to diagnose and monitor a disease and payment is not available when the test is used for screening purposes in clients who have no signs and symptoms. All the tests in the panel must be carried out when a BMP is prescribed.

Professional Considerations
Consent form NOT required.

Preparation

1. Tube: Red topped, red/gray topped, or gold topped and one blue topped.

2. Do NOT draw specimens during hemodialysis.

Procedure

1. Draw a 3- to 5-ml blood sample in each tube.

Postprocedure Care

1. None.

Client and Family Teaching

1. See individual test listings.

Factors That Affect Results

1. See individual test listings.

Other Data

1. See individual test listings.

Hepatitis A Antibody, IgM and IgG (HAV-Ab)—Blood

Norm. Negative.

Positive. Hepatitis A (formerly called infectious hepatitis) and jaundice.

Description. IgM is a marker for the hepatitis A virus that appears 2-4 weeks after exposure and is detectable for only 4-8 weeks. It does differentiate between an acute infection and a past or preexisting infection. Hepatitis A is never chronic, but acute relapses occur with an overall fatality of 0.2%. IgG replaces IgM, and these antibodies persist for life, providing immunity from reinfection of hepatitis A. Hepatitis A is usually transmitted through the fecal-oral route although it can be transmitted via blood transfusion. Hepatitis A is emerging in the Middle East region, especially in ages 5-14 years.

Professional Considerations

Consent form NOT required.

Preparation

1. See Client and Family Teaching.
2. Tube: Red topped, red/gray topped, or gold topped.
3. Screen the client for the use of herbal preparations or natural remedies such as Chinese *jin bu huan* ("gold-inconvertible," Jin Bu Huan Anodyne Tablets, patent medicine with misidentified constituents: essence of *t'ienchi* [*tianqi*] flowers, "Noto-ginseng"; also *kombucha*; also *Lycopodium serratum*, or club moss; but with plant alkaloid levotetrahydropalmatine, a potent neuroactive substance) and Bougainvillea Wild (Nyctaginaceae: *Bougainvillaea*).

Procedure

1. Draw a 2-mL blood sample.

Postprocedure Care

1. Remove the serum and freeze it if the blood will not be tested within 7 days.

Client and Family Teaching

1. Results may not be available for several days.
2. A person cannot be infected more than once with hepatitis A. Vaccination recommended for hospital workers.
3. Hepatitis A can be prevented by good handwashing. Wash your hands well with soap and water and with rapid scrubbing action after urinating or defecating.
4. Do not drink alcohol, beer, or wine or take medicine that contains acetaminophen or paracetamol for 3 weeks, or as specified by your physician.
5. Malfunction of other organs occurs in 30% of clients, including integumentary, musculoskeletal (joints), respiratory, cardiovascular, and digestive systems.

Factors That Affect Results

1. If using the radioimmunoassay technique, injection of radionuclides within the last week may falsely elevate results.
2. Herbs or natural remedies that may cause hepatitis include Chinese *in bu huan* (see above).
3. Herbs or natural remedies that decrease hepatitis are Bougainvillea Wild (Nyctaginaceae).
4. Peripheral stem cell transplant causes loss of antibodies in 14% of clients.

Other Data

1. This test requires 2 mL of serum.
2. The serum is stable at room temperature for 7 days and indefinitely if frozen.
3. In the United States, although more than 50% of the population is positive for anti-HAV IgG, it is clinically insignificant.
4. The presence of anti-HAV IgG does not rule out acute hepatitis B or non-A, non-B hepatitis.

5. Screening for HAV and HBV is recommended with elevated serum transaminase levels.
6. The vaccine Epaxal can be used as a booster, Havrix is a vaccine for hepatitis A with an 87% seroprotection rate and

Avaxim has a 90% 5-year protection rate. Substantial immune response occurs for at least 12 years to re-exposure.
7. Two-dose schedule (0 and 6 months) for combined hepatitis A and B elicits similar immunogenicity as the three-dose regimen.

Hepatitis B Core Antibody (Anti-HBc)—Blood

Norm. Negative.

Positive. Hepatitis B.

Description. Hepatitis B core antibody is the antibody marker that arises 1-2 weeks after contraction of the hepatitis B virus, increases during the chronic phase of the illness, and remains present for life. It is the most reliable test to determine the presence of hepatitis B infection in the absence of hepatitis B surface antibody and hepatitis B surface antigen.

Professional Considerations
Consent form NOT required.

Preparation

1. Tube: Red topped, red/gray topped, or gold topped.
2. Screen the client for the use of herbal preparations or natural remedies such as Chinese *jin bu huan* ("gold-inconvertible," Jin Bu Huan Anodyne Tablets, patent medicine with misidentified constituents: essence of *t'ienchi [tianqi]* flowers, "Noto-ginseng"; also *kombucha*; also *Lycopodium serratum*, or club moss; but with plant alkaloid levotetrahydropalmatine, a potent neuroactive substance), and Bougainvillea Wild (Nyctaginaceae: *Bougainvillaea*).

Procedure

1. Draw a 3-mL blood sample.

Postprocedure Care

1. Remove the serum and freeze it if the blood will not be tested within 7 days.

Client and Family Teaching

1. Results may not be available for several days.
2. Hepatitis B can be spread by blood and other body fluids, including the sharing of needles and sexual contact. An

infected mother can pass the infection to her baby.
3. Liver transplantation is associated with a high rate of viral transmission with carriers present in 16% liver donors (Italy) but recipients did not have a significant impact on graft survival. Donor race does not predict graft failure in liver transplantation.
4. To help prevent the spread of hepatitis B, wash your hands well with soap and water and use rapid scrubbing action after urinating or defecating.
5. Do not drink alcohol, beer, or wine or take medicine that contains acetaminophen or paracetamol for 3 weeks, or as specified by your physician.

Factors That Affect Results

1. If the radioimmunoassay technique is used, the injection of radionuclides within the last week may falsely elevate results.
2. Herbs or natural remedies that may cause hepatitis include Chinese *jin bu huan* (see above).
3. Herbs or natural remedies that decrease hepatitis are Bougainvillea Wild (Nyctaginaceae).
4. False positive in persons recently vaccinated for influenza.

Other Data

1. The serum is stable at room temperature for 7 days and indefinitely if frozen.
2. Wastewater treatment plant workers are at increased risk.
3. Two-dose schedule (0 and 6 months) for combined hepatitis A and B elicits similar immunogenicity as the three-dose schedule.
4. Clients with chronic GVHD are at significant risk for HBV reactivation.

Hepatitis B e Antibody (Anti-HBe, HBeAb)—Serum

Norm. Negative.

Positive. Hepatitis B.

Description. Hepatitis B e antibody is a serum marker for hepatitis B that appears 8-16 weeks after infection and indicates resolution of acute infection. The presence of this antibody in clients with chronic positive hepatitis B surface antigen indicates an asymptomatic, healthy carrier.

Professional Considerations
Consent form NOT required.

Preparation
1. See Client and Family Teaching.
2. Tube: Red topped, red/gray topped, or gold topped.
3. Screen the client for the use of herbal preparations or natural remedies such as *jin bu huan* ("gold-inconvertible," Jin Bu Huan Anodyne Tablets, patent medicine with misidentified constituents: essence of *t'ienchi* [*tianqi*] flowers, "Noto-ginseng"; also *kombucha*; also *Lycopodium serratum*, or club moss; but with plant alkaloid levo-tetrahydropalmatine, a potent neuroactive substance) and Bougainvillea Wild (Nyctaginaceae: *Bougainvillaea*).

Procedure
1. Draw a 2-mL blood sample.

Postprocedure Care
1. Remove the serum and freeze it if the blood will not be tested within 7 days.

Client and Family Teaching
1. Results may not be available for several days.

Factors That Affect Results
1. If the radioimmunoassay technique is used, injection of radionuclides within the previous week may falsely elevate results.
2. An herb or natural remedy that may cause hepatitis includes Chinese *jin bu huan* (see above).
3. An herb or natural remedy that decreases hepatitis is Bougainvillea Wild (Nyctaginaceae: *Bougainvillaea*).
4. Methylprednisolone and antilymphoglobulin for treating severe aplastic anemia can develop high levels of hepatitis B e antibody in patients.

Other Data
1. The serum is stable at room temperature for 7 days and indefinitely if frozen.
2. The test is more meaningful when measured in conjunction with hepatitis B e antigen.
3. The test should be prescribed only in clients with documented recent infection of hepatitis B.
4. Tenofovir in combination with emtricitabine is alternative treatment for hepatitis B patients on adefovir.

Hepatitis B e Antigen (HBeAg)—Blood

Norm. Negative.

Positive. Hepatitis B.

Description. Usually appearing within 4-12 weeks of infection, hepatitis B e antigen is one of the first indicators of hepatitis B infection, usually preceding symptoms and representing the greatest threat of transmission. It is usually present for only 3-6 weeks. Persistence of the antigen for greater than 3 months is suggestive of chronic liver disease or hepatocellular carcinoma of genotypes A through H; clients with genotype HBV/G or C more frequently have HBeAg.

Professional Considerations
Consent form NOT required.

Preparation
1. Tube: Red topped, red/gray topped, or gold topped.
2. Screen the client for the use of herbal preparations or natural remedies such as Chinese *jin bu huan* and Bougainvillea Wild.

Procedure
1. Draw a 2-mL blood sample.

Postprocedure Care
1. Remove the serum and freeze it if the blood will not be tested within 7 days.

Client and Family Teaching
1. Results may not be available for several days.

Factors That Affect Results

1. If the radioimmunoassay technique is used, injection of radionuclides within the previous week may falsely elevate results.
2. An herb or natural remedy that may cause hepatitis includes Chinese *jin bu huan* (see above).
3. An herb or natural remedy that decreases hepatitis is Bougainvillea Wild (Nyctaginaceae: *Bougainvillaea*).

Other Data

1. The serum is stable at room temperature for 7 days and indefinitely if frozen.

2. Clients with chronic positive tests should also be tested for the hepatitis B e core antibody, which indicates that the client is an asymptomatic, healthy carrier.
3. A hepatitis B vaccine is available and recommended for health care workers.
4. Tenofovir in combination with emtricitabine is alternative treatment for hepatitis B patients on adefovir.
5. Hepatitis B surface antigen <300 IU/mL and >1 log reduction at month 6 predicts sustained response.
6. Sustained response to interferon treatment is low in chronic hepatitis B patients with genotype D.

Hepatitis B Surface Antibody (HBsAb)—Blood

Negative. Limits of detection 2-10 U/L. Post vaccine testing >10 U/L or >10 mIU/mL confers protection.

Positive. Hepatitis B.

Description. This marker appears 2-16 weeks after hepatitis B surface antigen has disappeared. It usually represents clinical recovery and immunity to the virus. It will also be present during passive transfer in blood by transfusion or by administration of hepatitis B immune globulin (HBIG). Presence of the hepatitis B surface antibody along with the hepatitis B surface antigen indicates a poor prognosis.

Professional Considerations
Consent form NOT required.

Preparation

1. Tube: Red topped, red/gray topped, or gold topped.
2. Screen the client for the use of herbal preparations or natural remedies such as Chinese *jin bu huan* and Bougainvillea Wild (Nyctaginaceae: *Bougainvillaea*).

Procedure

1. Draw a 3-mL blood sample.

Postprocedure Care

1. Remove the serum and freeze it if the blood will not be tested within 7 days.

Client and Family Teaching

1. Results may not be available for several days.

Factors That Affect Results

1. If the radioimmunoassay technique is used, injection of radionuclides within the previous week may falsely elevate results.
2. An herb or natural remedy that may cause hepatitis includes *jin bu huan* (see above).
3. An herb or natural remedy that decreases hepatitis is Bougainvillea Wild (Nyctaginaceae: *Bougainvillaea*).

Other Data

1. The serum is stable at room temperature for 7 days and indefinitely if frozen.
2. There is a high prevalence of positive tests among intravenous drug abusers.
3. Reverse seroconversion of hepatitis B virus is common after autologous and allogeneic bone marrow transplants.
4. Hexavac vaccine was withdrawn in 2005 amidst concerns about long-term hepatitis B protection.

Hepatitis B Surface Antigen (HBsAg:HAA)—Blood

Negative. Limits of detection 0.02-1.0 ng/mL.

Positive. Hepatitis B.

Description. The hepatitis B surface antigen usually appears between 4 and 12 weeks of infection. It is indicative of active hepatitis B, either acute or chronic (HBsAg persists more than 6 months). It is the earliest indicator of hepatitis B, specificity of 99%, often preceding clinical symptoms. Chronic hepatitis B can occur without hepatitis B surface antigen detected due to variants as in genotype A. HBsAg is common in clients undergoing immunotherapy, chemotherapy, or bone marrow transplant. Presence of the hepatitis B surface antibody along with the hepatitis B surface antigen indicates a poor prognosis making this test useful to predict clinical and treatment outcomes.

This test, required by the Food and Drug Administration when clients wish to donate blood, has helped reduce the incidence of hepatitis.

Professional Considerations
Consent form NOT required.

Preparation
1. Tube: Red topped, red/gray topped, or gold topped.
2. Screen the client for the use of herbal preparations or natural remedies such as Chinese *jin bu huan* and Bougainvillea Wild (Nyctaginaceae: *Bougainvillaea*).

Procedure
1. Draw a 2-mL blood sample.

Postprocedure Care
1. Remove the serum and freeze it if the blood will not be tested within 7 days.

Client and Family Teaching
1. If the client is giving blood, explain the donation procedure.
2. Results may not be available for several days.

Factors That Affect Results
1. If the radioimmunoassay technique is used, injection of radionuclides within the previous week may falsely elevate results.
2. An herb or natural remedy that may cause hepatitis includes Chinese *jin bu huan* (see above).
3. An herb or natural remedy that decreases hepatitis is Bougainvillea Wild (Nyctaginaceae: *Bougainvillaea*).
4. Genotype A and other rare mutations produce false negative results.
5. False positive results in heparinized samples, pregnancy, autoimmune diseases, chronic liver disease, interferences with hemoglobin or bilirubin, persons recently given hepatitis B vaccine,

Other Data
1. The serum is stable at room temperature for 7 days and indefinitely if frozen.
2. This test does not screen for hepatitis A, hepatitis C, or non-A, non-B viruses.
3. HBsAg may also be present in more than 5% of clients with Down syndrome, hemophilia, Hodgkin's disease, and leukemia.
4. When HBsAg is found in donor blood, it must be discarded because it carries a 40%-70% chance of transmitting hepatitis.
5. Report confirmed viral hepatitis to public health authorities.
6. Potatoes have been used successfully to orally administer the vaccine.
7. Subgenotypes worldwide include: B1 Japan, B2 China, B3 Indonesia, B4 Vietnam, C1 Korea and China, C2 China and Bangladesh, C3 Oceania, C4 Aborigines Australia, and D1-D4 Europe, Asia, and Africa.

Hepatitis C Antibody—Serum

Norm. Negative.

Positive. Hepatitis C and non-A, non-B hepatitis and some post kidney transplant diabetes mellitus (PTDM) clients.

Description. An assay to identify antibodies of the IgG class to the hepatitis C virus (HCV), a newly identified gene to a ribonucleic acid (RNA) virus that does not have the qualities of either hepatitis A or hepatitis B; 20% of posttransfusion hepatitis falls into this category. Transmission is via exposure to contaminated blood via intravenous drug use and abuse, organ transplant (before 1992), transfusions (of blood before 1992, of clotting factors before 1987), dialysis, and needle sticks. Infants born to HCV-positive mothers are also at risk. Hepatitis C infects 200 million people worldwide and is responsible for up to 10,000 deaths each year. Clients with hepatitis C may carry the virus chronically and not develop active disease until many years after initial infection.

Professional Considerations
Consent form NOT required.

Preparation
1. Tube: Red topped, red/gray topped, or gold topped.
2. Screen the client for the use of herbal preparations or natural remedies such as Chinese *jin bu huan* and Bougainvillea Wild (Nyctaginaceae: *Bougainvillaea*).

Procedure
1. Draw a 2-mL blood sample.

Postprocedure Care
1. Remove the serum and freeze it if the blood will not be tested within 7 days.

Client and Family Teaching
1. If the client is giving blood, explain the donation procedure.
2. Results may not be available for several days.

Factors That Affect Results
1. If the radioimmunoassay technique is used, injection of radionuclides within the previous week may falsely elevate results.

2. An herb or natural remedy that may cause hepatitis includes Chinese *jin bu huan* (see above).
3. An herb or natural remedy that decreases hepatitis is Bougainvillea Wild (Nyctaginaceae: *Bougainvillaea*).
4. This test is 97% sensitive for detecting the presence of hepatitis C virus, but cannot differentiate between chronic, acute, and past/resolved infection.

Other Data
1. This test requires 0.5 mL of serum.
2. The serum is stable at room temperature for 7 days and indefinitely if frozen.
3. Notify public health authorities if the test results are positive.
4. Up to now, there has been no commercially available serologic test to detect hepatitis C antigen (HCAg).
5. The incidence in the United States is 1.8% and for chronic dialysis clients it is 9%.
6. Inner-city STD-infected obstetric clients are at high risk for hepatitis C, as well as clients whose alcohol intake is >40 g per day.

Hepatitis C Genotype (HCV Genotype)—Serum

Norm. Negative.

Usage. Genotyping of the hepatitis C virus (HCV)–affected RNA is utilized, in conjunction with the client's clinical presentation and other laboratory findings, to determine a treatment plan and the client's prognosis and to assist in identifying a cause for clients with a diagnosis of hepatitis C.

Increased. Identification of hepatitis C genotype subtype 1a, 1b,

Decreased. 1c, 2a, 2b, 2c, 3a, 3b, 4a-h, 5a, and 6a.

Positive. Individual tests may yield additional genotypes.

Description. HCV is a genus from the family Flaviviridae. Its RNA is single stranded and has heterogeneous subtypes. Nucleic acid sequencing of the viral genome determines the type and subtype of the viral genome. Treatment decisions are based on the specific genotype identified in the affected HCV RNA. Clients with chronic HCV are at a greater risk for development of

cirrhosis and hepatocellular carcinoma. Genotype I runs a more severe course and has a faster progression.

Professional Considerations
Consent form NOT required.

Preparation
1. Tube: Lavender or gold topped.
2. Specimens may not be drawn during hemodialysis.
3. Screen the client for the use of herbal preparations or natural remedies such as Chinese *jin bu huan* ("gold-inconvertible," *Jin Bu Huan* Anodyne Tablets, patent medicine with misidentified constituents: essence of *t'ienchi [tianqi]* flowers, "Noto-ginseng"; also *kombucha*; also *Lycopodium serratum*, or club moss; but with plant alkaloid levo-tetrahydropalmatine, a potent neuroactive substance) and Bougainvillea Wild (Nyctaginaceae: *Bougainvillaea*).

Procedure
1. Collect 2 mL of blood (minimum 0.5 mL).

2. Transport specimen in ice immediately to laboratory.

Postprocedure Care
1. None.

Client and Family Teaching
1. A complete history should be obtained before testing to identify possible causes of HCV.
2. Treatment options should be explained to client on receipt of the results. Special attention to the possible side effects of the antiviral agents should be provided.

Factors That Affect Results
1. Qualitative (detect circulating HCV RNA) and quantitative (measure the circulating HCV RNA) testing should be completed before genotyping. (Samples containing less than 1000 RNA copies/mL may not be suitable for genotype testing.)
2. HCV genotyping is not effective in clients with mixed hepatitis types (hepatitis A and B); the test will be read as indeterminate.
3. Heparinized collection tubes or clients receiving heparin will render the test

invalid and will be read as indeterminate.
4. An herb or natural remedy that may cause hepatitis includes Chinese *jin bu huan* (see above).
5. An herb or natural remedy that decreases hepatitis is Bougainvillea Wild (Nyctaginaceae: *Bougainvillaea*).

Other Data
1. Genotypes 1 and 4 are associated with more complicated disease and are less responsive to interferon treatment as compared to genotypes 2 and 3, especially in African-Americans with chronic hepatitis C.
2. The antiviral agent ribavirin may be an adjunctive therapy option in chronic HCV and may be considered in more complicated cases in addition to treatment with interferon.
3. Non-A, non-B HCV is most frequently the origin of parenterally induced hepatitis.
4. Genotype 4 is common in Eastern Mediterranean and Egypt; genotype 1 is common in Japan; genotype 3 is common in India.

Hepatitis Delta Antibody (Total Anti-HDV)—Serum

Norm. Negative.

Positive. Hepatitis D.

Description. An assay to identify total (that is, predominantly IgG) antibodies to the hepatitis D virus. Hepatitis D is an incomplete virus requiring the presence of HBsAg of the hepatitis B virus for replication and expression. It infects only clients concurrently infected with hepatitis B virus or those who have a preexisting hepatitis B virus infection. Hepatitis D virus is most common among intravenous drug abusers, hemophiliacs, and clients who have received multiple blood transfusions. It is a more severe form of hepatitis than hepatitis B alone, accounting for a higher incidence of chronic hepatitis and cirrhosis.

Clinically, hepatitis D virus cannot be distinguished from other types of hepatitis. Serologic tests must be positive for hepatitis B virus and total anti-HDV to make a diagnosis of hepatitis D. Hepatitis D virus is not a reportable disease in most of the United

States at the present time. Prevalence among health care workers is 8.6%. Incidence of hepatitis D has decreased markedly with use of HBV vaccine although increased prevalence seen in those with chronic HBV infection.

Professional Considerations
Consent form NOT required.

Preparation
1. Tube: Red topped, red/gray topped, or gold topped.
2. Screen the client for the use of herbal preparations or natural remedies such as Chinese *jin bu huan* ("gold-inconvertible," *Jin Bu Huan* Anodyne Tablets, patent medicine with misidentified constituents: essence of *t'ienchi [tianqi]* flowers, "Noto-ginseng"; also *kombucha*; also *Lycopodium serratum*, or club moss; but with plant alkaloid levotetrahydropalmatine, a potent neuroactive substance) and Bougainvillea Wild (Nyctaginaceae: *Bougainvillaea*).

Procedure

1. Draw a 3-mL blood sample.

Postprocedure Care

1. Remove the serum and freeze it if the blood will not be tested within 7 days.

Client and Family Teaching

1. Results may not be available for several days.

Factors That Affect Results

1. If the radioimmunoassay technique is used, injection of radionuclides within the previous week may falsely elevate results.
2. Clients with lipemia or high-titer rheumatoid factor may have false-positive results.
3. An herb or natural remedy that may cause hepatitis includes Chinese *jin bu huan* (see above).

4. An herb or natural remedy that decreases hepatitis is Bougainvillea Wild (Nyctaginaceae: *Bougainvillaea*).

Other Data

1. This test requires 2 mL of serum.
2. Serum is stable at room temperature for 7 days and indefinitely if frozen.
3. Blood is potentially infectious during all phases of active infection.
4. Clients who test positive for HBsAg are at risk for hepatitis D; however, immunity to hepatitis B virus provides immunity to hepatitis D virus.
5. Mortality is 30% in chronic cases.
6. In rare cases, HBsAg may be transiently undetectable in serum, resulting in an erroneous diagnosis of non-A, non-B hepatitis, unless specific testing for hepatitis D is performed.

Hepatobiliary Scan (HIDA Scan)—Diagnostic

Norm. Negative. Requires interpretation by a radiologist.

Normal anatomy and physiology of liver, spleen, and biliary tract as determined by a radiologist. Normal distribution of injectate: 86% in reticuloendothelial system (RES) of liver, 6% in spleen, 8% in RES of bone marrow.

Hepatobiliary (scan after IV injection of ^{99m}Tc-dimethylacetic acid): First-hour images show liver, cardiac, and vascular activity; gallbladder (GB) and common bile duct/bowel activity seen by 60 minutes. GB uptake should precede bowel visualization. An inflamed gallbladder will not take up radionuclide. In the presence of biliary tree obstruction, no radionuclide will be visualized beyond the point of obstruction.

Liver-spleen (scan after IV injection of technetium-99m radionuclide): Uniform uptake throughout liver and spleen. Decreased uptake, or "cold spots," seen in areas with space-occupying lesions such as in Caroli's disease. Increased blood flow to the liver will be evidenced by increased radionuclide uptake, or "hot spots".

Usage. Used to visualize biliary tract and to detect acute acalculous, acute cholecystitis, calculous cholecystitis (caused by obstruction of cystic ducts), bronchobiliary fistulas, gallbladder disease, hepatocellular disease, jaundice, liver cancer, liver metastasis, obstruction, and perihepatic abscess; used to study biliary kinetics (biliary dyskinesia, gallbladder ejection fraction); evaluates patency of biliary system and cystic duct, including postsurgically, and nonspecifically demonstrates focal disease as "cold spots" of nonuptake of the radionuclide. Detection of post liver transplant biliary complications. Evaluation of pediatric jaundice (choledocho cyst; biliary atresia versus neonatal hepatitis); congenital bronchobiliary fistula; conditions causing increased flow to the liver will appear as "hot spots". Diagnosing complication of gastric bypass called Roux-en-O configuration.

Description. The hepatobiliary scan is a radionuclide study that demonstrates hepatic parenchyma, extrahepatic bile ducts, gallbladder, and normal passage into the intestines as well as the position, size, and shape of the liver. Intravenously injected HIDA, a radionuclide, travels through the liver into the biliary system, enabling gamma camera imaging of the entire hepatobiliary system. The cells of the liver absorb the radionuclide within 30 minutes and can be observed on the scan before it is redeposited in the bloodstream and excreted. Dye is excreted in the bile, stored briefly in the gall-bladder, and eliminated through the intestine, all within 4 hours. Failure of the dye to appear in the intestines is indicative of obstruction.

Professional Considerations
Consent form IS required.

Risks
Infection.
Contraindications
During pregnancy or breast-feeding; in children.

Preparation
1. Establish intravenous access.
2. Have emergency equipment readily available.
3. See Client and Family Teaching.
4. Just before beginning the procedure, take a "time out" to verify the correct client, procedure, and site.

Procedure
1. The client is injected with radionuclide (usually ^{99m}Tc-IDA, the dose calculated by body weight) intravenously 30 minutes before the scan.
2. Delay imaging for 6-48 hours after injection for clients known to have hepatocellular disease.
3. The client is positioned supine on the scanning table during the scan.
4. A gamma camera is placed over the right upper quadrant of the abdomen.
5. Scintiphotos are obtained at 15, 30, 60, and 90 minutes after injection of the radiopharmaceutical.
6. The procedure is repeated at 2-6 hours and 24 hours if obstruction is suspected or when the biliary system was not visualized.

Postprocedure Care
1. For 24 hours after the procedure, wear rubber gloves when discarding urine.

Wash the gloved hands with soap and water before removing the gloves. Wash the hands again after the gloves have been removed.

Client and Family Teaching
1. Fast from food and fluids for 4-6 hours before the scan.
2. The scan takes 1.0-1.5 hours.
3. Report any sensations that might indicate an allergic reaction such as itching or difficulty in breathing.
4. Meticulously wash the hands with soap and water after each void for 24 hours after the procedure.
5. Results are normally available from the physician within 24 hours.

Factors That Affect Results
1. The scan must be performed promptly after the injection because radionuclides have a short transit time through the liver.
2. Do not schedule any other radionuclear scans within 24 hours of this scan.
3. If the client has just eaten, the gallbladder will be contracted and may not fill with HIDA, or if the client has not eaten for many hours, the gallbladder may be full of bile or sludge giving a false-positive study for acute cholecystitis.
4. Total parenteral nutrition may also result in impaired visualization of the gallbladder.
5. The presence of barium in the intestinal tract may inhibit gallbladder visualization.

Other Data
1. Health care professionals working in a nuclear medicine area must follow federal standards set by the Nuclear Regulatory Commission. These standards include precautions for handling the radioactive material and monitoring potential radiation exposure.
2. Most cases of chronic cholecystitis (range 28%-90%) present with normal HIDA scan findings.

HER-2/*neu* Oncogene (C-*erb*B-2, C-*erb*-S, Human Epidermal Growth Factor)—Specimen

Norm. Normally present in cell membranes as a single DNA copy. Must be interpreted by a pathologist.

Positive immunoassay (serum): >15 ng/mL or mcg/L.

Positive. Presence of either or both molecular genetic alterations:

Gene amplification	Multiple DNA copies, characterized by in situ fluorescence hybridization
Gene overexpression	Characterized by membrane immunostaining by immunohistochemistry

Negative. Absence of gene amplification or overexpression.

Usage. Determination of genetic abnormalities in effort to predict client response to hormonal therapy, adjuvant chemotherapy, and monoclonal antibody therapy.

Increased (Overexpressed). Brain cancer, breast cancer (found in 25%-30%, predictive of poor short-term prognosis, but can benefit from Herceptin therapy), bladder, cervical, colorectal cancer (predicts poor survival), endometrial carcinoma, esophageal cancer, hepatocellular, malignant mesothelioma, non–small-cell lung cancer, osteosarcoma (unfavorable prognosis) ovarian cancer, pancreatic adenocarcinoma, salivary duct, stomach, synovial sarcomas, uterine serous papillary carcinoma, and vulvar Paget disease. Contributes to tamoxifen resistance.

Description. HER-2/*neu* is an oncogene, located on long arm of chromosome 17, that codes for a transmembrane tyrosine kinase. Amplification of the gene product is noted in up to 30% of breast, ovarian, and endometrial carcinomas. High levels of the gene product are associated with low estrogen and progesterone receptor concentrations, and clients have little or no response to hormonal therapy. HER-2/*neu* overexpression is a phenotypic marker for comedocarcinoma, a subtype of intraductal carcinoma with necrosis. It is associated with increased risk of relapse and decreased survival time. Breast cancer clients with overexpression of HER-2/*neu* have a better response to doxorubicin HCl (Adriamycin)-based chemotherapy regimens. The predictive value of HER-2/*neu* is true only with node-positive disease. In clients with endometrial carcinoma, HER-2/*neu* is also associated with shorter overall survival. Testing for HER-2/*neu* overexpression is useful when one is predicting which clients will have a response to monoclonal antibodies directed against HER-2/*neu*. HER-2/*neu* is measured by several techniques including gene amplification, mRNA level, and immunohistochemical staining. Immunohistochemistry may be performed on serum, plasma, and fresh or paraffin-embedded tissue, but fresh tissue is the specimen of choice. Fluorescence in situ hybridization (FISH) is the gold standard for detecting HER-2/*neu* in breast cancer.

Professional Considerations

(See Biopsy, Site-specific—Specimen for technique steps for obtaining the tissue specimen.) The considerations that follow are specific to the correct processing of tissue to maximize accurate results.

Consent IS required if biopsy is performed; see Biopsy, Site-specific—Specimen for risks and contraindications. Informed consent is recommended for genetic testing.

Preparation

1. Obtain solid-tumor biopsy bottle for tissue specimen (fluorescent pink).
2. If paraffin block is to be made, obtain container with 10% formalin.

Procedure

1. Obtain tissue specimen by desired procedure or draw blood and place in appropriate container.
2. Cut tissue into small pieces and quick-freeze on dry ice, in cryostat, or in liquid nitrogen within 20 minutes of collection. Place in biopsy bottle or formalin if paraffin block to be made.
3. If paraffin block is to be assayed, it must be fixed for 12-24 hours, not to exceed 48 hours.

Postprocedure Care

1. Apply clean, sterile dressing to biopsy site.
2. Assess the site and vital signs for signs of bleeding. The frequency may vary with the physician. Generally, assess every 15 minutes the first hour, every 30 minutes the second hour, and then every hour × 4.
3. Observe for signs of infection (fever, chills, hypotension, tachycardia, inflammation at site) for 24-48 hours.

Client and Family Teaching

1. Provide emotional support to the client awaiting results.
2. If biopsy confirms cancer, additional tests will be prescribed to determine appropriate treatment.
3. Results may not be available for several days.

Factors That Affect Results

1. Dried specimens must be discarded.
2. Frozen tissue thawed.
3. Use of fixative other than 10% formalin.
4. Reagents with a high degree of sensitivity and specificity to HER-2/*neu* in paraffin-embedded tissues should be selected for this test, or the sensitivity of the reagent used should be characterized to correctly interpret the significance of the test results. Studies have shown wide variability in the efficacy of the various antibody reagents currently in use. The use of more than one antibody (that is, antibody "cocktails") may also improve immunostaining.
5. Refer to Appendix B, "Informed Consent for Genetic Testing".

Other Data

1. HER-2/*neu* E75 peptide vaccine stimulates specific immunity in disease-free breast cancer patients but immunity wanes with time requiring a booster.
2. On mammography calcifications were predictors of HER-2/*neu* overexpression.
3. Positive Her-2/*neu* places breast cancer patients at increased risk for recurrence so give trastuzumab. The FDA, in June 2011, approved Inform Duel ISH that measures the number of copies of HER2 gene in tumor tissue to determine if women with breast cancer are positive for HER2 and therefore candidates for Herceptin (trastuzumab).
4. The Genetic Information Nondiscrimination Act of 2008 prohibits health plans from using genetic family history or genetic test results from influencing eligibility or premiums for health insurance. It also prohibits employers from using this information to influence decisions about hiring, terminating employment, or employment pay, promotions or privileges.

Heroin—Urine

Norm. Negative.

Positive. With heroin use the concentration of heroin in the urine is >2 ng/mL.

Overdose Symptoms and Treatment

Symptoms. Bradycardia, euphoria, flushing, itching, hypotension, hypothermia, respiratory depression.

Treatment

NOTE: Treatment choice(s) depend(s) on client's history and condition and episode history.

1. Administer naloxone (Narcan).
2. Hemodialysis will NOT remove heroin.

Description. Heroin (diacetylmorphine), a drug of abuse, is made from morphine. The half-life is 1.7-4.5 hours. Heroin is rapidly metabolized back into morphine, and up to 67% of the dose is excreted in the urine as morphine or morphine glucuronides; 50% is excreted in the urine in the first 8 hours and 90% in the first 24 hours. Serum, plasma, hair, oral fluid, and sweat are other matrices for testing.

Professional Considerations

Consent form NOT required unless results may be used as legal evidence.

Preparation

1. Obtain clean urine cup.
2. If the specimen may be used as legal evidence, have the specimen collection witnessed.

Procedure

1. Obtain 50 mL of random urine in a clean container.

Postprocedure Care

1. Store samples at −20 degrees C.
2. If the specimen may be used as legal evidence, write the client's name, date, exact time of collection, and specimen source on the laboratory requisition. Sign, and have the witness sign, the laboratory requisition. Transport the specimen to the laboratory immediately in a sealed plastic

bag marked as legal evidence. All clients handling the specimen should sign and write the time of receipt on the laboratory requisition.

Client and Family Teaching

1. Refer clients with intentional overdose for crisis intervention.
2. Referrals to appropriate rehabilitation centers and therapeutic community programs should be offered to all addicted clients who may be interested.

Factors That Affect Results

1. False-positive results occur if the client ingested 20 mg of codeine cough syrup or 5-15 g of poppy seeds 24 hours before the sample was obtained.

2. Heroin is eliminated from the system in 2 days, but quinine, which is a nonnarcotic used as a diluent, may stay in the system for up to 1 week.

Other Data

1. Street heroin is generally 5%-10% actual heroin, with the usual euphoric dose taken by abusers equivalent to 10-20 mg of morphine.
2. Common complications of overdose are pulmonary edema, endocarditis, *Clostridium botulinum* infection, and septicemia.
3. Heroin is detected in 7% of all drivers having driving accidents.
4. 50% of persons in heroin maintenance programs still use heroin.
5. Meconin in urine may be a useful adjunct in detecting illicit opiate use.

Herpes Culture

See Viral Culture—Specimen.

Herpes Cytology—Specimen

Norm. Negative.

Positive. Genital herpes, herpes virus infection, meningitis, and vaginitis.

Description. Herpes simplex virus types 1 and 2 are two similar viruses but differ slightly in structure. Herpes simplex virus type 1 is generally found in the respiratory tract, eyes, or mouth (cold sores), and herpes simplex virus type 2 is found in the genitourinary tract (transmitted by sexual contact, or during childbirth for infants). Both viruses have been isolated in both locations. Cytology is the examination of cells under a microscope to establish the presence of the virus, which is seen as multinucleated epithelial cells with enlarged atypical nuclei. This can be performed using a Papanicolaou test and has an average sensitivity of 45%-50%.

Professional Considerations

Consent form NOT required.

Preparation

1. Obtain a sterile tongue depressor or swab, slides, and a 95% ethyl alcohol (ethanol) fixative.

Procedure

1. Scrape the lesion with the sterile tongue depressor.
2. Spread the scrapings evenly on the slide with the tongue depressor, or roll the specimen onto the slide using the swab.

Postprocedure Care

1. Fix the slide with the 95% ethyl alcohol fixative.
2. Deliver the specimen to the laboratory within 1 hour.
3. The final report for a negative culture takes 5 days.

Client and Family Teaching

1. If the client is pregnant, a cesarean section may be required if the virus is still present at the time of delivery. The risk of

miscarriage is higher than normal in women infected with genital herpes.

2. Pain from sores may be treated with mild analgesics, warm baths, or wet tea bags held over the site.

3. Safe sex practices to prevent transmission to partner(s):

a. Notify all sexual partners to be tested for the virus.

b. Do not have sex when blisters or sores are present. These usually take about 4 weeks to clear up completely.

c. Use a condom during all sexual activity, even if sores are not present. Spermicides containing nonoxynol-9 help kill the herpesvirus.

4. Antivirals may reduce viral shedding and relieve skin discomfort.

5. Lesions of confused clients should be covered with a dressing to prevent autoinoculation (spread from one site to another).

Factors That Affect Results

1. Air-drying or improper fixative will cause the laboratory to reject the specimen.

2. Smears with heavy inflammatory exudate are difficult to interpret because of the nonspecific staining technique.

Other Data

1. Viral serologic testing is more definitive, but serologic testing in herpes simplex virus is of little practical importance in clients with HIV because most are seropositive.

2. 50% of active lesions may not demonstrate herpes inclusions.

3. Lesions that are dry may be moistened with saline before being scraped.

Herpes Simplex Antibody—Blood

Norm. Negative, <0.25 by ELISA, or <1:10.

Positive. 1:10 to 1:100 indicates infection within 7 days; 1:100 to 1:500 current-to-late infection; >1:500 established latent infection.

Usage. Genital herpes, herpes simplex, and herpes zoster virus infection.

Description. See Herpes cytology—Specimen for a description of the virus characteristics. Peak antibody levels are reached 4-6 weeks after inoculation with the virus and decline and stabilize thereafter. The serum sample is incubated onto a solid phase, and enzyme activity is quantitated and compared to a set of controls.

Professional Considerations

Consent form NOT required.

Preparation

1. Tube: Red topped, red/gray topped, or gold topped.

Procedure

1. Draw a 10-mL blood sample.

Postprocedure Care

1. Deliver the sample to the laboratory within 1 hour.

Client and Family Teaching

1. See Herpes cytology—Specimen.

Factors That Affect Results

1. Hemolysis of the specimen invalidates the results.

2. Herpes simplex virus type 1, herpes simplex virus type 2, and varicella zoster may cross-react, but the antibody increase in the infecting virus usually exceeds that of the other antibodies.

Other Data

1. Diagnosis of a current infection should not be made based on the results of a single serum analysis. Collection of two samples, 10-14 days apart, is recommended.

2. 89% of people are seropositive (in the city of Amsterdam) with an increase in seropositive with age, people of Turkish and Moroccan origin, homosexual men, and low education level.

Herpes Virus Antigen, Direct Fluorescent Antibody—Specimen

Norm. Negative.

Usage. Cervicitis, encephalitis, and herpes simplex.

Description. See Herpes cytology—Specimen for a description of the characteristics of the virus. If emergent diagnosis is necessary (such as encephalitis), this is the most rapid and sensitive test if cytology findings are negative. The specimen is examined by immunofluorescence or immunoperoxidase technique.

Professional Considerations
Consent form NOT required.

Preparation
1. Obtain a sterile swab and a sterile specimen container or Culturette.

Procedure
1. Collect the specimen from the infected site as described previously.
2. Do NOT place the specimen in a fixative.

Postprocedure Care
1. Send the sample to the laboratory immediately or freeze it. This includes operative specimens and spinal fluid specimens.
2. This test should be performed immediately, day or night, and the laboratory should be notified of arriving specimens.

Client and Family Teaching
1. See Herpes cytology—Specimen.
2. Results are normally available within 24 hours.

Factors That Affect Results
1. Specimens will be rejected if placed in fixative.
2. Inflammatory exudate on specimens will cause nonspecific color development of the immunoperoxidase reagent.

Other Data
1. None.

Heterophile Agglutinins—Blood

Norm. Negative.

Positive. Cytomegalic inclusion disease (by cytomegalovirus), infectious mononucleosis (by Epstein-Barr virus), serum sickness, and toxoplasmosis.

Description. A heterophile antibody is capable of reacting with an antigen that is completely unrelated to the antigen originally stimulating its formation. This infectious mononucleosis screening procedure tests for the presence of agglutinins (indicated by clumping) reacting to the red blood cells of horses or sheep. Infectious mononucleosis is a viral infection characterized by fatigue, anorexia, swollen glands, fever, and sore throat. Symptoms may continue for up to 6 weeks. Mode of transmission is through person-to-person transmission of saliva through kissing, sneezing, or coughing. Generally, this test is positive 3-10 days after infection, peaks within 3 weeks, and can remain elevated for up to 1 year.

Professional Considerations
Consent form NOT required.

Preparation
1. Tube: Red topped, red/gray topped, or gold topped or lavender topped.

Procedure
1. Draw a 2.5-mL blood sample.

Postprocedure Care
1. None.

Client and Family Teaching
1. For clients testing positive:
   a. Drink plenty of fluids and eat a balanced diet, even if not hungry or thirsty.
   b. Use saltwater gargle for sore throat.
   c. Use the antipyretic recommended by the physician for fever.
   d. Get plenty of rest during the febrile period. Then limit physical activity for 5 weeks.
   e. Isolation is not necessary, but avoid coughing or sneezing on or near other persons as well as kissing other persons until cleared by the physician.

Factors That Affect Results
1. Hemolysis of the specimen invalidates the results.
2. This test may be falsely negative because of the occasional delay in the appearance of the agglutinins in the first 4 weeks after infection, despite the presence of clinical symptoms.
3. False-positive results (<2%) have been reported with Hodgkin's disease, lymphoma, acute lymphocytic leukemia, infectious hepatitis, pancreatic cancer,

H

cytomegalovirus, Burkitt's lymphoma, rheumatoid arthritis, malaria, and rubella.

Other Data

1. With infectious mononucleosis, heterophile antibodies appear in 60% of clients within 2 weeks and in 90% within 4 weeks. Most titers decline in 3-6 months.

2. 10% of true adult Epstein-Barr virus mononucleosis cases have negative heterophile agglutinins; the virus occurs more frequently in children. Epstein-Barr virus antibodies may occur in these cases.

3. See also Epstein-Barr virus, Serology— Blood.

Heterophile Screen

See **Monospot Screen**—Blood.

HFP

See **Hepatic Function Panel**—Blood.

HIDA Scan

See **Hepatobiliary Scan**—Diagnostic.

High-Density Lipoprotein (HDL) Cholesterol (HDL-C)—Blood

Norm.

High-Density Lipoprotein Cholesterol

Age (years)	Male		Female	
	mg/dL	SI Units mmol/L	mg/dL	SI Units mmol/L
Adults				
20-24	30-63	0.78-1.63	33-79	0.85-2.04
25-29	31-63	0.80-1.63	37-83	0.96-2.15
30-34	28-63	0.72-1.63	36-77	0.93-1.99
35-39	29-62	0.75-1.60	34-82	0.88-2.12
40-44	27-67	0.70-1.73	34-88	0.88-2.28
45-49	30-64	0.78-1.66	34-87	0.88-2.25
50-54	28-63	0.72-1.63	37-92	0.96-2.38
55-59	28-71	0.72-1.84	37-91	0.96-2.35
60-64	30-74	0.78-1.91	38-92	0.98-2.38
65-69	30-75	0.78-1.94	35-96	0.91-2.48
≥70	31-75	0.80-1.94	33-92	0.85-2.38
Children				
Cord blood	6-53	0.16-1.37	13-56	0.34-1.45
5-9 years	38-75	0.98-1.94	36-73	0.93-1.89
10-14 years	37-74	0.96-1.91	37-70	0.96-1.81
15-19 years	30-63	0.78-1.63	35-74	0.91-1.91

NOTE: Levels for African-Americans are approximately 10 mg/dL (0.26 mmol/L, SI units) higher than those listed above.

Increased. Alcoholism, chronic hepatitis, biliary cirrhosis (primary), familial hyperalphalipoproteinemia. Drugs include carbamazepine, chlorinated hydrocarbons, cimetidine, cyclofenil, estrogens (alone or with progesterone), ethyl alcohol (ethanol), fibric acid derivatives, lovastatin, niacin, nicotinic acid, phenobarbital, phenytoin, statins (modest effect), and terbutaline. Herbs or natural remedies: flaxseed, soybean, soy sauce. Dark chocolate, hazelnuts (>30 g/day), and walnuts.

Decreased. Arteriosclerosis, bacterial infections, cholestasis, coronary heart disease, Cushing syndrome, diabetes type 2, familial hypoalphalipoproteinemia or LCAT or CETP deficiencies, fish eye disease, hypercholesterolemia, hypertriglyceridemia, hypolipoproteinemia, liver disease, malignancy, metabolic syndrome, nephrotic syndrome, obesity (often), polycystic ovary syndrome (PCOS), renal disease, Tangier disease, type IV hyperlipoproteinemia, viral infections, welder occupation. Drugs include androgens, beta-adrenergic blockers, and intravenous immunoglobulin (IVIG). Diet high in carbohydrates.

Description. High-density lipoprotein (HDL) is a type of cholesterol carried by alpha-lipoprotein. HDL is believed to help protect against the risk of coronary artery disease and has been shown to be inversely related to the risk of coronary heart disease. HDL levels <35 mg/dL for men and <40 mg/dL for women are risk factors for coronary heart disease. HDL levels <40 mg/dL for males and <50 mg/dL for females are one of a group of indicators that together indicate the presence of metabolic syndrome.

Professional Considerations
Consent form NOT required.

Preparation
1. See Client and Family Teaching.
2. Tube: Lavender topped (2 tubes for lipid profile).

Procedure
1. Draw a 4-mL blood sample after patient has been sitting for 5 minutes.
2. Avoid prolonged use of tourniquet.

Postprocedure Care
1. Resume previous diet.

Client and Family Teaching
1. Fast for 12-14 hours before sampling. Nonfasting samples are acceptable if HDL-C is not part of lipid profile. Water is permitted.
2. For clients with low levels, provide information regarding the reduction of modifiable risk factors, that is, smoking, obesity, and physical inactivity.
3. A low-cholesterol diet includes avoidance of butter, lard, palm oil, coconut oil, pastries, waffles, avocados, olives, liver, bacon, luncheon meats, hot dogs, red meat, whole milk, cream, ice cream, and chocolate.

Factors That Affect Results
1. Consuming a diet high in carbohydrates or polyunsaturated fats or smoking cigarettes decreases the results.
2. Taking statins or other cholesterol-lowering medications. Fenofibrate therapy does NOT affect HDL cholesterol.

Other Data
1. For every 5 mg/dL decrease in HDL below the mean, the risk of coronary heart disease increases by 25%.
2. The National Cholesterol Education Program recommends all adults >20 years old be screened for coronary heart disease.
3. The National Lipid Association, the American Academy of Pediatrics, and the American Heart association recommend screening children as young as 2 years of age for familial hypercholesterolemia, which would be suspected with a fasting LDL of at least 160 mg/dL.
4. The AIM-HIGH trial of extended-release niacin found that there was no incremental benefit in people with low HDL and high triglycerides that reached target levels when treated with statins.
5. HDL deficiency linked to ABCA1 gene mutation.
6. See also Cholesterol—Blood; Low-density lipoprotein cholesterol—Blood.

High-Molecular-Weight Kininogen
See **Factor, Fitzgerald**—Plasma.

High-Resolution CT
See **Computed Tomography of the Body**—Diagnostic.

High-Sensitivity CRP

See **C-Reactive Protein**—Plasma or Serum.

His Bundle Electrography—Diagnostic

Norm. Atrial-to-His (A-H) interval = 50-120 msec; His-to-ventricular (H-V) activation = 35-55 msec.

Usage. Antidysrhythmic drug evaluation, precise location of bundle branch block, bypass tract physiology evaluation, decision-making about pacemaker implant, syncope evaluation, and differentiation of true AV (atrioventricular) block from concealed AV extrasystoles.

Description. His bundle electrography is the use of a bipolar catheter electrode system during right-sided heart catheterization for recording activity of rhythm and conduction in the bundle of His located in the heart. This test provides information on intra-atrial and intraventricular conduction that is not available with regular electrocardiography.

Professional Considerations
Consent form IS required.

Risks
Dysrhythmias, phlebitis, pulmonary emboli, thromboemboli, and hemorrhage.
Contraindications
Clients with coagulopathy and acute pulmonary embolism.

Preparation
1. Have emergency medication available for use in case a dysrhythmia develops.
2. See Client and Family Teaching.
3. Just before beginning the procedure, take a "time out" to verify the correct client, procedure, and site.

Procedure
1. A catheter is introduced through the femoral vein and guided by fluoroscopy to the right ventricle.
2. Leads I, II, and III placed on the limbs are recorded simultaneously with two intra-cardiac bipolar electrograms. One is in the high right atrium (HRA), and the other is over the septal leaflet of the tricuspid valve to record the bundle of His (HBE). The first deflection of the HBE represents right atrial activity. The second deflection represents His bundle activity. The third deflection represents ventricular activation.

Postprocedure Care
1. Monitor vital signs and lower extremity pulses and observe and palpate for hematoma at the catheter site every 15 minutes × 4 and then hourly × 4.
2. Maintain the extremity in extension until the frequent monitoring period has passed.
3. Assess the catheter site for bleeding every 30 minutes for 4 hours.

Client and Family Teaching
1. Fast from food and fluids for at least 6 hours.
2. The test takes 1-3 hours.
3. Results are available immediately.

Factors That Affect Results
1. Poor catheter positioning.

Other Data
1. See also Cardiac catheterization—Diagnostic for other care required.

Histamine Stimulation Test

See **Gastric Acid Secretion Test**—Diagnostic.

Histopathology—Specimen

Norm. Requires interpretation by pathologist.

Usage. *Histologic diagnosis*: Abortion, abscess, ache vulgaris, achlorhydria, actinomycosis, alcoholism, amenorrhea, amyloidosis, appendicitis, arthritis (osteoarthritis), brain tumors, cancers, cardiomyopathy, cervicitis, cholecystitis, cirrhosis,

Crohn's disease, Cushing's syndrome, cystitis, cytomegalovirus, dermatitis, diverticulitis, diverticulosis, duodenal ulcer, echinococcosis, ectopic pregnancy, eczema, emphysema, endometritis, epididymitis, esophagitis, esophagoscopy, fever of undetermined origin, fibrocystic breast disease, C-cell hyperplasia, ganglioneuroblastoma, gangrene, gastric ulcer, gastritis, genital herpes, giardiasis, glycogen storage disease, gynecomastia, hairy-cell leukemia, Hashimoto's thyroiditis, hemochromatosis, hepatitis, Hirschsprung's disease, histoplasmosis, Hodgkin's disease, hydatidiform mole, hyperaldosteronism, hyperparathyroidism, idiopathic thrombocytopenic purpura, infertility, insulinoma, intraductal breast papilloma, jaundice, kidney stone, legionnaires' disease, leprosy (Hansen's disease), lupus panniculitis, lymphogranuloma venereum, melanoma, metastasis, myocarditis, necrotizing granulomas (histoplasmosis), nephrolithiasis, neuropathy, pancreatitis, pelvic inflammatory disease, pemphigus, peptic ulcer, pericarditis, peripheral neuropathy, peritonitis, pleurisy, psoriasis, renal infarction, Reye's syndrome, rubeola, sarcoidosis, scleroderma, Sjögren's syndrome, stress ulcers, tumors, ulcerative colitis, vasculitis, Whipple's disease, and xerostomia.

Description. Specimen or tissue disorder involving gross and microscopic examination of biopsy sample and diagnosis by a qualified pathologist.

Professional Considerations
Consent form NOT required.

Preparation
1. Obtain a sterile container and fixative or formalin.
2. The requisition must include the operative diagnosis and the site of the specimen.

Procedure
1. The tissue or fluid sample is obtained by means of local or general anesthesia.
2. Label the specimen with the client's name, age, sex, room number, and operative diagnosis; the source of the specimen; and the surgeon and other physicians desiring a copy of the pathology report.

Postprocedure Care
1. Fresh tissue is fixed in phosphate-buffered formalin (5-20 times the bulk of the specimen) or submitted directly to a responsible party on saline-soaked sterile gauze.
2. Deliver the specimen to the laboratory within 1 hour.

Client and Family Teaching
1. The diagnosis will take 1 day or more.
2. See Biopsy, Site-specific—Specimen.

Factors That Affect Results
1. Poor sampling technique or contamination.
2. A sample that has become dried out will impair interpretation.

Other Data
1. Tissue fixed in formalin CANNOT be used for bacteriology, electron microscopy, estrogen or progesterone receptors, or histochemistry study.
2. See also Biopsy, Site-specific—Specimen.

Histoplasmosis Serology—Blood

Norm. Immunodiffusion test.

Negative. Complement fixation titer <1:4 (normal finding).

Positive. Histoplasmosis.

A positive Fungitell beta-glucan test has 87% sensitivity for histoplasmosis.

Complement fixation titer: Fourfold rise in titer indicates current infection.

Suspicious for infection: 1:8 to 1:16; diagnostic for active infection, >1:32.

Immunodiffusion test: Presence of H (active) and M (active, recent, or past) bands indicates infection.

Description. *Histoplasma capsulatum* is a soil saprobic fungus that resides in the intestines of birds and bats and causes a common respiratory, noncommunicable infection called "histoplasmosis." *H. capsulatum* spores are inhaled, enter the bloodstream, and spread through the reticuloendothelial system, causing breathing difficulty and enlargement of the spleen and lymph nodes. The antibody titers are usually elevated 6 weeks after infection, last weeks or months, and decline quickly, though they may remain elevated for up to 1 year.

Professional Considerations
Consent form NOT required.

Preparation
1. Tube: Red topped, red/gray topped, or gold topped.
2. Obtain travel history to identify exposure in high-risk endemic areas.
3. Ascertain if the client has been exposed to droppings of bats, chickens, pigeons, starlings, or blackbirds.
4. The sample should be drawn before the histoplasmosis skin test.

Procedure
1. Immunodiffusion: Draw a 4-mL blood sample.
2. Complement fixation: Draw a 2-mL blood sample.

Postprocedure Care
1. No special care required.

Client and Family Teaching
1. Signs and symptoms of histoplasmosis include flulike symptoms, pleuritic pain, pericarditis, pancytopenia, and hepatosplenomegaly.
2. HIV-positive clients should avoid travel to endemic areas (in the United States, these include the middle, central, and south central states).
3. Follow-up specimens should be drawn at 2- to 3-week intervals to identify fluctuating antibody levels.
4. A 3% solution of formalin sprayed on contaminated soil will destroy the fungi.

Factors That Affect Results
1. False-positive results can occur with aspergillosis, blastomycosis, and coccidioidomycosis.
2. A recent histoplasmosis skin test may falsely elevate titer.

Other Data
1. One third of all cases are in infants.
2. Histoplasmosis can cause pleural effusion.
3. Serum LDH levels of 600 IU/L or greater are suggestive of histoplasmosis.

Histoplasmosis Skin Test—Diagnostic

Norm. Negative as evidenced by no induration and erythema <5 mm in diameter.

Positive. Histoplasmosis.

Description. (See Histoplasmosis serology—Blood.) Skin tests become positive 2-3 weeks after infection and remain positive in 90% of the infected population for life.

Professional Considerations
Consent form NOT required.

Preparation
1. Travel history should be included as part of the client's health history to determine exposure to high-incidence endemic areas.
2. Obtain an alcohol wipe, a needle, a syringe, and histoplasmin—an antigen prepared from culture (usually commercially prepared).

Procedure
1. Histoplasmin is injected intradermally.
2. Record the location of the injection for reading.
3. The injection should follow a blood draw for serum titer.

Postprocedure Care
1. Read the test in 24-48 hours. An area of erythema and induration of >5-mm diameter is indicative of a positive reaction.

Client and Family Teaching
1. See Histoplasmosis serology—Blood.

Factors That Affect Results
1. Test may be falsely negative in 50% of people with disseminated histoplasmosis and 10% of people with cavitary histoplasmosis.
2. False-negative results may occur because of depressed immunologic status (not in HIV clients) or steroid therapy.
3. False-positive results may occur in people with blastomycosis (30%) or coccidioidomycosis (40%).

Other Data
1. Acutely ill clients may not have a positive skin reaction.
2. This test is not recommended because of the difficult interpretation and because it may cause the serology test to be falsely positive.

HIV Battery

See Acquired Immune Deficiency Syndrome Evaluation Battery—Diagnostic.

HIV Oral Test

See Oral Mucosal Transudate—Specimen.

HIV-1 P24 Antigen

See Acquired Immune Deficiency Syndrome Evaluation Battery—Diagnostic.

HLA B-27

See Human Leukocyte Antigen B-27—Blood.

Holter Monitor—Diagnostic

Norm. No dysrhythmias.

Usage. Brugada syndrome, cardiomyopathy, cerebral ischemia, dysrhythmias (detection), mitral valve prolapse, pacemaker function, palpitations, polyarteritis nodosa, sensing of atrial demand pacemaker failure, and syncope.

Description. A Holter monitor is a portable, miniaturized electrocardiographic amplifier coupled to a magnetic recorder. It is used to obtain a permanent recording of continuous electrocardiographic activity of a client for an extended period of time, such as 24-48 hours. The client wears the monitor continuously and must record all activity and symptoms experienced at the specific times of occurrence throughout the monitoring period. The resulting electrocardiographic recording is analyzed for abnormalities and correlated with the documented activities and symptoms to help diagnose or rule out abnormalities such as those listed under Usage.

Professional Considerations

Consent form NOT required.

Preparation

1. Explain purpose to client or family.
2. Obtain a diary and a pen or pencil, electrodes, and a Holter monitor.
3. The electrodes must be applied to skin free of hair (shaved) that has been cleansed with acetone.
4. See Client and Family Teaching.

Procedure

1. Assess for paper-roll availability with each monitor.
2. Maintain a diary of movements to assist the diagnostician in evaluating the heart rhythm.

Postprocedure Care

1. Remove all electrodes.

Client and Family Teaching

1. This monitor is used to identify abnormal heart rhythms that may occur for brief periods of time. Keeping a complete diary of times, activities, and sensations throughout monitoring helps pinpoint the cause of symptoms and the effect of activities on the heart.
2. Avoid bathing (other than sponge bath), magnets, metal detectors, high-voltage areas, and electric blankets because these may interfere with recording.

Factors That Affect Results

1. An incomplete diary interferes with accurate interpretation of findings.
2. Failure to apply electrodes correctly may cause an artifactual or incomplete signal.

Other Data

1. PVCs after remote MI often originate within scar tissue.
2. Paroxysmal atrial fibrillation present in 9.2% patients with stroke or TIA.
3. ST depression is associated with oxytocin during C-section.

4. Holters are useful in detecting cardiac disease in children with ADHD.

5. A wireless interface for and EEG/PSG Holter monitor exists.

Homocysteine—Plasma (Hcy) or Urine (HcySU)

Norm. NOTE: Studies are underway to establish reference levels. Norms below were taken from the findings of a variety of these initial studies. Higher homocysteine levels are almost always associated with low folate and vitamin B_{12} levels.

	SI Units
Plasma	
From the Hordaland Homocysteine Study:	
Norms in nonsmoking adults 40-42 years of age with high folate intake and who drink less than 1 cup of coffee per day	3.0-4.8 µmol/L
Findings from Other Studies:	
Preterm infants up to 48 hours of age	3.5-4.1 µmol/L
Term infants	4.8-7.4 µmol/L
12-19 years of age	
Male	4.3-9.9 µmol/L
Female	3.3-7.2 µmol/L
20-59 years	
Male	6.5-11.43 µmol/L
Female	5.35-9.95 µmol/L
>59 years	
Male	5.9-15.3 µmol/L
Female	5.3-15.3 µmol/L
Male and Female < 65 (Italy)	2.27-2.33 µmol/L
Male and Female > 65 (Italy)	2.84-2.96 µmol/L
>100 years	4.9-37.3 µmol/L
Urine	0-9 µmol/g of Creatinine

Increased. Aging, Alcohol ingestion, Alzheimer's disease, atherosclerosis, cancer, cardiovascular disease, carotid artery occlusion, cigarette smoking, coffee consumption, cognitive dysfunction, coronary artery ectasia, coronary syndrome (Severity), diabetes, diet high in polyunsaturated fatty acids and low in fiber, folate, and vitamin C, epilepsy, follicular phase of menstrual cycle, giant cell arteries, high protein meal (10%-15% at 6-8 hours after meal) homocystinuria, hypothyroidism, hypovolemia, inherited metabolic defects, Marfan syndrome, MI (severity), obesity, osteoporosis, ovarian syndrome, pancreatitis (chronic), panic disorder, peripheral artery disease (severity), polycystic polymyalgia rheumatica, pregnancy complications (pre-eclampsia, eclampsia), premature vascular disease, psoriasis, psychiatric disorders, renal failure (chronic), schizophrenia, sepsis, vitamin deficiency (ascorbic acid [vitamin C], cobalamin [vitamin B_{12}], folate-B_9, pyridoxine [vitamin B_6]), vitiligo (extensive). Drugs include androgens, cyclosporine (rat model), diuretics, fibric acid derivatives, isotretinoin (acne treatment), L-dopa, metformin, methotrexate, niacin, theophylline.

Decreased. Azoospermia, diet rich in wheat, Down syndrome, hyperthyroidism, pregnancy. Drugs include Betadine, celiprolol, estrogens, folic acid 5 mg daily, mesna, nebivolol, penicillamine, simvastatin, tamoxifen, vitamin B_{12} 1500 µg/day.

Description. Homocysteine is an amino acid that results from the metabolism of methionine by the B vitamins cobalamin, folate, pyridoxine, and riboflavin. The breakdown of methionine to homocysteine is counterbalanced by choline and betaine, coenzymes that convert homocysteine back into methionine. Although the exact function of homocysteine is not known, it is postulated that it may cause damage to the vascular endothelium or have a part in the causation of thrombi. Homocystinuria is an inherited disease in which persons who lack the enzymes that help control homocysteine levels demonstrate severe cardiovascular disease at a young age. Hyperhomocysteinemia has been established in recent years as an independent risk factor for cardiovascular disease, including atherosclerosis, carotid artery stenosis, coronary artery disease, stroke, peripheral vascular disease, and venous thrombosis. Elevated levels are also associated with fetal neural tube defects, recurrent spontaneous abortion, placental infarction, and reduced cognitive functioning in the elderly, and are considered to be a uremic toxin. Because firmly established reference ranges do not yet exist, homocysteine may often not be measured. Instead, physicians measure vitamin levels and, when vitamin deficiencies are found, infer elevated homocysteine levels. In other situations, homocysteine levels may be used as a functional test to determine folate deficiency because there exists an inverse relationship between the two values. The plasma test is best for this purpose and for assessment of cardiovascular risk. The urine homocysteine test should NOT be used in clients with renal failure, although it has been.

Professional Considerations
Consent form NOT required.

Preparation
1. *For plasma test*: Tube: lavender topped.
2. Obtain a clean, random urine specimen container and ice for urine test.

Procedure
1. *For plasma test:* Collect a 2-mL blood sample.

2. *For urine test*: Collect random urine sample from second morning void. Place specimen immediately on ice.

Postprocedure Care
1. Send specimen to the lab immediately.
2. Process specimen immediately (that is, within 30 minutes) to separate plasma. Specimen may be stored refrigerated or frozen up to 48 hours.

Client and Family Teaching
1. Fast from food and fluids for 8 hours before the test.

Factors That Affect Results
1. Levels are higher in smokers, coffee drinkers, diabetic clients, and persons who are obese or hypertensive.
2. Levels correlate directly with age and are higher in males than in females and in African-American women than in Caucasian women.
3. Falsely increased values will result if the specimen is allowed to sit without separation of the plasma because the red blood cells will continue to manufacture homocysteine in vitro.

Other Data
1. Folic acid and supplementation with vitamins B_{12} and B_6 are used to treat hyperhomocysteinemia.
2. Hyperhomocysteinemia is associated with a 4-fold increased risk of cerebral vein thrombosis and increased risk of stroke.
3. Increased levels are not a risk factor for cardiac events in metabolic syndrome patients.
4. No significant difference in values between vegetarian and non-vegetarian diets.

Homovanillic Acid (HVA)—24-Hour Urine

Norm. Measures of HVA and measures of creatinine as follows:

	µg of HVA/mg of Creatinine	SI Units µmol of HVA/mol of Creatinine
Adults	0.25-2.5 or <8 mg/24 hours	1-14 10-35 mol/24 hours
Children		
<1 year	1.2-35	7-192
1 year	4-23	22-126

Continued

	µg of HVA/mg of Creatinine	SI Units µmol of HVA/mol of Creatinine
2-4 years	0.5-14	3-77
5-9 years	0.5-9	3-49
10-14 years	0.25-12	1-66
15-18 years	0.5-2	3-11

Increased. Autistic children, brain tumor, Costello syndrome, ganglioneuroblastoma, occupational manganese exposure, neuroblastoma, and pheochromocytoma. Traffic police occupation. Drugs include aminosalicylic acid, disulfiram, levodopa, methocarbamol, pyridoxine, reserpine, and Robaxin. Increased urine levels in presence of DRD2 genotype of TaqIA1 allele, oral dietary supplement quercetin.

Decreased. Horner syndrome. Drugs include aminosalicylic acid, levodopa, methocarbamol, moclobemide, and monoamine oxidase inhibitors.

Description. Homovanillic acid is the major terminal metabolite of dopamine, one of the three catecholamines produced in the brain. Dopamine is broken down by the liver and excreted in the urine as homovanillic acid. Elevated levels can occur as a result of catecholamine-secreting tumors. Because urinary HVA levels fluctuate with creatinine excretion, results are normalized to the amount of creatinine present in the urine sample.

Professional Considerations
Consent form NOT required.

Preparation
1. Obtain a clean, 3-L container without preservative.
2. Write the beginning time of collection on the laboratory requisition.
3. See Client and Family Teaching.

Procedure
1. Discard the first morning urine specimen.
2. Save all urine voided for 24 hours in a refrigerated, clean, 3-L container to which 20 mL of hydrochloric acid (HCl) preservative has been added. Document the quantity of urine output during the collection period. Include the urine voided at the end of the 24-hour period. For catheterized clients, keep the drainage bag on ice and empty urine into the collection container hourly.

Postprocedure Care
1. Compare the urine quantity in the specimen container with the urinary output record for the test. If the specimen contains less urine than what was recorded as output, some of the sample may have been discarded, thus invalidating the test.
2. Document the quantity of urine output and the ending time for the collection period on the laboratory requisition.
3. Send the entire 24-hour urine specimen immediately to the laboratory for testing.

Client and Family Teaching
1. Avoid antihypertension agents, aspirin, caffeine, chocolate, coffee, fruit, onions, phenothiazine, tea, tomatoes and any vanilla-containing substances for 72 hours (3 days) before urine collection.
2. If taking levodopa medication, the physician may discontinue this medication for 2 weeks before the test.
3. Save all the urine voided in the 24-hour period and urinate before defecating to avoid loss of urine. If any urine is accidentally discarded, discard the entire specimen and restart the collection the next day.

Factors That Affect Results
1. Falsely elevated results may occur with excessive physical exercise or emotional stress.

Other Data
1. Homovanillic acid is usually measured simultaneously with metanephrine, normetanephrine, and vanillylmandelic acid to assist in differential diagnosis.
2. Relapse or progression of neuroblastoma cannot be detected reliably by tumor marker alone but a HVA/VMA ratio <1 or >2 has a poor prognosis.

Hormonal Evaluation, Cytologic—Specimen

Norm. Requires interpretation based on clinical status. Maturation index is reported as percentages of parabasal, intermediate, and superficial cells.

Usage. Amenorrhea, feminizing tumor, ovarian dysfunction, pituitary dysfunction, and virilizing tumor.

Description. Microscopic evaluation of cellular composition of the surface layers of the vaginal squamous epithelium, which reflects the balance of estrogen and progesterone.

Professional Considerations
Consent form NOT required.

Preparation
1. Obtain drapes, a sterile wooden spatula, a glass slide, and a fixative spray or 95% ethyl alcohol (ethanol).
2. The client should disrobe below the waist.
3. See Client and Family Teaching.

Procedure
1. Position the client in the dorsal lithotomy position, and drape her for privacy and comfort.
2. Use lubricating gel sparingly because excess will interfere with the cytologic examination.
3. Excess glove powder should be removed before the spatula is handled because starch granules make slide interpretation difficult.
4. Scrape the lateral vaginal wall with a sterile wooden spatula.

Postprocedure Care
1. Transfer the secretions to a glass slide and fix them with 95% ethyl alcohol or spray fixative.
2. Include on the laboratory requisition the date of the last menstrual period and history of radiation therapy or gynecologic surgery.

Client and Family Teaching
1. Do not douche for 24 hours before obtaining the smear.
2. The test is painless and takes only a moment.

Factors That Affect Results
1. A dried specimen caused by failure to apply fixative is cause for specimen rejection.
2. Agents that cause misleading desquamation include cortisone, digitalis, estrogen, and tetracycline suppositories.

Other Data
1. This test has limited value when applied to an individual because there is a great variation in normal values and between counters.
2. Smokers can have an absence of maturation of vaginal squamous cells as well as an earlier menopause.

HP

See Hypersensitivity Pneumonitis Serology—Blood.

HPRL

See Prolactin—Serum.

HPV

See Human Papillomavirus In Situ Hybridization—Specimen.

HRCT

See Computed Tomography of the Body—Diagnostic.

H

hsCRP

See **C-Reactive Protein**—Plasma or Serum.

hTau Antigen

See **Tau Test**—CSF.

Human Chorionic Gonadotropin (hCG), Beta Subunit—Serum

Norm.

		SI Units
Beta subunit	<2 ng/mL	<2 µg/L
	or <5 mIU/mL	<5 IU/L

Increased. Cancer (bladder, choriocarcinoma, colon, esophageal squamous cell, germ cell, gynecomastia, hepatoma, leiomyosarcoma, lung [NSCLC], osteosrcoma, [metastatic] ovarian, pancreas, pleomorphic, stomach, testicular, thymus), eclampsia, ectopic pregnancy, erythroblastosis fetalis, gynecomastia, hydatidiform mole, hyperreactio luteinalis, insulinoma, osteolytic meningioma, osteosarcoma, pregnancy, and seminoma.

Decreased. Abortion and ectopic pregnancy, nonviable in vitro fertilization, ruptured interstitial pregnancy, treatment success in ectopic pregnancy after MTX therapy.

Description. Human chorionic gonadotropin is a glycoprotein hormone with alpha and beta subunits, which are normally produced by a developing placenta and may be produced by some germ cell tumors. The alpha sequence is identical to the follicle-stimulating hormone, luteinizing hormone, and thyroid-stimulating hormone, and it can cause a false-positive pregnancy test if not tested along with the beta subunit. This test can detect pregnancy in as little as 1 week after conception. Serial monitoring is used to help determine gestational age. The beta subunit is often used to follow the status of neoplasms after surgery or chemotherapy. Elevated levels have been associated with a poor outcome in clients with colorectal cancer.

Professional Considerations

Consent form NOT required.

Preparation

1. Tube: Red topped, red/gray topped, or gold topped.
2. For females, write the date of the last menstrual cycle on the laboratory requisition.

Procedure

1. Obtain a 4-mL blood sample.

Postprocedure Care

1. Send the sample to the laboratory immediately. The sample can be kept at 2 to 8 degrees C for up to 24 hours. Additional delay in processing would require that the serum be frozen.

Client and Family Teaching

1. If the test is being used to determine pregnancy, results are normally available within 2 hours.
2. Additional samples will be drawn periodically to help determine fetal gestational age.

Factors That Affect Results

1. False-positive tests result from hemolyzed, lipemic, or icteric serum and pericardial cyst.
2. If the test is to be performed using radioimmunoassay, a radionuclide scan within 1 week of the test may falsely elevate results.
3. EDTA (ethylenediaminetetraacetate solution) and heparin anticoagulants decrease plasma levels and may cause false-negative results.
4. Values increase more slowly in ectopic than in normal pregnancies.

Other Data

1. Does not eliminate the possibility of pregnancy if results are low or borderline.
2. False-positive results have resulted in unnecessary treatment with chemotherapy

for suspected malignancy. One can confirm or exclude positive hCG tests by obtaining a quantitative urine hCG test. Assistance can be obtained from the hCG Reference Service when accuracy of results is questionable. (The hCG Reference Service is located at Yale University, New Haven, CT 06520.)

3. See also Pregnancy test, Routine—Serum.

Human Chorionic Gonadotropin (hCG, Pregnancy Test)

See **Pregnancy Test, Routine, Serum and Qualitative—Urine**.

Human Epidermal Growth Factor

See **HER-2/*neu* Oncogene—Specimen**.

Human Epididymis Protein 4 (HE4, WFDC2)—Blood

Norm. Reportable range: 30-854 pM. A change of greater than or equal to 25% is considered a significant change for the woman being monitored.

Premenopausal women: 95% of findings are less than 150 pM.

Postmenopausal women: 94% of findings are less than 150 pM.

Percent of Findings in Disease

	0-150 pM	>150 pM
Ovarian cancer	21%	79%
Benign gynecologic disease	93%	7%

Increased. Epithelial ovarian carcinoma, transitional cell urinary carcinoma (Xi, 2009).

Decreased. Not applicable.

Usage. Monitoring for recurrence (Anastasi, 2010a) of progressive disease in women who are undergoing or who have completed treatment for epithelial ovarian cancer. More sensitive than CA-125 for detecting stage I ovarian cancer. Helps distinguish epithelial ovarian carcinoma from benign disease of the ovaries.

Description. The HE4 ovarian cancer monitoring test is a quantitative test that measures the blood level of human epididymis protein 4 (HE4), which is produced by the WFDC2 (HE4) gene that is overexpressed when ovarian carcinoma is present. In comparison to CA-125, HE4 has fewer false-positive results when measured in women who do not have ovarian cancer. HE4 levels may help differentiate tumors of the ovary from endometriotic cysts of the ovary, because values are higher in malignancy.

Professional Considerations
Consent form NOT required.

Preparation
1. Tube: Red topped or a gel-barrier tube.

Procedure
1. Collect a 3-mL blood sample.
2. Separate serum.

Postprocedure Care
1. Refrigerate for up to 72 hours until testing. Test with the sample at room-temperature.

Client and Family Teaching
1. The HE4 protein is influenced by malignant and non-malignant conditions, thus additional confirmatory examinations and testing are needed when a significant change in values occurs.

Factors That Affect Results
1. HE4 is present in varying levels in ovarian, breast, endometrial, lung and gastrointestinal cancer; also present in healthy women (Anastasi, 2010b).
2. HE4 level is typically lower during pregnancy.
3. An elevated HE4 level can indicate recurrence of ovarian cancer, or benign gynecologic disease. Thus findings cannot be used alone for diagnosis of ovarian cancer.

4. HE4 levels are higher in older women and in women who began menstruating at an older age.

Other Data

1. Serial testing is recommended for monitoring ovarian cancer.

Human Immunodeficiency Virus

See Acquired Immune Deficiency Syndrome Evaluation Battery—Diagnostic.

Human Leukocyte Antigen (HLA) B-27—Blood

Norm. Requires clinical correlation.

Positive. Acute leukemia, ankylosing spondylitis (Marie-Strümpell disease), aortitis, arthritis (rheumatoid), Cogan's syndrome, congenital adrenal hyperplasia, Crohn's disease, erythema nodosum, Forestier's disease, gastroenteritis (joint pain), Goodpasture's syndrome, enthesitis, herpetic eye graft failure, HIV (low viral loads), IgA nephropathy, juvenile spondyloarthropathy, Ménière's disease (bilat), multiple myeloma, myelodysplastic syndrome, narcolepsy, pemphigus, periaortitis (chronic), psoriasis, reactive arthritis after salmonellosis, Reiter syndrome, sarcoidosis (pulmonary), sensorineural hearing loss, spondyloarthropathy, synovitis (chronic), thyroiditis (autoimmune, subacute), uveitis and viral diseases (EBV, HCV, HIV, HSV).

Negative. Normal finding.

Description. HLA-B27 is a major histocompatibility complex molecule whose primary function is to present endogenous peptides to T-cells and receptors on natural killer cells. The presence of B-27 antigen is highly correlated with ankylosing spondylitis and rheumatoid arthritis. There are currently (as of 2011) 75 alleles identified. Also see Human Leukocyte antigen typing—Blood for a description of the HLA tissue typing antigen.

Professional Considerations
Consent form NOT required.

Preparation

1. Tube: Green topped.
2. Preschedule this test with the laboratory.

Procedure

1. Draw a 10-mL blood sample.

Postprocedure Care

1. Send the specimen to the laboratory immediately; do not freeze it.

Client and Family Teaching

1. Results are normally available within 24 hours.

Factors That Affect Results

1. The test must be performed on live lymphocytes. If the cells have died, a new sample must be drawn.

Other Data

1. Clients who are HLA B-27 positive have a 120 times greater chance of developing ankylosing spondylitis than clients who are negative.
2. Potentially lethal inferior J-waves on ECG occur in 44% patients with ankylosing spondylitis.
3. HLA-B27 associated with high rate of spontaneous viral clearance in acute Hepatitis C patients of genotype 1 only.
4. Subtypes HLA-B 2707 and 2708 may be protective against ankylosing spondylitis.
5. HLA-B27 is a factor predisposing autosomal dominant PKD patients to insulin dependent diabetes post kidney transplant.

Human Leukocyte Antigen (HLA) Typing (Tissue Typing)—Blood

Norm. Interpretation required for tissue typing and determination of histocompatibility match or nonmatch. Ethnic alleles identified in the United States include: Caucasians DRB1*080101, African-Americans DRB1*080401, Asians DRB1*080302, and Hispanics DRB1*080201.

Usage. Paternity testing and transplants (to determine histocompatibility); selection of platelet donors for immunized clients. Those who carry the antigen have less erosive psoriatic arthritis. Used in determining IPEX (rare X-linked disorder) and echocardiography valve failure.

Description. Human leukocyte antigens (HLAs) are glycoproteins found on all nucleated cells. They result from four closely linked genes on chromosome 6 and are important to histocompatibility complement and immune response. The antigens are divided into A, B, C (Class I, derived from T cells), D, and DR (D-related, Class II, derived from B cells). There are multiple antigens of each type, meaning that the combinations of antigens that identify any individual are infinite. The HLAs are inherited as two sets (one from each parent) of six antigens. This test is most commonly used in bone marrow and renal transplantation. The antigens must match for transplantation to occur without organ rejection.

Professional Considerations
Consent form NOT required.

Preparation
1. Preschedule this test with the laboratory. The sample should be drawn before or 72 hours after a blood product transfusion.
2. *For donor specimen:* Tube: two green topped tubes.
3. *For recipient specimen:* Tube: red topped, red/gray topped, or gold topped.

Procedure
1. *Donor specimen:* Completely fill two green topped tubes with blood (7 mL each).
2. *Recipient specimen:* Completely fill a red topped tube with 7 mL of blood.

Postprocedure Care
1. Send the specimen to the laboratory for immediate testing.
2. Do not refrigerate or freeze the specimen or place the specimen on ice.

Client and Family Teaching
1. Encourage the client to express concerns regarding illness (such as awaiting a suitable donor, symptom management).

Factors That Affect Results
1. Refrigeration of or delay in processing specimens may result in inadequate lymphocytes for accurate testing.

Other Data
1. Samples that have been used for crossmatching should be frozen and stored for 1 year.
2. Bone marrow transplant clients or clients receiving chemotherapy with HLA-B51 or HLA-B52 who develop an infection at time of WBC nadir may develop ARDS.
3. Concentration of TNF-alpha in aqueous humor is significantly greater in HLA-B27–positive people.
4. See also Human leukocyte antigen B-27—Blood.

Human Papillomavirus (HPV) in Situ Hybridization—Specimen

Norm. Determination (by histopathologist) of absence of genetic changes consistent with the human papillomavirus.

Usage. Used to confirm HPV infection and to determine HPV type. Most specific for clients taking oral contraceptive pills to differentiate the mimicking of low-grade squamous intraepithelial lesions. Risk factor for oral cancer.

Description. Human papillomaviruses are DNA viruses that are known to cause Bowen's extragenital disease, warts, condyloma acuminatum, intraepithelial neoplasia, and anogenital, cervical, or oropharyngeal cancers. There are more than 70 different types of HPV, with about 20 of these types being associated with genital warts. Most genital warts are associated with the "low-risk" HPV types 6 and 11. Invasive carcinoma of the cervix, vulva, anus, and penis is associated with HPV types 16, 18, 33, 35, and 39. Endocervical carcinoma is associated with HPV 18. Although these specific associations exist, only a small proportion of HPV 16 and 18 lesions actually progress to a malignancy. In situ hybridization is a technique used to both confirm the presence of the HPV virus in a specimen and to type the HPV. DNA from the specimen is placed on a nitrocellulose membrane and fixed. The membrane can then be hybridized to a DNA sample of known sequence that is radioactively labeled. If the pathogenic DNA is present in the sample (such as HPV type 18), the sample DNA will hybridize to the known

DNA, producing a double-stranded DNA segment. The radioactive label is incorporated into the double-stranded DNA segment, allowing this segment to be detected by autoradiography.

Professional Considerations
Consent form IS required for the procedure used to obtain the specimen.

Risks
Bleeding, infection.
Contraindications
Bleeding disorder or anticoagulated state.

Preparation
1. Schedule collection from a female client when she is not menstruating, preferably 1 week after menses (especially important if a Pap smear is also being obtained).
2. A special collection kit is obtained from the laboratory that will be doing the hybridization. For *Detection and typing, HPV probe*, it is necessary to use the HPV collection kit (supplied by Roche).
3. Cervical swabs or biopsy specimens may be obtained from female client; urethral swabs are obtained from male clients.
4. Specimen collection cannot be performed after colposcopy if acetic acid is used.
5. If biopsy specimen is obtained, specimen should be approximately 3 mm in diameter. Specimen should immediately be placed in transport tube and frozen at ≈20 degrees C. If cervical (female) or urethral (male) swab is obtained, it is placed in a collection tube and may be stored at room temperature for up to 7 days.
6. Just before beginning the procedure, take a "time out" to verify the correct client, procedure, and site.

Procedure
1. *In situ hybridization:*
   a. Assist the client to the lithotomy position.
   b. A colposcope may be used to visualize the cervix and is inserted through the unlubricated speculum.
   c. Tissue sample(s) removed from any visible lesion(s) or doctor-selected site(s); enough for a minimum of eight 5-mm sections.
2. *DNA probe:*
   a. *Male*: Collect cells from the urethra using a swab. Place the collection device in the HPV transport tube for shipment to the lab.
   b. *Female*: Collect cervical cells from the endocervical canal and the exocervix using the HPV collection kit. Place a swab in the transport tube for shipment to the lab.

Postprocedure Care
1. Tissue: Submit the biopsy (frozen), 3 mm in diameter, in an HPV collection tube. Biopsy specimens must be shipped frozen at −20 degrees C.
2. Swab the cervix with silver nitrate to control bleeding after biopsy, and the examiner may insert a tampon if bleeding persists.
3. The tissue must be fixed with formalin solution immediately and then embedded in paraffin within 72 hours. Embed in paraffin in a way that the tissue section will fit into a 10-mm circle. The specimen must not remain in formalin beyond 72 hours.
4. Complete the laboratory requisition form, noting the number and appearance of tissue samples.

Client and Family Teaching
1. Rest for 8-24 hours after the procedure, avoiding heavy lifting or strenuous exercise.
2. Avoid douching and intercourse for 2 weeks or as directed by the physician.
3. An odorous, gray-green vaginal discharge is normal and may occur for up to 3 weeks after the procedure.
4. Some bleeding will occur normally, but inform the doctor if heavy bleeding (heavier than menstrual clots) occurs.
5. Mild discomfort during and after the procedure is normal. Take a nonaspirin analgesic as needed.
6. Results may not be available for several days.

Factors That Affect Results
1. Improperly fixed tissue cannot be used for this test.
2. An inadequate amount of tissue would cause specimen rejection.
3. Specimen has become thawed out.
4. Specimen was obtained after acetic acid application to biopsy or swab site.

Other Data

1. A DNA probe is used to aid in the diagnosis of sexually transmitted HPV infections, distinguishing between infections with types associated with low-grade squamous intraepithelial lesions (LSIL), types 6, 11, 42, 43, or 44, and types associated with SIL of all grades, including high-grade (HSIL), types 16, 18, 31, 33, 35, 45, 51, 52, and 56.
2. The 2006 National Cancer Institute Consensus Guidelines on HPV-Associated Cancer recommends that it is reasonable to obtain HPV genotyping assays in women who are at least 30 years of age and who have negative HPV cytology results. The polymerase chain reaction test for HPV detection can identify 9 specific types of the virus and FISH analysis is another method for detecting high risk HPV. Specimen collection and preprocedure and postprocedure care are essentially the same as for the in situ hybridization method.

Human Prolactin

See Prolactin—Serum.

Human Tumor Stem-Cell Assay—Diagnostic

Norm. Growth or inhibition of growth of tumor cells.

Usage. Determine the sensitivity or resistance of an individual's tumor cells to an anticancer drug.

Description. An in vitro test to determine responsiveness of tumor cells to specific drugs. A specimen of tumor is obtained from the individual. The cells are enzymatically dissociated, centrifuged, and placed into suspensions. Different anticancer drugs are added to each sample before being placed onto agar plates. The plates are examined microscopically twice each week for at least 2-3 weeks when cell growth is likely to have occurred. Growth of the cells implies resistance to the drug or irradiation, and lack of growth indicates some anticancer effect.

Professional Considerations

Consent form NOT required but IS required for the procedure used to obtain the specimen. See individual procedure for risks and contraindications.

Preparation

1. Prepare surgical instruments for tissue removal.

Procedure

1. Cells from the tumor are obtained and enzymatically dissociated in the laboratory.
2. The cells are examined microscopically twice a week for 2-3 weeks.

Postprocedure Care

1. Apply a sterile dressing to the incision site.
2. Observe the site for bleeding and symptoms of infection for 24-48 hours.
3. See Biopsy, Site-specific—Specimen.

Client and Family Teaching

1. Results take approximately 3 weeks but can help the physician select the treatment regimen most likely to be effective in destroying cancer cells.

Factors That Affect Results

1. Approximately 50% of tumors are unsuitable for in vitro growth, making the test difficult to interpret.

Other Data

1. Prediction of drug sensitivity is 40%-90% correct, and prediction of drug resistance is 90%-95% correct.

Hydrocephalus Radiologic Evaluation—Diagnostic

Norm. Absence of hydrocephalus.

Usage. Diagnosis of hydrocephalus and whether it is communicating or noncommunicating.

Description. Under computed tomography, radionuclide (usually technetium-99m) is tagged to albumin and injected into a lumbar puncture site. The radionuclide then travels upward into the brain, where it can be observed in terms of the amount of fluid and whether the fluid is able to travel into the ventricles (communicating). Noncommunicating hydrocephalus prevents the radionuclide from traveling into the ventricles.

Professional Considerations
Consent form IS required.

Risks
Increased intracranial pressure; allergic reaction to radiolabeled albumin (itching, hives, rash, tight feeling in the throat, shortness of breath, bronchospasm, anaphylaxis, death).

Contraindications
Previous allergy to radiolabeled albumin; increased intracranial pressure.

Preparation
1. Remove all metal objects from the client's head.
2. Obtain a lumbar puncture tray.
3. A CT scan is typically performed to rule out increased intracranial pressure before lumbar puncture in critically ill clients or those with changed mental status.
4. See Lumbar puncture—Diagnostic.

Procedure
1. Radiolabeled human serum albumin is given to demonstrate the flow of CSF from the point of the lumbar puncture up into the cranium.

Postprocedure Care
1. Assess vital signs every 15 minutes × 4.
2. Observe the client carefully for up to 60 minutes after the study for a possible (anaphylactic) reaction to the radionuclide.
3. For 24 hours wear rubber gloves when discarding urine after the procedure. Wash the gloved hands with soap and water before removing the gloves. Wash the ungloved hands after gloves are removed.

Client and Family Teaching
1. The test takes 1-2 hours.
2. Meticulously wash hands with soap and water after each void for 24 hours.

Factors That Affect Results
1. None.

Other Data
1. Health care professionals working in a nuclear medicine area must follow federal standards set by the Nuclear Regulatory Commission. These standards include precautions for handling radioactive material and monitoring of potential radiation exposure.
2. Technetium half-life is 6 hours.
3. MRI is an additional method for imaging CNS abnormalities in fetuses.
4. Hydrocephalus causes <5% cases of dementia.

Hydroxybutyrate Dehydrogenase (HBDH)—Blood

Norm. 140-350 IU/L.

Increased. Anemia (hemolytic or megaloblastic), carbon monoxide poisoning, hepatic cellular damage, leukemia, lymphoma, malignant melanoma, muscular dystrophy, myocardial infarction, nephrotic syndrome, and orthopedic hip surgery.

Decreased. Not clinically significant.

Description. Enzyme similar to lactate dehydrogenase 1 (LD1), which is found in the brain, heart muscle, kidney, and red blood cells. It is most generally used to diagnose myocardial infarction though levels may also be elevated when there is damage to other organs. HBDH levels are more specific and last longer than CK, AST, and total LD for diagnosing myocardial infarction.

HBDH levels rise within 8-10 hours of infarction, peak in 48-96 hours, and remain abnormal for 16-18 days. This test is primarily used in small laboratories where the complete LD isoenzyme battery is unavailable or because it is less costly and simpler to perform than LD electrophoresis.

Professional Considerations
Consent form NOT required.

Preparation
1. Tube: Red topped, red/gray topped, or gold topped.

Procedure
1. Draw a 7-mL blood sample, without hemolysis.

Postprocedure Care
1. Do not freeze the specimen.

Client and Family Teaching

1. Results are normally available within 24 hours.

Factors That Affect Results

1. Specimens may be falsely negative if frozen because enzyme activity is lost.

2. Traumatic venipuncture or hemolysis causes false-positive results.

Other Data

1. HBDH is stable at room temperature for 5 days and for 10 days refrigerated.

17-Hydroxycorticosteroids (17-OHCS)—24-Hour Urine

Norm.

		SI Units
Adult Female	2.5-10 mg/24 hours	6.9-27.6 μmol/24 hours
Adult Male	4.5-12 mg/24 hours	12.4-33.1 μmol/24 hours
Child		
0-1 year	0.5-1 mg/24 hours	1.4-2.8 μmol/24 hours
<12 years	1-4.5 mg/24 hours	2.8-12.4 μmol/24 hours

Increased. Acetonuria, acromegaly, chronic low back pain, Cushing's syndrome, fructosuria, glucosuria, hirsutism, hypertension (severe), insomnia, myelolipoma, obesity, pregnancy, stress, and virilization. Drugs include acetazolamide, ACTH, ascorbic acid, Atarax (hydroxyzine HCl), carbamazepine, cephalothin, cefoxitin, chloral hydrate, chlordiazepoxide, chlorpromazine, colchicine, cortisone acetate, digitalis glycosides, Doriden (glutethimide), erythromycin, etryptamine (alpha-ethyltryptamine), glutethimide, gonadotropins, hydrocortisone, hydroxyzine, iodides, mandelamine, meprobamate, methenamine, methicillin, methyprylon, oleandomycin, paraldehyde, quinidine, quinine, spironolactone, and troleandomycin.

Decreased. Addison's disease, anorexia nervosa, congenital adrenal hyperplasia, hypopituitarism, hypothyroidism, and workers exposed to polychlorinated biphenyls. Drugs include Apresoline (hydralazine HCl), carbamazepine, corticosteroids, dextropropoxyphene, estrogens, medroxyprogesterone, meperidine, morphine, oral contraceptives, pentazocine, phenothiazines, phenytoin, promethazine, reserpine (high doses), salicylates, and thiazide diuretics. Machiko et al (2003) found that levels decreased when clients relaxed by listening to their favorite music.

Description. 17-Hydroxycorticosteroids are carbon compounds that have a dihydroxyacetone group on the seventeenth carbon. In urine, the primary 17-OHCSs are breakdown products of cortisone and hydrocortisone, which can be used as a measure of their production (adrenocortical function).

Professional Considerations

Consent form NOT required.

Preparation

1. Obtain a 3-L plastic container with acetic, boric, or hydrochloric acid (HCl) additive.
2. Write the beginning time of collection on the laboratory requisition.
3. See Client and Family Teaching.

Procedure

1. Discard the first morning urine specimen.
2. Save all the urine voided for 24 hours in a clean, 3-L container (on ice) to which acetic acid, boric acid, or HCl preservative has been added. Document the quantity of urine output during the collection period. Include the urine voided at the end of the 24-hour period. For catheterized clients, keep the drainage bag on ice and empty urine into the collection container hourly.

Postprocedure Care

1. Compare the urine quantity in the specimen container with the urinary output record for the test. If the specimen contains less urine than what was recorded as output, some of the sample may have been discarded, thus invalidating the test.

2. Document the quantity of urine output and the ending time for the collection period on the laboratory requisition.
3. Send the entire 24-hour urine specimen to the laboratory for testing. Refrigerate or freeze the specimen after collection.

Client and Family Teaching

1. Stop all medications 24 hours before the collection of urine (with physician's approval).
2. Inform the physician ordering the test of any prescription or over-the-counter medications being taken.
3. Save all urine voided in the 24-hour period and urinate before defecating to avoid loss of urine. If any urine is accidentally discarded, discard the entire specimen and restart the collection the next day.

4. Resume medications after the 24-hour urine collection has been completed.

Factors That Affect Results

1. Increases in 17-OHCS levels can be caused by acute illness.
2. Methyprylon may interfere with the absorbance of both urinary 17-ketosteroids (using the Holtorff Koch modification of the Zimmerman reaction) and 17-hydroxycorticosteroids (using the modified Glenn-Nelson technique).

Other Data

1. Urinary free cortisol and serum cortisol levels are more sensitive and specific tests.
2. The specimen is stable up to 45 days if properly acidified and refrigerated.
3. See also Metyrapone test—Serum.

5-Hydroxyindoleacetic Acid (5-HIAA), Quantitative—24-Hour Urine

Norm. *Qualitative:* Negative, <131 μmol/24 hours.
Quantitative: 1-10 mg/24 hours (5.2-52 μmol/24 hours, SI units).

Increased. Carcinoid tumors (heart, foregut and midgut) and testicular tumors (when dietary sources of 5-HIAA are eliminated before testing), celiac sprue, diarrhea, endocarditis, ganglioneuroblastoma, oat cell carcinoma of bronchus, ovarian cancer, sperm motility and vitality is decreased, toxemia of pregnancy, tropical sprue, and ulcerative colitis. Drugs include acetaminophen, atenolol, cisplatin (peaks 6 hours after induction), diazepam, fluorouracil, glyceryl guaiacolate, melphalan, mephenesin carbamate, methocarbamol, naproxen, oxprenolol, phenacetin, pindolol, rauwolfia and reserpine. Plant seeds of *Griffonia simplicifolia* (treat depression/mood).

Decreased. Carcinoid tumors (rectal), depression, Hartnup disease, irritable bowel syndrome, mastocytosis, nonmetastatic carcinoid tumors, phenylketonuria, and small intestine resection. Drugs include acetic acid, corticotropin, dihydroxyphenylacetic acid, docetaxel, ethyl alcohol (ethanol), formaldehyde, gentisic acid, homogentisic acid, imipramine, isoniazid, lanreotide, levodopa, methenamine, methyldopa, monoamine oxidase (MAO) inhibitors, phenothiazines, salicylates, and sulfasalazine.

Description. 5-HIAA is a primary urinary metabolite of serotonin. Under normal conditions, serotonin is produced in the gastrointestinal tract and acts as a vasoconstrictor. Approximately 5% of serotonin is converted to 5-HIAA and excreted in the urine. Increased urinary 5-HIAA is reflective of overproduction of serotonin, which occurs with carcinoid tumors.

Professional Considerations

Consent form NOT required.

Preparation

1. Obtain a 3-L plastic container to which 12 g of boric acid or 25 mL of hydrochloric acid (HCl) has been added.
2. Write the beginning time of collection on the laboratory requisition.
3. See Client and Family Teaching.

Procedure

1. Discard the first morning urine specimen.
2. Save all the urine voided for 24 hours in a refrigerated, clean, 3-L container to which 12 g of boric acid or 24 mL of HCl has been added. Document the quantity of urine output during the collection period. Include the urine voided at the end of the 24-hour period. For catheterized clients, keep the drainage bag on ice and empty urine into the collection container hourly.

Postprocedure Care

1. Compare the urine quantity in the specimen container with the urinary output record for the test. If the specimen contains less urine than what was recorded as output, some of the sample may have been discarded, thus invalidating the test.
2. Document the quantity of urine output and the ending time for the collection period on the laboratory requisition.
3. Send the entire 24-hour urine specimen to the laboratory for testing.

Client and Family Teaching

1. Avoid the following foods 5 days before the test: alcohol, avocados, bananas, broccoli, cauliflower, eggplant, fish, kiwifruit, plums, plantain, pineapples, processed meat, seafood, tomatoes, and walnuts. These are sources of 5-HIAA.
2. Save all the urine voided in the 24-hour period and urinate before defecating to avoid loss of urine. If any urine is accidentally discarded, discard the entire specimen and restart the collection the next day.
3. Discontinue use of aspirin 5 days before urine collection.

Factors That Affect Results

1. Falsely elevated results may be caused by the ingestion of foods containing serotonin within 48 hours before specimen collection. Examples are avocados, bananas, eggplant, red plums, and tomatoes.
2. High triglyceride levels can cause lowering of urine 5-HIAA levels.
3. Prolonged-release lanreotide lowers urine 5-HIAA levels.
4. Iodine-131 MIBG used in imaging for carcinoid tumors decreases urine 5-HIAA significantly.
5. Marked variations occur with severity of diarrhea.

Other Data

1. Carcinoid tumors may cause increased excretion of tryptophan, 5-hydroxytryptophan, and histamine.

17-Hydroxyprogesterone (17-OHP)—Blood

Norm.

		SI Units
Adult Male	50-250 ng/dL	1.5-7.5 nmol/L
Adult Female		
Follicular phase	20-100 ng/dL	0.6-3.0 nmol/L
Midcycle peak	100-250 ng/dL	3.0-7.5 nmol/L
Luteal peak	100-500 ng/dL	3.0-15.5 nmol/L
PCOS diagnosis	0.37-0.97 ng/mL	
Children		
Cord blood	900-5000 ng/dL	27.3-151.5 nmol/L
Premature	26-568 ng/dL	0.8-17.0 nmol/L
Newborn	7-77 ng/dL	0.2-2.3 nmol/L
Child	3-90 ng/dL	0.1-2.7 nmol/L
Puberty, male	3-175 ng/dL	0.1-5.3 nmol/L
Puberty, female	3-265 ng/dL	0.1-8.0 nmol/L

Increased. Acne vulgaris, adrenal tumor, Antley-Bixler syndrome, congenital adrenal hyperplasia, germinoma, hirsutism, ovarian cysts, ovarian tumors, polycystic ovary syndrome (PCOS), and virilization. Drugs include steroids in preterm infants and metformin.

Decreased. Addison's disease, male pseudohermaphrodites. Drug betamethasone (used antenatally).

Description. 17-Hydroxyprogesterone (17-OHP), which is derived from progesterone, is the metabolic precursor of 11-deoxycortisol in cortisol biosynthesis. Elevated levels generally occur as a result of 21-hydroxylase or 11-hydroxylase deficiency. 17-OHP is converted and excreted as pregnanetriol.

Professional Considerations
Consent form NOT required.

Preparation
1. Tube: Red topped, red/gray topped, or gold topped; and ice.

Procedure
1. Draw a 1.5-mL blood sample. Place the sample immediately on ice.

Postprocedure Care
1. Deliver the sample to the laboratory within 30 minutes for immediate testing.

Client and Family Teaching
1. Results are normally available within 24 hours.

Factors That Affect Results
1. Recent radionuclide administration (within 48 hours) may cause false-positive results if the test is performed using radioimmunoassay technique.
2. False positives occur in neonates with CYP21 gene deficiency and very low birthweight infants with gestational age <32 weeks.
3. False negative values in severe salt wasting in children.

Other Data
1. Measurement of 11-deoxycortisol may help differentiate between 11- and 21-hydroxylase deficiencies.
2. Increased levels in preterm infants may be an indicator for early ICU care.

Hydroxyproline, Total—24-Hour Urine

Norm.

		SI Units
Adults		
18-21 years	20-55 mg/day	0.15-0.42 μmol/day
22-40 years	15-42 mg/day	0.11-0.32 μmol/day
41-55 years	15-43 mg/day	0.11-0.33 μmol/day
Children		
3 days	8-20 mg/day	0.06-0.15 μmol/day
1 month	32-63 mg/day	0.24-0.48 μmol/day
1-5 years	20-65 mg/day	0.15-0.49 μmol/day
6-10 years	35-150 mg/day	0.27-1.16 μmol/day
11-14 years	63-180 mg/day	0.48-1.37 μmol/day

Increased. Acromegaly, Albright's syndrome, bed rest, bone cancer, bone metastasis, bone osteopenia, burns (severe), congenital hypophosphatasia, diabetes mellitus, elderly, fibrous dysplasia, gastroenteritis, growth spurts, healing fracture, hyperparathyroidism, hyperpituitarism, hyperprolinemia type II, hyperthyroidism, Kashin-Beck disease, Marfan syndrome, multiple myeloma, osteomalacia, osteomyelitis, Paget's disease of the bone, psoriasis, rickets and sarcoidosis. Polluted areas with nitrogen dioxide. Drugs include growth hormone, parathyroid hormone, phenobarbital, sulfonylureas, thyroid hormone, and vitamin D. Herbal forms include Dan-Shao-Hua-Xian (DSHX), a Chinese herb.

Decreased. Hypoparathyroidism, hypopituitarism, hypothyroidism, malnutrition, and muscular dystrophy (chronic). Drugs include acetylsalicylic acid, antineoplastic agents, ascorbic acid, calcitonin, calcium gluconate, corticosteroids, diphosphonate, ergocalciferol, estradiol, estriol, glucocorticoids, mithramycin, and propranolol.

Description. Hydroxyproline is an amino acid found in collagen. Excretion of hydroxyproline in the urine is a useful measure of collagen turnover. It reflects bone resorption and is therefore a good test for monitoring the status of Paget's disease.

Professional Considerations
Consent form NOT required.

Preparation

1. Obtain a clean, 3-L container without preservative.
2. Write the beginning time of collection on the laboratory requisition.
3. See Client and Family Teaching.

Procedure

1. Discard the first morning urine specimen.
2. Save all the urine voided for 24 hours in a refrigerated, clean, 3-L container. Document the quantity of urine output during the collection period. Include the urine voided at the end of the 24-hour period. For catheterized clients, keep the drainage bag on ice and empty urine into the collection container hourly.

Postprocedure Care

1. Compare the urine quantity in the specimen container with the urinary output record for the test. If the specimen contains less urine than what was recorded as output, some of the sample may have been discarded, thus invalidating the test.
2. Document the quantity of urine output and the ending time for the collection period on the laboratory requisition.

3. Send the entire 24-hour urine specimen to the laboratory for testing and refrigerate it.

Client and Family Teaching

1. Avoid gelatin-containing foods and red meat, poultry, and fish 48 hours before urine collection, as this increases results.
2. Save all the urine voided in the 24-hour period and urinate before defecating to avoid loss of urine. If any urine is accidentally discarded, discard the entire specimen and restart the collection the next day.

Factors That Affect Results

1. Meat and gelatin may produce false-positive results.

Other Data

1. Normal range is higher in infancy, childhood, and adolescence, especially during growth spurts.
2. There is a diurnal variation in excretion, with higher levels excreted at night.
3. Urinary 3-hydroxyproline useful in cancer screening. Norms include 0.54-4.34 for males and 0.86-4.88 mg peptide/g creatinine for females.
4. Decreased 24-hour urine values for 4-hydroxyproline indicate Handigodu disease.

5-Hydroxytryptamine

See **Serotonin**—Serum or Blood.

Hypersensitivity Pneumonitis (HP) Serology—Blood

Norm. Negative or nondetected for the following: *Aspergillus flavus, Aspergillus fumigatus* #1, #2, #3, and #6, *Aureobasidium pullulans*, pigeon serum, *Micropolyspora faeni, Saccharomonospora viridis, Thermoactinomyces candidus, Thermoactinomyces sacchari*, and *Thermoactinomyces vulgaris* #1.

Positive. Asthma and farmer's lung. Workplace related to cockatiel, love-birds, pigeon, or chicken exposure, farming (mushroom/potato/onion), methotrexate exposure, methyl-methacrylate exposure to dental technicians, mold exposure (home, sausage), naphthalene-1,5-diisocyanate (NDI), working in the machining or plaster industry. Drugs include anagrelide with hydroxyurea, anthrax

vaccination, ciprofloxacin, dapsone, loxoprofen, or trofosfamide (Ixoten).

Description. Hypersensitivity pneumonitis (extrinsic allergic alveolitis) (HP) is an inflammatory, interstitial pneumonia that results from an immunologic reaction in response to over 200 inhaled antigens, resulting in dyspnea and coughing. Chronic HP can lead to irreversible pulmonary fibrosis. It is not clear if HP is immune complex-mediated or a cellular mediated disease although IL-17 is involved. Incidence is between 5% and 15% of the overall population. Genetic susceptibility in TAP1 and IL-6 genes. These antigens usually include organisms such as *Aspergillus fumigatus*,

Micropolyspora faeni, or *Thermoactinomyces vulgaris.* Other causes include triglycidyl isocyanurate, water-damaged buildings, dry cleaning exposure to tetrachloroethylene (TCE), exposure to hot tubs, stored maize corn, contaminated humidifier, or exposure to Esparto grass (Mediterranean).

Professional Considerations
Consent form NOT required.

Preparation
1. Tube: Red topped, red/gray topped, or gold topped.

Procedure
1. Obtain a 10-mL blood sample.

Postprocedure Care
1. None.

Client and Family Teaching
1. Results are normally available within 48 hours.

Factors That Affect Results
1. Reject hemolyzed, chylous, or contaminated samples.

Other Data
1. A client with no symptoms may produce a positive test, whereas a client with symptoms may produce a negative test. Careful correlation of clinical symptoms and laboratory results is mandatory.

Hyperventilation Test

Norm. No elevation in ST segment of ECG.

Usage. Provocative noninvasive diagnostic study used to identify coronary vasospasm as a causal agent in clients with variant angina and as an adjuvant test for anamnesis, epilepsy, panic disorder, and vegetative imbalance.

Positive. The hyperventilation test is positive when one of the following conditions is present on the ECG: ST-segment elevation ≥ 0.2 mV in two leads of the ECG during or after the test; ST-segment depression ≥ 0.1 mV in two leads after the completion of the test; inverted U wave not present on the baseline ECG; variant angina.

Description. Hyperventilation causes cellular alkalosis, which in turn promotes movement of calcium ions intracellularly, which leads to an increase in the tone of vascular smooth muscle in the coronary vasculature. The intent of this study is to induce vasoconstriction in the coronary arteries to determine alterations in myocardial tissue perfusion and oxygenation demonstrated on the ECG. Hyperventilation can facilitate induction of supraventricular tachycardia (SVT).

Professional Considerations
Consent form IS required.

Preparation
1. Test is best performed during the early morning hours between 0600 and 0800.
2. Vasodilators should not be administered 24-48 hours before the test.

Procedure
1. Perform baseline ECG.
2. Have client perform respirations of 35-40 breaths per minute × 6 minutes.
3. Arterial blood gas measurement should be completed at the end of the test to confirm an adequate alkalotic state (pH ≥ 7.55).

Postprocedure Care
1. Encourage client to rest after procedure.

Client and Family Teaching
1. Obtain a medical history before the test. Clients who have a history of pulmonary disease may be adversely affected or unable to tolerate the test and should be excluded.
2. Inform client to hold vasoactive medications before test.
3. Encourage client to verbalize any discomfort throughout and after the test.
4. Chest pain or ECG changes may not occur until completion of the 6 minutes of hyperventilation.
5. Dysrhythmias may occur, most commonly in test-positive clients.

Factors That Affect Results
1. Test becomes negative after abciximab administration.

Other Data
1. Calcium-channel blockers may be prescribed for clients having a positive hyperventilation test. Beta-adrenergic blockers should not be prescribed for clients having a positive hyperventilation test.

Hysterosalpingography (Uterosalpingography)—Diagnostic

Norm. Normal uterine cavity and fallopian tubes.

Usage. Identification of adhesions of peritoneum, hydrosalpinx, infertility, pelvic abscess or infection, tubal abnormality (44% of patients), tubal pregnancy, tubal ligation, and ureteroileal fistula confirmation.

Description. Using serial fluoroscopic radiographs, contrast medium (usually water-soluble diatrizoate or iothalamate) is inserted through the cervix so that the uterus, fallopian tubes, and lumens can be visualized. If laparoscopy is also used, the pelvic peritoneal space can be visualized. The test is used to identify malformations, foreign bodies, trauma, and fallopian-tube patency as well as fistulas or adhesions. Test has medium pain score of 5 (1-10 scale).

Professional Considerations

Consent form IS required.

Risks

Allergic reaction to dye (itching, hives, leukopenia, rash, tight feeling in the throat, shortness of breath, bronchospasm, anaphylaxis [severe], death); renal toxicity from contrast medium; uterine perforation; vascular injection of dye; and infection.

Contraindications

Previous allergy to iodine, shellfish, or radiographic dye; renal insufficiency; cervicitis; vaginal bleeding or infection; suspected pregnancy; and cardiopulmonary compromise.

Preparation

1. The test should be performed in the first part of the menstrual cycle.
2. Administer cleansing enemas.
3. Have emergency equipment readily available.
4. The client should disrobe and wear a gown and void just before the procedure.
5. Obtain a speculum, a uterine cannula, and dye (diatrizoate or iothalamate).
6. Measure and document baseline vital signs.
7. See Client and Family Teaching.
8. Just before beginning the procedure, take a "time out" to verify the correct client, procedure, and site.

Procedure

1. The client is positioned in the lithotomy position on a tilt table or regular procedure table.
2. A speculum is inserted into the vagina.
3. Under fluoroscopy, 6-10 mL (in 3-mL increments) of dye is injected into the cervical opening with a uterine cannula to fill the uterine cavity and fallopian tubes. The table is tilted (or the client is moved) to various positions to enable gravitational flow of the dye through the uterus and the fallopian tubes.
4. Radiographs are taken 8-24 hours later to help delineate delayed emptying when oily contrast medium is used.

Postprocedure Care

1. Assess for signs of gross bleeding or vaginal discharge.
2. Monitor vital signs every 15 minutes × 2 and then every 30 minutes × 2.
3. Small amounts of bloody vaginal discharge may be present up to 2 days postoperatively.

Client and Family Teaching

1. Take the prescribed laxative the night before the procedure. Cleansing enemas will be given before the procedure.
2. It is normal to experience cramping, similar to menstrual cramps, and dizziness during the procedure. Taking prostaglandin inhibitors such as ibuprofen before or after the procedure will lessen the cramping discomfort.
3. The procedure lasts about 45 minutes.
4. Avoid vaginal douching and sexual intercourse for 2 weeks after the procedure.

Factors That Affect Results

1. A normal fallopian tube may appear strictured if there is too much traction or if there is tubal spasm.
2. Fallopian tubes may appear normal in the presence of adhesions if too much traction is applied.

Other Data

1. Virtual hysterosalpingography is a non-invasive modality that combines hysterosalpingography techniques with multidetector CT scan.
2. See also Rubin's test—Diagnostic.

Hysteroscopy—Diagnostic

Norm. Uterine cavity normal.

Usage. Asherman's syndrome, endocervical biopsy, endometrial cavity evaluation, fibroid removal, hysterectomy, infertility, intrauterine adhesions, IUD or foreign body removal, septate uteri, and uterine arterial bleeding location.

Description. A 4-mm hysteroscope (telescope type of instrument) is inserted vaginally into the uterus to view the disorder within the uterine cavity that is sometimes missed by hysterosalpingography or curettage.

Professional Considerations
Consent form IS required.

Risks
Allergic reaction to Hyskon (32% solution of dextran 70 suspended in glucose) (itching, hives, rash, tight feeling in the throat, shortness of breath, bronchospasm, anaphylaxis, death); renal toxicity from contrast medium. Risks include infection, perforation, and a 1%-3% chance of developing PID. Possible life-threatening complications include disseminated intravascular coagulation (DIC) and acute respiratory distress syndrome (ARDS).

Contraindications
Previous allergy to Hyskon (if use is planned). Hysteroscopy is contraindicated in pelvic inflammatory disease (PID), inflamed cervix, and purulent vaginal discharge

Preparation
1. Schedule after menstrual bleeding has ceased and before ovulation.
2. Have emergency equipment readily available.
3. Have the client void before the procedure.

Procedure
1. A hysteroscope is inserted vaginally through the cervix into the uterus after the use of a speculum.
2. Carbon dioxide or Hyskon is instilled to distend the uterine cavity.
3. The interior walls of the uterus are closely examined for abnormalities, lesions, or bleeding, and photographs or biopsy specimens may be taken.
4. Just before beginning the procedure, take a "time out" to verify the correct client, procedure, and site.

Postprocedure Care
1. Assess for side effects from the use of carbon dioxide to distend the uterine cavity: shoulder pain, diaphoresis, nausea, and postoperative bleeding.
2. Assess for gas or air embolism, uterine perforation, and hemorrhage.
3. Assess for side effects of Hyskon: pulmonary edema, coagulation defects, and anaphylaxis.
4. Assess for hyponatremia and hypervolemia.
5. Assess for transient blindness if glycine is used as irrigation solution.

Client and Family Teaching
1. The procedure takes less than 30 minutes.
2. It is normal to experience cramping, similar to menstrual cramps, and dizziness during the procedure. Taking prostaglandin inhibitors such as ibuprofen before or after the procedure will lessen the cramping discomfort.
3. Carbon dioxide side effects (listed in option 1 under Postprocedure Care) may last for a few days. Use a mild analgesic to relieve discomfort.
4. Immediately report any nausea, pain, shortness of breath, or any other symptoms of discomfort after the procedure.
5. Avoid vaginal douching and sexual intercourse for 2 weeks after the procedure.
6. Infection rate following surgical hysteroscopy is low at 1.42%.

Factors That Affect Results
1. None found.

Other Data
1. Hysteroscopy did not improve the sensitivity of D&C in the detection of endometrial hyperplasia or carcinoma.
2. Paracervical anesthesia fails to reduce pain during outpatient hysteroscopy and endometrial biopsy.
3. Risk of vasovagal syndrome higher with use of rigid hysteroscope.

4. Uterine rupture can occur up to 1 year post hysteroscopy.
5. Peritonitis can occur from sorbitol used as a distending medium.
6. Saline contrast hysterosonography can replace hysteroscopy in evaluation of the uterine cavity.
7. High-volume surgeons have higher efficiency performing hysteroscopic myomectomy for fibroids.
8. Hysteroscopy is on the increase due to increased menorrhagia and postmenopausal bleeding.

Ibuprofen—Blood

Norm.

		SI Units
Therapeutic level	10-50 µg/mL	49-243 µmol/L
Toxic level	100-700 µg/mL	485-3395 µmol/L

Overdose Symptoms and Treatment

NOTE: Treatment choice(s) depend(s) on client's history and condition and episode history. *Symptoms.* The amount of ibuprofen ingested does not correlate well with symptoms. Ibuprofen overdose usually produces minimal symptoms of toxicity and is rarely fatal. Onset of symptoms generally occurs within 4 hours after ingestion, and clients with normal renal function usually recover completely within 24 hours with supportive care. Typical signs and symptoms include mild gastrointestinal symptoms such as nausea, anorexia, vomiting, and abdominal pain. Other signs and symptoms that may occur include gastrointestinal hemorrhage (especially in the elderly), headache, CNS depression (light-headedness, drowsiness, lethargy, coma), seizures, nystagmus, diplopia, tinnitus, hyperventilation, rash, hypotension, bradycardia, hypoprothrombinemia, hypothermia, hepatic failure, apnea, respiratory depression, and cardiac arrest. Renal insufficiency and secondary acute renal failure are generally reversible with supportive therapy.

Treatment of Overdose in Adults

Ingestion of <100 mg/kg	Encourage intake of milk or water to decrease gastrointestinal toxicity.
Ingestion of >100 mg/kg	Empty the stomach by emesis using ipecac syrup or gastric lavage. (Do NOT induce vomiting in clients with a decreased level of consciousness, clients with an absent or depressed gag reflex, or a client with a history of a seizure disorder.) After gastric emptying, a saline cathartic should be given.
Laboratory Monitoring	Renal function studies (BUN, creatinine, urinalysis): baseline and repeated in 1-2 weeks, ABG, CBC, liver function studies

Management of Specific Symptoms

Hypotension	IV fluids and dopamine if needed
Seizures (recurrent)	IV diazepam, followed by barbiturates
Symptomatic	Atropine for bradycardia
Severe metabolic	May treat with sodium bicarbonate (acidosis, pH <7.10)
Renal failure	Dopamine, dobutamine

1. The effectiveness of urine alkalinization to enhance urinary excretion is controversial.
2. Hemodialysis is not effective in the treatment of toxicity because of the high degree of protein binding of the drug.

3. Monitor for hematuria and proteinuria.
4. Observe and assess vital signs and neurologic status of symptomatic adults for 24 hours.
5. Asymptomatic adults should be observed for 4 hours.
6. Safety considerations and psychiatric consultation are indicated in intentional overdose.

Treatment of Overdose in Children

Amount Ingested	Treatment
<100 mg/kg	Generally unlikely to result in toxicity
	Home observation
	Caregiver education regarding signs and symptoms to monitor for any dangers of childhood poisoning
100-200 mg/kg	Empty the stomach by emesis and observe for 4 hours. (Do NOT induce vomiting in clients with a decreased LOC or an absent or depressed gag reflex, a child who ingested >400 mg/kg, or a client with a history of a seizure disorder.)
200-400 mg/kg	Gastric decontamination, followed by cathartic. Observe at least 4 hours.
>400 mg/kg	Immediate gastric lavage. Observe child carefully for seizure activity.

Usage. Ibuprofen blood levels are not generally indicated; however, they may be useful to identify drug concentrations when overdose, misuse, toxicity is suspected. Monitoring therapeutic levels in long-term ibuprofen use or when high doses are used in children with cystic fibrosis.

Description. Ibuprofen is a nonsteroidal anti-inflammatory drug (NSAID) that is also used for its antipyretic and analgesic activity. Its anti-inflammatory action is believed to be attributable to the inhibition of the synthesis or release of prostaglandins and to its antipyretic effect because of its action on the hypothalamus, with heat dissipation increased as a result of vasodilatation and increased peripheral blood flow. Ibuprofen is rapidly absorbed from the gastrointestinal tract and is 99% protein bound. It is metabolized in the liver and almost completely excreted in the urine 24 hours after ingestion. Half-life is 2-4 hours, with peak blood levels reached in 1-2 hours, though it may take up to 2 weeks to achieve therapeutic response for chronic inflammatory problems. Ibuprofen is used for rheumatoid arthritis and osteoarthritis, musculoskeletal disorders, fever, primary dysmenorrhea, gout, and dental pain. It can increase bleeding time by inhibiting platelet aggregation, though this action is reversible within 24 hours after the medication is discontinued. High-performance liquid chromatography is used to establish ibuprofen blood levels.

Professional Considerations
Consent form NOT required.

Preparation
1. Tube: Red topped. Plasma may be acceptable from tubes with heparin (green topped), EDTA (lavender topped), or sodium fluoride/potassium oxalate (gray topped). Use of gel tubes (red/gray topped) is NOT advised.

Procedure
1. Draw blood from opposite arm if client is receiving ibuprofen intravenously. Draw a 3-mL blood sample.
2. Refrigerated samples can be used for up to 2 weeks.

Postprocedure Care
1. If toxic levels are found, withhold the drug and notify the physician.

Client and Family Teaching
1. If overdose is suspected, prepare the client and family for supportive treatment outlined previously.
2. If overdose or toxicity occurred in child, instruct the child's parents or caregiver in safe, accurate administration of ibuprofen and review safety issues regarding prevention of accidental poisoning.
3. Refer clients with intentional overdose for crisis intervention.

Factors That Affect Results
1. None found.

Other Data

1. "STAT" ibuprofen blood levels are not widely available and are not frequently used in overdose or suspected toxicity cases. Because blood levels are not readily available during the relevant initial 4-hour period and there is little correlation between ibuprofen blood levels and symptoms, the management of ibuprofen overdose focuses on symptom management.
2. Ibuprofen blood levels are not generally monitored during routine ibuprofen therapy. Therapeutic response is monitored by evaluation of the degree of symptom relief.
3. Ibuprofen may decrease renal function because of the inhibition of renal prostaglandin synthesis. This is especially important in clients with decreased renal function or congestive heart failure, because renal prostaglandins may have a role in supporting renal perfusion in these clients. Serum BUN and creatinine levels should also be monitored in clients with impaired renal function, heart failure, or hepatic dysfunction, those receiving nephrotoxic drug concomitantly, dehydrated clients, and geriatric clients.
4. Liver-function studies should be monitored in long-term ibuprofen therapy.

IFN Gamma Assay

See RD1-Interferon Tests for Tuberculosis—Blood.

iFOBT

See Immunochemical Fecal Occult Blood Testing—Stool

IgA

See Immunoglobulin A—Serum.

IgD

See Immunoglobulin D—Serum.

IgE

See Immunoglobulin E—Serum.

IgG

See Immunoglobulin G—Serum.

IgM

See Immunoglobulin M—Serum.

¹²⁵I-Labeled Fibrinogen (Fibrinogen Uptake) Leg Scan—Diagnostic

Norm. No evidence of thrombi. No areas of abnormal concentration in the deep veins of the lower legs.

Usage. Used to monitor the development and progression of deep vein thromboses. Longitudinal screening for clients at risk for thrombotic processes.

Positive. Deep vein thrombosis, thrombophlebitis, and thrombosis.

Negative. Normal finding. Also negative after the active clotting process has stopped.

Description. Fibrinogen (factor I) is a complex polypeptide that converts to the insoluble polymer of fibrin after thrombin enzymatic action and combines with platelets to clot the blood. The ¹²⁵I-labeled fibrinogen leg scan is an invasive, nuclear medicine test involving the intravenous injection of radionuclide-labeled fibrinogen (fibrinogen labeled with radioactive iodine) and scanning with a well counter for subsequent incorporation of the radioactive material into a thrombus. The scan measures increased surface radioactivity (>20%), which indicates uptake by thrombi in the leg(s). The test is most useful in detecting actively forming thromboses of the calf; 85% of positive results are seen within the first 24 hours after the calf is injected with iodine-125.

Professional Considerations
Consent form IS required.

Risks
Infection, allergic reaction to radiolabeled fibrinogen (itching, hives, rash, tight feeling in the throat, shortness of breath, bronchospasm, anaphylaxis, death).

Contraindications
Anticoagulant therapy, bleeding disorders, thrombocytopenia, during pregnancy or breast-feeding, previous allergy to radiolabeled albumin.

Preparation
1. Ten drops of Lugol's solution in juice are given to block thyroid gland uptake of the radioactive tracer.
2. Establish 18-gauge intravenous access.
3. Have emergency equipment readily available.

4. Assess for swelling in the calf, tenderness, and cyanosis of the skin.
5. Assess for Homans' sign. Once it is determined to be positive, do NOT repeat Homans' sign assessment.
6. Elevate the legs during the imaging procedure, which takes about 10 minutes.
7. Just before beginning the procedure, take a "time out" to verify the correct client, procedure, and site.

Procedure
1. The client's legs are elevated during scanning to prevent pooling of blood in the veins of the legs.
2. ¹²⁵I-labeled fibrinogen is injected intravenously, and serial scans are performed on each leg 1, 4, 24, and 48 hours afterward. Surface radioactivity may be measured daily for as long as 2 days.
3. The extremity is marked in segments along the course of the vein tract.
4. Areas of fibrinogen incorporation into a thrombus are detected with the counter as areas exhibiting increased radioactivity, indicating increased concentration of radioactive tracer.

Postprocedure Care
1. Maintain bed rest if thrombi are detected.
2. Do not wash off markings on the extremity.
3. Assess the venipuncture site for infiltration.
4. Assess for swelling in the calf, tenderness, and cyanosis of the skin.
5. Observe the client carefully for up to 60 minutes after the study for a possible (anaphylactic) reaction to the radionuclide.
6. For 24 hours after the procedure, wear rubber gloves when discarding urine. Wash the gloved hands with soap and water before removing the gloves. Wash the ungloved hands after the gloves have been removed.

Client and Family Teaching
1. This test involves several leg scans after the client receives an intravenous tracer that shows up on the scan. Scanning may continue for up to 2 days after the injection.
2. The test poses no risk of radioactive damage to the client.

3. Maintain bed rest until deep venous thrombosis (DVT) has been ruled out.
4. Meticulously wash hands with soap and water after each void for 24 hours.

Factors That Affect Results
1. False-negative results may occur where active clot formation is completed, but the thrombus still remains.
2. Usually 1-2 days are required for enough radiolabeled fibrinogen to be incorporated into the clot before the clot can be detected.
3. Thrombi of the pelvis are difficult to detect with this test.
4. False-positive results may occur in clients with bacterial inflammatory conditions of the lower extremities.
5. A radioactive test within the previous 24 hours invalidates the results.

6. Up to 72 hours may elapse before the results become positive.

Other Data
1. Other tests to detect DVT are Doppler ultrasonography, venography, thermography, perfusion lung scan, gas ventilation lung scan, and pulmonary angiography.
2. This test is insensitive to upper thigh and pelvic vein thrombosis.
3. Rate of thrombosis is significantly less with laparoscopic intervention only.
4. Health care professionals working in a nuclear medicine area must follow federal standards set by the Nuclear Regulatory Commission. These standards include precautions for handling the radioactive material and monitoring of potential radiation exposure.
5. Iodine-125 half-life is 60 days.

Imipramine

See Tricyclic Antidepressants—Plasma or Serum.

Immune Complex Assay—Blood

Norm. Complexes not detected.
C1q binding: <13%.
Raji cell assay: <50 g of aggregated human gamma globulin equivalents (AHG).

Positive. Arthritis (rheumatoid), biliary cirrhosis, dengue fever, disseminated gonorrhea, endocarditis, glomerulonephritis, Hansen's disease (leprosy), Hodgkin's disease, leukemia, malaria, malignant melanoma, pulmonary fibrosis, schistosomiasis, serum hepatitis, serum sickness, Sjögren's syndrome, and systemic lupus erythematosus (SLE).

Description. Complements are proteins that, when activated, assist the cell lysis function of antibodies. Activation of complement by an antigen-antibody response is called the "classical pathway." Complement activation independent of antibody, initiated by complement binding to the surfaces of infectious organisms, is known as the "alternative pathway." Both pathways ultimately result in the complement cascade's formation of the membrane attack complex

(MAC). This radioimmunoassay (RIA) test is helpful in diagnosing autoimmune and infectious inflammatory disease processes.

Professional Considerations
Consent form NOT required.

Preparation
1. Tube: Red topped, red/gray topped, or gold topped.

Procedure
1. Draw a 2-mL blood sample.

Postprocedure Care
1. Write the collection time and date on the laboratory requisition.

Client and Family Teaching
1. Results are normally available within 2 days.

Factors That Affect Results
1. Reject specimens received more than 1 hour after collection.
2. Certain cryoglobulins, cold agglutinins, rheumatoid factors, and paraproteins may cause false-positive results.

Other Data

1. There are specific assays to measure different populations of immune complexes.
2. Also see Raji cell and immune complex assay—Blood.
3. Clinical information and physical findings may be the first sign of an immune complex disorder.
4. See also TA90 immune complex assay—Serum.

Immunochemical Fecal Occult Blood Testing (iFOBT, Fecal Immunochemical Testing, FIT)—Stool

Norm. Negative

Usage. Screening for colon cancer in average risk individuals. Not for use in individuals known to have an increased risk of colon cancer. Specific for detection of occult bleeding in the large colon.

Description. In contrast to traditional fecal occult blood testing, which detects the heme portion of red blood cells, immunochemical testing for blood in the stool uses of antibody binding to hemoglobin. Since globin from the upper gastrointestinal tract does not normally survive passage into the lower intestine, this test is specific for identifying lower gastrointestinal bleeding. iFOBT tests offer advantages over traditional FOBT for individuals (Allison and Potter, 2009) of average risk for colorectal cancer. The tests can detect bleeding in smaller amounts (as small as 0.3 ml/day) and are not affected by dietary intake or drugs such as NSAIDs or Vitamin C. In addition, they provide higher sensitivity (69%-100%) than traditional fecal occult blood testing (FOBT) (11%-68%) for detection of colorectal cancer and pre-cancerous adenomas in individuals of average risk for these conditions. Sensitivity can be less than traditional FOBT in individuals with an increased risk. Finally, test collection is simpler than other methods of fecal occult blood testing; thus, is well suited to self-collection of an at-home specimen.

Professional Considerations
Consent form NOT required.

Preparation

1. Obtain test kit.
2. No dietary restriction is needed.

Procedure

1. Place collection sheet or receptacle over the toilet.
2. Sample should be collected without allowing the stool sample to come into contact with the water in the toilet.
3. After defecation, twist open the cap of the sampling bottle, then scrape the stool in a circular motion with the testing probe. Make sure that the grooved portion of the probe is covered with stool, then insert the test probe into the sampling bottle, snapping the lid on tightly.
4. Flush the collection sheet and the remaining stool.

Postprocedure Care

1. Complete the label with individual identifying information. Then insert the sampling bottle into the mailing envelope and mail to the lab for testing.

Client and Family Teaching

1. Mail the sample promptly.
2. To reduce the chance of a false negative, daily samples collected over a 2-3 day period can be tested.

Factors That Affect Results

1. False negative results can occur when there is a delay in processing the specimen, or in the presence of colorectal cancer that does not or has not yet caused sufficient bleeding or that only bleeds intermittently.
2. Results are less likely than FOBT to be positive when the source of blood in the stool is from the upper gastrointestinal tract because the enzymes in the upper GI tract degrade globin, the target of this test.

Other Data

1. Because of the simplicity of sample collection, improved patient follow-through rates are seen when this test is used.
2. Colorectal cancer is the second highest cause of death from cancer in the United States. Populations that have lower than average rates of testing are those that have diabetes, are obese, or are current or former smokers.

3. Brand names of iFOBT tests include InSure (Enterix), Instant-View (Alpha Scientific Designs), immoCARE (Care Products, Inc.), MonoHaem (Chemicon International), and OC-Auto Micro (Polymedco).
4. See also ColoSure™ test—Stool; Occult blood—Stool.

Immunoelectrophoresis—Serum and Urine

Norm. *Serum:* No abnormal proteins present.
Urine: No abnormal proteins present; requires pathologist's interpretation.

Usage. Dysproteinemia, Hodgkin's disease, humoral immune deficiency, multiple myeloma, renal failure, and Waldenström's macroglobulinemia.

Description. A sample of serum or urine is placed on a slide containing agar gel, and an electrical current is passed through the gel, causing separation according to different electrical charges in each immunoglobulin: IgG, IgA, IgM, IgD, and IgE. Each immunoglobulin develops a band that has a certain curvature, position, and intensity of color. Abnormalities in any immunoglobulin cause the band for that precipitation to be displaced, bowed, lighter in color, thicker, or absent. After protein electrophoresis, antisera to immunoglobulins G, A, and M and to kappa and lambda light chains are applied to a urine sample to confirm and identify a suspected monoclonal protein or the presence of Bence Jones proteins (free kappa or lambda light chains).

Professional Considerations
Consent form NOT required.

Preparation
1. *For serum:* Tube: red topped, red/gray topped, or gold topped. *For urine:* Sterile urine collection container.

2. Record any vaccinations or immunizations within the previous 6 months on the laboratory requisition.
3. Record any blood or blood component therapy within the previous 6 weeks on the laboratory requisition.

Procedure
1. *For serum test:* Draw a 4-mL blood sample.
2. *For urine test:* Obtain a 12-mL urine sample in a sterile container.

Postprocedure Care
1. Refrigerate the urine; send it to the laboratory within 2 hours.

Client and Family Teaching
1. Results are normally available within 24 hours.

Factors That Affect Results
1. Anticoagulants, anticonvulsants, hydralazine, oral contraceptives, and phenylbutazone affect the thickness of the bands, causing difficult interpretation in serum tests.
2. Chemotherapy and radiation treatments affect color and thickness of the bands, adding difficulty to the interpretation of the serum test.

Other Data
1. This is a valuable initial screening tool for identifying diseases with altered protein fractions.
2. The urine test cannot be performed if urine protein is <60 mg/L or if urine protein electrophoresis is normal.

Immunofluorescence, Skin Biopsy—Specimen

Norm. Requires interpretation.

Positive. Collagen disease, dermatitis herpetiformis, immune complex glomerulonephritis, immune disorders of the lung, Kindler syndrome, lupus, malignant lymphoma, multiple myeloma, pemphigus, Waldenström's macroglobulinemia, Wegener's granulomatosis.

Negative. Keratinized tissue.

Description. This procedure uses fluorescent light to visualize tissue and subepidermal blood vessels for the presence of complement, immunoglobulins, and immune complexes containing antibodies and their antigens. Immune complexes are present in many autoimmune diseases, and identification of their presence in skin specimens can help to differentiate a diagnosis.

Professional Considerations

Consent form IS required for the procedure used to obtain the specimen. See Biopsy, Site-specific—Specimen for procedure-specific risks and contraindications.

Preparation

1. Obtain covered saline-soaked gauze or filter paper, a punch biopsy instrument, ice or a petri dish, and a local anesthetic.
2. The container must be labeled with the client's identification information and the date.
3. See Biopsy, Site-specific—Specimen.

Procedure

1. Local anesthetic may be injected into the biopsy site.
2. A 3-mm punch biopsy of tissue is collected and placed on ice or in a petri dish containing 0.9% saline.

Postprocedure Care

1. Send the moistened tissue sample to the laboratory immediately to be quickly frozen in liquid nitrogen.
2. The site may be left open to air or covered with a dry, sterile dressing.

Client and Family Teaching

1. Keep the site clean and dry and report any signs of infection, such as redness, pain (severe) for more than 24 hours, swelling, or purulent drainage.
2. Keep the site covered with a Band-Aid or gauze for 2 days, and then leave the site open to air.
3. Call the physician if there is bleeding amounting to more than a small area on the dressing, or bleeding that will not stop after pressure is applied for 5-10 minutes.
4. Use a mild analgesic as prescribed, if necessary, for site tenderness.

Factors That Affect Results

1. Reject specimens in a fixative or any that have dried out.

Other Data

1. Failure to detect IgG may be attributed to an infectious or inflammatory process in the sampled tissue.
2. Repeated biopsies may be necessary for diagnosis of dermatitis herpetiformis.
3. Skin biopsy in combination with histopathologic examination yields the best diagnostic results.
4. Submit an additional specimen in formalin for light microscopy.

Immunoglobulin A (IgA)—Serum

Norm.

		SI Units
Adults	90-400 mg/dL	0.9-4.00 g/L
Children		
Newborn	0-5 mg/dL	0-0.05 g/L
Infants, 25% of adults	0-11 mg/dL	0-0.11 g/L
1-3 months	7-34 mg/dL	0.07-0.34 g/L
4-6 months	10-46 mg/dL	0.10-0.46 g/L
7-12 months	19-55 mg/dL	0.19-0.55 g/L
13-24 months	26-74 mg/dL	0.26-0.74 g/L
25-36 months	34-108 mg/dL	0.34-1.08 g/L
3 years, 50% of adults		
3-5 years	66-120 mg/dL	0.66-1.20 g/L
6-8 years	79-169 mg/dL	0.79-1.69 g/L
9-11 years	71-191 mg/dL	0.71-1.91 g/L
12-16 years	85-211 mg/dL	0.85-2.11 g/L
>16 years	90-400 mg/dL	0.9-4.00 g/L

Increased. Arthritis (rheumatoid), autoimmune disorders, Berger's disease, carcinoma, chronic infections, cirrhosis, dysproteinemia, Henoch-Schönlein purpura, multiple myeloma, polio, sinusitis, and Wiskott-Aldrich syndrome.

Decreased. Bruton's disease, burns, childhood asthma, congenital IgA deficiency, hereditary ataxia telangiectasia, humoral immunodeficiency, hypogammaglobulinemia, nephrotic syndrome, and protein-losing enteropathies. Drugs include carbamazepine, dextran, estrogens, gold, methylprednisolone, oral contraceptives, penicillamine, phenytoin, and valproic acid.

Description. Immunoglobulin A (IgA) exists in both serum and secretory forms. IgA is the antibody effective against viruses and certain bacteria such as *Clostridium tetani*, *Corynebacterium diphtheriae*, and *Escherichia coli*. With an area of response localized primarily to mucosal membranes, it is the main immunoglobulin in colostrum, saliva, tears, and secretions of the bronchial, gastrointestinal, genitourinary, and respiratory tracts. IgA has been found in receptors on alveolar macrophages and on leukocytes and is most recently thought to perform a broad protective function in the respiratory tract. It protects by neutralizing invading viruses at the apical surface of endothelium after infection. In the blood, IgA normally constitutes 10%-15% of client's total serum immunoglobulins.

Professional Considerations
Consent form NOT required.

Preparation
1. Tube: Red topped, red/gray topped, or gold topped.
2. Write the client's age on the laboratory requisition.

Procedure
1. Draw a 4-mL blood sample.

Postprocedure Care
1. Refrigerate the specimen if it is not processed immediately.

Client and Family Teaching
1. Results are normally available within 24 hours.

Factors That Affect Results
1. Reject hemolyzed or turbid samples.

Other Data
1. IgA does not cross the placenta.
2. Clients with congenital IgA deficiency may develop anaphylaxis if transfused with blood products containing IgA.
3. Secretory IgA is under investigation for production rate in response to varying conditions. More than one study has found an increase in production of salivary IgA after subjects performed progressive relaxation techniques.

Immunoglobulin A (IgA) Antibodies—Serum

Norm. Antibody not present (negative).

Positive. Anaphylactic transfusion reaction in IgA-deficient individual; disease-specific IgA antibodies indicate past infection.

Description. Antibody formed against IgA when IgA is introduced into the bloodstream of a client with a congenital IgA deficiency. The IgA is recognized as a foreign antigen, with resultant action of IgG antibodies attacking it, causing anaphylaxis. Testing for IgA antibodies should be performed in all anaphylactic transfusion reactions. A particle gel immunoassay method being tested shows promise for rapid, sensitive, and reproducible detection of IgA antibodies, which can help to quickly confirm IgA transfusion reaction. Other uses for IgA antibody testing are to determine whether a client has had a past infection from a specific organism, such as *Actinomyces*, *Chlamydia pneumoniae*, *Entamoeba histolytica*, measles, polio, or *Toxoplasma gondii*.

Professional Considerations
Consent form NOT required.

Preparation
1. Tube: Red topped, red/gray topped, or gold topped.

Procedure
1. Draw a 4-mL blood sample.

Postprocedure Care
1. Give the client a wallet card, specifying the IgA deficiency.

Client and Family Teaching
1. If the test is positive, any future blood transfusions must be IgA deficient or else a severe allergic reaction will occur.

Factors That Affect Results
1. Temperature of specimen not held at 37 degrees C.

Other Data
1. None.

Immunoglobulin D (IgD)—Serum

Norm. Composes <1% of client's serum immunoglobulins.

		SI Units
Adult	0-8.0 mg/dL	5-30 μg/L
Newborn	<1.0 mg/dL	<10 μg/L

Increased. Chronic infections, connective tissue disease, dysproteinemia, and IgD myeloma.

Decreased. Acquired immunodeficiency syndrome. Drugs include phenytoin.

Description. Immunoglobulin D is a protein that may act as an autoimmune antibody in clients with collagen disease. The true biologic function of IgD is unknown but is suspected to play a role in the induction of humoral response and tolerance. The utility of this test is limited, because abnormal findings are rare.

Professional Considerations
Consent form NOT required.

Preparation
1. Tube: Red topped, red/gray topped, or gold topped.
2. Write the client's age on the laboratory requisition.

Procedure
1. Draw a 4-mL blood sample.

Postprocedure Care
1. None.

Client and Family Teaching
1. Results are normally available within 24 hours.

Factors That Affect Results
1. A chylous serum sample invalidates the results.

Other Data
1. 75% of IgD is in the intravascular compartment.
2. 90% of multiple myelomas are of the IgD type.

Immunoglobulin E (IgE)—Serum

Norm.

	IU/mL	U/mL	SI Units (μg/L)
Adults	3-423	4.2-592	10-1421
15-20 years	6.8-39.6	1.5-384	3.60-921.6
21-40 years	20.3-36.5	0.9-239	2.20-573.6
41-60 years	26-53	1.2-324	2.90-777.6
61-87 years	16.2-43.8	0.7-197	1.70-472.8
Children			
Cord blood	0.1-1.5	0.1-2	0.24-4.8
6 weeks	0.1-2.8	0.1-4	0.24-9.6
6 months	0.9-28	0.1-56	0.24-134.4
1 year	1.1-10.2	0.1-83	0.24-199.2
4 years	2.4-34.8	0.4-144	0.96-345.6
10 years	0.3-215	1.9-421	4.56-1010.4
14 years	1.9-159	1.6-456	3.84-1094.4

Increased. Alcohol intake (moderate or more), allergic rhinitis, asthma, atopic dermatitis, bronchopulmonary aspergillosis, eczema, food and (some) drug allergies, hay fever, IgE myeloma, insect sting allergy, occupations with high exposure to hairdressing chemicals, latex allergy, paracoccidioidomycosis, parasitic infections, pemphigoid, periarteritis nodosa, postoperatively (early phase, correlating with severity of surgical injury), sinusitis, visceral leishmaniasis, and Wiskott-Aldrich syndrome. Drugs include gold compounds. Herbal or natural remedies include documented reactions to garlic or *Echinacea*.

Decreased. Advanced carcinoma, agammaglobulinemia, alcoholics (after ethanol abstinence), ataxia-telangiectasia, and IgE deficiency. Drugs include phenytoin sodium. Herbal or natural remedies include *shoseiryu-to* ("minor blue dragon combination," *syo-seiryu-to, xiao-qing long-tang,* composed of *Pinellia, ma huang* [yellow vetch], peony, licorice, cinnamon bark, wild ginger [Asarum], schizandra [*Schisandra*], and ginger [*Panax*]).

Description. Immunoglobulin E is the antibody protein primarily responsible for allergic reactions such as hay fever, asthma, and allergies to foods and drugs, as well as atopic reactions such as latex allergies. When inhaled or ingested, IgE comes into contact with and activates the mast cells in the respiratory and gastrointestinal tracts and causes a histamine response in the body.

Professional Considerations
Consent form NOT required.

Preparation
1. Tube: Red topped, red/gray topped, or gold topped.
2. Write the client's age on the laboratory requisition.

Procedure
1. Draw a 4-mL blood sample.

Postprocedure Care
1. Handle the tube carefully because hemolysis invalidates the test.

Client and Family Teaching
1. IgE level is elevated in approximately half of people with allergies.

Factors That Affect Results
1. The test should not be performed if the client has undergone a radionuclide scan within the previous 72 hours.
2. Levels increase during allergic reactions and disease processes described previously, and decrease as symptoms subside and clinical conditions improve.

Other Data
1. 50% of IgE is intravascular.
2. Normal IgE levels do not exclude allergic phenomena.
3. IgE normally constitutes <0.1% of the client's immunoglobulins.
4. Among investigational treatments being studied for allergic conditions are an anti-IgE therapy using immunoglobulin directed against IgE and the use of disodium cromoglycate for reduction of IgE production.

Immunoglobulin G (IgG)—Serum

Norm. Normally constitutes 75% of client's total immunoglobulins.

		SI Units
Adults	565-1765 mg/dL	5.65-17.65 g/L
Children		
Cord blood	650-1600 mg/dL	6.5-16.0 g/L
1 month	250-900 mg/dL	2.5-9.0 g/L
2-5 months	200-700 mg/dL	2.0-7.0 g/L
6-9 months	220-900 mg/dL	2.2-9.0 g/L
10-12 months	290-1070 mg/dL	2.9-10.7 g/L
1 year	340-1200 mg/dL	3.4-12.0 g/L
2-3 years	420-1200 mg/dL	4.2-12.0 g/L
4-6 years	460-1240 mg/dL	4.6-12.4 g/L
>6 years	650-1600 mg/dL	6.5-16.0 g/L

Increased. Infections (chronic or recurrent), liver disease (chronic), malignancies (lymphomas), multiple myeloma, pulmonary tuberculosis, rheumatoid arthritis, sarcoidosis, systemic lupus erythematosus, toxoplasmosis, and Waldenström's disease. The IgG titer is usually elevated in clients with *Helicobacter pylori*, indicating active infection.

Decreased. Acquired immunodeficiency syndrome, aplastic anemia, humoral immunodeficiency, and Wiskott-Aldrich syndrome.

Description. Immunoglobulin G is comprised of four subclasses, IgG1 through IgG4, and constitutes 75% of all immunoglobulins in the bloodstream. IgG possesses antibody activity against viruses, some bacteria, and toxins. It is able to cross the placenta and provide immunity to a developing fetus and also serves as an activator of the complement system. IgG levels increase in response to infection and remain elevated, even if the infection becomes chronic. IgG is also important in autoimmune diseases because many of the autoantibodies belong in this class. This test evaluates humoral immunity and monitors therapy in IgG myeloma. Various forms of IgG assays are designed to pinpoint disease-specific IgG antibodies for a variety of infections. Subclass measurement and evaluation of IgG is not useful because clients with subclass deficiency often show normal IgG function.

Professional Considerations
Consent form NOT required.

Preparation
1. Tube: Red topped, red/gray topped, or gold topped.

2. Write the client's age on the laboratory requisition.

Procedure
1. Draw a 4-mL blood sample.

Postprocedure Care
1. None required.

Client and Family Teaching
1. Results are normally available within 24 hours.

Factors That Affect Results
1. Specimens should be stored at 37 degrees C.

Other Data
1. IgG is the only immunoglobulin that crosses the placenta.
2. Laboratory-based serology titers should be obtained to quantitate the antibody level and establish a baseline when treatment for *H. pylori* is planned. This allows for follow-up after therapy, which, if successful, will usually show a consistent fall in IgG titer levels.
3. A dipstick dye immunoassay is available to detect IgG and IgM antibodies in toxoplasmosis.

Immunoglobulin G (IgG) Synthesis Rate, Cerebrospinal Fluid

See **Cerebrospinal Fluid, Immunoglobulin G, Immunoglobulin G Ratios and Immunoglobulin G Index, Immunoglobulin G Synthesis Rate**—Specimen.

Immunoglobulin M (IgM)—Serum

Norm. Normally constitutes 5%-10% of the client's total immunoglobulins.

		SI Units
Adults	35-375 mg/dL	0.35-3.75 g/L
Children		
Cord	0-19 mg/dL	0.000.19 g/L
1-3 months	7-78 mg/dL	0.07-0.78 g/L
3-6 months	19-72 mg/dL	0.19-0.72 g/L
6-12 months	21-104 mg/dL	0.21-1.04 g/L
1-2 years	19-148 mg/dL	0.19-1.48 g/L
2-3 years	40-151 mg/dL	0.40-1.51 g/L
3-5 years	28-142 mg/dL	0.28-1.42 g/L
5-8 years	30-162 mg/dL	0.30-1.62 g/L
8-12 years	24-161 mg/dL	0.24-1.61 g/L
12-16 years	26-221 mg/dL	0.26-2.21 g/L
Pregnancy	IgM development during pregnancy occurs at an increase of 0.5 mg/dL per week of gestation.	

Increased. Biliary cirrhosis, collagen vascular disease, cutaneous leishmaniasis, cytomegalovirus, dysproteinemia, hyperimmunoglobulin M syndrome (HIGM), infection (bacterial, parasitic), leptospirosis, Lyme disease, reticulosis, rheumatoid arthritis, sarcoidosis, toxoplasmosis, trypanosomiasis parasite, and Waldenström's macroglobulinemia. Drugs include chlorpromazine.

Decreased. Humoral immunodeficiency, hypogammaglobulinemia, multiple myeloma IgA or IgG, and protein-losing enteropathy. Drugs include carbamazepine and dextran.

Description. Immunoglobulin M is the first antibody to appear after an antigen enters the body and is active against gram-negative organisms and rheumatoid factors. IgM forms the natural antibodies such as those to the ABO blood groups. The IgM molecule is too large to cross the placenta; thus it does not help provide fetal immunity to antigens. If levels are elevated in cord blood samples, it may indicate that the infant was infected before birth with organisms that can cause birth defects, such as *Toxoplasma gondii*, cytomegalovirus, or togavirus (causing rubella). This test is used to screen for congenital infections and to help diagnose and monitor infections.

Professional Considerations
Consent form NOT required.

Preparation
1. Tube: Red topped, red/gray topped, or gold topped.

Procedure
1. Draw a 4-mL blood sample.

Postprocedure Care
1. None.

Client and Family Teaching
1. Results are normally available within 24 hours.

Factors That Affect Results
1. Specimen storage at a temperature other than 37 degrees C may cause falsely decreased results.
2. IgM responses may remain positive for up to 20 years after a client has had Lyme disease.

Other Data
1. A dipstick dye immunoassay is available to detect IgG and IgM antibodies in toxoplasmosis. A dipstick assay that detects IgM antibodies in brucellosis is much less sensitive (28%) than the standard serum agglutination test (87%).

Indentation Tonometry
See **Tonometry Test for Glaucoma**—Screen.

Indican—Urine

Norm. <220 µmol in 24 hours, or negative.

Positive. Hartnup disease and ileal dysfunction.

Negative. Normal protein catabolism or intestinal absorption.

Description. Indican is a tryptophan metabolite that is excreted mostly in the feces but also in small amounts in the urine as a result of absorption and detoxification of indole produced by bacterial action on tryptophan in the intestines. The presence of indican in the urine indicates amino acid malabsorption.

Professional Considerations
Consent form NOT required.

Preparation
1. Obtain a sterile plastic container.
2. A sample from a first-morning void or an aliquot of a 24-hour collection is preferred.

Procedure
1. Collect at least a 6-mL or a random urine specimen in a sterile plastic container.

Postprocedure Care

1. Transport the specimen to the laboratory within 1 hour after collection and refrigerate until testing.

Client and Family Teaching

1. Results are normally available within 24 hours.

Factors That Affect Results

1. Results are invalid if the urine is not delivered to the laboratory within 1 hour after collection.

Other Data

1. Increased indican may cause the urine specimen to blacken in color over time.

Indirect Antiglobulin Test

See Coombs' Test, Indirect—Serum.

Infectious Mononucleosis Screening Test

See Heterophil Agglutinins—Blood.

Infertility Screen—Specimen

Norm.

Multiplex polymerase chain reaction test:	Negative
Antisperm antibody test:	Negative for sperm agglutinating antibody
Semen analysis:	*See Semen analysis—Specimen*

Usage. Evaluation for possible causes of infertility.

Description. The infertility screen includes tests of sperm function, antisperm antibody detection, and a genetic test to detect deletion of the Y chromosome long arm DAZ (deleted in azoospermia) gene. This screen may be done alone or as part of a full infertility evaluation that narrows down causes of infertility into the following common categories: abnormal sperm function, abnormal ovulation, tubal dysfunction, antisperm antibodies, and genetic causes. For *evaluation of sperm function*, semen is analyzed for the presence, number, volume, motility, morphology, and liquefaction time of sperm. *To test for the presence of antisperm antibodies*, spermatozoa, cervical mucus, and both male serum and female serum are analyzed using an enzyme-linked immunosorbent assay, mixed antiglobulin reaction (MAR) with or without immunobead-binding tests, which can identify IgG, IgA, and IgM anti–sperm antibodies. These antibodies have been linked to infertility and are believed to interfere with the interaction of the sperm and the egg and to block the sperm from passing through cervical mucus. Genetic testing includes identifying micro deletions from specific regions of the Y chromosome and identification of a congenital bilateral absence of the vas deferens, which is associated with the cystic fibrosis gene. Micro deletions are present to a greater extent in azoospermic men than in men with less severe spermatogenic infertility. Micro deletions reduce fertility. *Other testing* commonly included in infertility evaluation includes vaginal, endometrial, or semen culture for *Chlamydia trachomatis*, ovulation evaluation, laparoscopy, hysterosalpingography, the Sims-Huhner test, and postcoital testing. Less common testing methods sometimes used include hormonal testing, pelvic ultrasonography, hysteroscopy, cervical cultures, and endometrial biopsy.

Professional Considerations

Informed consent is recommended for genetic testing.

Preparation

1. Obtain a tube for each partner: Red topped, red/gray topped, or gold topped.
2. See Semen analysis—Specimen.
3. See Client and Family Teaching.

Procedure

1. Obtain a 7-mL blood sample from each partner.
2. See Semen analysis—Specimen.

Postprocedure Care

1. Explain that repeat testing may be necessary.
2. See Semen analysis—Specimen.

Client and Family Teaching

1. See Semen analysis—Specimen.
2. Refer to Appendix B, "Informed Consent for Genetic Testing".
3. Clients with positive genetic tests should be referred for follow-up genetic counseling.

Factors That Affect Results

1. Repeat testing may be necessary because results vary with samples.

Other Data

1. The infertility rate is about 15%, with the most frequent cause being of genetic origin in the male.
2. The Genetic Information Nondiscrimination Act of 2008 prohibits health plans from using genetic family history or genetic test results from influencing eligibility or premiums for health insurance. It also prohibits employers from using this information to influence decisions about hiring, terminating employment, or employment pay, promotions, or privileges.
3. See also Semen analysis—Specimen.

Influenza A and B Titer—Blood

Norm. Less than a fourfold increase in titer in paired sera. Less than 1:8 titer indicates previous exposure.

Positive. Influenza.

Negative. Bacterial infections.

Description. Influenza viruses are typed for epidemiologic surveys. Both viruses, A and B, cause major epidemics every 2-4 years, as antigenic shifts occur, leaving the population susceptible to reinfection by a different strain. Virus B usually is sporadic and local, whereas virus A spreads rapidly and to all population areas. The influenza titer evaluates the body's response to influenza immunization.

Professional Considerations

Consent form NOT required.

Preparation

1. Tube: Red topped, red/gray topped, or gold topped.

Procedure

1. Draw a 7-mL blood sample at the onset of symptoms.
2. Draw a convalescent sample 14 days later.

Postprocedure Care

1. None.

Client and Family Teaching

1. Return in 2 weeks for a second sample to be drawn. This helps monitor recovery.
2. Annual influenza vaccinations are recommended in the latter portions of each year for the elderly, health care workers, and others at high risk for exposure to the influenza virus.

Factors That Affect Results

1. Failure to collect a convalescent sample limits the value of the acute sample results.
2. Immune response to the vaccine is less in those that have received previous influenza vaccination than in those receiving it for the first time.
3. The immune response to the influenza vaccine is impaired in clients who have received liver transplants.

Other Data

1. Serologic diagnosis is not necessary during an epidemic but is valuable for epidemiologic purposes.
2. Influenza vaccination is typically not very effective in those ≥80 years old. One study found immune response in this population to be enhanced in those given nutritional supplementation. Another study found that in the elderly, vitamin E levels are significantly correlated with an intact immune response to influenza immunization.
3. Intranasal and intradermal vaccines have been found equivalent to the intramuscular route in stimulating the immune response.

Inhibition Level of Antibiotic

See **Schlichter Test**—Specimen.

INR

See **Prothrombin Time and International Normalized Ratio**—Blood.

Insulin and Insulin Antibodies—Blood

Norm. Free insulin: fasting ≤25 µIU/mL (<172.5 pmol/L, SI units). (Norms and standardization of the test method vary widely by laboratory.)

Insulin Level via Radioimmunoassay

		SI Units
Adult, fasting level	<17 µIU/mL or 1.00 mg/L	<117 pmol/L
Newborn	3-20 µIU/mL	21-139 pmol/L
Infant	<13 µIU/mL	≤89 pmol/L
Prepubertal child	<13 µIU/mL	≤89 pmol/L
Panic levels	>30 µIU/mL	>207 pmol/L
Last trimester, amniotic fluid	11.3 µIU/mL	78 pmol/L

Insulin Antibodies. Undetectable to less than 4% when using either bovine or porcine insulin as a reagent. Insulin antibodies have been shown to occur more frequently with aging and more in females than in males.

Panic Level Symptoms and Treatment

Symptoms. Diaphoresis, dizziness, faintness, pallor, weakness, progressing to stupor and seizures.

Treatment
NOTE: Treatment choice(s) depend(s) on client's history and condition and episode history.
1. Administer 50% dextrose in water (D₅₀W) by 50-mL IV injection, followed by carbohydrate and protein foods.
2. Follow with D₁₀W infusion if NPH or other long-acting insulin was taken.
3. Administer glucagon IV if the client has normal liver function.
4. Take bedside or laboratory glucose measurement hourly.
5. If serum potassium level is low or cardiac dysrhythmias are present, give KCl infusion.
6. Hemodialysis and peritoneal dialysis will NOT remove insulin.

Increased Insulin. Acromegaly, Beckwith-Wiedemann syndrome, beta-cell adenoma, Cushing's syndrome, dystrophia myotonica, familial fructose and galactose intolerance, hyperinsulinism, hypoglycemia, insulin-resistance syndromes, insulinoma, liver disease, metabolic syndrome, nesidioblastosis, non–insulin-dependent diabetes mellitus, obesity, overdose of insulin, pancreatic islet cell lesion, and pheochromocytoma. Drugs include albuterol, calcium gluconate in the newborn, estrogen, fructose, glucagon, glucose, insulin, levodopa, medroxyprogesterone, oral contraceptives, prednisolone, quinidine, quinine, spironolactone, sucrose, terbutaline, tolazamide, and tolbutamide.

Decreased Insulin. Diabetes mellitus, hyperglycemia, hypopituitarism, and pancreatectomy-induced diabetes. Drugs include asparaginase, beta-adrenergic blockers, calcitonin, cimetidine, diazoxide, ethacrynic acid, ether, ethyl alcohol (ethanol), furosemide, metformin, nifedipine, phenformin, phenobarbital, phenytoin, and thiazide diuretics.

Positive Insulin Antibodies. Factitious hypoglycemia, autoimmune insulin syndrome (AIS).

Negative Insulin Antibodies. Normal finding. Also negative in insulinoma.

Description. Insulin is a hormone that regulates carbohydrate metabolism. It is produced in the pancreas by the beta cells of the islets of Langerhans, and its rate of secretion is determined primarily by the level of blood glucose. The radioimmunoassay test measures endogenous insulin by using a series of tubes containing a fixed amount of antibody label and an aliquot of standard, control, or unknown. The client's unlabeled antigen in the blood competes with labeled antigen for antibody-binding sites. The percentage of antigen bound to antibody is related to the total antigen present and is reflected by the distribution of a radioactive label. Low immunoreactive insulin levels have been associated with a higher risk of developing degenerative diseases such as atherosclerosis, hypertension, and dyslipidemia. *Insulin antibodies*, also referred to as anti–insulin-Ab, may be present in diabetic clients treated for several weeks or more with conventional insulin. These antibodies may also be present in persons who have never received insulin but have autoimmune insulin syndrome (AIS), a rare condition characterized by hyperinsulinemia and hypoglycemia. For diabetic clients, this test may be used with C-peptide to determine whether hypoglycemia is caused by insulin abuse. Insulin antibodies are transferred through the placenta and are present in 30%-50% of children at the time of diagnosis before beginning insulin therapy.

Professional Considerations

Consent form NOT required.

Preparation

1. Tube: Red topped, red/gray topped, or gold topped. Also obtain ice.
2. Specimens MAY be drawn during hemodialysis.
3. See Client and Family Teaching.

Procedure

1. Draw a 7-mL blood sample. Place the sample immediately on ice.

Postprocedure Care

1. Resume diet and any medications held before the test.
2. Assess the client for signs of hypoglycemia, which could occur as a response to fasting.

Client and Family Teaching

1. This test is used to evaluate for insulin-producing neoplasm (islet cell tumor, insulinoma) or to evaluate insulin production in diabetes mellitus.
2. Fast from food and fluids (except water) for 8 hours before the test.
3. Do not take insulin before the test.
4. Review the procedure used to obtain the blood sample, including the fact that some discomfort may be experienced when the needle enters the skin.

Factors That Affect Results

1. Reject specimens if the client had a radioactive scan within 7 days before the test.
2. Hemodialysis destroys insulin.
3. Specimen hemolysis invalidates the results.
4. Falsely elevated results have been found when insulin antibodies are present in the blood when the radioimmunoassay testing method is used. More accurate results are obtained when the immunoradiometric assay testing method is used if insulin antibodies are suspected.
5. Values are higher in plasma samples than in serum.
6. Elevated levels have been found in men with elevated C-reactive protein levels.

Other Data

1. Serum insulin level is commonly prescribed with serum glucose level to confirm functional hypoglycemia, uncontrolled insulin-dependent diabetes mellitus, or fasting hypoglycemia of unknown cause.
2. The norms and standardization of the test method vary widely by laboratory.
3. Undetectable in amniotic fluid during the first trimester.
4. Complete absence of insulin during the last trimester of pregnancy is associated with intrauterine death.
5. Some studies evaluating the relationship of C-reactive protein, glucose, and Hb A_{1c} indicate a possible role of inflammation in insulin resistance.
6. When insulin antibodies are present, the test of choice is C-peptide to determine whether exogenous insulin administration is being abused. If C-peptide levels are not elevated, endogenous insulin secretion has not increased.

7. There is some discussion in the literature concerning possible increased stimulation of insulin antibodies when the inhaled route of insulin is used versus the subcutaneous route.

Insulin-like Growth Factor-I (IGF-I)—Blood

Norm. Standard reference ranges vary widely. Test result should include reference range.

	Male		Female	
	ng/mL	SI Units nmol/L	ng/mL	SI Units nmol/L
Children				
2 months–5 years	17-248	2.23-32.49	Same as male	
6-8 years	88-474	11.53-62.09	Same as male	
9-11 years	110-565	14.41-74.02	117-771	15.33-101.00
	Male		Female	
Teens/Young Adults				
12-15 years	202-957	26.46-125.37	261-1096	34.19-143.58
16-24 years	182-780	23.84-102.18	Same as male	
Adults				
25-39 years	114-492	14.93-64.45	Same as male	
40-54 years	90-360	11.79-47.16	Same as male	
≥55 years	71-290	9.30-37.99	Same as male	

Increased. Acromegaly, diabetic retinopathy, gigantism, hyperpituitarism, obesity, pituitary gigantism, precocious puberty, and pregnancy.

Decreased. Anorexia nervosa, chronic illness, cirrhosis, delayed puberty, diabetes mellitus, emotional deprivation syndrome, hepatoma, hypopituitarism, hypothyroidism, kwashiorkor, Laron dwarfs, liver disease, maternal deprivation syndrome, nutritional deficiency, and pituitary tumor.

Usage. Helps identify cause of abnormal growth. Used in conjunction with a growth hormone stimulation test in children with signs of deficient growth hormone. Use in conjunction with a growth hormone suppression test in children suspected of having gigantism or adults suspected of having acromegaly; helps evaluate pituitary function. Used to monitor status after removal of a growth hormone–producing tumor. Also used to monitor response to growth hormone therapy.

Description. Insulin-like growth factor-I (IGF-I) is a small polypeptide produced primarily in the liver, transported in the plasma, and bound by carrier proteins. Acting via cell membrane receptors, IGF-I directly stimulates growth and proliferation of normal cells and affects glucose metabolism and thus affects growth. Serum levels of IGF-I are regulated both by growth hormone levels and by nutritional status. Increased or decreased growth hormone in the bloodstream causes a directly correlated increase or decrease in the level of IGF-I. Thus this test may be used to confirm growth hormone deficiencies secondary to pituitary abnormalities. It may also be used when monitoring response to growth hormone treatment in growth hormone replacement therapy in adults or in pituitary dwarfism because levels are highest during growth spurts. IGF-I is also used to evaluate the severity of acromegaly.

Professional Considerations
Consent form NOT required.

Preparation
1. Tube: Lavender topped.
2. Specimens MAY be drawn during hemodialysis.
3. See Client and Family Teaching.

Procedure
1. Draw a 2-mL blood sample.

Postprocedure Care

1. Immediately separate and freeze serum. The specimen is stable for 30 days.

Client and Family Teaching

1. Fast from food and fluids from midnight before the test.
2. Results may not be available for several days.

Factors That Affect Results

1. Results may be falsely elevated if the client received a radioactive scan within the previous 7 days.
2. During puberty, levels may be 4-5 times higher than adult levels. IGF levels decrease with aging.
3. Norms in pregnant women are higher than those in nonpregnant women.

Other Data

1. IGF-I is now produced by recombinant DNA technology and may be useful in the treatment of acromegaly and certain types of dwarfism.
2. IGF-II is similar in structure to IGF-I and is believed to be an important regulator of embryonic and fetal growth. Its level remains fairly constant after an initial rise in the first year of life.
3. Recent studies of the interrelationship of IGF-I, insulin, and IGF-binding proteins indicate a possible correlation of increased bioavailability of IGF-I with increased risk of colon cancer.
4. The test was formerly known as somatomedin C.

InSure

See Immunochemical Fecal Occult Blood Testing—Stool.

Interferon Gamma Release Assays

See RD1-Interferon Tests for Tuberculosis—Blood.

International Normalized Ratio

See Prothrombin Time and International Normalized Ratio—Blood.

International Sensitivity Index

See Prothrombin Time and International Normalized Ratio—Blood.

Intraductal Ultrasonography

See Pancreas Ultrasonography—Diagnostic.

Intraocular Pressure Measurement

See Tonometry Test for Glaucoma—Diagnostic.

Intravascular Coagulation Screen

Norm.

D-Dimer (fibrin degradation fragment)	<1 µg/mL or <100 µg/L
Fibrinogen	
Adult	200-400 mg/dL
Newborn	125-300 mg/dL
Fibrin breakdown products	<10 µg/mL
Platelet count	
Adult	150,000-400,000/mm³
Newborn	84,000-478,000/mm³
Activated partial thromboplastin time (APTT)	25-35 seconds
Prothrombin time	
Adult	11-15 seconds
Newborn	2-35 seconds
Premature	3-5 seconds
Thrombin time	16-23 seconds

Usage. Differentiation of acute disseminated intravascular coagulation (DIC) from chronic DIC.

Description. Intravascular coagulation is a process in which multiple fibrin thrombi with micro infarctions lead to tissue and organ necrosis. This is caused by activation of the clotting mechanism and depletion of clotting factors and platelets with a secondary fibrinolysis that results in bleeding. In severe situations, the life-threatening condition of DIC can occur. DIC is triggered when the endothelial or other circulating cells release tissue factor, which activates systemic hemostasis. The systemic activation eventually overcomes natural inhibitor mechanisms, allowing more coagulation to occur. The ongoing coagulation depletes the supply of fibrinogen and platelets, leading to uncontrolled diffuse bleeding. Using a combination of coagulation tests that reveal different aspects of the systemic hemostasis mechanism is necessary to differentiate acute from chronic DIC. The following table lists typical findings for the intravascular coagulation screen in acute and chronic DIC.

Test	Acute DIC	Chronic DIC
D-Dimer	Increased	Increased
Fibrinogen	Decreased	Normal or increased
Fibrin breakdown	Positive	Positive
Platelet count	Decreased (or may appear normal if falling from a baseline high level)	Normal or increased
APTT	Increased	Normal
Prothrombin time	Increased	Normal
Thrombin time	Increased	Increased
Peripheral smear	Schistocytes present	

Professional Considerations

Consent form NOT required.

Preparation

1. Tubes: Three red topped, red/gray topped, or gold topped.

Procedure

1. Draw three 5-mL blood samples in the three tubes.

Postprocedure Care

1. Place a pressure dressing on the venipuncture site. Monitor closely for bleeding.

Client and Family Teaching

1. Clients with disseminated intravascular coagulation (DIC) may be in acute

crisis. Support the family; explain that there may be a need for blood product therapy.

Factors That Affect Results
1. Heparin increases clotting time.

Other Data
1. DIC is eliminated only by eliminating the underlying cause. Short-term symptomatic support includes administration of cryoprecipitate, platelet concentrates, and fresh frozen plasma.

Intravascular Ultrasonography
See Coronary Intravascular Ultrasonography—Diagnostic.

Intravenous Cholangiography—Diagnostic

Norm. Even filling of the hepatic and biliary ducts. Complete filling of the gallbladder occurs. Negative for stricture or filling defects.

Usage. Alternative to oral cholecystography when client cannot tolerate oral iodopaque tablets or in clients with active intestinal inflammation; and detection of calculi (or their movement), strictures, or leaking anastomosis or anastomoses in the biliary ductal system.

Description. Intravenous cholangiography involves taking a series of radiographs of the gallbladder and hepatobiliary duct systems over several hours after the intravenous administration of a radiographic contrast medium. The contrast medium is allowed to circulate to the liver through the hepatic artery and empty into the biliary tree. Strictures or stones cause defects in the pattern of filling and can be visualized on the radiograph. Strictures occurring in the hepatobiliary ducts may be congenital or caused by ductal damage during exploratory or therapeutic biliary surgery or may be caused by benign or malignant tumor or inflammation. Intravenous cholangiography carries a diagnostic accuracy of 99% for detection of stones in the common bile duct; however, it has NOT been shown to provide incrementally superior information than other tests used to evaluate the hepatobiliary system. Gallbladder and biliary system ultrasound, a noninvasive procedure, is the test of choice for evaluating the biliary system and has largely replaced the use of intravenous cholangiography.

See Endoscopic retrograde cholangiopancreatography—Diagnostic, Gallbladder and biliary system ultrasonography—Diagnostic.

These three tests that are used more commonly than intravenous cholangiography.

Professional Considerations
Consent form IS required.

Risks
Hypotension, infection, nausea, respiratory failure, tachycardia, vomiting, allergic reaction to dye (itching, hives, rash, tight feeling in the throat, shortness of breath, bronchospasm, anaphylaxis, death), renal toxicity from contrast medium.

Contraindications
Respiratory failure; previous allergy to iodine, shellfish, or radiographic dye; renal insufficiency; during pregnancy (because of radioactive iodine crossing the blood-placental barrier).

Preparation
1. A laxative or cathartic may be administered 24 hours before the procedure.
2. A cleansing or tap-water enema may be given the morning of the procedure.
3. Establish intravenous access.
4. Have emergency equipment readily available.
5. See Client and Family Teaching.

Procedure
1. The client is positioned supine on the scanning table.
2. A radiographic contrast medium is injected intravenously or infused by drip and allowed at least 30 minutes to circulate to the liver and become excreted into the bile ducts. Radiographs of the hepatic and bile ducts are taken at this time.

3. 2-3 hours are then allowed to pass to allow the gallbladder to fill with contrast medium. Radiographs may be taken of the gallbladder and biliary system at intervals for up to 8 hours after injection.

Postprocedure Care

1. Resume previous diet.
2. Assess for allergy to contrast medium for 24 hours.
3. Dysuria is not uncommon because the contrast medium is excreted in the urine.

Client and Family Teaching

1. Fast from food and fluids overnight before the test.
2. Morning insulin may be withheld for diabetics because the test may take up to 8 hours.
3. A burning or flushing sensation may be experienced when the dye is injected.
4. Bring something to read, if desired, because the test may take several hours.

5. Blockage of the gallbladder can be caused by stones formed from natural bile salts and substances similar in nature to cholesterol. A low-fat diet is generally recommended for clients with gallbladder disease.
6. In women who are breast-feeding, formula should be substituted for breast milk for 1 or more days after the procedure.

Factors that Affect Results

1. Hepatic failure with bilirubin >3.5 mg/dL (58 mmol/L, SI units) will interfere with gallbladder visualization. The dye must be processed in the liver before it passes into the gallbladder. The test will be canceled for a high bilirubin level.

Other Data

1. See also Endoscopic retrograde cholangiopancreatography—Diagnostic a test that is used more commonly than intravenous cholangiography.

Intravenous Pyelography (IVP, Excretory Urography)—Diagnostic

Norm. Normal renal pelvis, ureters, and bladder. No obstruction or masses.

Usage. Berger's disease, glomerulonephritis, hydronephrosis, renal cell cancer, renal failure, renal hypertension, tubular necrosis, and Wilms' tumor. Examination of the superior ureters during pregnancy as compared with ultrasonography (see Contraindications).

Description. An invasive test that uses contrast radiopaque dye to assess the ability of the kidneys to excrete dye in the urine. Radiographs are taken after dye injection to visualize the kidneys, ureters, and bladder to assess for obstruction, hematuria, stones, bladder injury, and renal artery occlusion of the renal pelvis. IVP is the first choice for evaluation for kidney stones, if noncontrast computed tomography is not available. IVP is primarily used to examine the upper urinary tract.

Professional Considerations

Consent form IS required.

Risks

Dysuria, nephrotoxicity, urinary tract infection, vasovagal response, allergic reaction to dye (itching, hives, rash, tight feeling in the throat, shortness of breath, bronchospasm, anaphylaxis, death), renal toxicity from contrast medium, weakness.

Contraindications

Dehydration, pregnancy (because of radioactive iodine crossing the blood-placental barrier), previous allergy to iodinated radiographic dye, renal insufficiency.

Preparation

1. Bowel preparation of orally administered evacuation preparation 24 hours before the test and evacuation enema 8 hours before test.
2. Assess for high-risk clients: dehydration, elderly, severe diabetes mellitus, renal insufficiency, or multiple myeloma.
3. Have emergency equipment readily available.
4. Just before beginning the procedure, take a "time out" to verify the correct client, procedure, and site.

Procedure

1. The client is placed in slight Trendelenburg position or supine.
2. A venipuncture is performed, and dye is injected into a vein.

3. Serial radiographs are taken periodically for the next 30 minutes.

Postprocedure Care

1. The client should drink at least three 8-ounce glasses of liquid to flush the kidneys of the dye (when not contraindicated).
2. Assess for signs of allergic reaction to the dye (listed under Risks) for 24 hours.

Client and Family Teaching

1. It is normal to feel flushed and warm and to notice a salty taste soon after the dye is injected. This will last only a few moments.
2. Stress the importance of drinking water after the test to flush dye from the body, prevent osmotic diuresis from the dye, and protect the kidneys.

3. In women who are breast-feeding, formula should be substituted for breast milk for 1 or more days after the procedure.

Factors That Affect Results

1. Poor bowel evacuation or poor renal perfusion will decrease the uptake of dye, leading to poor radiograph quality.

Other Data

1. Dosages of radiation range from 1047 to 1465 mR (milliroentgens).
2. The test Magnetic resonance urography—Diagnostic, although much more costly, is superior to renal ultrasonography in identifying pathology for clients with kidneys that do not opacify (such as those with renal transplants) during excretory urography.

Intrinsic Factor Antibody—Blood

Norm. Negative; none detected.

Positive. Graves' disease, insulin-dependent diabetes, megaloblastic anemia, and pernicious anemia.

Description. Intrinsic factor is produced by the parietal cells of the gastric mucosa and is required for the effective absorption of vitamin B_{12}. In some diseases, antibodies that bind the cobalamin-intrinsic factor complex are produced and prevent the complex from binding to receptors in the ileum.

Professional Considerations
Consent form NOT required.

Preparation

1. Tube: Red topped, red/gray topped, or gold topped.
2. Do not collect a sample if vitamin B_{12} was injected or ingested by client within 48 hours before the test.

Procedure

1. Draw a 3-mL blood sample.

Postprocedure Care

1. None.

Client and Family Teaching

1. If the test results show the presence of antibodies and a positive diagnosis is made of pernicious anemia, the client requires regular injections of vitamin B_{12} because of the body's inability to produce the intrinsic factor secreted by the parietal cells in the stomach lining.

Factors That Affect Results

1. Reject if the client had a radioactive scan within 7 days before the test.

Other Data

1. Causes of vitamin B_{12} deficiency include pancreatic insufficiency, parasitic infestations of the small intestine, regional enteritis, malnutrition, or transcobalamin protein abnormalities.

IRF

See Reticulocyte Count—Blood.

Iron (Fe)—Serum
Norm.

		SI Units
Adult female	40-150 µg/dL	7.2-26.9 µmol/L
Adult male	50-160 µg/dL	8.9-28.7 µmol/L
Newborn	100-250 µg/dL	17.9-44.8 µmol/L
Infant	40-100 µg/dL	7.2-17.9 µmol/L
Child	50-120 µg/dL	8.9-21.5 µmol/L
Panic level	>300 µg/dL	>54.05 µmol/L

Panic Level Symptoms and Treatment
Symptoms
1. 0-6 hours after ingestion: vomiting and diarrhea, abdominal pain, gastrointestinal bleeding/bloody diarrhea.
2. 6-24 hours after ingestion: may be asymptomatic.
3. 12-48 hours after ingestion: metabolic acidosis, shock, coma, seizures, purpura, renal failure.
4. Toxic/panic symptoms (risk with ingestion of over 60 mg/kg): shock and coma may be the first symptoms seen.

Treatment
1. Support airway, breathing, and circulation.
2. Gastric lavage is useful only if started within 1 hour of ingestion.
3. Perform whole bowel irrigation with polyethylene glycol (used with caution).
4. Induce chelation with intravenous deferoxamine. Start immediately, without waiting for other test results, if serious ingestion is verified.
5. Hemodialysis and peritoneal dialysis help remove ferrioxamine in clients who are anuric.

Increased. Acute hepatitis, aplastic anemia, blood transfusion, hemochromatosis, hemolytic anemia, hepatitis, lead poisoning, nephritis, pernicious anemia, polycythemia, sideroblastic anemia, thalassemia, and vitamin B_6 deficiency. Drugs include alcohol (wine, ethanol).

Decreased. Blood loss, burns, carcinoma, gastrectomy, infection, iron deficiency anemia, kwashiorkor, malabsorption, nephrosis, postoperative state, pregnancy, rheumatoid arthritis, schizophrenia (chronic), tetralogy of Fallot, and uremia. Drugs include metformin.

Description. Iron is an inorganic ion, found mostly in hemoglobin, that acts as a carrier of oxygen from the lungs to the tissues and indirectly aids in the return of carbon dioxide to the lungs. Although the primary source of body iron is food, only a small portion of that consumed from the diet is absorbed. Iron is stored in the liver and reticuloendothelial tissue in the form of ferritin and hemosiderin and is released from storage as needed to meet the body's demands. Although iron levels are assumed to be highest in the morning because of a diurnal variation, studies have not shown that restricting specimen collection to the morning improves the reliability of the result. Significant toxicity can occur with ingestions of over 20 mg/kg of iron.

Professional Considerations
Consent form NOT required.

Preparation
1. Tube: Red topped, red/gray topped, or gold topped.
2. Screen client for use of herbal medicines or natural remedies.
3. Document the date of the last blood transfusion on the laboratory requisition.
4. Do NOT draw specimens during hemodialysis.

Procedure
1. If using Vacutainer and venipuncture for multiple samples, draw this sample first to avoid mixing heparin with the sample. Draw a 7-mL blood sample.

Postprocedure Care
1. None.

Client and Family Teaching
1. The basic role of iron in hemoglobin formation is to allow blood to efficiently

carry oxygen to the tissues. Foods rich in iron include red meats and some green, leafy vegetables.

Factors That Affect Results

1. Hemolysis of the specimens invalidates the results.
2. Vitamin B_{12} ingested within 48 hours may increase the results.
3. Herbs that interfere with iron absorption include St. John's wort and saw palmetto, which contain tannic acids.
4. Iron levels in blood do not correlate well with the amount of iron ingestion. Therefore treatment should be based on

symptoms and on what is known about the amount of iron ingested.

Other Data

1. Adenocarcinoma of the gastrointestinal tract may be detected by iron deficiency.
2. Increased serum iron concentrations of 300-500 mg/dL (53.7-89.6 mmol/L, SI units) can be the result of one ingested iron tablet.
3. Increased ferritin levels frequently accompany neoplastic activity.
4. See also Ferritin—Serum; Iron and total iron-binding capacity/transferrin—Serum; Soluble transferrin receptor assay—Serum.

Iron (Fe) and Total Iron-Binding Capacity (TIBC)/Transferrin—Serum

Norm.

		SI Units
Adult female	40-150 µg/dL	7.2-26.9 µmol/L
Adult male	50-160 µg/dL	8.9-28.7 µmol/L
Newborn	100-250 µg/dL	17.9-44.8 µmol/L
Infant	40-100 µg/dL	7.2-17.9 µmol/L
Child	50-120 µg/dL	8.9-21.5 µmol/L
TIBC		
Adult	250-400 µg/dL	44.8-71.6 µmol/L
Infant	100-400 µg/dL	17.9-71.6 µmol/L
Transferrin saturation	20% to 45%	
Adult	200-400 mg/dL	2-4.0 g/L
Maternal	305 mg/dL	3.0 g/L
(Term)		
Fetal	190 mg/dL	1.9 g/L
Newborn	130-275 mg/dL	1.3-2.8 g/L

Increased TIBC. Hepatitis, microcytic anemia, and pregnancy. Drugs include iron salts and oral contraceptives.

Decreased TIBC. Cirrhosis, dysmenorrhea, hemochromatosis, hemorrhage, hepatitis, hypothyroidism, kwashiorkor, microcytic anemia, myocardial infarction, neoplasm, nephrosis, pernicious anemia, thalassemia, and uremia. Drugs include ACTH, asparaginase, chloramphenicol, corticotropin, cortisone, dextran, steroids, and testosterone.

Description. This test differentiates anemia secondary to iron deficiency from other diseases associated with variations in cellular oxidation. Iron is an element necessary for many body processes, including the

transport of oxygen to the tissues and for oxygen-carrying chromoproteins, hemoglobin, myoglobin, and enzymes such as xanthine oxidase and peroxidase. Transferrin is a plasma iron-transport protein, also called siderophilin, formed in the liver that has a half-life of 7-10 days. Transferrin is capable of binding more than its own weight in iron (that is, 1 g of transferrin can carry 1.43 g of iron). In normal clients, iron saturation of transferrin is between 20% and 45%. Transferrin saturation by iron demonstrates a diurnal pattern, with a morning peak and an early evening trough. The formula for transferrin saturation by iron is:

(Serum iron/TIBC)×100

= Transferrin saturation

TIBC is the maximum amount of iron that can be bound to transferrin. It is useful in distinguishing anemia (increased value) from chronic inflammatory disorders (normal value). In this test, iron is added to the client's serum until all transferrin-binding sites are bound with iron. Then the excess iron is removed, and the total amount of remaining (bound) iron is measured, giving an assessment of the ability of the individual's transferrin to bind iron.

Professional Considerations
Consent form NOT required.

Preparation
1. Tube: Red topped, red/gray topped, or gold topped; and 20-gauge or larger needle.
2. Document the date of the last blood transfusion on the requisition.
3. See Client and Family Teaching.

Procedure
1. Draw a 7-mL blood sample, without hemolysis.

Postprocedure Care
1. None.

Client and Family Teaching
1. Fast 12 hours before sampling. Water is permitted.
2. If the results indicate a low level of iron, eat foods rich in iron such as organ meats, eggs, and dried fruits.

Factors That Affect Results
1. Inflammatory states may decrease results below normal.
2. Hemolysis may cause falsely elevated iron values.

Other Data
1. A decrease in iron and an increase in TIBC are found in microcytic anemia.
2. Serum transferrin may be calculated from TIBC using the following formula:

$$0.8 \times TIBC - 43$$

3. See also Soluble transferrin receptor assay—Serum; Transferrin—Serum.

Iron Stain, Bone Marrow
See Bone Marrow Aspiration Analysis—Specimen.

ISI
See Prothrombin Time and International Normalized Ratio—Blood.

Isopropyl Alcohol
See Toxicology, Volatiles Group by GLC—Blood or Urine.

IVP
See Intravenous Pyelography—Diagnostic.

Ivy Bleeding Time
See Aspirin Tolerance Test—Diagnostic; Bleeding Time, Ivy—Blood.

Ketone, Semiquantitative

See **Ketone, Semiquantitative**—Urine.

Ketone Bodies

Norm. Negative or 0.3-2.0 mg/dL (<0.17 mmol/L, SI units).

Panic Level. >20 mg/dL (>3.44 mmol/L, SI units).

Panic Level Symptoms and Treatment

Symptoms. Fruity breath, acidosis, ketonuria, depressed level of consciousness.

Treatment

NOTE: Treatment choice(s) depend(s) on client's history and condition and episode history.
1. Perform blood glucose measurements every hour.
2. Infuse insulin.
3. Perform neurologic checks every hour.

Positive. After anesthesia, alcoholism, carbohydrate deficiency, diabetes mellitus, eclampsia, fasting, glycogen storage disease, high-fat (ketogenic) diet, hyperglycemia, isopropanol alcohol ingestion, ketoacidosis, pregnant diabetic woman, prolonged exercise, reducing diets, starvation, and von Gierke's disease. Drugs include methyldopa and propranolol (poisoning).

Negative. Not applicable.

Description. Ketones are synthesized by the liver from fatty acids when a lack of glucose causes the body to use fat for energy. In a low-insulin state such as diabetes, fat and fatty acids are metabolized less efficiently than normal, resulting in a buildup of serum ketones. Ketone bodies consist of acetone, acetoacetic acid, and beta-hydroxybutyric acid. Beta-hydroxybutyric acid is the predominant type of ketone body occurring in diabetic ketoacidosis. Extremely elevated levels in the bloodstream can lead to coma. This test only measures acetone and acetoacetic acid and is used in conjunction with the Beta-hydroxybutyrate—Blood test to help differentiate coma caused by a hyperosmotic state (in which a negative test would be expected) from coma caused by ketoacidosis.

Professional Considerations

Consent form NOT required.

Preparation
1. Tube: Red topped, red/gray topped, or gold topped; or capillary tubes.

Procedure
1. Draw a 4-mL blood sample in a tube or collect the specimen in capillary tubes, filling them as completely as possible. Either central venous or peripheral blood is acceptable.

Postprocedure Care
1. None.

Client and Family Teaching
1. Ketone bodies, a natural by-product of metabolism, can be dangerously elevated in some diseases.
2. Coma caused by diabetic ketoacidosis is usually reversible.

Factors That Affect Results
1. Hemolysis of the specimen invalidates the results.
2. A low-carbohydrate or low-fat diet may cause elevated results.
3. After 7 days of storage at −20 degrees C, levels of acetoacetate are about 40% lower than at the time of specimen collection. After 40 days, levels are 100% lower. The degradation of acetoacetate can be slowed by storing at −80 degrees C, resulting in 85% of the original acetoacetate still being present after 40 days.
4. This test is not useful for monitoring response to treatment in DKA, because acetoacetate levels tend to remain stable, even with treatment. The Beta-hydroxybutyrate—Blood test should be used for treatment monitoring.

Other Data
1. Elevated acetone with normal anion gap, bicarbonate, and plasma glucose levels is suggestive of rubbing alcohol (isopropanol) intoxication.
2. Ketones appear in the urine before there is a significant increase in the amount in the blood.
3. See also Beta-hydroxybutyrate—Blood; Anion gap—Blood.

Ketone, Semiquantitative—Urine

Norm. Negative.

Usage. Detection of ketones in the urine for carbohydrate deprivation, diabetes mellitus, diabetic ketoacidosis, or ketonuria.

Positive. Alcoholism, convulsions, diabetes mellitus, eclampsia, Fanconi syndrome, glycogen storage disease, ketoacidosis, ketogenic diet, and von Gierke's disease. Drugs include anesthetics, isopropyl alcohol (isopropanol), levodopa, and mesna.

Description. Ketone bodies consist of acetoacetic acid, beta-hydroxybutyric acid, and acetone and are by-products of fat and fatty acid metabolism. In a low-insulin state such as diabetes, fat and fatty acids are metabolized less efficiently than normal, resulting in a buildup of serum ketones. Elevated serum ketones are excreted through the kidneys into the urine. In this test, a dipstick is used for determining ketones in the urine. The reagent strip correlates only moderately well with quantitative acetoacetate in plasma and poorly with total blood ketones, but is a better screening test for diabetic ketoacidosis than the anion gap or serum bicarbonate tests. Semiquantitative results mean testing several different dilutions of each urine specimen to obtain a better degree of differentiation of ketone body products than can be obtained from qualitative testing.

Professional Considerations

Consent form NOT required.

Preparation

1. Obtain a clean, plastic specimen container.

Procedure

1. Instruct the client to void and then to drink a glass of water.
2. 30 minutes later, ask the client to void into the specimen container.
3. Dip the stick into the urine for 5 seconds.
4. Tap the edge of the stick against the container of urine to remove excess urine.

5. After 15 seconds, compare the color of the ketone section (buff or purple) with the appropriate color chart. Report the results of ketones that are positive as either small, moderate, or large.

Postprocedure Care

1. Send the specimen to the laboratory immediately. If the specimen cannot be tested immediately, refrigerate it. Cap the container tightly.
2. Testing must occur within 60 minutes of the specimen being obtained, for specimens kept at room temperature. Refrigerated urine may be tested later but must first be returned to room temperature.

Client and Family Teaching

1. Assess over-the-counter medications for drugs that may cause false positives.

Factors That Affect Results

1. The preservative 8-hydroxyquinoline, used in foods, may increase urine levels.
2. Drugs that may cause false-positive results include ascorbic acid, levodopa, phenazopyridine HCl (Pyridium), phthalein compounds given for liver or kidney tests, and valproic acid.
3. A low-carbohydrate or high-fat diet may cause elevated results.

Other Data

1. Ketones appear in the urine before serum elevations are seen.
2. Pentamidine therapy for AIDS may induce ketoacidosis in clients with diabetes mellitus.
3. Keto-Diastix assesses ketones only, not glucose.
4. Breath acetone testing is more practical than and as reliable as urine ketone testing when performing ongoing monitoring of ketone levels for clients receiving ketogenic diets for control of intractable seizures.

17-Ketosteroids

See **Metyrapone**—24-Hour Urine.

Ketostix

See **Ketone, Semiquantitative—Urine**.

KeyPath™ MRSA/MSSA Blood Culture Test—Blood

Usage. Used to distinguish whether there is methicillin susceptibility when a *Staphylococcus aureus* infection is present.

Description. A 5-hour test performed on a blood culture that contains *S. aureus*. This test, approved by the U.S. FDA in 2011, identifies *S. aureus* and uses phenotypic determination of methicillin resistance and susceptibility by identifying anti-bacteriophage antibodies. Rapid detection enables rapid treatment decisions, with the advantage of possibly avoiding overtreatment with broad-spectrum antibiotics.

Professional Considerations
Consent form NOT required.

Preparation
1. Obtain the MRSA/MSSA Blood Culture Test kit containing a detector and blue and red testing tubes.

Procedure
1. Add an existing sample of *S. aureus*-positive blood to each of two testing tubes. The blue tube identifies *S. aureus* and the red tube tests for susceptibility.
2. After incubation, drop a sample from each tube into the detector included in the test kit.
3. The presence of *S. aureus* is indicated by the development of a test line in the blue ID window of the detector. Susceptibility or resistance to methicillin is indicated on the test line in the red RS window of the detector.

Postprocedure Care
1. Not applicable.

Client and Family Teaching
1. None.

Factors That Affect Results
1. None.

Other Data
1. Not for use as a screening test.

Kidney Biopsy—Specimen

Norm. Interpretation required.

Usage. Alport's syndrome, childhood idiopathic nephrotic syndrome, diabetic glomerulosclerosis, glomerulonephritis, Goodpasture's syndrome, hematuria, Kimmelstiel-Wilson disease, nephrosis, nephrotic syndrome, renal failure, and toxemia. Also used for kidney transplantation to evaluate potential donor kidney's appropriateness for transplant and after kidney transplant to evaluate for subacute clinical rejection.

Description. The surgical or percutaneous needle biopsy resulting in the aseptic removal of a small quantity of kidney tissue. Before kidney transplantation, a histologic examination of a kidney biopsy specimen is performed to evaluate the extent of glomerulosclerosis, interstitial fibrosis, and vascular damage, which can reduce the long-term survival of the graft. After kidney transplantation, a biopsy of the transplanted kidney can provide evidence of subacute clinical rejection and chronic allograft nephropathy. This procedure is often performed under the guidance of ultrasound or computed tomography, but may also be an open (surgical) or a transjugular (transvenous) procedure. In the rare instance of pelvic kidney, a laparoscopy has been used to obtain the biopsy.

Professional Considerations
Consent form IS required.

Risks
Bleeding, infection, pneumothorax.
Contraindications
Percutaneous biopsy is contraindicated in uncooperative clients; in clients with bleeding diatheses, uncontrolled hypertension, or renal infection; or (usually) in clients

with a solitary functional kidney. Mendelssohn and Cole (1995) recommend conditions under which clients with solitary functional kidneys might be considered candidates for kidney biopsy.

Preparation
1. Before the biopsy, an intravenous pyelography test or renal scan should be performed to document bilateral renal function.
2. Obtain a biopsy tray, including a needle, sponges, lidocaine (Xylocaine), and slides or a sterile specimen jar.
3. See Biopsy, Site-specific—Specimen.

Procedure
1. A renal biopsy can be performed percutaneously with a special needle or under direct visualization during surgery.

Postprocedure Care
1. Send the specimen to the laboratory immediately.
2. Monitor vital signs every 15 minutes × 4.

3. Monitor for blood in the urine 8 hours after the biopsy.

Client and Family Teaching
1. This examination of renal tissue can provide valuable details in diagnosing kidney disease.
2. Report any pain in the flank or abdomen after the procedure.

Factors That Affect Results
1. None found.

Other Data
1. Indications for a renal biopsy are not clear-cut or universally agreed upon.
2. A 1-year creatinine measurement has been shown to be as useful, and less risky, than kidney biopsy for prediction of long-term kidney function after kidney transplant.
3. Histologic preparations using hematoxylin and eosin, periodic acid–Schiff, silver, or trichrome (Masson) stains are also routinely performed on the tissue sample.

Kidney Echography
See **Kidney Ultrasonography**—Diagnostic.

Kidney Profile
See **Basic Metabolic Panel**—Blood.

Kidney Scan
See **Renocystogram**—Diagnostic.

Kidney Stone Analysis—Specimen
Norm. Interpretation required.

Type of Stone	Prevalence	Characteristic	Condition
Calcium compounds such as calcium oxalate and calcium phosphate	80%	Appear black, gray, or white	Chronic dehydration (failure to routinely drink adequate amounts of water each day) Familial tendencies Hypercalcemia Hyperparathyroidism Hyperthyroidism Renal tubular acidosis Unknown cause (common) Vitamin D intoxication

K

Type of Stone	Prevalence	Characteristic	Condition
Calcium oxalate			Intake of diet high in oxalate-rich foods Methoxyflurane anesthesia Vitamin B deficiency
Cystine	<2%	Appear yellowish with flecks of shiny material	Renal tubular defects
Magnesium ammonium phosphate (struvite, staghorn stones)	5%-20%	Appearance similar to deer antlers	Urinary tract infection caused by *Proteus* type of bacteria
Uric acid	5%-10%	Difficult to visualize on x-ray	Cancer Gout Lymphoproliferative disorders

Usage. Hematuria, kidney stone, and nephrolithiasis. Determination of the chemical composition of kidney stones gives an indication as to the underlying cause and helps guide future preventive treatment.

Description. Kidney stones (renal calculi) are formed in up to 20% of people from urine particulates such as calcium oxalate, magnesium ammonium phosphate, uric acid, and cystine. The occurrence of kidney stones is higher in Caucasians than in African-Americans, and in males than in females. Kidney stones can be diagnosed via computed tomography or an intravenous pyelogram. Kidney stones for analysis are either passed naturally through the ureters into the urine, or removed via surgery. In this procedure, infrared spectroscopy is used to examine the kidney stone(s) after the specimen has been washed free of tissue and blood to determine the composition. The spectra of the stone(s) are compared to the known spectra of chemical compounds. Knowing the composition helps understand the underlying causes, which are listed above. Factors that increase a person's risk for kidney stones include having a personal or family history of kidney stones, being a 20-50 year old male, being on prolonged bed rest, sustaining a spinal injury that affects the bladder, having frequent urinary tract infections, or having inflammatory bowel disease.

Professional Considerations

Consent form NOT required but IS required for the procedure used to obtain the specimen. See the individual procedure for risks and contraindications.

Preparation

1. Obtain a clean specimen container.

Procedure

1. Send the stone in a plastic or glass container to the laboratory immediately.

Postprocedure Care

1. Encourage the intake of fluids.
2. A mild analgesic may be prescribed for use as needed.

Client and Family Teaching

1. Strain the urine for further stones if they are needed for analysis.
2. If the stone can be removed and the infection stopped, the client has a low probability of the condition returning.
3. A low-oxalate diet may help prevent kidney stones formed from calcium oxalate. A low-oxalate diet includes avoiding soybean products, wheat germ, grapefruit juice, strawberries, bananas, orange juice, canned pineapples or tomatoes, kidney beans, beets, spinach, carrots, celery, onions, sweet and white potatoes, green and waxed beans, cauliflower, cucumber, squash, broccoli, eggplant, cabbage, cashews, peanut butter and other nuts, cola beverages, and tea.

Factors That Affect Results

1. Do not apply tape to stones because adhesives interfere with infrared spectroscopy.

Other Data

1. Children commonly have stones from infection caused by calcium phosphate and magnesium ammonium phosphate.

2. Large doses of vitamin B$_6$ may reduce the risk of kidney stone formation in women.
3. Helical computed tomography has been shown to be helpful in identifying the fragility of kidney stones, and thus potential susceptibility to shock wave lithotripsy. See Computed tomography of the body—Diagnostic.

Kidney Ultrasonography (Kidney Echography, Kidney Ultrasound)—Diagnostic

Norm. Bilateral kidneys are properly located and are of normal size and shape. The outer contour is smooth. The kidney is surrounded by echoes reflected from perirenal fat. Intense echoes are reflected by the renal sinus. Absence of calculi, cyst, hydronephrosis, obstruction, or tumor.

Usage. Alternative to renal dye imaging tests for clients with allergy to radiographic dyes. Used for detection of hydronephrosis; diagnosis and localization of renal cysts, tumors, or calculi; evaluation of status after renal transplantation; and guidance for antegrade pyelography, biopsy, aspiration, or nephrostomy tube insertion. Also used to screen for preanal hydronephrosis. Although this procedure is inferior to intravenous pyelography when used alone, its advantages include the ability to detect some stones without the use of ionizing radiation. Disadvantages include risk of inaccurate measurement of calculus diameter, poor differentiation of true obstruction from nonobstructed dilatation, and inability to demonstrate the ureteral jet phenomenon at the uterovesical junction.

Description. Evaluation of the kidney structure by the creation of an oscilloscopic picture from the echoes of high-frequency sound waves passing over the flank area (acoustic imaging). The time required for the ultrasonic beam to be reflected back to the transducer from differing densities of tissue is converted by a computer to an electrical impulse displayed on an oscilloscopic screen to create a three-dimensional picture of the kidney. The kidney is imaged by use of the liver or spleen as an acoustic window. Renal cysts appear smooth, sonolucent, and spherical, with well-defined borders. In contrast, solid masses are of irregular shape with poorly defined borders and higher attenuation. Inflammatory cysts have thicker walls, have less well-defined borders, and contain low-level echoes. Early hematomas look like cysts and become more echogenic over time. Hydronephrosis is demonstrated by a large extrarenal pelvis, with renal parenchyma not detectable. In multicystic disease, the kidney is smaller than normal size, and the renal pelvis cannot be visualized. In polycystic disease, irregularly shaped cysts >1 mm in diameter are present in variable shapes and sizes. Because ultrasound cannot pinpoint obstruction, the presence of hydronephrosis requires additional confirmatory testing such as computed tomography, intravenous pyelography, or magnetic resonance urography.

Professional Considerations
Consent form NOT required.

Preparation
1. The client must be hydrated before the procedure.
2. This test should be performed before intestinal barium tests or after the barium is cleared from the system.
3. The client should disrobe below the waist or wear a gown.
4. Obtain ultrasonic gel or paste.

Procedure
1. The client is positioned prone in bed or on a procedure table. Very young children are positioned supine.
2. The flank area is covered with ultrasonic gel, and a lubricated transducer is passed slowly over the flank area at a variety of angles and at intervals about 1-2 cm apart.
3. Photographs are taken of the oscilloscopic display.

Postprocedure Care
1. Remove the lubricant from the skin.
2. If a biopsy is performed, see Biopsy, Site-specific—Specimen; Kidney biopsy—Specimen.
3. If an antegrade pyelography or a nephrostomy tube insertion is performed with

this test, see Antegrade pyelography—Diagnostic.

Client and Familyv Teaching
1. The procedure is painless and carries no risks (if kidney ultrasonography is not performed with invasive procedures).
2. This procedure takes about 30 minutes.

Factors That Affect Results
1. Dehydration interferes with adequate contrast between organs and body fluids.
2. Intestinal barium obscures results by preventing proper transmission and deflection of the high-frequency sound waves.
3. The more trunk fat present, the greater the attenuation (reduction in sound-wave amplitude and intensity), which interferes with the clarity of the picture. A lower frequency transducer should be used if a great deal of fat surrounds the kidney.
4. Magnetic resonance urography, while much more costly, is superior to kidney ultrasonography in identifying pathology for clients with kidneys that do not opacify (such as those with renal transplants) during excretory urography.
5. Proper hydration is essential for best detection. In clients who are not properly hydrated, up to 30% of obstructions and 25%-65% of hydronephrosis may not be detected.

Other Data
1. Further studies may include tomography or other radiographic imaging. Computed tomography is becoming the test of choice to detect kidney stones.
2. Contrast-enhanced ultrasonography of the kidney is being used investigationally and shows promise as an inexpensive test for detection of lesions, lacerations, hematomas, and infections of the kidney, pancreas, and liver.
3. See also Antegrade pyelography—Diagnostic.

Kidney Ultrasound
See **Kidney Ultrasonography**—Diagnostic.

Kidney-Ureter-Bladder (KUB)
See **Flat-Plate Radiography of Abdomen**—Diagnostic.

Kirsten
See **K-*ras***—Blood or Specimen.

Kleihauer-Betke Stain
See **Betke-Kleihauer Stain**—Diagnostic.

K-*ras* (Kirsten)—Blood or Specimen

Norm. Negative for K-*ras* mutations.

Usage. Colorectal cancer, adenocarcinoma of the lung, endometrial carcinoma (up to 33%), pancreatic and bile duct carcinoma (>75%). Used investigationally to determine its use in the detection, diagnosis, determination of response to therapy, and prognosis of colorectal cancer.

Description. The K-*ras* oncogene is one of three members of the *ras* family of oncogenes, along with H-*ras* and N-*ras*. This oncogene resides on chromosome 12p12 and is involved in protein coding that modulates cellular proliferation and differentiation. Mutations of the K-*ras* gene occur very early in tumorigenesis and are associated with more than 50% of colorectal adenocarcinomas and carcinomas, and in certain types of mutations, they may be predictive of eventual metastasis to the liver. A strong correlation has been demonstrated between the presence of mutated K-*ras* gene in the colorectal tumor and the presence of the mutated K-*ras* gene in the blood. The mutant K-*ras* protein p21*ras* can be detected in the blood by use of a DNA-extraction method, such as a polymerase chain reaction (PCR)–based assay that uses sequence-specific primers to amplify the mutant DNA, thus detecting the tumor cells in blood. It can also be detected in tissue specimens using immunohistochemical methods. The K-*ras* oncogene has the potential to be a specific and sensitive marker for colorectal cancer and has been associated with a poor prognosis when present in the blood. There have been incidents where clients with colorectal tumors containing the mutated K-*ras* gene did not have the K-*ras* gene identified in blood samples. These observations have been attributed to the possible genetic difference of metastatic lesions from the primary tumor, with the metastatic lesions either being lost or never possessing the K-*ras* mutation.

Professional Considerations

Informed consent is recommended for genetic testing.

Preparation

1. Tubes with the additives EDTA (lavender topped) or sodium citrate (blue topped). Heparinized tubes (green topped) have been used; however, there is some potential that heparin may inhibit the amplification assay. Confirm tube choice with the lab conducting the study. Clotted blood has been used. The mutated K-*ras* oncogene has been identified in serum and plasma samples.

Procedure

1. Amount of blood collected varies from 10 to 20 mL. Confirm amount of blood needed for the specimen with laboratory. A test has been conducted on serum and plasma stored in frozen state after several years.
2. Alternatively, tissue specimens may be obtained via biopsy. See Biopsy, Site-specific—Specimen.

Postprocedure Care

1. If biopsy is used, see Biopsy, Site-specific—Specimen.
2. None.

Client and Family Teaching

1. Refer to Appendix B, "Informed Consent for Genetic Testing".
2. Results may not be available for several days if testing is performed at a distant site.

Factors That Affect Results

1. None found.

Other Data

1. Generally, plasma or serum DNA mutations match the DNA mutations found in the primary tumor, leading to the assumption that the DNA mutations found in the blood are derived from the primary tumor.
2. K-*ras*–mutated DNA associated with colorectal cancer has been found in colorectal tumors and in the feces of clients with colorectal cancer, holding implications for use in screening for colorectal cancer.
3. The Genetic Information Nondiscrimination Act of 2008 prohibits health plans from using genetic family history or genetic test results from influencing eligibility or premiums for health insurance. It also prohibits employers from using this information to influence decisions about hiring, terminating employment, or employment pay, promotions, or privileges.

KUB (Kidney-Ureters-Bladder)

See Flat-Plate Radiography of Abdomen—Diagnostic.

Labile Factor

See Factor V—Blood.

La Crosse Virus Titer

See California Encephalitis Virus Titer—Serum.

Lactate Dehydrogenase (LD, LDH)—Blood

Norm. Highly method dependent.

		SI Units
Wróblewski Method	150-450 Units/L	72-217 IU/L
37 degrees C SCE method		Adult = 208-378U/L
Oxidoreductase method		Adult = 140-280 U/L; Neonate = 415-690 U/L.
Adult		
≤60 years	45-90 Units/L	45-90 U/L
>60 years	55-102 Units/L	55-102 U/L
Newborn	160-500 Units/L	160-500 U/L
Neonate	300-1500 Units/L	300-1500 U/L
Infant	100-250 Units/L	100-250 U/L
Child	60-170 Units/L	60-170 U/L

Increased Total LD. Alcoholism, anemia (hemolytic, megaloblastic, pernicious), anoxia, breast cancer (prognostic factor in skeletal metastasis), burns (electric, thermal), cancer, cardiomyopathy, cerebrovascular accident, cirrhosis, congestive heart failure (with myocardial infarction), convulsions, delirium tremens, dysrhythmias (ventricular), folic acid anemia, hepatic neoplasm, hepatitis (acute, toxic), hypothyroidism, infectious mononucleosis, intracardiac prosthetic valves, jaundice (obstructive), lactic acidosis, leukemia (granulocytic, acute), lymphoma, malaria, megaloblastic anemia, mononucleosis (infectious), muscular dystrophy, myocardial infarction, myxedema, nephrectomy, nephritis, nephrotic syndrome, ovarian dysgerminoma, pain (muscle and bone), peritonitis, pernicious anemia, pheochromocytoma, *Pneumocystis carinii* pneumonia, polymyositis, pulmonary embolism, pulmonary infarction, renal cortical infarction, renal infection, renal malignancy, rutile Fe-doping titanium dioxide nanorods in wastewater treatment (rat study, Nemmar et al, 2011), shock, sickle cell anemia, skeletal muscle necrosis, splenomegaly, sprue, toxic shock syndrome, trauma, tumors (malignant), and ulcerative colitis. Drugs include anesthetics, cephalosporins, chlorpromazine hydrochloride, clofibrate, codeine, dicumarol, ethyl alcohol (ethanol), floxuridine, fluorides, heparin, imipramine, lithium carbonate, lorazepam, meperidine, methotrexate, metoprolol tartrate, mithramycin, morphine and other narcotic analgesics, niacin, nifedipine, nitrofurantoin, piperacillin, procainamide hydrochloride, propranolol, quinidine, sulfonamides, thyroid hormone, and valproic acid.

Decreased Total LD. Irradiation therapy. Drugs include amikan, clofibrate, oxalates.

Description. Lactate dehydrogenase (LD) is an intracellular enzyme found in almost all body tissues and is released after tissue damage. The highest concentrations are found in organs such as the heart, liver, kidneys, and skeletal muscle cells as well as red blood cells. When body tissue is damaged from trauma, ischemia, or acid/base imbalance, LD is released into the bloodstream. The results of this test indicate that tissue damage has occurred but cannot pinpoint the specific location of damage. When total

LD is elevated to at least 130 IU/L, the test Lactate Dehydrogenase Isoenzymes—Blood should be performed to narrow down the source of tissue damage.

Professional Considerations
Consent form NOT required.

Preparation
1. Tube: Red topped, red/gray topped, or gold topped.
2. Do NOT draw during hemodialysis.

Procedure
1. Draw a 4-mL blood sample, without hemolysis.

Postprocedure Care
1. None.

Client and Family Teaching
1. This test is used to look for compounds commonly found in the body after some type of damage to the tissue. If the results are elevated, another test is usually performed on the same blood specimen to help determine which type of tissue has been damaged.

Factors That Affect Results
1. Reject hemolyzed, frozen, or refrigerated samples. Hemolysis elevates the LD_1 isoenzyme, which will elevate total LD results.
2. Heparin increases LD in one third of all clients being treated with heparin.
3. In burn clients, plasma LD activity is higher than in serum, possibly as a result of leakage from ruptured platelets.

Other Data
1. LD determination is recommended as a prognostic factor in colorectal carcinoma. Clients with an initially normal level versus those with an abnormal level had median survivals of 16 and 7 months, respectively. LD is also being studied for its use as a prognostic factor in myelodysplastic syndrome, with higher levels being associated with shorter survival.
2. See also Lactate dehydrogenase isoenzymes —Blood.

Lactate Dehydrogenase (LD) Isoenzymes—Blood

Norm.
LD_1 = 22%-36% cardiac and RBC origin
LD_2 = 35%-46% cardiac and RBC origin
LD_3 = 13%-26% lung, lymph, skeletal muscle, and spleen origin
LD_4 = 3%-10% hepatic and skeletal muscle origin
LD_5 = 2%-9% hepatic and skeletal muscle origin
$LD_2 > LD_1$
$LD_1:LD_2 \leq 1$
$LD_4 > LD_5$
$LD_5:LD_4 \leq 1:3$

Increased LD Total. Anemia (megaloblastic, hemolytic), cardiomyopathy, congestive heart failure, delirium tremens, hypothyroidism, inflammation, leukemia, muscle injury, myeloproliferative syndromes, myxedema, pulmonary infarction, and renal infarction. See Lactate dehydrogenase— Blood.

Increased LD_1. Folic acid anemia, germ cell tumors, hepatitis, megaloblastic anemia, myocardial infarction (rises 24 hours after injury, peaks at 72 hours, and returns to baseline level within 2 weeks), pernicious anemia, renal infarction, and testicular cancer.

Increased LD_2. Muscular dystrophy, pernicious anemia, renal (cortex) infarction, rhabdomyolysis, tumor.

Increased LD_3. Advanced cancer, collagen disease, infection (viral), lymphocytosis, pancreatitis, pericarditis, platelet destruction, pulmonary embolism, pulmonary infarct with hepatic congestion, pulmonary pneumonia, and skeletal muscle injury.

Increased LD_4. Hepatitis, infectious mononucleosis, lymphocytic leukemia, lymphoma, malignant ascites, ovarian carcinoma, platelet destruction, pulmonary embolism, and skeletal muscle injury.

Increased LD_5. Alcoholism, cirrhosis, congestive heart failure, hepatitis, infectious mononucleosis, malignant ascites, megaloblastic anemia, myocardial infarction, neonates, ovarian carcinoma, pulmonary infarct with hepatic congestion, and skeletal muscle injury.

Increased LD$_2$, LD$_3$, LD$_4$. Massive platelet destruction such as in pulmonary embolism, extensive blood transfusion, lymphatic involvement (infectious mononucleosis, lymphocytic leukemia, lymphoma).

Increased LD$_1$:LD$_2$ Ratio. Inverted, or "flipped," in anemia (hemolytic, megaloblastic, pernicious, sickle cell [acute]), cardiac hypoxia, folic acid deficiency, hemolysis, megaloblastic anemia, myocardial infarction, renal infarction.

Increased LD$_5$:LD$_4$ Ratio. Alcoholism.

Decreased. LD$_1$ is normally decreased in neonates and is also decreased in malignant ascites.

Description. See Lactate dehydrogenase—Blood. This test is normally conducted when total LD levels are elevated. Electrophoresis is used to separate the five isoenzymes of lactate dehydrogenase (LD), an enzyme that catalyzes the reversible oxidation of lactic acid to pyruvic acid. LD isoenzymes help pinpoint whether tissue damage is of cardiac, red blood cell, hepatic, or skeletal muscle origin. Sevinc et al (2005) found that examination of LD isoenzyme patterns was helpful in differentiating the origins of ascites. The study found that LD$_1$ was lower and LD$_4$ and LD$_5$ were higher in malignant ascites as compared to values found in nonmalignant ascites.

Professional Considerations
Consent form NOT required.

Preparation
1. Tube: Red topped, red/gray topped, or gold topped.

Procedure
1. Draw a 4-mL blood sample, without hemolysis. The test may also be performed on the original specimen sent for total LD measurement.

Postprocedure Care
1. Do not refrigerate or freeze the specimen.

Client and Family Teaching
1. This test is useful in diagnosing myocardial infarction, liver disease, tumors, and pulmonary embolus.

Factors That Affect Results
1. Reject hemolyzed specimens because this elevates LD$_1$.

Other Data
1. Isoenzymes should not be measured if total LD is <130 IU/L.

Lactic Acid—Blood

Norm.

		SI Units
Venous	0.5-2.2 mEq/L or 4.5-19.8 mg/dL	0.5-2.2 mmol/L
Arterial	0.5-1.6 mEq/L or 4.5-14.4 mg/dL	0.5-1.6 mmol/L

Increased.

Type A Lactic Acidosis (Inadequate Delivery of Oxygen to the Tissues)	Type B Lactic Acidosis (No Evidence of Inadequate Delivery of Oxygen to the Tissues) (Low Tissue Perfusion State May or May Not Be Present)
Conditions Causing Poor Tissue Perfusion to Hypoxia	B1 (caused by underlying disease or leading conditions)
Left ventricular failure	Cholera
Decreased cardiac output/cardiac arrest	Cirrhosis

Type A Lactic Acidosis	Type B Lactic Acidosis
Mesenteric ischemia	Diabetes mellitus
Shock	Hyperthermia
	Malaria
	Malignancy
Reduced Permeability of the Vasculature	
Reduced vascular tone	Organ failure (liver, kidney)
Decreased arterial oxygen	Panic attack
Hypoxemia	Sepsis
Severe anemia accompanied by poor perfusion	
CO poisoning	*B2 (Caused by Substances [e.g., Drug and Other Substance Toxicities])*
	Biguanides (e.g., phenformin), catecholamines, cocaine, cyanide, diethyl ether, ethanol, ethylene glycol, isoniazid, lactulose, methanol, nalidixic acid, niacin, nitroprusside, papaverine, paracetamol, paraldehyde, parenteral nutrition, salicylates, sorbitol, streptozotocin, theophylline, vitamin deficiency
Anaerobic Muscular Activity	*B3 (Caused by Inborn Errors of Metabolism)*
Exercise (strenuous)	Congenital lactic acidosis
Seizures (grand mal)	Enzyme deficiencies
	D-Lactic acid syndrome

From Cohen R, Woods H: *Clinical and biochemical aspects of lactic acidosis*, Oxford, 1976, Blackwell Scientific Publications.

Decreased. Hypothermia.

Description. Lactic acid is derived from carbohydrate metabolism and is used for muscle contraction when energy needs exceed oxygen supply (anaerobic metabolism). One fifth of the lactic acid produced is oxidized through the citric acid cycle, and the rest is converted in the muscle to glycogen. Lactic acid is involved in the body's automatic compensatory systems that maintain acid-base balance, increasing in response to compensate for respiratory alkalosis. Levels are elevated when the body is undergoing physiologic stress. Several classification schemes that differentiate types of lactic acidosis related to cause are presented in the literature and summarized in the preceding table.

Professional Considerations
Consent form NOT required.

Preparation
1. Tubes: Gray topped for the venous sample. Also obtain arterial puncture supplies and one heparinized tube.
2. Draw the blood sample without a tourniquet if possible.
3. Do NOT allow the client to clench and then unclench the hand before blood drawing.

Procedure
1. Obtain a 4-mL venous blood sample in a gray topped tube containing a glycolytic inhibitor.
2. Draw an arterial sample in a heparinized tube, place it on ice immediately, and transport it quickly to the laboratory. NOTE: Arterial samples are of little diagnostic value.

Postprocedure Care
1. Assess the arterial puncture site after applying pressure for 5 minutes.
2. Send the specimen to the laboratory immediately.

Client and Family Teaching
1. Pressure will be maintained on the area where the artery was accessed to avoid unnecessary bruising.

Factors That Affect Results
1. Reject specimens received more than 15 minutes after collection.
2. Intravenous infusions may affect acid-base balance.

Other Data
1. Lactic acidosis is accompanied by an increase in the anion gap.
2. Lactic acidosis has been successfully treated with dichloroacetate.

Lactic Acid, Cerebrospinal Fluid

See **Cerebrospinal Fluid, Lactic Acid**—Specimen.

Lactic Dehydrogenase (LDH)

See **Lactate Dehydrogenase**—Blood.

Laparoscopy (Peritoneoscopy)—Diagnostic

Norm. Negative.

Usage. Ascites, biopsy, cholangiography, cirrhosis, complex renal stones, dysmenorrhea, ectopic pregnancy, endometritis, fever of undetermined origin, gallbladder disease, identification of abdominal cavity adhesions, infertility, jaundice, lymphoma staging, malignancy staging, pancreatic disease, and pelvic inflammatory disease (PID). Used in conjunction with ultrasound to stage pancreatic cancer. Enables accurate staging of gastrointestinal malignancies; superior to other imaging methods for detecting superficial liver metastases; provides a diagnostic route with access for therapeutic surgical interventions if abnormalities are identified. Also used therapeutically for surgical procedures, such as colectomy and nephrectomy.

Description. Direct inspection of the surfaces of the internal organs such as the liver, gallbladder, pancreas, fallopian tubes, ovaries, uterus, and lymph nodes by use of a fiberoptic telescope inserted transabdominally into the abdominal cavity. Diagnostic laparoscopy prevents unnecessary surgical laparotomies by providing direct visualization inside of the abdominal cavity with a minimally invasive procedure. Surgical procedures such as cholecystectomy, biopsy, or tubal ligation may be performed by means of laparoscopy. Use of electronic power morcellators is a newer method for removal of tissue that reduces the risk of postprocedure hernia by minimizing fascia damage, but carries with it higher risk for internal organ damage. Other advances in technology include 3-dimensional views and high-resolution digital images.

Professional Considerations
Consent form IS required.

Risks
Hemorrhage, infection, intestinal or organ puncture or damage, myocardial ischemia, peritonitis, respiratory acidosis, subcutaneous emphysema.

Contraindications
Advanced abdominal wall malignancy, anticoagulant therapy, bleeding disorders, chronic tuberculosis, intra-abdominal hemorrhage, multiple surgical adhesions, peritonitis, thrombocytopenia.

Precautions
Use with caution during pregnancy. "The occurrence of a miscarriage, premature labor or fetal death appears to be related to the underlying pathology, independent of the operative intervention" (Al-Fozan and Tulandi, 2004). The use of CO_2 insufflation has been associated with cardiorespiratory deterioration in clients with preexisting respiratory problems.

Preparation
1. Assess for allergies.
2. Prepare the surgical site by removal of any hair.
3. Insert an indwelling urinary catheter.
4. Administer a cleansing enema 4 hours before the procedure.
5. The client should void just before the procedure.
6. Bandage inguinal and umbilical hernias.
7. See Client and Family Teaching.
8. Just before beginning the procedure, take a "time out" to verify the correct client, procedure, and site.

Procedure
1. Anesthesia may be given. Regional anesthesia is associated with less postoperative side effects and a shorter recovery period than is general anesthesia.

2. A small surgical incision is made in the abdomen just below the umbilicus.
3. Carbon dioxide is used to insufflate the abdominal cavity so that the organs are easily visualized.
4. The laparoscope is inserted and visualization begins.
5. Surgical specimens may be taken using electronic power morcellators.
6. The procedure takes about 30 minutes.

Postprocedure Care
1. Assess the surgical incision area for signs of infection for 24 hours.
2. Assess for signs and symptoms of hemorrhage as the major complication. Signs may include bleeding at the dressing site, increasing abdominal pain and firmness, and hypotension.
3. Monitor vital signs every 30 minutes × 4 and PRN.
4. Provide analgesia for incisional pain and for the pain caused by the carbon dioxide gas remaining in the peritoneal cavity.

Client and Family Teaching
1. Fast from food and fluids for 8-12 hours before the procedure.

2. A common complaint after this procedure is shoulder, scapular, and general discomfort in the upper torso caused by referred pain from the carbon dioxide gas remaining in the abdomen. This pain can last for several days but should decrease in severity as each day passes. Pain medicine will be prescribed to help ease the pain.
3. Avoid carbonated beverages for 1-2 days after the procedure because such beverages will add to the gas pains and may cause vomiting when added to the carbon dioxide left over from the procedure.
4. Minimize physical activity for 3-7 days, as instructed by the physician.
5. Notify the physician for increasing pain, redness, or drainage at the laparoscopy site.

Factors That Affect Results
1. Equipment should be in good working order.

Other Data
1. Nausea, puncture of the intestinal loop, infection, hemorrhage, and subcutaneous emphysema are possible complications of laparoscopy.

LASA

See Lipid-Associated Sialic Acid—Plasma or Serum.

Laxative Abuse Test

See Phenolphthalein Test—Diagnostic.

LD

See Lactate Dehydrogenase—Blood.

LDH

See Lactate Dehydrogenase—Blood.

LDL or LDL-C

See Low-Density Lipoprotein Cholesterol—Blood.

LE Cell Test

See **Lupus Test**—Blood.

LE Preparation

See **Lupus Test**—Blood.

LE Slide Cell Test

See **Lupus Test**—Blood.

LE Test

See **Lupus Test**—Blood.

Lead—Blood and Urine

Norm.

		SI Units
Whole Blood		
Adult	<20 μg/dL	<1.0 μmol/L
Child	<10 μg/dL	<0.5 μmol/L
Industrial exposure	<60 μg/dL	<2.9 μmol/L
Lead encephalopathy in children*	>100 μg/dL	>4.8 μmol/L
Urine	0.08 mg/mL	0.39 mmol/L
	120 mg/24 hours	

*The Centers for Disease Control and Prevention defines lead toxicity in children as a blood level of ≥25 μg/dL combined with erythrocyte protoporphyrin ≥35 μg/dL.

Poisoning Level Symptoms and Treatment

Symptoms. Early signs of lead poisoning include anorexia, apathy or irritability, headache, dizziness, sleep disturbances, fatigue, anemia, weight loss, and abdominal "lead colic." Characteristic toxic effects include encephalopathy and peripheral neuropathy (wrist drop) and seizures. Elevated erythrocyte protoporphyrins in the blood is also suggestive of lead poisoning. Aminoaciduria, glycosuria, and Fanconi syndrome have been demonstrated in children exposed to lead.

Treatment

NOTE: Treatment choice(s) depend(s) on client's history and condition and episode history.

1. For blood lead levels of 45-70 μg/dL, use chelation therapy with succimer.

2. For blood lead levels >70 μg/dL:
   a. Admit for hospitalization.
   b. Perform lavage of the stomach with magnesium sulfate or sodium sulfate.
   c. Control seizures with diazepam (Valium).
   d. Reduce cerebral edema with osmotic diuresis (mannitol) and corticosteroids.
   e. Administer possible chelation therapy that includes several injections of calcium disodium EDTA and dimercaprol (see Lead mobilization test—24-Hour urine).

Increased. Ataxia, iron deficiency in children, metal poisoning, microcytic anemia from lead poisoning, and neuropathy; drinking from earthen teapots that contain lead. Herbal or natural remedies include the Chinese fungus *Cordyceps sinensis*.

Description. Lead is a heavy metal that is used in paint, leaded gasoline, insecticides, pottery glaze, and illicit liquor and is found in the fumes of old painted wood. It is an electropositive metal that has an affinity for the negatively charged sulfhydryl group and inhibits three enzymes in the body: delta-aminolevulinic acid dehydrase, copropor-phyrinogen oxidase, and ferrochelatase. These enzymes are necessary for the production of heme, the iron-containing portion of hemoglobin. The majority of lead in the body is stored in the skeletal system and is thought to be released into the bloodstream in increasing amounts during periods of accelerated bone turnover and mineral loss. The acceptable levels for blood lead content have been gradually lowered over time as new information on lead's detrimental effects has become available. Lead measurements are performed on whole-blood specimens because whole-blood concentrations are 75 times higher than those of plasma or serum. Exposure of children to low levels of lead has been associated with reduced intellectual and neuropsychologic development. For this reason, many communities have in place routine screening for lead exposure of all schoolchildren. This test is the most appropriate test in screening for elevated lead levels in children and in workers in close contact with lead-containing substances.

Professional Considerations
Consent form NOT required.

Preparation
1. Tube: Lead-free, lavender topped or green topped for whole-blood sample. Samples MAY be drawn during hemodialysis.
2. Obtain a 3-L plastic, acid-washed urine collection container for the urine sample.
3. Screen client for use of herbal medicines or natural remedies.
4. See Client and Family Teaching.

Procedure
1. *Whole blood*: Draw a 3-mL blood sample.
2. *Urine*: Collect all the urine voided in a 24-hour period in a 3-L plastic container that has been washed with 10% hydrochloric acid (HCl) solution.

Postprocedure Care
1. *Urine*: Record starting and ending dates and times, as well as the total volume of urine, on the laboratory requisition.

Client and Family Teaching
1. Maintain on low-calcium diet for 3 days before collection of the 24-hour sample to mobilize lead from the bones and prevent false-positive results.
2. Save all the urine voided in the container provided and avoid contaminating the urine with stool or toilet paper. If any urine is accidentally discarded, discard the entire specimen and restart the collection the next day.
3. Avoid eating from old pottery bowls that may have been glazed with lead-based paint.
4. Some herbal medicines contain high levels of lead, which can cause lead poisoning. Do not use these products without first consulting your physician.

Factors That Affect Results
1. Anticoagulant other than heparin is found in the tube.
2. A high-calcium diet creates false-positive results in the urine test.
3. A fungal remedy that may increase lead levels and induce lead poisoning as a result of its lead content is *Cordyceps sinensis* powder.
4. There is some evidence that lactation increases the release of lead from bone storage into the bloodstream.
5. It is thought that conditions of high bone turnover such as pregnancy, menopause, and secondary hyperparathyroidism lead to increased release of lead into the bloodstream.

Other Data
1. Fingerstick specimens are not recommended. If they are used, positive results should be confirmed with venous whole-blood testing to rule out contamination of the fingerstick specimen.
2. Urine levels for lead toxicity may be normal when serum levels indicate lead toxicity.
3. Urine uric acid levels and blood erythropoietin levels may be elevated in lead exposure.

Lead Mobilization Test (Calcium Disodium EDTA Mobilization Test), 24-Hour—Urine

Norm.

		SI Units
Normal Lead Level Before Mobilization Test		
Adult	<150 μg/day	<0.73 μmol/day
Child	<100 μg/day	<0.48 μmol/day
Normal Lead Level After Mobilization Test		
Adult	<650 μg/day	<3.2 μmol/day
Child	<1 μg of Pb/mg of CaNa$_2$-EDTA administered over a 24-hour period	
Lead Level in Clients With a Higher-Than-Normal Body Burden of Lead After Mobilization Test		
Adult	>1000 μg/day	>4.9 μmol/day
Child	<1 μg of Pb/mg of CaNa$_2$-EDTA administered over a 24-hour period	

Usage. Diagnosis and treatment of lead poisoning. Used when blood lead levels are >100 mg/dL.

Description. Lead is an environmental trace metal of which the average client takes in 150-250 μg/day. Only a small fraction of that taken in is absorbed. Lead poisoning occurs when clients frequently come into contact with items or industries that contain large amounts of lead. Some examples are paint, batteries, gasoline, pottery, bullets, and printing materials and the mining, auto manufacturing, and welding industries. Lead affects many organs and tissues of the body, but most of it is stored in the bones. Symptoms of lead toxicity include gastrointestinal colic, vomiting, anorexia, anemia, and central nervous system abnormalities ranging from irritability, peripheral neuropathy, memory lapses, and impaired concentration to severe lead encephalopathy. *Calcium disodium EDTA* (calcium disodium edetate, CaNa$_2$-EDTA, calcium versenate) is one of three substances known to bind to lead or form tight complexes with lead, resulting in removal of lead from the body tissues and excretion of lead through the kidneys. The complex forms when lead displaces calcium from the drug molecule. The test involves administering calcium disodium EDTA intravenously or intramuscularly and assessing the change in urinary lead excretion for 24 hours. Half-life of the drug is 20-60 minutes intravenously and 90 minutes intramuscularly. This test is currently the most reliable index of the body burden of lead.

Professional Considerations
Consent form NOT required.

Risks and Precautions
This procedure should be used with caution in clients with renal impairment.
Contraindications
Severe lead encephalopathy, pregnancy, anuria, or severe renal disease.

Preparation
1. Assess for adequate urinary output.
2. Obtain a baseline 24-hour urine collection for lead level in a refrigerated, lead-free (polyethylene), 4-L container that has been rinsed with hydrochloric acid (HCl).
3. Obtain a baseline urinalysis; a urine coproporphyrin level; blood urea nitrogen and serum creatinine, calcium, and phosphorus levels; and repeat daily throughout the test.
4. Write the beginning time of the urine collection for the mobilization test on the laboratory requisition.
5. Uncomfortable intramuscular injection site pain may be minimized by the addition of 1 mL of 1% procainamide to each milliliter of drug.

Procedure

1. Begin a 24-hour urine collection in a lead-free, 4-L container that has been washed with HCl.
2. *Adults*: Perform the mobilization using one of the following three regimens:
   a. *Intravenous route*: Administer 1.0 g of $CaNa_2$-EDTA in 250-500 mL of 5% dextrose in water over 1-2 hours intravenously every 12 hours for no more than 5 days. Wait 2 full days before repeating the test, if necessary.
   b. *Intramuscular route*: Administer 2.0 g of $CaNa_2$-EDTA per day intramuscularly in divided doses (that is, 500 mg in each buttock, 12 hours apart).
   c. *Long-term mobilization*: Administer 1.0 g of $CaNa_2$-EDTA three times a week until the urine collection shows normal levels of lead excretion.
3. *Children*: Perform the mobilization using one of the following two regimens:
   a. *For mildly to moderately increased lead levels*: Administer $CaNa_2$-EDTA 500-1000 $mg/m^2/24$ hours intramuscularly (preferred) or intravenously every 12 hours for 3-5 days. Do not exceed 50 mg/kg/24 hours. Wait 4 full days before repeating the test, if necessary.
   b. *For severe lead intoxication*: Administer $CaNa_2$-EDTA 50 mg/kg/24 hours or 1500 $mg/m^2/24$ hours intravenously or intramuscularly in divided doses. Do not exceed 70 mg/kg/24 hours.
4. Continue urine collection for 24 hours. Encourage the oral intake of fluids throughout the collection period except for clients with lead encephalopathy (because of the risk of increasing intracranial pressure).

Postprocedure Care

1. Write the ending time and total urine output on the laboratory requisition.

2. Transport the entire specimen to the lab. The lead measurement is performed in a lead-free laboratory space on an aliquot of the 24-hour specimen.

Client and Family Teaching

1. Save all the urine voided in the container provided and avoid contaminating the urine with stool or toilet paper. If any urine is accidentally discarded, discard the entire specimen and restart the collection the next day.
2. Outline environmental sources of lead.
3. See also Lead—Blood and urine.

Factors That Affect Results

1. Clients who have reached the point of lead encephalopathy may not show clinical improvement after this procedure.
2. The higher the blood lead level, the greater the excretable amount of lead.

Other Data

1. Intake and output must be monitored during this test. Diminished urine output may result in symptoms of lead toxicity.
2. Other substances used to chelate lead include succimer, dimercaprol (British anti-Lewisite [BAL]) and D-penicillamine.
3. Dimercaprol (BAL) may be combined with $CaNa_2$-EDTA for clients with extremely severe lead intoxication.
4. As blood lead is chelated and excreted in the urine, levels may rise again as stored bone lead is mobilized. The mobilization test may be repeated in this circumstance.
5. There is some evidence that lead mobilized from the bones after chelation becomes redistributed to body organs, especially the brain and liver.
6. $CaNa_2$-EDTA is reported to also chelate some other heavy metals.

Lecithin/Sphingomyelin Ratio

See **Amniocentesis and Amniotic Fluid Analysis**—Diagnostic Routine Analysis.

LEEP

See **Colposcopy, Diagnostic; Pap Smear**—Diagnostic.

Legionella Antigen (*Legionella* Urine Antigen, LUA)—Urine

Norm. Negative.

Usage. Provides rapid diagnosis for infection with *Legionella pneumophila*.

Description. Approximately 80% of clients with *Legionella* serogroup 1 infection will shed soluble *Legionella* antigens in their urine. Thus this ELISA is the test of choice for rapid diagnosis of *Legionella* (serogroup 1) infection. However, the most accurate diagnosis is obtained using results from this test in combination with culture, serologic results, and antibody testing. Peak month for diagnosis is September.

Professional Considerations
Consent form NOT required.

Preparation
1. Obtain a sterile specimen collection container.

Procedure
1. Collect a 10-mL midstream or catheter urine specimen.

Postprocedure Care
1. None.

Client and Family Teaching
1. See *Legionella pneumophila*—Culture.

Factors That Affect Results
1. The sensitivity of this test for travel-associated *Legionella* infection is 95%, for community-acquired *Legionella* infection is 80%, and for nosocomial *Legionella* infection only 45% (Helbig et al, 2003).

Other Data
1. See *Legionella pneumophila*—Culture; *Legionella pneumophila*, Direct FA smear—Specimen; Legionnaires' disease antibodies—Blood.

Legionella pneumophila—Culture

Norm. Negative. No growth. A positive culture may be grown in 2-7 days.

Positive. Legionnaires' disease.

Description. A gram-negative, non–acid-fast bacillus that causes legionnaires' disease, a form of lobar pneumonia that causes symptoms of fever, headache, malaise, and diffuse alveolar damage. Concomitant symptoms of legionnaires' disease may also include cardiac inflammation (endocarditis, pericarditis), pancreatitis, perirectal abscess, peritonitis, pyelonephritis, sinusitis, and wound infection. Two forms of this disease are a mild, self-limiting flulike syndrome of malaise and muscle aches, and a more severe form in which pneumonia and septic shock can occur. If untreated, *Legionella* is fatal in up to 25% of immunocompromised clients. Because of its ability to thrive in water, outbreaks of legionnaires' disease have been attributed to community water supplies contaminated with *Legionella pneumophila*. In addition, strains have been found to persist for years in contamination of hospital water supplies. Symptoms develop 2-10 days after exposure to the organism. Clients at highest risk of developing this disease are asphalt workers, those who received cytotoxic chemotherapy or corticosteroids, those with preexisting pulmonary disease, passengers in a vehicle where windscreen wiper fluid does not contain added screenwash, professional drivers who drive through industrial areas, smokers, supermarket-associated mist machine contact, telephone manhole workers, and users of whirlpool spa. This test includes culture and direct fluorescent antibody (FA) smear of a fresh specimen, which may be obtained from a biopsy of the lung, pleural fluid, washings or brushings from the bronchi, transtracheal aspirates, blood, pus, or sputum.

Professional Considerations
Consent form NOT required for this test but IS required when bronchoscopy, lung biopsy, or lung aspiration is used to obtain the specimen. See the individual procedures for risks and contraindications.

Preparation
1. Obtain a sterile specimen container.

Procedure
1. The physician obtains a sterile specimen of tissue by bronchoscopy or biopsy or of pleural fluid by aspiration. Sterile

collections of sputum, blood, or pus may also be collected.
2. Send the specimen to the laboratory immediately.
3. Expectorated sputum will NOT have an FA smear.

Postprocedure Care
1. Results take 1-2 weeks.
2. Do not freeze the specimen.

Client and Family Teaching
1. Undue pain or shortness of breath should be reported.
2. Legionnaires' disease is treated with erythromycin (drug of choice) or rifampin if erythromycin does not eradicate the organism.

Factors That Affect Results
1. Contamination of the specimen will affect the results.
2. The sensitivity of the sputum sample results is improved when the sample is treated with an acid wash before being cultured.

Other Data
1. Lung biopsy provides the highest rate of identification (>90%), followed by sputum (80%-90%). The specificity of blood testing is only ≤30%.
2. A negative culture does not rule out the presence of *Legionella* because sensitivity of culturing methods may be 50%.
3. The most commonly used rapid diagnostic test for *Legionella* organism is *Legionella* antigen—Urine.

Legionella pneumophila, Direct FA Smear—Specimen

Norm. Negative.

Positive. Legionnaires' disease.

Description. See *Legionella pneumophila*—Culture for a description of legionnaires' disease. This test performs a direct fluorescent antibody microscopic examination of a specimen smear of lung tissue, pleural fluid, sputum, bronchial washing, or other body fluid. It provides rapid results (within 1-3 hours). The sensitivity of this test varies widely, from 24% to 80%, but has high specificity at >95%.

Professional Considerations
Consent form NOT required for the test but IS required for lung biopsy or lung aspiration by bronchial washing. See the individual procedure for risks and contraindications.

Preparation
1. Obtain the necessary sterile biopsy containers.

Procedure
1. Prepare for a lung biopsy, bronchial washing, pleural tap, or sterile sputum specimen.

Postprocedure Care
1. Send the specimen to the laboratory in the sterile container immediately after collection.

Client and Family Teaching
1. Report undue pain or shortness of breath.
2. Legionnaires' disease is treated with erythromycin (drug of choice) or rifampin if erythromycin does not eradicate the organism.

Factors That Affect Results
1. False-positive results are seen with tularemic pneumonia.
2. False-negative results may occur if a saliva specimen, rather than a sputum specimen, is sampled.

Other Data
1. There are several subgroups of *Legionella*: *L. bozemanii*, *L. dumoffii*, *L. gormanii*, *L. jordanis*, *L. longbeachae*, and *L. micdadei*.
2. The most commonly used rapid diagnostic test for *Legionella* organism is *Legionella*—Urine test.

Legionella Urine Antigen

See Legionella Antigen—Urine.

Legionnaires' Disease Antibodies—Blood

Norm. Negative or less than a fourfold change in titer between acute and convalescent samples.

A *fourfold rise in titer* >1:128 from the acute-to-convalescent sample provides evidence of recent infection.

A *single titer* ≥1:256 is evidence of infection at an undetermined time.

Positive. Legionnaires' disease.

Negative. Normal.

Description. See *Legionella pneumophila*—Culture for a description of legionnaires' disease. This test identifies specific antibodies produced after the body has been infected with the *Legionella* organism. In legionnaires' disease, antibody titers rise and fall at a predictable rate. Levels are low the first week, rise steadily at weeks 2-4, peak during week 5 of the disease, and then drop slowly and remain elevated for many years.

Professional Considerations
Consent form NOT required.

Preparation
1. Tube: Red topped, red/gray topped, or gold topped.

Procedure
1. Draw a 10-mL blood sample.

Postprocedure Care
1. Draw convalescent samples of blood 4-6 weeks after the onset of symptoms.

Client and Family Teaching
1. Legionnaires' disease is treated with erythromycin (drug of choice) or rifampin if erythromycin does not eradicate the organism.

Factors That Affect Results
1. Hemolysis of the specimen invalidates results.
2. False-positive results may be caused when the client has tuberculosis.
3. Clients with a history of *Legionella pneumophila* infection can have elevated titers for several years.
4. 10%-20% of clients with *L. pneumophila* infection have false-negative results.
5. False-positive results may occur in clients infected with gram-negative organisms and non–*L. pneumophila* infections.

Other Data
1. The most commonly used rapid diagnostic test for *Legionella* organism is *Legionella* antigen—Urine test.

Leiden Mutation

See **Factor V**—Blood; **Protein C**—Blood.

Leptospira Culture—Urine

Norm. Negative; no *Leptospira* isolated.

Positive. Leptospirosis.

Description. *Leptospira* is a pathogenic spirochete causing human infection (leptospirosis). Common hosts include cattle, dogs, foxes, mice, opossums, rats, raccoons, and skunks. Leptospirosis has traditionally been an occupational disease for veterinarians, animal caretakers, butchers, fish handlers, and dog wardens, who contract the disease through direct skin contact with the urine or tissue of infected animals. In recent years, it is becoming a significant health problem in urban slums in developing nations, where there is poor sanitation. Symptoms are flulike but may be as severe as meningitis, renal insufficiency, and hemolytic anemia. Culture for *Leptospira* is used to confirm findings from screening methods such as dipstick, IgM ELISA, and slide agglutination tests. Isolation of *Leptospira* in culture may occur in as little as 6-14 days or take as long as 28 days. Serum *Leptospira* serodiagnosis for antibody identification should always be performed concomitantly with urine culture.

Professional Considerations
Consent form NOT required.

Preparation

1. Obtain a sterile urine specimen container.
2. Alkalinization of the urine may reduce the chance of false-negative results.

Procedure

1. Collect a 50-mL midstream urine specimen in a sterile plastic container. See clean-catch collection instructions in the test Body fluid, Routine—Culture.

Postprocedure Care

1. Transport the specimen to the laboratory within 1 hour.

Client and Family Teaching

1. The clean-catch urine technique must be used to decrease the risk of specimen contamination. See clean-catch collection instructions in the test Body fluid, Routine—Culture.

2. Up to 4 weeks may be required for cultures to grow.

Factors That Affect Results

1. Repeat samples may be necessary if the sample is not tested immediately because acidic urine destroys *Leptospira* bacteria.

Other Data

1. Serum should always be obtained for antibody studies when the urine culture is obtained.
2. Leptospirosis is treated with penicillin or doxycycline.
3. Urine results are normally available in 4-8 weeks.
4. *Leptospira* cultures are difficult to grow and frequently give false-negative results when the specimen is not inoculated to medium within 30 minutes of being obtained.

Leptospira Serodiagnosis—Blood

Norm. Negative.

Positive. Jaundice, leptospirosis (fourfold increase in titer between acute and convalescent specimens), meningitis, and renal failure (acute).

Description. See *Leptospira* culture—Urine for a description of leptospirosis. This test is used to detect antibodies to *Leptospira* in the blood and can detect the antibodies when negative results are obtained from culture or dark-field examination for the *Leptospira* organism.

Professional Considerations

Consent form NOT required.

Preparation

1. Tube: Red topped, red/gray topped, or gold topped.

Procedure

1. Draw a 7-mL blood sample.

Postprocedure Care

1. Draw a convalescent sample of blood 14-21 days later.

Client and Family Teaching

1. Leptospirosis cannot be ruled out just because cultures were negative. This test can identify antibodies to the organism, even when cultures are negative. It is important to return for convalescent sampling in 2-3 weeks.

Factors That Affect Results

1. Hemolysis of the specimen invalidates the results.
2. A variety of rapid screening tests have demonstrated a low to high sensitivity during the first week of illness, when treatment decisions are crucial. Thus choice of methods used for rapid detection should be literature-based.

Other Data

1. None.

Leucine Aminopeptidase (LAP)—Blood

Norm. Males: 80 to 200 units/mL.
　　Females: 75 to 185 units/mL.

Increased. Cancer of the liver, pancreas, or head and neck; cholelithiasis; cirrhosis; jaundice (obstructive); liver damage or dysfunction; pancreatitis; pregnancy (third trimester).

Description. Leucine aminopeptidase (LAP) is an enzyme present in liver cells, blood, bile, and urine, and in the placenta. This test is helpful in the differential diagnosis of elevated alkaline phosphatase because the leucine aminopeptidase level is normal in clients with diseases of the bone. Because LAP is released into the bloodstream after liver damage and by liver tumors, it may serve as a marker for these conditions.

Professional Considerations
Consent form NOT required.

Preparation
1. Tube: Red topped, red/gray topped, or gold topped.
2. See Client and Family Teaching.

Procedure
1. Draw a 7-mL blood sample.

Postprocedure Care
1. None.

Client and Family Teaching
1. Fast, except for fluids, for 8 hours.

Factors That Affect Results
1. The last trimester of pregnancy increases the results.

Other Data
1. Maternal serum placental LAP was shown in one study to decrease in women who subsequently experienced preterm labor.

Leukocyte

See **Differential Leukocyte Count**—Peripheral Blood.

Leukocyte Acid Phosphatase

See **Tartrate-Resistant Acid Phosphatase Stain**—Specimen.

Leukocyte Alkaline Phosphatase (LAP, Neutrophil Alkaline Phosphatase, NAP)—Blood

Norm. Score: 20-100 out of a maximum of 400. Score is based on a 0 to 4+ rating of 100 neutrophils.

Increased. Age ≤14 days, agnogenic myeloid metaplasia, aplastic anemia, burns, Down syndrome, Hodgkin's disease, immediately postoperatively, leukemia (acute lymphocytic or hairy cell), myelofibrosis with myeloid metaplasia, polycythemia vera, pregnancy and during lactation, stress, thrombocytopenia infection, tissue necrosis, trauma. Drugs include ACTH, ethylene glycol (intoxication), and oral contraceptives.

Decreased. Anemia (aplastic, pernicious), leukemia (acute monocytic, chronic granulocytic, or chronic myelogenous), cirrhosis, collagen disease, congestive heart failure, diabetes mellitus, erythroleukemia, gout, hereditary hypophosphatemia, hypophosphatasia, idiopathic thrombocytopenic purpura, infectious mononucleosis (early), and paroxysmal nocturnal hemoglobinuria.

Description. Leukocyte alkaline phosphatase (LAP) is an enzyme present in neutrophilic granules from the metamyelocyte to the segmented stage and represents intracellular metabolism. Dye is added to a smear of blood, and a color reaction occurs, enabling the stained neutrophils to be identified by the appearance of red, blue, or purple granules viewed in the cytoplasm of mature leukocytes. The neutrophils are given a rating of 0 to 4, based on the intensity of the color reaction. The score is the sum of the ratings for each neutrophil, with a total possible score of 400. This test helps differentiate chronic myelogenous leukemia, which produces low scores, from three other myeloproliferative diseases—polycythemia vera, myelofibrosis, and essential thrombocytopenia—that produce higher scores. It also is useful for differentiating polycythemia vera from secondary polycythemia, in which normal scores would be found.

Professional Considerations

Consent form NOT required.

Preparation

1. Preschedule the test with the laboratory.
2. *For venous or arterial sample*: Tube: green topped or black topped. Also obtain foil.
3. *For capillary sample*: Obtain a lancet and six slides.

Procedure

1. Draw a 2-mL blood sample and wrap the tube in foil.
2. Alternatively, obtain a peripheral finger-stick or earlobe capillary sample and smear it onto six slides.

Postprocedure Care

1. Transport the specimen to the laboratory immediately. The slides must be fixed in 1:9 formalin/methanol for 30 seconds at 0 to 5 degrees C, washed in running water, and air-dried within 30 minutes.

Client and Family Teaching

1. Fast for 6 hours before the test.
2. Results are normally available within 4 hours.

Factors That Affect Results

1. Reject specimens collected in EDTA-anticoagulated (lavender topped) tubes because EDTA inhibits the activity of LAP.
2. Results are invalid if the client is neutropenic (that is, <1000/mm³ neutrophils).

Other Data

1. Values are normal in myelomonocytic leukemia, lymphosarcoma, multiple myeloma, relative polycythemia, sickle cell crisis, and viral infections.

Leukocyte Cytochemistry (Cytochemical Stain)—Specimen

Norm. Requires interpretation.

Increased. Cushing's disease, diphtheria, Down syndrome, eclampsia, hemolytic anemia, hemorrhage, Hodgkin's disease, leukemia (acute lymphocytic), leukocytosis (15,000-50,000/mL) associated with infection, lobar pneumonia, lymphoma, malaria, meningitis, mercury poisoning, myeloid metaplasia, multiple myeloma, polycythemia vera, pregnancy, stress, syphilis, tissue necrosis, tuberculosis, tumors, and trauma. Drugs include ACTH and oral contraceptives.

Decreased. Anemia (aplastic), collagen disease, hereditary hypophosphatasia, idiopathic thrombocytopenic purpura, leukemia (acute and chronic myelocytic, acute monocytic), myelosclerosis, paroxysmal nocturnal hemoglobinuria, and pernicious anemia.

Description. A staining of blood smears and bone marrow that estimates alkaline phosphatase enzyme activity in neutrophilic granules. A newer microarray technique enables extensive immunophenotyping into distinctive patterns that differentiate chronic lymphocytic leukemia (CLL), hairy cell leukemia, mantle cell lymphoma, acute myeloid leukemia, and T-cell acute lymphoblastic leukemia.

Professional Considerations

Consent form IS required for bone marrow biopsy. See Bone marrow aspiration analysis—Specimen for procedure risks and contraindications.

Preparation

1. Obtain a bone marrow biopsy tray, slides, a sterile container, an alcohol wipe, a tourniquet, a needle, a syringe, and a lavender topped tube.

Procedure

1. Draw a 2-mL or capillary (preferred) blood sample.
2. Obtain a bone marrow biopsy and place it in a sterile container. See Bone marrow aspiration analysis—Specimen.

Postprocedure Care

1. Apply a pressure dressing to the bone marrow site and assess it for bleeding every 5 minutes × 3.
2. Transport the specimen to the laboratory immediately.

Client and Family Teaching

1. Bone marrow specimens are usually taken from the hip (iliac crest) or sternum. The procedure is transiently painful and has been described as extremely painful but only for a short time.

Factors That Affect Results
1. Tubes containing EDTA inhibit the activity of leukocyte alkaline phosphatase.

Other Data
1. Normal levels found in kwashiorkor, leukemia (chronic lymphocytic, acute and chronic myelomonocytic), lymphosarcoma, and viral infections.
2. See also Bone marrow aspiration analysis—Specimen for care implications for the bone marrow biopsy procedure.

Leukocyte DNA—Specimen

Norm. DNA chain interpretation required.

Usage. Used in the establishment of genetic disorders, endocrinopathy, leukemias, myotonic dystrophies, prion encephalopathies, and cellular alterations such as tumors.

Description. DNA studies of all biologic specimens use a technique called "polymerase chain reaction" (PCR) to amplify the quantity of DNA being studied. The polymerase chain reaction technique has diverse applications in detecting mutations and rare sequences of DNA. The discovery of heat-stable polymerase led to the invention of the PCR machine. PCR has found its way into virtually all fields of biology, including medicine, evolutionary biology, and genetics.

Professional Considerations
Procedural consent MAY BE required, depending on the procedure used to obtain the specimen. Informed consent is recommended for genetic testing.

Preparation
1. Contact the laboratory for specific collection regimens, depending on the specimen required.

Procedure
1. For blood samples, obtain a 7-mL sample in a citrate-anticoagulated or EDTA-anticoagulated tube.
2. A reaction mixture consisting of specimen DNA, primers, DNA polymerase, nucleotides, and buffer containing magnesium is placed into the machine, which automatically runs through the cycles of heating and cooling. Generally 25-35 cycles are enough to amplify a single-copy genomic sequence by a factor of 10 million.

Postprocedure Care
1. Care is specific to the procedure used to obtain the specimen. See each individual procedure for care implications.

Client and Family Teaching
1. Refer to Appendix B, "Informed Consent for Genetic Testing".
2. Results may not be available for up to 2 weeks.

Factors That Affect Results
1. Anticoagulants mixed with samples invalidate the results.

Other Data
1. At this time, this technique has the highest sensitivity of all molecular techniques.
2. The Genetic Information Nondiscrimination Act of 2008 prohibits health plans from using genetic family history or genetic test results from influencing eligibility or premiums for health insurance. It also prohibits employers from using this information to influence decisions about hiring, terminating employment, or employment pay, promotions or privileges.

Lidocaine (Xylocaine)—Serum

Norm.

	Trough	SI Units
Norm	1.5-6.0 µg/mL	6.4-25.6 µmol/L
Panic Level	6-8 µg/mL	25.6-34.2 µmol/L
Toxic Level	>8 µg/mL	>34.2 µmol/L

Panic Level Symptoms and Treatment
Symptoms
Panic level: Slurred speech, central nervous system depression, cardiovascular depression.

Toxic level: Coma, convulsions, decreased cardiac output, muscle twitching, obtundation.

Treatment
NOTE: Treatment choice(s) depend(s) on client's history and condition and episode history.
1. Provide continuous ECG monitoring for bradycardia, heart block, dysrhythmias, or cardiac arrest.
2. Support airway, breathing, and hemodynamic stability.
3. Monitor temperature every hour for hyperthermia. Use cool room or hypothermia, or both, as needed.
4. Initiate seizure precautions.
5. Hemodialysis will NOT remove lidocaine.

Increased. Convulsions and drug abuse. Drugs include anesthetics, cimetidine, norepinephrine, propranolol. Dysrhythmias.

Decreased. Dysrhythmias. Drugs include anesthetics, norepinephrine, phenobarbital, phenytoin, and propranolol.

Description. Lidocaine is a class I antiarrhythmic and anesthetic drug used to treat ventricular tachycardia or defibrillation resistant to defibrillation. It is also used as a local anesthetic. Lidocaine suppresses automaticity of the His-Purkinje system and elevates the threshold of ventricle during diastole. Half-life is normally 70-140 minutes but in uremia is 77 minutes, in cirrhosis is 296 minutes, and in cardiac failure is 115 minutes. Because the half-life increases after 24-48 hours, the dose should be reduced after 24 hours when prolonged infusions are given. Lidocaine is metabolized in the liver and excreted in the urine. Steady-state levels are reached after 5-10 hours.

Professional Considerations
Consent form NOT required.

Preparation
1. Tube: Red topped, red/gray topped, or gold topped or lavender topped.
2. Draw the first sample 12 hours after starting lidocaine.
3. Specimens MAY be drawn during hemodialysis.

Procedure
1. Draw a 4-mL TROUGH blood sample. Obtain serial measurements at the same time each day.

Postprocedure Care
1. Observe for signs of lidocaine toxicity.

Client and Family Teaching
1. Toxic symptoms normally resolve within 12-24 hours after cessation of lidocaine therapy.

Factors That Affect Results
1. Cardiopulmonary bypass surgery decreases serum levels.
2. Do not collect in a serum separator tube because the separator gel may extract the lidocaine and cause falsely low results.

Other Data
1. Action of drug begins 10-90 seconds after intravenous administration.

Lipase—Serum

Norm. <200 U/L with triolein; <160 U/L with olive oil.

		SI Units
Adults	13-141 U/L	0.22-2.40 µKat/L
20-60 years	31-186 U/L	0.53-3.16 µKat/L
>60 years	≤302 U/L	≤5.13 µKat/L
>90 years	26-267 U/L	0.44-4.54 µKat/L
Children	20-136 IU/L	0.34-2.30 µKat/L
Infants	9-105 IU/L	0.15-1.78 µKat/L

Increased. Cholecystitis, cirrhosis, duodenal ulcers, eating disorders (pancreatitis), fat embolism, fructose malabsorption, gallstone colic, pain (abdominal), pancreatic carcinoma, pancreatic cholera, pancreatic trauma, pancreatitis, peritonitis, renal disease with impaired output, and strangulated bowel. Drugs include bethanechol, heparin, and narcotic analgesics.

Decreased. Gross lipidemia. Drugs include EDTA, heavy metals, and quinine.

Description. Lipase is a pancreatic enzyme that changes fats and triglycerides into fatty acids and glycerol. The pancreas is the only body organ that demonstrates significant lipase activity. In acute pancreatitis, serum lipase begins to increase in 2-6 hours, peaks at 12-30 hours, and remains elevated but slowly decreases for 2-4 days. Lipase rises and falls in tandem with amylase in acute pancreatitis but is a more specific marker than amylase for this condition.

Professional Considerations
Consent form NOT required.

Preparation
1. Tube: Red topped, red/gray topped, or gold topped.

Procedure
1. Draw a 4-mL blood sample.

Postprocedure Care
1. None.

Client and Family Teaching
1. Results are normally available within 12 hours.

Factors That Affect Results
1. Endoscopic retrograde cholangiopancreatography procedure (ERCP) may increase lipase activity.
2. Traumatic venipuncture can inhibit lipase activity.
3. Baseline levels increase during pregnancy.

Other Data
1. The sample is stable for several days at room temperature, longer if refrigerated or frozen.

Lipid-Associated Sialic Acid (Lipid-Bound Sialic Acid, LASA, LSA)—Plasma or Serum

Norm. *Serum*: <25 mg/dL.
Plasma: <20 mg/dL.

Increased. Cancer: breast, brain, cervix uteri, colon, head and neck, leukemia, liver, lung, melanoma, metastatic, neuroblastoma, ovarian, pancreatic, renal, and uterine; hypertriglyceridemia, postmyocardial infarction (first 3 days).

Decreased. Response in therapy from high tumor burden to low tumor burden.

Description. Lipid-associated sialic acid (LASA) is a derivative of neuraminic acid, a widely distributed sugar that attaches itself to proteins and lipids. This lipid-associated tumor marker is found in the serum of clients with malignant disease and is associated with higher tumor burdens as opposed to low and moderate tumor burdens. Theoretically, LASA levels are believed to be increased in cancer because LASA has the ability to identify cells with altered surface properties, such as cancer cells, and bind to the surfaces, making the tumor cells more susceptible to metastasis and probable lysis by activated macrophages. LASA is also elevated after myocardial damage and is a constituent of total sialic acid, which is an independent cardiac risk factor.

Professional Considerations
Consent form NOT required.

Preparation
1. Tube: Lavender topped. Obtain ice.

Procedure
1. Draw a 5-mL blood sample.

Postprocedure Care
1. Place the sample immediately on ice and deliver it to the laboratory for immediate spinning and freezing. The sample should be kept frozen until tested.

Client and Family Teaching
1. Results may take several days if the sample is sent off site to be tested.

Factors That Affect Results
1. None found.

Other Data

1. No significant difference has been found in LASA levels between survivors and nonsurvivors of persons with a myocardial infarction.

2. The amount of sialic acid present on the surface of malignant cells has been correlated directly with the ability to metastasize.

Lipid Profile—Blood

Norm. See individual test listings for age-specific norms, including norms for children.

		SI Units
Lipids, total	400-800 mg/dL	4.0-8.0 g/L
Triglycerides	10-190 mg/dL	0.2-4.8 mmol/L
HDL cholesterol		
Females	35-85 mg/dL	0.9-2.2 mmol/L
Males	30-65 mg/dL	0.8-1.7 mmol/L
LDL cholesterol	80-190 mg/dL	2.0-4.9 mmol/L
VLDL cholesterol (calculated)	≤30 mg/dL	<0.78 mmol/L
Total-to-HDL cholesterol ratio	Median = 5	

Condition	Triglycerides	Total Cholesterol	HDL	LDL
Alcoholism	Increase	Increase	Increase	Increase
Aortic aneurysm	Increase	Increase	Increase	Increase
Aortitis	Increase	Increase	Increase	Increase
Arteriosclerosis	Increase	Increase	Decrease	Increase
Diabetes mellitus	Increase	Increase	Increase	Increase
Glycogen storage	Increase	—	—	Increase
Hyperalimentation	Decrease	Decrease	Decrease	Decrease
Hypercholesterolemia	Increase	Increase	—	Increase
Hyperlipoproteinemia	Increase	Increase	Increase	Increase
Hypothyroid	Increase	—	Decrease	—
Malabsorption	Decrease	Decrease	Decrease	Decrease
Myxedema	Increase	Increase	Increase	Increase
Nephrotic syndrome	Increase	Increase	Increase	Increase
Pancreatitis	Increase	Increase	Increase	Increase

Description. Lipid profile is a battery of laboratory studies to help determine the risk factors in coronary artery disease. Blood lipids comprise cholesterol, triglycerides, and phospholipids. Fasting lipid profiles are recommended every 5 years in clients older than age 19. See individual test sections for further descriptions of the components of the lipid profile, as well as levels for which lifestyle changes and therapeutic drug regimens are recommended.

Total Cholesterol—Coronary Heart Disease Risk

	Desirable		Borderline High Risk		High Risk	
	Norm mg/dL	SI Units mmol/L	mg/dL	SI Units mmol/L	mg/dL	SI Units mmol/L
Adult	<200	<5.18	200-239	5.18-6.19	≥240	≥6.22
Child	<170	<4.40	170-199	4.40-5.15	≥200	≥25.18

HDL Cholesterol—Coronary Heart Disease Risk

	Very Low Risk		Low Risk		Moderate Risk		High Risk	
	mg/dL	SI Units mmol/L	mg/dL	SI Units mmol/L	mg/dL	SI Units mmol/L	mg/dL	SI Units mmol/L
Adults	>60	>1.554	45-59	1.16-1.53	35-45	0.91-1.16	<35	<0.91

Total to HDL Ratio

Coronary Heart Disease Risk	Average Risk	2 × Average Risk	3 × Average Risk
Male	5.0	9.6	23.4
Female	4.4	7.1	11.0

LDL Cholesterol—Coronary Heart Disease Risk

Low Risk				Moderate Risk		High Risk			
Optimal		Near Optimal		Borderline High		High		Very High	
mg/dL	SI Units	mg/dL	SI Units	mg/dL	SI Units	mg/dL	SI Units	mg/dL	SI Units
<100	<2.59	100-129	2.59-3.34	130-159	3.37-4.12	160-189	4.14-4.89	>190	>4.92

Professional Considerations

Consent form NOT required.

Preparation

1. Tubes: Two red topped, red/gray topped, or gold topped.
2. See Client and Family Teaching.

Procedure

1. Draw two 7-mL blood samples.

Postprocedure Care

1. None.

Client and Family Teaching

1. Maintain regular dietary habits for 2 weeks before the test.
2. Fast from food and fluids for 12 hours before the test.
3. Desirable levels and risk for coronary heart disease are shown in the table.

Factors That Affect Results

1. Oral contraceptives may increase the levels of lipids in the serum.
2. If the test was done on a non-fasting specimen, only the total cholesterol and HDL cholesterol results are valid.
3. Herbal or natural remedy effects: Many studies have conflicting results concerning garlic's effect on lowering serum lipid level, but there are more studies showing this effect than there are studies showing equivocal results. Kong et al (2004) showed a 29% decrease in serum cholesterol, 35% decrease in serum triglycerides, and 25% decrease in LDL cholesterol in clients given Berberine, a Chinese herb. An herbal powder containing guar gum, *meshasringi* (*Gymnema sylvestre, mesha shringi,* Indian milkweed vine), *methi* (fenugreek leaves), and *tundika* (*Coccinia indica*) has been shown to reduce total cholesterol and LD levels but to have no effect on HDL and VLDL levels. Long-term treatment with Chinese herbal drugs *Cordyceps sinensis* (a fungus), *dai-saiko-to* (Chinese: *da-chai hu-tang* 'major *Bupleurum* preparation': mixture of *Pinellia, Scutellaria, Zizyphus,* ginseng, licorice, and ginger), and *saiko-ka-ryukotsu-boreito* (Chinese: *chai hu-jia-long gu-mu li-tang* 'Bupleurum-with added-dragon bone-oyster-preparation,' composed of *Bupleurum, Pinellia,* ginger, *Scutellaria, Zizyphus,* cinnamon, China root fungus [*fu ling,* hoelen, *Poria cocos, P. sclerotium*], Codonopsis, Chinese rhubarb, ginseng, oyster shell, and fossil bone for calcium) has been shown to significantly increase HDL levels. Soy has been shown to reduce LDL, triglycerides, and total cholesterol as well as to increase HDL. The Ayurvedic herb *amla* (emblic, *Phyllanthus emblica,* Indian gooseberry) was shown to reduce total and LDL cholesterol in an uncontrolled study. Lethicin has been known to be used to lower cholesterol.

4. All levels except HDL are generally increased in obesity, whereas HDL levels are generally decreased.

Other Data

1. Risk factors for heart disease include high-saturated-fat diet, cigarette smoking, hypertension, obesity, high salt intake, diabetes mellitus, and left ventricular hypertrophy.
2. Risk for and incidence of coronary heart disease increase as the total-to-HDL cholesterol ratio increases.

3. The National Lipid Association, the American Academy of Pediatrics, and the American Heart Association recommend screening children as young as 2 years of age for familial hypercholesterolemia, which would be suspected with a fasting LDL of at least 160 mg/dL.
4. See also Cholesterol—Blood; High-density lipoprotein cholesterol—Blood; Low-density lipoprotein cholesterol—Blood; Triglycerides—Blood.

Lipoprotein-Associated Phospholipase A₂ (LpPLA, Lp-PLA₂, Platelet-Activating Factor Acetylhydrolase, PLA₂, PLAC)—Blood

Norm. Low risk: <200 ng/mL
Moderate risk: 200-235 ng/mL
High risk: >235 ng/mL

Usage. May be used in conjunction with other stroke risk evaluations, such as high-sensitivity C-reactive protein, to provide additional supportive evidence of risk for coronary heart disease and/or stroke as a consequence of atherosclerosis when an individual has low LDL-C.

Description. When vascular inflammation becomes chronic, it is thought that risk for coronary heart disease and/or stroke increases. Lipoprotein-associated phospholipase A₂ is a biomarker enzyme that elevates in the blood when vascular inflammation is present and is also present in the plaques of atherosclerosis. Therefore, it is thought to be pro-atheresclerotic and, in fact, has been found to be significantly correlated with the risk for coronary heart disease in disease-free women (Hatoum et al, 2011).

Professional Considerations
Consent form NOT required.

Preparation

1. Tube: Red-top, green-top heparin or lavender-top EDTA.

Procedure

1. Collect a 2-mL blood sample.

Postprocedure Care

1. None.

Client and Family Teaching

1. This test has not conclusively been shown to correlate with future incidence of stroke.

Factors That Affect Results

1. Results are up to 30% lower when the client is receiving antilipidemic therapies.

Other Data

1. This test is being used investigationally to determine whether it can help differentiate between acute myocardial infarction and pericarditis.
2. Also known as platelet-activating factor acetylhydrolase (PLAC).

Liquid Ecstasy

See **Gamma-Hydroxybutyric Acid**—Blood or Urine or Human Hair.

Liquid Pap Test

See **Pap Smear**—Diagnostic.

Lithium—Serum

Norm. Negative.

	Therapeutic Trough Levels	SI Units
Treatment of acute mania	0.8-1.6 mEq/L	0.8-1.6 mmol/L
Ongoing prophylaxis	0.5-1.0 mEq/L	0.5-1.0 mmol/L
Panic level	>2.0 mEq/L	>2.0 mmol/L

Panic Level Symptoms and Treatment
Symptoms

At levels = 1.5-2.5 mmol/L: Ataxia, coarse tremor, diarrhea, muscle weakness, sedation, and vomiting.

At levels = 2.5-4.0 mmol/L: Choreiform movements, confusion, convulsions, diminishing level of consciousness, increased deep tendon reflexes, muscle hypertonia, somnolence, stupor, T-wave flattening, renal toxicity accompanied by hypernatremia or hyponatremia.

At levels >4.0 mmol/L: Coma, death possible.

Treatment

NOTE: Treatment choice(s) depend(s) on client's history and condition and episode history.

1. Perform gastric lavage.
2. Whole bowel irrigation and/or administration of sodium polystyrene sulfonate (Kayexalate) will decrease absorption of sustained-release lithium.
3. Administer intravenous normal saline or ½ normal saline to force diuresis and renal elimination of lithium.
4. Both hemodialysis and peritoneal dialysis WILL remove lithium. Some references indicate that dialysis should be considered in clients on chronic lithium therapy who are stable when lithium level is >4 mmol/L, or who are unstable when lithium level is >2.5 mmol/L, or when a change in mental status is present.

Usage. Drug abuse, manic-depressive psychosis, metal poisoning, and monitoring for therapeutic levels during lithium therapy.

Increased. Lithium overdose, sodium restriction. Drugs include ACE inhibitors, fluoxetine, NSAIDs, and thiazide diuretics. In addition, concomitant drugs that increase the risk for lithium toxicity include methyldopa, metronidazole, and phenytoin.

Decreased. Drugs include sodium chloride. Herbal or natural remedies include psyllium (*Plantago psyllium, P. ovata*), fleawort (fleabane in Canada). In addition, acetazolamide, aminophylline, caffeine, sodium bicarbonate, and theophylline may increase lithium excretion.

Description. Lithium is an alkali metal salt used as a mood stabilizer mostly in the treatment of bipolar disorder (manic-depressive illness) and shows promise in the treatment of cluster migraine headaches. This drug is absorbed in the gastrointestinal tract, has a half-life of 17-36 hours and an onset of 5-10 days, and is excreted in the urine. Lithium alters the sodium transport in nerve and muscle cells, which assists in stabilizing mood.

Professional Considerations
Consent form NOT required.

Preparation
1. Tube: Green topped (not lithium-heparin).
2. Do NOT draw during hemodialysis.

Procedure
1. Draw a 2-mL TROUGH blood sample 8-12 hours after the last dose.

Postprocedure Care
1. Sodium, lithium, and fluid balance must be assessed weekly.

Client and Family Teaching
1. Periodic lithium level determination is necessary to identify and prevent lithium toxicity symptoms. Teach symptoms from the preceding list.
2. Clients with levels >2.5 mmol/L will require intensive care monitoring and intervention.
3. For intentional overdose, refer the client and family for crisis intervention.

Factors That Affect Results
1. Reject the results if the specimen was collected in lithium-heparin.

Other Data

1. The common side effects of lithium include elevated thyroid-stimulating hormone (TSH).
2. Levels correlate poorly with the appearance of toxic symptoms. Toxic symptoms may occur at normal lithium levels. Elderly clients show signs of toxicity at lower levels than do younger clients.
3. Higher lithium levels may be required in children than in adults to achieve therapeutic results.

Liver Battery (Liver Profile, Liver Function Tests)—Serum

Norm.

		SI Units
Alanine Aminotransferase (ALT, Formerly SGPT)		
Adult Female	4-35 U/L	4-35 U/L
Adult Male	7-46 U/L	7-46 U/L
Elderly	Slightly higher than adult	
Children		
<12 months	≤54 U/L	≤54 U/L
1-2 years	3-37 U/L	3-37 U/L
2-8 years	3-30 U/L	3-30 U/L
8-16 years	3-28 U/L	3-28 U/L
Alkaline Phosphatase (ALP)		
Adults (20-60 years)	44-147 U/L	44-147 U/L
Elderly	Slightly higher	
Newborn	1-4 times adult values	
Children	Values remain high until epiphyses close	
Females		
2-10 years	100-350 U/L	100-350 U/L
10-13 years	110-400 U/L	110-400 U/L
Males		
2-13 years	100-350 U/L	100-350 U/L
13-15 years	125-500 U/L	125-500 U/L
Aspartate Aminotransferase		
Adult females		
≤60 years	8-20 U/L	8-20 U/L
>60 years	10-20 U/L	10-20 U/L
Adult males		
≤60 years	8-20 U/L	8-20 U/L
>60 years	11-26 U/L	11-26 U/L
Children		
Newborn	16-72 U/L	16-72 U/L
Infant	15-60 U/L	15-60 U/L
1 year	16-35 U/L	16-35 U/L
5 years	19-28 U/L	19-28 U/L
Bilirubin (Total)		
1 Month to adult	<1.5 mg/dL	<25.65 µmol/L
Premature infant		
Cord	<2.8 mg/dL	<47.88 µmol/L
24 hours	1-6 mg/dL	17.1-102.6 µmol/L
48 hours	6-8 mg/dL	102.6-136.8 µmol/L
3-5 days	10-12 mg/dL	171-205.2 µmol/L

		SI Units
Full-term infant		
Cord	<2.8 mg/dL	<47.88 µmol/L
24 hours	2-6 mg/dL	34.2-102.6 µmol/L
48 hours	6-7 mg/dL	102.6-119.7 µmol/L
3-5 days	4-6 mg/dL	68.4-102.6 µmol/L
Bilirubin (direct)	0.0-0.3 mg/dL	1.7-5.1 µmol/L
Bilirubin (indirect)	0.1-1.0 mg/dL	1.7-17.1 µmol/L

Gamma-Glutamyltransferase/Gamma-Glutamyltranspeptidase (GGT/GGTP, Gamma-GT)

Adult females	4-25 U/L	4-25 U/L
3-33 U/L at 37°C	3-33 U/L at 37°C	
Adult males	7-40 U/L	7-40 U/L
9-69 U/L at 37°C	9-69 U/L at 37°C	
Children		
Cord blood	190-270 U/L at 37°C	190-270 U/L at 37°C
Premature infant	<140 U/L at 37°C	<140 U/L at 37°C
1-3 days	56-233 U/L at 37°C	56-233 U/L at 37°C
4-21 days	0-130 U/L at 37°C	0-130 U/L at 37°C
3-12 weeks	4-120 U/L at 37°C	4-120 U/L at 37°C
3-6 months, female	5-35 U/L at 37°C	5-35 U/L at 37°C
3-6 months, male	5-65 U/L at 37°C	5-65 U/L at 37°C
>6 months, female	15-85 U/L	15-85 U/L
>6 months, male	5-55 U/L	5-55 U/L
1-15 years	0-23 U/L at 37°C	0-23 U/L at 37°C
Hepatitis B Surface Antigen	Negative	Negative

Lactate Dehydrogenase (LD/LDH)

Wróblewski Method 30°C	150-450 U/L	72-217 U/L
Adults		
≤60 years	45-90 U/L	45-90 U/L
>60 years	55-102 U/L	55-102 U/L
Children		
Newborn	160-500 U/L	160-500 U/L
Neonate	300-1500 U/L	300-1500 U/L
Infant	100-250 U/L	100-250 U/L
Child	60-170 U/L	60-170 U/L

Leucine Aminopeptidase (LAP)

Female	75-185 U/mL	
Male	80-200 U/mL	
5'-Nucleotidase (5'-NT or 5'-N)	0-17 U/L	2-15 IU/L
Bodansky units	0-1.6 U	0.3-3.2

Protein Electrophoresis

Norms are dependent on laboratory procedure. Percentage values are for the agarose method and represent the percentage of total protein.

Adult (agarose method)		
Total protein	6.4-8.3 g/dL	5.90-8.00
Albumin	58%-74%	0.58-0.74
Alpha$_1$ globulin	2.0%-3.5%	0.02-0.04
Alpha$_2$ globulin	5.4%-10.6%	0.05-0.11
Beta globulin	7.0%-14.0%	0.07-0.14
Gamma globulin	8.0%-18.0%	0.08-0.18

Continued

		SI Units
Adult		
Total protein	6.0-8.0 g/dL	60-80 g/L
Albumin	3.3-5.0 g/dL	35-50 g/L
Alpha$_1$ globulin	0.1-0.4 g/dL	1-4 g/L
Alpha$_2$ globulin	0.5-1 g/dL	5-10 g/L
Beta globulin	0.7-1.2 g/dL	7-12 g/L
Gamma globulin	0.8-1.6 g/dL	8-16 g/L
Premature infant		
Total protein	4.4-6.3 g/dL	44-63 g/L
Albumin	3.0-4.2 g/dL	30-42 g/L
Alpha$_1$ globulin	0.11-0.5 g/dL	1.1-5 g/L
Alpha$_2$ globulin	0.3-0.7 g/dL	3-7 g/L
Beta globulin	0.3-1.2 g/dL	3-12 g/L
Gamma globulin	0.3-1.4 g/dL	3-14 g/L
Newborn		
Total protein	4.6-7.4 g/dL	46-74 g/L
Albumin	3.5-5.4 g/dL	35-54 g/L
Alpha$_1$ globulin	0.1-0.3 g/dL	1-3 g/L
Alpha$_2$ globulin	0.3-0.5 g/dL	3-5 g/L
Beta globulin	0.2-0.6 g/dL	2-6 g/L
Gamma globulin	0.2-1.2 g/dL	2-12 g/L
Infant		
Total protein	6.0-6.7 g/dL	60-67 g/L
Albumin	4.4-5.4 g/dL	44-54 g/L
Alpha$_1$ globulin	0.2-0.4 g/dL	2-4 g/L
Alpha$_2$ globulin	0.5-0.8 g/dL	5-8 g/L
Beta globulin	0.5-0.9 g/dL	5-9 g/L
Gamma globulin	0.3-0.8 g/dL	3-8 g/L
Child		
Total protein	6.2-8.0 g/dL	62-80 g/L
Albumin	4.0-5.8 g/dL	40-58 g/L
Alpha$_1$ globulin	0.1-0.4 g/dL	1-4 g/L
Alpha$_2$ globulin	0.4-1.0 g/dL	4-10 g/L
Beta globulin	0.5-1.0 g/dL	5-10 g/L
Gamma globulin	0.3-1.0 g/dL	3-10 g/L
Prothrombin Time		
Adult		10-15 seconds
Newborn		<17 seconds
Child		11-14 seconds

Usage. Workup for liver disease, biliary disease; hepatoma; liver metastasis; chronic active hepatitis; cirrhosis, including biliary cirrhosis; hepatic complications associated with medications or TPN.

Increased. See individual test listing.

Decreased. See individual test listings.

Description. Liver battery includes testing for several blood levels that reflect hepatic function. In general, a liver battery includes the following: Alanine aminotransferase—Serum; Alkaline phosphatase—Serum; Aspartate aminotransferase—Serum; Bilirubin—Serum; Gamma-glutamyl transpeptidase—Blood; Hepatitis B surface antigen—Blood; Lactate dehydrogenase—Blood; Leucine aminopeptidase—Blood; 5'-Nucleotidase—Blood; Protein electrophoresis—Serum; Prothrombin time and international normalized ratio—Blood. See individual test listings for specific descriptions.

Professional Considerations
Consent form NOT required.

Preparation
1. Obtain foil or a paper bag.
2. Tubes: Two red topped, red/gray topped, or gold topped, and one blue topped.

Procedure
1. Completely fill all three tubes with blood. Cover one red topped, the red/gray topped, and the gold topped with foil, or place them in a paper bag to protect them from light.

Postprocedure Care
1. Immediately spin the blue topped tube, and then refrigerate it. The testing should be performed within 4 hours.

Client and Family Teaching
1. See individual test listings.

Factors That Affect Results
1. See individual test listings.
2. Herbal or natural remedy: *Echinacea purpurea* may cause hepatotoxicity. The risk for this is increased when taken with other hepatotoxic drugs.

Other Data
1. See individual test listings.
2. Interpretation of LFTs is an art, not a science. There are no absolute rules regarding how mild, moderate, or severe liver damage is defined. When one is identifying abnormalities, the client's clinical condition and other diagnostic testing must be considered.
3. Consider herbal medicines as contributors in otherwise unexplained hepatic injury.

Liver Biopsy (Percutaneous Liver Biopsy)—Diagnostic

Norm. Normal liver cells and tissue. Negative for malignancy, fibrosis, inflammatory infiltrates, Mallory's hyaline, and steatosis.

Usage. Used in the past to diagnose liver disease. Today is used primarily to determine prognosis for liver disease and monitor client response to treatment after imaging and serologic testing have confirmed the diagnosis of hepatitis C and other liver disease. Fine-needle aspiration biopsy is the diagnostic procedure of choice for evaluation of liver lesions. Almost all fine-needle aspiration biopsies of the liver use interventional radiology, primarily ultrasonography and computed tomography. Used when the diagnosis or cause cannot be established by other means. Also indicated to evaluate liver transplant allografts.

Description. A liver biopsy is a relatively safe, simple, and valuable method of evaluating pathologic liver conditions. After the client is given local anesthetic, and while using an aseptic technique, a needle is inserted through the abdominal wall to the liver (percutaneous approach). Liver tissue is obtained by the needle biopsy for microscopic examination. The transjugular, laparoscopic, or intraoperative approaches may also be used. Liver biopsy may be performed in conjunction with ultrasound or computed tomography guidance.

Professional Considerations
Consent form IS required.

Risks
Follow-up studies have indicated a very low rate of serious complications (0.06%-0.32%) manifesting as pain, hemorrhage (1%-5% risk), bile peritonitis, liver cyst, penetration of abdominal viscera, and pneumothorax. Mortality is rare (0.006%-0.1%). The estimated rate of needle-tract seeding is small in fine-needle aspiration of the liver. Only three cases reported.

Contraindications
Uncorrectable bleeding diathesis. Prothrombin time in the anticoagulant range (2-3 seconds over control values); platelet count less than 50,000/mm³; other bleeding disorders; anemia and inability to tolerate major blood loss associated with inadvertent puncture of an intrahepatic blood vessel; pronounced ascites; obstructive jaundice caused by a possible bile leakage; infection of the biliary tract; infection in the right pleural space or right upper quadrant of the abdomen; a hemangioma; or an inability to cooperate during procedure

(such as remaining still and holding the breath during sustained exhalation). Sedatives are contraindicated in clients with central nervous system depression. See also Computed tomography of the body—diagnostic if CT will be used.

Precautions

See also Computed tomography of the body—Diagnostic if CT will be used.

Preparation

1. Obtain a biopsy tray, sterile gloves, slides, sterile sponges, and tape for dressing.
2. Ensure that all coagulation tests are normal.
3. Administer any sedative medications as prescribed.
4. A CT scan may need to be scheduled if the biopsy needle must be inserted under CT guidance to obtain tissue from a specific area of the liver.
5. See Client and Family Teaching.
6. Just before beginning the procedure, take a "time out" to verify the correct client, procedure, and site.

Procedure

1. The area of the liver suspected of being abnormal is noted.
2. The client is placed in the supine or left lateral position.
3. The skin area used for puncture is anesthetized locally.
4. The client is asked to exhale and hold the inhalation so that the liver descends and the possibility of a pneumothorax is decreased.
5. The biopsy needle is inserted by the physician into the liver during the client's sustained exhalation, and a liver tissue is obtained.
6. The needle is withdrawn from the liver.
7. A pressure dressing is applied.
8. The procedure takes approximately 30 minutes.

Postprocedure Care

1. Touch-prints on glass slides may be made before fixation and may be submitted for cytologic evaluation.
2. Needle rinses in 50% alcohol or saline may also provide helpful diagnostic material.
3. Direct slides from needle aspirates may be made, and the slides may be fixed immediately in 95% alcohol.

4. Tissue samples may be placed into a specimen bottle containing 10% formalin for fixation.
5. Send the specimens to the pathology department.
6. Assess vital signs frequently (every 15 minutes × 2) to determine evidence of hemorrhage (increased pulse rate and blood pressure) and peritonitis (increased temperature).
7. Assess the biopsy site for bleeding.
8. Place the client on the right side for 1-2 hours after the procedure. This position will compress the liver against the chest wall and will decrease the risk of hemorrhage or bile leak.
9. Bed rest with 24-hour observation after the biopsy is usually prescribed. Some studies have found no increase in adverse outcomes when discharging clients with no complications 1 hour after fine-needle aspiration liver biopsy.

Client and Family Teaching

1. Explain the purpose of the procedure.
2. Fast from food and fluids after midnight on the day of the test.
3. The procedure takes about 30 minutes. Local anesthetic is used to control pain.

Factors That Affect Results

1. False-negative results may occur, and localized liver disease may be missed, because a very small fragment of liver tissue, which is often partially destroyed, is taken in a random manner from a large organ. False-negative results may be attributable to (1) sampling error, because the detection rate of liver metastasis is approximately 60% with blind biopsy and about 85% using ultrasound guidance, and (2) degeneration or distortion, which has been caused by faulty preparation of the specimen.
2. False-positive results may be attributable to incorrect interpretation of very reactive hepatocytes.

Other Data

1. An experienced gastroenterologist or radiologist should perform the procedure.
2. Specimens for histologic and cytologic examination may be obtained using ultrasound radiologic guidance and a tissue-core biopsy needle, such as the

Menghini needle. Specimens for cytologic examination may be obtained only by use of a fine-aspirate needle.

3. Detection of portal vein tumor invasion in clients with hepatocellular carcinoma is important to determine therapy and prognosis. Fine-needle aspiration of a portal vein thrombus under ultrasonographic guidance helps to distinguish malignant from benign thrombus without resorting to laparotomy.

4. See also Hepatic function panel—Blood.

Liver Echography

See Liver Ultrasonography—Diagnostic.

Liver Function Tests

See Liver Battery—Serum.

Liver ^{131}I Scan—Diagnostic

Norm. Normal size, shape, and position of liver.

Usage. Cirrhosis, diffuse infiltrating processes affecting the liver (such as amyloidosis, sarcoidosis), granulomas, hepatic abscesses or cysts, hepatomas, jaundice, tuberculosis, and tumors. Also used as confirmatory test after other findings have been obtained.

Description. A nuclear medicine scan in which radioactive iodine is used to determine the uptake in the liver to outline and detect structural changes in the liver.

Professional Considerations
Consent form IS required.

Risks
Allergic reaction to dye (itching, hives, rash, tight feeling in the throat, shortness of breath, bronchospasm, anaphylaxis, death).
Contraindications
Previous allergy to iodine, shellfish, or radiographic contrast medium; renal insufficiency; during pregnancy (because of radioactive iodine crossing the blood-placental barrier) or breast-feeding.

Preparation
1. Have emergency equipment readily available.
2. Just before beginning the procedure, take a "time out" to verify the correct client, procedure, and site.

Procedure
1. The client is transported to the nuclear medicine department. For inpatients, a nuclear medicine technologist may administer the radionuclide at the bedside.
2. The client is injected intravenously with radioactive iodine-131.
3. A gamma-ray detector is placed over the right upper quadrant of the client's abdomen 30 minutes after the client has been injected.
4. The client is placed in lateral, prone, and supine positions, so that all the surfaces of the liver may be visualized.
5. Scans are taken of the liver at intervals.
6. The radionuclide image of the distribution of radioactive particles in the liver is recorded on either x-ray or Polaroid film.

Postprocedure Care
1. Assess vital signs every 15 minutes × 2.
2. Observe the client carefully for up to 60 minutes after the study for a possible (anaphylactic) reaction to the radionuclide.
3. For 24 hours wear rubber gloves when discarding urine after the procedure. Wash the gloved hands with soap and water before removing the gloves. Wash the ungloved hands after the gloves have been removed.

Client and Family Teaching
1. No fasting or premedication is required.

2. The IV injection of the radionuclide is the only discomfort associated with this procedure.

3. You will not be exposed to large amounts of radiation, because only tracer doses of ^{131}I are used.

4. This procedure is performed by a trained technologist in approximately 1 hour. A physician trained in nuclear medicine interprets the results.

5. Meticulously wash your hands with soap and water after each void for 24 hours after procedure.

6. Family members must wear rubber gloves when discarding the client's urine for 24 hours after procedure, if family will be providing this care.

7. Follow-up diagnostic tests (such as ultrasonography, CT scan, or biopsy) are needed to confirm the diagnosis.

Factors That Affect Results

1. Barium in the GI tract overlying the liver or spleen will produce defects on the scan, which may be mistaken for masses.

2. False-negative results may occur in clients with space-occupying lesions (such as tumors, cysts, abscesses) smaller than 2 cm because the scan can demonstrate only filling defects greater than 2 cm in diameter.

3. False-positive results may occur in clients with cirrhosis. Because of the distortion of the client's liver parenchyma, the scan may be incorrectly interpreted as positive for filling defects.

Other Data

1. Health care professionals working in a nuclear medicine area must follow federal standards set by the Nuclear Regulatory Commission. These standards include precautions for handling the radioactive material and monitoring of potential radiation exposure.

2. If "cold spots" (areas that do not take up the radionuclide) appear, then cysts, abscesses, and tumors may be suspected.

3. The half-life of iodine-131 is 8 days.

4. See also Hepatobiliary scan—Diagnostic.

Liver Scan

See Computed Tomography of the Body—Diagnostic; Hepatobiliary Scan—Diagnostic; Liver 131I Scan—Diagnostic.

Liver/Spleen Scan

See Hepatobiliary Scan—Diagnostic.

Liver ^{99m}Tc Scan of Blood Vessels

See Hepatobiliary Scan—Diagnostic.

Liver Ultrasonography (Liver Echography, Liver Ultrasound)—Diagnostic

Norm. Liver is of proper size, shape, and position and with a homogeneous soft echo pattern. Image indicates normal relationship to adjacent anatomic structures. Negative for intrahepatic duct dilatation, abscess, cyst, hematoma, or tumor.

Usage. Determine the cause of jaundice; differentiate between obstructive and nonobstructive jaundice; detect cirrhosis, hepatic abscess, cyst, hematoma, and tumors; differentiate cysts and abscesses from tumors; examine the shape and structure of intrahepatic ducts; visualize pleural effusion; evaluate hepatic hemodynamic flow balance; evaluate ascites; and monitor hepatic metastasis response to cancer therapy. Used before and after placement of a transjugular intrahepatic portosystemic shunt (TIPS). May be used before a liver biopsy or can help differentiate the constitution of abnormalities identified during hepatobiliary nuclear medicine scanning. It is useful with liver scanning to define the "cold spots." Serial scans may be used to determine the volume of the liver. Not reliable in detecting metastasis, especially when a client's liver is high and primarily under the rib cage. Without contrast, this procedure is a less sensitive alternative to hepatic dye imaging tests for clients with allergy to radiographic dyes. Advancements in contrast agents have led to contrast-enhanced ultrasound imaging that is comparable to CT and MRI results.

Description. With or without contrast enhancement, this procedure provides an evaluation of the liver, intrahepatic duct structure, and ancillary areas of the gallbladder and diaphragm. It creates an oscilloscopic picture from the echoes of high-frequency sound waves, which pass over the right upper quadrant of the abdomen (acoustic imaging). A computer converts the time required for the ultrasonic beam to be reflected back to the transducer from differing densities of tissue to an electrical impulse. This impulse is displayed on an oscilloscopic screen to create a three-dimensional picture of the liver. Hepatitis and fatty liver may be indicated by hepatomegaly. Fatty infiltration also causes brighter-than-normal echoes, with decreased amount of vascular structures. Hepatic fibrosis is demonstrated by a smaller-than-normal liver size and inhomogeneity of the liver tissue. Cysts appear sonolucent with borders that are easily defined, and they have an echo-free nature. Abscesses may contain internal echoes. Malignant neoplasm (such as adenocarcinoma and other primary liver tumors) may appear as a diffusely distorted parenchymal area, where homogeneity of tissue would be expected. The image pattern, which is produced by malignant neoplasms, is called a "bull's-eye." This is attributable to the dense central echo pattern that is surrounded by the less echo-producing halo.

Professional Considerations
Consent form NOT required.

Preparation
1. This test should be performed before intestinal barium tests or after the barium is cleared from the system.

2. Obtain ultrasonic gel or paste.
3. See Client and Family Teaching.

Procedure
1. The client is positioned supine in bed or on a procedure table.
2. The right upper quadrant of the abdomen is covered with ultrasonic gel, and a lubricated transducer is passed slowly over the area along the transverse plane at intervals 1 cm apart with the client in deep inspiration. This is followed by longitudinal scanning in 0.5- to 2-cm increments, moving from the umbilicus to the xiphoid process, with the transducer angled so that the sound waves pass under the rib cage. The client may be changed to a left lateral decubitus position to obtain lateral views of the liver by coronal scanning. If the client is dehydrated, he or she may be asked to expand the abdomen to enhance the smoothness of the anterior abdominal wall. The final views taken are right anterior oblique.
3. Photographs are taken of the oscilloscopic display.
4. The procedure takes less than 30 minutes.

Postprocedure Care
1. Remove the lubricant from the skin.

Client and Family Teaching
1. Fast from food and fluids, and refrain from tobacco smoking overnight before the test.
2. The procedure is painless and carries no risk.
3. Wear a gown during the test.
4. Findings of fatty liver increase the risk of developing type 2 diabetes mellitus within 5 years.

Factors That Affect Results
1. Dehydration interferes with adequate contrast between the organs and body fluids.
2. Intestinal barium, gas, or food obscures results by preventing proper transmission and deflection of the high-frequency sound waves.
3. Fatty liver causes scattering in the attenuation of the ultrasonic beam.
4. The more abdominal fat present, the greater is the attenuation (reduction in sound-wave amplitude and intensity), which interferes with the clarity of the picture.

5. Lung tissue may interfere with visualization of the liver dome in transverse views.
6. Rib artifacts may obscure images of the right lobe of the liver.

Other Data
1. See also Gallbladder and biliary system ultrasonography—Diagnostic.

Liver Ultrasound

See Liver Ultrasonography—Diagnostic.

Lorazepam

See Benzodiazepines—Plasma and Urine.

Low-Density Lipoprotein (LDL, LDL-C) Cholesterol—Blood

Norm.

Age (years)	Male mg/dL	Male SI Units mmol/L	Female mg/dL	Female SI Units mmol/L
Adults (optimum)	50-70	1.3-1.8 mmol/L	50-70	1.3-1.8 mmol/L
20-24	66-147	1.71-3.81	57-159	1.48-4.12
25-29	70-165	1.81-4.27	71-164	1.84-4.25
30-34	78-185	2.02-4.79	70-156	1.81-4.04
35-39	81-189	2.10-4.90	75-172	1.94-4.45
40-44	87-186	2.25-4.82	74-174	1.92-4.51
45-49	97-202	2.51-5.23	79-186	2.05-4.82
50-54	89-197	2.31-5.10	88-201	2.28-5.21
55-59	88-203	2.28-5.26	89-210	2.31-5.44
60-64	83-210	2.15-5.44	100-224	2.59-5.80
65-69	98-210	2.54-5.44	92-221	2.38-5.72
>70	88-186	2.28-4.82	96-206	2.49-5.34
Children				
Cord blood	20-56	0.52-1.45	21-58	0.54-1.50
5-9	63-129	1.63-3.34	68-140	1.76-3.63
10-14	64-133	1.66-3.44	68-136	1.76-3.52
15-19	62-130	1.61-3.37	59-137	1.53-3.55

LDL Cholesterol Levels and Recommendations

	Desirable Level mg/dL	Desirable Level SI Units mmol/L	Level for Diet Therapy and Increased Exercise mg/dL	Level for Diet Therapy and Increased Exercise SI Units mmol/L	Level for Drug Consideration mg/dL	Level for Drug Consideration SI Units mmol/L	Goal
Lower risk (Without CHD and with 0-1 risk factors* for CHD)	<160	<4.14	>160	>4.14	≥190	≥—4.92	Lower LDL-C to ≤160 mg/dL
Moderate risk (Without CHD and with 2 or more risk factors* for CHD, 10-year risk <10%)	<100-130	<2.59-3.37	>130	>3.37	≥160	≥4.14	30%-40% reduction

	Desirable Level		Level for Diet Therapy and Increased Exercise		Level for Drug Consideration		
	mg/dL	SI Units mmol/L	mg/dL	SI Units mmol/L	mg/dL	SI Units mmol/L	Goal
Moderate risk (Without CHD and with 2 or more risk factors* for CHD, 10-year risk 10%-20%)	<130	<3.37	>130	>3.37	≥130	≥3.37	30%-40% reduction
High risk (With CHD or CHD risk* equivalents) 10-year risk >20%	<100	<2.59	>100	>2.59	≥100-130	>2.59-3.37	50% reduction

Data from National Cholesterol Education Program Guidelines, 2004 update (Grundy et al, 2004).
*Framingham risk factors for myocardial infarction and death from coronary heart disease.

LDL Cholesterol Treatment Targets

	Target
Moderate risk	<115 mg/dL
High risk	<100 mg/dL
Very high risk	<70 mg/dL or if that cannot be obtained then reduce LDL cholesterol by at least 50%

Targets from The Task Force for the management of dyslipidaemias of the European Society of Cardiology (ESC) and the European Atherosclerosis Society (EAS): ESC/EAS Guidelines for the management of dyslipidaemias, *Atherosclerosis* 217S:S1–S44, 2001.

Usage. Predict risk of coronary heart disease (CHD); evaluate therapeutic response to diet, exercise, and/or drug therapy for hyperlipidemia.

Increased. Acute myocardial infarction, anorexia nervosa, coronary arterial atherosclerosis, Cushing's disease, diabetes mellitus, diet high in cholesterol and saturated fats, dysglobulinemia, eclampsia, hepatic disease, hyperlipidemia, type II hyperlipoproteinemia, hypothyroidism, Laënnec's cirrhosis, multiple myeloma, nephrotic syndrome, obesity (often), porphyria, pregnancy, and renal failure. High levels are associated with an increased risk for atherosclerotic heart disease. Drugs include androgens, aspirin, catecholamines, diuretics, glucogenic corticosteroids, oral contraceptives, phenothiazines, and sulfonamides.

Decreased. Abetalipoproteinemia, arteriosclerosis, chronic obstructive lung disease, type I hyperlipoproteinemia, hyperthyroidism, hypoalbuminemia, inflammatory joint disease, malabsorption, malnutrition, multiple myeloma, pulmonary disease, Reye's syndrome, stress, and Tangier disease. Drugs include aspirin, cholestyramine, clofibrate, cortisone, estrogens, fenofibrate, neomycin, nicotinic acid, probucol, tamoxifen, and thyroxine. Herbs or natural remedies include garlic (aged extract taken on an ongoing basis); soy; and herbal powder containing guar gum, *meshasringi* (*Gymnema sylvestre, mesha shringi*, Indian milkweed vine), *methi* (fenugreek leaves), and *tundika* (*Coccinia indica*). The Ayurvedic herb *amla* (emblic, *Phyllanthus emblica*, Indian gooseberry) was shown to reduce total and LDL cholesterol in an uncontrolled study. Diet rich in non-soy legumes.

Description. Very-low-density lipoproteins (VLDLs) carry the body's cholesterol and triglycerides in plasma from the liver to other parts of the body and deposit it in the peripheral tissues. As VLDLs are degraded, low-density lipoprotein remnants (LDLs) are left in the bloodstream. LDLs are oxidative and atherogenic and thus associated with an increased risk of arteriosclerotic heart and peripheral vascular disease. Beta-lipoproteins, or LDLs, are moderately high in protein and cholesterol but low in triglycerides. Much research has been done on the effect of hyperlipidemia, and U.S. national guidelines are available that help guide drug therapy for this condition. Results of randomized clinical trials have shown benefit in lowering LDL cholesterol to as low as 50 mg/dL. Thus recommended blood level targets for statin drug therapy have been reduced. VLDL is very hard to measure, and thus is usually estimated via calculation. LDL cholesterol may be directly measured, or it may be calculated. When calculated, LDLs can be derived from the formula:

$$LDL = Cholesterol \times (HDL + Triglycerides)/2$$

Professional Considerations
Consent form NOT required.

Preparation
1. Tube: Red topped, red/gray topped, or gold topped.
2. Indicate on the laboratory requisition any drugs that may affect the test results.
3. See Client and Family Teaching.

Procedure
1. Draw a 2-mL blood sample.

Postprocedure Care
1. None.

Client and Family Teaching
1. Fast from food for 14 hours before the test. Only water is permitted. Exception: No fasting is required if the client is a child aged 3 to 17 years.
2. Follow a regular diet for 2 weeks before the test.
3. For elevated levels, provide information regarding appropriate body weight and diet.
4. If cholesterol is still elevated after lifestyle modifications, prescription medication may be an option to discuss with the physician.

Factors That Affect Results
1. Results are invalid if the client has undergone a radioactive scan within 7 days before this test.
2. Consumption of alcoholic beverages within the previous 24 hours will affect the results.
3. Test results could be elevated by a diet high in saturated fats and sugar (such as butter, cream, fatty meats, bacon, and candy).
4. Binge eating can also alter lipoprotein values.

Other Data
1. Calculation is not valid for specimens >400 mg/dL or for clients with type III hyperlipoproteinemia.

Lower GI
See **Barium Enema**—Diagnostic.

LP Examination
See **Lumbar Puncture**—Diagnostic.

Lp-PLA and Lp-PLA$_2$
See **Lipoprotein-associated phospholipase A2**—Blood.

LSA
See **Lipid-Associated Sialic Acid**—Plasma or Serum.

LSD

See **LSD**—Blood or Urine.

L/S Ratio

See **Amniocentesis and Amniotic Fluid Analysis**—Diagnostic Routine Analysis.

LUA

See **Legionella Antigen**—Urine.

Lumbar Puncture—Diagnostic

Norm. See Cerebrospinal fluid, Glucose—Specimen; Cerebrospinal fluid, Immunoglobulin G, Immunoglobulin G ratios and immunoglobulin G index, Immunoglobulin G synthesis rate—Specimen; Cerebrospinal fluid, Lactic acid—Specimen; Cerebrospinal fluid, Heparin binding protein, Myelin basic protein, Oligoclonal bands, Protein, and Protein electrophoresis—Specimen; Cerebrospinal fluid, Routine analysis—Specimen; Cerebrospinal fluid, Routine—Culture and cytology.

Usage. To assist in the diagnosis of primary or metastatic brain or spinal cord neoplasm, cerebral hemorrhage, meningitis, encephalitis, degenerative brain disease, autoimmune diseases involving the central nervous system, neurosyphilis, and demyelinating disorders (such as multiple sclerosis, acute demyelinating polyneuropathy). Also, this procedure may be performed therapeutically to inject therapeutic or diagnostic agents, to administer spinal anesthetics, or to reduce/drain volume of CSF to a normal level in benign intracranial hypertension (pseudotumor cerebri, idiopathic intracranial hypertension). See individual test listings above for additional specific usage.

Description. An invasive sterile procedure that can be performed at the bedside. A needle is placed into the subarachnoid space of the spinal column. Cerebrospinal fluid (CSF) pressure is measured, and CSF is obtained for examination. The spinal fluid is analyzed to diagnose spinal cord and brain diseases. CSF protects the brain and spinal column from injury and transports products of neurosecretion and cellular metabolism. Under special circumstances, CSF may be obtained from a ventriculotomy or from cisternal or lateral cervical punctures.

Professional Considerations
Consent form IS required.

Risks
Bleeding causing epidural hematoma, cerebral and spinal herniation, brain shift, cranial neuropathy, headache (severe for 2 days), hematoma (spinal subdural or intracranial occipital), increased intracranial pressure, infection, low back pain, meningitis, nausea, nerve root irritation. Bloody or traumatic results decrease from 25% to 1% when using physicians who are trained and perform the procedure frequently.

Contraindications
Degenerative joint disease affecting the spine; an agitated or uncooperative client; infection near the L2-S1 site, which could carry the infective process into the CSF and change cytologic results; coagulation defects, low back pain, or spinal deformities; brain shift (usually characterized by headache and vomiting; papilledema may or may not be present).

Note: Comatose clients with high intracranial pressure but without brain shift may be candidates for lumbar puncture without prior CT when the need for the lumbar puncture diagnostic information is mandatory and urgent, such as in cases of suspected acute meningitis (van Crevel et al, 2002).

Preparation

1. See Client and Family Teaching.
2. If a prescheduled procedure, verify whether client has stopped taking anticoagulants for the length of time required per the physician.
3. Obtain a lumbar puncture or a spinal tap sterile tray, sterile drapes, 1%-2% lidocaine (Xylocaine), and a dry, sterile dressing.
4. If increased intracranial pressure is suspected, a computed tomographic scan of the brain should be performed to rule out this possibility before the lumbar puncture. Herniation of the brain may occur in such clients.
5. Assess the client's vital signs. Perform a baseline neurologic assessment of the legs by assessing strength, sensation, and movement.
6. Client should empty bowel and bladder before the procedure.
7. Just before beginning the procedure, take a "time out" to verify the correct client, procedure, and site.
8. EMLA topical anesthetic cream may be prescribed for application to puncture site 30 minutes before the start of the procedure for children in nonemergent situations.
9. In pediatric patients the ideal depth of needle insertion in centimeters = 10 [weight(kg)/height(cm)] + 1.

Procedure

1. Position the client in a lateral position with the knees drawn up to the abdomen, the chin placed on the chest, and hands clasped around the knees. Children should be in sitting position with flexed hips to maximally increase interspinous space of lumbar spine.
2. Assist the client in relaxing during the procedure by using soothing words and by instructing the client to breathe slowly and deeply with the mouth open. Give reassurance by using touch or holding the client's hand, unless this is opposed by the client. Children have reduced pain and anxiety with music therapy.
3. The puncture site is selected, usually in the lumbar sac at L3-L4 or at the L4-L5 site. A little bone at the L5-S1 interspace, the "surgeon's delight," facilitates selection of the puncture site.
4. The site is thoroughly cleansed with an antiseptic solution.
5. The surrounding area is draped carefully with sterile towels such that the towels do not obscure important landmarks.
6. A local anesthetic (usually lidocaine) is injected into the L3-L4 or L4-L5 spinal column area, creating a burning sensation.
7. A spinal needle, which contains an inner obturator (stylet), is placed through the skin and into the spinal canal. Postdural puncture headache may be decreased if the Sprotte atraumatic needle or a Quincke needle is used.
8. The subarachnoid space is entered. The client may feel the entry (a "pop") of the needle through the dura mater. Postdural puncture headache prevalence decreases when the smallest needle possible is used and when the bevel of the needle is inserted parallel (instead of perpendicular) to the dural fibers. NOTE: In children a rule of thumb to use for mean insertion depth is 0.03 × height of child (in centimeters).
9. The obturator is removed, and CSF will be seen slowly dripping from the needle.
10. The needle is attached to a sterile manometer.
11. Ask the client to relax and straighten the legs. This will reduce the intra-abdominal pressure, which will cause an increase in CSF pressure.
12. The opening CSF pressure is recorded.
13. Three numbered sterile polypropylene CSF transfer tubes are filled sequentially, with a total of 6-12 mL of CSF.
14. The Queckenstedt procedure is performed during a lumbar puncture if blockage in the CSF circulation in the spinal subarachnoid space is suspected. The jugular vein is temporarily occluded manually by digital pressure or by a medium-sized blood pressure cuff inflated to approximately 20 mm Hg. The CSF pressure should increase to 15-40 cm H_2O within 10 seconds of jugular occlusion. No rise after 10 seconds is suggestive of a complete obstruction in the spinal canal. The pressure should return promptly to normal within 10 seconds of release of pressure. A sluggish rise or fall of CSF

pressure is suggestive of partial blockage of CSF circulation.

15. The closing pressure of CSF is measured.

16. One may decrease a puncture headache by pointing the face of the bevel in the direction of the client's side, replacing the stylet, and rotating the needle 90 degrees before withdrawing the needle.

17. The procedure takes 30 minutes.

Postprocedure Care

1. Discard the first specimen, which is likely to be contaminated with blood. Label all test tubes immediately with the proper number (1, 2, 3), the client's name, the date, and the room number. Colored or very cloudy spinal fluid requires additional mixing with 0.5 mL of sterile sodium citrate per 5 mL of CSF to prevent clotting.

2. Transport the specimens to the laboratory immediately. Analysis must be performed promptly on freshly collected specimens. Refrigerate the CSF or store the specimens for culture in a bacteriologic incubator when prompt analysis is not possible.

3. Apply a dry, sterile dressing to the lumbar puncture site.

4. Monitor vital signs and assess for changes in level of consciousness, headache, and neurologic status every 15 minutes × 4, every 30 minutes × 4, and then hourly × 4.

5. Assess the client for numbness, tingling, and movement of the lower extremities; irritability; change in level of consciousness; nonreactive eye pupils; and ability to void.

6. Assess the puncture site for redness, swelling, drainage, and pain every 4 hours for 24 hours. Notify the physician of any unusual findings. Notify the physician immediately if there is a sign of leakage at the puncture site.

7. Encourage the client to drink increased amounts of fluid with a straw to replace CSF removed during the lumbar puncture, unless this is contraindicated.

8. Headache is common after lumbar puncture, usually beginning within 48 hours and may last up to 4 months, but it usually resolves within 1 week. The cause is thought to be related to CSF hypotension caused by spinal fluid leak. However, this is not proven. There is no correlation between amount of postprocedure bed rest and the duration of the headache; however, lying still typically reduces the severity of the symptoms. Treatment sometimes involves injection of a blood patch into the epidural space, as well as medication for pain. The incidence of post-puncture headache progressively decreases as needle gauge decreases (Evans et al, 2000).

Client and Family Teaching

1. Explain the procedure, potential risks and benefits, and postprocedural care. Allay the client's fears, and allow him or her time to verbalize concerns.

2. There will be a burning sensation with the injection of local anesthetic, and transient pain or pressure may occur during the lumbar puncture.

3. No fasting or sedation is required. Blood thinners may have to be stopped for preplanned procedures, depending on physician prescription.

4. Empty the bladder and bowels before the procedure.

5. You will have to lie on your side with your chin bent down onto your chest and clasp your hands around your knees. The knees should be drawn up to but not compress the abdomen so that the back bows. (A sitting position, with the client straddling a straight-backed chair and flexing the head to the chest, can also be used.)

6. It is important to lie very still throughout this procedure because movement may cause accidental injury. Do not hold your breath, strain, or talk during procedure.

7. Notify the physician or nurse if you are having severe back pain, numbness or tingling in the lower extremities, more than minor bleeding, headache that lasts more than 1 day, or a temperature higher than 101 degrees F (38.3 degrees C).

8. Headaches are common after this procedure. They usually resolve on their own within a week.

9. Avoid heavy lifting for 2 days after the procedure.

Factors That Affect Results

1. Contamination of the specimen will cause inaccurate results. The first tube could be contaminated with blood from

the spinal tap and should not be used for protein determination, cell count, or culture.

2. A traumatic spinal tap could cause blood to be present in the specimen, and this may be mistaken for a clinical problem.

3. Cloudy specimens may be caused by elevated white blood cells. Yellow specimens may be caused by elevated protein >100 mg/dL. Pink or red specimens may be caused by red blood cells. Turbid specimens may be caused by the presence of fungi.

4. Refrigeration will alter the test results if bacteriologic and fungal studies are done.

5. Certain drugs could cause a falsely increased CSF protein level, such as acetophenetidin (phenacetin), anesthetics, chlorpromazine (Thorazine), salicylates (aspirin), streptomycin, and sulfonamides.

6. CSF chloride level determination may be invalidated by IV fluid containing chloride.

7. Hyperglycemia could increase the CSF glucose level.

Other Data

1. Handle specimens cautiously to prevent self-contamination.

2. It is recommended that lumbar punctures continue to be performed in children with first febrile convulsions, especially if less than 18 months of age.

3. The total amyloid beta peptide (Abeta) protein in CSF has not been found to be a useful marker for current diagnosis of Alzheimer's disease.

4. The role of routine lumbar puncture in the initial evaluation of symptom-free infants for congenital syphilis is not recommended because of the low yield of reactive VDRL in CSF and to the similar CSF leukocyte and protein values in the syphilis group and control group.

Lung Function Test

See **Pulmonary Function Tests**—Diagnostic.

Lung Scan, Perfusion and Ventilation (V/Q Scan)—Diagnostic

Norm. Low probability for emboli or thrombus.

Perfusion scan: Uniform uptake of particles within the entire lung vasculature.

Ventilation scan: Equal gas distribution in the pulmonary airways.

Usage. Diagnosis of pulmonary embolism or thrombosis; determination of the percentage of lungs functioning normally; assessment of pulmonary vasculature supply by providing an estimate of regional pulmonary blood flow and identifying areas of shunting and areas where capillaries are absent (that is, emphysema); and diagnosis of asthma, atelectasis, bronchitis, chronic obstructive pulmonary disease, inflammatory fibrosis, lung cancer or tumors, and pneumonia.

Description. This is a nuclear medicine procedure. There are three types of lung scans: (1) the perfusion scan, (2) the ventilation scan, and (3) the inhalation scan. In the perfusion scan, blood flow to the lungs is evaluated by use of an intravenous injection of macroaggregated albumin (MAA) tagged with technetium (^{99m}Tc). The radiolabeled particles become temporarily lodged in the pulmonary vasculature because their diameter is larger than that of the pulmonary capillaries. A gamma-ray detector scans the client, and a scintillation camera records the distribution of particles within the pulmonary vascular supply. "Hot spots" are areas of normal blood flow. "Cold spots" are areas of low radioactivity uptake and indicate poor perfusion and emboli. Although the lung perfusion scan is sensitive, it is not specific because a variety of pathologic conditions can cause the same abnormal results. Therefore lung perfusion scans should be performed with a lung ventilation scan. This scan determines the patency of the pulmonary airways and detects abnormalities in ventilation (such as pneumonia, pleural fluid, emphysema). Ventilation scans will show a normal wash-in and wash-out of radioactivity from the embolized lung area in embolic disorders. Conversely, the wash-in and wash-out will be abnormal in parenchymal disease (such as pneumonia). Finally, a normal inhalation scan looks much like a perfusion scan, except that the trachea and major airways are more visible. Results are interpreted as high, indeterminate, or low probability of embolus or thrombus.

Professional Considerations
Consent form IS required.

Risks
Allergic reaction to iodine-131 if use is planned (itching, hives, rash, tight feeling in the throat, shortness of breath, bronchospasm, anaphylaxis, death).

Contraindications
Lung perfusion scanning is contraindicated in clients with primary pulmonary hypertension or right-to-left heart shunts. During pregnancy or breast-feeding. Previous history of allergy to iodine, eggs, or shellfish if iodine-131 will be used.

Precautions
In pregnant or lactating women; Chan et al (2002) conclude that pediatric risks are low when this procedure is performed during pregnancy.

Preparation
1. A chest radiograph should be obtained before or after a lung perfusion scan. Comparison of the perfusion scan with a chest radiograph can detect infiltrating disease.
2. Have emergency equipment readily available.
3. If iodine-131 is to be given (though this is rarely the case), give the client 10 drops of Lugol's solution several hours before the test. This will prevent iodine uptake by the thyroid gland.
4. Sedation may be prescribed for very young children or those who are unable to lie still for the scan.
5. Establish intravenous access.
6. Breathing methods are reviewed with the client before injection and imaging.
7. See Client and Family Teaching.
8. Just before beginning the procedure, take a "time out" to verify the correct client, procedure, and site.

Procedure
1. Transport the client to the nuclear medicine department.
2. In a perfusion scan, a radionuclide-tagged MAA is injected slowly intravenously over several respiratory cycles. Half is injected while the client is sitting up, and the other half while lying down. The client is placed in the supine, prone, and various lateral positions on the nuclear medicine table under the camera. Scanning with a gamma-ray detector is begun immediately. The scintillation camera takes several single stationary images of the anterior, posterior, and lateral areas of the chest. Perfusion imaging lasts about 45 minutes.
3. In a ventilation scan, the client inhales a mixture of air and radioactive gas (xenon-133, krypton-85, krypton-81m, or ^{99m}Tc-diethylenetriaminepentaacetic acid [^{99m}Tc-DTPA]) through the mouthpiece of a face mask. The radioactive gas follows the same pathway as the air in normal breathing. A nuclear scan is performed at three phases: during the buildup of gas, after the client rebreathes from a bag and the radioactivity reaches a steady level, and after removal of the radioactive gas from the lungs. Ventilation imaging lasts about 30 minutes.
4. In an inhalation scan, droplets of radioactive material can be administered by a positive-pressure ventilator. The aerosol is then inhaled through the mouthpiece of a face mask.

Postprocedure Care
1. Observe the client carefully for up to 60 minutes after the study for a possible (anaphylactic) reaction to the radionuclide.
2. When urine is being discarded, rubber gloves should be worn for 24 hours after the procedure. Wash the gloved hands with soap and water before removing the gloves. Wash the ungloved hands after the gloves have been removed.

Client and Family Teaching
1. Peripheral venipuncture is the only discomfort associated with this test.
2. A physician trained in diagnostic nuclear medicine interprets the results.
3. The total time for the procedure is approximately 2 hours.

4. No fasting or premedication is required.
5. The client will not be exposed to large amounts of radioactivity because only tracer doses of isotopes are used.
6. Remove jewelry around the chest area.
7. Meticulously wash your hands with soap and water after each void for 24 hours after procedure.
8. Family members must wear rubber gloves when discarding the client's urine for 24 hours after the procedure if the family will be providing this care.

Factors That Affect Results

1. Jewelry or metal objects in the x-ray field distort the results.
2. The client must lie motionless throughout the scan for the most accurate results.
3. Ventilation scans with ^{99m}Tc-DTPA require client cooperation with deep breathing and appropriate use of breathing equipment to prevent contamination with the radioactive gases.
4. The scan results of clients with pulmonary parenchymal disease (such as pneumonia, emphysema, pleural effusion, tumors) will appear to demonstrate perfusion defect and simulate pulmonary embolism. Ventilation scans are hard to interpret in obstructive airway disease

that interferes with the distribution of the radioactive gases.
5. False-positive scan results occur in vasculitis, mitral stenosis, and pulmonary hypertension and when tumors obstruct a pulmonary artery with airway involvement.

Other Data

1. In pulmonary emboli, perfusion is decreased but ventilation is maintained. Diagnosis of pulmonary embolus cannot be made on the basis of a lung perfusion scan alone.
2. In pneumonia, ventilation is absent.
3. The perfusion scan immediately follows the ventilation scan. However, ventilation scans using krypton can be performed before, during, or after perfusion scans.
4. Health care professionals working in a nuclear medicine area must follow federal standards set by the Nuclear Regulatory Commission. These standards include precautions for handling the radioactive material and monitoring of potential radiation exposure.
5. Technetium half-life is 6 hours.
6. See also Gas ventilation lung scan—Diagnostic.

Lung Volumes

See Pulmonary Function Tests—Diagnostic.

Lupus Anticoagulant

See Circulating Anticoagulant—Blood.

Lupus Erythematosus Cell Test

See Lupus Test—Blood.

Lupus Panel—Blood

Norm.

	SI Units
Antinuclear antibody titer (ANA)	<1:20 or none detected
Anti-DNA titer	<1:10

C3 Complement		SI Units
Adult	88-201 mg/dL	0.88-2.01 g/L
Child		
Cord blood	65.113 mg/dL	0.65-1.13 g/L
Birth-1 month	59-121 mg/dL	0.59-1.21 g/L
Between 1 and 2 months	55-129 mg/dL	0.55-1.29 g/L
Between 2 and 3 months	61-155 mg/dL	0.61-1.55 g/L
Between 3 and 4 months	67-136 mg/dL	0.67-1.36 g/L
Between 4 and 5 months	65-182 mg/dL	0.65-1.82 g/L
Between 5 and 6 months	67-174 mg/dL	0.67-1.74 g/L
Between 6 and 7 months	77-179 mg/dL	0.77-1.79 g/L
Between 7 and 9 months	78-173 mg/dL	0.78-1.73 g/L
Between 9 and 11 months	76-187 mg/dL	0.76-1.87 g/L
Between 1 and 2 years	87-181 mg/dL	0.87-1.81 g/L
Between 2 and 3 years	84-177 mg/dL	0.84-1.77 g/L
Between 3 and 5 years	80-178 mg/dL	0.80-1.78 g/L
Between 5 and 11 years	89-203 mg/dL	0.89-2.03 g/L
Between 12 and 18 years	88-201 mg/dL	0.88-2.01 g/L

C4 Complement		SI Units
Adult	15-45 mg/dL	0.15-0.45 g/L
Child		
Cord blood		
Birth-1 month	8-30 mg/dL	0.08-0.3 g/L
Between 1 and 2 months	9-33 mg/dL	0.09-3.3 g/L
Between 2 and 3 months	9-37 mg/dL	0.09-3.7 g/L
Between 3 and 4 months	10-35 mg/dL	0.1-0.35 g/L
Between 4 and 5 months	10-49 mg/dL	0.1-0.49 g/L
Between 5 and 6 months	9-48 mg/dL	0.09-0.48 g/L
Between 6 and 7 months	12-55 mg/dL	0.12-0.55 g/L
Between 7 and 9 months	13-48 mg/dL	0.13-0.48 g/L
Between 9 and 11 months	16-51 mg/dL	0.16-0.51 g/L
Between 1 and 2 years	16-52 mg/dL	0.16-0.52 g/L
Between 2 and 5 years	12-47 mg/dL	0.12-0.47 g/L
Between 5 and 11 years	12-52 mg/dL	0.12-0.52 g/L
Between 12 and 18 years	10-40 mg/dL	0.10-0.40 g/L

Positive. Dermatomyositis, discoid lupus, infectious mononucleosis, lupoid hepatitis, myasthenia gravis, polyarteritis, rheumatoid arthritis, scleroderma, Sjögren's syndrome, and systemic lupus erythematosus (SLE).

Negative. Normal finding; lack of SLE.

Description. Three distinct laboratory tests are used to verify the diagnosis of SLE. First, antinuclear antibody (ANA), which assesses tissue-antigen antibodies, is frequently used for diagnosing SLE. Antinuclear antibodies, which are gamma globulins, react with the nuclei of all organs of people or animals. These ANAs usually belong to more than one immunoglobulin class. Immuno-fluorescence detects ANAs and produces homogeneous and peripheral (RIM) staining patterns in clients with SLE. Second, anti-DNA, an antinuclear antibody, is almost always present in SLE and is present in lupus nephritis 95% of the time. Anti-DNA values may fluctuate according to the remission and exacerbation of the disease. Third, C3 and C4 complements are proteins that are activated into enzymes when IgG and IgM antibodies are combined with their specific antigens. These are measured during an acute or chronic inflammatory process. Both serum C3 and C4 complements will be decreased in clients with SLE.

Professional Considerations
Consent form NOT required.

Preparation

1. Tube: Red topped, red/gray topped, or gold topped.

Procedure

1. Draw a 5-mL blood sample.

Postprocedure Care

1. None.

Client and Family Teaching

1. Signs and symptoms of SLE include fatigue, fever, rash (butterfly over the nose), leukopenia, and thrombocytopenia.
2. If positive for SLE, have daily rest periods, which will help to decrease the symptoms.
3. Lupus Foundation of America, Inc., 2000 L Street NW, Washington, DC 20036, Toll-free 888-787-5380.

Factors That Affect Results

1. Hemolysis of the specimen invalidates the results.
2. Several drugs may cause positive tests for ANAs. For example, clients who are receiving hydralazine or procainamide may demonstrate ANAs at increased titers, even though they do not exhibit any signs of SLE.
3. Heat can destroy the complement components.
4. The serum value of C3 may decrease if the sample is left standing for 1-2 hours at room temperature.

Other Data

1. A positive (high) titer of ANAs does not necessarily indicate a disease process because ANAs are present in some apparently normal clients.
2. Some clients with connective tissue disease or who may develop such a disease at a later time have developed a positive titer of ANAs.
3. A negative test for total antinuclear antibody is strong evidence that the client does not have SLE.
4. Anti-DNA titer correlates with systemic lupus erythematosus and the occurrence of glomerulonephritis.
5. Other tests to confirm the diagnosis of SLE include (1) anti-SM, (2) CH_{50}, and (3) kidney or skin biopsy.

Lupus Test (LE Test, LE Cell Test, LE Preparation, LE Slide Cell Test, Lupus Erythematosus Cell Test, Lymphocyte Erythematous Cell Test)—Blood

Norm. Negative; no LE cells found.

Positive. Arthritis (rheumatoid), other rheumatic diseases, hepatitis, scleroderma, and systemic lupus erythematosus (SLE). Drugs include Azulfidine (salicylazosulfapyridine), chlorpromazine, ethosuximide, hydralazine, isoniazid, methyldopa, penicillamine, phenytoin, practolol, primidone, procainamide, and thiouracil.

Description. This is a serologic test used to diagnose SLE and to monitor its treatment. Clients with SLE have antibodies against the components of nuclei within their own cells. One usually performs this test by traumatizing white blood cells and exposing the nuclear material within them. Then the nuclear material is incubated with the client's serum. Neutrophils in the affected client's serum will phagocytize the traumatized nuclear material. The phagocytized complex appears as a blue-staining, amorphous mass distending the neutrophil's cytoplasm after the cells are stained with Wright's stain. When these neutrophils, which are now filled LE cells, are seen, the test is considered positive.

Professional Considerations

Consent form NOT required.

Preparation

1. Tube: Red topped, red/gray topped, or gold topped.
2. Avoid heparin therapy for 2 days before the test.

Procedure

1. Draw a 5-mL blood sample.
2. List on the laboratory requisition any drugs that may affect results (from the list above, under Positive, and from the list under Factors That Affect Results).

Postprocedure Care

1. None.

Client and Family Teaching

1. No fasting is required.

2. Discuss the signs of potential infection at the venipuncture site with the client because clients with SLE are often immunocompromised.

Factors That Affect Results

1. Drugs that may cause false-negative results include heparin and steroids.
2. Drugs that may cause false-positive results include acetazolamide, aminosalicylic acid, anticonvulsants (phenytoin, Mesantoin, chlorprothixene, chlorothiazide, clofibrate, griseofulvin, isoniazid (INH), hydralazine, methyldopa, methysergide, oral contraceptives, penicillin, phenylbutazone, procainamide, quinidine, reserpine, streptomycin, sulfonamides, and tetracyclines.
3. This is a nonspecific test. False-positive results have been reported in those having rheumatoid arthritis, scleroderma, and drug-induced lupus, which were related to tetracycline, phenytoin, and oral contraceptives.
4. Reject clotted specimens. Hemolysis of the blood sample could affect the results.

Other Data

1. The LE test is positive in only 60%-80% of acutely ill clients.
2. Use more sensitive tests, such as antinuclear antibodies or anti-DNA, to confirm SLE.

Luteinizing Hormone—Blood

Norm. Ranges vary among laboratories.

		SI Units
Adult Females		
Follicular phase	5-30 mIU/mL	5-30 Arb* units
Midcycle	75-150 mIU/mL	75-150 Arb units
Luteal phase	3-40 mIU/mL	3-40 Arb units
Postmenopausal	30-200 mIU/mL	30-200 Arb units
FSH:LH ratio	<3.1	<3.1
Adult Males	6-23 mIU/mL	6-23 Arb units
Female Children		
1-3 months	7.8-27 mIU/mL	7.8-27 Arb units
3-5 months	5.6-20.8 mIU/mL	5.6-20.8 Arb units
5-7 months	5.4-21.4 mIU/mL	5.4-21.4 Arb units
7-12 months	2.1-4.7 mIU/mL	2.1-4.7 Arb units
10-13 years	2-14 mIU/mL	2-14 Arb units
14-18 years	2-29 mIU/mL	2-29 Arb units
Male Children		
1-3 months	8.9-35.7 mIU/mL	8.9-35.7 Arb units
3-5 months	3.7-27.3 mIU/mL	3.7-27.3 Arb units
5-7 months	9.1-25.1 mIU/mL	9.1-25.1 Arb units
7-12 months	5.7-42.3 mIU/mL	5.7-42.3 Arb units
10-13 years	4-12 mIU/mL	4-12 Arb units
14-18 years	6-19 mIU/mL	6-19 Arb units

*Arb means arbitrary.

Usage. To evaluate infertility in women and men (high serum values of LH are related to gonadal dysfunction, and low values of LH are related to dysfunction or failure of the hypothalamus or pituitary gland); to evaluate hormonal therapy for inducing ovulation; and to evaluate endocrine problems related to precocious puberty in children.

Increased. Amenorrhea, anorchia (congenital absence of testicles), endocrine problems related to precocious puberty in children, hyperpituitarism, Klinefelter's syndrome (in prepubertal boys) (such as sex chromosome disorder), liver disease, menopause, ovarian or testicular failure (primary gonadal dysfunction), polycystic ovary syndrome, primary male hypogonadism,

Stein-Leventhal syndrome (polycystic ovary syndrome), tumors (pituitary, testicular), and Turner's syndrome (ovarian dysgenesis). Drugs include anticonvulsants, clomiphene, naloxone, and spironolactone. Herbs or natural remedies include *Unkei-to*.

Decreased. Adrenal hyperplasia or tumor, amenorrhea (pituitary failure, secondary gonadal insufficiency), anorexia nervosa, anovulation, eating disorders, hypophysectomy, hypopituitarism, hypothalamic disorder, luteinizing hormone deficiency, male hypogonadism, malnutrition, ovarian hypofunction (secondary, tertiary), pituitary disorder, prostate cancer and testicular failure (related to pituitary failure). Drugs include atrial natriuretic hormone (long-acting), digoxin, estrogen compounds, kaliuretic hormone, oral contraceptives, phenothiazines, progesterone, stanozolol, testosterone, and vessel dilator hormone administration.

Description. Luteinizing hormone (LH), a glycoprotein, is secreted by the anterior lobe of the pituitary gland in response to stimulation by the hypothalamic release of gonadotropin-releasing hormone. LH plays a critical role in regulation of ovulatory and reproductive function. In women, LH initiates luteinization in the ovary, and together with follicle-stimulating hormone (FSH) induces ovulation. A surge of LH in blood levels indicates that ovulation has occurred. In men, LH stimulates the secretion of androgens and increases the production of testosterone. Together with FSH, testosterone influences the development and maturation of spermatozoa. Luteinizing hormone levels peak at midcycle in women of childbearing age, surging when ovulation has occurred. In menopausal women, levels may be up to five times normal levels.

Professional Considerations
Consent form NOT required.

Preparation
1. Client may be asked to withhold estrogen-containing medications for 4 weeks before the test.
2. Tube: Red topped, red/gray topped, or gold topped.
3. Document client's age, date of last menstrual period, and whether client is menopausal or premenopausal (females) on laboratory requisition.
4. Discuss with physician whether to withhold medications that could interfere with the test results.

Procedure
1. In men, one single sample is taken. In women, daily blood samples must be taken at the same time each day. A series of daily blood specimens can establish the presence or absence of a midcycle peak in women with anovulatory fertility problems. Alternatively, several samples may be taken in one day, 20-30 minutes apart. This is because LH is released in a pulsatile manner with levels varying during the menstrual cycle.
2. Draw a 4-mL blood sample without hemolysis.

Postprocedure Care
1. None.

Client and Family Teaching
1. Encourage the client to express concerns related to infertility or other health problems to the nurse or the physician.
2. Episodic fluctuations in LH can be great; thus multiple blood samples are more reliable than a single sample.

Factors That Affect Results
1. Hemolysis of the specimen invalidates the results.
2. Drugs that could increase or decrease plasma LH levels. (Refer to relevant sections above.)
3. Women using oral contraceptives will have an absence of midcycle LH peak until the contraceptives are discontinued.
4. Collection of the daily specimen at different times in the day may cause inaccurate results.
5. Pulsatile secretion patterns may be disrupted in clients with seizure disorders.
6. Radiology tests involving injection of a radioactive tracer within 7 days before the test can invalidate the results.

Other Data
1. Follicle-stimulating hormone (FSH) level may be requested from the same specimen.
2. Progesterone, not luteinizing hormone, concentration at the time of ovum transfer is a significant variable associated with spontaneous abortion (miscarriage).

Luteinizing Hormone—Urine

Norm.

Adult Female	
Follicular phase	5-25 IU/24 hours
Midcycle	30-95 IU/24 hours
Luteal phase	2-24 IU/24 hours
Postmenopausal	40-100 IU/24 hours
Adult Male	5-25 IU/24 hours

Increased. See Luteinizing hormone—Blood.

Decreased. See Luteinizing hormone—Blood.

Description. See Luteinizing hormone—Blood. In addition, urine assays are used to monitor ovulatory cycles of clients undergoing in vitro fertilization.

Professional Considerations

Consent form NOT required.

Preparation

1. Obtain a specimen container for 24-hour urine collection. (The presence of a preservative eliminates the need for refrigeration.)
2. Label the container with the client's name, test, date, and time. For females, write the date of last menstrual period on the laboratory requisition. Note if the woman is menopausal, and record her age.

Procedure

1. Discard the first morning urine specimen.
2. Save all the urine voided for 24 hours in the collection container. Include the urine voided at the end of the 24-hour period.

For catheterized clients, keep the drainage bag on ice and empty the urine into the collection container hourly.

3. Refrigerate the urine if the 24-hour container does not contain a preservative.

Postprocedure Care

1. Compare the urine quantity in the specimen container with the urinary output record for the test. If the specimen contains less urine than what was recorded as output, some urine may have been discarded, thus invalidating the test.
2. Document the quantity of urine output for the collection period on the laboratory requisition.

Client and Family Teaching

1. Save all the urine voided in the 24-hour period and urinate before defecating to avoid loss of urine. If any urine is accidentally discarded, discard the entire specimen and restart the collection the next day.

Factors That Affect Results

1. Urine that is stored in a container without a preservative or urine that is not refrigerated will yield invalid results.

Other Data

1. The 24-hour urine collection will minimize the episodic "peak-and-valley" secretion of LH that may occur with blood serum specimens.
2. One or more blood samples of LH may also be evaluated.
3. One-step test strip kits for detection of LH in urine are available for use at home.

Lyme Disease Antibody—Blood

Norm. Within 4 weeks of symptom onset: negative ELISA and IgG Western blot and IgM Western blot.

Borrelia burgdorferi total antibodies, IgG and/or IgM by ELISA: Negative: 0.99 LIV or less; antibody not detected. Equivocal: 1.00-1.20 LIV. Perform repeat testing in 10-14 days on convalescent sample. Positive: ≥1.21 LIV. Probable presence of antibody to *Borrelia burgdorferi* detected. Follow up with IgG and/or IgM Western blot.

IgG Western blot assay: Positive when any five of the following bands are positive: 18, 23, 28, 30, 39, 41, 45, 58, 66, or 93 kDa.

IgM Western blot assay: Positive when any two bands of the following bands are positive: 23, 39, 41 kDa.

Increased. Indicative of recent infection or past exposure to Lyme disease.

Description. Lyme disease was first named because of its close geographic clustering in

Lyme, Connecticut, in 1975. Today it is found mostly in the northeastern, upper Midwestern, and western United States. This blood test identifies antibodies to the spirochete agent of Lyme disease, *Borrelia burgdorferi*. *B. burgdorferi* is carried by several tick vectors, primarily the deer tick *Ixodes dammini*, and is transmitted to humans through a tick bite. Lyme disease is an inflammatory disease involving multiple body systems and causing symptoms that mimic other diseases, beginning with a bull's eye rash and progressing to flulike symptoms and eventually to arthritis. If left untreated, Lyme disease can progress to symptoms as serious as encephalitis, cardiomegaly, and inflammation of the pericardium and sensory nerves. Levels of specific IgM antibodies peak during the third to sixth week after the onset of the disease and then gradually decline. Titers of specific IgG antibodies are usually low during the first several weeks of illness. The IgG antibodies will reach maximum levels months later and will often stay elevated for up to 20 years after the active disease has resolved. For clients with symptoms suggesting Lyme disease and with no prior history of it, an initial enzyme-linked immunosorbent assay (ELISA) should be done. Follow-up testing on serial samples is preferred and varies based upon the ELISA results and time since onset of symptoms, as described under Procedure. These methods are of limited use in certain clients; positive results will occur if the client has previously been vaccinated with the *B. burgdorferi* vaccine. Because 25% of those vaccinated fail to develop immunity, it is possible to become infected with Lyme disease even after vaccination. For previously vaccinated clients with current suspected Lyme disease, the *B. burgdorferi* C6 peptide antibody test—Serum should be used.

Professional Considerations

Consent form NOT required.

Preparation

1. Tube: Red topped, red/gray topped, or gold topped.
2. Ask the client if there has been any recent history of a tick bite.
3. Assess for a reddish, macular lesion at the site of the tick bite and elsewhere.

Procedure

1. Draw a 3-mL blood sample.
2. If results are negative, repeat the test 2-4 weeks later on the convalescent sample. If initial ELISA results are positive, follow up with an IgG and IgM Western blot confirmatory test if less than 8 weeks from onset or with an IgG Western blot confirmatory test if more than 8 weeks from onset.

Postprocedure Care

1. Transport specimen to laboratory immediately for serum/cell separation.

Client and Family Teaching

1. No fasting or special preparation is required.
2. Return as prescribed for serial specimen collection.
3. A reddish, macular lesion usually occurs about 1 week after the tick bite. The primary disease occurs 4-20 days after the initial bite. The secondary disease develops after 3-24 weeks of infection.
4. Wear clothing that covers all extremities when in areas infested by ticks and deer and when in the woods.
5. See a doctor immediately if bitten by a tick or if a macular lesion results from a tick bite. Antibiotic therapy will usually be started.

Factors That Affect Results

1. Reject specimens with low dilutions of serum.
2. False-negative results may occur when the client has recently undergone antibiotic therapy.
3. Sensitivity and specificity of testing is better in later stages of Lyme disease than in early stages.
4. Because of the cross-reactivity of *B. burgdorferi* with other organisms, false-positive results can occur if careful separation of the immune complexes from the serum is not done. Conditions in which false-positive results are possible include Rocky Mountain spotted fever, relapsing fever, ehrlichiosis, babesiosis, syphilis, mononucleosis, systemic lupus erythematosus, and rheumatoid arthritis.

Other Data

1. The organism may also be cultivated from cerebrospinal fluid or skin biopsy specimens.

2. Seronegativity usually rules out the diagnosis of Lyme disease.

3. The Lyme disease vaccine has been withdrawn from the market.

Lymph Node Biopsy

See Biopsy, Site-Specific—Specimen.

Lymphangiography (Lymphography, Lymphangiogram)—Diagnostic

Norm. Normal-sized vessels and nodes containing no filling defects.

Usage. Indicated in clients with edema of lower extremities with unknown cause, Hodgkin's disease, lymphadenopathy, lymphoma, prostate cancer, testicular malignancy, tumor metastatic to the lymphatic system. Used to stage clients with lymphoma, demonstrate the extent and level of lymphatic metastasis, and evaluate the effectiveness of chemotherapy or radiation therapy. Used in conjunction with fine-needle aspiration to obtain biopsy of suspected cervical malignancy. Largely replaced by CT for evaluation of the retroperitoneal lymph nodes, but is still used if CT results are inconclusive.

Description. Radiographic test of the lymphatic vessels and lymph nodes. A radiopaque iodine contrast oil, such as Ethiodol, is injected into the lymphatics of the foot or hand. The dye remains in the lymph nodes for 6 months to 1 year; thus repeat plain x-rays films can be performed for follow-up of disease progression or to determine the effectiveness of the cancer treatment.

Professional Considerations

Consent form IS required.

Risks

Allergic reaction to dye (itching, hives, rash, tight feeling in the throat, shortness of breath, bronchospasm, anaphylaxis, death); renal toxicity from contrast medium; lipid pneumonia (e.g., contrast dye causes micropulmonary emboli); lymphangitis; infection or cellulitis.

Contraindications

Previous allergy to iodized oil, iodine preparations, contrast dye used in other x-ray tests, or shellfish are relative contraindications. If allergies exist, the radiologist may prescribe a diphenhydramine and steroid preparation, which may be given before the procedure. Then a hypoallergenic, nonionic contrast medium will be used during the test. Other contraindications: severe chronic lung diseases, pregnancy (because of radioactive iodine crossing the blood-placental barrier), pulmonary insufficiency, cardiac disease, and severe renal or hepatic disease.

Preparation

1. Have emergency equipment readily available.
2. See Client and Family Teaching.
3. Just before beginning the procedure, take a "time out" to verify the correct client, procedure, and site.

Procedure

1. In the radiology department, the client is positioned supine on the examination table.
2. An oil-based dye is injected intradermally between each of the first three toes of each foot to outline the lymphatic vessels. (The stain can also be injected into the web of the skin between the fingers.)
3. Under local anesthesia, a 1- to 2-inch incision is made in the dorsum of each foot (or hand) about 15-30 minutes later.
4. The lymphatic vessel is identified. This will be easily visualized after the stain is absorbed.
5. A 30-gauge lymphangiographic needle with polyethylene tubing is carefully inserted into the identified lymphatic vessel. A low-rate infusion pump is used to administer an extremely low-pressure, slow injection (1-1.5 hours) of iodine contrast material.
6. The flow of iodine dye is followed by fluoroscopy.
7. When the contrast material reaches the level of the third and fourth lumbar

vertebrae, the injection is stopped. This usually occurs in about 1½ hours.

8. Radiographs are then taken of the chest, abdomen, and pelvis. This will demonstrate the filling of the lymph nodes.

9. The cannula is removed, and the incision is closed with sutures after the injection of contrast is completed. The entire procedure takes about 3 hours.

10. A second set of x-ray films is often made in 24-48 hours.

Postprocedure Care

1. Elevate legs to prevent swelling for 24 hours if prescribed. Keep the client on bed rest for 24 hours or as prescribed.

2. Assess for signs of oil embolism every 4 hours for 24 hours (such as dyspnea, pain, and hypotension).

3. Observe injection and incision sites for evidence of cellulitis (such as redness, drainage, swelling, pain). Monitor temperature every 4 hours for 48 hours after the procedure.

4. The dressing is usually not changed for the first 48 hours.

5. Allow the client to rest after the procedure.

6. Monitor for complications, such as delayed wound healing or infection at the site of the incision or injection; edema of legs; allergic dermatitis; headache; sore mouth and throat; skin rashes; transient fever; lymphangitis; or oil embolism, which could occur if the contrast medium causes micro pulmonary emboli and could produce lipid pneumonia.

Client and Family Teaching

1. No fasting or sedation is required.

2. Discomfort may be felt when the stain is injected and when the feet are anesthetized.

3. It is important to lie very still during the injection of the contrast dye. X-ray filming usually takes about 30 minutes.

4. The dye will turn the urine and stool blue for 48 hours. Also, IV administration of the lymphatic stain or excessive infiltration of the stain may impart a transient bluish tint to the entire skin surface.

5. Inspect the injection and incision sites for redness, swelling, and pain if the client will be returning home after the procedure.

6. Sutures should be removed 7-10 days after the test.

Factors That Affect Results

1. Inability to cannulate lymphatic vessels.

Other Data

1. To visualize axillary and supraclavicular nodes, injections are made in each hand.

Lymphocyte

See **Differential Leukocyte Count**—Peripheral Blood.

Lymphocyte Erythematous Cell Test

See **Lupus Test**—Blood.

Lymphocyte Marker Studies

See **T- and B-Lymphocyte Subset Assay**—Blood.

Lymphocyte Subset Enumeration

See **Acquired Immunodeficiency Syndrome Evaluation Battery**—Diagnostic.

Lymphocyte Subset Typing

See **T- and B-Lymphocyte Subset Assay**—Blood.

Lymphocyte Assay

See T- and B-Lymphocyte Subset Assay—Blood.

Lymphogranuloma Venereum Titer (LGV)—Blood

See Chlamydia Culture and Group Titer—Specimen.

Lymphography

See Lymphangiography—Diagnostic.

Lymphs

See Differential Leukocyte Count—Peripheral Blood.

LSD (Lysergic Acid Diethylamide)—Blood or Urine

Norm. Negative.

Positive. Drug abuse.

Overdose Symptoms and Treatment
Symptoms. Hypertension, tachycardia, piloerection, and suicidal tendency. LSD-related violent behavior includes suicide, homicide, and accidental death. See also Client and Family Teaching.
Treatment. There is no systematic program of treatment for LSD ingestion. A quiet environment and diazepam may be effective in controlling the individual. Hemodialysis and peritoneal dialysis are unlikely to remove lysergic acid from the bloodstream.

Description. A potent hallucinogen derived from ergot, a fungus that spoils rye grain. It is equally effective by the intravenous route as by the oral route, is metabolized in the liver and excreted in the bile, and affects both parasympathetic and sympathetic nervous systems. May produce hallucinations years after ingestion, without warning.

Professional Considerations
Consent form NOT required unless the specimen is collected as part of legal evidence.

Preparation
1. Tube: Light-protected (usually amber), nonglass transport tube (for the blood and urine samples).
2. Obtain a sterile specimen container (for the urine sample).

Procedure
1. Draw a 7-mL blood sample or obtain 4 mL of urine. Transfer specimen immediately to light-protected tube.

Postprocedure Care
1. If the results are to be used as legal evidence, the chain of possession must remain unbroken from the time the specimen is collected until court testimony.
2. Refrigerate or freeze specimen until testing.

Client and Family Teaching
1. This drug may cause delirium, delusions, and hallucinations.
2. Clients who experience palinopsia (prolonged afterimages, visual perseveration) during LSD intoxication may continue to be symptomatic up to 3 years after they cease to ingest the drug. Some studies show clonazepam as useful in helping to control these symptoms.

Factors That Affect Results
1. Levels may be decreased if stored at room temperature.

2. The use of Stealth adulterant in the urine sample will cause negative results in a positive sample.

Other Data

1. None.

Lysozyme

See **Muramidase**—Serum and Urine.

Magnesium—Serum

Norm.

	Normal Serum Levels	SI Units
Newborn	1.2-2.9 mEq/L	0.6-1.45 mmol/L
Child	1.6-2.6 mEq/L	0.8-1.3 mmol/L
Girls		0.75-1.0 mmol/L
Boys		0.76-1.0 mmol/L
Adult	1.3-2.5 mEq/L or 1.8-3.0 mg/dL	0.65-1.25 mmol/L
Panic level	<0.5 mEq/L or >3.0 mg/dL	<0.25 or >1.23 mmol/L
Toxic level	>12.0 mEq/L	>6 mmol/L

Panic Level Symptoms and Treatment

High Magnesium Symptoms. Lethargy, drowsiness, flushing, nausea, vomiting, slurred speech, hypotension, weak or absent deep tendon reflexes, electrocardiogram changes (such as prolonged P-R and Q-T intervals, widened QRS, bradycardia), respiratory depression.

Treatment

NOTE: Treatment choice(s) depend(s) on client's history and condition and episode history.

1. Administer magnesium salts intravenously (8-16 mmol of magnesium sulfate in 10-100 mL of D_5W over 10-15 minutes, followed by 40 mmol of magnesium sulfate in 500 mL of D_5W over 5 hours).
2. Reduce auditory, mechanical, and visual stimuli.
3. Monitor for respiratory depression and areflexia if intravenous magnesium sulfate is given.
4. Monitor for diarrhea and metabolic alkalosis if oral magnesium replacement is given.

Increased. Addison's disease, adrenalectomy, ataxia, dehydration (severe), diabetes (uncontrolled diabetes, diabetic acidosis before treatment, controlled diabetes in an older client), dysrhythmias, hypercalcemia, hypophosphatemia, hypothyroidism, kidney stone, leukemia (lymphocytic and myelocytic), mood disorders, nephrolithiasis, parenteral nutrition, renal insufficiency or failure. Drugs include antacids containing magnesium (such as Maalox, Mylanta, Aludrox, DiaGel, Milk of Magnesia), calcium-containing medications, cathartics, Epsom salt gargle, laxatives (such as Epsom salt, magnesium citrate), lithium, and thyroid medications.

Decreased. Acute tubular necrosis (diuretic phase), alcoholism (chronic), aldosteronism, Bartter syndrome, bone fractures, bowel resection complications, convulsions, diabetic ketoacidosis, diarrhea (chronic), dysrhythmias, eating disorders (laxatives, impaired nutritional status), excessive lactation, excessive sweating, hepatic cirrhosis, hepatic insufficiency, hepatitis, hungry bone syndrome, hypokalemia, hypercalcemia, hyperthyroidism, hypoparathyroidism, intravenous solutions without magnesium, ketoacidosis, kwashiorkor (severe malnutrition), laxative abuse, magnesium-deficiency tetany syndrome, pancreatitis (chronic, acute), phosphate depletion, postoperatively, primary hyperaldosteronism, prolonged gastric drainage, reduced magnesium absorption (specific magnesium malabsorption, generalized malabsorption syndrome, excessive bowel resection, diffuse bowel disease or injury), reduced magnesium intake, renal defect of magnesium resorption, renal disease (chronic), renal transplantation, renal tubular acidosis, status post obstructive diuresis, stress states with catecholamine excess, tetany, toxemia of pregnancy, ulcerative colitis, volume expansion (extracellular fluid). Drugs include alcohol, amphotericin B, some antibiotics (neomycin, aminoglycosides), calcium gluconate, cisplatin, citrates, corticosteroids, cyclosporin A, diuretics (loop, thiazide, such as furosemide, ethacrynic acid, hydrochlorothiazide), gentamicin, glucose, laxatives, insulin, mannitol, proton pump inhibitors (PPIs, long-term use), and urea.

Description. Measurement of magnesium levels is used as an index to (1) metabolic activity in the body (such as carbohydrate metabolism, protein synthesis, nucleic acid synthesis, contraction of muscular tissue) and (2) renal function, because 95% of magnesium that is filtered through the glomerulus is reabsorbed in the tubules. Most of the body's magnesium, which is an electrolyte, is concentrated in the bone, cartilage, and the cell itself. In addition, magnesium is needed in the blood-clotting mechanism. Magnesium regulates neuromuscular irritability, acts as a cofactor that modifies the activity of many enzymes, and has a significant effect on the metabolism of calcium.

Professional Considerations
Consent form NOT required.

Preparation
1. Tube: Red topped, red/gray topped, or gold topped or green topped.
2. Do NOT draw during hemodialysis.
3. See Client and Family Teaching.

Procedure
1. Draw a 4-mL blood sample without hemolysis.

Postprocedure Care
1. Separate serum from the red blood cells as soon as possible. Allow serum to clot completely.
2. Serum separated from the cells is stable for 7 days at room temperature or refrigerated. Stable for 1 year if frozen.

Client and Family Teaching
1. No special diet or fasting is required before sampling.

2. Eat foods rich in magnesium (such as seafood, meats, green vegetables, whole grains, and nuts) if magnesium level is low.
3. Avoid constant use of antacids or laxatives containing magnesium, if magnesium level is high. Check drug labels to identify magnesium-containing formulations.
4. Magnesium lactate contains both calcium and magnesium where 84 mg = 7 meq.

Factors That Affect Results
1. Hemolysis of the specimen will create falsely elevated levels of magnesium.
2. Glucuronic acid therapy will interfere with the color reaction in some laboratory methods and will produce falsely decreased results.
3. Prolonged intravenous fluid therapy, hyperalimentation, exchange blood transfusions, or prolonged nasogastric suctioning may yield falsely decreased results.
4. Prolonged use of magnesium products (such as antacids, laxatives), lithium compounds, or salicylate therapy will cause falsely increased levels, especially if renal damage is present.
5. Hyperbilirubinemia interferes with serum magnesium levels, resulting in misleadingly low levels.
6. High-phosphate diet suppresses both magnesium and calcium absorption.
7. Levels may decrease from baseline in women taking oral contraceptives, and may increase from baseline in women taking injectable contraceptives.

Other Data
1. Nutritional status is important to the interpretation of the test results.
2. If hypocalcemia is present, magnesium should also be measured. Magnesium deficiency may cause apparently unexplained hypocalcemia and hypokalemia.
3. Respiratory failure and death are possible when magnesium levels exceed 12 mEq/L. Magnesium level may be decreased after surgery for hyperparathyroidism.
4. A high serum Ca/Mg ratio may increase recurrent breast cancer.
5. A diet of Omega-3 and -6 fatty acids, magnesium and zinc decreases symptoms of ADHD.
6. Familial hypomagnesemia is linked to mutations in the caludin-16/19 complex.

Magnesium—24-Hour Urine

Norm. Normal values vary with different test methods:

5-16 mEq/24 hours (2.5-8.0 μmol/24 hours)

12-199 mg/24 hours

7.3-12.2 mg/dL (random sample)

Increased. Alcoholism, Bartter syndrome, hypermagnesemia, and nephrolithiasis. Drugs include aldosterone, cisplatin, corticosteroids, diuretics (ethacrynic acid), and thiazides.

Decreased. Renal disease, kidney stones, magnesium deficit, osteoporosis, and syndrome of inappropriate antidiuretic hormone secretion (SIADHS).

Description. A 24-hour urine test is useful in evaluation of renal disease and magnesium deficiency. In magnesium deficiency, urine magnesium decreases before serum magnesium. See also Magnesium—Serum.

Professional Considerations
Consent form NOT required.

Preparation
1. Obtain a 3-L, acid-washed, metal-free urine collection container without preservatives, and a container of ice.

Procedure
1. Instruct the client to void and discard the initial specimen.

2. Collect all the urine voided in a 24-hour period in the above container. Maintain the specimen on wet ice throughout the collection period. Do not collect urine in a metal bedpan or urinal.

Postprocedure Care
1. Record total 24-hour urine volume and exact beginning and ending times of collection on the container and the laboratory requisition.
2. Send the specimen to the laboratory on wet ice.
3. Specimen is stable at room temperature or refrigerated for 1 week and for 1 year if frozen.

Client and Family Teaching
1. Save all the urine you void for 24 hours in the plastic container provided. If any urine is accidentally discarded, throw out the entire specimen and restart the collection the next day.

Factors That Affect Results
1. Reject any urine specimen that has had contact with metal.
2. Increased blood alcohol level increases urine magnesium excretion.

Other Data
1. Urinary excretion of magnesium is diet-dependent.

Magnetic Resonance Angiography (MRA)—Diagnostic

Norm. Anatomy of normal vessels are well visualized, and blood flow is unobstructed.

Usage. Evaluate vascular structure; evaluate blood flow, especially in the venous system, for possible aneurysms, stenosis, thromboses, or blockages; determine tumor vascularity; assess for evidence of direct tumor involvement of vascular structures; evaluate clients with carotid stenosis preoperatively so that the carotid artery endarterectomy is performed with decreased complication; assist in diagnosis of cerebrovascular disease, cardiovascular disease, cerebral arteriovenous malformations, congenital heart disease, renal or hepatic vasculature disorder, trigeminal neuralgia; assess effectiveness of various therapeutic interventions related to vascular structure and blood flow.

Description. Magnetic resonance angiography (MRA) is a noninvasive vascular imaging technique. This procedure is performed by use of the magnetic resonance imaging (MRI) scanner equipment, and MRA may be performed with MRI. MRA provides structural evaluation of arteries and veins and the image of blood flow. The two types of MRA are time of flight (TOF) and phase contrast (PC). TOF angiography uses a process described as "flow-related enhancement," which relies on the inflow of fully magnetized blood into the imaging plane. PC angiography directly measures flow by generating vascular images. These images detect changes in the phase of the blood's transverse magnetization as it moves along a magnetic field gradient. Therefore it relies on alterations in spin phase for image contrast. Both of these methods emphasize the signals in the structures, which contain blood flow, and reconstruct only those structures with flow. The computer subtracts images of other structures, which are of lesser interest, from the image. Both of these methods can obtain two- or three-dimensional images. MRA can be performed without injection of contrast medium or radiation exposure. However, some radiologists prefer using a contrast, such as gadolinium chelate or gadolinium-DTPA, to enhance the visualization of venous flow.

Professional Considerations
Consent form IS required.

Risks
See Risks, Magnetic resonance imaging—Diagnostic.
Contraindications
See Contraindications, Magnetic resonance imaging—Diagnostic.
Precautions
See Precautions, Magnetic resonance imaging—Diagnostic.

Preparation
1. See Preparation, Magnetic resonance imaging—Diagnostic.

Procedure
1. See Procedure, Magnetic resonance imaging—Diagnostic.

Postprocedure Care
1. If the client has been sedated for the procedure, make certain that he or she is fully awake before ambulating, and follow institutional protocol for postsedation monitoring.

Client and Family Teaching
1. This procedure may take 15-30 minutes to perform.
2. See Client and Family Teaching, Magnetic resonance imaging—Diagnostic.

Factors That Affect Results
1. See Factors That Affect Results, Magnetic resonance imaging—Diagnostic.
2. False-positive and false-negative results in cerebral aneurysm evaluation can be caused by vessel tortuosity and susceptibility artifacts (which occur at the interfaces of structures with different magnetic susceptibilities).

Other Data
1. The same MRI scanner equipment, with different software and pulse sequences, is used to perform MRA.
2. The results of MRA are beginning to guide medical management and determine the extent of surgical intervention.
3. The use of MRA versus conventional angiography remains controversial. Gadolinium-enhanced MRA is more sensitive and specific, as well as less risky, than conventional arteriography for detection of renal artery stenosis. Risk for false results with MRA exists with cerebral aneurysms. MRA has been found to be as accurate as arteriography for carotid artery stenosis in large vessels, but not in smaller vessels such as the terminal carotid branch.

Magnetic Resonance Cholangiopancreatography (MRCP)—Diagnostic

Norm. Requires interpretation. Normal images of liver, biliary tree, and pancreas.

Usage. Used when more invasive procedures such as endoscopic retrograde cholangiopancreatography (ERCP) are contraindicated or have not been successful. Can detect choledocholithiasis, obstruction and dilation of the bile and pancreatic ducts because of malignancies, abnormal anatomy, or pancreatitis. Used preoperatively to depict the anatomy of the ductal system before surgical drainage. Used postoperatively to evaluate the hepatobiliary system after gastrointestinal surgery. Superior to ERCP in visualizing dilated ducts proximal to an obstruction. The diffusion-weighted technique is particularly helpful in detecting early ischemic stroke and multiple sclerosis, and in differentiating neoplasm from brain abscess.

Description. Magnetic resonance cholangiopancreatography (MRCP) is a noninvasive, noncontrast procedure for evaluating the gallbladder, biliary tract, and pancreatic duct. MRCP is able to visualize extrahepatic bile ducts and central intrahepatic ducts. Because these structures contain fluid, they appear as bright images under magnetic resonance imaging. Because this procedure can be performed in about 10 minutes, can visualize the entire hepatobiliary system, and does not use risky contrast material, it is being used more often as a replacement for the traditional ERCP procedure. MRCP may be enhanced with the use of the breath-hold method, using intravenous gadolinium (Gd).

Professional Considerations
Consent form IS required.

Risks
See Risks, Magnetic resonance imaging—Diagnostic.
Contraindications
See Contraindications, Magnetic resonance imaging—Diagnostic.
Precautions
See Precautions, Magnetic resonance imaging—Diagnostic.

Preparation
1. See Preparation, Magnetic resonance imaging—Diagnostic.

Procedure
1. The client is positioned supine on the MRCP table and an antenna is coiled around the abdomen.

2. *Noncontrast method:*
   a. A scout MRCP is performed to locate the biliary tract and pancreatic duct and then is used as a guide to acquire multiple images of the bile and pancreatic ducts.
   b. A regular MRI of the abdomen may follow.
3. *Breath-hold method:*
   a. An intravenous injection of 10 mL of gadolinium chelate is followed by fast-spoiled, gradient echo sequences acquired during breath-holding at 5, 10, and 15 minutes.
   b. The collecting system is evaluated according to a scale of 0 to 3.

Postprocedure Care
1. See Postprocedure Care, Magnetic resonance imaging—Diagnostic.

Client and Family Teaching
1. MRCP is used to evaluate whether there are obstructions in the area of the gallbladder, liver, and pancreas.
2. See Client and Family Teaching, Magnetic resonance imaging—Diagnostic.

Factors That Affect Results
1. See Factors That Affect Results, Magnetic resonance imaging—Diagnostic.

Other Data
1. None.

Magnetic Resonance Imaging (MRI)—Diagnostic

Norm. Description of normal tissue, structure, and blood flow.

Usage. To detect abscesses, abnormalities in blood flow through coronary branches and through extremities, acute tubular necrosis, adenopathy, Alzheimer's (diffusion tensor imaging), aortic and ventricular aneurysm, atrial and ventricular septal defects, avascular necrosis, blood clots, brain contusion, cancer and tumors (brain, bone, disk herniation, epidural hematoma on spine, extra-axial, head, intracardiac, hilar, mediastinal, neck, parenchymal, pericardiac, pituitary, pulmonary, renal, sarcoma, spinal cord and vagina), cavernous hemangioma, cerebral infarction, congenital heart disease, Cushing's disease (differentiation from Cushing's syndrome), cysts, dementia, demyelinating disease, edema, epilepsy, focal viral encephalitis, Gaucher disease, glomerulonephritis, hemorrhage, hydronephrosis, hyperparathyroidism, infection, intervertebral disk abnormalities, knee abnormalities, Marfan syndrome, Mullerian duct anomalies, myocardial infarction (and afterward to detect scars, aneurysms, pseudoaneurysms, septal defects, mural thrombi and valvular regurgitations), multiple sclerosis, muscular disease, osteomyelitis, plaque formation, pulmonary atresia, renal transplants, renal vein thrombosis, seizures, shoulder abnormalities, skeletal abnormalities, soft-tissue infections, spinal cord compression or injuries, subarachnoid hemorrhage, subdural hematoma, temporomandibular joint abnormalities, tumor invasion (inferior vena cava and seminal vesicles), and tumor staging (cervix, large hydronephroma, prostate, urinary bladder, and uterus). MRI is superior to computed tomography and ultrasound for its sensitivity in detection of changes in soft tissue. MRI is the standard in the diagnosis of most abnormalities of the brain and spine (except trauma). The ability of MRI to support the diagnosis of multiple sclerosis declines with increasing age of the client. MRI eliminates the need for many knee arthroscopies and has virtually replaced arthrography. Unlike computerized axial tomographic (CAT) scans, MRI can evaluate cerebral infarction within hours of the event. MRI virtually eliminates the need for myelography. MRI is more effective than CT in identifying white matter brain disease, such as multiple sclerosis.

Description. MRI is a noninvasive diagnostic tool that enables visualization of the body's tissues, structure, and blood flow. It uses a strong magnetic field in conjunction with radiofrequency waves to transmit signals from the body's cells to a computer that produces cross-sectional images. MRI actually stimulates the body to produce a signal that causes the cell's nuclei to react as tiny magnets in the presence of a strong external magnetic field (MRI). The signal density of the multiple body-plane images depends primarily on the tissue characteristics, pulse sequence, and timing parameters. Newer enhancements of MRI include the use of diffusion-weighted imaging, functional MRI, and fast MRI. In *diffusion-weighted or diffusion tensor MRI*, the intracellular and extracellular spaces are compared for the degree of diffusion of water molecules contained within them and is helpful in discerning Alzheimer's from normal aging. Brighter areas indicate restricted diffusion, such as in ischemic cell damage or blockage by tumor. In *functional MRI (fMRI)*, successive images are taken in rapid succession while the client follows commands. The images are compared for signal intensity and cerebral blood flow to help evaluate brain function in pathologic brain deterioration and psychiatric disorders and can also be used to evaluate the auditory system. Research uses for fMRI include identifying patterns in brain images that help predict which clients are likely to respond to specific drugs, such as antidepressants. *Fast MRI*, which has become possible through software advances, allows shortened breath-holding timeframes, better resolution, and procedure completion in 30 minutes or less. Fast MRI is used for evaluation of fetal anatomy or pathology when ultrasound does not yield enough information, and is also showing promise for evaluation of heart failure and screening for metastases. In addition, the newest equipment, called *dual mode imaging*, combines MRI with functional imaging modalities such as PET or SPECT for improved imaging results (see Dual modality imaging—Diagnostic). MRI is painless and has no known side effects.

Professional Considerations
Consent form IS required. 1%-2% of people refuse MRI because of claustrophobia.

Risks
Critical injury to the client could result from ferrous metal in the body (e.g., flecks of ferrous metal in eye could cause retinal hemorrhage).

Contraindications
Intraocular metal foreign bodies; heart valves manufactured before 1964 and middle ear prosthetics (these can be tested by obtainment of a duplicate, which is then placed into the bore, and if no torque is experienced, the test may be safely performed); nerve-stimulating devices may be a contraindication.

Precautions
Some older versions of aneurysm clips may not be ferromagnetic; verify this from manufacturer or hospital records. MRI uses non-ionizing radiation, and thus is considered the least risky of radiographic procedures during pregnancy, and there is no evidence of teratogenic or developmental abnormalities associated with this procedure. However, the literature recommends that pregnant women should not be scanned unless absolutely necessary. Radiologists and operators must be informed

M

of the presence of cardiac pacemakers, implanted cardioverter-defibrillators and implanted venous access devices, and cochlear implants, though they are rarely a contraindication. Most stainless-steel orthopedic implants and prosthetic devices are not ferromagnetic and are not affected by MRI. Clients with tattooed eyeliner may experience skin irritation or swelling around the eyes caused by the MRI's effects on ferrous pigments in the tattoo. Use of sedatives during this test is contraindicated in clients with central nervous system depression.

Preparation

1. See Client and Family Teaching.
2. Screen the client for cardiac pacemaker, artificial heart valve, brain aneurysm clips or any type of surgical clip or staple, shunt, neurostimulation (TENS unit), implanted insulin pump, implanted venous access infusion devices, bone growth stimulator, internal electrodes, embolic spring coil, eye implant surgery (with staples), cochlear implant, hearing aid, foil or metallic medication patches, any orthopedic item(s) (such as pins, wires, rods, screws, clips, plates), artificial limb or joint, dental braces, any type of removable dental item, IUD, metallic eye makeup, metal fragments (in head, eye, skin), history of work in the machine tool industry, history of work with a metal lathe, or history of any accidents with metal or ferromagnetic objects (e.g., beebee [BB] guns, flecks of ferrous metal in eye). These items may be hazardous to the client's safety.
3. Screen the accompanying adult for the above items if the client undergoing the procedure is a pediatric client.
4. Remove any loose metal objects (such as hairpins, barrettes, watches, jewelry, pen clip, steel-toed shoes or clothing with metal snaps or zippers) because they can become projectile in the magnetic force.
5. Inform the physician if the client is using an IV controller pump or computerized equipment because the magnets in the MRI can disrupt the function of the machine (such as IV flow).
6. Determine if client has any problems with claustrophobia. Interventions to reduce claustrophobia include, as appropriate, the following:
   a. Relaxation techniques or a sedative may be used.
   b. Determine availability of an "open MRI."
   c. Interact with client in an unhurried, relaxed manner.
   d. Provide a thorough explanation of the procedure, including methods to reduce anxiety, such as relaxation or controlled breathing techniques.
   e. Suggest that the client keep his or her eyes closed throughout the procedure.
   f. Offer a cool cloth to be placed over the eyes.
   g. Point out that the ends of the scanner are always open.
   h. Offer to have client remove his or her shoes and be covered with a light sheet.
   i. Keep room temperature cool. Use compressed air through a cannula positioned to blow past the client's face during the procedure.
   j. Arrange for family member to enter the scanner room to speak with the client between scans.
7. If the client is very young or unable to follow directions, sedation may be indicated to complete the scan.
8. Start an IV line if contrast medium is to be given.
9. Just before beginning the procedure, take a "time out" to verify the correct client, procedure, and site.

Procedure

1. The client is positioned on a padded table and moved into the cylinder-shaped scanner (such as a magnet bore).
2. Contrast medium may be administered before the procedure if prescribed.
3. The technologist will operate controls determining image-signal density, pulse sequence, and timing parameters.
4. If blood flow is to be determined in an extremity, the arm or leg to be examined is placed into a cradle-like support. The technologist will mark reference sites to be imaged on the arm or leg. Then the extremity is moved into a flow cylinder.
5. If a functional MRI is being done, the client may be asked to watch a display of images and press a button when certain images or patterns of images are noted.

6. The MR image is interpreted by a specially trained radiologist.

Postprocedure Care

1. Continue the assessment of respiratory status after receiving sedation. If deep sedation was used, follow institutional protocol for post-sedation monitoring. Typical monitoring includes continuous ECG monitoring and pulse oximetry, with continual assessments (every 5-15 minutes) of airway, vital signs, and neurologic status until the client is lying quietly awake, is breathing independently, and responds to commands spoken in a normal tone.
2. Remove the IV line if one was inserted for injection of the contrast medium.

Client and Family Teaching

1. For pelvic or abdominal scans, do not eat or drink for 6 hours before the procedure.
2. You will lie on a flat, narrow, padded surface and will be rolled into a cylinder-shaped scanner. The scanner will be around the area of the body that is being scanned.
3. You will hear various noises from the test, including a muffled drumbeat sound. You may bring in earplugs for the test or use the earplugs that are available. In an open MRI machine, there are no loud noises.
4. You can communicate with MRI personnel, who will be in another room, by means of an intercom system.
5. It is important to remain completely still during the scan.
6. Remove jewelry, watches, hairpins, glasses, and any metal objects. The magnetic field can damage watches.
7. Do not approach the MRI unit if you have a cardiac pacemaker.
8. You will not be exposed to radiation during this procedure. The contrast medium that may be used is not an iodinated contrast.
9. The procedure may take 45-90 minutes to scan the head or chest area and approximately 15 minutes to scan an arm or leg. In fast MRI, the procedure will take 30 minutes or less.

Factors That Affect Results

1. The image will be distorted by movement during the procedure.
2. Metal, whether ferrous or nonferrous, may produce artifacts that degrade the images if the metal is in proximity to the area of the body that is being scanned.
3. Because of the possibility of loss of data contained on magnetic recording media, MRI systems are normally contained within a restricted magnetic range, from 15 to 50 gauss.
4. MRI does not use ionizing radiation; therefore there are none of the hazards found in x-rays.

Other Data

1. Intravenous gadolinium-DTPA contrast, which is a commercially available contrast medium, may be necessary for some examinations at the discretion of the radiologist. This contrast is chemically unrelated to the iodinated contrast, which is used in conventional radiography.
2. Magnetophosphenes (flickering lights in the visual field), which can occur with MRI, are completely reversible and have no known long-term health effects.
3. The Food and Drug Administration (FDA) has classified MRI devices into class II, which includes low-risk devices.
4. Tissue plasminogen activator (tPA) intervention is effective more than 4 hours after stroke.
5. Less functional MRI activity and APOE 4 status identifies individuals at risk for developing cognitive decline over a brief time period.

Magnetic Resonance Neurography (MRN, Neurography)—Diagnostic

Norm. Description of normal nerve structure.

Usage. Helps diagnose and evaluate peripheral nerve tumors, carpal tunnel syndrome, ulnar nerve compression, thoracic outlet syndrome, brachial plexus injuries (including birth injuries), sciatica with no convincing spinal cause, any suspected nerve impingement, accidental injury to peripheral nerves, postirradiation neuritis, chronic nerve compression, and pain syndromes when an anatomic lesion is suspected. In the evaluation of clients with spinal problems, it can also be used as a follow-up or adjunct test to MRI, CT, and myelogram when there are ambiguous test results or if the client has clinical symptoms that are not confined to a single dermatome. MRN may also be useful in surgical planning to localize and determine the resectability of tumors through accurate depiction of the relation of the tumor to the nerve fascicles or presence of nerve laceration.

Description. MRN provides longitudinal and cross-sectional fascicular images of nerves. It is a noninvasive imaging technique that uses a magnetic resonance imaging (MRI) scanner that has been modified with a spin-echo pulse sequence combined with fat suppression and diffusion weighting to generate neurographic images. MRN images show the nerves as the most prominent feature, providing detail of the internal fascicular structure. The cross-sectional images can be viewed individually or reconstructed to provide fully isolated nerves and nerve structure (longitudinal views).

Professional Considerations

Consent form IS required.

Risks

See Risks, Magnetic resonance imaging—Diagnostic.

Contraindications

See Contraindications, Magnetic resonance imaging—Diagnostic.

Precautions

See Precautions, Magnetic resonance imaging—Diagnostic.

Preparation

1. See Preparation, Magnetic resonance imaging—Diagnostic.

Procedure

1. See Procedure, Magnetic resonance imaging—Diagnostic.
2. Contrast medium is not used in this test.

Postprocedure Care

1. See Postprocedure Care, Magnetic resonance imaging—Diagnostic.

Client and Family Teaching

1. See Client and Family Teaching, Magnetic resonance imaging—Diagnostic.
2. There is no contrast agent used and there are no injections.
3. The test takes about 30-40 minutes.

Factors That Affect Results

1. See Factors That Affect Results, Magnetic resonance imaging—Diagnostic.
2. Variable sensitivity occurs in imaging very small nerves. Decreased sensitivity is associated with imaging small nerves that traverse multiple anatomic planes, such as those in the pelvis (that is, the ilioinguinal nerve).
3. It is important that clinical evaluation correlate with abnormal findings of MRN. It has been reported that up to 60% of the population with no pain has been found to have a herniated disk, bone spurs, or narrowing of spinal canals. In a symptomatic client, these "commonly occurring" abnormalities may be inaccurately diagnosed as the cause of the symptoms when in actuality the pathologic condition is located at a more distal nerve site.

Other Data

1. At this time, MRN cannot be accomplished by means of the "open" MRI machines. The magnet-field gradient required for MRN imaging cannot be maintained with the open MRI equipment.

Magnetic Resonance Spectroscopy (MRS)—Diagnostic

Norm. Qualitative and quantitative cellular biochemical data, such as steady-state cellular concentrations of metabolites, are visible with MRS.

Usage. Provide follow-up study and prognosis for clients with AIDS dementia and lesions, Alzheimer's disease, Canavan disease, cancer and tumors, diabetes mellitus, hepatic encephalopathy, intracranial mass, metabolic disorders, neurodegeneration, renal failure, stroke, systemic lupus erythematosus (SLE); detect degeneration, inflammation, and necrosis in tissues; differentiation of high-grade from low-grade brain tumors; differentiation of recurrence of cerebral neoplasm from radiation therapy injury; monitor and evaluate therapeutic interventions in conjunction with MRI; evaluate biochemical basis for neuropsychiatric disorders and dementias. Future application may include detection of changes at the cellular level that precede morphologic changes detected with MRI or other radiologic imaging modalities.

Description. Magnetic resonance spectroscopy (MRS) is a noninvasive vascular imaging technique. This procedure is performed by use of the magnetic resonance imaging (MRI) scanner equipment and different software. Two types of MRS include the proton MRS and phosphorus-31 (^{31}P) MRS. The MRS describes the molecular state of water—the chemical environment of cells and tissues—and the qualitative and quantitative states of intermediary metabolism. It can produce specific metabolite profiles in various pathologic conditions.

Professional Considerations

Consent form IS required.

Risks

See Risks, Magnetic resonance imaging—Diagnostic.

Contraindications

See Contraindications, Magnetic resonance imaging—Diagnostic.

Precautions

See Precautions, Magnetic resonance imaging—Diagnostic.

Preparation

1. See Preparation, Magnetic resonance imaging—Diagnostic.

Procedure

1. See Procedure, Magnetic resonance imaging—Diagnostic.
2. MRS always needs to be performed before contrast medium is added because a contrast medium may affect the expression of metabolites.
3. To obtain the best image, the areas to be avoided in MRS include frontal and ethmoid sinuses, temporal bones, deep-in-posterior fossa, subcutaneous fat, and areas of high flow or hypervascular disorder.

Postprocedure Care

1. See Postprocedure Care, Magnetic resonance imaging—Diagnostic.

Client and Family Teaching

1. See Client and Family Teaching, Magnetic resonance imaging—Diagnostic.

Factors That Affect Results

1. See Factors That Affect Results, Magnetic resonance imaging—Diagnostic.
2. Many factors influence the profile of the MR spectra, including magnetic-field uniformity and interclient variability, age, and developmental stage. Normal metabolite ratios change substantially during development, particularly from birth to 2 years of age. Quantification of metabolites is difficult as a result of the complexity of the spectra.

Other Data

1. None.

Magnetic Resonance Urography—Diagnostic

Norm. Requires interpretation.

Usage. Identification of urinary tract dilation, particularly after transplantation; detection of neurogenic bladder dysfunction, ectopic ureters in children; alternative to intravenous pyelography and computed tomography in renal-impaired clients for whom excretory urography is contraindicated, such as those with uremia and renal impairment or those with no excretory function. Helpful during pregnancy and in those clients allergic to contrast medium, because

of the noninvasive nature of the procedure. Other usage should be reserved for those clients in which less expensive testing has proven inconclusive.

Description. Magnetic resonance urography (MRU) is a costly but extremely accurate, noninvasive, and noncontrast method of identifying renal conditions which are not well identified with other technology such as computed tomography, pyelography, and ultrasound. In MRU, urine appears white, and so the adequacy of the excretory route and obstructive impairments can be evaluated. The MRU may be enhanced with the use of the breath-hold method, using intravenous gadolinium (Gd).

Professional Considerations
Consent form IS required.

Risks
See Risks, Magnetic resonance imaging—Diagnostic.

Contraindications
See Contraindications, Magnetic resonance imaging—Diagnostic.

Precautions
See Precautions, Magnetic resonance imaging—Diagnostic.

Preparation
1. See Preparation, Magnetic resonance imaging—Diagnostic.
2. Client must be well hydrated before the procedure.

Procedure
1. The client is positioned supine on the MRU table and an antenna is coiled around the abdomen.
2. *Noncontrast method:*
   a. A scout MRU is performed to locate the kidneys and ureters and then is used as a guide to acquire multiple images of the urinary system.
3. *Breath-hold method:*
   a. An intravenous injection of 10 mL of gadolinium chelate is followed by fast-spoiled, gradient echo sequences acquired during breath-holding at 5, 10, and 15 minutes.
4. The collecting system is evaluated according to a scale of 0 to 3.

Postprocedure Care
1. See Postprocedure Care, Magnetic resonance imaging—Diagnostic.

Client and Family Teaching
1. MRU is used to evaluate whether there are obstructions in the kidneys and ureters.
2. See Client and Family Teaching, Magnetic resonance imaging—Diagnostic.

Factors That Affect Results
1. See Factors That Affect Results, Magnetic resonance imaging—Diagnostic.
2. Insufficient hydration will reduce the quality of the results.

Other Data
1. MRU with contrast has been used to evaluate renal tumors and to evaluate the upper urinary tract in children.

Malaria Smear (Giemsa Stain)—Blood

Norm. Negative.

Positive. Malaria (one of four *Plasmodium* species: *P. falciparum, P. vivax, P. malariae, P. ovale*) and trypanosomiasis.

Description. Malaria is a contact disease caused by a *Plasmodium*. The parasites, which are in the salivary glands of the anopheline mosquito, are introduced into the bloodstream of the human by means of mosquito bites. The parasites enter the cells of the liver, where they multiply without causing recognizable disease. A few days later, spores multiply asexually and fill red blood cells, destroying them and leading to fever and chills in the human. Malaria is most common in rural areas such as Central and South America, India, and Africa, but also exists in Eastern Europe. In the latter 1990s, over 1200 cases per year were reported in the United States and were attributed to acquisition of the disease when out of the country. Early detection via smear is essential so that treatment can be initiated and critical complications such as anemia, renal failure, pulmonary edema, disseminated intravascular coagulation, coma, and even death can be avoided. In this procedure, a thick and/or thin smear is collected. The thick smear only detects whether any of the *Plasmodium* species are present, whereas the thin smear is the only test that can pinpoint the specific *Plasmodium* species.

Professional Considerations
Consent form NOT required.

Preparation
1. Tube: Lavender topped or pink topped EDTA.
2. Obtain a lancet and 10 glass slides.
3. Monitor the client's temperature every 4 hours or as indicated.

4. Report chills and fever to the physician.
5. Obtaining specimens before fever spike is preferable.
6. Include on the laboratory requisition any recent travel, including country and dates.

Procedure

1. Draw a 5-mL blood sample.
2. Obtain fresh fingersticks (five each of thick and thin film on glass slides). Both thick and thin smears may be collected on the same slide, if necessary. Thick smears are prepared by spreading 10-20 μL of whole blood in a dime-sized area on the slide.

Postprocedure Care

1. Transport tube of blood and unstained, unfixed slides to the laboratory within 24 hours. Allow to dry completely before fixing with Giemsa stain.
2. Testing must be performed within 48 hours of collection.

Client and Family Teaching

1. Inform the nurse when having chills.

Factors That Affect Results

1. Hemolysis of the specimen invalidates the results.
2. The level of parasitemia varies from hour to hour (especially for *Plasmodium falciparum* infections).

Other Data

1. Blood samples are usually drawn when fever and chills are present daily for 3 days at specified times, such as every 6 or 12 hours.
2. The smear is considered positive if ≥2%-30% of the red blood cells are infected.
3. Blood should be examined several times a day for 2-3 days because results are seldom greater than 2% of the total cells.
4. In *P. falciparum* malaria, severe parasitemia is 10% total infected cells and may reach levels of 20%-30% or more.
5. Clinical signs and symptoms may include myalgias, arthralgias, chills, fever of unknown origin, drenching sweat, fatigue, nausea, vomiting, abdominal pain, diarrhea, splenomegaly, hepatomegaly, and jaundice.
6. American trypanosomiasis (Chagas disease) and African trypanosomiasis (sleeping disease) are two diseases caused by trypanosomes, which are flagellated protozoans.
7. A new nonradioactive DNA diagnostic procedure is available to detect malaria infection, which may aid in determining the diagnosis.

Mammography (Mammogram, Screen Film Mammography [SFM])—Diagnostic

Norm. Radiographic image of normal breast tissue. Calcification, if present, is evenly distributed. Normal duct contrast with gradual narrowing of branches of the ductal system is evident.

Positive. Benign or malignant masses in the breast tissue or nipple. Radiographic signs of breast cancer include asymmetric density; a poorly defined spiculated mass; fine, stippled clustered calcifications, which are seen as white specks on the x-ray film; and skin thickening. Malignant cancers are irregular and poorly defined and tend to be unilateral.

Negative. Normal finding.

Usage. Indicated to detect tumors that are clinically nonpalpable in women over age 40 as part of routine annual screening; to survey the opposite breast after mastectomy; to screen for breast cancer in clients at high risk for breast cancer; to evaluate breasts when symptoms are present, such as skin changes, nipple or skin retraction, nipple discharge or erosion, breast pain, "lumpy" breast (such as multiple masses or nodules); to rule out breast cancer in a client with adenocarcinoma of undetermined site; to localize a mass before a biopsy is performed; to follow up after a previous breast biopsy or cancer treatment to determine its effectiveness. Used to diagnose benign breast masses, cysts, or abscesses; benign breast calcifications; breast cancer; fibrocystic breasts; intraductal papilloma of the breast; occult cancer (such as client with metastatic disease and unknown primary tumor); suppurative mastitis; and Paget's disease of the breast.

Description. Mammography is a soft-tissue x-ray examination of the breast. Careful interpretation of these x-ray films can detect cancer, even before a lesion becomes palpable. Accuracy of breast cancer detection is approximately 85% and gives less than 10% false-positive diagnoses. It is believed that survival rates are improved with early detection of breast cancer. A *xeromammogram* provides the same information as a routine mammogram and has the same risks and benefits. However, xeromammograms are positive prints, unlike regular radiographs, which are negative prints. This test has four views: oblique, lateral, craniocaudal, and chest wall. At least two views of each breast should be performed, one of which should be of the chest wall. A newer digital technique called *full-field digital mammography* (FFDM) is approved for use in screening for breast cancer. Digital mammography has improved detection in clients with dense breasts, usually younger women. Use of computer aided detection in mammography as a decision support has <10% false positive rate.

Professional Considerations
Consent form IS required.

Risks
Breast implant rupture (Brown et al, 2004). The U.S. National Cancer Institute estimates the risk of mammographically induced carcinogenesis at 3.5 cancers/1 million women/yr/rad for Western women over age 30 at the time of exposure after a latent period of 10 years. About 13% of women have a palpable breast cancer mass within 1 year of a normal mammogram.

Precautions
During pregnancy, risks of cumulative radiation exposure to the fetus from this and other previous or future imaging studies must be weighed against the benefits of the procedure. Although formal limits for client exposure are relative to this risk:benefit comparison, the United States Nuclear Regulatory Commission requires that the cumulative dose equivalent to an embryo/fetus from occupational exposure not exceed 0.5 rem (5 mSv). Radiation dosage to the fetus is proportional to the distance of the anatomy studied from the abdomen and decreases as pregnancy progresses. For pregnant clients, consult the radiologist/radiology department to obtain estimated fetal radiation exposure from this procedure.

Contraindications
In clients who are pregnant because of the risk of fetal damage.

Preparation
1. Ask client to identify areas of lumps or thickening, if any.
2. Ask the client if she is pregnant.
3. Record client history of prior biopsies or breast surgeries or treatments.
4. Have the lactating mother breastfeed or pump milk just prior to the mammogram. This reduces the density of breast tissues and makes the mammogram easier to read.
5. See Client and Family Teaching.

Procedure
1. The client is taken to the radiology department and stands or is seated in front of the mammography machine.
2. The breast(s) is (are) exposed, and one breast is placed on the x-ray plate.
3. The x-ray cone is brought down on top of the breast to compress it firmly between the broadened cone and the x-ray plate.
4. The x-ray film is exposed. This creates the craniocaudal view.
5. The x-ray plate is turned perpendicularly to the floor and then is placed laterally on the outer aspect of the breast.
6. The broadened cone is brought in medially, and the breast is gently compressed. This is the lateral, or axillary, view.
7. Occasionally a third view, the oblique view, is required. At least two views of each breast should be performed.
8. For clients with implants, the implant is pushed back and extra views are taken.
9. This procedure is performed in 10-20 minutes by a radiologic technician.
10. A hand-held scanner helps detect early breast cancer that cannot be identified with conventional mammography.

Postprocedure Care
1. In the United States, the Mammography Quality Standards Act, phased in the 1990s, established standards for reporting of findings to the client within 5 days after

the procedure if the findings may indicate malignancy and within 30 days after the procedure for findings not suggestive of malignancy.

Client and Family Teaching

1. The mammogram takes 10-20 minutes for both breasts to be x-rayed.
2. Mammography is the best method for detecting breast cancer in a curable stage.
3. Some discomfort is experienced when the breast is compressed. Compression allows better visualization. Discomfort is minimized if the test is scheduled during the week after your menstrual period ends.
4. Mammography does not affect the milk in lactating women. It is safe to breast-feed after mammography.
5. Do not use any powder, deodorant, perfume, or ointments in the underarm area. Residue on the skin from these agents can obscure the visualization.
6. A minimal radiation dose will be used during the test.
7. Wear a blouse with a skirt or slacks, rather than a dress, because you will need to remove clothing from the upper half of the body.
8. If experiencing painful breasts, refrain from coffee, tea, cola, and chocolate 5-7 days before testing.
9. American Cancer Society mammography screening guidelines: screening mammogram by age 40 and then annually thereafter.
10. Call your doctor for results if you have not received a written or telephone test result within 10 days after the procedure.
11. Perform a monthly breast self-examination if 20 years of age or older and have a clinical breast examination by a health care provider at least every 3 years until age 40 and then every year. Breast self-examination should be performed after each menstrual period.
12. 80% of lumps found by a mammogram are benign.

Factors That Affect Results

1. False-positive mammograms are more common in younger women and may result from calcifications of fibrocystic changes, calcification-like deposits in the skin secondary to tattoos, sebaceous gland secretions, and talcum powder.
2. False-negative results are possible. Up to 25% occur in women 40-49 years of age, and up to 10% occur in women 50-69 years of age. The principal cause of false-negative mammograms is dense parenchymal tissue because masses show up more clearly in fatty breasts.
3. Postoperative and postradiotherapy changes may be mistaken for carcinomas.
4. Jewelry worn around the neck can preclude total visualization of the breast(s).
5. More breast tumors (55%) are missed when implants are present than in women without implants (33%) (Miglioretti et al, 2004). The scintimammography test may pose lower risk for rupture and better chance of detection for women with implants.

Other Data

1. Magnification mammography is limited because of its higher radiation doses, but it can be useful in postoperative and post-radiotherapy examinations, possibly preventing unnecessary biopsy.
2. Mammography immediately after stereotaxic breast biopsy is suboptimal for establishment of a new baseline view as a result of the frequent finding of hematoma.
3. According to one study, women undergoing mammography preferred to have their doctor call them into their office if the results were abnormal.
4. Calcifications are predictors of HER-*2/neu* overexpression.
5. National organizations have discrepant recommendations for screening mammography. The American College of Obstetricians and Gynecologists in 2011 recommended screening every year for women age 40 and older. The United States Preventive Services Task Force recommended in 2009 that screening start at age 50 and be repeated every 2 years.
6. A 2011 study (Bennett et al) concluded that adding computer-aided detection to a mammogram offers no benefit in enhancing the accuracy of diagnosis and, in fact, leads to more recalls for further testing.

Mantoux Skin Test (PPD Test, Purified Protein Derivative Test, Tb Test, Tuberculin Skin Test, TST, Tuberculosis Test)—Diagnostic

Norm. Negative.

Positive. The appropriate criterion for defining a positive skin test reaction depends on the population being tested. For adults and children with HIV infection, close contacts of infectious cases, and those with fibrotic lesions on chest radiograph, a reaction of ≥5 mm is considered positive. For other at-risk adults and children, including infants and children younger than 4 years of age, a reaction of ≥10 mm is positive. Persons who are unlikely to be infected with *Mycobacterium tuberculosis* should generally not be skin tested. If a skin test is performed on a person without a defined risk factor for tuberculosis infection, ≥15 mm is positive.

Negative. Normal finding; lack of redness or induration of skin at site of skin test; zone of redness and induration <5 mm.

Usage. Screening is used to identify infected persons at high risk of disease who would benefit from preventive therapy and to find persons with clinical disease in need of treatment. As a screening tool, tuberculin skin testing is the standard method of identifying persons infected with active *M. tuberculosis*. It is indicated for clients with signs suggestive of current tuberculosis (TB) disease (such as abnormality in mediastinum on radiograph) or symptoms (such as cough, hemoptysis, weight loss); recent contact with clients with confirmed or suspected cases of TB; clients with abnormal chest radiographs compatible with past TB; clients with medical conditions that increase the risk of TB (such as diabetes, immunosuppressive therapy, AIDS); groups at high risk for developing TB. For clients with previous BCG vaccination or in clients at risk for latent TB infection, the CDC as of 2005 no longer recommends Mantoux testing, and instead recommends use of newer interferon tests. (See RD1-interferon tests for tuberculosis—Blood.)

Description. An intradermal skin test to detect tuberculosis infection (active or dormant). Tuberculin, a protein fraction of tubercle bacilli, is injected intradermally in the human. A localized thickening with redness indicates an accumulation of small, sensitized lymphocytes, which occurs as a result of active or dormant tuberculosis. Clients at high risk for tuberculosis (HIV-infected persons, the very young and the very old, the malnourished, alcoholics, drug abusers, and the chronically ill) should be screened with the tuberculin skin test. Clients with human immunodeficiency virus infection are at increased risk for developing tuberculosis infection and should be screened with the tuberculin skin test. Other clients at high risk for becoming infected with *Mycobacterium tuberculosis* include the very young and the very old, those who are malnourished, alcohol and drug abusers, and the chronically ill. Newer interferon tests called "IFN gamma assays" have been approved in Europe and the United states to help detect latent tuberculosis infection. See RD1-interferon tests for tuberculosis—Blood for more information on these tests.

Professional Considerations
Consent form IS required.

Risks
It is not known whether the test can cause fetal harm or affect reproductive capacity.
Contraindications
The test should be given to pregnant women only if clearly indicated. The test should not be given if the client has had a previous positive test.

Preparation
1. Assess for previous history of positive purified protein derivative (PPD) reaction. (The test should not be administered in this case.)
2. Obtain a tuberculin syringe and PPD.
3. Draw up PPD in a tuberculin syringe, following the manufacturer's directions. Use a ½-inch, 26- or 27-gauge needle.

Procedure
1. Cleanse the injection site on the lower dorsal surface of the forearm with alcohol, and allow the area to dry.
2. Stretch the skin taut.
3. Inject intradermally 0.1 mL of a solution containing 0.5 tuberculin unit of PPD.

Injection should be made with a disposable needle and syringe just under the surface of the skin, with the needle bevel facing upward to provide a discrete, pale elevation of the skin (a wheal) 6 to 10 mm in diameter. Discard used needles and syringes in a puncture-resistant container (do not recap needles).

Postprocedure Care

1. Mark the test area to locate it for reading.
2. Read the test area 48-72 hours later. Examine the site, using good light. Inspect the skin for induration. Induration ≥5 mm diameter generally indicates infection. Rub lightly from the area of normal skin to the indurated area. Circle the induration with a pencil.
3. An induration of ≥5 mm diameter should be interpreted as a positive reaction if the client has known contact with an individual with active tuberculosis or if there is a chest radiograph with findings consistent with tuberculosis. Isoniazid therapy is recommended to decrease the risk of developing the disease in positive reactors.
4. A chest radiograph is necessary with all positive reactions.
5. Epinephrine hydrochloride solution (1:1000) should be readily available for use in the event of anaphylaxis.

Client and Family Teaching

1. The skin test does not distinguish between current disease and past infection.
2. The skin test should not be administered to known tuberculin-positive reactors because of the possibility of severe reactions (vesiculation, ulceration, and necrosis).

Factors That Affect Results

1. Tuberculin must be stored as recommended by the manufacturer. Tuberculin solution should be stored between 2 and 8 degrees C (35 and 46 degrees F). It should be exposed to light only when being withdrawn and administered. An open vial may be used only for 1 month.
2. Subcutaneous rather than intradermal injection will nullify the test.
3. Cross-reactions with nontuberculous mycobacteria may cause false-positive results.
4. Serial testing may cause false-positive results.
5. Vaccination with the bacille Calmette-Guérin (BCG) has a variable effect on the skin test reaction. However, a history of BCG vaccination should not alter interpretation of the skin test. The newer RD1-interferon tests for tuberculosis—Blood are the test of choice instead of Mantoux testing for these clients.
6. False-negative reactions may occur in the following instances: bacterial infections, immunologic defects, immunosuppressive agents, live virus vaccinations (BCG, measles, mumps, polio, and rubella), malnutrition, old age, overwhelming tuberculosis, renal failure, and viral infections (chickenpox, measles, and mumps).
7. False-negative results can occur, even in the presence of active TB, whenever sensitized T lymphocytes are temporarily depleted in the body.

Other Data

1. See also RD1-interferon tests for tuberculosis—Blood.

MAP Kinase

See Mitogen-Activated Protein Kinase—Specimen.

MAPK

See Mitogen-Activated Protein Kinase—Specimen.

Maprotiline

See Tricyclic Antidepressants—Plasma or Serum.

Marijuana

See Cannabinoids, Qualitative—Blood or Urine.

Maximum Bactericidal Dilution

See Schlichter Test—Specimen.

MBD

See Schlichter Test—Specimen.

MCA

See Mucin-Like Carcinoma-Associated Antigen—Blood.

MCH

See Blood Indices—Blood.

MCHC

See Blood Indices—Blood.

MCV

See Blood Indices—Blood.

Mean Corpuscular Hemoglobin

See Blood Indices—Blood.

Mean Corpuscular Hemoglobin Concentration

See Blood Indices—Blood.

Mean Corpuscular Volume

See Blood Indices—Blood.

Mean Platelet Volume (MPV)—Blood

Norm.

Preterm infants	7.5-9.5 fL
Term infants (0-1 month)	7.6-9.9 fL
1 month-48 months	6.3-8.9 fL
48 months-12 years	7.0-9.0 fL
12 years-adult	5.9-9.8 fL

Usage. Evaluates platelet abnormalities; improves detection of platelet-related diseases when the platelet count is normal; determines the platelet changes associated with exercise and hyperthyroidism; predicts hypertensive crisis in pregnancy; predicts the presence of sepsis in neonates; and predicts hemorrhage in clients with rheumatoid arthritis who are experiencing thrombocytopenia as a side effect of parental gold therapy. In screening clients with preexisting coronary artery disease, MPV over 11.6 fL was associated with an increased risk of subsequent myocardial infarction.

Increased. Acute poststreptococcal glomerulonephritis (APSGN), arterial disease (angina, atherosclerotic disease), coagulase-negative staphylococcal sepsis in neonates, cyanotic congenital heart disease, diabetes, hyperthyroidism, iron-deficiency anemia, ITP (idiopathic thrombocytopenic purpura), myeloproliferative disorders, myocardial infarction, pregnant women with preeclampsia, renal failure, rheumatic heart disease, smokers, splenomegaly, states of increased platelet production, and thrombocytopenia.

Decreased. Active inflammatory bowel disease; clients with rheumatoid arthritis who are receiving parental gold therapy.

Description. The MPV is an automated measurement of the average volume of platelets. It is the arithmetic mean volume of the platelet population derived from the platelet histogram on automated Coulter counters. Increased MPV may reflect either increased platelet activation or increased numbers of large, hyperaggregable platelets. Because the MPV increases during conditions of rapid platelet turnover, it can signify the release of larger, younger platelets into the circulation. When the MPV is low, the platelets are generally smaller. The MPV is expressed in femtoliters (fL).

Professional Considerations
Consent form NOT required.

Preparation
1. Tube: Lavender topped.

Procedure
1. Leaving a tourniquet in place less than 1 minute, draw a 5-mL blood sample.
2. Gently invert the tube two or three times.

Postprocedure Care
1. Send the specimen to the laboratory within 1 hour.

Client and Family Teaching
1. Results are normally available within 4 hours.

Factors That Affect Results
1. When potassium EDTA is used as an anticoagulant, platelets demonstrate a progressive increase in mean platelet volume with storage, as measured by the Coulter counter. This increase is most noticeable within the first 2 hours but continues at a slower rate subsequently.

Other Data
1. The mean platelet volume (MPV) is comparable to the mean corpuscular volume (MCV) of red blood cells.
2. Younger platelets are larger than older platelets. Larger platelets are functionally and metabolically more active than smaller ones, contain more granules, and express more enzymatic activity in vitro.
3. Increases in MPV can occur, even though thrombocytopenia has developed.
4. The MPV may be normal in central thrombocytopenic diseases, such as aplastic anemia and acute leukemia.

Meat Fibers—Stool

Norm. Negative.

Positive. Gastroenteritis, intestinal lymphoma, malabsorption syndrome, pancreatic insufficiency, severe ulcerative colitis, surgical removal of section of intestine, and Whipple's disease.

Description. Examination of stool for yield of meat fibers correlates with the amount of fat secretion in the stool. Meat fibers found in stool result from multiple abnormalities in absorption of nutrients. These include defects in the intestinal lumen that result in inadequate fat hydrolysis, inadequate proteolysis, altered bile salt metabolism, and defects in mucosal epithelial cells or intestinal lymphatics that affect absorbing surfaces and interfere with the transport of nutrients. This test is performed by examining a stained specimen under a microscope to detect fecal meat fibers.

Professional Considerations

Consent form NOT required.

Preparation

1. Barium procedures or laxatives should be avoided for 1 week before specimen collection.
2. Obtain an enema apparatus and warm saline, or a prepackaged enema, and a sterile plastic specimen container
3. See Client and Family Teaching.

Procedure

1. Obtain a 5-g (1 g for pediatrics) stool specimen by giving the client a warm saline enema or a prepackaged enema.
2. Collect the stool specimen in a sterile plastic container.

Postprocedure Care

1. None.

Client and Family Teaching

1. Include at least 3 ounces of red meat per day for 24-72 hours before the test.
2. Results are normally available after 24 hours.

Factors That Affect Results

1. Reject specimens collected with enemas other than saline or Fleets (such as mineral oil, bismuth, or magnesium compounds).

Other Data

1. Serum protein level should be determined because hypoproteinemia is the major clinical feature of protein-losing enteropathy.
2. Biopsy of the intestinal mucosa is more useful than other diagnostic tests for definitive diagnosis of intestinal mucosal abnormalities.

Meckel's Scan—Diagnostic

Norm. Negative; no increased uptake of radionuclide in the right lower quadrant of the abdomen.

Usage. Detection of Meckel's diverticulum, including double Meckel's diverticulum, which contains ectopic gastric mucosa, in clients with abdominal pain or occult gastrointestinal bleeding.

Description. A nuclear medicine scan in which a radioisotope, ^{99m}Tc (technetium)-pertechnetate, is injected intravenously. The radioisotope is concentrated in the normal gastric mucosa within the stomach and in the ectopic gastric mucosa in Meckel's diverticulum. This is a very sensitive and specific test for this congenital abnormality.

Professional Considerations

Consent form IS required.

Risks

Hematoma, infection.

Contraindications

During pregnancy or breast-feeding.

Preparation

1. Assure the client that nuclear medicine personnel will remain within hearing range and will be able to see the client throughout the study.

2. A histamine (H_2)-receptor antagonist (such as cimetidine orally every 6 hours for 24 hours) is usually administered for 1-2 days before the test. This drug inhibits acid secretion and allows for improved visualization of the Meckel's diverticulum.
3. See Client and Family Teaching.
4. Just before beginning the procedure, take a "time out" to verify the correct client, procedure, and site.

Procedure

1. In the nuclear medicine department, the client lies in a supine position.
2. ^{99m}Tc-pertechnetate is administered intravenously 15 minutes before imaging.
3. An anterior body-image view is obtained with a rectilinear scanner or scintillation (gamma) camera. Images are taken at 5-minute intervals for 1 hour.
4. During the scan, the client may be asked to lie on the left side to increase the amount of radioisotope present in the intestines.
5. Total examining time is 60 minutes.

Postprocedure Care

1. Observe the client carefully for up to 60 minutes after the study for a possible (anaphylactic) reaction to the radionuclide.
2. Ask the client to void after the procedure, and a repeat image may be obtained.

3. Rubber gloves should be worn for 24 hours after the procedure when urine is being discarded. Wash the gloved hands with soap and water before removing the gloves. Wash the ungloved hands after the gloves are removed.

Client and Family Teaching

1. It is necessary to lie still for 60 minutes for this scan. There is no pain associated with this test.
2. Refrain from eating or drinking anything for 6-12 hours before the test.
3. Void before the study to increase the visibility of the intestines.
4. Meticulously wash your hands with soap and water after each void for 24 hours after the procedure.
5. Family members must wear rubber gloves for 24 hours after the procedure when discarding the client's urine if the family will be providing this care.

Factors That Affect Results

1. A positive scan is dependent on an adequate amount of gastric mucosa within Meckel's diverticulum. Only 25% of clients with Meckel's diverticulum will have sufficient ectopic gastric mucosa to produce a positive scan.
2. Meckel's scan is unreliable for evaluation of gastrointestinal bleeding.
3. Other radionuclide studies performed within the previous 24 hours will interfere with this test.
4. A waiting period that is either too short or too long after the radionuclide injection will alter the results.
5. Premedication with pentagastrin and a histamine (H_2)-receptor blocker (Zantac) may increase the sensitivity of the test.
6. Barium in the small or large bowel may mask the radionuclide concentration.
7. False-positive result can be from inflammation from the periumbilical laparoscopic port site.

Other Data

1. Health care professionals working in a nuclear medicine area must follow federal standards set by the Nuclear Regulatory Commission. These standards include precautions for handling the radioactive material and monitoring of potential radiation exposure.
2. The half-life of technetium is 6 hours.

MeCP2 Full Gene Sequencing—Blood

Norm. Negative.

Usage. Used to confirm the diagnosis when Rett syndrome is suspected; helps identify MeCP2 mutation when pre-conception testing is done for couples where a family member has mental retardation.

Description. The MeCP2 gene affects how other genes function; thus defects in the MeCP2 gene can cause abnormal expression of a variety of other genes, leading to a wide array of symptoms. Rett syndrome is an x-linked, autosomal dominant disorder that occurs when an x-chromosome contains a defect in methyl-CpG-binding protein 2 (MeCP2). Rett syndrome is a genetic disorder characterized by rapid regression of motor skills and language capabilities, after the infant has developed normally for 6 to 18 months (Noah, 2011). Because the defect occurs on the x-chromosome, it is almost never seen in males, this being because the defect leads to miscarriage, stillbirth or newborn/infant death. Rett syndrome is almost always seen in females, since the second x-chromosome may be normal, and allow survival of the fetus. When Rett syndrome develops, a floppiness of the extremities first appears, followed rapidly by apraxia, language development deterioration, drooling, disrupted sleep patterns, reduced interactivity with others, seizures and breathing problems (Noah, Budeck, Patwari, Weese-Mayer, 2011). Children with Rett syndrome require close medical attention and support. Survival into young or middle-adulthood is common, with death caused by complications of the symptoms.

Professional Considerations

Informed consent is recommended for genetic testing.

Preparation

1. Tube: Lavender, pink, or yellow top.

Procedure

1. Obtain a 3-mL blood sample.

Postprocedure Care

1. Store refrigerated for up to 1 week before testing. Do not freeze.

Client and Family Teaching

1. Refer to Appendix B, "Informed Consent for Genetic Testing."
2. Rett syndrome incidence occurs once per 10-15,000 live births of females.
3. There is less than a 1% chance of passing the defect on to a child.
4. The severity of the symptoms is proportional to the amount of cells that carry the defective gene.

Factors That Affect Results

1. Sensitivity and specificity of this test are both 99%.

2. This test cannot identify deep intronic mutations and large deletions/duplications.

Other Data

1. Because not all individuals with Rett syndrome carry the defective MeCP2 gene, diagnosis is most often made based on displayed symptoms.
2. The Genetic Information Nondiscrimination Act of 2008 prohibits health plans from using genetic family history or genetic test results from influencing eligibility or premiums for health insurance. It also prohibits employers from using this information to influence decisions about hiring, terminating employment, or employment pay, promotions or privileges.

Mediastinoscopy—Diagnostic

Norm. Normal mediastinal structure and lymph nodes; no evidence of disease process.

Usage. To detect lymphoma (such as Hodgkin's disease), lung metastasis to mediastinal lymph nodes, granulomatous infection, mediastinal tuberculosis, sarcoidosis; to obtain biopsy specimen of mediastinal lymph nodes or intrathoracic lesions; to determine staging of bronchogenic carcinoma; treatment for severe superior vena cava syndrome; and to evaluate tumor spread or intrathoracic diseases. Used when fine-needle aspiration biopsy of the thoracic structures has not yielded a diagnosis.

Description. Mediastinoscopy is a surgical endoscopic procedure performed with the client under general anesthesia. A small incision is made at the suprasternal notch, and a mediastinoscope is inserted into the mediastinum. The purpose of this procedure is to visualize the mediastinal structure and lymph nodes and to obtain a biopsy sample of lymph nodes or other lesions. The lymph nodes in the mediastinum receive lymphatic drainage from the lungs. A mediastinoscopy is usually performed when radiographs, sputum cytologic evaluation, and lung scans (CT and nuclear) have not confirmed a diagnosis. Mediastinoscopy is an invasive procedure and is performed with the client under general anesthesia because of the pain and coughing that result from the manipulation of the trachea.

Professional Considerations

Consent form IS required.

Risks

Perforation of the trachea, esophagus, aorta, or other blood vessels; pneumothorax; laryngeal nerve damage; and infection.

Contraindications

Previous mediastinoscopy (caused by adhesions); clients who are not candidates for general anesthesia.

Preparation

1. See Client and Family Teaching.
2. Complete preoperative checklist, and perform routine preoperative care, which is the same as with any other surgical procedure. Check if the client's blood needs to be typed and cross-matched.
3. Measure and record baseline vital signs.
4. Ask the client if he or she is allergic to any anesthetic medicine.
5. Encourage the client and family members to express concerns about the procedure. Answer questions and refer those that you cannot answer to appropriate health care professionals.
6. Administer preprocedural medication approximately 1 hour before the test, as prescribed.
7. Just before beginning the procedure, take a "time out" to verify the correct client, procedure, and site.

Procedure

1. The client is transported to an operating room and general anesthesia is administered.
2. A small incision is made in the suprasternal fossa, and a mediastinoscope is passed through this neck incision, along the anterior course of the trachea, and into the superior mediastinum.
3. The area is visualized. Photographs of specific areas and structures may be taken. Biopsies of the lymph nodes may also be performed.
4. The mediastinoscope is withdrawn, and the incision is sutured.

Postprocedure Care

1. Assess vital signs every 15 minutes × 2, then every 30 minutes × 2, then hourly × 4, and then every 4 hours until 24 hours after the procedure. Report changes in vital signs (such as increase in pulse rate or respiratory rate, decrease in blood pressure).
2. Auscultate lung sounds, and assess for any respiratory abnormalities, such as dyspnea.

3. Check for bright red blood or increased blood on the dressing. Observe the wound for symptoms of infection.
4. Provide comfort measures as needed (such as position change, medication).
5. Send biopsy specimens to the pathology laboratory immediately.

Client and Family Teaching

1. Refrain from eating or drinking for 8-12 hours before the procedure.
2. Void before the surgical procedure.
3. This procedure will take approximately 1 hour and is performed by a surgeon.
4. You will be asleep during the procedure.

Factors That Affect Results

1. Phenytoin hypersensitivity may result in a "pseudolymphoma," causing false-positive cytologic results.

Other Data

1. Thoracotomy is advisable in the instance of negative cytologic characteristics in lesions likely to be malignant.

Melanin—Urine

Norm. Negative.

Positive. Malignant melanoma.

Description. Urine test to detect biochemical markers of melanoma progression. Melanin, which is the main pigment in the body, is synthesized by the melanocytes primarily in the skin and eyes. It is highly elevated in malignant melanoma. Both eumelanin (brown-black pigment) and pheomelanin (yellow-red pigment) are produced, with dihydroxyindole (DHI) and cysteinyldopa (CD) being the major precursors. Melanin metabolites are often released in the urine of clients with disseminated melanoma metastasis (melanuria). These metabolites include a pheomelanin metabolite, 5-S-CD, and a eumelanin metabolite, 6-hydroxy-5-methoxyindole-2-carboxylic acid (6H5MI2C). Melanogen, a colorless precursor of melanin, is also excreted in the urine of 25% of people with melanin-producing tumors.

Professional Considerations
Consent form NOT required.

Preparation

1. Obtain a sterile, plastic, light-protected (amber) specimen container and ice.

Procedure

1. Obtain a 2-mL freshly voided urine specimen.

Postprocedure Care

1. Place container on ice and transport specimen immediately to the lab for immediate testing. Freeze specimen if it cannot be tested immediately.

Client and Family Teaching

1. Results are normally available within 24 hours.

Factors That Affect Results

1. Drugs that may cause false-positive results include salicylates.
2. Results are invalidated if the specimen remains at room temperature or is refrigerated or is exposed to light.

Other Data

1. The test is more frequently positive in people with hepatic metastasis.

2. Plasma 6H5MI2C levels are usually high (>1.75 ng/mL) in clients with metastatic malignant melanoma, and it produces a more sensitive and reliable test than the melanin (5-S-CD) urine test.

3. Elevated urine melanin in test results is a high-risk factor for metastatic malignant melanoma.

Melanocyte-Stimulating Hormone (MSH)—Blood and Urine

Norm. *Blood:* Norms vary by laboratory and are provided with the test result.
Urine: Negative for melanin.

Positive. Addison's disease, hyperpituitarism, melanoma, and liver metastasis.

Description. Melanocyte-stimulating hormone (MSH) is part of the melanocortin system, which helps regulate the body's balance of energy via the hypothalamus. Alpha, beta, and gamma MSH subtypes exist and are thought to adhere to special melanocortin receptors, resulting in differing functions. Alpha MSH is thought to be involved in the body's stress response and in mediation of hyperthermia. Alpha MSH has also been shown to suppress appetite in conjunction with leptin, leptin receptors, and neuropeptide Y. It is also the most influential subtype in causing darkening of skin in humans, providing skin protection from ultraviolet rays. Gamma MSH is thought to have a role in sodium metabolism and hypertension involving sodium levels. MSH levels are closely linked to ACTH secretion, and experimental studies demonstrate body fat reduction after treatment with exogenous MSH/ACTH.

Professional Considerations
Consent form NOT required.

Preparation
1. Hold steroids, ACTH, and antihypertensives for 18 hours before collection, when not contraindicated.
2. Tube: Red topped or lavender topped for blood.
3. Obtain a sterile, plastic specimen container for urine.

Procedure
1. Draw a 5-mL blood sample.
2. Obtain a freshly voided urine specimen in a sterile, plastic container.

Postprocedure Care
1. Transport specimen to the laboratory immediately. Freeze specimen if it cannot be tested immediately.

Client and Family Teaching
1. Results are normally available after 24 hours.

Factors That Affect Results
1. The secretion of MSH is increased when levels of circulating cortisol are low.

Other Data
1. None.

Mendelian Inheritance in Genetic Disorders—Diagnostic

Norm. Negative for genetic disorders.

Usage. Used prospectively for genetic counseling to predict the probability that future offspring will inherit a genetic disorder; used retrospectively to determine or confirm the presence of a Mendelian disease.

Description. This procedure is an analysis of gene sequences on a client's DNA and RNA to detect the presence of genetic disorders in the family history or in the client. More than 4000 Mendelian diseases obey statistical laws and exist in a family. Examples are breast cancer, colon cancer, color blindness, congenital malformations, cystic fibrosis, hemophilia, Marfan syndrome, and sickle cell anemia. As genetic techniques improve, Mendelian testing is becoming more commonly used for population-based screening, such as in screening newborns for phenylketonuria and other disorders. Screening carries with it legal and ethical dilemmas concerning confidentiality, privacy, discrimination, and interventions taken based on findings.

Professional Considerations
Informed consent is recommended for genetic testing.

Preparation
1. Provide teaching.

Procedure
1. A family pedigree analysis is performed, including generational continuity of the disorder, sex relationship, and segregation (Mendelian) ratio.

Postprocedure Care
1. Genetic counseling and referral for follow-up study.

Client and Family Teaching
1. Inform the client about the reasons for genetic counseling. Refer to Appendix B, "Informed Consent for Genetic Testing."

Factors That Affect Results
1. Gene-mapping is most accurate in identifying simple genetic disorders, such as those caused by a single abnormal gene. Newer techniques are being developed to help identify genetic causes of more complicated diseases.

Other Data
1. Other disorders can mimic Mendelian disorders, such as chromosomal disorders, congenital infections, and mental retardation.
2. The Online Mendelian Inheritance in Man (OMIM) databases, available on the Internet, provide up-to-date information on gene mutation findings.
3. The Genetic Information Nondiscrimination Act of 2008 prohibits health plans from using genetic family history or genetic test results from influencing eligibility or premiums for health insurance. It also prohibits employers from using this information to influence decisions about hiring, terminating employment, or employment pay, promotions or privileges.

Mephenytoin (Mesantoin)—Blood

Norm. Negative.

		SI Units
Mephenytoin Therapy		
Therapeutic level of mephenytoin	1-5 μg/mL or mg/L	4.6-23 μmol/L
Therapeutic level of mephenytoin and parent drug 5-phenyl-5-ethylhydantoin metabolite	25-40 μg/mL or mg/L	115-184 μmol/L
Panic level	>20 μg/mL or mg/L	>92 μmol/L
Normephenytoin	15-35 μg/mL or mg/L	69-161 μmol/L
Panic level	>50 μg/mL or mg/L	>230 μmol/L

Overdose Symptoms and Treatment
Symptoms. Ataxia, blood dyscrasias, coma, drowsiness, dysarthria, hypotension, nystagmus, and unresponsive pupils may be seen.

Treatment
1. There is no specific treatment.
2. Refer to a physician.
3. Give general supportive care: lavage and maintenance of airway and blood pressure.
4. Hemodialysis WILL remove mephenytoin and is used especially with drug toxicity in children.

Increased. Overdose. Drugs include chloramphenicol and methsuximide.

Decreased. Convulsions, inadequate dosage, and noncompliance with therapeutic regimen.

Description. Mephenytoin (Mesantoin) is an anticonvulsant used to treat grand mal, tonic-clonic, psychomotor, temporal lobe, focal, and Jacksonian seizures. It is metabolized in the liver and excreted in the urine.

Professional Considerations
Consent form NOT required.

Preparation
1. Tube: Red topped, red/gray topped, gray topped, green topped, or pink topped.
2. Do NOT draw during hemodialysis.

Procedure
1. Draw a 5-mL blood sample.

Postprocedure Care

1. Transport specimen to the laboratory and refrigerate until testing.

Client and Family Teaching

1. Explain overdose symptoms and treatment (see above) as appropriate.
2. Drug levels should be monitored routinely during therapy.

3. Refer clients with intentional overdose for crisis intervention.

Factors That Affect Results

1. Compliance with administration.

Other Data

1. Trade name is Mesantoin.

Meprobamate—Blood

Norm. Negative.

Meprobamate Therapy		SI Units
Therapeutic level	5-20 µg/mL or mg/L	23-92 µmol/L
Toxic level	>35 µg/mL or mg/L	>160 µmol/L
Panic level	>50 µg/mL or mg/L	>229 µmol/L
Lethal level*	>100 µg/mL or mg/L	>458 µmol/L

*Death has been reported with as little as 12 g, and survival with as much as 40 g.

Overdose Symptoms and Treatment

Symptoms. Drowsiness, lethargy, stupor, ataxia, hemolytic toxicity symptoms (fever, sore throat, bruising, bleeding), coma, shock, vasomotor and respiratory collapse, and death may occur.

Treatment

NOTE: Treatment choice(s) depend(s) on client's history and condition and episode history.

1. Maintain patent airway and support breathing with mechanical ventilation, if needed.
2. Support blood pressure with vasopressors.
3. If seizing, comatose, or lacking a gag reflex, perform gastric lavage only with an endotracheal tube in place with cuff inflated to prevent aspiration.
4. If fully awake with intact gag reflex, induce emesis and follow with instillation of activated charcoal and gastric lavage.
5. Monitor urine output and avoid overhydration.
6. Both hemodialysis and peritoneal dialysis WILL remove meprobamate.
7. Osmotic diuresis with mannitol has also been effective.
8. Avoid dehydration.

Increased. Drug abuse and overdose.

Decreased. Noncompliance with therapeutic regimen.

Description. Meprobamate is a sedative-hypnotic used to treat anxiety disorders. It is a central nervous system depressant that is metabolized in the liver and excreted in urine and feces. Meprobamate is a metabolite of carisoprodol (Soma), a muscle relaxant that some consider a suspect drug of abuse.

Professional Considerations

Consent form NOT required.

Preparation

1. Tube: Red topped, red/gray topped, lavender topped, pink topped, green topped, or gray topped.
2. Do NOT draw during hemodialysis.

Procedure

1. Draw 5-mL blood sample.

Postprocedure Care

1. None.

Client and Family Teaching

1. Explain overdose symptoms and treatment (see above) as appropriate.
2. For intentional overdose, refer for crisis intervention and counseling. Referrals to appropriate rehabilitation centers and

therapeutic community programs should be offered to all clients who may be interested.

Factors That Affect Results

1. Onset of action is within 1 hour after oral dosage. Peak concentration is 2 hours from dosage, half-life is 6-17 hours, and steady-state levels occur in 1.5-4.0 days.

Other Data

1. An alternative method of determining meprobamate levels is by gas chromatography. This method is accurate and precise and is particularly suitable for toxicology studies.

Mercury—Blood and Urine

Norm.

		SI Units
Blood	≤0.06 µg/mL or ≤60 ng/mL	≤0.3 nmol/L
Critical value	>0.6 µg/mL	>3 nmol/L
Panic value	>100 µg/mL	>500 nmol/L
Urine	0-10 µg/L (random urine)	0-0.05 µmol/L
	≤10 µg/24 hours	≤0.05 µmol/day
Panic value	>50 µg/24 hours	>0.25 µmol/day

Panic Level Symptoms and Treatment

Symptoms. Symptoms appear when levels reach 600 µg/L (3 µmol/L, SI units). Signs of chronic poisoning include difficulty concentrating, short-term memory loss, irritability, fatigue, ataxia, muscle spasms, gingivitis, tremors, joint pain, and paresthesias. Signs of acute poisoning include cardiovascular collapse, renal failure, and severe damage to the gastrointestinal tract, as well as headache, fever, chills, tremors, dyspnea, and chest tightness.

Treatment

NOTE: Treatment choice(s) depend(s) on client's history and condition and episode history. The first step is to eliminate the source.

1. Chelation with penicillamine or succimer has been used, but is not approved for chelation therapy. No definitive studies exist that demonstrate the effectiveness of chelation therapy.
2. Monitor behavior and neurologic status closely.

Increased. Mercury poisoning.

Description. Mercury exists in elemental, inorganic, and organic forms. Elemental mercury—the type that exists in thermometers, thermostats, and dental amalgam—is the only metal that is liquid at room temperature. Inorganic mercury found in mercury salts is poorly absorbed by the body. Organic mercury is found in some fish, and industrial wastes. The more common sources of mercury poisoning are industrial inhalation of mercury vapors from paints and other materials and direct contact with mercury from broken thermometers or from dental fillings. Mercury is primarily absorbed by inhalation but can also be absorbed through the skin and gastrointestinal tract. It is then distributed to the central nervous system and kidneys and excreted in the urine, having a half-life of up to 25 days. This test is used to evaluate for mercury toxicity. Urine is the recommended specimen for measuring inorganic mercury and mercury secondary to dental amalgam fillings Hair is the recommended specimen for measurement of mercury levels secondary to seafood consumption. Saliva is not recommended as a substrate for mercury testing.

Professional Considerations

Consent form NOT required.

Preparation

1. For blood sample: Tube: lavender topped, EDTA tube.
2. For urine specimen: Obtain a 3-L, acid-washed plastic specimen container without preservative.
3. Assess the possible causes of mercury poisoning: occupational activities, hobbies

(such as painting ceramics), target shooting, home renovation, and auto repair.

4. Screen client for use of herbal preparations or natural remedies.

Procedure

1. *Blood*: Draw a 3-mL blood sample.
2. *Urine*: Collect all the urine voided in a 24-hour period in a 3-L, acid-washed plastic container without preservative.

Postprocedure Care

1. For increased levels, encourage fluids and monitor urine output because mercury is nephrotoxic.

Client and Family Teaching

1. *Urine*: Save all the urine voided in the 24-hour period and urinate before defecating to avoid loss of urine. If any urine is accidentally discarded, discard the entire specimen and restart the collection the next day.
2. Some Chinese herbal medicines and remedies contain high levels of mercury. Do not use these preparations without first consulting your physician.

Factors That Affect Results

1. Drugs that may cause falsely low levels include iodine-containing medications.

Other Data

1. High mercury levels found in fish in Brazil (Lemire et al, 2006), Canada (Innis et al, 2006), and children from poor inner city neighborhoods in the United States (Sexton et al, 2006).

Mesantoin

See **Mephenytoin**—Blood.

Metanephrines, Total, 24-Hour—Urine and Free-Plasma

Norm.

	Normal	Diagnostic for Pheochromocytoma*
Plasma-Free Metanephrines		
Normetanephrine	<0.90 nmol/L	>1.5 pmol/L
Metanephrine	<0.50 nmol/L	>1.4 pmol/L
Urine Metanephrines		
Normetanephrine	50-650 µg/day	
Metanephrine	30-350 µg/day	>2000 µg/day

*Diagnostic for pheochromocytoma: More than 4-fold normetanephrines and 2.5-fold metanephrines above the upper reference limits indicate a pheochromocytoma with 100% specificity.

Increased. Adrenal mass, brain tumors, chemodectomas, ganglioneuroblastoma, ganglioneuroma, hypertension with pheochromocytoma, malignant pheochromocytoma, metastasis (widespread), myasthenia gravis, neuroblastoma, pheochromocytoma, progressive muscular dystrophy, sepsis, and severe stress.

Description. This is a test to evaluate adrenomedullary function. Metanephrine testing is usually performed when a client with hypertension is suspected of having pheochromocytoma, which is a tumor of the chromaffin cells of the adrenal medulla. (Fewer than 1% of clients with hypertension have pheochromocytoma.) Metanephrines (such as normetanephrine and metanephrine) are one of the principle substances formed by the adrenal medulla, released into the bloodstream, and excreted into the urine. These substances contain a catechol nucleus and an amine group; therefore they are referred to as catecholamines. The traditional method for testing has been a 24-hour urine test (sensitivity 89%-100%) because blood testing had too many interfering factors. The newest techniques for plasma testing provide an almost 100% sensitivity and specificity. Plasma metanephrine testing also provides the advantages of lower susceptibility to changing catecholamine levels resulting from posture changes, exercise, or surgical stress; closer correlation with tumor size; less interference by medications; and insight into ongoing (long-term) production of catecholamines. Metanephrine testing is the best test for the diagnosis of pheochromocytoma because levels are unaffected by the many factors that affect catecholamine levels.

Professional Considerations
Consent form NOT required.

Preparation
1. *Plasma*: Obtain a lavender topped tube and ice.
2. *Urine*: Obtain a 3-L plastic container with 20-25 mL of hydrochloric acid (HCl) preservative. Label the container with the client's name, the test, and the date.
3. Discuss with the physician if any drugs are to be discontinued 3-7 days before the test.
4. See Client and Family Teaching.

Procedure
1. *Plasma test*: Obtain a 7-mL blood sample. Place specimen immediately on ice.
2. *Urine*: Collect all the urine voided in a 24-hour period in a refrigerated, 3-L plastic container to which 20-25 mL of HCl preservative has been added. For specimens collected from an indwelling urinary catheter, keep the drainage bag on ice, and empty urine into the refrigerated collection container hourly. Document urinary output throughout the collection period.

Postprocedure Care
1. Write the beginning and ending times of collection and total urinary output (container quantity should match output record) on the laboratory requisition and on the specimen container.
2. Send the urine specimen to the laboratory refrigerator after the 24-hour collection is completed. Metanephrines are stable for at least 1 week.

Client and Family Teaching
1. Save all the urine voided in the 24-hour period and urinate before defecating to avoid loss of urine. If any urine is accidentally discarded, discard the entire specimen and restart the collection the next day.
2. Avoid caffeine, coffee, tea, cocoa products, bananas, vanilla products, aspirin, and phenothiazine-containing medications for 48 hours before collecting urine and during the urine collection.
3. Encourage the client to rest, take in adequate food and fluids, and avoid stress during the test.

Factors That Affect Results
1. Drugs that interfere with test results in unpredictable ways include acetaminophen, aminophylline, amphetamines, appetite suppressants, bromocriptine, buspirone, caffeine, chloral hydrate, chlorpromazine, clonidine, dexamethasone, diuretics, dopamine, epinephrine, ethanol (alcohol), guanethidine, hydralazine, hydrocortisone, imipramine, insulin, isoetharine, levodopa, lithium, methyldopa (Aldomet), MAO (monoamine oxidase) inhibitors, nalidixic acid, nicotine, nitroglycerin, nose drops, phenacetin, phenobarbital, phenylephrine, propafenone (Rythmol), reserpine, salicylates, tetracycline, theophylline, tricyclic antidepressants, and vasodilators.
2. False negative results may occur when catecholamine release is intermittent and no attack occurs during testing.
3. Dietary intake high in bananas may cause falsely increased results.
4. Vigorous exercise may cause an increase in catecholamine levels.
5. The 24-hour urine collection is problematic for practical reasons and for client compliance. Improper specimen collection may lead to falsely increased results.

Other Data
1. Urinary catecholamines and vanillylmandelic acid (VMA) are often measured with urine metanephrines.
2. If a positive plasma result is followed by a negative result in repeat testing, pheochromocytoma can be ruled out. This is because metanephrines are continuously secreted by the tumor.
3. Guller et al (2006) found that the most sensitive tests for diagnosing pheochromocytoma are the total urinary normetanephrine test (96.9% specificity) and the platelet norepinephrine test (93.8% specificity) and I-MIBG scintigraphy. The MIBG scan—Diagnostic is recommended to improve accuracy of diagnosis if catecholamine levels are normal, but pheochromocytoma is suspected.

Methacholine Challenge Test (Bronchial Challenge Test, Bronchial Provocation Test)—Diagnostic

Norm. Negative.

Usage. Most useful in excluding the diagnosis of asthma. Use in diagnosing asthma is most effective when pretest probability of asthma is 30%-70% (American Thoracic Society, 2000). Often used after a negative exercise challenge test when asthma is suspected. This test with altered cutoff points of 10% or 15% may be used in chronic asthma to monitor response to therapy. Also used to diagnose airway hyper-reactivity in children post stem cell transplant where a decline of 51% in specific airway conductance is considered positive.

Description. The methacholine challenge test involves measurement of lung volumes before and after inhalation of methacholine chloride, a bronchial constrictor. This test is useful in demonstrating bronchial hyperreactivity (BHR), which is a characteristic of asthma. However, a single negative test is not sufficient to rule out asthma; therefore the test should be performed using both a direct and an indirect stimulus. Clients with symptoms suggestive of asthma often have normal resting pulmonary function test results but are more sensitive than healthy people to the bronchoconstrictive effects of methacholine (Anderson, Brannan, 2011). The test may be performed with tidal breathing and/or with deep inhalation, and it uses the lowest concentration of methacholine needed to achieve a 20% reduction in FEV_1 (also known as provocation concentration 20 or PC_{20}). Test is significantly higher in winter and spring.

Professional Considerations
Consent form IS required.

Risks
Bronchospasm and its potential complications. This risk is greater in small children than in adults.

Contraindications
Not appropriate for those under school-age. Also contraindicated when severe airflow limitation is present (e.g., FEV_1 <50% predicted or <1 L) or in clients with a myocardial infarction or stroke within the prior 3 months, in clients with known aortic aneurysm, and in clients with uncontrolled hypertension. Relative contraindications include nursing mothers, pregnant clients, clients taking cholinesterase inhibitors for myasthenia gravis, clients with moderate airflow limitation (e.g., FEV_1 <60% predicted or <1.5 L), and in those clients unable to perform spirometry using proper technique.

Preparation

1. Verify with physician and instruct client to avoid the following medications before the test: short-acting inhaled bronchodilators (8 hours), medium-acting inhaled bronchodilators (24-48 hours), oral bronchodilators (24-48 hours), cromolyn sodium, nedocromil, hydroxyzine (3 days), cetirizine (3 days), and leukotriene modifiers (24 hours).

2. Instruct client to avoid caffeine or chocolate the day of the test.

3. Just before beginning the procedure, take a "time out" to verify the correct client, procedure, and site.

4. Obtain nebulizer and methacholine chloride. Prepare increasing concentrations of methacholine. Vials should be at room temperature for testing.

   a. For the 2-minute tidal breathing protocol, use the following concentrations: 0.031 mg/mL, 0.0625 mg/mL, 0.125 mg/mL, 0.5 mg/mL, 1 mg/mL, 2 mg/mL, 4 mg/mL, 8 mg/mL, 16 mg/mL.

   b. For the five-breath dosimeter protocol, use the following concentrations: 0.0625 mg/mL, 0.25 mg/mL, 1 mg/mL, 4 mg/mL, 16 mg/mL.

5. Verify that resuscitation equipment (including oxygen, nebulizer, sphygmomanometer, pulse oximeter) and personnel able to manage severe bronchospasm are immediately available. Medications to treat bronchospasm should also be immediately available and include epinephrine, subcutaneous atropine, albuterol, and ipratropium.

6. Inform client that cough or mild chest tightness may be experienced and that occasionally severe breathing problems occur, but that equipment and personnel prepared to handle these complications are readily available.

Procedure

1. Position the client in a seated position.
2. Baseline spirometry is performed and target FEV_1 is calculated. The target would indicate a 20% fall in FEV_1.
3. *Two-minute tidal breathing protocol:*
   a. A nose clip is applied and the client breathes the lowest of five concentrations of methacholine through a nebulizer for 2 minutes and then the nebulizer is removed.
   b. The FEV is remeasured in 30 seconds and again in 90 seconds after stopping the nebulizer. The highest FEV_1 is recorded.
4. *Five-breath dosimeter protocol:*
   a. The client inhales through the nebulizer slowly and deeply for five breaths. Each inhalation should take about 5 seconds.
   b. The FEV is remeasured in 30 seconds and again in 90 seconds after the end of the fifth inhalation. The highest FEV_1 is recorded.
5. If the FEV does not fall at least 20% from baseline, the test is repeated with a higher dose of methacholine. Twofold increases in concentration are used for the 2-minute tidal breathing method and fourfold increases are used for the five-breath dosimeter method. These steps may be repeated as needed to achieve a 20% fall from baseline FEV, until the highest concentration of methacholine has been reached.
6. If the FEV falls at least 20% from baseline, the test is stopped. Record client symptoms. Then administer inhaled albuterol and repeat the test.
7. Failure to achieve a 20% reduction in the FEV is considered a negative test.

Postprocedure Care

1. Monitor respiratory status.

Client and Family Teaching

1. Symptoms suggestive of asthma include cough, chest tightness, and dyspnea.
2. In patients with previous physician-diagnosed asthma, only a single methacholine challenge test is required to confirm asthma.

Factors That Affect Results

1. Inability to follow directions and comply with instructions yields invalid results.
2. Inhaled heparin may have an inhibitory role on methacholine bronchial challenge, possibly through a direct effect on smooth muscle.
3. Clients with mild airway hyperresponsiveness may demonstrate false-negative results with the deep inhalation method of this test.
4. Inhaling the methacholine too quickly will reduce measured PC_{20}.
5. False-negative tests occur in asthmatic clients with a PC_{20} greater than 8-25 mg/mL.
6. A positive test may indicate asthma, airway injury, or exercise-induced bronchospasm.

Other Data

1. This test has a positive predictive value of 60%-88% and a negative predictive value of 100% to rule out asthma.
2. Some experimental work is being conducted to evaluate the usefulness of a skin-prick test with methacholine in shortening the MCT. One study found that a negative skin-prick test reduced the chances of low-to-moderate risk clients having asthma by 10-20 fold.
3. Histamine is sometimes used in place of methacholine for the bronchial challenge test, but is associated with increased side effects.

Methanol

See **Toxicology, Volatiles Group by GLC**—Blood or Urine.

Methaqualone (Quaalude, Mandrax)—Blood

Norm. Negative.

		SI Units
Therapeutic level	2-3 µg/mL	8-12 µmol/L
Panic level	>8 µg/mL	>32 µmol/L
Toxic level	>10 µg/mL	>40 µmol/L

Panic Level Symptoms and Treatment

Symptoms. Pronounced drowsiness, confusion, dilated pupils, delirium, coma, restlessness, hyperexcitability, hypertonia, convulsions, shock, and cardiopulmonary failure may occur. Spontaneous vomiting with increased secretions may cause aspiration pneumonia or respiratory obstruction. Swelling, fluid retention, and abnormal bleeding may also occur. Death may occur from doses >5 g (20 mmol).

Treatment

NOTE: Treatment choice(s) depend(s) on client's history and condition and episode history.

1. Maintain patent airway.
2. Support blood pressure.
3. Perform gastric lavage and evaluation of gastric contents by lavage after airway has been ensured.
4. Monitor neurologic, cardiac, and respiratory status closely.
5. Be prepared to mechanically ventilate and to treat bradycardia or cardiac arrest.
6. Analeptics are contraindicated.
7. Hemodialysis and peritoneal dialysis will NOT remove methaqualone.
8. Use psychotropic analgesic nitrous oxide to treat acute withdrawal following "white pipe" use.

Usage. Drug abuse and therapeutic monitoring. Smoking methaqualone is a serious problem in South Africa and when combined with cannabis is called "white pipe."

Description. Methaqualone (Quaalude) is a nonbarbiturate, sedative-hypnotic agent with an unknown mechanism of action. It is absorbed from the gastrointestinal tract, metabolized in the liver, and excreted in the urine, bile, and feces. This drug has a high abuse potential. The minimum lethal dose of methaqualone is 5 g (20 mmol).

Professional Considerations

Consent form NOT required.

Preparation

1. Tube: Red topped, red/gray topped, or gold topped or lavender topped.
2. If the client may also have taken diazepam or chlordiazepoxide, indicate this on the laboratory requisition.
3. Specimens MAY be drawn during hemodialysis.

Procedure

1. Draw a 5-mL blood sample.

Postprocedure Care

1. None.

Client and Family Teaching

1. Explain the procedure and the reason for drawing the specimen.
2. Explain the overdose symptoms and treatment (see above), as appropriate.
3. Withdrawal symptoms may not appear for 2-3 days, and convulsions may occur on the eighth or ninth day after cessation of the drug.
4. For intentional overdose, refer client and family for crisis intervention.
5. Referrals to appropriate rehabilitation centers and therapeutic community programs should be offered to all clients who may be interested.

Factors That Affect Results

1. The peak level of methaqualone is 2 hours after dose. Half-life is 33-38 hours, and steady-state levels occur in 7-8 days.
2. Results are unreliable with concurrent administration of diazepam or chlordiazepoxide when the spectrophotometric method is used.
3. Adulterants such as household chemicals, hand soap, and glutaraldehyde invalidate test results.

Other Data

1. Monitor coagulation studies carefully if the client is taking an anticoagulant.

2. Methaqualone can be detected in the urine for up to 7 days. False negative results are found with use of glutaraldehyde (G-cide) and Perle hand soap. Invalid test results occur with use of ethanol, isopropanol, or peroxide.

Methemoglobin—Blood

Norm.

% of Total Hemoglobin		SI Units
≤2%	≤0.02 g/dL	≤3.1 µmol/L

Methemoglobinemia Signs and Symptoms

Symptoms. Clients suspected of having methemoglobinemia may experience symptoms of anoxia or cyanosis, without evidence of cardiovascular or pulmonary disease:

Normal po_2 with decreased pco_2
Decreased calculated oxygen saturation
Decreased HCO_3^-
>15% *methemoglobin*: Chocolate cyanosis (pale blue-gray skin, brownish lips and mucous membranes)
>30% *methemoglobin*: Dizziness, fatigue, headache, tachycardia, weakness
>45% *methemoglobin*: Signs of central nervous system (CNS) depression
>55% *methemoglobin*: Acidemia, bradycardia, dysrhythmias, respiratory compromise
>70% *methemoglobin*: Death secondary to hypoxia; fatal dose of nitroglycerin or sodium nitrite is reported to be 2 g.

Treatment

NOTE: Treatment choice(s) depend(s) on client's history and condition and episode history.

1. Support symptoms: Protect airway, administer 100% oxygen, check neurologic status every hour.
2. Perform continuous pulse oximetry.
3. Do NOT induce emesis in clients with no gag reflex or with CNS depression or excitation.
4. Perform gastric lavage if it can be done soon after ingestion.
5. Draw arterial blood gas with measured oxygen saturation.
6. Methylene blue must be administered with caution when methemoglobin level is >30%. Methylene blue reverses the process of methemoglobin formation by reducing methemoglobin back to hemoglobin. This treatment should not be used in the presence of G6PD deficiency.
7. Give blood exchange transfusion(s).
8. Administer hyperbaric oxygen therapy.
9. Forced diuresis and urine alkalinization are NOT helpful.
10. Do NOT acidify urine.

Increased. Acquired or hereditary methemoglobinemia, carbon monoxide poisoning, ionizing radiation, malaria (cerebral), pregnancy (high risk), sepsis or septic shock, smoking. Drugs include acetanilid, aniline dyes, benzene derivatives, benzocaine, Bromo-Seltzer, chlorates, chloroquine, dapsone, hydrogen peroxide (dialysis treatment during hospital water disinfection of water supply), isoniazid, lidocaine, metoclopramide, nitrates, nitrites (including silver nitrate topical ointment), phenacetin, resorcinol, and sulfonamides.

Decreased. Pancreatitis.

Description. This test is used to help detect the adverse effects of drugs containing nitrates or nitrites, such as nitroglycerin. Methemoglobin is formed when the iron in the heme portion of deoxygenated hemoglobin is oxidized to a ferric form as a result of a hereditary deficiency of the enzyme nicotinamide adenine dinucleotide-diaphorase or as a result of exposure to chemicals and drugs. In the ferric form, oxygen and iron cannot combine. This is a normal process, and it is balanced by the reduction of methemoglobin to hemoglobin. However, when a high concentration of methemoglobin is produced in the red blood cells (RBCs), the capacity of RBCs to combine with oxygen is reduced, and anoxia and cyanosis result.

Methemoglobinemia occurs when greater than 1% of the blood hemoglobin has been oxidized to the ferric form; it is a rare but potentially dangerous condition in which the oxygen-carrying capacity of blood is compromised. Infants are more susceptible to methemoglobinemia than adults because fetal hemoglobin is more easily converted to methemoglobin than is adult hemoglobin.

Professional Considerations
Consent form NOT required.

Preparation
1. Tube: Green topped. Also obtain ice.

Procedure
1. Draw a 2-mL venous blood sample.

Postprocedure Care
1. Place the specimen on ice and deliver immediately to the laboratory. Specimens must be tested within 1 hour of collection.

Client and Family Teaching
1. Review with the client and family potential sources that may have caused methemoglobinemia and identify corrective measures for removal of the exposure.
2. Pregnant women with methemoglobin level blood sample >1.5g/L had children with jaundice, hyperbilirubinemia, heart murmurs and learning and memory impairments.

Factors That Affect Results
1. The intestinal flora of nursing infants is capable of converting significant amounts of inorganic nitrate (such as well water) to the nitrite ion, which can produce serious toxicity.
2. Amyl nitrite ingestion increases methemoglobinemia.
3. Falsely elevated results occur when there is a delay of more than 1 hour after collection before the test is performed.
4. Falsely low results may occur when the sample is not kept on ice until testing.
5. Symptoms will appear at lower than the above scale in clients who are anemic.
6. Dental use of benzocaine or prilocaine can cause methemoglobinuria.

Other Data
1. Hidden sources of nitrates, which could cause methemoglobinemia, include spinach and Polish sausage, which is rich in nitrite and nitrate, and drinking well water, which contains nitrite. Nitrate can be absorbed from topical applications, such as silver nitrate (used to treat serious bums). It must be used sparingly when applied to infants to avoid serous conversion of nitrate to nitrite.
2. Poisoning is reportable to public health authorities if secondary to occupational or environmental causes.
3. See also CO-oximeter profile, Arterial or venous—Blood.

Methicillin-Resistant *Staphylococcus aureus* (MRSA)—Culture

Norm. Negative.

Usage. Infections. Test is used in the differential diagnosis of clients with skin and soft tissue infections, or with suspected necrotizing pneumonia, osteomyelitis, and other necrotizing conditions and preoperatively.

Description. MRSA is a strain of *Staphylococcus aureus* that is resistant to methicillin, the antibiotic most commonly used to treat staphylococcal infections. MRSA organism is most commonly acquired in hospitals and is known for increasing length-of-stay in intensive care units. The death rate is high in clients with grafts infected with MRSA after vascular surgery and post-op orthopedic surgery. A community-acquired strain of MRSA (CA-MRSA) is particularly virulent, faster growing, and genetically distinct from the hospital strain. CA-MRSA can cause necrotizing skin infections and necrotizing pneumonia that can be fatal within 24 hours of onset. Both types of MRSA are spread via the contact method of transmission. Rapid test kits are available that are less expensive, quicker to use, and highly sensitive and specific. PCR screening upon admission to critical care units provides quicker results in MRSA positive patients.

Professional Considerations
Consent form NOT required.

Preparation

1. Obtain a sterile cotton-tipped Culturette swab with sodium chloride medium.

Procedure

1. Culture a specific site, using a rotating motion for 10 seconds and using one swab per site.
2. Place the swab in the sodium chloride medium.

Postprocedure Care

1. Transport the sample to the laboratory within 8 hours.

Client and Family Teaching

1. Results are normally available within a few days.
2. Patients who are nasal carriers need to be treated before orthopedic surgery to decrease post-op infection risk.

Factors That Affect Results

1. Detection is enhanced by incubation at 30 to 35 degrees C and the use of sodium chloride medium.

Other Data

1. Methicillin-resistant staphylococci are considered resistant to all cephalosporins and imipenem. Vancomycin is used for treatment.
2. 0.3% triclosan (Bacti-Stat), used as a hand-washing soap, has eradicated MRSA outbreaks in hospitals.
3. One study (Itoh et al, 2000) found remission of MRSA in clients treated with the herb *hochu-ekki-to*.
4. MicroPhage test uses 2 tubes of blood, 1 to see if you have *S. aureus* is in the blood and the other to determine if it's MRSA. This test detects *S. aureus* within hours, not days as in usual plating.
5. 67% of persons who work in ambulatory healthcare clinics are positive for MRSA.
6. A 2011 study (Matheson et al) found that individuals who consume hot tea or coffee are likely to have half the rate of MRSA in nasal secretions as compared to the U.S. population.
7. See also KeyPath MRSA/MSSA blood culture test—Blood.

---

p-Methoxyamphetamine

See Amphetamines—Blood.

Methsuximide

Norm. Negative.

Therapeutic Range		SI Units
Methsuximide	<1 µg/mL	
Normethsuximide	10-40 µg/mL	53-212 µmol/L
Total	10-40 µg/mL	53-212 µmol/L
Toxic level (of metabolite)	>60 µg/mL	>318 µmol/L
Panic level (of metabolite)	>150 µg/mL	>793 µmol/L

Panic Level Symptoms and Treatment

Symptoms. CNS symptoms (ataxia, confusion, dizziness, drowsiness, slurred speech, tremor, decreased level of consciousness) and GI symptoms (anorexia, abdominal pain, diarrhea, nausea, vomiting) are most common. Other symptoms include hypotension, severe depression, skin rash, periorbital edema, urinary frequency, vaginal bleeding, pancytopenia, hepatotoxicity, neuropathy.

Treatment

NOTE: Treatment choice(s) depend(s) on client's history and condition and episode history.

1. Administer saline cathartic unless client has an ileus.
2. Administer sorbitol.
3. Perform gastric lavage if possible soon after ingestion.
4. Protect airway and support breathing.
5. Perform neurologic checks every hour.

M

6. Forced diuresis is not helpful.
7. Charcoal hemoperfusion may be helpful in removing the methsuximide metabolite in comatose clients. No information was found on the effectiveness of any type of dialysis in removing methsuximide.

Increased. Overdose ingestion.

Decreased. Convulsions and epilepsy. Drugs include valproic acid.

Description. Anticonvulsant for "absence seizures," also known as petit mal seizures, that depresses nerve transmission to the motor cortex, thereby decreasing paroxysmal spike-and-wave patterns. Methsuximide is also used to supplement other medications in clients with intractable seizures. Plasma half-life is 2-4 hours. Methsuximide is metabolized in the liver and excreted in urine.

Professional Considerations
Consent form NOT required.

Preparation
1. Tube: Red topped, lavender topped, or pink topped, green topped, or gray topped.
2. Do NOT draw specimens during hemodialysis.

Procedure
1. Draw a 5-mL blood sample before the next dose of medication.

Postprocedure Care
1. Refrigerate specimen until testing.

Client and Family Teaching
1. Explain overdose symptoms and treatment (see above) as appropriate.
2. For an intentional overdose, refer the client and family for crisis intervention.
3. Referrals to appropriate rehabilitation centers and therapeutic community programs should be offered to all clients who may be interested.

Factors That Affect Results
1. Obtaining specimens after medication has been ingested will cause increased results.
2. Hepatic or renal dysfunction may cause increased results.

Other Data
1. This drug may cause a positive albumin result in the urine and an elevated BUN.
2. In pediatric clients, the C/D ratio (plasma concentration and dose per kilogram of weight) is less sensitive to both age and associated therapy.
3. Methsuximide decreases valproic acid levels.

Methylenedioxyamphetamine
See Amphetamines—Blood.

Methylphenidate—Serum
Norm. Negative.
Therapeutic level: 0.01-0.04 mg/mL (0.04-0.17 mmol/L, SI units).

Overdose Symptoms and Treatment
Symptoms. Agitation, hyperactive, talkative, sleepless for days, paranoia, hallucinations, violent behavior possible, confusion, dryness of mucous membranes, headache, mydriasis, hypertension, rapid and irregular pulse, sweating, vomiting, cerebral hemorrhage, seizures, convulsions, and coma.

Treatment
NOTE: Treatment choice(s) depend(s) on client's history and condition and episode history.
1. Perform gastric lavage.
2. Perform forced diuresis.
3. Acid urine hastens excretion.
4. Administer cathartic.
5. Acidify urine.
6. Support symptoms.
7. Take precautions to prevent self-injury.

8. Treatments administered outside a health care facility should be used as directed by a poison control center.
9. Dialysis is unlikely to remove methylphenidate.

Usage. Monitor levels of methylphenidate, which is used in the treatment of hyperkinetic disorders (such as ADHD, hyperactivity associated with minimal brain dysfunction), narcolepsy, mild depression, senile behavior, and children with perceptual problems; methylphenidate also counteracts overdose from depressant drugs.

Increased. Overdose and stimulant drug abuse.

Decreased. Subtherapeutic dose.

Description. Methylphenidate (Ritalin) is a central nervous system (CNS) stimulant and antidepressant that presumably activates brainstem and cortex arousal. Methylphenidate is well absorbed from the gastrointestinal tract and is distributed throughout the body. Its actions appear in about 1 hour after ingestion and last up to 6 hours. The drug is completely metabolized in the liver to inactive products that are excreted in urine.

Tolerance to the CNS and peripheral effects develops with continued use.

Professional Considerations
Consent form NOT required.

Preparation
1. Tube: Red, lavender, pink, or gray topped. Also obtain ice.
2. Do NOT draw specimens during hemodialysis.

Procedure
1. Draw a 7-mL blood sample. Place specimen on ice.

Postprocedure Care
1. Transport specimen immediately to the laboratory. Separate plasma or serum, and then freeze.

Client and Family Teaching
1. Counsel regarding proper dosing as needed.
2. For intentional overdose, refer client and family for crisis intervention.

Factors That Affect Results
1. None found.

Other Data
1. None.

Methyprylon—Serum

Norm. Negative.

		SI Units
Therapeutic level	8-10 µg/mL	44-55 µmol/L
Panic level	>30 µg/mL	>164 µmol/L

Panic Level Symptoms and Treatment
Symptoms. Apnea, ataxia, bradycardia, central nervous system depression, confusion, hypotension, weakness, pulmonary edema, convulsions, shock, coma. Death has occurred after ingestion of 6 g.

Treatment
NOTE: Treatment choice(s) depend(s) on client's history and condition and episode history.
1. Perform diuresis with IV fluids.
2. Give gastric lavage if possible soon after ingestion.
3. Give supportive therapy.
4. Hemodialysis, peritoneal dialysis, and hemoperfusion WILL remove methyprylon.

Usage. Monitoring for therapeutic drug level.

Description. Methyprylon is a sedative-hypnotic that induces sleep within 45 minutes by increasing the threshold of the arousal centers of the brain. Plasma half-life is 3-6 hours. It is conjugated in the liver and excreted in the urine. Addiction and physical dependence can occur.

Professional Considerations
Consent form NOT required.

Preparation
1. Tube: Red or lavender topped.
2. Do NOT draw specimens during hemodialysis.

Procedure
1. Draw a 7-mL blood sample.

Postprocedure Care
1. None.

Client and Family Teaching
1. Counsel regarding proper dosing as appropriate.
2. For intentional overdose, refer client and family for crisis intervention.

3. Referrals to appropriate rehabilitation centers and therapeutic community programs should be offered to all clients who may be interested.

Factors That Affect Results
1. Interferes with urine diagnostics for 17-KS and 17-OHCS.

Other Data
1. The trade name is Noludar.

Metyrapone (Cortisol) Test—Serum
Norm.

		SI Units
11-Deoxycortisol	>7 µg/dL	>202 nmol/L
Cortisol	<3 µg/dL	<83 nmol/L

Increased. Adrenal carcinoma, Cushing's syndrome, diabetic acidosis, fever, hepatic disease, hyperthyroidism, hypoalbuminemia, obesity, pain, pregnancy, renal disease, and stress. Drugs include estrogens, oral contraceptives, and spironolactone.

Decreased. Addison's disease, fungal invasion, hemorrhage, hepatic disease, hypopituitarism, hypothyroidism, low–birth-weight infants, respiratory distress syndrome, and tuberculosis. Drugs include amitriptyline, androgens, chlordiazepoxide, glucocorticoids, methysergide, oral contraceptives, phenobarbital, phenothiazines, phenytoin, progestins, rifampin, and steroids.

Description. The metyrapone test is a diagnostic test for secondary adrenal insufficiency. Metyrapone is an inhibitor of 11β-hydroxylase that prevents the conversion of 11-deoxycortisol to cortisol in the adrenal glands. The diminished level of cortisol stimulates the pituitary to produce adrenocorticotropic hormone (ACTH) in a negative-feedback mechanism. In normal individuals, more ACTH is produced.

Professional Considerations
Consent form NOT required.

Preparation
1. Tube: Red topped, red/gray topped, or gold topped or green topped. Also obtain ice.

2. Metyrapone, 30 mg/kg (range 2-3 g), is given orally, usually with milk, at 11 PM.
3. Assess for a history of heroin addiction or use and methadone maintenance because this test may induce a narcotic withdrawal-like syndrome.

Procedure
1. Draw a 4-mL blood sample at 8 AM the following morning.

Postprocedure Care
1. Specimens should be placed on ice.

Client and Family Teaching
1. Return tomorrow at approximately 8 AM for a repeat blood draw.

Factors That Affect Results
1. Reject the specimen if the client had a radioactive scan within 7 days of the test.
2. Specimens should be frozen if the test is not performed within 24 hours.
3. Results are highly dependent on the time of day the specimen is obtained (circadian variation).

Other Data
1. Do NOT perform this test if primary adrenal insufficiency is likely.
2. Long-term treatment with metyrapone can cause hypertension.
3. See also Cortisol—Plasma or serum; Metyrapone—24-Hour urine.

Metyrapone (Cortisol)—24-Hour Urine

Norm. *17-Hydroxycorticosteroids (17-OHCS):* 2-4 times base level.

17-Ketogenic steroids (17-KGS): 2.5-3.0-fold rise but at least 10 mg/dL (35 μmol/day, SI units).

17-Ketosteroids (17-KS): >2 times base level.

Increased. Acute alcohol intoxication, Cushing's syndrome, ectopic adrenocorticotropic hormone (ACTH) syndrome, hepatic disease, hyperthyroidism, obesity, and stress (children, adults). Drugs include amphetamines, corticosteroids, morphine, phenothiazines, and reserpine.

Decreased. Addison's disease, adrenogenital syndrome, and pituitary insufficiency.

Description. Diagnostic test for secondary adrenal insufficiency. An inhibitor of 11β-hydroxylase that prevents the conversion of 11-deoxycortisol to cortisol. The diminished levels of cortisol stimulate the pituitary to produce more ACTH in a negative-feedback mechanism. In normal individuals, more ACTH is produced, which results in an increase in urinary hydroxysteroids and ketosteroids.

Professional Considerations

Consent form NOT required.

Preparation

1. Assess for history of heroin addiction and use or methadone maintenance because this test may cause narcotic withdrawal-like symptoms.
2. Administer metyrapone to adults in doses of 750 mg every 4 hours × 6 doses. In the child, the dose is 300 mg/m².
3. Begin administration at 11 PM.

Procedure

1. Begin a 24-hour urine collection at 8 AM the morning after the drug was ingested.
2. Collection container must be acidified with either hydrochloric or acetic acid as a preservative.

Postprocedure Care

1. Write the beginning and ending date and time as well as total urine voided in the 24-hour period on the laboratory requisition.
2. Record the total dose and the time metyrapone was given on the laboratory requisition.

Client and Family Teaching

1. Minimize stress levels before urine collection.
2. Save all the urine voided in the 24-hour period and urinate before defecating to avoid loss of urine. Keep the specimen on ice or refrigerate it during the collection period. If any urine is accidentally discarded, discard the entire specimen and restart the collection the next day.

Factors That Affect Results

1. Inaccurate collection of urine.
2. When possible, hold all medications for several days before testing. Drugs that may interfere with results include estrogens, glucose, meprobamate, penicillin, and radiographic contrast materials.
3. Obesity, pregnancy, and stress may affect results.

Other Data

1. Hospitalization may be required to ensure accuracy of the 24-hour urine collection.
2. Long-term treatment with metyrapone can cause hypertension.
3. The 24-hour urine specimen reflects cumulative levels rather than circadian variation.
4. See also Cortisol—Urine; Metyrapone test—Serum.

MIBG (^{131}I-*m*-Iodobenzylguaidine) Scan—Diagnostic

Norm. The adrenal glands will not be visualized. There is variable physiologic uptake by the bladder, colon, heart, spleen, and uterus.

Usage. Location and diagnosis of primary and metastatic pheochromocytoma (limited to use in patients with negative cross-sectional imaging and those with recurrent

M

or metastatic disease), adrenal medullary hyperplasia, multiple endocrine neoplasia (MEN), von Hippel-Lindau disease, von Recklinghausen's disease, neuroblastoma, paraganglioma, medullary carcinoma of thyroid, and other neuroendocrine tumors. Chronic heart failure patients with a delta-washout rate ≥50% predicts cardiac death.

Description. An MIBG scan is a nuclear medicine scan of the whole body after injection of the radioactive tracer ^{131}I-MIBG for the purpose of detecting areas of increased uptake by hyperactive endocrine tissue or tumor. MIBG is a catecholamine analog, similar to noradrenaline. Various organs and tumors uptake the tracer to varying degrees. A series of scans is conducted at 24 and 48 hours following injection of radioisotope. The isotope is concentrated in hyperactive endocrine tissue, such as pheochromocytoma tissue, and appears on the scan as a "hot spot."

Professional Considerations
Consent form IS required.

Risks
Allergic reaction to tracer (itching, hives, rash, tight feeling in the throat, shortness of breath, anaphylaxis).

Contraindications
Previous allergy to MIBG or iodine solution (Lugol's solution or SSKI) or shellfish; pregnancy (because of radioactive iodine crossing the blood-placental barrier); breast-feeding; anuria; dialysis.

Preparation
1. See Client and Family Teaching.
2. Assess client for history of allergy to iodine or shellfish.
3. A prescribed dose of potassium iodide (SSKI) or Lugol's solution will be started 24 to 48 hours before the injection of the radioisotope to prevent uptake of radioisotope by the thyroid.
4. Women of childbearing age should have a pregnancy test within 48 hours before the test.
5. A bowel prep may be prescribed.
6. Have emergency equipment readily available.

7. Remove jewelry and metal objects before each scan.
8. Just before beginning the procedure, take a "time out" to verify the correct client, procedure, and site.

Procedure
1. Position client in lying position and take baseline BP.
2. Slowly inject radioisotope intravenously over 1-2 minutes.
3. Monitor BP during injection and 20 minutes following injection.
4. A scan may be done 4, 24, 48, and possibly 72 hours following the injection of the isotope. For the scan, the client is positioned supine on the imaging table and the whole body is scanned using a gamma camera.

Postprocedure Care
1. SSKI or Lugol's solution will be given throughout the test period and will continue for 4-7 days following the injection of MIBG.
2. Check with institutional policy regarding special instructions for discarding urine for 24 hours following isotope injection.

Client and Family Teaching
1. Many prescribed and over-the-counter medications can interfere with the results of this test. Be sure to inform physician of any medications that are being taken.
2. Medications that may need to be discontinued up to 4-6 weeks before the test include labetalol, reserpine, loxapine, tricyclic antidepressants (doxepin, amitriptyline and derivatives, imipramine and derivatives, amoxapine), sympathomimetics (phenylephrine, phenylpropanolamine, pseudoephedrine), calcium channel blockers, SSRIs, catecholamine receptor agonists and antagonists, phenothiazines, butyrophenones (i.e., haloperidol), guanethidine, phenoxybenzamine.
3. Inform the physician if pregnant or breast-feeding, or if young children are in the household.
4. No fast is required for this test.
5. You will need to lie still during the procedure. Young children may need to be sedated.
6. There is no discomfort associated with the scan.

7. SSKI or Lugol's solution will be taken for 4-7 days, beginning 1-2 days before the injection of the radioisotope. This medication can be diluted in a glass of water or juice.
8. Despite the use of thyroid-blocking medication, the thyroid may be affected for a short period of time. Prolonged feelings of fatigue, temperature irregularities, or changes in heart rate should be reported to the physician.
9. The scan takes approximately 1-2 hours.

Factors That Affect Results
1. Many medications can impact the results of this test. Refer to Client and Family Teaching.

2. False positive MIBG reported in diagnosed pneumonia.

Other Data
1. During the scan, the kidneys may be localized in relation to the adrenal glands by obtaining a correlative image of the kidneys using a renal tracer.
2. MIBG is excreted by the kidneys. The half-life is 8 days.
3. Health care professionals working in a nuclear medicine area must follow federal standards set by the Nuclear Regulatory Commission. These standards include precautions for handling the radioactive material and monitoring of potential radiation exposure.

Microalbumin

See **Albumin**—Serum, Urine, and 24-Hour Urine.

Microfilariae—Peripheral Blood

Norm. Negative or no parasite identified. An indirect hemagglutination titer of 1:128 as well as a bentonite flocculation titer of 1:5 are considered minimally significant titers.

Positive. *Brugia, Dipetalonema, Loa loa, Mansonella,* and *Wuchereria.*

Description. Filariae make up a large group of parasitic worms that produce an embryo known as a microfilaria (intermediate stage between egg and larva). These parasites invade the lymphatics, causing lymphedema and elephantiasis. Microfilariae are the smallest forms of filariae.

Professional Considerations
Consent form NOT required.

Preparation
1. Tube: Green topped.
2. Include the client's recent travel history on the laboratory requisition.

Procedure
1. Draw a 4-mL blood sample.
2. Repeat the test to obtain daytime and nighttime specimens.

Postprocedure Care
1. Transport specimens to the laboratory immediately. Specimens should NOT be clotted.

Client and Family Teaching
1. Two specimens, drawn preferably 12 hours apart, are necessary.

Factors That Affect Results
1. One negative result does not rule out a parasitic infection.
2. Circulating microfilariae may NOT be detected in blood for 6-12 months after transmission occurs.

Other Data
1. Because *Wuchereria* and *Brugia* are nocturnal, the optimal blood sample time would be 10 PM to 2 AM.
2. Because *Loa loa* is diurnal, the optimal time for the blood sample would be 12 PM (noon).
3. Treatment of choice is combination of ivermectin and albendazole or diethylcarbamazine.
4. Among immigrants from high-risk Central and West Africa, 1.8% were found to be positive mostly for loiasis (disease from mangrove fly, Chrysops).

Microhemagglutination *Treponema pallidum* (MHA-TP) Test—Serum

Norm. Titer <1:160 or nonreactive.

Usage. Serologic confirmation of syphilis when nontreponemal antibody tests (RPR or VDRL) are positive.

Description. Syphilis is a complex, sexually transmitted disease characterized by a wide range of symptoms that imitate other diseases and is caused by the organism *Treponema pallidum*. In this test, the client's serum is heat treated and mixed with *T. pallidum*–sensitized sheep red blood cells, incubated, and compared with a control. A positive result occurs when agglutination occurs in the test sample but not in the control. This test is less sensitive than the fluorescent treponemal antibody, absorbed double stain (FTA-Abs DS) test for primary syphilis. Positive results will occur in treponemal diseases of bejel, pinta, syphilis, or yaws.

Professional Considerations
Consent form NOT required.

Preparation
1. See Client and Family Teaching.
2. Tube: Red topped.

Procedure
1. Draw a 4-mL blood sample.

Postprocedure Care
1. Send the specimen to the laboratory and refrigerate until tested.

Client and Family Teaching
1. Fast overnight before the test.
2. The use of condoms significantly reduces the risk of sexually transmitted diseases.
3. A referral for HIV testing may be indicated and should be discussed and offered to interested clients.
4. If testing is positive:
   a. Notify all sexual contacts from the previous 90 days (if early stage) to be tested for syphilis.
   b. Syphilis can be cured with antibiotics. These may worsen the symptoms for the first 24 hours.
   c. Do not have sexual contact for 2 months and until after repeat testing has confirmed that the syphilis is cured. Use condoms after that for 2 years. Return for repeat testing every 3-4 months for the next 2 years to make sure the disease is cured.
   d. Do not become pregnant for 2 years because syphilis can be transmitted to the fetus.
   e. If left untreated, syphilis can damage many body organs, including the brain, over several years.

Factors That Affect Results
1. False-positive results may be attributable to autoimmune disorders, connective tissue diseases, infectious mononucleosis, leprosy, or systemic lupus erythematosus.
2. Testing errors may be associated with dusty or improper plates and pipetting errors.

Other Data
1. This test may remain positive indefinitely for clients previously infected with syphilis. Thus it is not useful for monitoring clinical response to treatment for syphilis.
2. Test results may become negative after treatment. Therefore negative results do NOT necessarily exclude a history of syphilis.
3. There is a significant correlation between the diagnosis of syphilis and seropositive HIV.
4. See also Fluorescent treponemal antibody–absorbed double-stain test—Serum; Rapid plasma Reagin test—Blood; Venereal disease research laboratory test—Serum.

MicroPhage, Blood
See Methicillin-Resistant *Staphylococcus aureus*—Culture.

MicroPhage Test
See KeyPath MRSA/MSSA Blood Culture Test— Blood.

Microsomal Antibody

See Thyroid Peroxidase Antibody—Blood.

Microsatellite Instability Testing—Specimen

Norm. There are no normal findings, since this test is performed on tumor tissue.

Classification of findings:

Stable = MSI not detected. (Microsatellite regions of the tumor match the microsatellite regions of the patient's normal cells.)

Unstable High = changes in 2 or more regions; suggestive of HNPCC syndrome

Unstable Low = changes in 1 region

Usage. Differentiation of colorectal cancer to aid selection of appropriate treatment and to confirm or rule out hereditary nonpolyposis colorectal cancer (HNPCC) syndrome. Relatives of individuals with confirmed HNPCC mutation should have heightened surveillance for colorectal cancer (Lindor, 2009).

Description. A test performed on colon, endometrial or other cancer tissue to identify HNPCC syndrome. This syndrome accounts for the most common form of hereditary colorectal cancer, accounting for approximately 5% of cases. It is an autosomal dominant condition that occurs at a relatively young age, usually before age 50 for the first family member diagnosed. HNPCC syndrome, also known as "Lynch Syndrome," carries a 50%-60% risk of developing colorectal cancer. Once cancer develops, it progresses rapidly—from polyp to invasive cancer within 3 years. Thus, relatives of individuals with confirmed HNPCC mutation should have heightened surveillance for colorectal cancer. Other cancers associated with the HNPCC mutation are small bowel and endometrial cancers as well as cancer of the ureter or renal pelvis.

Testing for HNPCC identifies mutations in any of 5 genes responsible for repairing mismatched DNA in region called "microsatellites". Cancer with this type of mutation demonstrates microsatellite instability in the region of the DNA associated with each of the 5 genes.

Bethseda criteria for testing or HNPCC and microsatellite instability include (Umar et al, 2004):

• Colorectal cancer diagnosed in a patient who is less than 50 years of age.

• Presence of synchronous, metachronous colorectal, or other HNPCC-associated tumors, regardless of age.

• Colorectal cancer with the MSI-H histology diagnosed in a person younger than age 60.

• Colorectal cancer diagnosed in one or more first-degree relatives with an HNPCC-related tumor, with one of the cancers being diagnosed in a person under 50 years of age.

• Colorectal cancer diagnosed in two or more first- or second-degree relatives with HNPCC-related tumors, regardless of age.

Professional Considerations

Informed consent is recommended for genetic testing.

Preparation

1. Formalin, paraffin-embedded tissue block.
2. Tube: lavender top or yellow top.

Procedure

1. Obtain a tissue block of the tumor. Fix with formalin.
2. Obtain 2-mL of whole blood.

Postprocedure Care

1. Keep tissue block and blood at room temperature. Do not freeze specimen.

Client and Family Teaching

1. Refer to Appendix B, "Informed Consent for Genetic Testing."
2. Heightened surveillance activities to detect colorectal cancer when HNPCC is present include:
   a. Bi-annual full colonoscopy, beginning at age 21 (or 10 years earlier than the earliest occurrence of HNPCC in the family); then annually after age 40.
   b. Annual pelvic exam and transvaginal ultrasound.
   c. Annual CA-125 blood test for women.

d. Urine cytology every 12-24 months.

e. Endometrial biopsy as symptoms arise.

3. Test results will be available in 4 to 20 weeks.

Factors That Affect Results

1. MSI is often absent when the tumor is associated with the MSH6 mutation.

2. As many as 10% of patients with HNPCC syndrome have negative results. Those with negative results, yet a history suggestive of HNPCC syndrome, should have further immunohistochemical testing for DNA repair genes mutation indicating Lynch syndrome.

Other Data

1. About half of individuals with HNPCC syndrome have what is known as "Lynch syndrome," which is defined as a hereditary predisposition to colorectal and other cancers as a result of a hereditary gene mutation known as germline mismatch repair (MMR). Those without the germline mismatch repair are referred to as having "Familial colorectal cancer type X."

2. The Genetic Information Nondiscrimination Act of 2008 prohibits health plans from using genetic family history or genetic test results from influencing eligibility or premiums for health insurance. It also prohibits employers from using this information to influence decisions about hiring, terminating employment, or employment pay, promotions or privileges.

Midazolam

See **Benzodiazepines**—Plasma and Urine.

Milk Precipitins—Blood

Norm. Negative.

Increased. IgA deficiency, celiac disease, infantile diarrhea, mongolism, pulmonary hemosiderosis, and Wiskott-Aldrich syndrome.

Description. Milk precipitins are antibodies found occasionally in children who are sensitive to milk. This test involves adding blood to an agar gel and waiting for a specific antibody concentration to develop in a line formation. The distance of the precipitin line from the point of application of the blood is directly proportional to the concentration of antigens in the client's bloodstream.

Professional Considerations
Consent form NOT required.

Preparation

1. Tube: Red topped, red/gray topped, or gold topped.

Procedure

1. Draw a 7-mL blood sample.

Postprocedure Care

1. Results are normally available within 48 hours but may take several days if the test is performed off-site.

Client and Family Teaching

1. The test does not differentiate between sensitivity and allergy.

Factors That Affect Results

1. Gross contamination.

2. A positive test does not necessarily mean that the child is allergic to milk because milk sensitivity may also produce a positive test.

Other Data

1. None.

Mini–Mental State Exam (MMSE)—Diagnostic

Norm. *Perfect score* (normal for clients with twelfth grade or higher education and no cognitive impairment): 30 points.

Cognitive impairment: ≤24 points.

Usage. Detection and tracking of cognitive impairment.

Description. The Mini–Mental State Exam (MMSE) tests for cognitive impairment by evaluating orientation, registration, attention and calculation, recall, and language. The MMSE has demonstrated an 85% specificity and 87% sensitivity for identifying cognitive impairment in hospitalized clients.

Professional Considerations
Consent form NOT required.

Preparation
1. Examination may be done at the client's bedside.
2. Obtain copy of examination and a clipboard.
3. Observe client's level of consciousness, educational level, visual impairments, and any physician-imposed limitations.

Procedure
1. Inform client that a series of questions will be asked. Instruct client to attempt to answer all the questions.

Postprocedure Care
1. None.

Client and Family Teaching
1. Retesting should be done after 6 months if score is borderline (23-25 points).

Factors That Affect Results
1. Clients with less than a fourth-grade education do poorly on the reading and writing portions of this examination but may not be cognitively impaired.
2. Medical conditions such as reduced vision ability, memory impairment, stroke, and diabetes have been associated with cognitive deterioration.
3. Better self-care ability is related to better results on the simple processing items (registration, naming, repetition, commanding) and attention/memory functions such as time/place orientation, recall, and attention.

Other Data
1. None.

Miraluma

See **Scintimammography**—Diagnostic.

Mitogen-Activated Protein Kinase (MAP Kinase, MAPK)—Specimen

Norm. Requires interpretation.

Usage. Prostate cancer, colon cancer, breast cancer. Use of MAPK in the detection, diagnosis, and determination of response to therapy for these conditions is in the research arena.

Description. MAP kinases act as transducers of extracellular signaling, by means of tyrosine kinase–growth factor regulators, to regulate a variety of transcription factors. MAP kinases are unique in that phosphorylation of both threonine and tyrosine residues is required for activation of the MAPK pathway cascade. One MAPK pathway is stimulated by serum growth factors that target extracellular-regulated kinases (ERKs), resulting in cellular proliferation or differentiation. Another MAPK pathway is activated by stressors (that is, radiation or ultraviolet radiation), ultimately triggering apoptosis (organized cellular death). It is believed that various overexpressed or mutated oncogenes activate MAPK pathways and are responsible for stimulating tumor growth. Some of these oncogenes involved in the MAPK pathways include *ras*, *raf*, and *src*. MAPK activity is tested using the immune complex assay. When compared to normal or noncancerous tissue, hyperexpression of MAP kinase is associated with carcinomas.

Professional Considerations
Consent form IS required for the procedure, that is, tumor resection or biopsy used to obtain the specimens used for this test. (See Biopsy, Site-specific—Specimen for procedure-specific risks and contraindications.)

Preparation
1. See Biopsy, Site-specific—Specimen; Client and Family Teaching.
2. Obtain a sterile container and fixative or formalin.

3. The requisition must include the operative diagnosis and the site of the specimen.

Procedure

1. The tissue sample is obtained with use of local or general anesthesia.
2. Label the specimen with the client's name, age, sex, room number, and operative diagnosis; the source of the specimen; and the surgeon and other physicians desiring a copy of the pathology report.
3. A freshly frozen tissue sample may be used. See Frozen tissue section—Diagnostic as appropriate.

Postprocedure Care

1. Fresh tissue may be fixed in phosphate-buffered formalin. Confirm preferred tissue handling with physician.

2. Deliver the specimen to the laboratory promptly.
3. See Biopsy, Site-specific—Specimen.

Client and Family Teaching

1. See Biopsy, Site-specific—Specimen.
2. Call the physician for signs of infection at the procedure site: increasing pain, redness, swelling, purulent drainage, or temperature >101 degrees F (>38 degrees C).

Factors That Affect Results

1. Poor sampling technique or contamination.

Other Data

1. None.

Mixed Leukocyte Culture (Mixed Lymphocyte Culture)—Specimen

Norm. Requires interpretation.

Usage. Aplastic anemia, immune deficiency (detection of T-lymphocyte abnormalities), transplants, and tuberculosis.

Description. Mixed leukocyte culture is performed to determine whether the mononuclear cells of a prospective tissue transplant recipient will react against a potential donor's leukocyte antigens. This histocompatibility test may be performed in two ways. In a one-way test, the potential donor sample is irradiated or treated with mitomycin C, which prevents the sample from blast formation in reaction to mixture with the prospective recipient sample. This allows measurement of prospective recipient blast formation only. In a two-way test, blast formation of both samples is monitored by comparison of the amount of blast formation in the combined sample with that of each separate sample in combination with controls.

Professional Considerations
Consent form NOT required.

Preparation

1. Preschedule the test with the laboratory.
2. Tube: Two green topped tubes.

Procedure

1. Draw a 7-mL blood sample from the prospective transplant donor. Label the tube "donor sample."
2. Repeat the test for the prospective recipient. Label the tube "recipient sample."

Postprocedure Care

1. Send the specimens to the laboratory within 2 hours.
2. Specimens must be tested the same day.

Client and Family Teaching

1. Results are normally available in 7-10 days.

Factors That Affect Results

1. Reject any specimen that was not collected using a sterile procedure, not drawn in a heparinized tube, or has arrived in the laboratory more than 2 hours after collection.
2. False-negative results may occur if the prospective recipient is severely immunocompromised.

Other Data

1. May be helpful in predicting graft survival.
2. This test should be repeated for several days.

MJD GENE
See **SCA Gene Test**—Diagnostic.

MMSE

See Mini–Mental State Exam—Diagnostic.

Monocytes

See Differential Leukocyte Count—Peripheral Blood.

Monos

See Differential Leukocyte Count—Peripheral Blood.

Monospot Screen (Heterophil Screen)—Blood

Norm. Negative.

Positive. Adenovirus, Burkitt's lymphoma, cytomegalovirus, Epstein-Barr virus, herpes simplex virus, HIV, Hodgkin's disease, infectious mononucleosis, Izumi fever, leukemia, malaria, pancreatic cancer, rheumatoid arthritis, rubella virus, sarcoidosis, serum sickness, systemic lupus erythematosus, and viral or infectious hepatitis.

Negative. Normal finding or infection of bacterial cause.

Description. The monospot screen, a screening test that rapidly detects heterophil agglutinins, is performed on two slides, each containing serum and horse red cells, with one slide also containing guinea pig kidney and the other slide containing beef red cell stroma. Agglutination that occurs on only the slide with guinea pig kidney is diagnostic of infectious mononucleosis. Heterophil agglutinins can appear in serum approximately 6-10 days after contact. Detection may remain for up to 1 year and peaks between 4 and 8 weeks after exposure.

Professional Considerations

Consent form NOT required.

Preparation

1. Tube: Red topped, red/gray topped, or gold topped or lavender topped.

Procedure

1. Draw a 2-mL blood sample (red topped, red/gray topped, or gold topped) or a 3-mL blood sample (lavender topped).

Postprocedure Care

1. Specimens should be refrigerated before being tested.

Client and Family Teaching

1. Results are normally available within 72 hours.

Factors That Affect Results

1. A hemolyzed or chylous sample invalidates the results.
2. About 10% of adults (more for children) produce false-positive or false-negative results.

Other Data

1. The monospot screen has a 99% specificity and an 86% sensitivity in helping to diagnose infectious mononucleosis.
2. In the presence of infectious mononucleosis, 10%-25% atypical lymphocytes may be observed in the differential cell count.
3. If mononucleosis is suspected based on clinical symptoms but the screening test is negative, more sensitive tests, such as heterophil antibody, cytomegalovirus, or *Toxoplasma* antibodies, should be considered.
4. See also Heterophile agglutinins—Blood.

Morphine

See Toxicology, Drug Screen—Blood or Urine.

M

Morphine—Urine

Norm. Negative.

Panic Levels		SI Units
Hydromorphone	>0.1 mg/dL	>0.2 μmol/L
Methadone	>0.2 mg/dL	>10 μmol/L
Morphine	>0.005 mg/dL	0.2 μmol/L

Panic Level Symptoms and Treatment

Symptoms. Bradycardia, itching, hypotension, bradypnea, hypoxia, muscle spasms, pinpoint (miotic) pupils, dilated pupils in mixed drug overdose or severe acidosis, coma.

Treatment

NOTE: Treatment choice(s) depend(s) on client's history and condition and episode history.

1. Administer naloxone 0.4-2 mg IV every 2-3 minutes in adults.
2. Administer naloxone 0.01 mg/kg IV every 2-3 minutes in children.
3. Provide respiratory support.
4. Hemodialysis and peritoneal dialysis will NOT remove morphine. High-permeability dialysis WILL remove morphine.

Increased or Positive. Drug use or abuse (especially heroin).

Description. Morphine is a narcotic analgesic used for pain relief. It relieves anxiety and tension and causes sedation. It is habit-forming and addictive. Overdose may cause bradycardia, hypotension, and severe respiratory and central nervous system depression. Although morphine may be a potentially addictive or abused narcotic, two derivatives of morphine (heroin and codeine) are more commonly abused. Ninety percent of a morphine dose is excreted in the urine within 24 hours of administration, but levels may be detected for up to 7 days after heroin use.

Professional Considerations

Consent form NOT required unless the specimen is collected as legal evidence.

Preparation

1. Supervise the client when obtaining the sample if results may be used as medico-legal evidence.

2. Obtain a sterile, preservative-free plastic or silanized (SiH₄)-glass specimen container.
3. MAY be drawn during hemodialysis.

Procedure

1. Obtain a 25-mL random urine specimen.

Postprocedure Care

1. If the results are to be used as legal evidence, the chain of possession must remain unbroken from the time the specimen is collected until court testimony.

Client and Family Teaching

1. For intentional overdose, refer client and family for crisis intervention.
2. Referrals to appropriate rehabilitation centers and therapeutic community programs should be offered to all addicted clients who may be interested.
3. Behavior and level of consciousness may be significantly altered under the influence of opiates.
4. Signs and symptoms of withdrawal may include agitation, anorexia, anxiety, diaphoresis, disorientation, hallucinations, insomnia, seizures, and tremors.

Factors That Affect Results

1. Poppy seed ingestion may produce false-positive results with the immunoassay method for up to 60 hours after ingestion.
2. Morphine, 10 mg intravenously, is detectable in the urine for up to 84 hours.
3. One measurement method identified endogenous morphine excreted in the urine at a level of 0.71 pg/mL (2.5 fmol/mL, SI units).
4. The use of Stealth adulterant in the urine sample will cause negative results in a positive sample.

Other Data

1. Heroin is rapidly deacetylated to morphine in the human body.

2. Hydromorphone is a semisynthetic phenanthrene derivative structurally similar to morphine. Hydromorphone has an 8-10 times more potent analgesic effect compared to morphine.

3. Codeine is a phenanthrene derivative of opium made by methylation of morphine.

4. Morphine levels can be measured in corpses for several days after death.

5. Infants with hypoxic ischemic encephalopathy have reduced morphine clearance.

6. See also Toxicology, Drug screen—Blood or urine.

Motile Sperm, Wet Mount—Diagnostic

Norm. Negative.

Usage. Reported sexual assault.

Description. Fresh vaginal specimen examined microscopically for presence of sperm.

Professional Considerations

Consent form or verbal consent IS usually required because specimens may be used as legal evidence.

Preparation

1. Obtain a speculum, a wooden Pap-smear stick, normal saline with a 60-mL syringe, a sterile specimen cup, and slides with frosted tips on which to label client information.

2. See Client and Family Teaching.

Procedure

1. Have the specimen collection witnessed if the specimen may be used as legal evidence.

2. Do NOT lubricate the speculum; this may inhibit sperm mobility.

3. Obtain a vaginal specimen by vaginal wash with normal saline or a Pap-smear stick.

4. Avoid cotton-tipped applicators.

Postprocedure Care

1. Write the client's name, the date, exact time of collection, and specimen source on the laboratory requisition. Sign, and have the witness sign, the laboratory requisition.

2. Transport the specimen to the laboratory immediately in a sealed plastic bag marked as legal evidence. All clients handling the specimen should sign and mark the time of receipt on the laboratory requisition.

Client and Family Teaching

1. The client may urinate before the procedure but should not wipe the vulva afterward; this may eliminate sperm.

2. Survivors of sexual assault should be referred to appropriate crisis counseling agencies as well as for gynecologic follow-up study.

3. Referral for HIV testing should be reviewed and offered to all sexual assault victims.

4. Preventive treatment for chlamydiosis, gonorrhea, and syphilis should be provided to all survivors of sexual assault.

5. The option of a postcoital contraceptive should be reviewed with all survivors of sexual assault.

Factors That Affect Results

1. Avoid extreme temperature change or direct sunlight on slides when en route to the laboratory or a legal agency.

2. Delayed delivery of the specimen or use of a condom may decrease the number of viable sperm.

3. Treatment with acetyl carnitine, L-arginine, and ginseng improves sperm motility.

4. High lipopolysaccharides (indicative of stress, bacterial infection, and chronic inflammatory disease) revealed reduction in sperm counts and motility.

5. Overweight and obese men, those with increased body mass index, have lower sperm counts and motility.

Other Data

1. The presence of sperm is not proof of rape because the definition of rape is a legal matter. Low levels do not exclude intercourse.

2. Normal postcoital cervical mucosa reveal at least 10 motile sperm per high-power field.

3. Federal and local laws, regulations, customs, and procedures must be known.

4. A new Sperm Motility Analysis System (SMAS) from Japan has high reliability in estimating sperm concentration and motility.

MPV

See **Mean Platelet Volume**—Blood.

MRA

See **Magnetic Resonance Angiography**—Diagnostic.

MRCP

See **Magnetic Resonance Cholangiopancreatography**—Diagnostic.

MRI

See **Magnetic Resonance Imaging**—Diagnostic.

MRN

See **Magnetic Resonance Neurography**—Diagnostic.

MRSA

See **Methicillin-Resistant** *Staphylococcus aureus*—Culture.

MRU

See **Magnetic Resonance Urography**—Diagnostic.

MSLT

See **Polysomnography**—Diagnostic.

Mucin Clot Test—Specimen

Norm. Firm clot formation with surrounding fluid appearing clear.

Usage. Helps differentiate the types of joint diseases.

Description. The mucin clot test reflects the polymerization of synovial fluid hyaluronate and correlates with viscosity except in acute effusions. Test is normal with degenerative joint disease, rheumatic fever, and systemic lupus erythematosus. An abnormal test demonstrated by a friable clot and turbid surrounding fluid occurs in a wide variety of inflammatory joint diseases such as arthritis of acute bacterial, rheumatoid, septic, or tuberculous origin, and gout. The addition of acetic acid to synovial fluid causes a mucin clot that is graded good, fair, poor, or very poor. If normal, a firm clot forms surrounded by a clear solution. A soft clot formed in a slightly turbid solution is graded as fair. A friable clot formed in a turbid solution and shredding on agitation is graded as poor. No clot formation is graded as very poor.

Professional Considerations
Consent form IS required for synovial fluid aspiration. See Biopsy, Site-specific—Specimen for procedure-specific risks and contraindications.

Preparation
1. Obtain a sterile aspiration tray.
2. Tube: Lavender topped or any sterile tube containing 20 mL of 5% acetic acid.
3. A local anesthetic should be considered before aspiration of synovial fluid.

Procedure
1. Aspirate the synovial fluid into a sterile tube while using sterile technique.
2. Add 5 mL of fluid into 20 mL of 5% acetic acid. Normally a clot will form in 60 seconds.

Postprocedure Care
1. Refrigerate specimens if not tested within 5 hours.

Client and Family Teaching
1. Monitor the site for bleeding, drainage, or inflammation for 24-48 hours.
2. A mild analgesic may be required for pain control.
3. Call the physician for signs of infection at the procedure site: increasing pain, redness, swelling, purulent drainage, or temperature >101 degrees F (>38.3 degrees C).

Factors That Affect Results
1. Lack of synovial fluid aspirate.

Other Data
1. Results are nonspecific alone and are not diagnostic of a single pathologic entity.

Mucin-like Carcinoma–Associated Antigen (MCA-Ag)—Blood

Norm. <11 U/mL.

Increased. Breast cancer, cirrhosis of the liver, gastrointestinal cancer, hepatitis, lung cancer, mammary dysplasia, metastasis, and ovarian cancer.

Decreased. Not clinically significant.

Description. Mucin-like carcinoma–associated antigen (MCA) is a high-molecular-weight glycoprotein product of the MUC1 gene containing many side chains of carbohydrate. Small amounts of MCA are normally produced by epithelial cells that line the respiratory, gastrointestinal, and genitourinary tracts. Exocrine tissues such as mammary, salivary, and sweat glands will also produce small amounts of MCA. MCA can be useful as a serial marker for metastasis, in monitoring therapeutic responses to cancer treatment, in detecting relapse metastasis, in enhancing specificity of bone scintigraphy, and for tumor staging. Several cancer antigens are classified as "mucin-like" because they contain the same core MUC1 gene, with different variations of glycosylation. They include CA 15-5 commonly used for monitoring ovarian cancer, CA 19-9 used for monitoring gastrointestinal cancer, CA 50 used for monitoring lung and gastrointestinal cancers, CA 72-4 used for monitoring gastrointestinal and ovarian cancers, CA 125 used for monitoring breast and ovarian cancers, CA 549, newly identified as a marker for breast cancer, and carcinoma-associated mucin antigens (CA M) 28 and 29. CA M 28 and CA M 29 were found in one study to be superior to both CA 15-5 and CA 549 in detecting metastatic breast cancer disease. None of these markers are useful for detecting small tumor masses or early disease. See also CA 549—Blood.

Professional Considerations
Consent form NOT required.

Preparation
1. Tube: Red topped, red/gray topped, or gold topped for serum samples. Lavender topped for plasma samples.

Procedure
1. Draw a 0.5-mL blood sample.

Postprocedure Care
1. If the specimen is not tested immediately, it can be refrigerated for up to 48 hours. If testing is delayed beyond 48 hours, the specimen should be frozen.

Client and Family Teaching
1. Results are normally available within 72 hours.

Factors That Affect Results
1. MCA is normally elevated in the second trimester of pregnancy and will steadily rise until the postpartum period. Thus in pregnant women, MCA is useful for monitoring breast cancer only in the early stages of pregnancy.
2. When MCA is used to monitor therapeutic response to cancer treatment, it is necessary to consistently measure

either serum or plasma samples; they should not be interchanged.

3. Specimens should be rejected if 48 hours have passed since specimen collection and the specimen is not frozen.

Other Data

1. Performance characteristics of testing have NOT been established.

2. Two thirds of all clients with breast or ovarian cancer have elevated MCA levels.

3. Single MCA levels are NOT helpful when one is screening women for breast cancer.

4. MCA has a 72% sensitivity in detecting reoccurrence of cancer in high-risk populations.

Mucopolysaccharides, Qualitative—Urine

Norm. Negative.

Positive. Atrial myxoma, Beta-glucuronidase syndrome, Hunter's syndrome, Hurler's syndrome, Maroteaux-Lamy syndrome, Morquio's syndrome, Sanfilippo syndrome, and Scheie's syndrome. Drugs include heparin.

Description. Mucopolysaccharidoses are a group of inherited, autosomal recessive diseases. These inborn errors of metabolism result in an increased excretion of urinary mucopolysaccharides because of a lysosomal enzyme deficiency of alpha-L-iduronidase, sulfoiduronate sulfatase, chondroitin sulfate, or arylsulfatase B.

Professional Considerations

Consent form NOT required.

Preparation

1. Obtain a sterile specimen container.

Procedure

1. Obtain a 20-mL random urine specimen in a sterile container without preservative.

Postprocedure Care

1. The specimen is stable for 1 week at 4 degrees C.

Client and Family Teaching

1. Results are normally available within 72 hours.

Factors That Affect Results

1. Increased turbidity of urine causes positive results.

Other Data

1. False-negative results can be as high as 32%.

Multigated Equilibrium Heart Scan (MUGA)—Diagnostic

See **Heart Scan**—Diagnostic.

Multiple Sleep Latency Test

See **Polysomnography**—Diagnostic.

Mumps Antibody—Blood

Norm. Negative or titer <1:8.

Mumps virus antibody IgG: negative, 0.89 index value (IV) or less; equivocal, 0.90-1.09 IV; antibody detected, >1.10 indicates current or past exposure, which indicates immunity in the absence of symptoms.

Mumps virus antibody IgM: negative, <0.90 IV; equivocal, 0.91-1.09 IV; antibody detected, >1.10 indicates current or recent mumps infection.

Mumps specific antibody titers (median in children): 729 IU/mL, with girls having higher titers than boys.

Positive. Viral mumps. Recent infection with the virus is indicated by a fourfold rise in titer between the acute and convalescent specimens, with the ratio of viral (V) to soluble (S) titer increasing.

Description. Mumps (infectious parotitis) is an acute, self-limiting, contagious, febrile disease that causes inflammation of the parotid glands and other salivary glands. Peak infection rates occur in the winter and spring months. Symptoms include fever, malaise, chills, headache, pain below the ear, and swelling of the parotid glands. In clients who have passed puberty, it may cause orchitis, oophoritis, and inflammation of many vital organs. Mumps virus contracted in the first trimester of pregnancy may be associated with a higher risk of congenital anomalies. Maternal immunity lending lasts up to infancy. Mumps is caused by the mumps paramyxovirus that is spread from client to client through droplet spray or direct contact with the saliva of an infected client. This test for IgG and IgM antibodies supports recent mumps virus infection or previous exposure to it. Besides mumps, this virus has been known to cause meningitis and encephalitis.

Professional Considerations

Consent form NOT required.

Preparation

1. Tube: Red topped, red/gray topped, or gold topped.

Procedure

1. Draw a 5-mL blood sample. Label the tube as the acute sample.
2. Repeat the test in 7-14 days, and label the tube as the convalescent sample.

Postprocedure Care

1. Place the specimens on ice.

Client and Family Teaching

1. Return in 1-2 weeks for drawing of a convalescent sample.
2. If mumps is suspected, the client should be isolated for 9 days after parotid gland swelling appears, until the period of communicability has passed. The incubation period is between 16 and 18 days.
3. Infection confers lifelong immunity.
4. There is no specific treatment for mumps after it has been acquired. Vaccination is available for clients who have not had the infection.
5. There is no advantage in delaying MMR2 vaccine from kindergarten to middle school.

Factors That Affect Results

1. Reject hemolyzed or chylous serum specimens.
2. Failure to collect a convalescent sample limits the value of the acute sample results.
3. Low levels of IgM antibody sometimes persist for up to 1 year after mumps infection.
4. Lower mumps antibody titers found in HLA-DQB1*0303 alleles.
5. Children treated for ALL (leukemia) respond less to mumps vaccine than to diphtheria and tetanus toxoid vaccines.

Other Data

1. Increased hemagglutination-inhibition titer indicates either mumps or another parainfluenza virus.

Muramidase (Lysozyme)—Serum and Urine

Norm.

		SI Units	
Serum			
Gel diffusion assay	0.4-1.3 mg/dL	4-13 μg/mL	4-13 mg/L
Nephelometric	0.36-0.78 mg/dL	3.6-7.8 μg/mL	3.6-7.8 mg/L
Radial immunodiffusion	0.9-1.7 mg/dL	9-17 μg/mL	
Radioimmunoassay	0.46 ± 0.08 mg/dL	4.6 ± 0.8 μg/mL	4.6 ± 0.8 mg/L
Turbidimetric	0.27-0.93 mg/dL	2.7-9.3 μg/mL	2.7-9.3 mg/L
Urine			
Random		<3 μg/mL	0-2.9 mg/L
24-hour			1.3-3.6 mg/24 hours

Increased Serum and Urine Levels. Desquamative interstitial pneumonia, glomerulonephritis, Hodgkin's disease, leukemia (acute myelomonocytic, chronic myelomonocytic [CMML], chronic myelocytic [CML]), nephrosis, pleurisy (tuberculous type), pyelonephritis, renal insufficiency (severe), renal transplant rejection, urinary tract infection.

Increased Serum Levels. Anemia (megaloblastic), atherosclerotic heart disease, Crohn's disease, infection (acute bacterial), sarcoidosis, ulcerative colitis, tuberculosis.

Decreased. Neutropenia secondary to bone marrow hypoplasia.

Description. Muramidase (lysozyme) is an enzyme present in numerous body fluids (blood, saliva, sweat, tears, urine) and renal cells that is released into the bloodstream as a result of degradation of granulocytes and monocytes. Thus it is a marker of mononuclear phagocytic cells. It normally functions in the process of gram-positive bacterial destruction. The proximal tubule of the kidney is the site of catabolism and reabsorption. Muramidase measurement may be used to differentiate lymphatic leukemia from myelogenous and monocytic leukemias because muramidase is not produced when lymphocytes are degraded. Because levels drop when myelogenous leukemia and monocytic leukemia are successfully treated, muramidase can also provide an indicator of disease remission progress. The level of serum lysozyme has also been used as an indicator of central nervous system involvement associated with leukemia. Urine muramidase is excreted in renal tubular disease but not in glomerular disease. With normally functioning kidneys, serum levels must exceed three times the normal range before the enzyme will appear in the urine. However, in renal damage, serum levels may be normal in the presence of elevated urine levels.

Professional Considerations
Consent form NOT required.

Preparation
1. Tube: Red topped, red/gray topped, green topped, or gold topped or lavender topped.
2. Urine test should be prescheduled with the laboratory. Obtain a sterile, preservative-free plastic specimen container.

Procedure
1. Draw a 4-mL blood sample or collect a 5-mL random urine specimen.

Postprocedure Care
1. Separate the serum and freeze it immediately in a plastic vial on dry ice.
2. Freeze the urine specimen on dry ice if the specimen is not tested immediately.

Client and Family Teaching
1. Blood test results are normally available within 1 week. Urine results are normally available within 3 days.

Factors That Affect Results
1. Urine not maintained on ice after collection invalidates the results.
2. Clients who are menstruating should be rescheduled for the urine test. Blood in the urine may produce falsely elevated results.
3. Bacteria in the urine may produce falsely low results.

Other Data
1. Urinary lysozyme is not useful in detecting pre-eclampsia.

Muscle Biopsy—Specimen

Norm. Interpretation by a pathologist is required.

Usage. Cytochrome oxidase deficiency, Danon disease, dermatomyositis, glycogen storage disease II (Pompe's disease), hereditary myopathy with early respiratory failure (HMERF), Kennedy's disease, muscular dystrophy (Becker's, Duchenne's, oculopharyngeal), myalgia, myopathy (mitochondrial, myofibrillar), polymyositis, primary thymic carcinoma, neurogenic atrophy, pain (muscle and bone), trichinosis, and vasculitis.

Description. Microscopic examination of a piece of muscle for evaluation, diagnosis, or classification of muscular disease. The technique may be done via open muscle biopsy or via percutaneous fine-needle aspiration muscle biopsy. The presence of hypercontracted fibers must be differentiated for cause. If accompanied by inflammation, hypercontracted fibers are indicative of pathology. If no inflammation is present, hypercontracted fibers are attributed to strenuous exercise before the biopsy procedure. The quadriceps femoris is recommended for generalized diseases, and the gastrocnemius is suggested as a distal muscle for biopsy. The deltoid is not suitable for enzyme histochemistry. Optimally a specimen should be taken from a muscle with known disease that has NOT reached end-stage atrophy.

Professional Considerations
Consent form IS required.

Risks
Bleeding, bruising, hematoma, infection.
Contraindications
Anticoagulant therapy, bleeding disorders, thrombocytopenia.

Preparation
1. Tests that may be helpful before biopsy include serum creatine kinase (CK) level, 24-hour urine for creatine and serum creatinine levels, erythrocyte sedimentation rate (ESR), serum aldolase level, and thyroid profile.
2. Obtain a biopsy tray, sterile drapes, a sterile jar of sterile 0.9% saline, a sterile specimen container of formalin, and a sterile container of glutaraldehyde.
3. Just before beginning the procedure, take a "time out" to verify the correct client, procedure, and site.

Procedure
1. Obtain a biopsy specimen, using sterile procedure. Biopsies for simple histologic examination may be obtained using thin-needle aspiration. Tissue should be obtained from a relaxed, noncontracted isometric muscle. Fine-needle aspiration may also be used for ocular muscle biopsy. To estimate capillary supply, a sample sufficient to yield at least 50 muscle fibers is recommended.

2. If histochemistry is desired, do not use epinephrine with lidocaine or procaine in securing the biopsy.
Postprocedure Care
1. Place the biopsy specimen in a sterile jar containing sterile saline. For histopathologic evaluation, place the specimen in formalin, and for electron microscopy, submit a small or minced specimen that is placed into glutaraldehyde.
2. Label the container with the client's name and room number, date, and site of specimen collection.
3. The specimen should be delivered to the pathology department within 30 minutes. If the specimen cannot be delivered within 30 minutes, freeze it quickly, using liquid nitrogen.
4. Turnaround time is between 48 hours and 3 weeks.

Client and Family Teaching
1. Call a physician for signs of infection at the biopsy site over the next 24-48 hours: increasing pain, redness, swelling, purulent drainage, or for temperature >101 degrees F (38.3 degrees C).
2. Mild pain should be expected at the biopsy site. Severe pain should be reported to a physician.
3. A mild analgesic may be required for pain control.
4. Monitor for signs and symptoms of infection until the site is healed.

Factors That Affect Results
1. Results are invalidated if the wrong fixative is used, if the specimen dries out, or if the specimen is received without a label.
2. Muscle that has been recently injected or undergone electromyographic studies may not be suitable for microscopic examination.

Other Data
1. Specimens for histologic examination are commonly stained with hematoxylin-eosin. This allows for the assessment of inflammatory processes.

Muscle Profile
See Aldolase—Serum; Aspartate Aminotransferase—Serum; Creatine Kinase—Serum; Differential Leukocyte Count—Peripheral Blood; Lactate Dehydrogenase—Blood; Myoglobin—Serum; Thyroid Test: Thyroxine—Blood; Thyroid Test: Thyroxine Free—Serum; Thyroid Test: Triiodothyronine—Blood; Thyroid Test: Free Thyroxine Index—Serum.

Mycobacteria, Cerebrospinal Fluid

See **Cerebrospinal Fluid, Routine**—Culture and Cytology.

Mycoplasma Enzyme Immunoassay

Norm. Current technology does not provide a recommended reference standard. There are inconsistencies in various test methodologies, laboratories, and manufacturers.

Reference ranges are often determined by individual labs for each run. Interpretations of ARUP laboratories are in the following table.

M. pneumoniae Antibody	Acute Specimen	Convalescent Specimen	ARUP Interpretation
IgG	≤0.20 U/L	>0.32 U/L	Current or recent infection
	≤0.20 U/L	≤0.32 U/L	Antibody change not significant
	>0.32 U/L	<0.20 U/L	Indicates past infection
IgM	<0.76 U/L		Negative
	0.77-0.95 U/L		Low positive; collect convalescent specimen in 2 weeks
	≥0.96 U/L		Positive

Usage. Pneumonia, pertussis. Two *M. pneumoniae*–specific antibody levels, IgG and IgM, are typically used to evaluate the occurrence of current or past *M. pneumoniae* infection. The immune status of an individual can be determined with a single specimen. The use of paired samples, acute and convalescent, aids in the confirmation of the diagnosis of a recent or current infection. Testing should be done when clinical symptoms are present or exposure is suspected.

Description. *M. pneumoniae* are aerobic bacteria, unique in that they do not have cell walls. *M. pneumoniae* infection may be asymptomatic or produce an upper respiratory tract disease or atypical pneumonia. *M. pneumoniae* is transmitted from an infected person in close contact with another person through respiratory droplets, and thus is a common cause of community-acquired pneumonia. Signs and symptoms include nonproductive cough, sore throat, low-grade fever, malaise, middle-ear involvement, scattered rales and rhonchi, and cervical adenopathy. Extrapulmonary symptoms, such as gastrointestinal symptoms and skin rashes, may also occur. *M. pneumoniae* infection is difficult to differentiate from viral diseases by clinical symptoms alone. Differentiation of the organism is important because the typical empirical treatment of

respiratory tract infections with beta-lactam antibiotics is not effective with *M. pneumoniae*. This test involves an IgG and an IgM enzyme immunoassay and is often carried out in conjunction with a polymerase chain reaction test on a nasopharyngeal sample. Together, these findings represent the most sensitive, specific, and rapid diagnosis for *M. pneumoniae*.

Professional Considerations
Consent form NOT required.

Preparation
1. Tube: Red topped, lavender topped, green topped, red/gray topped, or yellow topped.
2. Obtain a specimen swab if a nasopharyngeal specimen will also be tested.

Procedure
1. Collect 6 mL of blood (2-4 mL for children). Label sample clearly as "acute" or "convalescent." Acute samples should be collected as soon as possible after the onset of symptoms and no later than several days after onset. The second, or convalescent, sample should be collected 14 to 21 days after the acute specimen was collected.
2. Obtain a nasopharyngeal specimen using the swab.
3. Transport to laboratory immediately. Unacceptable samples include those that

are severely lipemic, hemolyzed, or contaminated.
4. Paired samples of acute and convalescent samples should be run together.

Postprocedure Care

1. Stability of sample after separation from clot: ambient (2 to 8 degrees C), 2 days; refrigerated (4 degrees C), 2 weeks; frozen, 1 year. Avoid repeated freeze-thaw cycles.

Client and Family Teaching

1. Results are normally available in 3-5 days.

Factors That Affect Results

1. A single positive serum result indicates prior exposure to *M. pneumoniae*. The antibody level in a single specimen does not typically indicate disease severity.
2. *M. pneumoniae*–specific IgM antibodies become elevated 7 days after the onset of symptoms, and levels peak at 2-3 weeks. A single elevated IgM level is often used to support the diagnosis of a *M. pneumoniae* infection; however, low IgM levels can remain for years after an infection. The evaluation of paired sera—acute and convalescent samples—for an increasing IgM level is recommended if a more definitive diagnosis is necessary. The absence of *M. pneumoniae*–specific IgM antibody in the blood 10-20 days after the onset of symptoms has strong negative predictive value for the presence of a current *M. pneumoniae* infection.
3. *M. pneumoniae*–specific IgG antibody levels increase 7-14 days after the onset of symptoms and can remain elevated for years. Use of paired IgG levels—acute and convalescent—or comparison of IgG levels to IgM levels is recommended for definitive diagnosis of acute *Mycoplasma* infection.

4. False-positive results may occur in clients with *Ureaplasma*, *Mycoplasma hominis*, *Mycoplasma genitalium*, pancreatitis, bacterial meningitis, and other acute inflammatory disease. The prevalence of *M. pneumoniae* IgG antibodies in the general population is high.
5. False-negative results may occur if samples are drawn too early after the onset. Some individuals may never generate detectable antibody levels. Decreased production of specific IgM antibodies is associated with increased age and reinfection with *M. pneumoniae*.
6. Results are invalidated if the specimen is severely lipemic, icteric, or hemolyzed; if the specimen is contaminated; or if the specimen was not kept refrigerated.

Other Data

1. *M. pneumoniae* infection can have a long incubation period, and reinfection may occur.
2. Elevated cold agglutinins are associated with but not specific to *M. pneumoniae* infections. Other associated lab data include elevated WBC count (exceeds 10,000/μL in approximately 30% of cases) and greatly elevated erythrocyte sedimentation rates. Culturing this bacterium is difficult because the organism requires special growth media and the incubation time is 5-20 days, which is 6-20 times slower than that of most bacteria.
3. *M. pneumoniae*–specific IgM and IgG antibodies play an important role in the ability of immunocompetent individuals to eliminate the infection in 10-14 days with the use of antimicrobial agents. Macrolides or tetracyclines are generally effective in reducing the duration of the illness.
4. See also *Mycoplasma* titer—Blood.

Mycoplasma Titer—Blood

Norm. Negative or complement fixation (CF) <1:64 and Seradyn Color Vue (SCV) agglutination <1:320.

Positive. Diarrhea and mycoplasmal pneumonia.

Description. *Mycoplasma* organisms are of the pleuropneumonia type that can pass through tiny bacteriologic filters, the smallest ranging from 125 to 250 nm. *Mycoplasma* bacteria are the smallest free-living organisms, characteristically have no cell wall, and are dependent for survival on a host, which is most commonly a child. The mechanisms by which *Mycoplasma* interact with the immune defenses of the host are elusive. Commonly causing upper respiratory tract infection in children, newer research is linking *M. pneumoniae* together with *Chlamydia pneumoniae* as significant causative organisms in pneumonias of the lower respiratory tract in those under 5 years of age. There is no quick method for pinpointing the organism as a source of infection. Therefore diagnosis and treatment are often based on clinical symptoms, with the *Mycoplasma* serologic titer, immunoassay, or polymerase chain reaction.

Professional Considerations
Consent form NOT required.

Preparation
1. Tube: Red topped, red/gray topped, or gold topped.

Procedure
1. Draw a 3-mL blood sample.

Postprocedure Care
1. Draw a convalescent sample of blood 10-14 days later.

Client and Family Teaching
1. Return in 10-14 days to have another blood sample drawn from the vein to obtain accurate results.

Factors That Affect Results
1. False-positive results may occur in clients with acute pancreatitis or streptococcal infection.
2. A diet of green, leafy vegetables may produce false-positive results.

Other Data
1. High titers are not significant for recent infection, because antibodies may persist >1 year and repeated infections occur.
2. Mycoplasmal pneumonia is treated with tetracycline or erythromycin.
3. Serologic confirmation is desirable, because *Mycoplasma* is difficult to culture. See *Mycoplasma* enzyme immunoassay—Blood.

Myelin Basic Protein

See Cerebrospinal Fluid, Heparin Binding Protein, Myelin Basic Protein, Oligoclonal Bands, Protein, and Protein Electrophoresis—Specimen.

Myelogram—Diagnostic

Norm. Normal cervical, lumbar, or thoracic myelogram. Normal spinal subarachnoid space with no obstructions.

Usage. Arachnoiditis, back pain, disk rupture, spinal problems (especially degenerative), accidental injury, tumors of the spine, degenerative disease of the spine, nerve plexus lesions, cancer metastasis to the spine.

Description. Myelography is a radiographic study of the spinal cord and nerve roots by using contrast dye, contrast oil, or air injected by way of spinal needle into the spinal subarachnoid space. Myelography use is declining because magnetic resonance imaging (MRI) can usually match the findings of myelography with less risk to the client. Myelography is more often reserved for conditions that cannot be evaluated via MRI or CT, such as weight-bearing flexion

and extension views, or walking views. Use of oil contrast has the disadvantage of tissue irritation and poor absorption by the subarachnoid spaces. Air contrast may be used instead of oil, but in this case, tomography is essential to improve visualization.

Professional Considerations
Consent form IS required.

Risks
Allergic reaction to dye (itching, hives, rash, tight feeling in the throat, shortness of breath, bronchospasm, anaphylaxis, death); contrast-induced renal failure; intramedullary cord injection, seizure. Multiple sclerosis may be worsened by this procedure.

Contraindications
Previous allergy to dye, iodine, or shellfish; renal insufficiency; bleeding abnormalities

or clients receiving anticoagulants; increased intracranial pressure; low back pain; spinal deformities; infections near the puncture site; pregnancy (because of radioactive iodine crossing the blood-placental barrier).

Preparation

1. Sedation or narcotic analgesia should be considered before this procedure.
2. Shave the lumbar area if necessary.
3. Obtain a lumbar puncture tray, sterile drapes, 1%-2% lidocaine (Xylocaine), iodized Pantopaque oil or water-soluble iodine metrizamide contrast medium, antiseptic, and sterile gauze.
4. If metrizamide is to be used as a contrast dye, discontinue the use of phenothiazines 48 hours before the procedure.
5. Obtain baseline vital signs.
6. Have emergency equipment readily available.
7. If increased intracranial pressure is suspected, a CT of the brain should be performed before lumbar puncture to rule out this condition.
8. See Client and Family Teaching.
9. Just before beginning the procedure, take a "time out" to verify the correct client, procedure, and site.

Procedure

1. The client is positioned on the side with the knees drawn up toward the abdomen and the chin on the chest for the lumbar puncture.
2. The lumbar puncture is verified by fluoroscopy.
3. Spinal fluid is generally obtained for analysis.
4. 5-15 mL of iodized Pantopaque oil dye or water-soluble iodine metrizamide contrast is injected into the subarachnoid space in the lumbar area or into the cisterna magna.
5. The client is tilted to maneuver oil up and down the spine.
6. Radiographic films are taken.
7. Oil is removed by aspiration after the procedure.

Postprocedure Care

1. Cleanse the puncture site with antiseptic and cover with a dry, sterile dressing.

2. See Lumbar puncture—Diagnostic.
3. Do not administer phenothiazines for nausea or vomiting if water-soluble contrast was used.
4. A blood patch may be used for unrelieved headache after the procedure.
5. Results are normally available within 48 hours.

Client and Family Teaching

1. The client should fast from food and fluids for 4-8 hours before the procedure.
2. If you have a seizure disorder, check with your doctor about disconuing anti-seizure medications prior to the myelogram.
3. Other drugs that are usually stopped 24-48 hours before myelography include long-acting anticoagulants, antipsychotics, antidepressants, and diabetes drugs such as metformin. Phenothiazines are discontinued when certain contrast material will be used.
4. The procedure takes 1 hour.
5. Review activity limitations.
6. Drink 6-8 glasses of water or other fluids each day for 2 days (when not contraindicated) to hasten removal of any contrast medium.
7. Potential side effects or complications include arachnoiditis, headache, nausea and vomiting, seizures, spinal infection, subarachnoid bleeding, and tingling at the puncture site.
8. Observe the puncture site for bleeding, hematoma, or swelling for 24-48 hours after the procedure.
9. A mild analgesic may be required for pain control.
10. Monitor the lumbar puncture site for signs and symptoms of infection until the site is healed.

Factors That Affect Results

1. Conditions such as convulsions, pain, stiffness of the neck, and stupor may interfere with the procedure.
2. Severe kyphosis or scoliosis may prohibit completion of this procedure.

Other Data

1. Dye usage affects preparation and postprocedure care.

Myoglobin, Qualitative—Urine

Norm. Negative or <20 ng/mL.

Positive. Acute alcohol intoxication with delirium tremens, acute or chronic muscular disease, barbiturate toxicity, burns (severe), diabetic acidosis, glycogen and lipid storage diseases, hyperthermia, hypokalemia, hypophosphatemia, hypothermia, muscular dystrophy, myocardial infarction, poisoning, polymyositis, renal failure, rhabdomyolysis, surgical procedure, trauma, and viral or bacterial infection. Herbs or natural remedies include licorice (*Glycyrrhiza glabra*), which can cause intoxication.

Description. Myoglobin is a heme-containing, oxygen-binding, low-molecular-weight protein similar to hemoglobin that is exclusive to striated and nonstriated skeletal or cardiac muscle. It functions in short-term oxygen storage, carrying the muscle from one contraction to the next. It is released into the interstitial fluid as early as 3 hours after any muscle injury including a myocardial infarct and remains detected in the urine for up to 7 days later.

Professional Considerations
Consent form NOT required.

Preparation
1. Obtain a sterile specimen container.

Procedure
1. Collect a 10-mL random urine specimen in a sterile plastic container without preservatives.
2. Collection time should be early morning when possible.

Postprocedure Care
1. Specimens should be refrigerated.

Client and Family Teaching
1. Results are normally available within 72 hours.

Factors That Affect Results
1. False-negative results are likely if the test is used for screening.
2. The presence of hypochlorite or microbial peroxidase or other oxidizing contaminants may cause false-positive results.
3. Clients should not receive isotopes 7 days before testing.
4. High concentrations of vitamin C decrease the sensitivity of this test.

Other Data
1. Because myoglobin is excreted by the kidney, renal function should be assessed.
2. Serum levels are preferred to urine levels when one is obtaining myoglobin values.
3. See also Myoglobin—Serum.

Myoglobin—Serum

Norm. Normal levels may be higher in men compared to women but increase in both sexes with age.

	Serum Myoglobin	SI Units
Male	28-72 ng/mL	1.43-3.67 nmol/L
Female	25-58 ng/mL	1.28-2.96 nmol/L

Usage. In combination with other tests, helps diagnose myocardial ischemia; serial values are used to monitor for reinfarct, success of thrombolytic treatment, and myocardial injury during open-heart surgery.

Increased. Acute alcohol intoxication with delirium tremens, acute coronary syndrome (myoglobin ≥200 ng/mL predictor of all cause mortality), after cardioversion (possible increase), after open-heart surgery, angina (possible increase), burns (severe), cocaine users, congestive heart failure (possible increase), dermatomyositis, divers during competitive breath holding ("packing blackout"), dysrhythmias (possible increase), glycogen and lipid storage diseases, hyperthermia, hypothermia, muscular dystrophy, myocardial infarction (increased levels are detected 2-3 hours after injury, peak at 6-9 hours, and return to baseline level within 36 hours), polymyositis, renal failure, rhabdomyolysis, shock, skeletal muscle injury or extreme skeletal muscle exertion, surgical procedure, systemic lupus erythematosus (SLE), trauma, and viral or bacterial infection. Drugs include ethyl alcohol (ethanol) (heavy use). Herbs or natural remedies include licorice (*Glycyrrhiza glabra*), which can cause intoxication.

Description. Myoglobin is a heme-containing, oxygen-binding protein similar to hemoglobin that is exclusive to striated and nonstriated skeletal or cardiac muscle. It functions as short-term oxygen storage, carrying the muscle from one contraction to the next. It is released into the interstitial fluid with elevated serum levels detected as early as 30-60 minutes after a myocardial infarct or damage to any muscle tissue. Serum myoglobin is generally detected earlier than traditional cardiac enzymes (total creatinine kinase [CK] or isoenzyme creatinine kinase–MB [CK-MB]). Because myoglobin is contained in both skeletal and cardiac muscle, it is not used alone to diagnose myocardial infarction. Tests used in combination with myoglobin for this purpose include troponin and CK-MB, with or without carbonic anhydrase III (a marker for skeletal muscle damage). Serum myoglobin may lack specificity in the diagnosis of myocardial infarct. Elevated levels are also observed after angina, chest trauma, cocaine use, electrical accidents, exercise, intramuscular injection, muscular injury of any type, and renal failure. Within 8 hours of symptoms, myoglobin specificity is 97.9% for acute MI, as opposed to CK-MB, which has 100% specificity.

Professional Considerations
Consent form NOT required.

Preparation
1. Tube: Red, green, lavender, or pink topped.
2. Clients should have no isotopes 7 days before testing.

Procedure
1. Draw a 2-mL blood sample.

Postprocedure Care
1. Specimens should be refrigerated.
2. Specimens may be frozen and stored for up to 2 years.

Client and Family Teaching
1. Results are normally available within 48 hours.

Factors That Affect Results
1. Hemolysis of the specimen invalidates the results.
2. False-negative results are likely if the test is used for screening.
3. Serum levels must be obtained within 2-12 hours of the onset of symptoms of a myocardial infarct to be useful in assessing myocardial injury.
4. Hypertriglyceridemia or postprandial specimens may affect the results.
5. Serum myoglobin levels have been found to increase proportionally with the size of muscle damage.
6. Glomerular filtration rate influences myoglobin when concentration is >40.1 ng/mL.

Other Data
1. Increased levels should be correlated with client signs and symptoms.
2. Myoglobin can be measured by a variety of approaches, including fluorometric measurement, latex agglutination, and nephelometric and turbidimetric assay. Each approach has its own reference range.
3. IM injections, bicycle exercise, and cardiac catheterization should NOT increase levels.
4. Patients with rhabdomyolysis with blood myoglobin >3865 ng/mL are at high risk for acute renal failure.
5. As myoglobin increases in critically ill patients so does mortality. Values >500 microg/L have 82% mortality.
6. See also Myoglobin, Qualitative—Urine.

Mysoline
See **Primidone**—Serum.

NAP
See **Leukocyte Alkaline Phosphatase**—Blood.

Narcotics Drug Screen

See Toxicology, Drug Screen—Blood or Urine.

Nasal Culture, Swab

See Culture, Routine.

Nasopharyngeal Culture, Swab

See Culture, Routine.

Natriuretic Peptides, Atrial (ANP, Atrial Natriuretic Hormone, Atrial Natriuretic Factor), Pro-Brain Natriuretic Peptide (NT-Pro-BNP), B-Type (BNP, Beta), C-Type (CNP)—Plasma

Norm

	Immunofluorescence Assay	SI Units
ANP		
Adults	20-77 pg/mL	20-77 ng/L
Children		
10-15 years	>55 pg/mL	>55 ng/L
Infants		
3 days	165-185 pg/mL	165-185 ng/L
1 week	165-185 pg/mL	165-185 ng/L
10 days	98-122 pg/mL	98-122 ng/L
30-60 days	52-72 pg/mL	52-72 ng/L
BNP	>100 pg/mL is diagnostic of congestive heart failure	
Male		
<45 years	<25 pg/mL	<25 ng/L
45-54 years	<4 pg/mL	<4 ng/L
55-64 years	<73 pg/mL	<73 ng/L
65-74 years	<64 pg/mL	<64 ng/L
≥75 years	<79 pg/mL	<79 ng/L
Female		
<45 years	<48 pg/mL	<48 ng/L
45-54 years	<73 pg/mL	<73 ng/L
55-64 years	<82 pg/mL	<82 ng/L
65-74 years	<96 pg/mL	<96 ng/L
≥75 years	<181 pg/mL	<181 ng/L
NT-Pro-BNP		
≤75 years	≤124 pg/mL	<124 ng/L
>74 years	≤449 pg/mL	<449 ng/L
CNP	Norms not established. Consult reference range provided with test results.	

Usage. Helps distinguish heart failure from other causes of dyspnea; under investigation for usefulness in assessing prognosis for long-term survival of clients with heart failure and acute myocardial infarction.

Increased ANP. Atrial fibrillation, congestive heart failure (acute), cardiovascular disease accompanied by increased preload, cerebral salt-wasting syndrome, dysrhythmia (paroxysmal atrial tachycardia), hyperthyroidism, lactate-induced panic attacks, left ventricular enlargement, myocardial ischemia, myotonic dystrophy, pacemaker (atrial), sleep apnea, SIADHS, small cell lung cancer, subarachnoid hemorrhage, ventricular pacing.

Increased BNP and NT-Pro-BNP. Cardiovascular disease accompanied by increased preload, cerebral salt-wasting syndrome, congestive heart failure (acute), hyperthyroidism, lactate-induced panic attacks, left ventricular enlargement, myocardial ischemia, myotonic dystrophy, pacemaker (atrial), renal failure, SIADHS, sleep apnea, small cell lung cancer, subarachnoid hemorrhage, ventricular pacing.

Increased CNP. Has been found to increase in response to local inflammation.

Decreased ANP. Congestive heart failure (chronic). Drugs include prazosin, urapidil, and xipamide.

Decreased BNP and NT-Pro-BNP. BNP has been found to return to normal levels after successful treatment of volume overload.

Decreased CNP. Not established.

Description. Natriuretic peptides are substances produced by the body that function in regulation of fluid balance through feedback mechanisms from and to the renin-angiotensin-aldosterone system. *Atrial natriuretic peptide* (ANP) is released by cardiac cells in the atria of the heart, and brain or *B-type natriuretic peptide* (BNP) is released by cardiac cells in the ventricles of the heart. Both ANP and BNP are secreted in response to the stimulation of the heart's volume receptors by the stretch from increased blood volume. ANP is also released in response to atrial fibrillation and supraventricular tachycardia. ANP and BNP reduce renal reabsorption of sodium, thus having diuretic and antihypertensive effects. They also reduce blood pressure by blocking the secretion of aldosterone and renin and inhibiting the action of angiotensin II. The net effect is reduced preload, afterload, and blood volume, and a reduction in systemic hypertension. Measurement of ANP and BNP helps identify subnormal levels as a cause of chronic congestive heart failure. *Pro-brain natriuretic peptide* (NT-Pro-BNP) is secreted by the heart's left ventricle, is more stable in serum samples, and is more

sensitive but less specific than BNP for CHF. *C-type natriuretic peptide* (CNP) is produced in the brain, by most of the major endocrine glands, and locally from endothelial tissue and from macrophages; CNP is not considered to be a cardiac peptide. CNP is thought to contribute to local neuroendocrine regulation.

Professional Considerations
Consent form NOT required.

Preparation
1. Tube: Lavender or pink topped. Also obtain ice.
2. For dialysis clients, collect the sample AFTER dialysis and on the same day of the week as prior samples.

Procedure
1. Draw a 5-mL blood sample.

Postprocedure Care
1. Place the specimen immediately on ice and deliver it to the laboratory for immediate spinning.

Client and Family Teaching
1. Results are normally available within 24 hours.

Factors That Affect Results
1. Results are invalidated if the sample is hemolyzed or is not kept on ice until it is spun and frozen.
2. Females >75 years have a greater prevalence of false-positive results.

Other Data
1. Secretion of ANP and vasopressin by small cell lung cancer may be a contributing factor to hyponatremia.
2. Natriuretic peptides are relatively new in medical knowledge. ANP was first identified in 1984 and BNP was not identified until 1988.
3. Recombinant natriuretic peptides such as nesiritide (Natrecor) are being used for treatment of acute decompensated congestive heart failure.
4. Prosen et al (2011) found that adding lung ultrasound to the Pro-BNP test provides high diagnostic accuracy for differentiating the underlying cause of dyspnea. When the comet tail sign is present on lung ultrasound, heart failure can be excluded when the NT ProBNP in a client with a history of heart failure is greater than 1,000 pg/mL.

Near-Infrared Spectroscopy

See Transcranial, Near-Infrared Spectroscopy—Diagnostic.

Needle Aspiration—Diagnostic

Norm. Nonmalignant, or negative.

Usage. Essential to diagnosing malignancies and benign growths. Also used to evaluate tissue for reaction to hormones; these results assist in selecting appropriate therapy for cancer. Help diagnose actinomycosis, HIV lymphadenopathy, and mycetoma.

Description. Surgical procedure in which a sample of body tissue or fluid is removed transcutaneously through a needle and then examined microscopically for abnormal cells or tested in a hormone receptor assay. This procedure can be performed on an ambulatory surgery basis under local anesthesia and can help prevent unnecessary surgery.

Professional Considerations
Consent form IS required.

Risks
Infection at needle aspiration site, mediastinitis.

Contraindications
Previous allergy to local anesthetic. Cutaneous infection at site, platelet count of less than 100,000/mm^3, prothrombin time longer than 15 seconds.

Preparation
1. Obtain 1%-2% lidocaine (Xylocaine) for local anesthesia, a cutting needle, a sterile cup with normal saline, and a heparinized tube.
2. Just before beginning the procedure, take a "time out" to verify the correct client, procedure, and site.

Procedure
1. Position the client supine.
2. Under local anesthesia, a cutting needle (such as a Cope's needle or Vim-Silverman needle) is inserted into the suspected area, and a core of tissue is removed and placed into normal saline, or fluid is aspirated and placed into a heparinized tube.

Postprocedure Care
1. Apply a dry, sterile dressing to the site.
2. Label the specimens and transport them to the laboratory promptly.
3. Assess vital signs every 15 minutes × 2.
4. Monitor the site every 2 hours × 3 for bleeding, inflammation, or drainage.
5. Results are normally available in 48-72 hours.

Client and Family Teaching
1. Monitor for drainage and inflammation for 24-48 hours.
2. A mild analgesic may be required for pain control.
3. Call the physician for signs of infection at the procedure site: increasing pain, redness, swelling, purulent drainage, or for temperature >101 degrees F (38.3 degrees C).

Factors That Affect Results
1. Failure to obtain adequate sample(s) or a sample from a nonsuspect site or to properly prepare the smear can result in a false-negative finding.

Other Data
1. Permanent microscopic sections are preferred to frozen sections because permanent sections have more clarity.
2. A negative result does not always exclude the diagnosis of cancer.

Neisseria gonorrhoeae Smear—Specimen

Norm. Negative.

Positive. Gonorrhea.

Description. *Neisseria gonorrhoeae* is a pyogenic, gram-negative, oxidase-positive cocci that is an obligate parasite of humans.

N. gonorrhoeae inhabits the mucous membranes of the genital tract, causing gonorrhea. Symptoms include dysuria, fever, pharyngitis, peripheral skin lesions, proctitis, and purulent urethral discharge. It may also cause inflammation of any of the mucous membranes of the body. Females are often asymptomatic. Left untreated, gonorrhea leads to skin lesions, arthritis, meningitis, and reproductive problems. *N. gonorrhoeae* is most often found in the urethra of males and the endocervical canal of females. This test is performed using nucleic acid amplification, a method with improved sensitivity and higher cost than older methods. It is often performed in conjunction with testing for *Chlamydia trachomatis*, another sexually transmitted organism.

Professional Considerations
Consent form NOT required.

Preparation
1. Determine the potential infected area(s): anus, cervix, conjunctivae, endocervix, skin lesion, throat, and urethra.
2. Wait 1 hour after urination to collect urethral specimens.
3. Obtain a wooden scraper or swab and a glass slide with frosted edges.

Procedure
1. Obtain a sterile microbiologic smear. With a swab, swab the potential infected area for 10 seconds.
2. Apply to a glass slide and allow to air-dry.
3. Label the slide.

Postprocedure Care
1. Place the air-dried slide in a sterile container and send it to the laboratory.
2. Results are normally available immediately or within 24 hours.

Client and Family Teaching
1. The client should be referred for medical follow-up examination after the treatment is concluded. Repeat cultures or smears may be necessary to assess response to treatment.
2. The use of condoms significantly reduces the risk of sexually transmitted diseases.

3. Gonorrhea infection is treatable with antibiotics.
4. If results are positive, provide the client with the appropriate information on sexually transmitted diseases:
   a. Notify all sexual partners from the previous 90 days to be tested for gonorrhea infection.
   b. Do not have sexual relations until the physician confirms that the infection is gone.
   c. Referral for HIV testing should be reviewed and offered to all clients.
5. Do not use feminine hygiene sprays or douche during treatment.
6. Wear underpants and pantyhose that have a cotton lining in the crotch.
7. Take showers instead of tub baths until the infection is gone.

Factors That Affect Results
1. False-positive results occur in 50% of endocervical specimens because normal flora have similar morphologic appearance.
2. Insufficient specimen volume.

Other Data
1. DNA probe assay (Gen-Probe, San Diego) is an alternative test that can be used to diagnose *N. gonorrhoeae*.
2. A culture is necessary to confirm diagnosis.
3. *N. gonorrhoeae* is 37%-100% resistant to fluoroquinolone (ciprofloxacin, ofloxacin, lomefloxacin) treatment and 71%-79% to penicillin treatment.
4. High levels of azithromycin resistance to *N. gonorrhoeae* found in the United Kingdom results from mutation A2059G of the 23S rRNA gene.
5. Effective treatments include injectable sepctinomycin and ceftriaxone (most reliable).
6. See also Genital, *Neisseria gonorrhoeae*—Culture.

Nephrotomography—Diagnostic

Norm. Normal kidney size, shape, and position.

Usage. Adrenal tumor, carcinoma of the kidney, nephrolithiasis, polycystic kidney disease (diagnostic when used in conjunction with ultrasound), and renal laceration.

Description. Radiographic examination of a single plane of renal tissue. It is a routine procedure performed during urography. Delineates renal borders and aids in distinguishing cystic from solid lesions. Precisely locating the kidneys, however, can be difficult. Nephrotomography may be performed with excretory urography (intravenous pyelography). The use of this test for detection of nephrolithiasis is decreasing as the newer technique of three-dimensional spiral computed tomography equals the accuracy of nephrotomography for this purpose.

Professional Considerations
Consent form IS required.

Risks
Radiation exposure, allergic reaction to contrast media (itching, hives, rash, tight feeling in the throat, shortness of breath, bronchospasm, anaphylaxis, death), contrast-induced renal failure.

Contraindications
Pregnancy; previous allergy to dye, iodine, or shellfish; pregnancy (because of radioactive iodine crossing the blood-placental barrier); renal insufficiency.

Preparation
1. Have emergency equipment readily available.
2. Residual barium from prior studies should be completely cleared from the gastrointestinal tract before this test is performed.
3. See Client and Family Teaching.

Procedure
1. A plain film of the kidneys is taken.
2. Contrast medium is injected intravenously, the first half in 5 minutes (rapid phase) and the next half in 10 minutes (slow phase).
3. Serial tomograms are initiated as soon as the slow phase begins.
4. The procedure takes 1 hour.

Postprocedure Care
1. Monitor vital signs and urinary output every 4 hours for 24 hours.

Client and Family Teaching
1. Fast from food and fluids for 8 hours before the procedure.
2. Be alert for an allergic reaction to the dye for 24 hours (itching, hives, shortness of breath, hypotension). Call the physician immediately if these symptoms occur or go to the nearest emergency department.

Factors That Affect Results
1. Residual barium interferes with visualization.

Other Data
1. Perform this procedure with caution on individuals who have severe cardiovascular disease, multiple myeloma, asthma, pheochromocytoma, or myasthenia gravis.
2. This test is routinely performed with an intravenous pyelogram (IVP).
3. See also Intravenous pyelography—Diagnostic.

Nerve Biopsy—Diagnostic

Norm. Negative.

Usage. Primarily used to aid diagnosis of infiltrative neuropathies (amyloid infiltration, hypertrophic polyneuropathy, peripheral neuropathy) and vasculitis. Also used in the diagnosis of amyloid infiltration, demyelination, inflammation axonal degeneration, lepromatous leprosy lesions, metachromatic leukodystrophy, and sarcoidosis when other testing is inconclusive.

Description. Removal of peripheral nerve tissue for electromicroscopic, biochemical, histochemical, or virologic examination to establish a diagnosis for neuropathies when

radiologic evaluation and direct inspection have been inconclusive. Findings must be used in conjunction with clinical history and assessment findings for the most accurate diagnosis.

Professional Considerations
Consent form IS required.

Risks
Bruising, infection.

Contraindications
Anticoagulant therapy, bleeding disorders, thrombocytopenia.

Preparation

1. Prepare for local anesthesia and obtain biopsy instruments and a 3- × 5-inch index card.
2. Consult laboratory personnel for special handling of the specimen if electron microscopic examination is required.
3. Just before beginning the procedure, take a "time out" to verify the correct client, procedure, and site.

Procedure

1. Place a 1.5-cm portion of nerve on cardboard with the firmness of a 3- × 5-inch index card and then straighten and slightly stretch it.
2. Allow the specimen to adhere to the cardboard for 1 minute.
3. Keep the handling of specimens to a minimum.
4. Submerge the specimen in 0.05 mol/L phosphate-buffered glutaraldehyde.

Postprocedure Care

1. Transport specimens to the laboratory immediately.

Client and Family Teaching

1. Monitor for drainage and inflammation for 24-48 hours.
2. A mild analgesic may be required for pain control.
3. Call the physician for signs of infection at the procedure site: increasing pain, redness, swelling, purulent drainage, or for temperature >101 degrees F (38.3 degrees C).

Factors That Affect Results

1. Drying out of samples invalidates the results.

Other Data

1. The nerve where the biopsy specimen was taken will not regenerate.
2. The most common nerve used for biopsy is the superficial peroneal sensory nerve.

Nerve Conduction Studies—Diagnostic

Norm. Maximum conduction velocity = 40-80 msec for those 3 years of age and older. Distal latency <4 msec and amplitude 13.2 mV. Values decreased by half for infants and elderly. Equipment and technique vary; thus laboratories establish their own norms.

Usage. Carpal tunnel syndrome, Kennedy's disease (bulbospinal muscular atrophy), organophosphate poisoning, peripheral entrapment neuropathies, tarsal tunnel syndrome, and thoracic outlet syndrome.

Description. Percutaneous stimulation of peripheral, sensory, or mixed sensory/motor nerve fibers. Recording of muscle and sensory action potentials distinguishes between disease processes that cause both segmental demyelinative lesions and axonal losses.

Professional Considerations

Consent form IS required.

Risks

Pain at needle-electrode sites.

Contraindications

Nicotine-patch drug users.

Preparation

1. Shave the area for better conduction if needed.

Procedure

1. An electrode is applied to the specific nerve area.
2. Electrical current is passed through and read distally to determine nerve conduction time.

Postprocedure Care

1. Assess the skin area for irritation.

Client and Family Teaching

1. Results are normally available within 48 hours.

Factors That Affect Results

1. Poor conduction of electrodes from use of outdated electrodes, improper site preparation, or movement during the procedure.
2. Lower amplitudes are demonstrated in obese clients than in thin clients.

Other Data

1. Professional interpretation must follow the results of the study.
2. Supplements electromyographic studies.

Neurography

See Magnetic Resonance Neurography—Diagnostic.

Neuron-Specific Enolase (NSE)—Serum

Norm. 3.7-12.5 µg/mL.

Cord blood: 4.8-19.4 µg/L.

Increased. Adrenocortical carcinoma (overexpression of p53 gene), brain cell distress (e.g., secondary to seizure, tumor, cerebral edema, traumatic brain injury), medullary carcinoma of the thyroid, neuroblastoma (marker, elevated in >90% of children with advanced condition) that is metastatic, pancreatic islet cell tumor, small cell carcinoma of the lung, seizures (7.4-22.54 ng/dL), stroke (12.9-60.9 g/L), and uremia. Drug imipramine.

Decreased. Not applicable.

Description. Neuron-specific enolase (NSE) is an isoenzyme of a glycolytic enzyme found in neuronal and neuroendocrine cells of the central and peripheral nervous system. NSE is produced by adult T-cell leukemia and other tumor cells and is a sensitive tumor marker used to monitor response to therapy or detect neuroendocrine cell destruction disease progression because there is a strong correlation between disease state and concentration. NSE levels correlate with outcome in neuroblastoma and SCLC. Interpretation of results is unreliable unless accompanied by an estimate of red cell disruption.

Professional Considerations

Consent form NOT required.

Preparation

1. Tube: Red topped, red/gray topped, or gold topped. Also obtain ice.

Procedure

1. Collect a 2-mL blood sample. Place the specimen in a container of ice.

Postprocedure Care

1. Send the specimen to the laboratory immediately. Serum must be separated and refrigerated within 45 minutes of collection. The specimen should be frozen at −70 degrees C if not tested the same day.

2. A compensating factor due to effect of hemolysis on measurement of NSE is (H × 0.30 microg/L) where this should be subtracted from the measured NSE concentration..

Client and Family Teaching

1. Results may not be available for as long as 7 days.

Factors That Affect Results

1. Serum is not separated after collection.

Other Data

1. This test is not useful in screening for early stages of neoplasms.

2. Clients with NSE >15 ng/mL are likely to have metastatic small cell lung cancer. Sensitivity for this condition is about 80% and specificity is about 80%-90%.

Neut

See Differential Leukocyte Count—Peripheral Blood.

Neutrophil Alkaline Phosphatase

See Leukocyte Alkaline Phosphatase—Blood.

Neutrophils

See Differential Leukocyte Count—Peripheral Blood.

NH₃

See **Ammonia**—Blood and Urine.

Nipple Discharge Cytology

See **Cytologic Study of Nipple Discharge**—Diagnostic.

NIRS

See **Transcranial Near-Infrared Spectroscopy**—Diagnostic.

Nitrite, Bacteria Screen—Urine

Norm. <0.1 mg/dL, <100,000 organisms/mL, or negative.

Usage. Cystitis, differentiation between acute bacterial infections and viral or tuberculosis (TB) infections, dysuria, pyelonephritis, shigellosis, and urinary tract infection.

Description. Humans normally oxidize ingested nitrite and excrete it as nitrate. The presence of nitrite in urine indicates a urinary tract infection caused by organisms that reduce nitrate back to nitrite.

Professional Considerations
Consent form NOT required.

Preparation
1. Cleanse the urethral orifice with a sterile wipe.
2. Obtain a sterile plastic container.

Procedure
1. Collect a first morning void of 12 mL of urine, or a specimen collected at least 4 hours after the client last voided, in a sterile plastic container.

Postprocedure Care
1. Refrigerate the sample within 2 hours.

Client and Family Teaching
1. Results are normally available within 72 hours.

Factors That Affect Results
1. Incidence of false-positive results is 12%-34% as a result of age less than 2 months, *Candida albicans* and *Nocardia* infections, echovirus, hemophilia A, Hodgkin's disease, lymphoma, malaria, and parasitic infections.
2. Incidence of false-negatives is 5%-9% as a result of agammaglobulinemia, diabetes mellitus, localized infection, sickle cell anemia, and systemic lupus erythematosus.
3. Drugs that may cause false-positive results include oral contraceptives and phenazopyridine.
4. Drugs that may cause false-negative results include antibiotics, anti-inflammatories (corticosteroids and phenylbutazone), and ascorbic acid concentration >25 mg/dL in specimens containing <0.03 mg/dL of nitrite ions.
5. Diuresis, delay of several hours without refrigeration of specimen, and contamination in obtaining specimen invalidate the results.
6. Dipsticks stored in ambient humidity may produce false-negative results.
7. Another degree of color development on the reagent test strip is NOT proportional to the number of bacteria present.
8. Bacteria infections are less likely to be detected when the urine output is high.
9. An increased urine specific gravity will decrease the sensitivity of this test.

Other Data
1. Urinary tract infections may be caused from organisms that will not produce a positive nitrite test.
2. If nitrites are positive on the dipstick or are negative but the client is symptomatic, a urine culture should be performed.

Nitroglycerin Scan

See **Heart Scan**—Diagnostic.

Nocardia **Culture, All Sites**—Specimen

Norm. Negative.

Positive. Human immunodeficiency virus, immune deficiency, leukemia, lymphoma, lymphoreticular malignancy, pulmonary alveolar proteinosis, tuberculosis, and wounds. Drugs include corticosteroids and chemotherapeutic agents.

Description. Microscopic examination to detect gram-positive filamentous branching bacteria that may segment into reproductive bacillary fragments. *Nocardia* is found in soil, grass, grain, straw, and decaying matter. The human infections produced are primary skin lesions (rare), lung (60%-80%), and brain (20%-40%). Brain abscess is the most fatal complication of *Nocardia*. *Nocardia*, a primary pathogen for organ transplant clients, is an uncommon infection, with approximately 500-1000 cases reported annually in the United States. *Nocardia* is extremely difficult to culture. It grows on various media but may take 3-30 days or more to appear. A modified acid-fast stain is helpful in the diagnosis of *Nocardia*.

Professional Considerations

Consent form NOT required.

Preparation

1. Preschedule the test with the laboratory.
2. Obtain a sterile Culturette or a sterile plastic container.

Procedure

1. Obtain a sterile culture from a suspected site (tissue, fluid, aspirate, or respiratory specimen). Place specimen in an air-tight container.

Postprocedure Care

1. Send the specimen to the laboratory within 1 hour.

Client and Family Teaching

1. Results are normally available from 72 hours to 30 days.

Factors That Affect Results

1. A contaminated culture invalidates the results.

Other Data

1. Sulfonamides or minocycline is the treatment of choice.

Nocturnal Penile Tumescence Testing

See **Polysomnography**—Diagnostic.

Non–Stress Testing

See **Fetal Monitoring, External, Non–Stress Testing**—Diagnostic.

Norepinephrine

See **Catecholamines**—Plasma.

Norpace

See **Disopyramide Phosphate**—Serum.

Nortriptyline

See **Tricyclic Antidepressants**—Plasma or Serum.

Nose Culture

See Culture, Routine.

NST

See Fetal Monitoring, External, Non–Stress Testing—Diagnostic.

NT-Pro-BNP

See Natriuretic Peptides, Atrial—Plasma.

5′-Nucleotidase (Five Prime Nucleotidase)—Serum

Norm. 2-15 IU/L, 0-17 U/L, 0-1.6 U, or 0.3-3.2 Bodansky units.

Increased. Alcoholism, cirrhosis, craniocerebral trauma, drug-induced cholestasis, extrahepatic obstruction, granulomatous infiltrative disease, hypercoagulation, liver dysfunction, liver failure, liver metastasis, rheumatoid arthritis inflammation, sickle cell anemia, and surgery. Drugs include acetaminophen, aspirin, narcotics, phenothiazines, and phenytoin. Herbals include *Syzygium cumini*.

Decreased. Hepatitis.

Description. A plasma membrane enzyme that is an isozyme of alkaline phosphatase that is found in hepatic parenchyma and bile ductal cells. This test aids differential diagnosis between bone and liver cancer because 5′-nucleotidase is rarely elevated in bone cancer. When coupled with elevated alkaline phosphatase, the levels are indicative of liver metastasis.

Professional Considerations
Consent form NOT required.

Preparation
1. Tube: Red topped, red/gray topped, or gold topped or blue topped.

Procedure
1. Draw a 2-mL blood sample.

Postprocedure Care
1. The sample remains stable for 5 days at room temperature, 1 week when refrigerated, and 1 month when frozen.

Client and Family Teaching
1. Results are normally available within 72 hours.

Factors That Affect Results
1. Contaminated sample and hemolysis.

Other Data
1. Liver enzyme studies should be evaluated with results.

O₂ Sat

See Blood Gases, Arterial—Blood.

O-Banding—CSF or Plasma

Norm. Negative.

Usage. Burkitt's lymphoma, cerebellar ataxia, cortical multifocal action myoclonus, cryptococcal meningitis, multiple sclerosis, myoclonic ataxia, neurosyphilis, polyneuropathy, rubella panencephalitis of progressive nature, and subacute sclerosing panencephalitis.

Description. Serum electrophoresis to diagnose inflammatory and autoimmune central nervous system (CNS) diseases that produce quantitative changes in oligoclonal proteins in the serum. O-banding can also be performed on cerebrospinal fluid (CSF) by electrophoresis and is detected in virtually all MS patients. Two or more definite bands with no counterparts is considered positive identification.

Professional Considerations
Consent form NOT required.

Preparation
1. Tube: Red topped, red/gray topped, or gold topped.
2. See also Lumbar puncture—Diagnostic.

Procedure
1. If both plasma and CSF are being evaluated, they should be drawn at approximately the same time.
2. Draw a 4-mL blood sample and/or a 5-mL CSF sample.

Postprocedure Care
1. Plasma or CSF specimens should be frozen if testing is delayed.
2. See Lumbar puncture—Diagnostic.

Client and Family Teaching
1. Results are normally available within 72 hours.
2. See also Lumbar puncture—Diagnostic.

Factors That Affect Results
1. Unlabeled specimens.

Other Data
1. These bands are not seen in vascular disease, brain tumors, or other nonimmunologic brain disorders.
2. O-banding is not a significant prognostic factor in heart transplant recipients, HIV infections, or multiple sclerosis.
3. This test has a 90% sensitivity level.

Obstetric Ultrasonography (Obstetric Echogram, Obstetric Ultrasound)—Diagnostic

Norm. Fetus(es) and sac are of normal size for gestational date. No fetal abnormality detected.

Usage. Evaluate amniotic fluid volume, cleft lip, fetal age, fetal occiput position, size, or viability for proper timing of induced or cesarean delivery; fetal abnormality detection; and multiple gestation determination. Helps diagnose abruptio placentae, cloacal malformations, ectopic tubal pregnancy, endometriosis, fetal death, molar pregnancy, ovarian size, ovarian torsion, pelvic inflammatory disease, placenta previa, skeletal dysplasias in fetus, uterine size or rupture; provides guidance for amniocentesis, cervical cerclage placement, fetoscopy, or intrauterine procedures. Used for tumor detection, localization, characterization, and staging; can identify Down syndrome structural markers (duodenal atresia, cardiac abnormalities, brachycephaly, mild ventriculomegaly, macroglossia, abnormal facies, nuchal edema, echogenic or hyperechoic bowel, pyelectasis, and shortening of the limbs), indicating the need for genetic karyotyping.

Description. Evaluation of size, status, and location of fetus, fetal sac, and pelvic organs by the creation of an oscilloscopic picture from the echoes of high-frequency sound waves passing over the pregnant abdomen (acoustic imaging). The time required for the ultrasonic beam to be reflected back to the transducer from differing densities of tissue is converted by a computer to an electrical impulse displayed on an oscilloscopic screen to create a three-dimensional picture of the pelvic contents. Two-dimensional ultrasound has been found to be superior to the three-dimensional technology for evaluation of both healthy and malformed fetuses. Digital pelvic examination for determining fetal head position during labor is not accurate, but ultrasound with progression angle is the most accurate.

Professional Considerations
Consent form IS required. Although the procedure does not pose physical risks, informed consent information should include the diagnostic accuracy of this procedure for detecting fetal abnormalities.

Preparation
1. This test should be performed before intestinal barium tests or after barium is cleared from the system.
2. The client should disrobe below the waist or wear a gown.
3. Obtain water-soluble gel, a transducer for the ultrasound machine, a camera,

and videotape, with or without an oscilloscope.

4. See Client and Family Teaching.

Procedure

1. The client is positioned supine.
2. The pelvic and abdominal areas are coated with water-soluble gel.
3. A lubricated transducer is passed slowly and firmly over the abdominal and pelvic areas at a variety of angles.
4. Photographs are taken of the images transmitted to the oscilloscopic screen.
5. The procedure should take approximately 30-60 minutes.

Postprocedure Care

1. Wipe the gel off the abdominal and pelvic areas.
2. Instruct the client to empty her bladder immediately.

Client and Family Teaching

1. The client should drink 1 quart of water 1 hour before the procedure because a full bladder is needed to define pelvic organs by serving as an acoustic window for transmission of the sound waves. The full bladder also properly positions the uterus so that it is perpendicular to the transducer. Do not void until the test is completed.
2. Lying supine may cause shortness of breath. This may be relieved by elevation of the upper body or by lying on either side.

Factors That Affect Results

1. Miscalculation of the conception date.
2. Dehydration interferes with adequate contrast between the organs and body fluids.
3. Intestinal barium or gas obscures the results by preventing the proper transmission and deflection of the high-frequency sound waves.
4. Although a full bladder is recommended, during the first trimester one that is overfilled may compress the uterus, making it difficult to obtain adequate pictures of the early embryonic and extra-embryonic structures.

Other Data

1. An abnormal echo pattern may indicate a multiple pregnancy.
2. This procedure has a 98% accuracy rate for identifying the placental site.
3. In the first trimester of pregnancy, a transvaginal approach to ultrasonography may be preferred. This method requires an empty bladder and the passage of a small transducer gently into the vagina. This process eliminates the interference of transverse abdominal tissue, allowing for more detailed visualization.
4. A chaperone should be present during transvaginal ultrasonography.

Obstetric Ultrasound

See **Obstetric Ultrasonography**—Diagnostic.

OC

See **Osteocalcin**—Plasma or Serum.

OCA 125 Antigen

See **CA 125**—Blood.

Occult Blood, Gastric Contents

See **Gastric Analysis**—Specimen.

Occult Blood—Stool (Hemoccult, Hemoccult II and Hemoccult SENSA)

Norm. Negative.

Positive. Alcohol abuse, colon cancer, Crohn's disease, diverticulitis, esophageal varices, gastric ulcer, gastritis, gastrointestinal bleeding, hemorrhage, intussusception, pancreatic carcinoma, peptic ulcer, stress ulcers, tumors, and ulcerative colitis. Drugs include aspirin, boric acid, bromides, colchicine, indomethacin, iodine, iron preparations, potassium preparations, reserpine, salicylates, steroids, and thiazide diuretics.

Description. Rapid method for qualitative detection of red blood cells in stool, based on pseudoperoxidase reaction between hemoglobin, the developer (hydrogen peroxide and denatured ethyl alcohol), and guaiac. The methodology used is testing of a sample of stool. Specimens obtained via digital rectal exam are considered unsuitable for fecal occult blood testing because of a risk of false-negative results. Occult blood detection has long been used to screen for colorectal cancer, the second highest cause of cancer deaths, though its sensitivity is low. However, this method is underused because of public expectation of discomfort. Newer methods of screening include detection of molecular markers, such as the K-*ras* oncogene mutation, which holds promise for becoming a more sensitive and specific test than fecal occult blood testing for screening for colorectal cancer. See K-*ras*—Blood or Specimen. The new immunofecal occult blood test (IFOBT) is specific for human hemoglobin, does not require dietary restrictions, and can detect precancerous lesions and colorectal cancer in early stages. Its positive predictive value and sensitivity is better for males.

Professional Considerations

Consent form NOT required.

Preparation

1. See Client and Family Teaching.
2. Obtain a guaiac-impregnated card for occult blood testing and a wooden applicator.
3. Check the developer and the slides for expiration dates.

Procedure

1. Obtain a stool sample that is not contaminated with toilet water.
2. Open the front flap of the guaiac-impregnated slide.
3. Using the applicator provided, apply a thin smear of stool in each box. Use a separate sample from a different part of the stool specimen for each smear.
4. Close the slide cover.
5. Open the flap on the back of the slide. Apply two drops of developer to each box and to the quality control monitor.
6. Read the results after 30 seconds and within 2 minutes. Any trace of blue color is positive for occult blood.
7. Repeat for three consecutive bowel movements.
8. Test stools within 48 hours of collection.

Postprocedure Care

1. Assess the rectal area for irritation.

Client and Family Teaching

1. Follow a meat-free, high-residue diet for 24-72 hours before the test. The diet should also be free of vegetables with high peroxidase activity (including bananas, beets, broccoli, cantaloupe, cauliflower, grapes, horseradish, mushrooms, parsnips, and turnips). Does NOT apply to IFOBT test.
2. The client may perform the guaiac test at home following the same procedure stated above. Slides should be mailed to the physician's office or to the laboratory as instructed.
3. Factors that may interfere with results should be reviewed with the client and avoided before testing.
4. False-negative results can occur in the presence of colorectal cancer that does not or has not yet caused sufficient bleeding; also with consumption of Vitamin C.

Factors That Affect Results

1. Specimens will be positive if contaminated by menstrual or hemorrhoidal blood or povidone-iodine solution.
2. Diets rich in meats, green and leafy vegetables, poultry, and fish may produce false-positive results. Drugs include alcohol, anti-inflammatory agents, ascorbic acid (vitamin C), ethanol, and nonsteroidal anti-inflammatory agents.
3. Ascorbic acid (vitamin C) may also produce false-negative results.

4. Inadequate stool on the slide may produce false-negative results.
5. False-positives occur in about 10% of tests.
6. Sensitivity increases with serial collection and testing of 2 or 3 daily specimens.

Other Data
1. See also ColoSure™ test—Stool, and Immunochemical fecal occult blood testing—Stool.

O

Occult Blood—Urine

Norm. Negative, <5000-10,000 RBCs/mL or 2-3 RBCs per high-power field.

Positive. Benign familial hematuria, benign prostatic hypertrophy, bladder cancer, burns, cystitis, dysuria, glomerulonephritis, Goodpasture's syndrome, heavy exercise, hematuria, hemophilia, nephrolithiasis, thrombocytopenia, transfusion reaction, trauma, and urinary tract infection. Drugs include heparin, salicylates, and warfarin.

Description. Screening by dipstick or examination of urine sediment for asymptomatic hematuria, which may be associated with a serious urologic disease, or the presence of active bleeding with a hematologic disorder.

Professional Considerations
Consent form NOT required.

Preparation
1. Obtain a plastic specimen container and a centrifuge tube. If testing is to be performed immediately, obtain reagent strips with the manufacturer's instructions.

Procedure
1. Cleanse the genital area with soap and water.
2. Collect a 10-mL random urine specimen in a centrifuge tube and send the tube to the laboratory, or collect a specimen in a clean plastic cup for dipstick usage as directed by the manufacturer.

Postprocedure Care
1. Perform a dipstick reading according to the manufacturer's directions immediately, or send the specimen to the laboratory within 2 hours.

2. Write the collection time on the laboratory requisition.

Client and Family Teaching
1. Results are normally available within 24 hours.

Factors That Affect Results
1. Reject specimens received more than 2 hours after collection because leaving a specimen standing destroys red blood cells.
2. The presence of urinary bacteria may cause false-positive results; large amounts of ascorbic acid or formaldehyde in the urine will also cause false-positive results.
3. False-positives may also be caused by contact of the specimen with povidone-iodine solution, bleach, menstrual blood, or hemorrhoidal blood.
4. Failure to mix the sample, resulting in no RBCs in the supernatant and high levels of nitrite, may cause false-negative results.
5. Vitamin C may cause false-negative results, and ethyl alcohol (ethanol) may cause false-positive results.
6. Do NOT use a reagent strip to test urine if the client is receiving tetracycline (Panmycin), oxytetracycline (Terramycin), bromides, or copper because these create false-positive results.

Other Data
1. Sensitivity of reagent strips decreases with age and if urine contains high protein or high specific gravity readings.
2. Reagent strips are more sensitive to free hemoglobin than to intact red blood cells.

OCT

See Fetal Monitoring, External, Contraction Stress Test and Oxytocin Challenge Test—Diagnostic.

Octreotide Scan (Somatostatin-Receptor Scintigraphy)—Diagnostic

Norm. Physiologic tracer uptake demonstrates normal size, shape, and position of liver, spleen, bladder, and kidney.

Usage. Location and diagnosis of primary and metastatic cancers (NOT soft tissue lesions) arising from the neuroendocrine system that express somatostatin receptors, such as carcinoid tumors, gastrinomas of pancreas and duodenum, thymoma, thymic carcinoma, pheochromocytoma, pituitary adenomas (growth hormone, TSH tumors), islet cell tumors (insulinoma, glucagonoma), neuroblastoma, small cell carcinoma of the lung, paragangliomas, medullary carcinoma of thyroid, meningioma, astrocytoma, lymphoma, Merkel cell tumor, and breast cancer; staging of Hodgkin's disease; may help in client selection for clinical trials using somatostatin analogs in the treatment of neuroendocrine cancers. Not recommended for adjunct tumor staging, surveillance after resection or detectng bone lesions (unless it would change management and treatment plan). Used in conjuction with SPECT and CT scans.

Description. An octreotide scan is a nuclear medicine scan of the whole body after injection of a radioactive tracer, [^{111}In-DTPA-D-Phe]octreotide or [^{123}I-Thy3]octreotide, for the purpose of detecting areas of increased uptake by somatostatin-receptor tumors. The octreotide tracer is a somatostatin analog. Various organs and tumors uptake the tracer at varying degrees. The tracer radiation is emitted as gamma rays and is detected by gamma cameras. A series of images are taken from various angles around the client and compiled by single-photon emission computed tomography (SPECT). Cross-sectional and three-dimensional imaging can be accomplished. A series of scans are conducted at 4 and 24 hours following injection of radioisotope. Additional scans may be done.

Professional Considerations
Consent form IS required.

Risks

Octreotide may produce severe hypoglycemia in clients with insulinomas. An intravenous line is recommended for clients with suspected insulinomas for the administration of glucose solution as needed.

Contraindications
Women who are breast-feeding.

Precautions
During pregnancy, risks of cumulative radiation exposure to the fetus from this and other previous or future imaging studies must be weighed against the benefits of the procedure. Although formal limits for client exposure are relative to this risk:benefit comparison, the United States Nuclear Regulatory Commission requires that the cumulative dose equivalent to an embryo/fetus from occupational exposure not exceed 0.5 rem (5 mSv). Radiation dosage to the fetus is proportional to the distance of the anatomy studied from the abdomen and decreases as pregnancy progresses. For pregnant clients, consult the radiologist/radiology department to obtain estimated fetal radiation exposure from this procedure.

Preparation
1. See Client and Family Teaching.
2. Octreotide acetate therapy should be discontinued 24-48 hours before the scan, while monitoring client for signs of withdrawal.
3. Jewelry and metal objects should be removed before scanning.
4. A bowel prep such as GoLYTELY (CoLyte) or MagCitrate™ (magnesium citrate) may be recommended for the evening of the injection, before the 24-hour scan.
5. The client should be well hydrated.

Procedure
1. Intravenous radioactive tracer is administered $3\frac{1}{2}$ to 4 hours before the first scan.
2. The client should drink two glasses of water immediately following the injection and continue to increase fluid intake for the next 2 days.
3. The client is placed in a supine position and the whole body is scanned with a gamma camera.
4. A bowel prep such as GoLYTELY (CoLyte) or MagCitrate™ (magnesium citrate) may be recommended for the evening of day 1.
5. Repeat scan will be done 24 hours later.

6. Repeat scans may be done on days 3 and 4.

Postprocedure Care
1. Continue to maintain hydration throughout test period.

Client and Family Teaching
1. Fasting is NOT required for this test.
2. You may feel a warm sensation when the radioisotope is injected into your vein.
3. The level of radiation exposure is low and not associated with any significant risks.
4. You will need to lie still on a hard table during the procedure.
5. Each scan takes 1-2 hours and is painless.
6. Drink plenty of fluids during the 2 days following the injection of the isotope.

Factors That Affect Results
1. Reduced sensitivity of octreotide imaging may occur in clients receiving therapeutic doses of octreotide acetate (Sandostatin) therapy.

Other Data
1. The radioisotope tracer is primarily excreted by the kidney. Studies have not been conducted in clients with poor renal function. It is not known if octreotide can be removed by dialysis.
2. The physical half-life of [^{111}In-DTPA-D-Phe]octreotide is 2.8 days.
3. The scan is often used to identify tumors unrevealed by CT or MRI scans.
4. Uptake of the octreotide tracer may indicate the client is a candidate for octreotide injections to treat the cancer.
5. Health care professionals working in a nuclear medicine area must follow federal standards set by the Nuclear Regulatory Commission. These standards include precautions for handling the radioactive material and monitoring of potential radiation exposure.

Ocular Cytology—Specimen

Norm. Negative.

Usage. Adenovirus infection, *Chlamydia*, conjunctivitis, dry eye conditions, Kaposi's sarcoma, keratitis, and metastatic cancer from the breast or melanoma.

Description. An ocular smear or cellulose acetate filter paper impression is histologically evaluated for the presence of polymorphs or other inflammatory cells. Mapping of the ocular surface can be done from the impression specimen, providing information about changes in the surface cells of the eye, mucus production, and tear function. This test commonly includes staining by either Papanicolaou or Giemsa stain.

Professional Considerations
Consent form IS required for the fine-needle aspiration technique.

Risks of Fine-Needle Aspiration Technique
Infection, unilateral blindness.
Contraindications of Fine-Needle Aspiration Technique
Central retinal artery occlusion.

Preparation
1. For fine-needle aspiration, obtain a sterile fine-needle aspiration tray, a sterile plastic container, a sterile 2- × 2-inch gauze or sterile cotton-tipped applicator approved for microbiologic use, two glass slides, and a spray fixative.
2. For the impression technique, obtain 5-mm-thick half-circular cellulose acetate filter paper.
3. Just before beginning the procedure, take a "time out" to verify the correct client, procedure, and site.

Procedure
1. *Needle aspiration technique:* A fine-needle biopsy specimen is taken from the eye or by a cotton-tipped applicator, or a scraping is obtained. Place the smears on two clean glass slides, and immediately fix one slide with the spray and let the other slide air-dry.
2. *Impression technique:* Place filter paper in the upper and lower quadrants around the limbus, and press lightly against the surface. Remove filter paper and place in a sterile container. Topical anesthesia is not used.

Postprocedure Care
1. Assess the aspiration area every 5 minutes × 4 for bleeding, edema, or redness.
2. Results are normally available in 24 hours.

Client and Family Teaching
1. Monitor ocular site for inflammation or redness for 24-48 hours.
2. A mild analgesic may be required for pain control.

3. Monitor ocular site for signs and symptoms of infection until the site is healed.

Factors That Affect Results
1. A contaminated sample of the aspirate invalidates results.

Other Data
1. None.

Oculoplethysmography (OPG)—Diagnostic

Norm. Negative, or all pulses should occur simultaneously.

Usage. Ataxia, status after carotid endarterectomy, syncope, and transient ischemic attacks.

Description. Noninvasive test that measures ocular artery pressure by comparing pulse arrival times in the eyes with the ears, which reflects the adequacy of cerebrovascular blood flow in the carotid arteries.

Professional Considerations
Consent form IS required.

Risks
Corneal abrasion.
Contraindications
Clients who have had eye surgery within 2-6 months, cataract, conjunctivitis, diabetes mellitus, uncontrolled glaucoma, enucleation, history of retinal detachment or lens implantation, clients who are hypersensitive to local anesthetic, or uncooperative and combative clients.

Preparation
1. Obtain anesthetic eye drops, an eyecup, and photoelectric cells.

Procedure
1. Instill the anesthetic eye drops and apply the eyecup to the corneas with light suction (40-50 mm Hg).
2. Apply the photoelectric cells to earlobes.

3. Record the cyclic changes in volume on a graphic machine.

Postprocedure Care
1. Observe for ocular pain or photophobia, which may indicate corneal abrasion.

Client and Family Teaching
1. Do not rub the eyes or insert contact lenses for 30 minutes after the test.
2. Anesthetic eye drops may cause slight temporary burning.
3. It is not unusual to experience blurred vision for a short period after this procedure.
4. Continued blurred vision or pain should be reported to the physician.
5. The procedure takes a few minutes.

Factors That Affect Results
1. Constant blinking, nystagmus, or poor cooperation prevent accurate measurement.

Other Data
1. A 20-msec or greater delay in the pulse wave in the ophthalmic artery is abnormal, signifying stenosis.
2. Delayed arrival of the ocular pulse is associated with ipsilateral carotid stenosis.
3. This test does NOT distinguish between a completely occluded internal carotid artery and one that is nearly occluded.
4. This procedure is extremely useful for evaluating deep orbital circulation.
5. See also Color duplex ultrasonography—Diagnostic.

Oculopneumoplethysmography (OPPG)—Diagnostic

Norm. Difference between ophthalmic artery pressures should be <5 mm Hg. Ophthalmic artery pressure divided by the higher brachial systolic pressure should be >0.67.

Usage. Ataxia, carotid bruits of asymptomatic origin, carotid endarterectomy monitoring, carotid occlusive disease, syncope, and transient ischemic attacks.

Description. A vacuum applied to the sclera allows adjustment of intraocular pressure and a recording of ocular pressure waveform. Ophthalmic artery pressures are compared with the higher brachial pressure and with each other.

Professional Considerations
Consent form IS required.

Risks
Corneal abrasion, erythema, hematoma (scleras).

Contraindications
Anticoagulant therapy, conjunctivitis, enucleation, retinal detachment or history, uncontrolled glaucoma, eye surgery within the previous 2-6 months, increased intracranial pressure.

Preparation
1. Obtain anesthetic eye drops such as 0.5% proparacaine, an eyecup, suction vacuum apparatus, a plethysmograph, a sphygmomanometer, and a stethoscope.

Procedure
1. Instill the anesthetic eye drops.
2. Attach the eyecup to the scleras of the eyes.
3. Apply a vacuum of 300 mm Hg to each eye so that the pulse disappears. Then gradually release the suction until the pulse returns.
4. Take both brachial pressures.
5. The higher systolic brachial pressure is compared with the ophthalmic artery pressures.

Postprocedure Care
1. Observe for ocular pain or photophobia, which may indicate corneal abrasion.

Client and Family Teaching
1. Transient loss of vision when suction is applied is not unusual.
2. Anesthetic eye drops may cause slight temporary burning.
3. Do not rub the eyes or insert contact lenses for 2 hours after the test.
4. Continued pain should be reported to the physician.

Factors That Affect Results
1. Constant blinking, hypertension, nystagmus, and poor cooperation prevent accurate measurement.
2. Results may be difficult to interpret if the client has a history of hypertension.
3. Cardiac dysrhythmias may alter the results.

Other Data
1. This method is more accurate than oculoplethysmography.
2. See also Oculoplethysmography—Diagnostic.

OKT-3 Cells, OKT-4 Cells, OKT-8 Cells

See Acquired Immune Deficiency Syndrome Evaluation Battery—Diagnostic.

Oligoclonal Bands, Cerebrospinal Fluid

See Cerebrospinal Fluid, Heparin Binding Protein, Myelin Basic Protein, Oligoclonal Bands, Protein, and Protein Electrophoresis—Specimen.

Oligoclonal Bands

See O-Banding—CSF or Plasma.

OMT

See Oral Mucosal Transudate—Specimen.

Oncofetal Fibronectin

See Fetal Fibronectin—Specimen.

One-Step

See Glucose Monitoring Machines—Diagnostic.

One Touch

See Glucose Monitoring Machines—Diagnostic.

OPN

See Osteopontin—Serum.

Oral Cavity Cytology—Specimen

Norm. Negative.

Usage. Cancers of the tongue, gum, or mouth; *Candida albicans*; herpesvirus infection; human immune deficiency virus; Klinefelter's syndrome; pemphigus; trisomy 13, 18, and 21; and Turner's syndrome.

Description. Microscopic examination of cells scraped from the oral cavity surface.

Professional Considerations
Consent form NOT required.

Preparation
1. Obtain a glass of water, a spatula or tongue blade, a glass slide, a specimen container of 95% ethyl alcohol (ethanol) or spray fixative, and a light source.
2. Label the slide with the client's name and the specimen source.

Procedure
1. The client should rinse the mouth vigorously with water several times before the scraping is performed.
2. The lesion or oral surface is scraped with a spatula or tongue blade.
3. Smear the scraping on a labeled glass slide and fix it immediately in 95% alcohol or spray fixative.

Postprocedure Care
1. The requisition should include age; physical findings; history of smoking, dentures, skin lesions, and reverse smoking; and history of chemotherapy, immunotherapy, or radiation therapy.

Client and Family Teaching
1. Results are normally available in 24-48 hours.

Factors That Affect Results
1. Failure to fix specimens invalidates the results.

Other Data
1. Occasional diagnosis of palatal salivary gland neoplasm occurs.

Oral Mucosal Transudate (OMT, HIV Oral Test)—Specimen

Norm. Negative AIDS battery, nonreactive.
   Antibody detection: Negative for HIV antibodies.

Usage. Used in combination with a modified ELISA and salivary Western blot assay. Offers clinical and outreach advantage to health care personnel who provide counseling and testing. It is an alternative for clients with poor venous access or who are unwilling to donate a blood sample.

Description. Oral mucosal transudate is a serous fluid that derives from transudation at the gingival crevice. The OMT method detects the presence of HIV antibodies using a micro–enzyme-linked immunosorbent assay similar to the ELISA. Samples collected are placed in a nontoxic stabilizing preservative that prevents bacterial growth and degradation of IgG by bacterial protease. Modifications in collection technology and immunosorbent assays have improved the detection of HIV-1 antibodies in oral specimens. The EpiScreen HIV-1 Oral Specimen Collection device is currently the only FDA-approved oral HIV antibody test and is restricted to testing with the oral fluid Vironostika HIV-1 Microelisa System (Organon Teknika Corp., Durham, NC). The salivary Western blot is an in vitro qualitative assay developed specifically for oral mucosal transudate (Epitope, Inc.) The OraSure Specimen Collection Device (Epitope, Inc.) is an FDA-approved device that looks similar to a toothbrush, with a padded end that is used for collection of oral specimens for HIV testing. Oral mucosal specimens follow the algorithm recommended for blood samples by the Centers for Disease Control and Prevention.

Professional Considerations
Consent form NOT required.

Preparation
1. Only properly trained personnel may test using the oral specimen kits according to the manufacturer's directions.
2. Wear gloves and have timer available.

Procedure
1. OMT: A fiber pad is treated with a hypotonic salt solution. The client rubs the pad between the lower gum and cheek several times and then holds the pad in place for a minimum of 2 minutes to a maximum of 5 minutes. The OraSure Specimen Collection Device may also be used to collect the sample.
2. The time must be verified by the collector. The client immediately places the pad in the provided container. Follow the manufacturer's instructions.

Postprocedure Care
1. Dispose of the equipment in the room.
2. Specimen may be stored at room temperature.

Client and Family Teaching
1. Each client is given the pamphlet provided with the kit, and the purpose of the test, the procedure for collection, and the alternative of giving a blood specimen is explained.
2. The test might leave a slightly salty taste in your mouth.
3. Results may not be available for several days.
4. If the results are positive, it is recommended to follow with serum samples for ELISA and serum for Western blot or immunofluorescence assays.
5. Assess client understanding of safe sex practices and provide counseling as needed.

Factors That Affect Results
1. False-positive ELISA results may be seen in pregnant women in the first trimester because of immunoglobulin reaction and sloughing of epithelial tissue.
2. False-positive ELISA results have been documented in clients with anticoagulation therapy, an oral pathologic condition, autoimmune disease other than AIDS, and with monoclonal or polyclonal gammopathy.
3. False-negative results may occur as a result of the absence of antibodies to HIV-1 in the early phase of the infection.

Other Data
1. OMT testing is not intended for use in clients under 13 years of age.
2. This test is not designed to screen blood donors.

OraQuick Rapid HIV Tests (OraQuick Multispot HIV-1, HIV-2 Rapid Test, OraQuick Rapid HIV-1 Antibody Test)—Specimen

Norm. Negative. Negative results are indicated by the appearance of a single reddish-purple line in the device indicator window.

Positive. Preliminarily positive results are demonstrated by TWO reddish-purple lines in the device indicator window. Because there is a 0.4% chance of a false-positive result, confirmatory serologic testing should be done if results are not negative. See Acquired immune deficiency syndrome evaluation battery—Diagnostic.

Usage. Routine screening for human immunodeficiency virus type 1 (HIV-1), the most common type found in the United States. Also screens for HIV-2. Used in cases of occupational exposure and labor and delivery patients.

Description. The OraQuick Rapid HIV tests are a group of tests that were approved for use in the United States in 2004 and 2005; these tests are simple to perform. This test has a 93.1% sensitivity, 95.3% specificity and positive predictive value of 77%. This test is less sensitive on oral fluid (86.5%) than on fingerstick blood (94.5%) samples and had its best sensitivity on serum samples (97.5%).

Professional Considerations
Consent form NOT required.

Preparation
1. For fingerstick, obtain an alcohol wipe, a lancet, and the OraQuick collecting loop. For whole blood, obtain a tube for whole blood or plasma. For oral specimen, obtain the OraQuick oral swab device.
2. Obtain the OraQuick vial of developing solution.

Procedure
1. Fingerstick: Cleanse the fingertip with an alcohol wipe and allow to dry. Obtain a drop of blood by using the lancet on the side of the fingertip.
2. Whole blood: Obtain a 4-mL blood sample.
3. Using the OraQuick collecting loop, transfer the blood to the vial of

developing solution. Gently invert the tube several times to mix.
4. For oral specimens, gently swab the Ora-Quick device around the upper and lower outer gums, and then insert it into the vial of developing solution.
5. Wait 20 minutes before interpreting results. Results are preliminarily positive if the device indicator window displays two reddish-purple lines.

Postprocedure Care
1. Apply pressure to site.

Client and Family Teaching
1. Test limitations should be explained. Clients with preliminary positive results should be scheduled for confirmatory testing.
2. Counsel clients regarding HIV transmission risk reduction.
3. Advise clients with negative results to return for testing in 3 months if there is any chance that HIV could have been contracted in the prior 90 days.

Factors That Affect Results
1. False-negative HIV-1 blood antibody results may occur in HIV-1-infected clients exposed less than 90 days before testing.
2. More false-positive results occur with the oral test than with the blood test.

Other Data
1. Test is classified as "waived" testing by CLIA.
2. In Washington, D.C., USA, the overall HIV rate is 14.1% in homosexual men, with Blacks more likely positive than Whites, Latinos, Asians, and others.
3. A new test called Aware™ assay is 92.3% sensitive and 96.6% specific with a positive predictive value of 82.7%.

Ornithine Carbamoyltransferase (OCT)—Blood

Norm. 0-500 sigma units/mL, or 0-16 U/L.

Increased. Acute viral hepatitis, cholecystitis, cirrhosis, enteritis, hepatic necrosis, hepatotoxicity caused by drugs or alcoholism (rare), infectious mononucleosis, liver dysfunction, obstructive jaundice, metastatic liver carcinoma, and prolonged exercise. Drugs include all hepatotoxic drugs, heavy alcohol use, and oral contraceptives.

Decreased. Congenital hyperammonemia. Drugs include mercuric salts, p-(chloromercuri)benzoate, and 2,3-dimercaptopropanol.

Description. Ornithine carbamoyltransferase (OCT) is an enzyme found in the liver and to a lesser extent in the intestinal mucosa that is involved in urea metabolism of the Krebs cycle. An elevation specifically and sensitively indicates liver cell disease. Insufficient production of OCT is an inherited X-linked dominant genetic defect that leads to neurologic damage. The exact occurrence of the inherited X-linked genetic defect is unknown but has been estimated to be 1:80,000, with males more affected.

Professional Considerations
Consent form NOT required.

Preparation
1. Tube: Red topped, red/gray topped, or gold topped.

Procedure
1. Draw a 7-mL blood sample.

Postprocedure Care
1. None.

Client and Family Teaching
1. Results are normally available within 72 hours to 1 week.

Factors That Affect Results
1. Hemolysis of the specimen invalidates the results.

Other Data
1. The test is more sensitive than AST (SGOT) or ALT (SGPT) in assessing liver function.
2. The test does not distinguish between hepatic and biliary diseases.

Osmolality, Calculated Test (Osmolar Gap)—Blood

Norm.

		SI Units
Serum osmolality	280-300 mOsm/kg H_2O	280-300 mmol/kg H_2O
Critical low	≤230 mOsm/kg H_2O	≤230 mmol/kg H_2O
Critical high	≥375 mOsm/kg H_2O	≥375 mmol/kg H_2O
Osmolar gap	<10 mOsm/kg H_2O	<10 mmol/kg H_2O

Increased. Alcoholism, azotemia, burns, convulsions, dehydration, diabetes insipidus, diarrhea, hyperaldosteronism, hyperlipidemia, hyperproteinemia, presence of hyperosmolar substances such as ethyl alcohol (ethanol) or methanol or lactic acid, syndrome of inappropriate antidiuretic hormone secretion (SIADHS), thirst, and uremia. Drugs include mannitol.

Decreased. Hyponatremia and overhydration.

Description. Osmolality refers to a solution's concentration of solute particles per kilogram of solvent and is expressed in milliosmoles per kilogram (mOsm/kg). In the laboratory, it is measured by an osmometer. However, it is possible to calculate serum osmolality using serum measurements of sodium, glucose, and urea (BUN) according to the formulas listed under Procedure. The osmolar gap is the difference between the laboratory serum osmolarity value and the calculated osmolar value. Assessing this gap is most important in the diagnosis of ethyl alcohol (ethanol) or methanol poisoning.

Professional Considerations
Consent form NOT required.

Preparation
1. None, other than locating the results of serum sodium, glucose, and BUN levels.

Procedure
1. Calculate osmolality as follows:

$(1.86 \times [\text{Sodium}]) + ([\text{Glucose}]/18) + (\text{BUN}/2.8)$

2. Rounded formula:

$(2 \times [\text{Sodium}]) + ([\text{Glucose}]/18) + (\text{BUN}/2.8)$

3. Dr. Weisberg's formula:

$(2 \times [\text{Sodium}]) + ([\text{Glucose}]/20) + (\text{BUN}/3)$

4. Calculated osmolar gap:

$(1.86 \times [\text{Sodium}] + [\text{Glucose}] + \text{BUN})/182.8$

Postprocedure Care
1. Calculated osmolality may be compared to laboratory-measured osmolality.

Client and Family Teaching
1. Results are normally available within 72 hours.

Factors That Affect Results

1. Hemolysis of specimens used to obtain sodium, glucose, and BUN values invalidates results.
2. Herbal or natural remedy goldenseal (*Hydrastis canadensis*) causes increased renal water loss, whereas sodium is spared. This may increase osmolality.
3. Sodium (Na) concentration may decrease by 1 mEq/L for every 4.6 g/L of plasma lipids, causing pseudohyponatremia.
4. Na^+ concentration may decrease by 1.6 mEq/L for every 100 mg/dL increase in plasma glucose concentration because of an osmotic shift of water into the bloodstream.

Other Data

1. A difference between measured and calculated serum osmolality (osmolar gap) of >10 mOsm/kg of H_2O may indicate pseudohyponatremia. Causes of an osmolar gap may include the following:
   a. A decrease in serum water content (as by displacement because of severe hyperlipidemia).
   b. Hyperproteinemia, as occurs in macroglobulinemia and multiple myeloma.
   c. The presence of low-molecular-weight solutes such as ethyl alcohol (ethanol), methanol, ethylene glycol, isopropanol, or mannitol in the blood.
   d. In diabetic clients when hyperglycemia is present.
   e. In clients with chronic renal failure when dialysis is needed.
2. Abnormal calculated results should be confirmed by a serum osmolality test.
3. See also Osmolality—Serum.

Osmolality—Serum

Norm.

		SI Units
Adult	280-300 mOsm/kg H_2O	280-300 mmol/kg H_2O
Child	270-290 mOsm/kg H_2O	270-290 mmol/kg H_2O
Panic levels	<240 mOsm/kg H_2O	<240 mmol/kg H_2O
	>320 mmol/kg H_2O	>320 mOsm/kg H_2O

Panic Level Symptoms and Treatment

Symptoms. Poor skin turgor or interstitial edema, listlessness, acidosis by decreased pH, shock, seizures, coma, cardiopulmonary arrest. Respiratory arrest may occur when value exceeds 360 mOsm/kg H_2O.

Treatment

NOTE: Treatment choice(s) depend(s) on client's history and condition and episode history.

1. Assess electrolytes.
2. Administer IV fluids in specific osmotic concentrations to shift fluid into or out of the intravascular space as appropriate.
3. Add corrected electrolytes as needed.
4. Monitor for side effects of fluid and electrolyte imbalance.
5. Possibly conduct cardiac monitoring, depending on electrolyte values.
6. Perform neurologic checks every 1-4 hours.
7. Implement seizure precautions (the client is at risk for intracerebral edema or brain cell dehydration, depending on the relative serum osmolality in comparison with intracellular osmolality).
8. Treat gastrointestinal symptoms supportively.
9. Identify and correct cause.

Increased. Acidosis, advanced liver disease, alcoholism, burns, dehydration (associated with diabetes insipidus because too much antidiuretic hormone causes the kidney to excrete large amounts of water), diabetic ketoacidosis, hyperbilirubinemia, hypercalcemia, hyperglycemia, hyperglycemic hyperosmolar nonketotic coma, hypernatremia, high-protein diet, hypovolemic shock, lung function of adults includes decreased forced expiratory volume in one second (FEV-1) and forced vital capacity (FVC), Ménière's disease, methanol poisoning, nephrogenic diabetes insipidus, thirst.

Decreased. Acute renal failure; Addison's disease; hyponatremia; overhydration; syndrome of inappropriate antidiuretic hormone secretion (SIADHS), which is often associated with cancers (especially oat cell of the lung) or medications such as chemotherapy, oral agents for diabetes mellitus and tricyclic antidepressants, and narcotics; and disorders of the posterior pituitary gland.

Description. Osmolality is a measure of the concentration of particles in the serum per kilogram of water. Osmolarity is nearly the same as osmolality but measures the concentration per liter of water. Used to assess the fluid state of the client and determine the cause of fluid and electrolyte imbalances, particularly in endocrine disorders. The normally functioning osmoregulation system maintains the serum osmolality (the concentration of the blood) within a tight normal range. Receptors in the hypothalamus adjust the level of antidiuretic hormone from the posterior pituitary, which affects the free water excreted from the kidney. Disorders of the hypothalamus, the posterior area of the pituitary, or the kidney may alter serum osmolality. Dehydration from any cause increases osmolality. Overhydration decreases serum osmolality. Either is dangerous to the client. Urine osmolarity is usually obtained with serum osmolality because the comparison gives the true picture of the fluid-balance state. The set of serum electrolytes (especially sodium and glucose) will also be assessed.

Professional Considerations
Consent form NOT required.

Preparation
1. Tube: Red topped, red/gray topped, or gold topped.

2. Do NOT draw samples during hemodialysis.

Procedure
1. Draw a 4-mL blood sample.

Postprocedure Care
1. Measure the intake and output every hour until the results are within normal limits.

Client and Family Teaching
1. Results are normally available within 4 hours.
2. Clients with adrenocortical insufficiency should consult a physician about the continuation of steroid therapy.

Factors That Affect Results
1. The specimen is stable for only 10 hours if refrigerated.
2. The use of mineralocorticoids, osmotic diuretics, insulin, or mannitol may increase values because of the effect on fluid balance.
3. Hemolysis of specimens invalidates the results.
4. Lipemic serum may alter the results.
5. Herbs or natural remedies, such as *che qian zi* ("cart-before-seeds," seeds of *Plantago major*, var. *asiatica*, ribgrass), *fu ling* (*hoelen*, *Poria cocos*, *P. sclerotium*, China root fungus), goldenseal (*Hydrastis canadensis*), *ze xie* ("marsh-purge," *Alisma orientale*, water plantain), and *zhu ling* ("pig-fungus," *Polyporus umbellatus*, pore fungus), increase osmolality because of their aquaretic (orally absorbable, non-peptidergic competitive ADH antagonistic) or diuretic effects.

Other Data
1. See Osmolality, Calculated test—Blood, for information on osmolar gap.

Osmolality—Urine

Norm. See range below; the concentration of urine has a wide range as the body adjusts to varying fluid intake and requirements.

		SI Units
13 months to adult	200-1200 mOsm/kg H$_2$O	200-1200 mmol/kg H$_2$O
0-12 months	50-600 mOsm/kg H$_2$O	50-600 mmol/kg H$_2$O

The comparison of urine osmolality to serum osmolality is important for determining the significance of the urine osmolality.

Increased. Acidosis, Addison's disease, congestive heart failure, high-protein diet, hyperglycemia, hypernatremia, hypovolemia, intracellular dehydration, renal disease, shock, and syndrome of inappropriate antidiuretic hormone secretion (SIADHS), in which the serum osmolality will be decreased.

Decreased. Aldosterone insufficiency, diabetes insipidus (levels <200 mOsm/kg H_2O), diabetic ketoacidosis, diuretic therapy, hypokalemia, hyponatremia, nephrogenic diabetes insipidus, overhydration with intravenous D_5W, psychogenic polydipsia, renal disease that affects the kidneys' ability to concentrate urine. Drugs include lithium (long-term treatment).

Description. Measure of the number of osmotically active particles in a given urine volume, which reflects the kidney's concentrating ability. Normal fluid balance is achieved by the action of the posterior pituitary (ADH secretion) and properly functioning kidneys. Fine adjustments are made continuously to maintain normal fluid and electrolyte balance. The kidney is able to adjust the urine concentration over a wide range to maintain a normal serum concentration, or osmolality. Normally, when the client becomes even slightly dehydrated, the urine will become more highly concentrated. Therefore if there is high fluid intake, the urine will become more dilute in ridding the body of the excess fluid.

Professional Considerations
Consent form NOT required.

Preparation
1. The collection may be random or the client may be required to fast from food and fluids from midnight before the collection the next day.
2. Obtain a sterile, plastic specimen container.

Procedure
1. Collect a 10-mL random or morning urine specimen in a sterile, plastic container without preservatives.

Postprocedure Care
1. Send the specimen to the laboratory for immediate processing.
2. Intake and output (I & O) should be measured until the results are normal.

Client and Family Teaching
1. Results are normally available within 24 hours.
2. Clients with adrenocortical insufficiency should consult a physician about the continuation of steroid therapy.

Factors That Affect Results
1. Anesthetics, antibiotics, carbamazepine, chlorpropamide, detergent, dextran, diuretics, glucose, mannitol, and radiographic contrast agents affect the urine volume and therefore cause abnormal results.
2. Herbs or natural remedies, such as *che qian zi* ("cart-before-seeds," seeds of *Plantago major*, var. *asiatica*, ribgrass), *fu ling* (hoelen, *Poria cocos, P. sclerotium*, China root fungus), goldenseal (*Hydrastis canadensis*), *ze xie* ("marsh-purge," *Alisma orientale*, water plantain), and *zhu ling* ("pig-fungus," *Polyporus umbellatus*, pore fungus), increase urine osmolality because of their aquaretic (orally absorbable, nonpeptidergic competitive ADH antagonistic) or diuretic effects.

Other Data
1. Urine osmolality is considered a better measurement than specific gravity to assess for the state of hydration.

Osmolar Gap
See Osmolality, Calculated Test—Blood.

Osteocalcin (Oc, Bone Gla Protein, BGP)—Plasma or Serum

Norm. NOTE: No standardized reference norms exist for this marker. Reference ranges below are provided for guidance only. Refer to individual lab reference norms provided with test results.

Adult males	1.1-10.8 ng/mL
Adult females (premenopausal)	0.7-6.4 ng/mL

Usage. The identification of women at risk of developing osteoporosis; monitoring bone metabolism in clients with growth hormone deficiency, hypothyroidism, hyperthyroidism, and chronic renal failure; monitoring women during perimenopause and postmenopause and during hormone replacement therapy; treatment of premenopausal women with LH-RH agonists; monitoring glucocorticoid-induced suppression of bone turnover; monitoring renal osteodystrophy therapy.

Increased. Carotid calcification, diet of milk with whey and low minerals, hyperparathyroidism, rapid bone growth in children (peak levels occur between ages of 10 and 16), postmenopausal females, low estrogen production, low calcium intake, low physical activity, osteomalacia, osteoporosis, Paget's disease, hyperthyroidism (decreases with treatment), fractures (for up to 1 year), renal failure with dialysis (if assay includes measurements of Oc fragments). Drugs include bisphosphonates, 1,25-dihydroxyvitamin D, calcitriol, and rosuvastatin.

Decreased. Coronary heart disease, hypercalcemia associated with malignancy, hypoparathyroidism, liver cirrhosis, metabolic syndrome, multiple myeloma, obesity or overweight, umbilical cord blood of mothers who smoke. Drugs include glucocorticoids, heparin, warfarin, tamoxifen, postmenopausal hormone replacement therapy.

Description. Osteocalcin is a gamma-carboxylated protein of bone matrix that is used as a serum marker of bone turnover because it is specifically produced by the osteoblast. Oc is an integral part of the bone formation process; however, a small amount of Oc does enter the circulation. The circulating levels of Oc are a specific indicator of recent bone turnover.

Professional Considerations
Consent form NOT required.

Preparation
1. Serum separator tube: 3 or 7 mL; confirm type of collection tube with laboratory.
2. Fasting is not generally required.

Procedure
1. Draw a 2-5 mL blood sample between 0800 and 1100. Avoid hemolysis.

2. If serial samples are drawn, collect the samples at the same time of day.

Postprocedure Care
1. Send specimen immediately to the laboratory. Refrigerate the specimen immediately if not taken immediately to the laboratory.

Client and Family Teaching
1. The results are usually available in 3-5 days.

Factors That Affect Results
1. The tube additive EDTA may invalidate the results, depending on the analytical method used. Confirm correct sample collection tube with lab.
2. The serum samples are relatively unstable, especially when at room temperature
3. With RIA, very high osteocalcin levels (>5000 ng/mL) may exceed the highest standard concentration and appear as low values due to the "hook" effect. If this occurs, the test should be repeated with a diluted sample.
4. Because of the variety of evaluation methods available for measuring osteocalcin levels, there can be significant differences in the normal range between labs.
5. Diurnal variations in Oc levels have been reported, peaking in early morning (4 AM).
6. Menstrual cycle phase: highest level occurs during luteal phase.
7. Serum osteocalcin has a short half-life and is easily fragmented. Some assays detect only intact Oc, while others also detect Oc fragments. Because Oc is sensitive to in vitro degradation, assays that measure only intact Oc may provide lower values and assays that detect fragments may provide higher Oc values.

Other Data
1. Vitamin K (phylloquinone) is required for the carboxylation of Oc, which is essential for the synthesis of mature Oc. Low serum concentrations of vitamin K are associated with increased levels of undercarboxylated Oc. Undercarboxylated Oc can be measured by some assays, providing information regarding bone quality.

O

OsteoGram

See **Radiography of the Skull, Chest, and Cervical Spine**—Diagnostic.

Osteopontin (OPN)—Serum

Norm. There are no universal standards established. Use the reference values provided by the laboratory that provides the test results.

Usage. Malignant ovarian cancer, breast cancer, prostate cancer, lung cancer, colon cancer. Research is currently being conducted to determine the use of OPN in the detection, diagnosis, monitoring, and/or staging of these and other cancers. Research has indicated that OPN may be useful in determining the prognosis and guiding therapy in clients with head and neck squamous cell carcinoma.

Increased. Aortic valve calcification and stenosis, atherosclerosis, cancer (breast, colon, gastric, hepatocellular, lung, ovarian, prostate), carotid stenosis, diabetes mellitus, granulomas, HIV, multiple sclerosis, pelvic inflammatory disease (PID), sarcoidosis.

Decreased. Resection of non-small-cell lung cancer. Drugs include etanercept.

Description. Osteopontin is an acidic glycoprotein synthesized by preosteoblasts, osteoblasts, and osteocytes, and is incorporated into bone. It is also found in many other areas of the body, including the brain, kidney, and placenta. It is a chemotactic factor for macrophages and T cells. An overexpression of OPN has been associated with tumorigenesis and metastasis in several cancers. OPN level is measured with ELISA.

Professional Considerations
Consent form NOT required.

Preparation
1. See Client and Family Teaching.
2. Clarify type of collection tube needed with institutional lab.

Procedure
1. Clarify amount of blood required with institutional lab.
2. Transport specimen to the laboratory immediately.

Postprocedure Care
1. None.

Client and Family Teaching
1. Fasting is NOT required for this test.
2. The use of OPN as a tumor biomarker is currently under research.

Factors That Affect Results
1. Research has indicated that inflammatory and noninflammatory disease processes may reflect an overexpression of OPN, decreasing the specificity of OPN as a tumor marker.

Other Data
1. Biomarker for glioblastoma and risk marker for cardiovascular disease in patients with CKD. Increased serum levels correlate with poor prognosis of cancer (glioblastoma, NSCLC).
2. Increased levels in sepsis are risk factor for death (mice study).
3. Increased levels confer >4 times risk of renal insufficiency and CAD in patients with type 2 diabetes mellitus.

Otoscopy, Video—Diagnostic

Norm. Normal structure, absence of inflammation, infection, growths, or obstruction.

Usage. Anatomy and physiology of the ear canal, visualization of the tympanic membrane. Any trauma causing bleeding may be diagnosed as well as vascular tumors of the middle ear. Using pneumatic video-otoscopy, the mobility of the tympanic membrane is observed. Video recordings can be made during surgery.

Description. This technique combines the standard methods of ENT endoscopy with a small, handheld video camera for viewing and recording the examination and ENT procedure. It can be used with the ears, nose,

O

or larynx. The advantage of the video is in the visual record of the anatomy and physiology, which can be carefully studied at a later time without further discomfort to the client. The video can also be used in consultations with other physicians and can serve as an excellent teaching tool. The recording is stored as part of the client record. Prevalence of otitis media in children is 20% with peaks in December and March.

Professional Considerations
Consent form IS required.

Risks
Infection.

Contraindications
Sedatives are contraindicated in clients with central nervous system depression.

Preparation
1. Obtain a video camera, a light source, a video cassette recorder, a video printer, a monitor and an enhancer, and film.
2. Obtain an endoscope: Hopkins 4.0 mm for adults and Hopkins 2.7 mm for children.
3. Use anesthetic spray and sedation as prescribed. Monitor respiratory status closely throughout the procedure if sedation is given.
4. Obtain instruments to remove wax and superficial hairs from the ear.
5. See Client and Family Teaching.
6. Just before beginning the procedure, take a "time out" to verify the correct client, procedure, and site.

Procedure
1. Wax and hair are removed.
2. A topical anesthetic is applied to the canal.
3. Sedatives may be given intravenously.
4. The client is placed in an upright or supine position, and the endoscope is inserted.
5. The video recording may begin at the time of insertion.

Postprocedure Care
1. Continue the assessment of the respiratory status. If deep sedation was used, follow institutional protocol for post-sedation monitoring. Typical monitoring includes continuous ECG monitoring and pulse oximetry, with continual assessments (every 5-15 minutes) of airway, vital signs, and neurologic status until the client is lying quietly awake, is breathing independently, and responds to commands spoken in a normal tone.
2. Assess for postoperative complications, including bleeding and pain.

Client and Family Teaching
1. The procedure should take less than 1 hour.
2. The client should be very still during the procedure.

Factors That Affect Results
1. The client must be able to sit still for an extended length of time.

Other Data
1. Videos are also used in rhinoscopy and laryngoscopy.

Ova and Parasites (O & P)
See **Parasite Screen**—Stool.

OVA1 Score
See OVA1™ Ovarian Tumor Triage Test—Serum

OVA1™ Ovarian Tumor Triage Test—Serum
Norm.

Pre-menopausal	Low probability of malignancy	OVA1 <5.0
	High probability of malignancy	OVA1 ≥5.0
Post-menopausal	Low probability of malignancy	OVA1 <4.4
	High probability of malignancy	OVA1 ≥4.4

Usage. Used as an adjunct to other diagnostic tests such as a physician examination and x-rays to help identify ovarian cancer when a pelvic mass is present. Indicated preoperatively (Abraham, 2010) only for adult women who already have a known adnexal ovarian mass, suspicious of ovarian cancer. A high score means ovarian cancer is likely present; thus the woman should be directed to an oncologist with a specialization in gynecologic surgery, which improves survival rates.

Description. A qualitative immunoassay test that produces a 0 to 10 score based on changes identified in 5 biomarker proteins (transthyretin, apolipoprotein A1, β2-microglobulin, transferrin, and CA-125 II cancer antigen) that increase when ovarian malignancy is present. Test results use the OvaCalc™, a proprietary method to combine the results of the serum levels of the 5 proteins into a single score indicating risk of malignancy. Sensitivity is highest (96%) in women who are postmenopausal, and lowest (89%) in women who are premenopausal. In all women, sensitivity is 92%. Sensitivity of 89% for OVA1 is higher than CA-125 (60%), and specificity is low (43%). This could result in referrals of benign conditions to gynecologic oncology surgeons; however, it would not cause added risk to the client. A major benefit of using OVA1 over CA-125 is that the increased sensitivity identifies more than 70% of malignancies not identified using American College of Obstetricians and Gynecologists guidelines for referral of patients with a pelvic mass (Ueland, 2010; Ware Miller, Smith, 2011; Ueland, 2011).

Professional Considerations
Consent form NOT required.

Preparation
1. Patient criteria for testing: This test is approved by the FDA for women who:
   • Are at least 18 years old
   • Have an ovarian adnexal mass
   • Have surgery planned
   • Have not yet been referred to an oncologist
   • Have not had cancer in the past five years
   • Have a rheumatoid factor of less than 250IU/ml
2. Tube: Red topped serum separator tube.

Procedure
1. Obtain a 3-ml blood sample.

Postprocedure Care
1. Refrigerate sample until testing. Specimen is stable for 5 days, if refrigerated or for 63 days, if frozen.

Client and Family Teaching
1. This test will help determine whether ovarian cancer is present in conjunction with the pelvic mass.

Factors That Affect Results
1. Of the 5 markers that the Ova1 test measures, CA-125 has the most impact on the score.

Other Data
1. The Ova1 test is not intended for use as a screening test, and is not intended to be used as the only test for detecting the presence of ovarian cancer.
2. There is no evidence that survival is lengthened as a result of using the Ova1 test.
3. The cost of this test is $600-$700.

Ovarian Cancer Antigen 125
See **CA 125**—Blood.

Ovarian Function Tests
See **Estradiol**—Serum; **Follicle-Stimulating Hormone**—Serum; **Luteinizing Hormone**—Blood; **Progesterone**—Serum. See also **Androstenedione**—Serum; **Estrogens**—Serum and 24-Hour Urine; Hormonal Evaluation, Cytologic—Specimen; **17-Hydroxyprogesterone**—Blood; **Metyrapone**—24-Hour Urine; **Pregnanetriol**—Urine.

Oxalate—24-Hour Urine

Norm.

		SI Units
Male		
≥13 years	7-44 mg/day	78-488 mmol/24 hours
<13 years	13-38 mg/day	144-422 mmol/24 hours
Female		
≥13 years	4-31 mg/day	44-344 mmol/24 hours
<13 years	13-38 mg/day	144-422 mmol/24 hours

Increased. Celiac disease, cirrhosis, Crohn's disease, diabetes mellitus, diabetes mellitus type 2, ethylene glycol poisoning, fat malabsorption (severe), hyperoxaluria (primary), kidney stone, nephrolithiasis, pancreatic insufficiency, sarcoidosis, vitamin B_6 deficiency. Drugs include megadoses of ascorbic acid and calcium. Also ingestion of certain oxalate-rich foods—see Client and Family Teaching. Sorbitol in whites and xylitol in blacks.

Decreased. Gastrointestinal disease or surgery that affects absorption; hyperglycinemia, hyperglycinuria, renal failure. Drugs include calcium citrate with meals, Vitamin C.

Description. Oxalate is an end product of metabolism that is excreted through the urine. It may accumulate in the soft and connective tissues of the kidneys and bladder and cause renal calculi and chronic inflammation and fibrosis.

Professional Considerations
Consent form NOT required.

Preparation
1. Obtain a 3-L plastic container to which 30 mL of 6 N hydrochloric acid (HCl) has been added.
2. See Client and Family Teaching.

Procedure
1. Collect all the urine voided in a 24-hour period in a refrigerated, 3-L plastic container to which 30 mL of 6 N HCl has been added. For specimens collected from an indwelling urinary catheter, keep the drainage bag on ice and empty the urine into the collection container hourly. Document the quantity of urinary output throughout the collection period. Not all laboratories require refrigeration.

Postprocedure Care
1. Write the beginning and ending dates and times as well as the total 24-hour urine output on the collection container and the laboratory requisition.
2. Transport the specimen to the laboratory and refrigerate it until testing.

Client and Family Teaching
1. For 48 hours before testing, maintain a diet that avoids increasing oxalate levels by avoiding soybean products, wheat germ, grapefruit juice, strawberries, rhubarb, bananas, orange juice, canned pineapples or tomatoes, kidney beans, beets, spinach, carrots, tomatoes, celery, onions, sweet and white potatoes, green and waxed beans, cauliflower, cucumber, squash, broccoli, eggplant, cabbage, spinach, cashews, chocolate, cocoa, gelatin, peanut butter and other nuts, cola beverages, and tea. Also refrain from taking vitamin C supplements during this time and use of turmeric.
2. Urinate before defecating and avoid contaminating the urine with the stool or toilet tissue. If any urine is accidentally discarded, discard the entire specimen and restart the collection the next day.
3. A high-calcium diet may promote the development of kidney stones. Consult a dietitian.
4. Results are normally available within 24 hours.

Factors That Affect Results
1. Failure to include all urine voided in the 24-hour period invalidates the results.
2. Ascorbic acid may interfere with the testing process. It does not affect the level of oxalate excretion.
3. Certain foods need to be avoided because they raise oxalate levels (see #1 under Client and Family Teaching).

Other Data

1. Studies show that stone formation is not age specific or gender specific.

2. Grapefruit juice ingestion has been found to increase urinary oxalate excretion.

Oxazepam

See **Benzodiazepines**—Plasma and Urine.

Oximetry (Pulse Oximetry, SpO₂)—Diagnostic

Norm. Adult arterial blood saturation is 94%-100%; newborn arterial blood saturation, 40%-92%, is dependent on lung development and altitude.

Usage. Any clinical situation in which adequate oxygenation is potentially compromised. Particularly helpful when used between arterial blood gas (ABG) determinations, to reduce both the number of blood draws and costs when the accuracy and correlation are known to the clinicians. *Advantages*: Is quick, noninvasive, and continuous; can detect variations in saturation that may not be noted with ABGs. *Disadvantage*: Provides only one of the determinants of the ABG and may be of only limited value when single readings are obtained. Must be carefully correlated with the clinical situation (see #8 under Factors That Affect Results). Conditions when it is used include acute myocardial infarction, acute respiratory distress syndrome (ARDS), anesthesia monitoring, asthma, cerebrovascular accident, chronic obstructive pulmonary disease, congenital heart defects, congestive heart failure, cor pulmonale, cystic fibrosis, emphysema, head trauma, intraoperatively, lung cancer, oxygen therapy, postoperatively, premature infant monitoring, pulmonary edema, pulmonary emboli, sickle cell anemia, tuberculosis, ventilator dependence, and weaning from mechanical ventilation.

Description. Pulse oximetry involves the spectrophotometric estimate of functional oxygen saturation of hemoglobin. This is a noninvasive measurement of oxygen saturation (see Blood gases, arterial—Blood), a percentage representing the ratio of arterial hemoglobin that is capable of transporting (saturated with) oxygen. Measurement is performed by means of a spectrophotometer probe usually connected to the adult's finger, temporal area, or bridge of the nose, or to an infant's foot or toe. The probe emits red and infrared light that passes through the body part and is directed at a photodetector that determines the amplitude of the transmitted light and isolates the blood's pulsatile flow. This enables calculation of SpO₂ through measurement of light absorption based on known amounts absorbed by saturated and reduced hemoglobin. Oxygenated hemoglobin absorbs more infrared light than red light. Pulse oximetry equipment is available with motion-resistant capabilities, which improves the consistency and accuracy of readings through reduction of motion artifact. The type of technology used in these pulse oximeters is called "3-wavelength reflectance."

Professional Considerations

Consent form NOT required.

Preparation

1. Cleanse the area with water and dry it before attaching the probe.
2. Know the child's or adult's weight, as correct sensor size is determined by patient's weight.
3. For clients with impaired tissue perfusion, use a nasal probe or a temporal probe. If a finger probe must be used, apply a warm pack around the hand and the extremity for 10 minutes before the probe application. The newest equipment uses centrally-placed forehead sensors that deliver improved sensitivity and rapid detection of hypoxemia.

Procedure

1. The skin should be clean and dry before placement. Remove nail polish and acrylic nails.
2. Attach the probe (NOTE: probes are machine specific and should not be interchanged) to the toe or foot for infants; the finger (ring finger has less movement and

recommended site), earlobe, temporal area, or bridge of the nose for adults; and the bridge of the nose for obese clients. Nasal probes should be placed over cartilage for best results. In males the tip of the penis can be used for emergency or spot readings.

3. Avoid placing sensor on edematous tissue or same extremity used for automated noninvasive BP monitoring. Ensure all connections are secure.

4. Activate the pulse oximeter and set low and high alarm limits according to the manufacturer's instructions.

5. Note SpO$_2$ after allowing at least 30 seconds for the reading to stabilize.

6. For continuous or periodic oximetry, observe for downward trends in SpO$_2$. Generally, decreased SpO$_2$ below 90%-92% must be addressed by thorough assessment of the client and clinical status.

7. With disposable sensors, assess site every 2-4 hours and replace sensor every 24 hours or before if dirty. Reusable sensor sites should be assessed every 2 hours, changed every 4 hours, and disinfected when dirty or at least every 24 hours.

Postprocedure Care

1. Remove the probe. Clean nondisposable probes according to the manufacturer's instructions.

2. Wash the area with soap and water.

3. Evaluate area each hour because electrical burns have occurred.

Client and Family Teaching

1. Results are normally available immediately.

2. Alarms are normally set to sound for a trend downward in values. Keeping the probe covered with a cloth improves signal clarity.

3. In cases of lung disease, discuss smoking cessation programs and strategies if applicable.

4. Continuous monitoring indicated in critical patients, pre- and post-surgery, receiving conscious sedation, lung dysfunction, obesity, sleep apnea, cardiac disorder, postanesthesia, during hemodialysis.

Factors That Affect Results

1. Hyperbilirubinemia, hypotension, hypothermia, variant hemoglobin presence, use of vasopressor medications, impaired tissue perfusion, seizures, shivering, venous pulsations associated with tricuspid regurgitation or intraaortic balloon pump, or cold extremities may result in no reading or a falsely low reading, necessitating use of ABG SpO$_2$. Desaturation by pulse oximetry may be used as a sign of severe hypotension, requiring evaluation.

2. Failure to place the probe properly may result in no reading or a falsely low or high reading.

3. Very bright light surrounding the probe may make obtaining a reading difficult. If so, cover the probe with a sheet or other opaque material.

4. Falsely elevated results may occur in the presence of dyshemoglobins (carboxyhemoglobin, >3%; methemoglobin, 1.5 g/dL; sulfhemoglobin, 0.5 g/dL), necessitating periodic validation with ABG SaO$_2$.

5. Falsely decreased results may be caused by hyperbilirubinemia >20 mg%, which may necessitate periodic validation with ABG SaO$_2$.

6. Unreliable results may occur with the injection of certain radiographic dyes within 20 minutes of use (methylene blue, indocyanine green, indigo carmine), necessitating periodic validation with ABG SaO$_2$.

7. Results may not be accurate in clients with rapid oxygen desaturation, low perfusion states (cardiac dysrhythmias, heart failure, PVD, hypotension, smoking, sickle cell disease vasooclusive crisis), or hypothermia.

8. Clients who are anemic may have misleadingly high saturation of hemoglobin and still be hypoxemic because of decreased oxygen-carrying capacity.

9. Intra-arterial injection of Patent Blue lowers the pulse oximeter reading.

Other Data

1. Accurate between SaO$_2$ levels of 85% and 100%.

2. Some pulse oximeters give slightly false higher readings in dark-skinned clients, but use after validation with ABG is not affected.

3. In healthy volunteers, significant delays in the detection of acute hypoxemia by pulse oximetry occur when pulse oximeters are placed at the toe as compared with probes at either the ear or the hand.

4. Rosati et al (2005) found routine pulse oximetry useful in screening asymptomatic newborns after the first 24 hours of life; they determined that an SpO_2 less than 96% was indicative of critical congenital cardiovascular malformations (CCVMs) that require surgical correction. Follow-up cardiac ultrasonography revealed that the pulse oximetry screening had a 66.7% sensitivity and 100% specificity, a 50% positive predictive value, and a 100% negative predictive value for CCVMs.

5. Terminology: hypoxemia refers to subnormal oxygenation of arterial blood whereas hypoxia refers to subnormal oxygenation of tissue.

6. SpO_2 level above 95% correlates to PaO_2 value in normal range of 80-100 mmHg, and an $SpO_2 \leq 90$ correlates to PaO_2 below 60 mmHg.

7. Pulse oximetry should not be used during cardiopulmonary resuscitation, during adjustment of ventilatory support, or in patients with hypovolemia as these conditions warrant blood gas analysis.

Oxygen Saturation

See **Blood Gases, Arterial**—Blood; **Blood Gases, Capillary**—Blood; **Blood Gases, Venous**—Blood.

Oxyhemoglobin Dissociation Curve

See **Blood Gases, Arterial**—Blood.

Oxytocin Challenge Test

See **Fetal Monitoring, External, Contraction Stress Test and Oxytocin Challenge Test**—Diagnostic.

P-50

See **Blood Gases, Arterial**—Blood.

PALB

See **Transthyretin**—Serum or Vitreous Fluid.

p-ANCA

See **Antineutrophil Cytoplasmic Antibody Screen**—Serum.

Pancreas Ultrasonography (Pancreas Echogram, Pancreas Ultrasound)—Diagnostic

Norm. The pancreas is properly located and positioned and is of normal size and shape, with a regular border, and a homogeneous pattern that is of finer texture than that of the peritoneum, more intense than area soft tissue, and less intense than the liver. Major supporting arteries and veins as well as the pancreatic duct are visible and normal.

Usage. Aids diagnosis of idiopathic chronic pancreatitis (coinheritance of p.R75Q with SPINK1 gene variants), pancreatic inflammation, pseudocyst, or tumor (weight loss and jaundice strongest correlation to malignancy); guidance for needle biopsy of pancreas; and ongoing monitoring of pancreatic carcinoma response to therapy (that

P

is, change in the size of a tumor). Work-up of abdominal pain, particularly in clients with alcoholism, blunt abdominal trauma, gallbladder stones, and known hyperlipidemia because they are more prone to pancreatitis. The endoscopic/intraductal method using mini probes with or without fine-needle aspiration is used experimentally to identify intraductal papillary-mucinous tumor and cystic lesions of the pancreas (see Endoscopic ultrasonography—Diagnostic).

Description. Evaluation of pancreatic structure by the creation of an oscilloscopic picture from the echoes of high-frequency sound waves passing over the epigastric area (acoustic imaging). A variation of the technique involves moving the probe intraductally via endoscopic ultrasonography (see Endoscopic ultrasonography—Diagnostic). The time required for the ultrasonic beam to be reflected back to the transducer from differing densities of tissue is converted by a computer to an electrical impulse displayed on an oscilloscopic screen to create a three-dimensional picture of the pancreas. An advantage of this test is that it can help diagnose acute pancreatitis retrospectively. In acute pancreatitis, the pancreas appears larger than normal and is less echogenic than the liver. The edema may cause compression of the inferior vena cava, and the pancreatic duct may appear enlarged. In chronic pancreatitis, calculi, shadows, strictures, or stenoses may be viewed in the pancreatic duct as well as calcified areas in the body of the pancreas. An abscess may appear as an irregular-shaped, highly echogenic structure with thick walls. Adenocarcinoma may cause the gland to appear enlarged, with an irregular border and absence of normal parenchymal echo pattern. True cysts may be differentiated from pseudocysts by their spherical, sonolucent appearance. Pseudocysts are nonspherical and may contain scattered echoes caused by debris contained within them.

Professional Considerations
Consent form NOT required.

Preparation
1. See Client and Family Teaching.
2. This test should be performed before intestinal barium tests, or after the barium is cleared from the system.

3. If the pancreas alone will be studied, a full stomach improves visualization of the posterior portion of the pancreas. The client should drink 500-1000 mL of tomato or orange juice or a cellulose suspension to distend the stomach. Alternatively, glucagon (1 mg) or a cellulose suspension may be administered intravenously, with 500 mL of water ingested a few minutes later to reduce stomach peristalsis. This causes the stomach to function as a fluid-filled window for scanning for up to 60 minutes.
4. The client should wear a gown.
5. Obtain ultrasonic gel or paste.

Procedure
1. The client is positioned supine in bed or on a procedure table.
2. The area of the abdomen overlying the pancreas is covered with conductive gel, and a lubricated transducer is passed slowly and repeatedly over the pancreas. Scanning begins with transverse views taken at 1-cm intervals with the client in full inspiration. Scanning is started at the level of the xiphoid process and proceeds until the presence of intestinal gas hinders the view. The client may then be changed to a rising position, which moves gastric air to the fundus and distends the abdominal veins to provide landmarks for identifying the pancreas. This is followed by sagittal scanning, which alternates moving from midline to the right and then midline to the left, at 1-cm intervals. The client may be asked to suspend breathing on inhalation or exhalation to reduce motion artifact.
3. Photographs of the oscilloscopic display are taken.

Postprocedure Care
1. Remove the gel from the skin.
2. If a biopsy is performed, see Biopsy, site-specific—Specimen.

Client and Family Teaching
1. This transabdominal procedure is painless and carries no risks.
2. If the biliary system will also be examined, a fast from food and fluids for 7 or 8 hours before the test is required.
3. Oral ingestion of 500-700 mL of fluids 10-15 minutes before the procedure is for stomach distention that aids in the visualization of the pancreas.

4. It is important to lie still during the procedure. You may be asked to stop breathing for a few seconds during the procedure.
5. The procedure takes less than 60 minutes, and results are normally available within 48 hours.

Factors That Affect Results

1. Dehydration interferes with adequate contrast between the organs and body fluids. Dehydration may cause the duodenum to be mistaken for the pancreas.
2. Intestinal barium, gas, or food obscures the results by preventing proper transmission and deflection of the high-frequency sound waves.
3. The more abdominal fat present, the greater is the attenuation (reduction in sound-wave amplitude and intensity), which interferes with the clarity of the picture. Abdominal muscles and cartilage may have the same effect, necessitating repositioning of the client.
4. The stomach may interfere with views of the pancreatic anatomy in transverse scans.
5. If the left lobe of the liver is very small (<2 cm), it will function poorly as an acoustic window.

Other Data

1. Severe dehydration, especially when combined with obesity, has the potential to impair visualization of the pancreas and the surrounding area.
2. See also Endoscopic ultrasonography—Diagnostic.

Pancreatic Secretory Trypsin Inhibitor (PSTI)—Serum (TATI)

Norm. 16.6 ± 0.7 ng/mL. In pancreatic juice <25000 ng/mL.

Increased. Citrin deficiency (PSTI >29 ng/mL), colostrum, Crohn's disease, pancreatitis, severe infection of the GI tract, cell destruction in the mucosal layers of the GI tract, intraductal papillary mucinous neoplasm of pancreas (IPMN). Considered a marker for malignant pancreatic endocrine tumors. The related TATI tumor-associated trypsin inhibitor is considered a marker for certain cancers such as lung and ovarian. Levels may increase with rejection of transplanted pancreas. It is considered a marker for threatened organ rejection. Drugs: misoprostol (Cytotec).

Decreased. Alcoholic chronic pancreatitis with SPINK1 gene IVS3+2T>C mutation.

Description. PSTI is a potent protease inhibitor found in the pancreas, in the mucus-secreting cells of the gastrointestinal tract, and in the breasts, lungs, and kidneys. It is believed to be involved in healing after injury because it inhibits the proteolytic breakdown of mucus. It may also be capable of promoting growth activity. Newer studies suggest than PSTI gene alteration may be associated with the risk of developing chronic pancreatitis. PSTI is absorbed into the bloodstream and therefore can be measured by immunoradioassay. Absorbed PSTI is excreted in the urine. This test is performed by radioimmunoassay.

Professional Considerations

Consent form NOT required.

Preparation

1. Tube: Red topped, red/gray topped, or gold topped.
2. No fasting required.

Procedure

1. Draw 5 mL of blood.

Postprocedure Care

1. No special handling of the specimen is known.

Client and Family Teaching

1. Results will not be available for up to 5 days.

Factors That Affect Results

1. Radioisotope testing within the previous week invalidates the results.
2. Hemolysis of blood samples invalidates the results.
3. Oral contraceptives and steroids have a possibility of interfering with test results.

Other Data

1. None.

PAP

See **Prostatic Acid Phosphatase**—Blood.

Pap Smear (Papanicolaou Test)—Diagnostic

Norm. Results are reported according to the Bethesda System in a descriptive statement regarding the adequacy of the sample, followed by a descriptive diagnosis. Abnormalities are described as benign, low-grade squamous, high-grade squamous, glandular, or severe dysplasia with carcinoma in situ.

Abnormal. Terms used to describe abnormal cells include the following:

Term	Meaning	May Also Be Called
Atypical squamous cells of undetermined significance (ASCUS)	May indicate need for further diagnostic evaluation	
Dysplasia, mild, moderate, or severe	Appearance of cells is abnormal; no invasion of healthy tissue; cells may develop into early cervical cancer SIL, CIN 3	Mild: low-grade SIL, CIN 1 Moderate: high-grade SIL, CIN 2 Severe: high-grade
Squamous intraepithelial lesion (SIL), low grade or high grade	Abnormal appearance of cervical surface cells, which appear thin and flat	
Cervical intraepithelial neoplasia (CIN)	Presence of abnormal cell growth in cervical surface cells; may be further described with numbers 1 to 3 to indicate how much of cervix contains abnormal cells	
Carcinoma in situ	Presence of preinvasive cancer cells on surface of cervix	High-grade SIL, CIN 3

Previous Terminology

Class I	Normal
Class II	Probably normal
Class III	Doubtful (may be malignant)
Class IV	Probably malignant
Class V	Malignant

Positive. Abnormal cells indicative of endocrine disorders, cancer (uterine), endometriosis, lymphogranuloma venereum, tumors (cervical), and vaginal adenosis or inflammation that could lead to cancer.

Negative. Normal cervical cells.

Usage. This test is primarily used in the early detection of cervical and vaginal carcinomas and scrapings from the uterus. The *smear technique* can also be used to detect cancerous cells of the breast (aspiration of mammary gland tissue), lung (bronchial brushing and washing from bronchoscopy or coughed-up sputum), stomach (aspirated gastric secretions), and renal system (urine sediment). It is indicated as routine screening and for workup of disorders of reproduction function. Pap testing is not indicated for detecting recurrent cervical or endometrial cancer because efficacy (0%-7%) in these situations is very low.

Description. The Pap smear, the most widely used cancer-screening tool, is a cytologic examination of desquamated epithelial tissue to differentiate normal from anaplastic cells. Both a traditional slide method and a newer liquid method are described here. In the traditional method, one prepares the smears by scraping or aspirating cells from the tissue to be examined (that is, the cervix) and fixing them on glass slides, using ether and 95% ethyl alcohol (ethanol) solution. Slides are then dried, stained, and examined under a microscope by a pathologist or cytotechnologist. In the newer liquid Pap method, the tissue scrapings are placed in liquid to remove mucus and debris, which can interfere with the view through the microscope. Many studies have found that most human cervical cancers harbor types of high-risk human papillomavirus (HPV). For this reason, studies are being conducted to evaluate whether circulating HPV DNA in the plasma can serve as a marker for cervical cancer. (See Human papillomavirus in situ hybridization—Specimen.)

Professional Considerations
Consent form NOT required.

Preparation
1. See Client and Family Teaching.
2. Interview the client; record age, date of last menstrual period, prior history of abnormal Pap smear results, and pregnancy status.
3. Obtain a glass slide, a sterile Ayre spatula (for the ectocervix), a cytobrush (for the endocervix), a tongue blade, a pipette, a sterile cotton swab, sterile gloves, ether/95% alcohol solution (1:1), spray fixative, a graphite pencil, and a speculum. Using the graphite pencil, label the frosted ends of the slide with the client's name and the collection site. For liquid procedure, obtain ThinPrep.
4. The client should disrobe below the waist.
5. Position the client recumbent on a gynecologic examination table in the lithotomy position, and drape for comfort and privacy.

Procedure
1. *Liquid Pap Method*: Follow the steps below, substituting "transfer of the specimen to the ThinPrep Pap container" to "transfer of the specimen to a slide."
2. Note: Fixative must be applied to the slide before any drying of the specimen occurs. If a two-step specimen is taken, fixative should be applied after each step. Remove excess mucus by placing a 2- × 2-inch gauze pad over the cervix and gently peeling it away after a few seconds.
3. *Endocervical Smear:*
   a. Aspirate endocervical secretions from the cervical os as through a pipette. Spread the secretions onto a glass slide. Dip or spray the slide with the prepared fixative and dry it.
   b. Insert a cytobrush into the cervical os and rotate it 360 degrees, using one continuous motion. Smear the scrapings onto a glass slide, using a single continuous stroke to avoid traumatizing the cells. Fix immediately as described above.
4. *Ectocervical Scraping*: Using a wooden tongue blade or the blunt side of a wooden Ayre spatula inserted into the cervical os, rotate or scrape the entire surface at the squamocolumnar junction. Remove the tongue blade and smear onto a glass slide. Fix immediately as described above.
5. *Cervical Scraping*: Insert the pointed edge of a wooden Ayre spatula into the cervical os and rotate the spatula 360 degrees. Spread the cervical scrapings on a glass slide, fix it with an ether/95% ethyl alcohol solution, and dry the slide. A Cervex-Brush sampling device may be used, and it is recommended to be rotated a full 180 degrees to improve the sampling for abnormal cervical cells.
6. *Vaginal Pool*: Using the blunt side of a wooden Ayre spatula, scrape the vaginal floor behind the cervix. Spread the vaginal pool secretions on a glass slide, spray or soak them in fixative, and dry the slide. Vaginal fluid is obtained for suspected endometrial cancer or for a hormonal evaluation.
7. *Vulva Smear*: Using the blunt side of a wooden Ayre spatula, directly scrape the vulvar lesion. Spread the scraping on a glass slide and fix it immediately with spray fixative.

Postprocedure Care
1. On the laboratory requisition, write the client's age; the reason for the study; the date of the last menstrual period; any chemotherapy or hormonal medications; and history, including any previous abnormal Pap smears and treatment for cancer or abnormal vaginal bleeding.
2. Send the slides to the cytology laboratory.

Client and Family Teaching
1. For clients of childbearing age, test should be done 10-20 days after the first day of the last menstrual period.
2. Do NOT douche for 18-72 hours before the procedure.

3. It is customary practice for the client to be informed of the results, either positive or negative. The method of information exchange needs to be arranged with the client's physician.

4. 1 week is needed for result.

5. Further testing may be needed, including a repeat Pap (Salani, Backes, Fung, 2011), endometrial biopsy, or colposcopy. This decision will be made when the results of the test are received.

Recommended Cervical Pap Frequency Age (Years)	Regular (Traditional) Pap	Liquid-Based Pap (ThinPrep by Quest Diagnostics)
<21	No screening, regardless of sexual history	Same
21-29	Every 3 years	Every 2 years
30-65	Every 3 to 5 years; May also include testing for HPV	Same
65-70	Consider discontinuation of screening if last three tests were normal AND if there were no abnormal results in last 10 years AND if 2 or more HPV tests have been negative.	Same
After subtotal hysterectomy	Same as above	Same as above
After total hysterectomy because of invasive cervical disease	Every 3 months × 2 years, then every 6 months	
After total hysterectomy not necessitated by cancer or precancerous conditions	Not needed unless client has risk factors for cervical cancer	Same

Factors That Affect Results

1. Smears that dry before fixative is applied cannot be properly interpreted.
2. Do not lubricate the speculum; such lubrication distorts cells.
3. Use of formalin as a fixative invalidates the results.
4. Water or lubricant on the specimen can distort the cells.
5. A smear taken any time other than in the midmenstrual cycle can result in abnormal findings. The best time for a cervical cytology study is 5-6 days after menses.
6. Inadequate specimens may require retesting.
7. Tetracycline or digitalis preparations can affect the look of squamous epithelium.
8. Blood, mucus, or pus on the slide makes accurate specimen interpretation difficult. The presence of infection in the cervical area may contribute to the absence of endocervical cells.
9. Cells that are damaged from excessive manipulation during collection may be interpreted as atypical.

Other Data

1. False-positive Pap smear results requiring a repeat test in 6-12 weeks, as is standard, may be avoided if a culture for *Chlamydia* and *Neisseria gonorrhoeae* and wet-mount slides are examined at the time of the examination.
2. False-negative results can be minimized by obtaining double scrapings and smear cultures.
3. See also Pap smear, Ultrafast and fine-needle aspiration—Diagnostic.
4. Precancerous cervical cells often take up to 5 years to become cancerous. The American Cancer Society revised its recommendations for frequency of cervical cancer screening via Pap smear to reflect studies that have shown that less frequent testing only slightly increases the risk of missing precancerous conditions, but reduces the likelihood of detecting and subsequently overtreating benign cervical conditions.
5. Many studies have found that most human cervical cancers harbor the

high-risk human papillomavirus (HPV) types. For this reason, studies are being conducted to evaluate whether circulating HPV DNA in the plasma can serve as a marker for cervical cancer.

6. Persons who are older, lower education and have public health insurance are least likely to obtain a PAP smear.

Consensus Guidelines of the American Society for Colposcopy and Cervical Pathology (ASCCP) Recommended Follow-up for Abnormal Pap Smears

Finding	Recommended Follow-up
Atypical squamous cells (ASCs) of undetermined significance (ASCUS)	Two repeat cytology tests OR Immediate colposcopy with loop electrosurgical excision procedure (LEEP) (see Colposcopy—Diagnostic) OR DNA testing for high-risk types of human papillomavirus (preferred choice, if method used for Pap testing was liquid-based cytology); see Human papillomavirus in situ hybridization—Diagnostic
Finding cannot exclude high-grade squamous intraepithelial lesion (HSIL; ASC-H)	Immediate colposcopy with loop electrosurgical excision procedure (LEEP)
Low-grade squamous intraepithelial lesion or atypical glandular cells	Immediate colposcopy with loop electrosurgical excision procedure (LEEP)

Pap Smear (Papanicolaou Test), Ultrafast (UFP) and Fine-Needle Aspiration—Diagnostic

Norm. Normal cells and structure for the area biopsied. Absence of tumor cells or abnormalities of the cell nucleus.

Usage. Adenocarcinoma, of various organs; squamous cell carcinoma; neuroendocrine carcinomas; clear cell–type renal cell carcinoma; schwannoma; lymphoid hyperplasia, with small round lymphocytes, small cleaved lymphocytes, large noncleaved lymphocytes, and histiocytes (macrophages). Breast-tissue lesions, thyroid lesions, Hürthle cell carcinoma, and colloid nodule with hemorrhagic degeneration.

Description. This procedure involves fine-needle aspiration for cytologic evaluation and may be performed intraoperatively or during a colposcopic examination (see Colposcopy—Diagnostic). The ultrafast technique is particularly useful when a quick result is important. The method is particularly advantageous for looking at the cell nucleus because it provides the cytologist or histologist with a clear, stained view of the cell and organelles.

Professional Considerations
Consent form IS required for all fine-needle aspiration biopsy procedures. For specimens taken during surgery, the client gives consent for the surgical procedure.

Preparation
1. Obtain clear glass slides, a syringe, and 18-gauge needles; Coplin jars; normal saline; and 95% ethyl alcohol for storage and transport to the laboratory.
2. Notify the laboratory for on-site processing, staining, handling, and consultative interpretation of the specimen.
3. Just before beginning the procedure, take a "time out" to verify the correct client, procedure, and site.

Procedure
1. Depends on the body site and location of the area for biopsy. Some clients will be

prepared for surgery and taken to an operating room.
2. Ambulatory care and ward procedures may require local anesthesia.
3. The skin is prepared for the procedure.
4. Needle aspiration of the tissue is obtained; sometimes a special procedure such as fluoroscopy or isolation of a nodule is required. The specimen is taken with a sterile technique, and smears are made on the clear microscope slides. It is air-dried and processed for 30 seconds in normal saline and then in 95% ethyl alcohol and sent immediately to the laboratory for processing, or the cytologist present during the procedure handles the specimen. The developers suggest that fine-needle aspirations for cytology follow this procedure: (1) prepare several clear glass slides and air-dry; (2) stain and process the ultrafast slide; (3) save the other slides for laboratory use for other methods such as the Diff-Quik stain, which has other advantages for the final diagnosis.

Postprocedure Care
1. The specimen is carefully labeled and transported immediately to the cytology laboratory.
2. Apply a dry, sterile dressing over the site.
3. Monitor for bleeding at the site.
4. Give postsurgical care as appropriate.

Client and Family Teaching
1. Call the physician for signs of infection at the procedure site: increasing pain, redness, swelling, purulent drainage, or for temperature >101 degrees F (38.3 degrees C).
2. Results are normally available within 24 hours.

Factors That Affect Results
1. Inappropriate processing.

Other Data
1. Total turn-around time for these specimens may be as little as 30 minutes.
2. See also Pap smear—Diagnostic.

Paracentesis (Peritoneal Fluid Analysis)—Diagnostic

Norm.

Appearance	Clear, serous, light yellow
Amount	<50 mL
Protein	<4.1 g/dL
Glucose	70-100 mg/dL (equals serum)
Amylase	140-400 U/L (equals serum)
Ammonia	
Alkaline phosphatase	
Adult female	45-250 U/L
Adult male	90-240 U/L
Red blood cells	Negative
White blood cells	<300/mL
Culture	Negative
Cytologic result	No malignant cells
CEA and CA 125	Negative
Fungus	Negative

Usage. Used diagnostically to remove and examine small amounts of fluid for undiagnosed causes of abdominal effusion. May be used to instill and remove saline lavage to examine for the presence of blood if blunt trauma to the chest and abdomen is suspected.

Abnormal Appearance
Bloody: Trauma (or traumatic tap).
    Turbid (cloudy): Infection, pancreatitis, intestinal perforation, and cirrhosis.
    Milky: Chylous ascites.

Increased Protein. Cancer, tuberculosis, peritoneal carcinomatosis, and peritonitis.

Increased Amylase. Pancreatitis and intestinal strangulation, necrosis (intestinal), pancreatic pseudocyst, pancreatic trauma.

Increased Alkaline Phosphatase. Intestinal strangulation and ruptured intestine.

Increased Red Blood Cells. Intra-abdominal trauma, neoplasm, and tuberculosis.

Increased White Blood Cells. Infection and chylous ascites, cirrhosis, and peritonitis. Granulocyte count of >250 cells/mL is diagnostic for infection.

Increased CEA and CA 125. Malignancy. NOTE: An elevated CA 125 without elevation in CEA indicates primary malignancy is ovarian or endometrial.

Decreased Glucose Below Serum Level. Malignancy or TB peritonitis.

Description. Paracentesis is the transabdominal removal of fluid from the peritoneal cavity for analysis of electrolytes, red blood cells, white blood cells, bacterial and viral cultures, and cytology studies. The procedure may be done in conjunction with endoscopic ultrasound guidance, particularly when used to reach small areas of effusion. Paracentesis may also be used therapeutically to remove ascitic fluid when the accumulation is large and disabling (e.g., interferes with venous return, normal breathing, appetite, and activities of daily living) such as in ascites attributable to hepatic encephalopathy or other causes.

Professional Considerations

Consent form IS required.

Risks

Abdominal wall infection, hemorrhage, perforated bowel, increased peritonitis.

Contraindications

This procedure should be used with caution during pregnancy and in clients with coagulation abnormalities or bleeding tendencies.

Preparation

1. Have the client urinate or empty the bladder by catheterization. This will help prevent accidental bladder trauma.
2. Measure abdominal girth, weight, and baseline vital signs. Monitor vital signs every 10-15 minutes during the procedure.
3. Obtain povidone-iodine solution, sterile gauze sponges, 1%-2% lidocaine (Xylocaine), 10- and 30-mL syringes, 22- and 24-gauge needles, sterile gloves, sterile drapes, a trocar with a cannula, a sterile vacuum collection bottle, plastic tubing, a scalpel, suture, a needle holder, and tape.
4. Just before beginning the procedure, take a "time out" to verify the correct client, procedure, and site.

Procedure

1. Position the client sitting on the edge of a bed or examination table with the back supported and the feet resting on a stool.

The procedure may also be performed with the client lying supine.

2. Cleanse the client's abdomen with povidone-iodine solution and allow it to dry; then cover the areas surrounding the site with a sterile drape.
3. Numb the area with 1%-2% lidocaine (Xylocaine), first using a 22-gauge needle locally and then changing to a 24-gauge needle and anesthetizing the area deeper.
4. A scalpel is used to make a stab wound into the peritoneal cavity midway between the umbilicus and the symphysis pubis. Alternatively, the insertion may be through the iliac fossa, through the flank, or in each abdominal quadrant. The trocar-cannula is threaded through the incision. An audible sound may be heard when the needle pierces the peritoneum. The trocar is removed, and plastic tubing is attached to the cannula; the other end of the tubing is placed in the collection receptacle (usually a 500- to 1000-mL vacuum bottle). The fluid is slowly drained from the abdominal cavity. The client may need to be repositioned to improve drainage.
5. Inoculate ascitic fluid into blood culture bottles at the bedside.
6. Do not drain more than 5 L at a time. If hypovolemia occurs as a result of rapid drainage, raise the bottle to slow the drainage rate or clamp the drainage tube. To reduce risk of infection, do not leave drain in place longer than 6 hours.
7. When the fluid collection is complete, remove the cannula and suture the incision if necessary.

Postprocedure Care

1. Apply a dry, sterile dressing to the site.
2. Observe the site for bleeding or drainage.
3. Measure abdominal girth and weight.
4. Monitor vital signs for evidence of hemodynamic changes every 30 minutes for 2 hours, every hour for 4 hours, and then every 4 hours for 24 hours.
5. Write any recent antibiotic therapy on the laboratory requisition. Send the samples to the laboratory for analysis immediately.
6. Document in the client's record the time of the procedure; the name of the physician; the color, consistency, and amount

of fluid withdrawn; and the client's response to the procedure.

7. Monitor daily sequential multiple analyzer (SMA7) blood work.

8. Observe for hematuria caused by bladder trauma. If this is suspected at the time of the procedure, a BUN and creatinine value obtained on the paracentesis fluid should be sent to confirm the condition.

Client and Family Teaching

1. Notify the physician immediately if you notice bloody, pink, or red urine.

2. Results are normally available within 72 hours.

Factors That Affect Results

1. Inadvertent internal organ injury, including female organs, may contaminate the sample with bile, blood, urine, or feces or with bacterial flora.

2. Delay in analysis may cause inaccurate results.

3. Care must be taken to ensure a sterile technique, especially in handling specimens for culture and Gram stain.

Other Data

1. Frequently, salt-poor albumin or mannitol is infused for 24 hours after paracentesis for clients with ascites and poor nutrition, which increase the third spacing of fluid into this cavity.

2. Transient initial bloody fluid may result from a traumatic tap.

Paracentesis, Fluid Analysis

See **Paracentesis**—Diagnostic.

Parasite Screen—Blood

Norm. Negative. Acute parasitic infection is strongly indicated when titers increase fourfold (for most organisms) between acute and convalescent sera.

Usage. Nonspecific detection of parasitic infection.

Positive. Chagas disease, small protozoa of malaria (*Plasmodium falciparum, P. malariae, P. ovale,* and *P. vivax*), cysticercosis, *Babesia, Echinococcus, Entamoeba histolytica, Fasciola hepatica,* filariasis (*Wuchereria bancrofti*), *Giardia, kala-azar* (leishmaniasis), *Paragonimus, Strongyloides, Taenia solium, T. saginata,* toxoplasmosis (*Toxoplasma gondii*), trichinosis, trypanosomiasis (*Trypanosoma brucei* and *T. brucei rhodesiense*), and VLM (*Ascaris* and *Toxocara*).

Description. Parasites are organisms that must live in or on a host to survive and often require different hosts at different stages of development. Parasitic infections in humans may be acquired from the fecal-oral route or from contaminated food, animals, and some arthropods. Some parasites survive on the host by changing antigenic characteristics or becoming coated with host immunoglobulins, so that they are no longer recognized as foreign by the immune system. The most accurate method of diagnosing a blood-borne parasitic infection is to identify the actual parasite in a Giemsa-stained thick or thin film of blood. This is not always easy, however, because the amount of blood-borne parasites present at any given time may vary depending on the parasitic stages and cycles. The parasite screen is used when the presence of the actual parasite cannot be established. This screen involves several laboratory procedures that help to detect the presence of parasite antigen-antibody complexes in a sample of blood. Three of the methods typically used to identify parasitic infection are complement fixation, hemagglutination inhibition, and immunodiffusion. Results are reported in titers as the highest dilution of serum that tests positive for parasitic antibodies.

Professional Considerations

Consent form NOT required.

Preparation

1. Tube: Red topped, red/gray topped, or gold topped or pink topped, or Corvac tube.

Procedure

1. Parasite screen the fresh blood for filariae and trypanosomes, which should be collected between 2200 (10 PM) and 2400 (12 AM) hours.
2. Draw a 5-mL blood sample.
3. Avoid causing hemolysis.
4. An acute sample should be drawn as soon as possible after a parasitic infection is suspected.
5. Draw a convalescent sample in 2-4 weeks.

Postprocedure Care

1. None.

Client and Family Teaching

1. Return in 2-4 weeks to have a follow-up sample drawn.
2. Avoid donating blood until the results are known.

Factors That Affect Results

1. Hemolysis of the specimen may cause false-negative results.
2. A single test has little significance unless the results are extremely high.
3. For several of the parasites, false-negative results may be caused by the presence of antibodies from past infection.

Other Data

1. Even with positive results, diagnosis of a parasitic infection cannot be confirmed without recovery of the parasite.

Parasite Screen (Ova and Parasites, Tape Test)—Stool

Norm. Negative. No parasite, ova, or larvae identified.

Usage. Diagnosis of parasitic infestation of the intestinal tract.

Positive. *Ancylostoma duodenale* (hookworm), *Ascaris lumbricoides* (roundworm), *Balantidium coli, Blastocystis hominis, Capillaria philippinensis, Chilomastix mesnili, Clonorchis sinensis, Cryptosporidium* spp., *Dientamoeba fragilis, Diphyllobothrium latum* (fish tapeworm), *Dipylidium caninum* (tapeworm), *Endolimax nana, Entamoeba histolytica, E. hartmanni, E. polecki, Enterobius vermicularis* (pinworm), *Enteromonas hominis, Escherichia coli, Fasciola hepatica, Fasciolopsis buski, Giardia lamblia, G. helminths, G. protozoa, Heterophyes, Hymenolepis diminuta* (tapeworm), *Hymenolepis nana* (dwarf tapeworm), *Iodamoeba bütschlii, Isospora belli, Metagonimus yokogawai, Necator americanus* (hookworm), *Opisthorchis sinensis, Paragonimus westermani* (long fluke), *Retortamonas intestinalis, Sarcocystis* spp., *Schistosoma mansoni* (blood fluke ova), *Strongyloides stercoralis* (threadworm), *Taenia saginata* (beef tapeworm), *T. solium* (pork tapeworm), *Trichinella spiralis, Trichomonas hominis, Trichostrongylus* spp., and *Trichuris trichiura* (whipworm).

Description. Microscopic examination of stool to detect parasites at various stages of development from ova through mature or motile forms. A parasite screen is performed on a stool sample when a parasitic infection is suspected as evidenced (usually) by diarrhea of unknown origin. A parasite is an organism that survives at the expense of a host organism. Frequently, protozoa, amebas, and worms infect the gastrointestinal tract from contaminated food and water sources. Parasites, larvae, or ova may not be continuously present in fecal specimens; thus at least three samples, spaced 2-3 days apart, or as prescribed, are taken. For a screen, the laboratory will need to know travel information and will likely perform screens based on the parasites usually found in that location. Laboratory preparations for each parasite to be identified may vary.

Professional Considerations

Consent form NOT required.

Preparation

1. Question the client carefully about any recent travel and about hygiene practices.
2. Clarify whether a preservative is needed by contacting the laboratory that will be performing the test. If a preservative is to be used, stools for ova and parasite examination should be preserved in 5% formalin or polyvinyl alcohol solutions. Specimens should be diluted in a 3:1 stool-to-preservative ratio.

3. Obtain a clean plastic, waxed cardboard, or glass container and a tongue blade; or obtain clear cellophane tape, a tongue blade, a glass slide, and a clean container. If protozoa, amebas, or flagella are suspected, the specimen must be taken "stat" to the laboratory for examination.
4. See Client and Family Teaching.

Procedure

1. *Stool collection*: Collect three random stool samples, each 2-3 days apart. The specimens should be collected in a plastic, waxed cardboard, or glass container with a tight-fitting lid. The client should defecate directly into the container or into a clean, sterile bedpan. If a bedpan is used, lift 2 tablespoons of stool into the container with a wooden tongue blade, being cautious not to contaminate the outside of the container. Apply the lid tightly.
2. *Collection of pinworm or tapeworm eggs*: Collect the specimen between 2200 (10 PM) and 2300 (11 PM) hours or early in the morning before bath or bowel movement. Wrap clear cellulose tape around the end of a tongue blade and firmly press it against three or four separate portions of the perianal area, close to the anus. Do not insert the tongue blade into the anus. Remove the tape and, using a cotton ball, press it lightly onto a glass slide with the gummed side against the glass. Place the slide in a clean container for transport to the laboratory.
3. *Collection of tapeworm*: If tapeworm is suspected, send the entire stool so that the head of the tapeworm can be identified.

Postprocedure Care

1. Write the collection time, travel history, and suspected diagnosis on the laboratory requisition.
2. Send the specimen to the laboratory within 1 hour of collection. Unformed stools should have a preservative added.
3. Several specimens are usually prescribed: three specimens are usually standard.

Client and Family Teaching

1. Collect the stool specimen according to the procedure described above and avoid contaminating it with urine.
2. Cook food properly, boil water, and wash hands thoroughly if contamination is suspected.
3. Have water analyzed, especially well water.
4. With diarrhea, avoid milk, milk products, greasy foods, and spicy foods. Drink clear fluids with electrolytes.

Factors That Affect Results

1. Fresh, room-temperature stool samples provide the best specimens. Do not incubate, refrigerate, or freeze the specimens.
2. Reject specimens contaminated with urine, toilet paper, diapers, or toilet water.
3. Mineral oil or magnesium antacids, MOM, kaolin, antimalarial drugs, or bismuth may interfere with accuracy.
4. Specimens obtained by means of saline or phospho soda enemas are acceptable. Often the first stool after the enema is discarded, and the subsequent stools are examined.
5. Stool samples should be collected during laboratory hours so that they can be promptly examined.
6. Antimicrobial or antiamebic therapy within 5-10 days before specimen collection may cause false-negative results.
7. Residual barium from recent gastrointestinal studies may interfere with microscopic examination. Wait 1 week after barium procedures or laxative administration before collecting stool samples.
8. Drugs and other substances that interfere with microscopic examination of fecal samples include antacids, antibiotics, barium, bismuth, castor oil, enemas, iron, magnesia, Metamucil, and tetracyclines.

Other Data

1. Use caution when handling the sample because some parasitic infections are very contagious.
2. One negative result does not rule out a parasitic infection.
3. A 24-hour stool collection may be requested to obtain an estimated egg count in known parasitic infestation.
4. Information about travel is of utmost importance to the laboratory in detecting the suspected parasite because different techniques are used to analyze stool when one is looking for specific parasites or ova.
5. TF-Test (Immunoassay Com. Ind. Ltda, Sau Paulo, Brazil) is a practical, economical and sensitive kit for diagnosis of intestinal parasites.

P

Parathyroid Hormone (PTH)—Blood

Norm. NOTE: Norms vary by test method used. Check laboratory-specific norms.

		SI Units
Plasma or Serum		
Parathyroid hormone, biointact	10-47 pg/mL	10-47 ng/L
Parathyroid hormone, intact	15-75 pg/mL	15-75 ng/L
Midmolecule and C-Terminal (Serum)		
1-16 years	51-217 pg/mL	51-217 ng/L
Adults	50-330 pg/mL	50-330 ng/L
N-Terminal (Serum)		
2-13 years	14-21 pg/mL	14-21 ng/L
Adults	8-24 pg/mL	8-24 ng/L

Usage. Primarily in the evaluation of abnormal calcium states to assist with the diagnosis of hyperparathyroid or hypothyroid disease. An ionized calcium is usually drawn with the parathyroid hormone (PTH) sample. Levels are also followed in chronic renal clients to identify the development of hyperthyroid function caused by phosphate retention and to monitor clients treated for same.

Increased. As a response to low serum calcium levels caused by calcium malabsorption, chronic renal failure, dietary vitamin D deficiency, osteomalacia, and renal dialysis. Also, ectopic production of PTH, lactation, parathyroid adenoma, parathyroid carcinoma, parathyroid hyperplasia, pregnancy, primary hyperparathyroidism, pseudohypoparathyroidism (sometimes), renal hypercalciuria, rickets (vitamin D dependent, vitamin D deficient), secondary hyperparathyroidism, and squamous cell carcinoma (kidney, lung, ovary, pancreas). PTH levels increase with the aging process. PTH levels increased in surgical site irrigation fluid is associated with postoperative hypocalcemia.

Decreased. As a response to high calcium levels (i.e., cancer patients), autoimmune disease or cancer, Graves' disease, hypomagnesemia, hypoparathyroidism, parathyroidectomy (transient decrease), sarcoidosis, and vitamin A and D intoxication. Drugs include thiazide diuretics.

Description. Parathyroid hormone (PTH) is measured by radioassay using competitive protein-binding agents to identify and measure several molecular forms of PTH: intact and midmolecule fragments. N-terminal fragments and C-terminal fragments may be tested in some laboratories. Intact PTH is secreted by the parathyroid gland and is metabolized by the liver and kidneys into N-terminal fragments and C-terminal fragments. The intact and N-terminal fragments are helpful in identifying acute conditions, whereas C-terminal fragments indicate chronic disturbances of PTH metabolism. Parathyroid hormone is directly responsible for the plasma regulation of calcium and phosphorus. When the body's normal autoregulatory mechanism senses a decrease in serum calcium level, the parathyroid gland is stimulated to secrete PTH. The elevated serum PTH triggers the release of calcium from bone and stimulates the renal tubules to increase reabsorption of calcium ions in the distal convoluted tubules and to decrease reabsorption of phosphorus in the proximal convoluted tubules. When the serum calcium concentration again becomes adequate, the parathyroid gland decreases PTH secretion. In the presence of primary parathyroid tumor or hyperplasia, the PTH-calcium autoregulation fails. As PTH secretion increases, so does the serum calcium level, ultimately resulting in a hypercalcemic condition that can be life-threatening. Assessment of radioassayed PTH is helpful in differentiating parathyroid causes from nonparathyroid causes of hypercalcemia. Other causes of hypercalcemia generally display normal to slightly high or low PTH secretion. Thus PTH should always be evaluated in conjunction with serum ionized calcium levels.

Professional Considerations

Consent form NOT required.

Preparation

1. Tube: Red topped, red/gray topped, or gold topped or lavender topped; and ice.
2. A morning fasting sample is recommended because there is a diurnal variation in PTH levels.
3. Do NOT draw during hemodialysis.
4. See Client and Family Teaching.

Procedure

1. Completely fill the red topped, red/gray topped, or gold topped tube with blood.
2. Some laboratories require that the sample be packed in ice.
3. Some laboratories request 7 mL of blood in a lavender topped tube as well.

Postprocedure Care

1. Send the specimen to the laboratory immediately.
2. Resume previous diet.
3. Assess for signs of hypercalcemia: lethargy, headache, thirst, increased urinary output, decreased muscle tone, nausea, thirst, and flank pain.
4. Assess for signs of hypocalcemia: lethargy, nausea, cramps, dysrhythmias, shallow breathing, tetany, and Chvostek's and Trousseau's signs.

Client and Family Teaching

1. Fast overnight before sampling.
2. A change in diet may be needed, based on results. A diet either low or high in calcium may be indicated. Consider consulting a dietitian.
3. Calcium is important to your body. It helps with blood clotting, bone strength, and heart contraction.

Factors That Affect Results

1. Reject lipemic specimens or specimens not received on ice.
2. Ingestion of milk before the test may cause falsely low values.
3. Radioisotope testing within the last 7 days may alter the results.

Other Data

1. A neck venipuncture PTH level should be compared to a peripheral venipuncture PTH level if the test is performed to rule out parathyroid adenoma. The neck vein technique may help to confirm the diagnosis of hyperparathyroidism if the PTH level is much higher than that from a peripheral site.

Parathyroid Hormone Radioimmunoassay

See **Parathyroid Hormone—Blood**.

Parietal Cell Antibody—Blood

Norm. Negative. None detected, or titer <1:120.

Abnormal. Weakly positive, titer 1:120 to 1:140.

Positive. Titer >1:180.

Usage. Aids in differential diagnosis of autoimmune gastritis and pernicious anemia. Not as widely accepted as in the past for the diagnosis of pernicious anemia.

Positive. Autoimmune atrophic gastritis or pernicious anemia and thyroiditis. Parietal cell antibodies are also found in (but are not diagnostic of) Addison's disease, gastric ulcer, juvenile diabetes mellitus, iron deficiency anemia, myasthenia gravis, and Sjögren's syndrome.

Description. Parietal cells are located among the epithelial cells of the stomach and secrete hydrochloric acid (HCl), which is essential for protein breakdown. Many adults who suffer from alterations in gastric acid stimulation (such as pernicious anemia) have an autoimmune response with circulating parietal cell antibodies or other antibodies. Parietal cell antibodies are present in 20%-30% of people who have other autoimmune disorders. They are occasionally present in people who have gastric cancer or ulcers and are also found in up to 2% of normal children and 20% of older adults, particularly the siblings of clients with pernicious anemia. Some researchers believe that there may be a genetic component to pernicious anemia or gastric ulcer with parietal cell antibody activity. The antibodies can be detected with indirect immunofluorescence.

Professional Considerations
Consent form NOT required.

Preparation
1. Tube: Red topped, red/gray topped, or gold topped.

Procedure
1. Draw a 10-mL blood sample.

Postprocedure Care
1. None.

Client and Family Teaching
1. Results are normally available within 72 hours.

Factors That Affect Results
1. One study found that the levels increased with increasing severity of atrophic gastritis in clients positive for *Helicobacter pylori*.

Other Data
1. It has not been shown that parietal cell antibodies affect a person's ability to absorb B vitamins.

Paroxetine

See Selective Serotonin Reuptake Inhibitors—Blood.

Partial Thromboplastin Time

See Activated Partial Thromboplastin Time and Partial Thromboplastin Time—Plasma.

Paternity Testing

See Human Leukocyte Antigen Typing—Blood. See also Banding in Genetic Disorders—Diagnostic.

PCG

See Phonocardiography—Diagnostic.

PCHE

See Pseudocholinesterase—Plasma.

---

pco$_2$

See Carbon Dioxide, Partial Pressure—Blood; Blood Gases, Arterial—Blood.

PCP

See Phencyclidine, Qualitative—Urine.

PCT

See Procalcitonin—Plasma or Serum.

Pelvic Echogram

See **Gynecologic Ultrasonography**—Diagnostic.

Pelvic Ultrasonography

See **Gynecologic Ultrasonography**—Diagnostic.

Pelvimetry and Pelvicephalography—Diagnostic

Norms.

Pelvic Inlet (Anteroposterior Diameters)

Diagonal conjugate	12.5 cm
Obstetric conjugate	11.0 cm
True conjugate	11.5 cm

Pelvic Cavity (Midpelvis)

Midplane	12.75 cm
Anteroposterior diameter	11.5-12.0 cm
Posterior sagittal diameter	4.5-5.0 cm
Transverse diameter	10.5 cm

Pelvic Outlet

Anteroposterior diameter	9.5 cm
Obstetric anteroposterior diameter	11.5 cm
Transverse diameter	8.0 cm
Suprapubic angle	85-90 degrees

Usage. Evaluation of pelvic adequacy for vaginal delivery when any of the following conditions are present: labor has been dysfunctional or slow; fetal positioning is breech, the fetal head fails to engage, or other abnormal positioning in labor occurs, especially in primigravidas, when maternal pelvic adequacy is questioned; history of pelvic fracture or injury or congenital deformity or disease, such as rickets, polio, or hip dysplasia, may affect the bony pelvis or hips. Examination of very small women or those with kyphoscoliosis or dwarfism. May be indicated when the physician is considering oxytocin administration. It is not the pelvic measurements alone but the pelvic measurements in relation to the size of the fetal head that are important to ensure safe delivery for these indicators. Pelvimetry measurements may be used when previous deliveries have been difficult or have produced large infants or in previous deliveries with an unplanned forceps delivery or nonelective cesarean

section before another pregnancy. The radiographic tests are not performed as often as they were a decade ago. A trial of labor is usually permitted, regardless of the results of clinical pelvimetry.

Description. Pelvimetry is measurement of the internal dimensions of the bony pelvis, usually to determine the adequacy and shape of the maternal pelvis in relationship to fetal size and positioning for or during vaginal delivery. Estimates of pelvic measurements may be performed digitally during the physical examination by an obstetrician, nurse midwife, or trained obstetrical nurse (see pelvic measurements under Pelvimetry—Diagnostic). Other methods for more specific measurements of the pelvic outlet capacity and the fetal head size may be performed by radiography, CT scan, or MRI. Ultrasound pelvimetry is not considered accurate at this time. Pelvicephalography is a measurement of the fetal head diameters by a radiologic measurement. It is performed with special methods used to correct for radiographic distortion and magnification. Pelvimetry by radiography, ultrasonography, or computed tomography requires a physician's prescription.

Precautions

During pregnancy, risks of cumulative radiation exposure to the fetus from this and other previous or future imaging studies must be weighed against the benefits of the procedure. Although formal limits for client exposure are relative to this risk:benefit comparison, the United States Nuclear Regulatory Commission requires that the cumulative dose equivalent to an embryo/fetus from occupational exposure not exceed 0.5 rem (5 mSv). Radiation dosage to the fetus is proportional to the distance of the anatomy studied from the abdomen and decreases as pregnancy progresses. For pregnant clients, consult the radiologist/radiology department to obtain estimated fetal radiation exposure from this procedure.

Professional Considerations
Consent form NOT required.

Preparation
1. Prepare the client for transport to the appropriate radiology department.

Procedure
1. Radiographic pelvimetry is completed in the radiology department. The client is positioned carefully for an erect lateral view of the pelvis and a supine AP view of the pelvis. It is important that exact measurement of the woman's position and distance from the film at the time of radiography be taken for a correction factor used in the computation of pelvic measurements. The disadvantages include radiation hazards to the fetus and the fact that radiography alone is no longer considered reliable as a tool to diagnose problems with labor and delivery.
2. Computed tomographic pelvimetry is considered more accurate and easier to perform. There is less radiation exposure to the fetus and less chance of distortion if the woman is positioned correctly on the table. Three views are taken: anterior, lateral, and axial. Electronic calipers are used to take the numerical pelvic measurements. CT is particularly useful in women with a history of pelvic fractures and before delivery for any situation except those in which a cesarean section is already planned.
3. Ultrasonography is not yet clinically helpful. A radiograph is also required, and a fetal pelvic index that estimates proportion or disproportion for vaginal delivery must be computed.

4. MRI is considered quite accurate and allows for imagery of the complete fetus as well as the mother's pelvis and pelvic measurements. The MRI has the advantage of evaluation of the soft tissues of the pelvic region as reasons for dystocia and uses NO radiation to the fetus. MRI is costly and difficult to access in emergency situations.
5. Cephalopelvic proportion is use of the above radiographic techniques late in the pregnancy or during a difficult labor to assess the mother's pelvic dimensions as relates specifically to the size of the fetal head and position.
6. Knowledge of the course of normal labor and delivery and full understanding of the correction factors for radiographic pelvimetry are essential.
7. For digital examination, the lengths of the first two fingers on either hand of the examiner are measured in centimeters. These fingers should be used for obtaining all measurements.

Postprocedure Care
1. Assist the woman to a position of comfort.
2. Assess the parents' readiness for new roles; include information on feeding, supplies, safety, and referral agencies.

Client and Family Teaching
1. The procedure takes 15 minutes.
2. The client must remove clothes and put on a gown.
3. Explain the relationship of the results to the type of delivery—vaginal versus cesarean.

Factors That Affect Results
1. None.

Other Data
1. Emotional support is more likely needed during this test than at other times during pregnancy.

Pelvimetry (Pelvic Examination, Digital)—Diagnostic

Norm. *Pelvic inlet:* 11.0 cm.
　Pelvic outlet: 8.0 cm.

Usage. Evaluation of the pelvic adequacy for vaginal delivery. Clinical, noninvasive estimations of the important pelvic measurements in pregnancy. If there have been

pelvic injuries, known bony abnormalities, or a previous difficult labor, a radiograph or a CT scan is needed to fully assess the adequacy for vaginal delivery.

Description. Digital pelvimetry may be performed by the physician or nurse midwife during pregnancy or nearing delivery to estimate the adequacy of the woman's pelvic measurements for vaginal delivery. Any abnormality noted with this method is confirmed by other methods, and pelvicephalography is used to fully assess the prospects of normal delivery. The utility of this procedure has been questioned in the literature, as retrospective reviews indicate that a trial of labor is permitted, regardless of the pelvimetry findings (Wong et al, 2003).

Professional Considerations
Consent form not required.

Preparation
1. Obtain rubber gloves, lubricant, and a ruler or Thom's pelvimeters.
2. Position the woman on the examination table in the dorsal lithotomy position with her feet supported in stirrups.

Procedure
1. The lengths of the first two fingers on either hand of the examiner are measured in centimeters. These fingers should be used for obtaining all measurements.
2. *Pelvic inlet measurement:* The examiner inserts these fingers into the vagina, using the middle finger to locate the lower border of the symphysis pubis and the sacral promontory. To measure the diagonal conjugate, the other hand is used to indicate where the pubis makes contact with the proximal part of the hand. This distance is calculated in centimeters. The obstetric conjugate is calculated by subtraction of 1.5 cm from the length of the diagonal conjugate. The true conjugate is calculated by subtraction of 1.0 cm from the diagonal conjugate. Because the obstetric conjugate is the narrowest anteroposterior diameter through which the fetus must travel, radiographic examination for accurate measurement is helpful. To measure the obstetric conjugate on radiographic film, locate the inner point of the symphysis and measure back to the sacral promontory. This distance should be approximately 11.0 cm.
3. *Pelvic capacity measurement:* The sagittal posterior diameter is the only midpelvis diameter that can be palpated. The fingers are inserted into the vagina, locating the sacrospinous ligament. This ligament is traced by palpation from the ischial spines

to the sacrum. The sacrospinous ligament is usually three fingerbreadths long, or 4-5 cm. The capacity of the midpelvis, particularly the midplane, will give the examiner an idea of how labor will progress, if at all.

4. *Pelvic outlet measurement:* The pelvic outlet is the area in which the fetal head crowns and extends for delivery. The pelvic outlet measurements can be obtained by palpation. The most important diameter is the obstetric anteroposterior outlet diameter. The flexibility and mobility of this diameter are usually assessed by palpation of the coccyx. With the finger inserted into the rectum while the thumb externally grasps the coccyx, the examiner attempts to move the coccyx downward. An immobile coccyx indicates a decreased outlet diameter. The anteroposterior outlet diameter is obtained by insertion of two fingers into the vagina and locating the tip of the sacrum and externally locating the symphysis pubis with the other hand. The distance between the fingers is marked. The suprapubic angle is estimated by placement of the thumbs, side by side, at the symphysis border. The fingers are then separated from the thumbs and placed flat against the thighs. The angle at which the fingers are able to separate from the thumbs is the suprapubic angle. If the suprapubic angle is narrow, minimal finger-thumb separation will occur. Another way to measure the suprapubic angle is to insert one finger into the vagina, locating the internal margin, while the other hand externally palpates the top of the symphysis pubis. An imaginary line is drawn between the two points and assessments of the depth and bend of the symphysis pubis are made. From these calculations, an estimate of the angle is made. Preferably the symphysis pubis is short and continues inward, allowing for an adequate obstetric conjugate. If it were bony and elongated, the fetus might have difficulty extending the head during delivery. The transverse outlet diameter is measured with the fist on Thom's pelvimetry position between the ischial tuberosities. Pelvimetry outlet measurements are important in the assessment of the potential for fetal head injuries and

perineal tearing during the final stages of labor.

Postprocedure Care
1. Assist the woman to a position of comfort.

Client and Family Teaching
1. The procedure takes 15 minutes.
2. Explain the implications of the findings in relation to the type of delivery anticipated.

Factors That Affect Results
1. The accuracy of the results depends on the skill and performance technique of the examiner.

Other Data
1. Outlet dystocia is a narrowing of the pubic arch and may make it difficult for the fetus to extend its head, resulting in the need for a forceps delivery.

Pemphigus Panel—Blood

Norm.

	Normal	Borderline/ Indeterminate	Positive for Pemphigus Disease
IgG cell surface antibodies	Negative		
Desmoglein 1 IgG antibodies	Negative (<14 U)	14-20 U	>20 U (predominant in pemphigus foliaceus)
Desmoglein 3 IgG antibodies	Negative (<9 U)	9-20 U	>20 U (predominant in pemphigus vulgaris)

Usage. Confirmation of diagnosis and management of pemphigus and pemphigoid. Diagnosis is usually made by clinical findings and biopsy with findings of a histologic picture of disruption of the epidermal intercellular connections (which is called "acantholysis") and microscopic deposits of IgG.

Description. Pemphigus and pemphigoid are autoimmune blistering diseases of the skin and mucus membranes. Its cause is unknown, and it occurs in middle-age or older adults. Initial lesions are located in the mouth or on the scalp. After the blisters break, secondary infections may occur in the raw, eroded areas. Before the discovery of steroid therapy, the disease was fatal in 95% of cases. Pemphigus is an autoimmune disease, with cause unknown, in which the autoantibodies cause a separation of the epidermal cells, especially after even mild trauma to a specific area. The circulating IgG antibodies can be detected by indirect immunofluorescence. In addition, Desmoglein antibodies can be measured in clients with pemphigus and correlate with disease activity.

Professional Considerations
Consent form NOT required.

Preparation
1. Tube: Red topped, red/gray topped, or gold topped.

Procedure
1. Draw a 3-mL blood sample.

Postprocedure Care
1. None.

Client and Family Teaching
1. Pemphigus is treatable with immunosuppressive drugs, intravenous immunoglobulins, monoclonal antibodies (etanercept, rituximab) and/or steroid and nonsteroid (pimecrolimus 1%) drugs. These drugs can cause side effects that include slow healing, weight redistribution, and psychoses. It is important to watch for signs of these changes and tell the doctor about them. Treatment of refractory pemphigus can include allogeneic stem cell transplant.
2. Pemphigus is a risk factor for periodontitis and osteoporosis.
3. Anesthetic mouth rinses may reduce oral pain, especially before eating as 94.6% have pharyngeal, laryngeal or nasal lesions.
4. Secondary infection and fluid and electrolyte losses are the most common complications and causes of mortality. Worse

outcomes include persons <40 years of age or of Sephardic Jewish origin.

Factors That Affect Results

1. False-positive results may occur in the presence of lupus, burns, or drug reactions.

Other Data

1. Pemphigus may be drug induced by penicillamine or captopril.

Penicillin Skin Test—Diagnostic

Norm. Absence of immediate wheal and flare.

Usage. Determination of hypersensitivity to penicillin after previous history of allergic sensitivity.

Description. After a period of time, many people stop expressing IgE sensitivity to beta-lactam antibiotics (that is, penicillin), particularly if the reaction occurred during childhood or while the drug was taken orally. This test is used for individuals with a previous history of hypersensitivity to penicillin and who require the drug to treat a particular infection. By injecting small amounts of Pre-Pen (Kremer-Urban), benzylpenicilloyl polylysine, or benzylpenicillin G intradermally and examining for evidence of an enlarged wheal with erythema, one can identify many individuals at risk for developing anaphylaxis.

Professional Considerations
Consent form NOT required.

Risks
Allergic reaction to intradermal injection (itching, hives, rash, tight feeling in the throat, shortness of breath, bronchospasm, anaphylaxis, death).
Contraindications
Previous anaphylactic reaction to penicillin.

Preparation

1. Withhold antihistamines for 24-48 hours before the test.
2. *Emergency readiness*: The test should be completed in an area where appropriately trained ACLS personnel and emergency medical equipment are available because of the possibility of anaphylactic reaction.
3. Obtain 0.9% saline for the injection, Pre-Pen or benzylpenicillin G, alcohol, tuberculin syringes, and 25-gauge ½-inch needles for intradermal injection.

Procedure

1. Initially prick or scratch the skin on a distal extremity with Pre-Pen or benzylpenicillin G.
2. Wait 15 minutes to examine the area for evidence of wheal and flare.
3. If these are not evident, proceed with one of the following procedures:
   a. *Pre-Pen* test: Inject 0.02-0.04 mL of Pre-Pen reagent intradermally to make a 3-mm bleb on the forearm. At the same time, inject the same amount of 0.9% saline intradermally near the same area, making the same-sized bleb for use as a control site. After 15-20 minutes, examine the forearm for wheals. Measure the wheals, if present, in millimeters. A positive result will be >5 mm in diameter, with or without a surrounding erythematous area.
   b. *Benzylpenicillin G test*: Inject a small bleb of benzylpenicillin G, 100 U/mL, intradermally in the forearm. At the same time, inject the same amount of 0.9% saline intradermally near the same area, making the same-sized bleb for use as a control site. If no reaction occurs after 15-30 minutes, repeat the procedure, using benzylpenicillin G, 1000 U/mL. If no reaction occurs after 15-30 minutes, repeat the procedure using benzylpenicillin G, 10,000 U/mL. A 0.9% saline control should be administered with each successive dose. After 15-20 minutes, examine the forearm for wheals. Measure the wheals, if present, in millimeters. A positive result will be >5 mm in diameter, with or without a surrounding erythematous area.
   c. If the procedure is to be repeated using several strengths of penicillin, start with the lowest concentration.

Postprocedure Care

1. Keep the area uncovered and open to air.

Client and Family Teaching

1. Call the physician immediately if symptoms of a delayed allergic reaction (listed above, under Risks) occur, and seek immediate medical attention if any difficulty in swallowing or breathing occurs.
2. The penicillin skin test allows assessment only for immediate or accelerated hypersensitivity reactions. There is no test to assess for risk of delayed reactions.
3. Clients with a positive skin test to penicillin: about 2% are also generally reactive to first-generation cephalosporins.

Factors That Affect Results

1. Recent administration of antihistamines may cause false-negative results.

Other Data

1. A positive skin test indicates a 67%-73% risk of immediate to accelerated reaction to penicillin therapy.
2. 4% of the population is allergic to penicillin; 83% are females and 17% are males. Of clients with negative penicillin skin test results, 2%-6% have anaphylactic reactions with the administration of penicillin.
3. Repeat skin testing should be performed before reinitiation of penicillin therapy if the initial test was negative and the first course of the drug has been completed.
4. It is not necessary to withhold corticosteroids before penicillin skin testing.
5. Clients with a negative skin test should still be given penicillin cautiously; IV administration may quickly resensitize the client to the drug.

Pepsinogen I (Pepsinogen A, PGI) and Pepsinogen II (PGII)—Blood

Norm.

		SI Units
Pepsinogen I		
Adults	124-142 ng/mL	124-142 µg/L
Women at delivery	116-138 ng/mL	116-138 µg/L
Children		
Cord blood	24-28 ng/mL	24-28 µg/L
Premature infants	20-24 ng/mL	20-24 µg/L
<12 months	72-82 ng/mL	72-82 µg/L
12 months to ≤2 years	90-106 ng/mL	90-106 µg/L
3-6 years	80-104 ng/mL	80-104 µg/L
7-10 years	77-103 ng/mL	77-103 µg/L
11-14 years	96-118 ng/mL	96-118 µg/L
Pepsinogen II	3-19 ng/mL	3-19 mg/L
PGI:PGII Ratio	4:1	
Atrophic gastritis	<2.5	

Increased Pepsinogen I. Diseases or situations in which gastric acid is increased: duodenal ulcer (30%-50% of clients with duodenal ulcer have increased pepsinogen levels); gastrinomas; gastritis, acute and chronic; *H. pylori* with cag PAI gene, hypergastrinemia; and hypertrophic gastropathy. It is associated with chronic renal failure, *Helicobacter pylori* infection, and Zollinger-Ellison syndrome. May be inherited autosomal dominant trait. Drugs include omeprazole.

Increased Pepsinogen II. Acute and chronic superficial gastritis and duodenal ulcers, *H. pylori* infection, and Zollinger-Ellison syndrome. Drugs include omeprazole.

Decreased Pepsinogen I. Diseases or conditions in which there is a decrease in the mass of chief cells: Addison's disease, atrophic gastritis, gastric cancer, hypopituitarism, myxedema, pernicious anemia, and after vagotomy. Absence of pepsinogen I is seen with achlorhydria with pernicious anemia. Drugs include gastric inhibitory polypeptides (GIPs), anticholinergics, and histamine (H_2)-antagonists.

Decreased Pepsinogen II. Addison's disease, gastric neoplasia, gastric resection, gastritis, myxedema, status post gastrectomy.

Usage. Pepsinogen levels, especially pepsinogen II, are useful to help diagnose atrophic gastritis and as a clinical monitor to assess the efficacy of the treatment of gastric ulcer disease.

Description. The term *pepsinogen I* (PGI) encompasses five of the eight fractions of pepsinogen found in the bloodstream. Pepsinogen I (PGI) is an inactive precursor of the proteolytic enzyme pepsin and is produced by the chief cells of the gastric glands. Pepsinogen secretion is stimulated by the vagus nerve as well as hormonal activity of gastrin, secretin, and cholecystokinin. When the pH of the stomach is acidic, pepsinogen I is converted to pepsin, which acts on amino acids in the first step of protein digestion. Activated pepsin is capable of converting additional pepsinogen(s) to active enzymes. The remaining related pepsinogens are collectively termed "*pepsinogen II.*" Pepsinogens group II are related to the pepsinogen I group but are found in Brunner's gland and pyloric glands in the gastric antrum and proximal portion of the duodenum. The PGI:PGII ratio decreases linearly with the severity of atrophic gastritis, and decreased ratio has been associated with an increased risk of gastric cancer. A small amount of pepsinogen (1%) is absorbed into the bloodstream and can be assayed.

Professional Considerations
Consent form NOT required.

Preparation
1. Preschedule this test with the laboratory. The sample should be a fasting morning specimen.

2. Tube: Red topped, red/gray topped, or gold topped.
3. See Client and Family Teaching.

Procedure
1. Draw a 10-mL blood sample.
2. Send the sample to the laboratory for evaluation or storage (frozen) immediately.

Postprocedure Care
1. Begin meals as prescribed.

Client and Family Teaching
1. Fast overnight before the test.
2. High pepsinogen concentration is considered a risk factor for duodenal ulcer. High serum pepsinogen II level is a risk factor for developing gastric ulcers.
3. High pepsinogen I levels and low pepsinogen I:II ratios are associated with *H. pylori* infection, which is now associated with ulcer disease.
4. Results are normally available within 48 hours.

Factors That Affect Results
1. Impaired renal function causes elevated results.
2. Pepsinogen levels may increase with age.
3. There is a diurnal pattern to pepsinogen II secretion; failure to obtain an early-morning specimen may affect the interpretation of results.

Other Data
1. Endoscopy is considered of more use in diagnosing gastric and duodenal abnormalities than is the pepsinogen I level.
2. A diagnosis of chronic atrophic gastritis is recommended if the PGI level is less than 70 ng/mL and the PGI:PGII ratio is less than 3.0.
3. In pernicious anemia, pepsinogen I is decreased, while pepsinogen II is normal.
4. See also Pepsinogen I antibody—Blood.

Pepsinogen I Antibody—Blood

Norm. Negative.

Usage. Method of detection of autoantibodies of pepsinogen I in the serum.

Positive. Pernicious anemia (some gastric lesions and some duodenal lesions).

Description. One performs this test by using the enzyme-linked immunosorbent assay to detect the occurrence of autoantibodies against pepsinogen. Pepsinogen I antibody has been shown to be a major chief cell antigen. Its presence may indicate the presence of a gastric or duodenal lesion that destroys the mucosa of the surrounding area. This destruction is believed to trigger the production of autoantibodies against the pepsinogen cell contents not recognized as self by the immune system.

Professional Considerations
Consent form NOT required.

Preparation
1. Tube: Red topped, red/gray topped, or gold topped.

Procedure
1. Draw a 7-mL blood sample.

Postprocedure Care
1. None.

Client and Family Teaching
1. Results are normally available within 48 hours.

Factors That Affect Results
1. Renal failure may enhance positive results.

Other Data
1. This test may serve as a subclinical marker of clients with ulcer tendencies.
2. See also Pepsinogen I and pepsinogen II—Blood.

Peptavlon Stimulation Test
See Gastric Acid Analysis Test—Diagnostic.

Percutaneous Liver Biopsy
See Liver Biopsy—Diagnostic.

Perfusion Lung Scan
See Lung Scan, Perfusion and Ventilation—Diagnostic.

Pericardiocentesis—Diagnostic
Norm.

Feature	Normal Findings
Quantity of fluid	10-50 mL
Appearance	Clear, straw-colored
Bacteria	Absent
Glucose	Approximates blood glucose level
Erythrocytes	Absent
Leukocytes	Absent

Feature	Abnormal Findings
Blood streaks	Tuberculosis or tumors
Turbid	Infection, pericarditis, or malignancy
Grossly bloody	Traumatic tap, cardiac rupture, or bleeding disorders
Blood obtained on pericardiocentesis	If blood clots, heart has been entered; if it does not clot, sample is from pericardium
Milky	Lymphatic drained into pericardium, chylopericardium
Chemistry	
Low glucose compared to serum levels	Bacterial infection or malignancy
CEA levels	Tumor—correlate with cytology studies

Usage. Effusion (pericardial), emergency treatment for pericardial tamponade, and removal of pericardial fluid for diagnostic testing.

Description. Pericardiocentesis is the aspiration of fluid surrounding the heart and contained within the pericardial sac. The procedure involves the transthoracic insertion of a needle through the intercostal space into the pericardium and may be done with guidance from transesophageal echocardiography, when the effusions are small and harder to locate. Excess fluid may accumulate because of pericarditis, after cardiac surgery, heart transplant rejection, cardiac trauma, myocardial rupture, acute rheumatic fever, metabolic diseases (fluid will likely be clear), or tumor. If the amount is greater than 50 mL or accumulates rapidly, it may result in restricted ventricular filling and stroke volume, which progresses to elevated venous blood pressure, tachycardia, and, eventually, cardiac tamponade. Other less common causes of pericardial effusion are blunt chest trauma in children, sarcoidosis and other connective tissue disorders, and AIDS. Cases of chylopericardium after aortic valve surgery or coronary artery bypass grafting have been recorded.

Professional Considerations

Consent form IS required unless the procedure is performed as an emergency.

Risks

Air embolism, cardiac arrest, cardiac tamponade, coronary artery laceration, dysrhythmias, gastric puncture, hemorrhage, hemothorax, hepatic puncture (0.3%), hydropneumothorax, infection, laceration of coronary artery, left ventricular dysfunction (transient), left ventricular pseudoaneurysm, peritoneal puncture, pneumopericardium, pneumothorax, puncture of cardiac chamber, vasovagal arrest, ventricular puncture (0.8%), ventricular fibrillation, and ventricular perforation.

Contraindications

Anticoagulant therapy, bleeding disorders, thrombocytopenia.

Preparation

1. Obtain baseline vital signs and neurologic check, and monitor closely throughout the procedure. The procedure will likely be performed in the cardiac catheterization laboratory or an intensive care unit.

2. Have an emergency cart, a defibrillator, and a 12-lead ECG machine at the bedside, with appropriate personnel trained in ACLS.

3. Establish intravenous access.

4. Obtain 1%-2% lidocaine (Xylocaine), sterile gloves, povidone-iodine solution, and a sterile pericardiocentesis tray. The tray should include a short-beveled, 14- to 18-gauge, 4- to 5-inch cardiac needle or Cath-Over needle (spinal needle); a 25-gauge needle; a 35- to 50-mL syringe; a three-way stopcock; red topped, green topped, and lavender topped tubes; sterile gauze; a Kelly clamp; ground wire; and an alligator clip.

5. Perform continuous ECG monitoring before, during, and after the procedure. Observe for development of potentially life-threatening dysrhythmias.

6. See Client and Family Teaching.

7. Just before beginning the procedure, take a "time out" to verify the correct client, procedure, and site.

Procedure

1. Position the client semirecumbent with the head of the bed elevated between 30 and 60 degrees.

2. Cleanse the skin of the chest from the xiphoid process to the left costal margin with povidone-iodine solution.

3. The subxiphoid insertion site is injected with 1%-2% lidocaine.

4. A sterile alligator clip is used to attach ECG lead V to the aspiration needle, or an echocardiogram is used to guide the needle insertion. In emergency situations, in cardiac arrest, the needle insertion is performed "blind."

5. An open three-way stopcock with a 50-mL syringe attached is connected to the cardiac needle. The needle is then inserted into the subxiphoid area, between the xiphoid process and the costal margin.

6. The ECG (grounded) is used to monitor and to guide the needle insertion as follows: The appearance of an acute increase in the QRS complex indicates pericardial penetration. Epicardial ventricular contact by the needle is indicated by elevation of the ST segment and ventricular ectopy, and atrial contact by the needle is indicated by elevation of the PR segment. An abnormally shaped QRS

complex may indicate myocardial perforation. Echocardiography is increasingly used, especially in the nonemergency situation to guide pericardiocentesis.

7. When the pericardium is penetrated, pericardial fluid should appear in the syringe. Grossly bloody aspirate will occur if a cardiac chamber is perforated. At this point, a Kelly clamp applied to the needle at the point of insertion stabilizes the position. The remainder of the pericardial fluid is aspirated.

8. The Kelly clamp and syringe are then removed, and a gauze pad is applied with pressure to the site for 3-5 minutes.

9. The pericardial fluid is measured and injected into the red topped, green topped, and lavender topped tubes.

Postprocedure Care

1. Label the specimen tubes with the site and time of collection. Write the diagnosis and any recent antibiotic therapy on the laboratory requisition. Send the specimens to the laboratory.

2. The client is usually maintained in the intensive care unit to monitor ECG continuously for 24 hours after the procedure.

3. Assess vital signs every 15 minutes × 4, then every 30-60 minutes for 2 hours, and then every 4 hours for 24 hours if the client is hemodynamically stable.

4. Monitor for symptoms of cardiac tamponade for at least 24 hours. Beck's triad, the classic symptoms of cardiac tamponade, includes neck vein distention,

hypotension, and heart sounds that are muffled and distant. The narrowing of pulse pressure (when the systolic and diastolic blood pressure values begin to approach one another) may also be a sign of cardiac tamponade.

Client and Family Teaching

1. Inform the client and family about the procedure and the seriousness of the condition. They should, if possible, understand the procedure and the need for ICU care before consent.

2. It is important to lie motionless throughout the procedure.

3. Ensure that the client and family fully understand the condition related to the pericardiocentesis.

4. Signs and symptoms to report to the physician include chest pain, shortness of breath, and dizziness or lightheadedness.

5. The catheter may be left in place if there is a need for further fluid drainage.

6. The family should be approached on CPR readiness and given resources on how to learn CPR.

Factors That Affect Results

1. Before pericardiocentesis, echocardiographic localization of the effusion helps to minimize the chance of complications from the procedure.

Other Data

1. Pericardiocentesis with cisplatin instillation is effective for pericardial malignant effusion and tamponade.

Peritoneal Fluid Analysis

See Paracentesis—Diagnostic.

Peritoneoscopy

See Laparoscopy—Diagnostic.

Persantine-Sestamibi Stress Test and Scan

See Heart Scan—Diagnostic.

PET Scan

See Positron Emission Tomography—Diagnostic.

PET/CT Scan

See **Dual Modality Imaging**—Diagnostic.

PFT

See **Pulmonary Function Test**—Diagnostic.

pH

See **Blood Gases, Arterial**—Blood; **Blood Gases, Capillary**—Blood; **Blood Gases, Venous**—Blood.

pH—Stool

Norm.

Adult	7.0-7.5
Newborn	5.0-7.0
Bottle-fed infant	Neutral to slightly alkaline pH of 7.0-8.0
Breast-fed infant	Slightly acidic

Increased. Colitis, protein breakdown, and villous adenoma. Drugs include loperamide.

Decreased. Breast-fed infants, celiac disease, diabetes mellitus, disaccharidase deficiency, lactose intolerance, malabsorption (carbohydrates, fats), malnutrition, nontropical sprue (adult celiac disease), tropical sprue, and wheat bran diet. Drugs include antibiotics, senna.

Description. The pH of stool is used to screen clients with gastrointestinal tract disorders for malabsorption of carbohydrates and fats and disaccharide intolerance. Stools with pH >6.0 are indicative of disaccharide intolerance, whereas those with pH <6.0 indicate malabsorption of sugars and fats.

Professional Considerations

Consent form NOT required.

Preparation

1. The client should not have undergone barium procedures or taken laxatives for 1 week before specimen collection.

2. Obtain a bedpan, a stool specimen container with a lid, a tongue blade, and pH paper.

Procedure

1. Collect a random stool specimen in a bedpan or collection container. Mix the specimen with water to make a suspension. Test it with commercially prepared pH paper as directed.

Postprocedure Care

1. Refrigerate the specimen if the test cannot be performed promptly.

Client and Family Teaching

1. Results are normally available within 24 hours.
2. Do not contaminate the stool with urine or other secretions or with toilet paper.

Factors That Affect Results

1. Reject specimens mixed with urine, toilet paper, or toilet water.

Other Data

1. Acidic stools will have a sickly sweet odor in both adults and children.
2. Stool pH may be one factor related to the development of cancers of the gastrointestinal tract.

pH—Urine

Norm. Normal values have a wide range because the renal system acts as a buffer for the body and adjustments in urine pH provide homeostasis. Urine pH should be evaluated with other data and client information.

Adult

Early-morning specimen	pH 5-6
Random	4.5-8.0 as body adjusts acid base
Average	5-6
Newborn	5.0-7.0

Increased. As a response to alkali overdose, a diet high in vegetables and fruits (especially citrus), and after meals. Also occurs with metabolic alkalosis without potassium loss, Fanconi syndrome, prolonged gastric suction or vomiting, hyperaldosteronism, hypokalemia, renal insufficiency, respiratory alkalosis, and urinary tract infection with *Proteus* or *Pseudomonas*. Drugs include acetazolamide, aldosterone, amiloride, amphotericin B, carbenoxolone, epinephrine, mafenide acetate, niacinamide, phenacetin, potassium citrate, and sodium bicarbonate. Increased pH levels may be associated with renal calculi.

Decreased. Diets high in meat protein and cranberries or starvation diets; achlorhydria, alkaptonuria, diabetes, or other metabolic acidosis; severe diarrhea caused by potassium depletion; kidney stones; methanol poisoning; obesity; phenylketonuria; renal tuberculosis; respiratory acidosis; and uric acid calculi. Drugs include acid phosphate, ammonium chloride, ascorbic acid, corticotropin, diazoxide, hippuric acid, mandelate, methenamine, and methionine. Herbal or natural remedies include cranberry juice.

Description. Measurement of free hydrogen-ion excretion in urine. Urine pH is reflective of plasma pH and is an indicator of renal tubular function. Playing a role in acid-base balance, normally functioning kidneys will excrete excess hydrogen ions in the urine.

Professional Considerations
Consent form NOT required.

Preparation
1. Early-morning voids are preferred for urine pH testing.
2. Obtain a clean specimen container with a lid.

Procedure
1. Have the client urinate into a 50- to 100-mL collection container. A fresh specimen may be taken from a urinary drainage bag.
2. pH results should be read immediately. If urine is to be tested with a commercially prepared test reagent, follow the manufacturer's directions.

Postprocedure Care
1. Cover the container tightly and send the specimen to the laboratory if it is not tested immediately with a commercially prepared test reagent.

Client and Family Teaching
1. Notify the nurse immediately after you have collected the sample.
2. Results are normally available within 24 hours.

Factors That Affect Results
1. Urine pH testing must be performed on a freshly collected specimen. Urine left to stand will falsely raise the pH.
2. Urine with glucose may have falsely low pH caused by bacterial activity.
3. Bacterial infections can alter the pH in either direction.

Other Data
1. Urine pH is related to diet and may be one factor in the development of renal stones.

Phencyclidine (PCP, Angel Dust), Qualitative—Urine

Norm. Negative.

Nonfatal level	0.2 μg/L
Fatal level	1-5 μg/L

Overdose Symptoms and Treatment
Symptoms of Phencyclidine Use
1. *Stage I.* Psychiatric signs: drunken or euphoric with possible ataxia, muscle spasms, fever, tachycardia, flushing, small pupils, diaphoresis, salivation, nausea, and vomiting. Infant with obtundation, tongue thrusting.
2. *Stage II.* Stupor, convulsions especially after stimulation, hallucinations, and progressive increases in heart rate, fever, and blood pressure. CNS stimulation or depression may occur.

3. *Stage III.* Increases in heart rate and metabolism progress to cardiac and respiratory failure and multisystem organ failure.

Treatment

NOTE: Treatment choice(s) depend(s) on client's history and condition and episode history.

1. Provide respiratory support if needed.
2. Administer a cathartic such as sorbitol, followed by gastric lavage and suction for oral ingestion.
3. Administer benzodiazepines or haloperidol for severe agitation.
4. Treat seizures as needed.
5. Give IV nutrition and fluid and electrolyte support as needed.
6. Acidification of urine will increase the rate of phencyclidine excretion.
7. If rhabdomyolysis occurs, IV fluids, mannitol, and diuretics are required.
8. Maintain close observation of electrolytes, respiratory, and circulatory status until the client returns to baseline level.
9. Chronic abusers may become increasingly psychotic after the drug wears off.
10. Drug counseling and psychiatric counseling are advised.

Usage. Screening for drug abuse or PCP toxicity, and psychosis or coma (unexplained), which may be related to PCP use. Metabolites of abused drugs are excreted and can be detected in the urine for several days after ingestion. PCP is just one of the drugs screened for in urine toxicology screening as recommended by the National Institute of Drug Abuse (NIDA) for new-job physicals, criminals, and after industrial accidents.

Description. Phencyclidine is a highly addictive, illegal, hallucinative drug designed for use as an anesthetic and a veterinary tranquilizer. It causes euphoria by accelerating the metabolism of the body. Phencyclidine is available in powder or capsule form and can be smoked, snuffed, injected, or swallowed. It is excreted by the kidneys and is detectable in the urine for 7 days. The effects of PCP can be observed at concentrations as low as 12 ng/mL.

Professional Considerations

Consent form NOT required.

Preparation

1. Obtain a clean plastic container.

Procedure

1. Obtain a 100- to 125-mL random urine sample in a clean plastic container. A fresh specimen may be taken from a urinary drainage bag.

Postprocedure Care

1. Send the specimen to the laboratory. For screening for known drug abusers: Special care MUST be taken in obtaining the specimen and in specimen handling to avoid falsification of results. Documentation of observed collection and handling may be required.

Client and Family Teaching

1. Obtain a past and recent history of drug abuse.
2. For intentional overdose, refer client and family for crisis intervention.
3. Referrals to appropriate rehabilitation centers and therapeutic community programs should be offered to all addicted clients who may be interested.

Factors That Affect Results

1. Peak serum concentrations occur within 15 minutes after smoking phencyclidine. Half-life is 11 hours.
2. Drugs that may cause false-positive results include ketamine hydrochloride, venlafaxine.

Other Data

1. Qualitative urine testing identifies the presence of phencyclidine but does not indicate toxic levels.
2. PCP can be detected in blood samples stored at 4 or 20 degrees C for up to 3 years.

Phendimetrazine

See **Amphetamines**—Blood.

Phenmetrazine

See **Amphetamines**—Blood.

Phenobarbital

Norm. Negative. Therapeutic levels are relative. For control of seizures, the clinical picture is important.

		SI Units
Therapeutic Levels		
Adults	10-40 µg/mL	43-173 µmol/L
Infants 0-2 months	15-30 µg/mL	65-129 µmol/L
Children ≥3 months	15-40 µg/mL	65-172 µmol/L
Toxic Level		
Infants 0-2 months	≥40 µg/mL	≥172 µmol/L
Children ≥3 months	≥50 µg/mL	≥215 µmol/L
Panic Levels		
Coma with reflexes	65-117 µg/mL	280-504 µmol/L
Coma without reflexes	>90 µg/mL	>430 µmol/L

Panic Level Symptoms and Treatment

Symptoms. Cold, clammy skin; ataxia; CNS depression; hypothermia; hypotension; cyanosis; Cheyne-Stokes respirations; tachycardia; coma. Toxicity may cause severe renal impairment.

Treatment

NOTE: Treatment choice(s) depend(s) on client's history and condition and episode history.

1. Perform gastric lavage, followed by a slurry of multiple-dose-activated charcoal (MDAC) with cathartic.
2. Urine alkalinization is no longer recommended, as MDAC has been found to be more effective alone than in combination with urinary alkalinization.
3. Protect the client's airway.
4. The client may require intubation and mechanical ventilation, especially during gastric lavage if the gag reflex has been affected by the barbiturates.
5. Monitor closely for hypotension.
6. Hemodialysis, peritoneal dialysis, and hemoperfusion all WILL remove phenobarbital. Charcoal hemoperfusion is very effective in removing phenobarbital.

Usage. Suspected drug toxicity or abuse in clients with symptoms of lethargy, dizziness, ataxia, and diplopia. Monitoring therapeutic levels of phenobarbital especially for seizure disorders during puberty, after weight gain or loss, and if renal failure develops.

Increased. Drug (barbiturate) abuse and renal failure in clients treated with phenobarbital. Drugs that can increase levels for clients taking phenobarbital include monoamine oxidase (MAO) inhibitors, sodium valproate, and valproic acid.

Decreased. (Below therapeutic range.) Inadequate therapy, noncompliance, and malabsorption (oral doses).

Description. A long-acting, schedule IV barbiturate most commonly used for its anticonvulsant effect and occasionally used as a sedative. It is widely distributed throughout the body and metabolized by the liver, and 50% is excreted unchanged in the urine. The half-life is normally 50-120 hours in adults and 40-70 hours in children. Allowance of time for steady-state levels after changes in dosage should be considered, with monitoring of therapeutic blood levels. For rapid detection, the fluorescence polarization assay method can be used.

Professional Considerations

Consent form NOT required.

Preparation

1. Tube: Red topped, red/gray topped, or gold topped or black topped.

2. Do NOT draw specimens during hemodialysis.

Procedure

1. Draw a 4-mL blood sample.

Postprocedure Care

1. None.

Client and Family Teaching

1. Discuss the schedule and dose of taking medication.
2. Results are normally available within 24 hours.
3. Return for serum reevaluation within 7 days for long-term phenobarbital therapy.
4. If activated charcoal was given for elevated levels, the client should drink 4-6 glasses of water each day for 2 days to prevent constipation. Activated charcoal will cause stools to be black for a few days.

5. Consult physician before taking any herbal or natural remedies or medicines because some may lower seizure threshold when taken with anticonvulsants.

Factors That Affect Results

1. Draw the specimen within 1 hour before the next dose for ongoing monitoring.
2. Remeasure the phenobarbital level 7 days after dosage change for long-term therapy.

Other Data

1. Mephobarbital is metabolized to phenobarbital.
2. Peak levels occur 6-18 hours after dose.
3. Herbal or natural remedy concomitant ingestion of evening primrose (family Onagraceae) oil and borage (*Borago officinalis*) may lower seizure threshold.

Phenolphthalein Test (Laxative Abuse Test)—Diagnostic

Norm. Negative.

Usage. Anorexia nervosa (laxative use for weight loss), chronic self-prescribed laxative use, and unexplained diarrhea.

Description. The phenolphthalein test is a toxicologic screening for evidence of recent laxative use. Phenolphthalein is the active ingredient of many over-the-counter laxative preparations (banned by FDA in the United States in 1999). It causes stool evacuation by enhancing fluid and electrolyte accumulation in the intestines. After ingestion, phenolphthalein is excreted in both the feces and the urine and is detectable for up to 32 hours. It may also have laxative effects for up to 4 days and cause fluid and electrolyte abnormalities. This test is performed on an aliquot of a 24-hour urine sample to detect the presence of phenolphthalein by thin-layer chromatography.

Professional Considerations

Consent form NOT required.

Preparation

1. Preschedule this test with the laboratory.
2. Obtain a clean, 3-L container without preservative.
3. Write the beginning time of collection on the laboratory requisition.

Procedure

1. Discard the first morning urine specimen.
2. Begin to time a 24-hour urine collection.
3. Save all the urine voided for 24 hours in a refrigerated, clean, 3-L container. Document the quantity of urine output during the specimen collection period. Include the urine voided at the end of the 24-hour period. For catheterized clients, keep the drainage bag on ice and empty the urine into the collection container hourly.

Postprocedure Care

1. Compare the urine quantity in the specimen container with the urinary output record for the test. If the specimen contains less urine than what was recorded as output, some of the sample may have been discarded, thus invalidating the test.
2. Document the quantity of urine output and the ending time for the 24-hour collection period on the laboratory requisition.
3. Send the entire 24-hour urine specimen to the laboratory for testing. The test is performed on a 20-mL aliquot of the 24-hour specimen.

Client and Family Teaching

1. Save all the urine voided in the 24-hour period and urinate before defecating to avoid loss of urine. If any urine is accidentally discarded, discard the entire specimen and restart the collection the next day.
2. Results are normally available within 24 hours.
3. Discuss psychologic and rehabilitation services if laxative abuse is determined.

Factors That Affect Results

1. Repeating the collection on consecutive days for a total of three 24-hour

specimens increases the likelihood of detecting laxative abuse.

Other Data

1. Methods are available to test for a wide range of laxative ingredients in urine.
2. Complications of laxative abuse may include diarrhea, abdominal pain, hypokalemia, hypermagnesemia, cathartic colon, and the development of ammonium urate renal calculi.

Phenothiazines

Norm. Negative.

Quantitative Tests		SI Units
Chlorpromazine (Thorazine)		
Adults	50-300 ng/mL	157-942 nmol /L
Toxic level	>500 ng/mL	>1570 nmol/L
Children	30-80 ng/mL	94-251 nmol/L
Toxic level	≥200 ng/mL	≥630 ng/mL
Fluphenazine (Prolixin)	0.2-2.0 ng/mL	0.4-4.0 nmol/L
Perphenazine	0.8-2.4 ng/mL	
Prochlorperazine (Compazine)	<0.5 µg/mL	
Panic level	>1.0 µg/mL	
Thioridazine (Mellaril)	1.0-1.5 µg/mL	2.7-4.1 µmol/L
Panic level	>10 µg/mL	>27 µmol/L
Trifluoperazine (Stelazine)	<500 ng/mL	<1040 nmol/L
Panic level	>1000 ng/mL	>2080 nmol/L

Overdose Symptoms and Treatment

Symptoms. Extrapyramidal symptoms (including with injection of depot risperidone), central nervous system (CNS) depression, hyperkalemia, hyperprolactinemia, hypogonadism, menstrual disturbance, respiratory depression. Sodium-channel blockade manifesting as early prolonged QRS interval, rightward axis of 40 msec, and presence of an R wave in aV_R lead and an S wave in leads I and aV_L. Prolongation of QTc in overdose of thioridazine. CNS and respiratory depressive effects are worse when alcohol or antihypertensives are concomitantly ingested.

Treatment

NOTE: Treatment choice(s) depend(s) on client's history and condition and episode history.

1. Monitor for CNS and cardiac depression.
2. Perform ECG monitoring.
3. Perform gastric lavage for oral doses or a saline cathartic for oral spansules.
4. Do not induce vomiting.
5. Hemodialysis and peritoneal dialysis will NOT remove chlorpromazine or trifluoperazine and are unlikely to significantly remove fluphenazine, perphenazine, prochlorperazine, and thioridazine. There are no data available on the effect of high-permeability dialysis on phenothiazine drug levels.

Increased. Phenothiazine abuse and phenothiazine overdose (highest human blood concentrations include 927 ng/mL women and 733 ng/mL men). Drugs that may increase levels above therapeutic for clients on various phenothiazines include mono-amine oxidase (MAO) inhibitors.

Decreased. Inadequate therapy. Drugs include antacids, antidiarrheals, anticholinergics, barbiturates, CNS depressants, and lithium carbonate. Thorazine absorption from the gut is pH dependent, and so H_2 antagonists may decrease steady-state levels for the client on Thorazine therapy.

Description. A group of drugs with antipsychotic, antihistaminic, antipruritic, and antiemetic effects that act centrally on the reticular activating system and peripherally with anticholinergic and alpha-adrenergic blocking effects. Phenothiazines are widely distributed in body tissues, metabolized by the liver, and excreted by the kidney, with a half-life of 20-40 hours. Correlation of therapeutic effectiveness with blood levels is poor. This test is mainly used to determine whether or not the phenothiazine is being taken or for the diagnosis of possible overdose. Fatalities from large doses are rare.

Professional Considerations
Consent form NOT required.

Preparation
1. Tube: Red topped, red/gray topped, or gold topped.

2. Chlorpromazine levels MAY be drawn during hemodialysis.

Procedure
1. Draw a 7-mL blood sample. Protect specimen from light.

Postprocedure Care
1. Send the specimen to the laboratory immediately and refrigerate it until tested.

Client and Family Teaching
1. Evaluate the need for psychologic and rehabilitation support if an overdose is involved. Referrals to appropriate rehabilitation centers and therapeutic community programs should be offered to all addicted clients who are interested.

Factors That Affect Results
1. For therapeutic monitoring, draw samples within 1 hour before the next dose and at least 3 hours after the last dose.

Other Data
1. Newer phenothiazines include triflupromazine (Vesprin), perphenazine (Trilafon), fluphenazine (Prolixin), and mesoridazine (Serentil).

Phentermine

See **Amphetamines**—Blood.

Phenylalanine

Norm. Blood spot phenylalanine in newborn <240 mol/L.

Plasma Phenylalanine		SI Units
Infant 0-11 months	<4 mg/dL	<272 μmol/L
Newborn	1.2-3.4 mg/dL	73-206 μmol/L
Premature or low birth weight	2.0-7.5 mg/dL	121-454 μmol/L
Adult	0.8-1.8 mg/dL	48-109 μmol/L
Adult—monitored for diet compliance	1.3-3.4 mg/dL	78-204 μmol/L

Positive Test (Increased Result). Phenylketonuria (PKU) is diagnosed and confirmed by:
1. Greater than 4 mg/dL serum phenylalanine.
2. Association with low tyrosine levels of less than 0.6 mg/dL.
3. Urinary excretion of phenylpyruvic acid.

Description. Phenylketonuria (PKU) occurs in approximately 1 in every 15,000 infants born in the United States and is caused by an autosomal recessive gene. Infants with PKU lack the ability to produce the enzyme phenylalanine hydroxylase, which converts phenylalanine to tyrosine. The resulting buildup of phenylalanine in blood and tissues is correlated to low IQ and leads to severe mental retardation. The carrier rate for PKU is 2% in the United States. This test is performed when either a urine screening or Guthrie test screening for PKU has been positive or as the PKU screening test in newborns. Increased levels also found in HIV positive patients, obesity, ovarian cancer, sepsis, and trauma. Decreased levels found in bariatric surgery.

Professional Considerations
Consent form NOT required.

Preparation
1. Mark the birth date and the date of initiation of feedings on the laboratory requisition.
2. Tube: Green topped.

Procedure
1. Draw a 0.5-mL blood sample. Do not use cord blood.

Postprocedure Care
1. None.

Client and Family Teaching
1. Refer parents with PKU infants for genetic counseling.
2. Clients with PKU may be monitored for serum phenylalanine levels for life. The client must follow a low-protein diet, which is effective treatment but not a cure.

3. Level of mental capacity has been shown to be related to serum levels. Range is 2-6 mg/dL for best control.
4. Results are normally available within 48 hours.

Factors That Affect Results
1. False-negative results may occur with other tests for PKU before the third day of feeding, but the serum phenylalanine test for PKU has the advantage that it is usually accurate in the first 24 hours of life, especially in breast-fed babies because colostrum has a high protein content.
2. Phenylalanine clearance has been shown to be delayed in elderly males.
3. Do not use cord blood.
4. Fasting is not needed even for monitoring of older PKU clients.
5. The presence of antibodies in the sample makes results uninterpretable.

Other Data
1. Diagnosis of PKU may be made with concomitant urine testing and a plasma level >2 mg/dL (121 mol/L, SI units) on consecutive tests.
2. Male infants with PKU increase levels of phenylalanine at a faster rate than affected females.
3. Sapropterin therapy stabilizes blood phenylalanine levels in BH4-responsive PKU.
4. See also Guthrie test for phenylketonuria —Diagnostic (Filter paper test).

Phenylpropanolamine

See **Amphetamines**—Blood.

Phenytoin (Total and Free)—Serum

Norm.

Total Phenytoin	Trough	SI Units
Therapeutic range	10-20 µg/mL	40-79 µmol/L
Toxic level	>30 µg/mL	>120 µmol/L
Panic level	>60 µg/mL	>237 µmol/L
Free Phenytoin		
Therapeutic range	1.0-2.0 µg/mL	4-7.9 µnol/L
Toxic level	>3.5 µg/mL	>14 µmol/L
Percent Free Phenytoin	8%-14%	

Panic Level Symptoms and Treatment
Symptoms. Double vision, nystagmus, lethargy, upper facial dyskinesia. Central nervous system depression: drowsiness, confusion, slurred speech, coma, and respiratory depression.

Treatment

NOTE: Treatment choice(s) depend(s) on client's history and condition and episode history.

1. Support airway and breathing. Administer oxygen as needed.
2. Provide ECG monitoring (for levels >75 μg/mL), although the risk for arrhythmias is minimal.
3. Measure phenytoin levels every 4 hours.
4. Administer activated charcoal (multiple dose) every 2-6 hours as needed.
5. Administer IV fluids and vasopressor, as needed, for hypotension.
6. Administer a saline cathartic.
7. The use of sorbitol cathartic has NOT been shown to increase clearance values of phenytoin.
8. Peritoneal dialysis will NOT remove phenytoin. One study found hemodialysis over 6 hours removed 47% of phenytoin and another study found that direct hemoperfusion WILL remove phenytoin at a rate of about 20% per session. There are no data on the effect of high permeability of dialysis on phenytoin levels.

Increased. Paralytic ileus (changes absorption), phenytoin abuse, phenytoin overdose, renal disease in clients on maintenance phenytoin (Dilantin), undernourishment and genotypes CYP2C9, CYP2C19, ABCB1. Drugs that may increase phenytoin levels for clients on chronic treatment include acenocoumarol, allopurinol, amiodarone, anticoagulants (oral), benzodiazepines, chloramphenicol, chlordiazepoxide, cimetidine, diazepam, disulfiram, estrogens, ethyl alcohol (acute intake), ethosuximide, glutamine (in children), fluoxetine, H_2 antagonists, isoniazid, methsuximide, methylphenidate, phenacemide, phenothiazines, phenylbutazone, salicylates, sulfonamides, thiazides, tolbutamide, trazodone, trimethoprim, and vinblastine sulfate.

Decreased. Inadequate phenytoin therapy; noncompliance. Drugs that may alter (speed up) metabolism of phenytoin, leading to lower serum levels for clients receiving Dilantin, include carbamazepine, diazoxide, ethyl alcohol (chronic intake), folic acid, loxapine, methotrexate, sulfonylureas, theophylline, reserpine, sucralfate, and calcium-containing medications. Herbs include the Ayurvedic preparation *shankhapushpi* (often misspelled *shankapulshpi*, from Sanskrit *shankha-pushpi*, feminine form of 'conch-flower,' that is, [1] *Canscora decussata*, of the Gentianaceae family and containing iridoids and possible cyanogens and saponins/sapogenins, or [2] *Convolvulus microphyllus* [synonym *Convolvulus pluricaulis*], bindweed, containing various alkaloids). Enteral tube feedings may decrease absorption of oral phenytoin. Drugs that may *either increase or decrease* levels: phenobarbital, sodium valproate, and valproic acid.

Description. A hydantoin-derivative anticonvulsant also used as an antidysrhythmic. Phenytoin is widely distributed throughout the body, metabolized by the liver, and excreted in bile and urine, with a half-life of approximately 22 hours for oral administration. Five or 6 days of therapy are required to reach steady-state levels in adults, and 2-5 days are necessary in children. For rapid detection, the fluorescence polarization assay method can be used. Because phenytoin is highly protein-bound, free phenytoin levels are only useful in clients with abnormal or inconsistent protein binding. Examples are during pregnancy, in the elderly, and in hypoalbuminemia or hyperalbuminemia.

Professional Considerations

Consent form NOT required.

Preparation

1. Tube: Red topped, red/gray topped, or gold topped.
2. Specimens MAY be drawn during hemodialysis.
3. Screen client for the use of herbal preparations or medicines or natural remedies.

Procedure

1. Draw a 4-mL TROUGH blood sample. Obtain serial specimens at the same time each day.

Postprocedure Care

1. None.

Client and Family Teaching

1. Explore the reasons for inappropriate ingestion of phenytoin if appropriate.
2. If activated charcoal was given for elevated levels, the client should drink four to six glasses of water each day for 2 days

to prevent constipation. The activated charcoal will cause stools to be black for a few days.

3. Consult physician before taking any herbal or natural remedies or medicines because some may lower seizure threshold when taken with anticonvulsants.

4. For intentional overdose, refer client and family for crisis intervention.

5. Referrals to appropriate rehabilitation centers and therapeutic community programs should be offered to all clients who may be interested.

6. Chronic exposure to phenytoin throughout gestation disrupts hippocampal development which leads to impaired developmental function in adulthood.

Factors That Affect Results

1. Tube feedings should be held before and up to 2 hours after oral phenytoin administration.

2. Peak levels should be drawn 3-9 hours after oral administration of phenytoin. Trough levels should be drawn just before the administration of the next dose.

3. Five days should be allowed before measurement of phenytoin level after a change in dose.

4. Postmortem levels are not stable and were found to drop significantly in one study.

5. Levels may be significantly lower in clients with acquired immune deficiency syndrome. It is believed that this may be a result of the hypoalbuminemic state that accompanies this condition.

6. An herbal or natural remedy used to control seizures, *shankhapushpi* (see above), has been shown to decrease phenytoin concentrations in rats when given in multiple coadministered doses.

7. Hypoalbuminemia and concurrent valproic acid administration may increase free phenytoin levels. Clients with both conditions are at risk for exceeding the therapeutic range, even at normal dosages.

Other Data

1. Susceptibility to side effects and toxic effects, including Stevens-Johnson syndrome, may be increased in clients with head injuries or those with intracranial lesions, especially if irradiation is used as a treatment modality.

2. Herbal or natural remedy: Concomitant ingestion of evening primrose (family Onagraceae) oil and borage (*Borago officinalis*) may lower seizure threshold.

3. Free phenytoin levels are not meaningful when levels are less than 3.0 μg/mL.

4. Pharmacologic parameters do not differ significantly if drug received through a nasogastric tube or orally.

5. Purple glove syndrome (incidence 0%-6%) is a soft tissue injury after peripheral IV phenytoin administration or oral overdose. Symptoms are purple discoloration, edema, pain, decreased range of motion, and in severe cases abscess, skin loss, compartment syndrome. Treatment includes immediate interruption of phenytoin injection, splinting, elevation, close observation and surgical intervention for compartment syndrome.

Phlebography

See **Venography**—Diagnostic.

Phonocardiography (PCG)—Diagnostic

Norm. Normal S_1 and S_2 appear as spikes above the baseline on phonocardiograph paper. Absence of abnormal heart sounds as recorded by the phonocardiogram.

Usage. Aids diagnosis of cardiac valve abnormalities, hypertrophic cardiomyopathy, and left ventricular failure. May be performed and retained for reference as part of the client's permanent record as a visual representation of the intensity and loudness of murmurs and other abnormal heart sounds. Excellent teaching tool because it allows the learner to visualize the different heart sounds.

Description. A pictorial recording of the cardiac sounds heard on auscultation. A phonocardiogram uses microphones to transduce and amplify the sound into electrical impulses that are graphically recorded as a waveform by a high-speed recording apparatus. Generally, PCG is performed simultaneously with an electrocardiograph (ECG). S_1 and S_2 and any additional sounds, including S_3, S_4, murmurs, and clicks, are recorded. By comparing the ECG and PCG, one can locate normal and abnormal heart sounds and cardiac events and time them during the cardiac cycle. Phonocardiography with the addition of echocardiography is becoming a valuable noninvasive diagnostic tool. Newer phonocardiography technology may soon be available to noninvasively study coronary artery flow as well as estimate great vessel pressures, provide more reliable diagnosis, and stratify the severity of cardiac value dysfunction. A new phonocardiography-based fetal telemonitoring system allows long-term measurements at home of the pregnant women and the signal is transmitted by mobile network and internet.

Professional Considerations

Consent form NOT required.

Preparation

1. Obtain electrodes and alcohol.
2. Clip the hair from the electrode sites before placement.
3. Fetal telemonitoring at home requires a mobile network and internet.

Procedure

1. The client is positioned supine. The electrode sites should be cleansed with alcohol and lightly scraped with the edge of an electrode before placement.

2. After the heart apex and base are located with a stethoscope, a microphone is strapped (or secured with suction cups) in place over each site.
3. Both an ECG and a PCG are recorded simultaneously for four complete cardiac cycles of sinus rhythm. For dysrhythmias, 7 to 10 cardiac cycles are recorded. The procedure is repeated with the client changed to upright and left-lateral oblique positions. The client may be asked to change his or her breathing patterns (that is, hold breath or perform deep inspiration and expiration).

Postprocedure Care

1. Remove the electrodes and the residual electrode gel.

Client and Family Teaching

1. Cooperation is imperative throughout the procedure.
2. Phonocardiography is noninvasive and takes about 30 minutes.

Factors That Affect Results

1. Failure to obtain secure electrode placement causes an artifact in the electrocardiographic recording.
2. Careful calibration is needed for the results to be diagnostic and generalizable.

Other Data

1. Phonocardiography with esophageal echocardiography provides a valuable permanent and comparable record of cardiac valve murmurs. The progress of the disease process can be followed using serial recordings.

Phospholipids—Serum

Norm. Males > females except during pregnancy.

All	180-320 mg/dL
Adult ≤65 years	125-275 mg/dL
Adult >65 years	196-366 mg/dL
Birth	75-170 mg/dL
Infant	100-275 mg/dL
Child	180-295 mg/dL

Usage. Evaluation of fat metabolism. Used less often today because there are other specific tests for the plasma phospholipids. Levels are increased or decreased in the diseases listed below with more specific diagnostic tests available for most. Amniotic fluid levels of phospholipids reflect the surfactant level and give an indication of fetal lung maturity.

Increased. Diabetes mellitus, biliary cirrhosis, cholestasis, diet of low fat high carbohydrates, LCAT deficiency, hypothyroidism, ethanol cirrhosis, obstructive jaundice, nephrotic syndrome with breast cancer, chronic pancreatitis, and steatohepatitis. Drugs include estrogens, epinephrine, and some phenothiazines.

Decreased. Primary hypolipoproteinemia, Tangier disease, abetalipoproteinemia, and a dietary restriction of fat intake. Drugs include antilipemic agents such as clofibrate.

Description. Phospholipids, also known as "compound lipids," are the largest and most soluble of the lipid elements of the blood. Phospholipids (which contain phosphorus, fatty acids, and nitrogen) are needed for lipid transport and are essential components in cellular membranes. Serum phospholipid determinations may be monitored when disorders in lipid metabolism are suspected; however, cholesterol levels are more often prescribed and evaluated for this purpose.

Professional Considerations
Consent form NOT required.

Preparation
1. Tube: Red topped, red/gray topped, or gold topped.
2. See Client and Family Teaching.

Procedure
1. Draw a 5-mL fasting blood sample in the morning before any medications are administered.

Postprocedure Care
1. Note any medications taken on the laboratory requisition.
2. Specimens should be taken to the laboratory immediately.

Client and Family Teaching
1. Do NOT drink alcohol for 24-48 hours before sampling.
2. Consume a low- to moderate-fat evening meal on the day before the test.
3. Fast from midnight before sampling.

Factors That Affect Results
1. Hemolysis of the specimen invalidates results.
2. Recent intravenous injection of radiographic dye invalidates results.
3. Significant weight changes within 2 weeks before the test invalidate results.

Other Data
1. This test is not included in a routine assay of a "lipid profile."
2. APOA5-1131C allele carriers have higher CAD risk.

Phospholipid Antibodies

See Antiphospholipid Antibodies—Serum.

Phosphorus (Inorganic Phosphate)—Serum
Norm.

		SI Units
Adults ≤60 years	2.7-4.5 mg/dL	0.87-1.45 mmol/L
Females >60 years	2.8-4.1 mg/dL	0.90-1.30 mmol/L
Males >60 years	2.3-3.7 mg/dL	0.74-1.20 mmol/L
Children and infants		
Cord blood	3.7-8.1 mg/dL	1.20-2.62 mmol/L
Premature infant	5.4-10.9 mg/dL	1.74-3.52 mmol/L
Newborn	4.5-9 mg/dL	1.45-2.91 mmol/L
Infant (10 days-24 months)	4.5-6.7 mg/dL	1.45-2.16 mmol/L
Child (24 months-12 years)	4.5-5.5 mg/dL	1.45-1.78 mmol/L

Increased. >4.7 mg/dL or 1.3 mmol/L fasting: acromegaly, acute or chronic renal disease (associated mortality in chronic kidney disease), bone tumors or metastases, diabetic ketoacidosis, fulminant hepatic failure in children (indicator of poor prognosis), healing bone fractures, hyperthyroidism, hypoparathyroidism, lactic and respiratory acidosis, leukemia (myelogenous), magnesium deficiency, malignant hyperpyrexia after anesthesia, massive blood transfusions, metastatic bone tumors, milk-alkali (Burnett's) syndrome, multiple blood transfusions, multiple myeloma, Paget's disease, portal cirrhosis, postmenopausal, pseudohypoparathyroidism, pulmonary embolism, renal failure, sarcoidosis, secondary hypoparathyroidism, sickle cell, smokers, uremia, and vitamin D toxicity. Drugs include androgens, beta-adrenergic blockers, chemotherapy, diphosphates, ethyl alcohol (ethanol), furosemide (Lasix), growth hormone, hydrochlorothiazide, methicillin, parathormone, phenytoin, phosphate enemas or infusions, phosphate laxative abuse, steroids, and tetracycline (nephrotoxicity). Herbal or natural remedies include products containing aristolochic acids (*Akebia* spp., *Aristolochia* spp., *Asarum* spp., birthwort, *Bragantia* spp., *Clematis* spp., *Cocculus* spp., *Diploclisia* spp., Dutchman's pipe, *Fang chi, Fang ji, Guang fang ji, Kan-Mokutsu, Menispermum* spp., *Mokutsu, Mu tong, Sinomenium* spp., and *Stephania* spp.).

Decreased. <0.8 mg/dL, panic <0.3 mg/dL: acute alcoholism, burns (diuretic phase), Crohn's disease (caused by vomiting and diarrhea), diabetic ketoacidosis, dialysis, eating disorders, Fanconi syndrome (renal tubular defects), gout, hyperalimentation (without phosphorus supplement), hypercalcemia (severe), hyperinsulinism, hyperparathyroidism, hypokalemia, hypomagnesemia, hypothermia, hypovolemia, malabsorption, malnutrition, nasogastric suction, osteomalacia, respiratory alkalosis, rickets (primary or familial hypophosphatemia), salicylate poisoning, septicemia (gram-negative bacterial), sprue, and vitamin D deficiency. Drugs include acetazolamide, albuterol, amino acids, anesthetic agents, antacids (aluminum-containing and phosphate-binding), anticonvulsants, calcitonin, carbamazepine, corticosteroids, diuretics, epinephrine, estrogens, glucagon, glucocorticoids, glucose IV, insulin, isoniazid, magnesium hydroxide, niacin, oral contraceptives, phenytoin, Renagel (phosphate binder).

Description. The majority (85%) of phosphorus is stored in the bones in organic compounds. The remainder exists inorganically as phosphate anions within the soft tissue cells of the body and in the bloodstream. Phosphate functions in urinary acid-base buffering, energy storage and release, and metabolism of carbohydrates and lipids. Phosphorus is absorbed in the small intestine with the help of vitamin D, and phosphorus levels in the blood, along with calcium levels, are regulated by parathyroid hormone, calcitonin, vitamin D, and the renal phosphate excretion rate. An inverse relationship of calcium and phosphorus blood levels exists.

Professional Considerations
Consent form NOT required.

Preparation
1. The client must fast for 8-12 hours.
2. Tube: Red topped, red/gray topped, or gold topped.
3. Do NOT draw samples during hemodialysis.
4. See Client and Family Teaching.

Procedure
1. Draw a 4-mL blood sample.

Postprocedure Care
1. Send the specimen to the laboratory for immediate spinning.

Client and Family Teaching
1. Foods high in phosphorus include beans, chicken, eggs, fish, milk, and milk products.
2. Avoid excessive antacid intake and laxatives or enemas containing sodium phosphate.
3. For low phosphorus levels, avoid other persons with infections because phosphorus interferes with the functioning of the white blood cells.

Factors That Affect Results
1. Hemolysis of the specimen causes falsely elevated results.
2. Serum levels vary throughout the day and are lowest in the morning.
3. Eating before the test may falsely lower the phosphate level. Note that serum phosphorus concentration is weakly related to dietary phosphorus.
4. Hemodialysis will reduce phosphate levels.
5. Drugs that cause falsely decreased results include citrates, mannitol, oxalates, tartrate, and phenothiazines.

6. Levels may decrease from baseline in women taking oral contraceptives, and may increase from baseline in women taking injectable contraceptives.
7. Levels may be higher in blacks than whites.

Other Data
1. Calcium levels should also be measured to aid interpretation of results.
2. Hyperphosphatemia is related to LOW calcium levels and associated symptoms: tetany, dysrhythmias, and seizures.
3. Hypophosphatemia is associated with muscle weakness, difficult-to-wean chronic ventilator clients, encephalopathy, poor platelet function, decreased cardiac contractility, and paresthesias.
4. A 24-hour urine test for phosphate may be helpful in the workup of low phosphate levels.
5. Phosphorus and potassium requirements are greater for patients with traumatic brain injury.
6. Preoperative elevated serum phosphorus associated with cardiovascular mortality 30 days after major vascular surgery and long-term mortality.
7. In diabetics a serum phosphorus level >3.9 mg/dL is associated with cardiovascular mortality.

Phosphorus—Urine
Norm.

		SI Units
Adults	0.4-1.3 g/24 hours	13-42 mmol/day
	400-1300 mg/24 hours	
Restricted diet	<1.0 g/24 hours	<32 mmol/day
	<100 mg/24 hours	
Girls 7-17 years: phosphorus normalized to creatinine, P/Cr	0.85-1.44 mg/mg	
Boys 7-17 years: phosphorus normalized to creatinine, P/Cr	0.87-1.68 mg/mg	

NOTE: Restricted diet contains 0.9-1.5 g (29-48 mmol) of phosphorus and 10 mg (0.25 mmol) of calcium per day.

Increased. Bone fractures (transiently), familial hypophosphatemia, Fanconi syndrome (renal tubular damage), hyperparathyroidism, nonrenal acidosis (because phosphate excretion is a buffering mechanism), paraplegia, stone formers (associated with high dietary intake of calcium, phosphorus, and macronutrients), vitamin D–resistant rickets, and vitamin D toxicity. Drugs include acetazolamide, asparagine, bicarbonate, bismuth salts, calcitonin, corticosteroids, dihydrotachysterol, diuretics, hydrochlorothiazide, metolazone, phosphates (increased intake), PTH, valine, and vitamin D. Herbal or natural remedies include products containing aristolochic acids (*Akebia* spp., *Aristolochia* spp., *Asarum* spp., birthwort, *Bragantia* spp., *Clematis* spp., *Cocculus* spp., *Diploclisia* spp., Dutchman's pipe, *Fang chi, Fang ji, Guang fang ji, Kan-Mokutsu, Menispermum* spp., *Mokutsu, Mu tong, Sinomenium* spp., and *Stephania* spp.).

Decreased. Hypoparathyroidism or parathyroidectomy, pseudohypoparathyroidism. Drugs include aluminum-containing antacids; alanine in the obese, fasting client; Renagel, a phosphate binder; decreased urinary phosphate excretion in rats.

Description. See Phosphorus—Serum.

Professional Considerations
Consent form NOT required.

Preparation
1. Obtain a clean, detergent-free, 3-L urine container to which acetic acid wash has been added.
2. Write the beginning time of collection on the laboratory requisition.

Procedure
1. Discard the first morning urine specimen.
2. Save all the urine voided for 24 hours in a clean, refrigerated, 3-L container.

Document the quantity of urine output during the specimen collection period. Include urine voided at the end of the 24-hour period. For catheterized clients, keep the drainage bag on ice and empty the urine into the collection container hourly.

Postprocedure Care

1. Compare the urine quantity in the specimen container with the urinary output record for the test. If the specimen contains less urine than what was recorded as output, some of the sample may have been discarded, invalidating the test.
2. Document the quantity of urine output and the ending time on the laboratory requisition.
3. Hydrochloric acid is added in the laboratory on arrival for preservation.

Client and Family Teaching

1. Save all the urine voided in the 24-hour period and urinate before defecating to avoid loss of urine and to avoid contaminating the urine with stool. If any urine is accidentally discarded, discard the entire specimen and restart the collection.

Factors That Affect Results

1. All urine voided for the 24-hour period must be included to avoid a falsely low result.

Other Data

1. Because phosphorus levels vary throughout the day, this test is most informative if performed on a 24-hour urine sample.
2. Poor creatinine clearance will invalidate the results.

Pinworm

See **Parasite Screen**—Stool.

PIR

See **Pulse Volume Record Testing of Peripheral Vasculature**—Diagnostic.

PKU

See **Phenylalanine**.

PLA₂

See **Lipoprotein-Associated Phospholipase A2**—Blood

PLAC

See **Lipoprotein-Associated Phospholipase A2**—Blood

Plasma Free Metanephrines

See **Metanephrines, Total, 24-Hour**—Urine and Free-Plasma.

Plasma Renin Activity

See **Renin Activity**—Plasma.

Plasminogen Activity—Blood

Norm. 70%-113%.

Increased. Anxiety, congenital defect in the release of plasminogen inhibitors, deep-vein thrombosis, infancy, infection, inflammation, malignancy, myocardial infarction, pregnancy, stress, and surgery. Drugs include oral contraceptives.

Decreased. Cirrhosis, congenital defect in the release of plasminogen activators, disseminated intravascular coagulation, fibrinolysis, hyaline membrane disease, hypofibrinogenemia (acquired), liver disease, mesenteric ischemia (arterial and venous), nephrosis, surgery (coronary artery bypass graft, postoperatively), and thrombosis. Drugs include alteplase, L-asparaginase, streptokinase, and urokinase.

Description. Plasminogen is a beta-globulin protein found in fibrin clots of blood vessels, soft tissue, and any body cavity lined with endothelial cells. When healing or cellular repair has occurred, endothelial cell enzymes trigger the conversion of plasminogen to the fibrinolytic enzyme plasmin, and lysis of the fibrin clot begins. Plasminogen has a biologic half-life of 2 days. Plasminogen activity assays are used in the evaluation of fibrinolysis and increased fibrin-fibrinogen degradation products and in the diagnosis of the source of hypofibrinogenemia.

Professional Considerations
Consent form NOT required.

Preparation
1. Clarify with the laboratory whether this test must be prescheduled for processing.
2. Tube: blue topped; also obtain ice.

3. Do not use plasma collected in the presence of fluoride, EDTA, or heparin.
4. Specimens without lipidemia or hemolysis are preferred.
5. Specimens MAY be drawn during hemodialysis.

Procedure
1. Draw and discard a 2-mL blood sample and discard the syringe, leaving the needle in place. Perform venipuncture and withdraw 2 mL of blood into a syringe or vacuum tube. Remove the syringe or tube, leaving the needle in place. Attach a second syringe, and draw a sample quantity of 2.4 mL for a 2.7-mL tube and 4.0 mL for a 4.5-mL tube. Immediately place the specimens in a container of ice.

Postprocedure Care
1. Write the collection time on the laboratory requisition.
2. Send the specimens to the laboratory and refrigerate them if not processed within 8 hours.

Client and Family Teaching
1. If results are elevated, the client may need to change from oral contraceptives to other forms of birth control.

Factors That Affect Results
1. Reject hemolyzed or clotted specimens.

Other Data
1. Clients with decreased plasminogen concentration may be prone to developing recurrent thromboses.
2. Plasminogen concentrations are decreased with acquired or secondary hypofibrinogenemia and remain normal when congenital causes exist.

Platelet Activating Factor

See Lipoprotein-Associated Phospholipase A2—Blood

Platelet Adhesion Test—Diagnostic

Norm. Glass bead retention: 50%-95% (most commonly, 90%-95%).

Increased. Aging, atherosclerosis, burns, carcinoma, diabetes mellitus, exertion, homocystinuria, hypercoagulability, hyperlipemia,

infection (acute), multiple sclerosis, pregnancy, surgery, thrombosis, and trauma. Drugs include oral contraceptives.

Decreased. Afibrinogenemia, anemia (severe), azotemia, Bernard-Soulier syndrome,

Chédiak-Higashi syndrome, congenital heart disease, Glanzmann's thrombasthenia, glycogen storage disease, macroglobulinemia, multiple myeloma, myeloid metaplasia, myeloproliferative disorders, plasma cell dyscrasia, platelet release defect, storage pool disease, thrombasthenia, thrombocytopathy, uremia, and von Willebrand's disease. Drugs include vitamin E and dietary fish oil supplementation. Herbs or natural remedies include garlic (aged extract taken on an ongoing basis).

Description. This test evaluates the ability of platelets to adhere to foreign bodies during blood clotting by running blood through a collection of glass beads and counting the number of platelets adhering to the beads.

Professional Considerations
Consent form NOT required.

Preparation
1. Preschedule this test with the laboratory.
2. Tube: Red topped, red/gray topped, or gold topped.
3. Specimens MAY be drawn during hemodialysis.

4. Screen client for the use of herbal preparations or medicines or natural remedies.
5. See Client and Family Teaching.

Procedure
1. Draw a 10-mL blood specimen.

Postprocedure Care
1. None.

Client and Family Teaching
1. Do not take drugs that inhibit platelet adhesion within 10 days before the test.
2. Do not take drugs that decrease platelet levels within 10 days before the test (see Platelet count—Blood).
3. Fast for 8 hours before this test.
4. If results are elevated, the client may need to change from oral contraceptives to other forms of birth control.

Factors That Affect Results
1. Reject clotted specimens or specimens with an extremely low platelet count.
2. Platelet adhesiveness is increased during the spring season.
3. Platelet adhesiveness is highest during the afternoon hours.

Other Data
1. This test is difficult to standardize.

Platelet Aggregation—Blood; Platelet Aggregation, Hypercoagulable State—Blood

Norm. 60%-100% or according to specific laboratory.
  ADP: Normal.
  Collagen: Normal.
  Arachidonic acid: Normal.
  Ristocetin: Normal.
Hypercoagulable state: Normal values are reported in descriptive terms of rate of spontaneous platelet aggregation of samples as compared to rate of platelet aggregation of control, evaluation of a second wave of aggregation with adenosine diphosphate (ADP) reagent, and platelet response to serial dilutions of epinephrine.

Increased. Atheromatosis, cholangiocarcinoma, depressed patients, diabetes mellitus, hypercoagulability, hyperlipemia, polycythemia vera, smoking. Drugs include thiopental.

Decreased. Afibrinogenemia, anemia (sideroblastic), Bernard-Soulier syndrome (ristocetin test), beta-thalassemia major, Chédiak-Higashi syndrome, cirrhosis, Glanzmann's thrombasthenia (ADP, epinephrine, and collagen test), gray platelet syndrome (ADP, epinephrine, thrombin, collagen tests), Hermansky-Pudlak syndrome, homocystinuria, idiopathic thrombocytopenic purpura (ADP, collagen, epinephrine), macroglobulinemia, myeloid metaplasia, plasma cell dyscrasia, platelet release defects (ADP, second phase; epinephrine, second phase; and collagen tests), preleukemia, scurvy, snakebite, storage pool disease (ADP, second phase; epinephrine, second phase; and collagen tests), thrombasthenia (ADP, epinephrine, collagen), thrombocythemia (hemorrhagic), uremia, von Gierke's disease, von Willebrand's disease (ristocetin test), and Wiskott-Aldrich syndrome. Drugs include alphaprodine, antibiotics, anticoagulants, antihistamines, aspirin, azlocillin, bisoprolol, carbenicillin indanyl sodium, carvedilol, cephalothin sodium, chlordiazepoxide, chloroquine hydrochloride, chloroquine phosphate, clofibrate, clopidogrel, cocaine hydrochloride, corticosteroids, cyproheptadine hydrochloride, dexibuprofen, dextran, dextropropoxyphene, diabenol, diazepam, diphenhydramine hydrochloride, dipyridamole, eptifibatide, escitalopram, flufenamic acid, flurbiprofen, furosemide, gentamicin sulfate, glibenclamide, gliclazide, guaifenesin, heparin calcium, heparin sodium, ibufenac, ibuprofen, iloprost (aerosolized), imipramine, indomethacin, interferon alpha 2b, ketamine, marijuana, mefenamic acid, naproxen sodium, nebivolol, nitric oxide, nitrofurantoin, nortriptyline hydrochloride, oxyphenbutazone, penicillin G benzathine, penicillin G potassium, penicillin G procaine, phenothiazines, phenylbutazone, promethazine hydrochloride, propranolol, pyrimidine compounds, sibrafiban, statin drugs, sulfinpyrazone, theophylline, ticlopidine hydrochloride, tricyclic antidepressants, vitamin E, volatile general anesthetics (methoxyflurane, halothane, nitrous oxide), and zomepirac. Herbs or natural remedies include *Aesculus hippocastanum L.* (horse chestnut), *Ardisia elliptica* Thunberg (Myrsinaceae), *Cordyceps sinensis, dan shen* ('red-ginseng,' *Salvia miltiorrhiza*), feverfew, *Ganoderma lucidum* (a bracket fungus), garlic (aged extract taken on an ongoing basis), Ligustrazine isolated from Chuangxiong, Pycnogenol, tetramethylpyrazine (at high concentrations of 1.0 mmol). Other: Red wine is thought to exert cardioprotective effects through inhibition of platelet aggregation polyphenol resveratrol, one of its constituents.

Description. The platelet aggregation test assesses the ability of platelets to adhere to each other by mixture of the client's platelets in solution with substances that induce aggregation and measurement of the amount of light that passes through the solution after clumping has occurred. Substances that induce aggregation include arachidonic acid, ADP, epinephrine, ristocetin, collagen, and thrombin. The platelet aggregation test for a hypercoagulable state is a modification of

the standard platelet aggregation test. This test assesses the ability of platelets to adhere to each other in the following ways. First, the rate and amount of spontaneous platelet aggregation of the sample are compared to a known normal control sample. Second, the platelet-aggregating reagent ADP is added to the client's sample, which is then observed for evidence of a second wave of aggregation. Third, serial dilutions of epinephrine, another platelet-aggregating reagent, are added to the sample and the sample is studied for an enhanced platelet response.

Professional Considerations
Consent form NOT required.

Preparation
1. Preschedule this test with the laboratory.
2. Tube: Blue topped.
3. Do NOT draw specimens during hemodialysis.
4. Screen client for the use of herbal preparations or medicines or natural remedies.
5. See Client and Family Teaching.

Procedure
1. Draw nine 5-mL samples in blue topped tubes and one 5-mL sample in a lavender topped tube.
2. Traumatic venipuncture may cause contamination, thereby increasing aggregation.

Postprocedure Care
1. Write the specimen collection time on the laboratory requisition.
2. Deliver the specimen to the laboratory immediately. Do not refrigerate it. Testing should be performed within 2 hours after collection. Keep the specimen stable at room temperature for 1-3 hours.

Client and Family Teaching
1. Do not take drugs that inhibit platelet aggregation within the previous 10 days unless the test is being used to evaluate the drug effect on platelet function.
2. Do not eat or drink caffeine-containing products within 12 hours of the test.

Factors That Affect Results
1. Reject hemolyzed or clotted specimens or specimens received more than 2 hours after collection.
2. Platelet count <100,000/mm^3 causes inaccurate results.

3. A delay in testing may cause a loss of platelet ability to aggregate.
4. Lipemia may interfere with accurate measurement.
5. There is some evidence that red wine inhibits platelet aggregation.
6. Females have greater aggregability than males. The reason is hypothesized to be related to sex-related differences in testosterone levels.
7. Caucasian women are more prone to platelet aggregation.

Other Data

1. von Willebrand's disease may be ruled out by a normal response to ristocetin aggregating agent. Platelet aggregation inhibition caused by ingestion of aspirin may be ruled out by an inhibited response to arachidonic acid aggregating agent. Gray platelet syndrome may be ruled out when aggregation occurs with ristocetin but not with other aggregating agents.

Platelet Antibody—Blood

Norm. Negative or <1000 molecules of IgG per platelet.

Positive. Neonatal alloimmune thrombocytopenia (NATP), thrombocytopenia resulting from platelet autoantibodies causing idiopathic thrombocytopenic purpura (ITP), posttransfusion purpura, platelet refractoriness, isoimmune purpura, drug-induced (quinidine, quinine, furosemide, sulfonamides), or caused by platelet isoantibodies after receipt of multiple transfusions.

Description. The platelet antibody test is performed to detect the presence of platelet autoantibodies and platelet isoantibodies (alloantibodies). Platelet autoantibodies are IgG immunoglobulins of autoimmune origin and are present in all cases of ITP. A quantitative antiglobulin consumption test or other methods may be used to detect platelet autoantibodies. Platelet isoantibodies develop in clients when they become sensitized to platelet antigens of transfused blood. This results in destruction of both donor and native platelets and shortened survival time of platelets in the transfusion recipient. A complement fixation test (or other methods) may be used to detect platelet isoantibodies.

Professional Considerations

Consent form NOT required.

Preparation

1. Preschedule this test with the laboratory.
2. Tubes: Two blue topped.
3. Do NOT draw during hemodialysis.

Procedure

1. Completely fill two sodium citrate–anticoagulated, blue topped tubes with a blood sample.
2. If testing will be delayed, collect the sample into tubes containing acid citrate dextrose obtained from the laboratory.

Postprocedure Care

1. Send the specimens to the laboratory. Plasma should be separated from the red cells and frozen in a plastic tube at 25 degrees C.
2. For specimens collected into acid citrate dextrose, store the sample as collected at 4 degrees C.
3. Specimens may be frozen up to 3 years.

Client and Family Teaching

1. If thrombocytopenia is present, avoid rough physical activity and bumping into furniture. Use a stool softener and avoid straining to have a bowel movement. Use a soft toothbrush and watch for and report signs of bleeding: bruising, petechiae, blood in the stool/urine/sputum, bleeding from invasive lines, bleeding gums, abnormal or excessive vaginal bleeding.

Factors That Affect Results

1. Reject hemolyzed or clotted specimens.

Other Data

1. Samples with mean fluorescence greater than 2 standard deviations above the mean of the negative control sample are considered positive.

Platelet (Thrombocyte) Count—Blood

Norm.

Platelets (PLT)		SI Units
Adults	150,000-400,000/µL	150 to 400 × 10⁹/L
Critical low	<30,000/µL	<30 × 10⁹/L
Critical high	>1,000,000/µL	>1000 × 10⁹/L
Children		
Cord	100,000-290,000/µL	100 to 290 × 10⁹/L
Premature	100,000-300,000/µL	100 to 300 × 10⁹/L
Newborn	100,000-300,000/µL	100 to 300 × 10⁹/L
Neonate	150,000-390,000/µL	100 to 390 × 10⁹/L
3 months	260,000/µL	260 × 10⁹/L
Infant	200,000-473,000/µL	200 to 473 × 10⁹/L
1-10 years	150,000-450,000/µL	150 to 450 × 10⁹/L
Critical low	<20,000/µL	<20 × 10⁹/L
Critical high	>1,000,000/µL	>1000 x 10⁹/L

Increased. After splenectomy, anemia (hemolytic, iron-deficiency, post menorrhagic, sickle cell), asphyxia, asplenism, carcinoma, cirrhosis, collagen disease, cryoglobulinemia, exercise, fractures, heart disease, hemorrhage (acute), idiopathic thrombocythemia, infection (acute), inflammation, leukemia (chronic granulocytic, chronic myelogenous), malignancy, multiple myeloma, myelofibrosis, myeloproliferative disease, pancreatitis (chronic), polycythemia vera, postoperatively, postpartum, pregnancy (more in twin than single pregnancies), pseudothrombocytosis, reticulocytosis, rheumatoid arthritis, surgery, and tuberculosis. Drugs include epinephrine, epinephrine bitartrate, epinephrine borate, epinephrine hydrochloride, and oral contraceptives.

Decreased. After splenectomy (2 months), anemia (aplastic, megaloblastic, pernicious), aplastic or hypoplastic bone marrow, autoimmune disorders, Bernard-Soulier syndrome, blood transfusion (incompatible, large amounts), burns (severe), carcinoma (metastatic), cirrhosis, clostridial infection, collagen diseases, defibrination syndrome, diphtheria, disseminated intravascular coagulation, extracorporeal circulation, Gaucher disease, hemolytic disease of the newborn, hemorrhage, heparin therapy, histoplasmosis, hypersplenism, idiopathic thrombocytopenic purpura, infections (acute), irradiation, leukemia (acute granulocytic, acute lymphocytic, monocytic), lymphoproliferative disease, malaria, May-Hegglin anomaly, megakaryocytic hypoplasia, menstruation, multiple myeloma, myelofibrosis, radiation, regular plateletpheresis donors, septicemia, typhoid fever, uremia, and Wiskott-Aldrich syndrome. Drugs include acetazolamide, acetohexamide, amidopyrine, aminosalicylic acid, amphotericin B, ampicillin, antimony, antimony potassium tartrate, antineoplastics, arsenicals, aspirin, aurothioglucose, barbiturates, brompheniramine maleate, carbamazepine, chloramphenicol, chloroquine hydrochloride, chlorpropamide, chloroquine phosphate, chlorothiazide, colchicine, diazoxide, digitoxin, ethacrynate sodium, ethacrynic acid, ethoxzolamide, furosemide, gold sodium thiomalate, hydroxychloroquine sulfate, indomethacin, iothiouracil, isoniazid, mefenamic acid, meprobamate, methazolamide, methimazole, methyldopa, methyldopate hydrochloride, oral hypoglycemics, organic insecticides (some), oxyphenbutazone, oxytetracycline, oxytetracycline calcium, oxytetracycline hydrochloride, penicillamine, penicillins, phenylbutazone, phenytoin, phenytoin sodium, pyrimethamine, quinidine gluconate, quinidine polygalacturonate, quinidine sulfate, quinine sulfate, rifampin, salicylates, streptomycin sulfate, sulfonamides, thiazides, tolbutamide, tricyclic antidepressants, and vaccines. Herbal or natural remedies include the Chinese bracket fungus *Ganoderma lucidum*.

Description. Platelets are nonnucleated, disk-shaped cells that function in hemostatic plug formation, clot retraction, and coagulation factor activation. They are produced by the bone marrow from megakaryocytes released into the bloodstream to function in hemostasis.

Professional Considerations
Consent form NOT required.

Preparation

1. Tube: Lavender topped.
2. Do NOT draw specimens during hemodialysis.

Procedure

1. Leave a tourniquet in place less than 1 minute.
2. Draw a 5-mL blood sample.
3. Gently invert the tube two or three times.

Postprocedure Care

1. Send the specimen to the laboratory within 1 hour.
2. Closely monitor the site for bleeding in clients with known thrombocytopenia.

Client and Family Teaching

1. If thrombocytopenia is present, avoid rough physical activity and bumping into furniture. Use a stool softener and avoid straining to have a bowel movement. Use a soft toothbrush and watch for and report signs of bleeding: bruising, petechiae, blood in the stool/urine/sputum, bleeding from invasive lines, bleeding gums, abnormal or excessive vaginal bleeding.

Factors That Affect Results

1. Reject hemolyzed specimens or specimens received more than 1 hour after collection.
2. High altitudes, chronic cold weather, and exercise increase platelet counts.

Other Data

1. The serum sample is stable at room temperature for 10 hours, may be refrigerated for up to 18 hours, and should not be frozen.
2. Feverfew is an herb or natural remedy that may inhibit platelet activity and increase bleeding.

Plethysmography

See Pulse Volume Recorder Testing of Peripheral Vasculature—Diagnostic.

p-Methoxyamphetamine

See Amphetamines—Blood.

Pneumocystis Immunofluorescent Assay—Serum

Norm. Antibodies <1:16. No organisms observed.

Usage. Diagnosis of *Pneumocystis* pneumonia associated with acquired immune deficiency syndrome (AIDS), immunosuppressed cancers, and organ transplants.

Description. *Pneumocystis carinii* are protozoan bacteria that produce an inflammatory infection within the lungs known as *Pneumocystis* pneumonia. This type of pneumonia does not generally develop in humans unless they are immunocompromised by steroid therapy or cell-mediated immunodeficiencies. The alveolar exudate produced by *Pneumocystis* is a proteinaceous material pervaded with cysts and trophozoites. The antigens present in the bacterial cell walls produce antibodies that circulate in the blood. These antibodies can be examined under a microscope when stained with immunofluorescent dyes and examined under ultraviolet radiation.

Professional Considerations
Consent form NOT required.

Preparation

1. Tube: Red topped or pink topped, or Corvac tube.
2. Specimens MAY be drawn during hemodialysis.

Procedure

1. Draw a 10-mL blood sample.

Postprocedure Care

1. Handle the specimen with caution because of potential cross-infection.

Client and Family Teaching

1. Results are normally available within 24 hours.

Factors That Affect Results

1. Immunofluorescent antibody titers are elevated in only about 30% of clients with *Pneumocystis*.
2. Serum antibody or antigen detection is not reliable for definitive diagnosis of *P. carinii*.

Other Data

1. A diagnostic bronchoscopy for tissue brushings should be performed if the serum specimen is positive for *P. carinii*.

Pneumotonometry

See **Tonometry Test for Glaucoma**—Screen.

Poliomyelitis 1, 2, 3 Titer—Blood

Norm. <1.8 is normal. A fourfold increase in the antibody titer between the acute and convalescent blood specimens is diagnostic for poliomyelitis. Presence of a high IgM titer may also indicate recent infection.

Usage. Identification and diagnosis of the enterovirus poliovirus and differentiation of the serotype (1 = Brunhilde, 2 = Lansing, 3 = Leon).

Description. Poliomyelitis is an extremely contagious systemic infection resulting in necrotic and inflammatory lesions of the motor and autonomic neurons of the brain and spinal cord. The risk is low in immunized populations. Poliomyelitis usually manifests as a systemic viremia with headache, fever, vomiting, and back and neck pain progressing in severity to a prominent paralysis and possibly death. Immigrant and adopted children may present with monomelic amyotrophy. The virus is transmitted by ingestion of contaminated water or food. The virus incubates and replicates in the lymphoid tissue of the tonsils, Peyer's patches, pharynx, and alimentary tract. Enteroviruses (polioviruses) are excreted in the feces and can remain active outside of the human cells for months. The incubation period for poliomyelitis is 5-35 days, with acute symptoms occurring 7-12 days after exposure. Both acute and convalescent

blood samples are tested to detect an increase in titer levels. Antigen-neutralization tests quantitate titers and serotype the virus from centrifuged serum. Type 1, Brunhilde poliovirus, is associated with paralysis, chronic cardiomyopathy, diabetes, fetal malformation, myocarditis, and pericarditis. Orally administered vaccines available since the 1950s have decreased the incidence of this disease worldwide. A global poliomyelitis eradication initiative that began in 1998 has reduced the cases worldwide by over 99%. As of 2012, only 3 countries remain polio-endemic: Afghanistan, Nigeria, and Pakistan.

Professional Considerations

Consent form NOT required.

Preparation

1. Tube: Red topped, red/gray topped, or gold topped.
2. Specimens MAY be drawn during hemodialysis.

Procedure

1. Draw an 8- to 10-mL (adults) or a 3- to 4-mL (pediatric) blood sample.

Postprocedure Care

1. None.

Client and Family Teaching

1. Strict isolation precautions may be instituted if serum titers indicate

infection secondary to the extreme contagiousness.

Factors That Affect Results
1. In 50% of people with poliomyelitis, the serum titers have already peaked before testing.

Other Data
1. Use extreme caution when handling or transporting samples and wash hands well after handling a sample.
2. Poliovirus is human specific.

Polysomnography (PSG, Cardiopulmonary Sleep Study, CPAP Titration Study, Multiple Sleep Latency Test, MSLT, Sleep Apnea Study, Sleep Oximetry, Sleep Study)—Diagnostic

Norm. No abnormal patterns of sleep or breathing.

Usage. Routinely indicated for the diagnosis of sleep-related breathing disorders (such as obstructive sleep apnea which is highly prevalent in women with PCOS), suspicion of periodic limb movement sleep disorders, narcolepsy, evaluation of insomnias, atypical parasomnias and violent sleep behaviors, Wilson's disease. Also part of a CPAP titration study (treatment for obstructive sleep apnea), narcolepsy. May also be used to help diagnose disorders of arousal (sleepwalking, night terrors), rapid eye movement (REM) behavioral disorder, dissociative disorders, nocturnal seizures, nocturnal reflux, nocturnal pain syndromes and restless legs syndrome.

Description. Polysomnography (PSG) is a procedure that takes recordings of the electric potentials generated by the cerebral cortex of the brain during sleep. Electrical potentials demonstrated on PSG are of six types: (1) those generated by eye movements, (2) surface electrical potentials generated by chin muscle activity, (3) surface electrical potentials generated by the heart, (4) surface electrical potentials generated by the muscles in the leg (anterior tibialis), (5) nasal and oral airflow (each separately or combined), and (6) respiratory effort of chest and abdomen by piezoelectric or inductance belts. In special instances additional sensors are placed either on the head or on the abdomen, or are used to measure penile erections. This study can be coordinated with a multiple sleep latency test when an evaluation of excessive daytime sleepiness (that is, narcolepsy) is desired. The use of computerized digital monitoring provides objectivity in scoring of sleep-related events.

Professional Considerations
Consent form is NOT required.

Preparation
1. See Client and Family Teaching.
2. Document the client's current medications, and his or her height and weight.
3. Verify with the physician whether certain medications should be withheld before the test.
4. Review and complete the pretest questionnaire with the client.

Procedure
1. Sensor placement:
   a. The client sits on a bed or chair and electrodes are placed on the scalp (see Electroencephalography—Diagnostic, Description), around the eyes, and under the chin.
   b. The airflow monitors are placed near the mouth and nose, and the respiratory belts are placed around the chest and abdomen.
   c. Electrodes are placed on the chest to measure the ECG and on the legs to measure movements. For *nocturnal penile tumescence testing*, a mercury strain gauge will be placed at the base and tip of the penile shaft.
   d. Other sensors, such as a pH probe, are placed as necessary.
2. The client is asked to follow several commands to ensure that the sensors are functioning properly. This includes eye blinking, looking right, looking left, breath holding, right and left leg movements. This is known as "biocalibration."
3. The client then sleeps, and the PSG recordings are taken. A technician is continuously monitoring the recordings and client to detect lead detachment. For nocturnal penile tumescence testing, pressure

is placed on the head of the penis with a pressure plate to determine at what pressure the penis will buckle.

4. Recordings:
   a. The data obtained from a polysomnogram include the amount of sleep during the test, the amount of each stage of sleep, any events occurring during sleep, the number of arousals, the number of respiratory events, and the degree of desaturation.
   b. Apneas are defined as a complete cessation of breathing, whereas hypopneas are a partial cessation of breathing. These are usually reported as the number of respiratory events (apneas plus hypopneas) for an hour. This is known as the RDI, respiratory distress index, or the AHI, apnea hypopnea index.

5. CPAP titration studies:
   a. CPAP (continuous positive air pressure) is a treatment for obstructive sleep apnea and is essentially an air splint. Room air is blown through a mask covering the nose. The air pressure opens the posterior area of the pharynx eliminating the obstruction and snoring.
   b. The air pressure is titrated throughout the night, usually being slowly increased until both the obstructive respiratory events and the snoring are eliminated.
   c. Occasionally a bi-level machine that provides separate inspiratory and expiratory pressures is used.

6. "Split-night" studies:
   a. In these studies the first half of the night is used to confirm the existence of significant sleep-disordered breathing. The second half of the night is used to titrate CPAP. The use of "split-night" studies is still controversial. Not all laboratories will perform them.

7. The multiple sleep latency test (MSLT):
   a. The MSLT measures the degree of daytime sleepiness.
   b. Usually only the brain waves (EEG), eye movements (EOG), chin muscle activity (EMG), and heart activity (ECG) are measured during the (MSLT).
   c. The MSLT consists of five naps taken throughout the day, each 2 hours apart.
   d. The client is given up to 20 minutes to fall asleep on each nap. If the client falls asleep, he or she is given 15 minutes to sleep.
   e. Two results are obtained: The first is the average time to fall asleep on the five naps, known as the "mean sleep latency." The second is the number of naps on which REM is seen, known as "sleep-onset REMs."

Postprocedure Care

1. The various sensors are removed, and the conductive medium is removed from the scalp.
2. Every sleep lab should have facilities available for a client's morning toilet.

Client and Family Teaching

1. Often a pretest questionnaire is filled out the night of this study or mailed to the client before the study.
2. You will sleep all night in the sleep lab, and a video will be taken of you while you sleep. If the PSG will be followed by a multiple sleep latency test, you will spend the day in the sleep laboratory.
3. You will have wires and sensors attached to you, which are needed to perform the sleep study. The wires and sensors receive signals from your brain waves, muscle movement, heart, and breathing patterns that help evaluate your sleep patterns.
4. For clients who will have a CPAP titration study: A CPAP mask might be used for part or all of the test to determine whether it will help reduce sleep apnea. This mask fits very snugly over your nose and mouth. It delivers air into your lungs under pressure, and so it might be uncomfortable until you get used to it. You will be able to select the mask that is most comfortable for you.
5. You will be able to perform normal daily activities after the test.
6. Your test results will be sent to your referring physician, who will explain the results to you.

Factors That Affect Results

1. The use of caffeine or other stimulants before the test.
2. The client's normal sleep-wake cycle.
3. The client's information before the study and comfort sleeping in an unusual situation.

4. Nocturnal penile tumescence testing results may be inconclusive because of the client's anxiety, embarrassment, or startle response during testing, as well as sleep disorders that cause a reduction in the amount of REM-type sleep. Most penile nocturnal erections occur during REM sleep.

5. CPAP titration studies: A client's success in using CPAP is highly dependent on the skill of the sleep technician. The degree of client education about CPAP before the study of CPAP is a factor that can affect how well the client is able to tolerate the CPAP mask while sleeping. The technicians should be aware of the presence of any claustrophobia or difficulties the client might have by having things on the face.

Other Data

1. Even moderate weight reduction reduces the incidence of sleep-disordered breathing in obese clients with obstructive sleep apnea.

2. Plasma cystine levels are elevated in obstructive sleep apnea, range 412-555 mol/L, and decrease after effective apnea treatment.

3. Circadian rhythm sleep disorders which contribute to excessive daytime sleepiness include delayed sleep phase disorder, advanced sleep phase disorder, shift work disorder, and jet lag disorder. Polysomnography is NOT indicated for any of these conditions, unless a concomitant condition, such as restless legs syndrome or obstructive sleep apnea, is suspected.

Porphyrins, Quantitative—Blood

Norm.

		SI Units
Total erythrocyte porphyrins	<36 µg/dL	<0.05 µmol/L
ALA	<1 mg/dL	
Coproporphyrin	0.5-2.3 mg/dL	
Zinc protoporphyrin		<15 nmol/L
Uroporphyrin	Negative to trace	Negative to trace

Increased ALA. Chemical toxicity, cirrhosis (alcoholic), lead poisoning, and porphyrias.

Increased Coproporphyrin. Anemia (hemolytic, pernicious, sideroblastic), cirrhosis (alcoholic), coproporphyria (erythropoietic), erythroid hyperplasia, exercise (extreme), fever, hemochromatosis, Hodgkin's disease, lead poisoning, leukemia, myocardial infarction (acute), poliomyelitis (acute), porphyria (congenital erythropoietic), protoporphyria (erythropoietic), thyrotoxicosis, and vitamin deficiencies.

Increased Protoporphyrin. Anemia (hemolytic, sideroblastic), carbon tetrachloride and benzene toxicity, erythropoiesis, infection, iron deficiency, lead poisoning, protoporphyria (erythropoietic), and thalassemia.

Increased Uroporphyrin. Cirrhosis, lead poisoning, and porphyria (acute, intermittent, congenital erythropoietic).

Decreased ALA. Not applicable.

Decreased Coproporphyrin. Not applicable.

Decreased Protoporphyrin. Anemia (megaloblastic).

Decreased Uroporphyrin. Not applicable.

Description. Porphyrins are compounds necessary for heme synthesis in hemoglobin metabolism. ALA (delta-aminolevulinic acid) is the basic building block of porphyrins and is involved in the synthesis of coproporphyrin and protoporphyrin. Coproporphyrin is the main porphyrin found in urine, whereas protoporphyrin is the main porphyrin found in erythrocytes. When iron is added to protoporphyrin, the final heme molecule is formed. As the hemoglobin is eventually broken down, these products used for heme synthesis again appear in the blood, urine, and stool as hemoglobin-breakdown products. Clients with one of the congenital or acquired diseases classified as the "porphyrias" secrete and excrete increased amounts of these compounds. The diseases are characterized by neurologic abnormalities, acute abdominal pain, acute cutaneous pain, photosensitivity, or psychiatric disturbances. This test is used most frequently with the measurement of urine porphyrin levels to differentiate the cause and type of porphyria present.

Professional Considerations

Consent form NOT required.

Preparation

1. Tube: Green topped, lavender topped, or black topped.
2. Do NOT draw specimen during hemodialysis.
3. See Client and Family Teaching.

Procedure

1. Draw a 3-mL blood sample without hemolysis.

Postprocedure Care

1. None.

Client and Family Teaching

1. Do not drink alcohol for 24 hours before testing.
2. Clients with positive test results should avoid ethyl alcohol (ethanol), barbiturates, and anticonvulsants that might cause an acute attack of neurologic or psychotic porphyria (elevated ALA).
3. Clients with positive test results should avoid sunlight.
4. Genetic counseling may be necessary for the inherited form of porphyria.

Factors That Affect Results

1. Hemolysis of the specimen invalidates the results.
2. Increased levels may occur during menstruation or pregnancy.

Other Data

1. See also Protoporphyrin, Free erythrocyte —Blood; Coproporphyrin—Urine.

Positrace Imaging

See **Dual Modality Imaging**—Diagnostic.

Positron Emission Tomography (PET)—Diagnostic

Norm. Requires interpretation according to the type of study being performed.

Usage. Enables noninvasive regional tissue physiology study of metabolic changes in body tissues. Comparison of cerebral blood flow and energy metabolism; evaluation for leakage of the blood-brain barrier; study of brain pharmacology; evaluation of brain hemodynamics in cerebrovascular disease and psychiatry (affective disorders, dementia, schizophrenia, substance abuse); localization of seizure foci in clients with focal seizures; evaluation of regional myocardial blood flow, metabolism, and thus viability; study of the distribution of pulmonary edema; study of solid tumor proliferation, blood flow, glucose, and oxygen utilization alone and in response to therapy; diagnosing, staging, and restaging of cancer (lung, colorectal, lymphoma, melanoma, head and neck, and esophageal) along with monitoring therapy response. Used investigationally with Flutemetamol tracer to identify pathologic levels of amyloid associated with Alzheimer's disease.

Description. Positron emission tomography (PET) is a noninvasive radiographic method for studying blood flow and metabolic changes occurring in specific organs or regions of the body tissues. It involves the injection or inhalation of gamma ray–emitting, biologically compatible radioisotopes and the creation of images of radioisotope distribution in the body. As the radioisotopes disintegrate, they emit positrons, which are positively charged particles similar to electrons. As the positrons are captured by electrons, both are destroyed, resulting in the emission of two photons, which travel outward in opposite directions. The photons are detected simultaneously by the PET camera, an event known as a "coincidence." The summation of these coincidences allows for the creation of a continuous map of the metabolic activity of the body. A computer then creates pictures of cross-sections of the body area studied, which show brighter areas according to the amount of radioisotope present.

Some examples of radioisotopes include oxygen-15, nitrogen-13, carbon-11, and fluorine-18, which are labeled onto substances such as water, carbon dioxide, or glucose. Because the radioisotopes are biologically compatible, they take the place of the body's chemical elements (such as oxygen, nitrogen, or fluorine), and the resulting scan gives a true representation of the physiologic function of the body processes. The choice of radioisotope and material to be labeled is based on the body function to be studied. For example, blood flow is studied using ^{15}O-labeled HÖ⁻, glucose metabolism is studied using ^{18}F-labeled glucose, tissue perfusion is studied using ^{13}N-labeled NH_2, and anaerobic metabolism is studied using ^{11}C-labeled acetate. Some conditions in which the use of PET has been studied include Alzheimer's disease, asthma, brain tumors, cerebral atrophy, cerebrovascular disorders, chronic obstructive pulmonary disease, coronary artery disease, epilepsy, head trauma, Huntington's disease, myocardial infarction, obsessive compulsive disorder, pulmonary edema, schizophrenia, and unstable angina.

The newest equipment, called "Dual Mode Imaging," combines PET with structural imaging modalities such as Ultrafast CT or MRI for improved anatomical and malignant focus (bone, CNS, germ cell, lymphoma, neuroblastoma and soft-tissue tumors) imaging results. See Dual modality imaging—Diagnostic.

Professional Considerations
Consent form MAY be required.

Risks
Hematoma, infection, radiation exposure.

Precautions
During pregnancy, risks of cumulative radiation exposure to the fetus from this and other previous or future imaging studies must be weighed against the benefits of the procedure. Although formal limits for client exposure are relative to this risk:benefit comparison, the United States Nuclear Regulatory Commission requires that the cumulative dose equivalent to an embryo/fetus from occupational exposure not exceed 0.5 rem (5 mSv). Radiation dosage to the fetus is proportional to the distance of the anatomy studied from the abdomen. Conventional radiation dose is 127-169 mSv, which shortens children's life span between mean of 177-185 days, but new 18FDG PET/CT doses of 64-69 mSv has mean shortened lifespan of 68-103 days (Murano et al, 2010).

Preparation
1. About 30%-50% of all diagnostic imaging procedures are partially or totally inappropriate (Picano, 2008). Evaluate benefit:risk and aim at reducing useless imaging tests.
2. A premedication may be prescribed to be given before transport to the nuclear medicine department.
3. Diuretics should be withheld before the study unless an indwelling urinary catheter is present or will be inserted.
4. If pelvic imaging is to be performed, an indwelling urinary catheter should be inserted.
5. The client should have a meal before the procedure. Diabetic clients should be given their morning insulin before the procedure.
6. If abdominal imaging is indicated, a bowel preparation may be prescribed.
7. See Client and Family Teaching.

Procedure
1. The client is placed in a supine position on the scanning table, with an arm supported in extension.
2. Intravenous access is established.
3. A heparin flush solution is slowly infused.
4. An arterial line may be inserted for some procedures.
5. For brain scans, a polymer clay (Polyform)-molded face mask is placed over the temporal level of the face and secured to the headrest to immobilize the client's head. The mask is marked with a reference point to ensure exact repeat positioning for any necessary future PET studies.
6. The scanning table is moved into position within the lumen of the positron emission scanner.

7. Once the client is positioned, he or she must remain motionless throughout the study.
8. Some studies are conducted by having the client inhale the radioisotope. Others use intravenous injection.
9. An example of the steps involved in one type of scan follows.
10. *Cardiac PET:*
    a. ^{15}O-labeled HO$^-$ is injected intravenously, and a 15-minute test scan is conducted to verify proper positioning.
    b. A 30-minute transmission scan is then performed to correct for the attenuation of the chest and lungs.
    c. ^{13}N-labeled NH_2 is injected intravenously and allowed to equilibrate for 3 minutes. Then a PET study is performed for approximately 30 minutes to study cardiac tissue perfusion.
    d. Finally, glucose metabolism of the heart is studied. If the client has diabetes, with a glucose level >150 mg/dL, insulin may be given before this step. If the client has a low blood glucose level, either orally administered glucose or intravenous 50% dextrose in water will be given. Fluorodeoxyglucose (FDG) is injected intravenously to study glucose metabolism of the heart. After waiting 30 minutes for the FDG to circulate, one performs a 30-minute PET study.

Postprocedure Care

1. The arterial line, if inserted for the PET study, is discontinued, and the site should be monitored for the development of hematoma.

Client and Family Teaching

1. You must remain motionless in an enclosed space for 1-3 hours.
2. Wear comfortable clothing to the test.
3. You may bring a music player to listen to during the study.
4. Do not drink large quantities of fluid or caffeine-containing beverages within 2 hours before the study unless you have been informed that an indwelling catheter will be inserted.
5. Have a meal before the procedure.
6. You may need a bowel preparation if abdominal imaging is indicated.
7. Lactating women should not breast-feed for at least 20 hours after the scan.

Factors That Affect Results

1. Hypoglycemia may alter the results of PET glucose metabolism.
2. Movement more than about 1 cm may blur the resulting pictures. The ability of the client to remain motionless in an enclosed space affects whether an accurate study can be obtained.
3. Clients with insulin-dependent diabetes must have insulin administered the day of the study if glucose metabolism will be a focus of PET.
4. Anxiety in the client that causes tension in the neck area can cause increased uptake of the fluorine type of isotope, which can be misinterpreted as metastases.

Other Data

1. PET takes 1-3 hours. The half-life of the specific radioisotope used affects the length of the study.
2. Claustrophobia may occur during the procedure.

Potassium—Plasma or Serum

Norm. NOTE: Plasma levels are typically 0.2 to 0.3 mmol/L lower than serum levels. Plasma measurements are indicated when the client has thrombocytosis/high platelet counts.

	Serum levels	SI Units
Adult	3.5-5.3 mEq/L	3.5-5.3 mmol/L
Panic values	<2.5 mEq/L	<2.5 mmol/L
	or >6.6 mEq/L	or >6.6 mmol/L
Premature Infant		
Cord blood	5.0-10.2 mEq/L	5.0-10.2 mmol/L
2 days	3.0-6.0 mEq/L	3.0-6.0 mmol/L

	Serum levels	SI Units
Full-Term Newborn		
Cord blood	5.6-12.0 mEq/L	5.6-12.0 mmol/L
Newborn 0-7 Days	3.2-5.5 mEq/L	3.2-5.5mmol/L
Newborn, panic value	<2.5 mEq/L or >8.1 mEq/L	<2.5 mmol/L or >8.1 mmol/L
Infant 8-30 days	3.4-6.0 mEq/L	3.4-6.0 mmol/L
Infant 2-6 Months	3.5-5.6 mEq/L	3.5-5.6 mmol/L
Infant 7-11 months	3.5-6.1 mEq/L	3.5-6.1 mmol/L
Child	3.3-5.0 mEq/L	3.3-5.0 mmol/L

Panic Level Symptoms and Treatment

NOTE: Treatment choice(s) depend(s) on client's history and condition and episode history.

Hyperkalemia Symptoms. Irritability, diarrhea, cramps, oliguria, difficulty speaking, cardiac dysrhythmias including peaked T waves and progressing to refractory ventricular fibrillation with tachycardia.

Hyperkalemia Treatment
1. Provide continuous ECG monitoring.
2. Administer sodium polystyrene sulfonate (Kayexalate).
3. Administer intravenous insulin and dextrose.
4. Administer sodium bicarbonate.
5. Administer calcium chloride or gluconate.
6. Both hemodialysis and peritoneal dialysis WILL remove potassium.

Hypokalemia Symptoms. Malaise, thirst, polyurea, anorexia, weak pulse, low blood pressure, vomiting, decreased reflexes, ECG changes, including depressed T waves and ventricular ectopy.

Hypokalemia Treatment. Potassium replacement.

Increased. Acidosis, Addison's disease, adrenocortical insufficiency, anemia (hemolytic), anxiety, asthma, burns, dialysis (hemodialysis or peritoneal), diet (excessive potassium intake), dysrhythmia, hemolysis, hypoventilation, increased osmolality, infection (acute), ketoacidosis, leukocytosis, malignant hyperthermia (early), massive rapid red blood cell transfusion, metabolic acidosis, muscle necrosis, near-drowning, obstruction (intestinal), ostomies, pneumonia, pseudohypoaldosteronism, renal failure, renal hypertension, sepsis, shock, status epilepticus, syndrome of inappropriate antidiuretic hormone secretion (SIADHS), thrombocytosis, tissue trauma, uremia, and Waterhouse-Friderichsen syndrome. Drugs include aldosterone antagonists, amiloride, aminocaproic acid, antineoplastic agents, beta-adrenergic blockers, calcium, captopril, cyclophosphamide, cyclosporine, digoxin, enalapril, ephedrine, ephedrine sulfate, epinephrine, estrogens, heparin calcium, heparin sodium, histamine, hydrochlorothiazide, ibuprofen, indomethacin, isoniazid, lithium, mannitol, methicillin, methicillin sodium, nonsteroidal anti-inflammatory agents, potassium bicarbonate, potassium chloride, potassium citrate, potassium gluconate, potassium salts of penicillin, phenformin, propranolol, rofecoxib, salt substitutes, spironolactone, succinylcholine, tetracyclines, timolol maleate, triamterene, tromethamine, and valsartan.

Decreased. After sigmoidoscopy, acute tubular necrosis (diuretic phase), alcoholism, aldosteronism (primary), alkalosis, anorexia, barium intoxication, Bartter syndrome, bradycardia, cancer (colon), cerebral palsy, cholera, cirrhosis (chronic), congestive heart failure, Crohn's disease, Cushing's disease, dehydration, diabetes insipidus, diabetes mellitus, diarrhea, dumping syndrome, dysrhythmias, eating disorders, Fanconi syndrome, fever, fistulas, folic acid deficiency, hyperaldosteronism, hyperalimentation, hypercorticoadrenalism, hypertension, hypomagnesemia, hypothermia, hypovolemia, hysterectomy, ketoacidosis, kwashiorkor, laxative abuse, lymphoma, malabsorption, malignant hyperthermia (late-stage), metabolic alkalosis, nephritis, organic brain syndrome, ostomies, pancreatitis (acute), paralytic ileus, pseudoaldosteronism, pyelonephritis (chronic), pyloric obstruction, renal tubular acidosis, salicylate intoxication, salt-losing nephropathy, starvation, stress, suction (gastric),

P

surgery (postoperatively), sweating, toxic shock syndrome, ureterosigmoidostomy, villous adenoma, vipoma, vomiting, and Zollinger-Ellison syndrome (with diarrhea). Drugs include acetazolamide, albuterol, ammonium chloride, amphotericin B, aspirin, barium, beta-2 agonists, bicarbonate, bisacodyl, bronchodilators, carbenicillin, carbenoxolone, chlorthalidone, cisplatin, corticosteroids, corticotropin, digoxin, diuretics, EDTA, ethacrynic acid, furosemide, gammahydroxybutyrate (GHB), gentamicin sulfate, glucose, insulin, laxatives, mercurial diuretics, penicillin G, piperacillin, risperidone, salicylates, sodium bicarbonate, sodium chloride, succinylcholine chloride (in children), theophylline, thiazides, thiopental, ticarcillin, and trimethaphan camsylate. Herbs or natural remedies include aloe (long-term use), licorice (*Glycyrrhiza glabra*), which can cause intoxication, and products containing aristolochic acids (*Akebia* spp., *Aristolochia* spp., *Asarum* spp., birthwort, *Bragantia* spp., *Clematis* spp., *Cocculus* spp., *Diploclisia* spp., Dutchman's pipe, *Fang chi, Fang ji, Guang fang ji, Kan-Mokutsu, Menispermum* spp., *Mokutsu, Mu tong, Sinomenium* spp., and *Stephania* spp.).

Description. Potassium (K) is the major intracellular cation. The body obtains potassium through dietary ingestion, and the kidneys either preserve or excrete it depending on cellular need. Potassium is responsible for the regulation of cellular water balance, electrical conduction in muscle cells, and acid-base homeostasis. Although the majority of potassium is stored and used within tissue cells, serum potassium analysis can be helpful in evaluating electrolyte balance. Serum potassium levels are used in the evaluation of clients with cardiac dysrhythmias, renal dysfunction, mental confusion, gastrointestinal distress, and intravenous replacement therapy.

Professional Considerations
Consent form NOT required.

Preparation
1. Tube: Red topped, red/gray topped, or gold topped or green topped.
2. Do NOT draw specimens during hemodialysis.
3. Instruct client not to clench fist or exercise the arm prior to or during venipuncture.

Procedure
1. Draw the 4-mL venous specimen without using a tourniquet.
2. Using a 20-gauge or larger needle, draw a 4-mL blood sample.
3. Do not aspirate strongly or push the plunger into the vacuum tube too forcefully.
4. Avoid hemolysis.

Postprocedure Care
1. Write the collection time on the laboratory requisition.
2. Note on the laboratory requisition if the client is receiving potassium by pill, liquid, or intravenously.
3. Send the specimen to the chemistry laboratory for spinning within 1 hour of collection. Specimen is stable after separation for 2 weeks if refrigerated.
4. Serum and plasma must be separated from the red cells, or elevated results may occur.

Client and Family Teaching
1. The client must follow the prescribed dosage of potassium.
2. Foods high in potassium are apricots, bananas, meats, potatoes, prunes, and tomatoes.

Factors That Affect Results
1. Reject hemolyzed specimens or specimens received more than 1 hour after collection.
2. Use of a tourniquet and pumping the hand before obtaining a venous sample can increase the laboratory value by up to 20%.
3. Do NOT draw the specimen from a site where an intravenous infusion exists.
4. Clients with elevated white blood cell counts and platelet counts may have falsely elevated serum potassium levels.
5. Incomplete separation of the serum from the clot may cause falsely elevated results.
6. Acidemia causes potassium to move from cells into the extracellular fluid in exchange for hydrogen ions moving intracellularly.
7. Values are 0.2-0.4 mEq/L higher in samples collected in the afternoon and early evening.

Other Data

1. For elevated potassium levels, an arterial blood gas should be evaluated for acidemia.
2. Both systolic and diastolic blood pressure readings decrease after oral potassium.
3. Green et al (2002) found a higher risk for stroke in clients with low potassium intake (<2.5 g/day) and in clients on diuretics with lower potassium levels (<4.1 mEq/L or <4.1 mmol/L).
4. The 2011 Third National Health and Nutrition Examination Survey (NHANES III), a prospective cohort study of 12,267 U.S. adults, found that a dietary sodium/potassium ratio of <1 is protective in that it is associated with a decreased rate of mortality.

Potassium—Urine

Norm.

		SI Units
Adult	25-123 mEq/24 hours (intake-dependent)	25-123 mmol/day
Child	17-57 mEq/24 hours	17-57 mmol/day

Increased. Alkalosis, Cushing's disease, dehydration, diabetic ketoacidosis, diet (excessive potassium intake), fever, head trauma, hyperaldosteronism, hypokalemia, renal failure (chronic), renal tubular acidosis, salicylate intoxication, and starvation. Drugs include acetazolamide, ammonium chloride, amphotericin, fosinopril, glucocorticoids, loop diuretics, mercurial diuretics, penicillin, potassium, and thiazide diuretics. Herbs include Orthosiphon stamineus extract.

Decreased. Addison's disease, diarrhea, hyperkalemia, hypomagnesemia, malabsorption syndrome, nephrotic syndrome, potassium deficiency, renal failure (acute), and syndrome of inappropriate antidiuretic hormone secretion (SIADHS). Drugs include laxatives, epinephrine, levarterenol, and general anesthetic agents.

Description. Potassium (K) is the major intracellular cation. The body obtains potassium through dietary ingestion, and the kidneys either preserve or excrete it, depending on cellular need. Potassium is responsible for the regulation of cellular water balance, electrical conduction in muscle cells, and acid-base homeostasis. A 24-hour urine collection is obtained to determine excreted potassium levels. Urine potassium levels are helpful in the assessment of endocrine abnormalities and renal tubular function.

Professional Considerations

Consent form NOT required.

Preparation

1. Obtain a 3-L container without preservatives, or a pediatric urine collection device/bag and tape.
2. Write the beginning time of the collection on the laboratory requisition.
3. Note diuretic or glucocorticoid therapy on the laboratory requisition.

Procedure

1. Discard the first morning urine specimen.
2. Save all urine voided for 24 hours in a refrigerated, clean, 3-L container without preservatives. Document the quantity of urine output during the specimen collection period. Include urine voided at the end of the 24-hour period. For catheterized clients, keep the drainage bag on ice and empty urine into the collection container hourly.
3. *Pediatric/infant specimen collection:*
   a. Place the child in a supine position with the knees flexed and the hips externally rotated and abducted.
   b. Cleanse, rinse, and thoroughly dry the perineal area.
   c. To prevent the child from removing the collection device/bag, a diaper may be placed over the genital area.
   d. *Females:* Tape the pediatric collection device/bag to the perineum. Starting at the area between the anus and vagina,

apply the device/bag in an anterior direction.

e. *Males:* Place the pediatric collection device/bag over the penis and scrotum and tape it to the perineal area.

Postprocedure Care

1. Compare the urine quantity in the specimen container with the urinary output record for the test. If the specimen contains less urine than what was recorded as output, some of the sample may have been discarded, invalidating the test.
2. Document the quantity of urine and the collection ending time on the laboratory requisition.
3. Send the specimen to the laboratory and refrigerate it.

Client and Family Teaching

1. Save all the urine voided in the 24-hour period and urinate before defecating to avoid loss of urine. If any urine is accidentally discarded, discard the entire specimen and restart the collection the next day.

Factors That Affect Results

1. All urine voided for the 24-hour period must be included to avoid a falsely low result.

Other Data

1. Urine potassium levels exhibit a diurnal variation, with higher levels occurring at night.

Potassium Hydroxide Preparation (KOH Wet Mount)—Specimen

Norm. Negative. No fungus elements identified.

Usage. Identification and diagnosis of fungal dermatitis and infections.

Description. Fungi are slow-growing, eukaryotic organisms that can grow on living and nonliving organic materials and are subdivided into yeasts and molds. Only a few fungi species infect humans. The KOH preparation allows for direct microscopic examination of skin, nail, hair, sputum, abscess exudate, or biopsy tissue for the presence of fungal fragments. A 10%-20% KOH solution mixed with the specimen clears away debris, making visualization of mycelial filaments, hyphae, spores, spherules, and budding yeast cells possible under a low-power microscope.

Professional Considerations

Consent form NOT required.

Preparation

1. Obtain KOH preparation, methylene blue, a clear glass slide, a glass coverslip, a teasing needle, and a heat source.

Procedure

1. Place one drop of 10%-20% KOH preparation and, if indicated, methylene blue on a clear glass slide.
2. Using a needle or scalpel, gently scrape the skin, nails, tissue, or wound, or gather several strands of hair for a specimen and place them on a glass slide.
3. Using a teasing needle, separate the specimen to make a thin preparation on the slide.
4. Cover the specimen with a coverslip and pass the slide over a low flame two or three times. Gently press on the coverslip several times with a teasing needle until the specimen lies flat on the slide.
5. Allow the slide to cool.

Postprocedure Care

1. Write the specimen source on the laboratory requisition and send the specimen to the microbiology laboratory.

Client and Family Teaching

1. Antifungal medication may be prescribed if results are positive.
2. Deep coughs are necessary to produce sputum, rather than saliva. To produce the proper specimen, take several breaths in, without fully exhaling each, and then expel sputum with a "cascade cough."

Factors That Affect Results

1. False-positive results may occur if the specimen is contaminated with cotton fibers, cellulose fibers, or cholesterol deposits, which may be mistaken for hyphae.

Other Data

1. Handle the specimen with care to prevent self-contamination.
2. Dimethyl sulfoxide (DMSO) should be added to the slide if a nail specimen is being examined.

3. Adding glycerol to the KOH will enable preservation of the slide for a few days if it cannot be examined promptly.

4. Gram stain and potassium hydroxide preparation should be performed in cases of neonatal pustular disorders.

PPD

See **Mantoux Skin Test**—Diagnostic.

PRA

See **Renin Activity**—Plasma.

Prazepam

See **Benzodiazepines**—Plasma and Urine.

Prealbumin-Thyroxine Binding

See **Transthyretin**—Serum or Vitreous Fluid.

Precipitin Test Against Human Sperm and Blood—Vaginal Swab

Norm. Negative.

Usage. Used to identify the presence of semen or blood of human origin from vaginal secretions after sexual assault or rape.

Description. Human semen contains specific antibodies that are unique to the species. When vaginal secretions containing semen or blood are mixed with antisera solution, an antigen-antibody reaction or linkage will occur if the source is human sperm. The reaction is the result of the antigen binding to the antibody and forming an insoluble precipitate. One can perform this test by mixing the vaginal aspirate with antisera solution in a test tube or capillary tube. If an antigen-antibody reaction occurs, the cells will clump and fall to the bottom of the test tube, an indication that semen or blood present in the sample is from a human source. The result of the semen precipitation test is recorded as permanent evidence that coital relations occurred. Vaginal aspirations can also be tested for hemagglutination of ABO blood typing.

Professional Considerations
Consent form NOT required.

Preparation
1. Obtain a rape examination tray.
2. Use a speculum rinsed with 0.9% saline for examination and specimen collection.

Procedure
1. The collection of specimens is governed by the laws of each state.
2. Follow the directions in the "sex evidence kit" according to the requirements of the state.

Postprocedure Care
1. Follow directions in the "sex evidence kit" for the proper chain of command of evidence.
2. The specimen is generally given to the police and forwarded to the proper authorities for evidence testing.

Client and Family Teaching
1. Vaginal douching or bathing decreases the likelihood of obtaining positive results.
2. Survivors of sexual assault should be referred to appropriate crisis counseling agencies as well as for gynecologic follow-up examination.

3. Referral for HIV testing should be reviewed and offered to all sexual assault victims.
4. Preventive treatment for chlamydiosis, gonorrhea, and syphilis should be provided to all survivors of sexual assault.
5. The option of postcoital contraceptive should be reviewed with all survivors of sexual assault.

Factors That Affect Results

1. The laboratory must receive vaginal washing immediately, or else the specimen should be frozen.

Other Data

1. No universal threshold exists for evidence of intercourse or rape. A decrease in acid phosphatase after intercourse varies from hours to 4 days.

Pregnancy Test (hCG) Routine, Serum and Qualitative—Urine

Norm. NOTE: Norms are greatly dependent on test method used.

		SI Units
hCG—Serum		
Males	<3.0 mIU/mL	<3.0 IU/L
Females		
Nonpregnant	<3.0 mIU/mL	<3.0 IU/L
Pregnancy, first 6 weeks	Values double about every 2 days	
10 weeks of gestation	100,000 mIU/mL	
≥14 weeks of gestation	Levels trend downward	
hCG, Qualitative—Urine	Negative	

Increased. Breast cancer, bronchogenic carcinoma, choriocarcinoma, embryonal carcinoma, gastric carcinoma, hepatocarcinoma, hydatidiform mole, in vitro maturation day 12-13 (range 295-391 IU/L), malignant melanoma, multiple myeloma, pancreatic cancer, pregnancy, seminoma, teratoma, and trophoblastic tumor.

Decreased. Abortion (threatened, actual) and ectopic pregnancy.

Description. Human chorionic gonadotropin (hCG) is a hormone uniquely secreted by the placenta of a fertilized ovum implanted in the uterine wall. hCG production begins 8-10 days after conception or during days 21-23 of the cycle. It reaches peak concentration at 8-12 weeks of gestation and then gradually decreases until returning to normal within 3-4 days after normal full-term delivery. This test can be most accurately performed from 2 days to 3 weeks after missed menses.

Serum testing is performed by incubation of serum with anti-human chorionic gonadotropin (anti-hCG). If hCG is present in the sample, it combines with the anti-hCG antibodies and inactivates them. When these inactivated antibodies are exposed to

the indicator, which is red or latex cells coated with hCG, clumping of the cells does not occur, resulting in a positive pregnancy test. If clumping does occur, the test is negative.

Professional Considerations

Consent form NOT required.

Preparation

1. Tube: Red topped, red/gray topped, or gold topped for serum test.
2. Obtain random urine collection container for urine test.
3. Serum specimens MAY be drawn during hemodialysis.
4. See Client and Family Teaching.

Procedure

1. Draw a 4-mL blood sample for serum test.
2. Obtain a 4-mL random urine specimen.

Postprocedure Care

1. None.

Client and Family Teaching

1. May help differentiate actual pregnancy from an ectopic pregnancy in conduction with an ultrasonogram.
2. Avoid medications such as anticonvulsants, antiparkinsonian agents, hypnotics,

and tranquilizers, which may cause a false-positive result in the serum test.

Factors That Affect Results
1. False-positive results may be caused by incorrect performance or handling of the test, excessive production of luteinizing hormone (LH) of the pituitary gland, absence of gonadal hormones in menopausal women, hCG-producing tumors, multiple myeloma (due to hCG beta-chain production), passive transfusion of beta-human chorionic gonadotropin from donor red blood cells, or tubo-ovarian abscess.

2. False-negative results may occur when the test is performed very early in pregnancy.

Other Data
1. Although not usually present in healthy males or nonpregnant females, elevated levels of hCG may be detected in these clients with certain malignant tumors.
2. Urine sample mixture of equal amounts (500 microliters) of gold nanoparticle solution and urine samples produces pink color in pregnancy-positive and gray color in pregnancy-negative patients.
3. See also Human chorionic gonadotropin, Beta subunit—Serum.

Pregnanetriol—Urine
Norm.

		SI Units
Adult female	0.5-2.0 mg/24 hours	1.5-5.9 mmol/day
Adult male	0.4-2.4 mg/24 hours	1.2-7.1 mmol/day
Child		
<6 years	<0.2 mg/24 hours	<0.6 mmol/day
7-16 years	0.3-1.1 mg/24 hours	0.9-3.3 mmol/day

Increased. Adrenogenital syndrome, congenital adrenocortical hyperplasia, hirsutism, Stein-Leventhal syndrome, 21-hydroxylase deficiency, tumor (ovarian, adrenal cortex), and virilization.

Description. Pregnanetriol, a metabolite of 17-hydroxyprogesterone, is involved in the synthesis of adrenal corticoids and is normally excreted in the urine in only small amounts. Increased urinary excretion is caused by a deficiency in the enzyme that converts 17-hydroxyprogesterone to cortisol. The decreased cortisol production results in increased adrenocorticotropic hormone (ACTH), which leads to increased serum hydroxyprogesterone. This in turn stimulates the release of adrenal androgens. As the increased amounts of hydroxyprogesterone are metabolized, urine pregnanetriol levels increase. This test is most commonly abnormal in adrenogenital syndrome, which results in symptoms of hypertension, craving for salt, premature physical development of sexual characteristics in males, failure to

thrive in infants, and pseudohermaphroditism (females with male genitalia).

Professional Considerations
Consent form NOT required.

Preparation
1. Obtain a clean, 3-L container without preservative or to which acetic acid preservative has been added.
2. For pediatric/infant specimens, obtain a pediatric urine collection device/bag and tape.
3. See Client and Family Teaching.

Procedure
1. Discard the first morning urine specimen.
2. Save all the urine voided for 24 hours in a refrigerated, clean, 3-L container without preservative or to which acetic acid preservative has been added. Document the quantity of urine output during the specimen collection period. Include urine voided at the end of the 24-hour period. For catheterized clients, keep the

drainage bag on ice and empty the urine into the collection container hourly.

3. *Pediatric/infant specimen collection:*

    a. Place the child in a supine position with the knees flexed and the hips externally rotated and abducted.

    b. Cleanse, rinse, and thoroughly dry the perineal area.

    c. To prevent the child from removing the collection device/bag, a diaper may be placed over the genital area.

    d. *Females*: Tape the pediatric collection device/bag to the perineum. Starting at the area between the anus and vagina, apply the device/bag in an anterior direction.

    e. *Males*: Place the pediatric collection device/bag over the penis and scrotum and tape it to the perineal area.

Postprocedure Care

1. Compare the urine quantity in the specimen container with the urinary output record for the test. If the specimen contains less urine than what was recorded as output, some of the sample may have been discarded, invalidating the test.

2. Document the urine quantity on the laboratory requisition.

Client and Family Teaching

1. Save all the urine voided in the 24-hour period and urinate before defecating to avoid loss of urine. If any urine is accidentally discarded, discard the entire specimen and restart the collection the next day.

2. Avoid muscular exercise before or during the specimen collection period.

Factors That Affect Results

1. All the urine voided for the 24-hour period must be included to avoid a falsely low result.

2. Results are invalid if the specimen was not refrigerated throughout the collection period.

3. Exercise during the collection period causes increased androgen release.

Other Data

1. In 21-hydroxylase deficiency, there is also an increase in serum 17-hydroxyprogesterone and urinary 17-ketosteroids.

Prekallikrein

See Factor, Fletcher—Plasma.

Prenatal Screen

See ABO Group and Rh Type—Blood; Coombs' Test, Indirect—Serum.

Primidone (Mysoline)—Serum

Norm. Negative.

Therapeutic Levels	Trough	SI Units
Adults	5-12 μg/mL	23-55 μmol/L
Children <5 years	7-10 μg/mL	32-46 μmol/L
Panic level	>24 μg/mL	>110 μmol/L

Panic Level Symptoms and Treatment

Symptoms. Decreased level of consciousness, ataxia, anemia.

Treatment

NOTE: Treatment choice(s) depend(s) on client's history and condition and episode history. Discontinue primidone.

1. Protect airway.
2. Support hemodynamics.
3. Hemodialysis WILL remove primidone. High-permeability dialysis is likely to remove primidone. No data are available to indicate the effect of peritoneal dialysis on removal of primidone.

4. Treat anemia with folic acid or vitamin B$_{12}$.
5. Drugs that may accelerate the conversion of primidone to its metabolite phenobarbital include phenytoin and phenytoin sodium.

Usage. Monitoring the effectiveness of primidone therapy and prevention of primidone toxicity.

Increased. Drugs include carbamazepine, isoniazid, monoamine oxidase (MOA) inhibitors, phenobarbital, and sodium valproate.

Decreased. Subtherapeutic treatment. Drugs include acetazolamide and methsuximide.

Description. Primidone is an anticonvulsant used in the treatment of temporal lobe epilepsy and other grand mal seizures that are resistant to other anticonvulsants. When metabolized by the liver, it breaks down into phenobarbital and phenylethylmalonamide. These two metabolites have a synergistic ability to raise the seizure threshold. The metabolites of primidone are excreted by the kidneys. Half-life is 4-12 hours in adults and 4-6 hours in children. Peak time varies from 0.5 to 0.9 hours. Steady-state levels are reached after 16-60 hours in adults and after 20-30 hours in children. For rapid detection, the fluorescence polarization assay method can be used.

Professional Considerations

Consent form NOT required.

Preparation
1. Tube: Red topped or green topped.
2. Do NOT draw during hemodialysis.

Procedure
1. Draw a 5-mL blood TROUGH sample. Obtain serial specimens at the same time each day.

Postprocedure
1. Monitor for panic level symptoms (see above).
2. Monitor for convulsions if the drug is discontinued.

Client and Family Teaching
1. Take medication as prescribed and report any adverse side effects such as sedation, dizziness, nausea, vomiting, nystagmus, and loss of libido.
2. For accidental overdose, teach the client and family early warning symptoms of overdose (see above).
3. For intentional overdose, refer the client and family for crisis intervention.

Factors That Affect Results
1. Reject hemolyzed or lipemic specimens to avoid falsely elevated results.
2. Peak levels occur 2-4 hours after the oral dose.

Other Data
1. Data indicate there is no evidence of good seizure control with levels >10 mg/mL.

Proaccelerin

See **Factor V**—Blood.

Pro-BNP

See **Natriuretic Peptides, Atrial**—Plasma.

Procainamide—Serum

Norm. Negative.

	Trough	SI Units
Procainamide	4.9-12 µg/mL	20.7-50.8 µmol/L
Toxic level	>12 µg/mL	>50.8 µmol/L
Panic level	>20 µg/mL	>84.6 µmol/L
Procainamide + NAPA	6-20 µg/mL	25.3-84.5 µmol/L
Toxic level	>30 µg/mL	>126.7 µmol/L

Toxic Level Symptoms and Treatment

Toxic symptoms occur in 10% of people with levels >12 µg/mL. Serious toxicity occurs in 40% of people with levels >16 µg/mL.

Symptoms. Sodium-channel blockade manifesting as early prolonged QRS interval, rightward axis of 40 msec, presence of an R wave in aV_R lead and an S wave in leads I and aV_L. Torsades de pointes, nausea, vomiting, hepatic disturbances, agranulocytosis. In pediatrics, nausea, vomiting, antimuscarinic findings, blurred vision, dry mouth, odynophagia, pupils dilated, sluggishly reactive, and seizure.

Treatment

NOTE: Treatment choice(s) depend(s) on client's history and condition and episode history.

1. Protect airway.
2. Support hemodynamic stability.
3. Force emesis. Avoid Ipecac.
4. Perform gastric lavage. Charcoal therapy or whole bowel irrigation with polyethylene glycol solutions could be considered in patients ingesting the sustained-release forms of procainamide.
5. Administer infusion of a molar sodium lactate solution.
6. 12-lead ECG. Manage Torsade de pointes with Mg+ and K+ supplementation, isoproterenol infusion or pacer mediated increased intrinsic heart rate.
7. Treat hypotension with fluids and if refractory with inotropes or vasoconstrictors as guided by pulmonary catheter readings.
8. Seizures best treated with benzodiazepines or barbiturates.
9. Hemodialysis, hemoperfusion, or continuous arteriovenous hemofiltration WILL, but peritoneal dialysis WILL NOT, remove procainamide. High-permeability hemodialysis is likely to remove procainamide.

Increased Procainamide. Hepatic dysfunction. Drugs include amiodarone.

Increased Procainamide and NAPA. Renal dysfunction. Drugs include quinidine.

Decreased. NAPA: hepatic dysfunction. Drugs include midazolam.

Description. Procainamide is an antidysrhythmic used in the treatment of atrial and ventricular dysrhythmias. It is most commonly administered as an oral or intravenous drug and metabolized by the liver. 25% of procainamide is metabolized to N-acetylprocainamide (NAPA) by the liver; 60% of the dose is excreted via the kidneys, with a half-life of 3-4 hours. Procainamide's primary metabolite is NAPA, which has similar antidysrhythmic properties and a half-life of approximately 6 hours but is not metabolized by the liver. The differences in the half-lives result in slightly high NAPA levels until both reach stabilization approximately 18 hours after initiation of therapy. At this time, a 1:1 ratio exists between procainamide and NAPA. An increase or decrease in this ratio can alter the therapeutic effectiveness or result in toxicity. Therefore when procainamide is assayed, NAPA levels should be monitored simultaneously. Steady-state levels of procainamide are reached after 11-20 hours. Steady-state levels of NAPA are reached after 22-40 hours.

Professional Considerations
Consent form NOT required.

Preparation
1. Tube: Red topped, red/gray topped, or gold topped.
2. Do NOT draw specimens during hemodialysis.

Procedure
1. Draw a 4-mL TROUGH blood sample. Obtain serial measurements at the same time each day.

Postprocedure Care
1. Monitor for panic level symptoms (see above).

Factors That Affect Results
1. Reject hemolyzed or lipemic specimens.

Client and Family Teaching
1. Take medication as prescribed.
2. Report side effects such as anorexia, nausea, and vomiting.
3. For intentional overdose, refer client and family for crisis intervention.

Other Data
1. For the initial evaluation, draw a trough level just before the next dose of

procainamide and draw a peak level 75-90 minutes after oral administration or immediately after the loading dose and at 2, 6, 12, and 24 hours for intravenous administration.

2. For continuous therapeutic drug monitoring, three normal-range levels within one dosing interval are required initially. Then only trough levels are required unless toxicity is suspected.

Procalcitonin (ProCT, PCT)—Plasma or Serum

Norm.

	Procalcitonin
Adults	Nondetectable or <0.5 ng/mL
Children	Nondetectable or <0.5 ng/mL
Infants >2 days old	Nondetectable or <0.5 ng/mL
Neonates	
0-6 hours	<2 ng/mL
6-12 hours	<8 ng/mL
12-18 hours	<15 ng/mL
18-30 hours	<21 ng/mL
30-36 hours	<15 ng/mL
36-42 hours	<8 ng/mL
42-48 hours	<2 ng/mL

Increased. Bacterial meningitis, Crohn's disease, fever due to infectious cause, fungal infections, H1N1 related pneumonia, hematological disorders (acute leukemia), neonates post-op day 1, migraine, sepsis, vasculitis, wound dehiscence.

Value	Interpretation	Suggestions
<0.5 ng/mL	Not likely to be septic.	Repeat testing in 6-24 hours if sample <6 hours after infection was drawn and sepsis is suspected.
≥0.5 to <2 ng/mL	Bacterial infection or sepsis may be present. Other causes may include the following: neonates <2 days old; immediately following major trauma, burns, major invasive surgical procedures; OKT3 antibody administration; small cell lung cancer; C-cell carcinoma of thyroid-18; extended or severe cardiogenic shock; extended or severe low perfusion states.	Moderate risk for severe sepsis to develop. Client should be closely monitored and PCT repeated in 6-24 hours. Mortality 45.3% in septic patients with PCT >0.85ng/mL.
≥2 to <10 ng/mL	Systemic bacterial infection is probably present, unless other conditions present.	High risk for severe sepsis to develop.
≥10 ng/mL	Highly indicative of sepsis.	Severe sepsis most likely present.

For differentiation of types of lower respiratory tract conditions, highly sensitive measurements of ProCT concentrations are recommended with the following interpretation:

Value of ProCT	Interpretation	Suggestions
<0.1 ng/mL	No indication of bacterial infection.	Consider other diagnoses.
≥0.1 to <0.25 ng/mL	Bacterial infection most likely not present. >0.1 mcg/L = + blood culture	Antibiotic therapy discouraged.
≥0.25 to <0.5 ng/mL	Bacterial infections may be present. ≥ 0.31 microg/L = VAP	Antibiotic therapy suggested.
≥0.5 ng/mL	Bacterial infection most likely present.	Implement antibiotic therapy.

Decreased (<0.5 ng/mL). Bacterial infections may be present with low PCT levels during the early course of the infection (<6 hours, in which case the test should be repeated in 6-24 hours), in cases of localized infections, subacute infectious endocarditis, viral infections, chronic inflammatory disorders, autoimmune processes. Drugs include Prometheus.

Description. ProCT is a protein compound consisting of 116 amino acids. It is produced and secreted by the thyroid gland and is normally undetectable in the blood of healthy individuals. In response to infection and systemic inflammation, increased levels of ProCT are secreted into the bloodstream, and in combination with proteolytic enzymes are cleaved into the active hormone calcitonin. After infection occurs, ProCT increases within 3 hours, peaks within 12-24 hours, and has a half-life of 22-29 hours. When inflammation is caused by bacterial infection, the presence of ProCT is particularly pronounced as it is also released by the liver, kidney, lung, muscle, and adipose tissue, causing serum levels to increase drastically above normal. Thus ProCT is useful to help differentiate bacterial infections from other conditions and has been shown to be more sensitive and specific for this purpose than C-reactive protein. For example, ProCT is useful in differentiating lower respiratory tract bacterial infections from other conditions such as COPD, pneumonia, and acute bronchitis. ProCT also correlates with the severity of the infection and is useful to identify severe bacterial infection in children.

Professional Considerations
Consent form NOT required.

Preparation
1. Tube: Red topped or serum separator for serum. Lavender topped for plasma.

Procedure
1. Obtain a 5-mL blood sample.

Postprocedure Care
1. ProCT molecule is resilient in serum; no special handling and storage procedures are indicated.

Client and Family Teaching
1. Results normally available in 1 hour.

Factors That Affect Results
1. May be <0.5 ng/mL in persons without bacterial infection (see above).

Other Data
1. Helpful for monitoring response to therapy. Recommended frequency of measurement is once daily.
2. Helpful for establishing needs for antibiotic therapy.
3. Failure of the ProCT level to fall and normalize after initiation of therapy indicates very poor prognosis.

Prochlorperazine

See Phenothiazines.

Proconvertin

See Factor VII—Blood.

Pro-CT
See **Procalcitonin**—Plasma or Serum.

Proctoscopy—Diagnostic

Norm. The rectal lining is continuous, reddish, and free of lesions, abscesses, inflammation, ulcerations, and polyps. The anal lining appears grayish tan and smooth.

Usage. Melena or bleeding from the anorectal area, persistent diarrhea, changes in bowel habits, passage of pus and mucus, suspected chronic inflammatory bowel disease, bacteriologic and histologic studies, surveillance of known rectal disease or after rectal surgery, rectal pain, screening for suspected polyps or tumors, foreign-body removal, or adjunct to barium enema.

Description. A proctoscopy is the endoscopic, direct visual examination of the lining of the rectum and anal canal using a rigid, lighted proctoscope. Specimens for biopsy, cytologic evaluation, or culture may be taken during the procedure. Proctoscopy is usually performed with flexible sigmoidoscopy for clients demonstrating unexplained anemia, unexplained diarrhea, or the presence of blood in the stool.

Professional Considerations
Consent form IS required.

Risks
Bowel perforation, hemorrhage, peritonitis.
Contraindications
Severe necrotizing enterocolitis, toxic megacolon, painful anal lesions, or severe cardiac dysrhythmias.

Preparation
1. A tap-water, hypertonic phosphate, or saline enema may be prescribed. Clients with ulcerative colitis or acute diarrhea can be examined without an enema.
2. Obtain drapes, gloves, 1%-2% lidocaine (Xylocaine), a proctoscope with an obturator, and a light source. If a biopsy is to be performed, obtain a specimen container of 10% formalin. If cytology slides are to be prepared, obtain cytology slides and a Coplin jar of 95% ethyl alcohol (ethanol). If cultures are to be performed, obtain sterile swabs with culture tube.
3. See Client and Family Teaching.
4. Just before beginning the procedure, take a "time out" to verify the correct client, procedure, and site.

Procedure
1. The client is placed in a left-lateral or knee-to-chest position and draped for comfort and privacy.
2. The physician inserts a lubricated finger through the anus to assess for patency and the presence of obstruction.
3. After patency is determined, the lubricated proctoscope with obturator is inserted fully into the rectum through the anus, and the obturator is removed.
4. After a light is inserted, the physician carefully inspects the interior lining of the rectum and anal canal as the proctoscope is slowly withdrawn.
5. If biopsy specimens are taken, the site may be anesthetized first with 1%-2% lidocaine or another local anesthetic.
6. Any liquid drainage is removed with suction during the procedure.

Postprocedure Care
1. Send the specimens to the laboratory immediately.
2. The client should lie flat for 10-15 minutes following the procedure.
3. Monitor for signs of fatigue, abdominal pain or distention, fever, hypotension, or rectal bleeding.
4. Bloody stools are normal for 1-2 days after a rectal biopsy.
5. No enemas or barium studies for 1 week after rectal biopsy secondary to the increased risk of perforation.

Client and Family Teaching
1. Client may be asked to follow a clear liquid diet for 2 days or fast for 8 hours.
2. Try to defecate before the procedure.
3. An urge to defecate may be felt during the procedure, and slow, controlled deep breathing may help to diminish this feeling.

Factors That Affect Results

1. Residual barium from prior testing will impair visualization.
2. The presence of stool in the rectum impairs visualization.

Other Data

1. Complications of proctoscopy include rectal perforation, minimal bleeding from lacerations, transient abdominal discomfort, and cardiac dysrhythmias.

ProGastro™ Cd assay

See *C-difficile* Amplified Probe—Stool.

Progesterone—Serum

Norm.

		SI Units
Female		
Follicular phase	0.2-0.6 ng/mL	<2 nmol/L
Luteal phase	6-30 ng/mL	19-95 nmol/L
Midluteal phase	5.7-28.1 ng/mL	18-89 nmol/L
Oral contraceptives	0.1-0.3 ng/mL	<2 nmol/L
Postmenopause	0-0.2 ng/mL	<2 nmol/L
Pregnancy		
1-12 weeks	9-47 ng/mL	28-149 nmol/L
13-24 weeks	16.8-146 ng/mL	53-464 nmol/L
25 weeks to term	55-255 ng/mL	175-811 nmol/L
Male	0.1-0.3 ng/mL	<2 nmol/L
Child (Prepubertal)	7-52 ng/mL	0.2-1.7 nmol/L

Usage. Assessment of corpus luteum formation and placental function, and assistance in determining the day of ovulation.

Increased. Adrenal hyperplasia (congenital, males), ALS, congestive heart failure, corpus luteum cyst, in vitro fertilization failure, lipid ovarian tumors, molar pregnancy, multiple fetal pregnancies (e.g., twins), ovarian chorionepithelioma, ovarian neoplasms, placental tissue (retained after parturition), precocious puberty, theca-lutein cyst and varicose veins in pregnant women. Drugs include adrenocortical hormones, estrogens, and progesterones (oral or vaginal application). Herbal (Chinese) Zhuyun-III (ZYIII).

Decreased. Abortion (first trimester if progesterone <15 ng/mL), adrenogenital syndrome, amenorrhea, anovular menstruation, dermatomyositis (juvenile), fetal abnormality or death, luteal deficiency, menstrual abnormalities, ovarian failure, panhypopituitarism, placental failure or insufficiency, preeclampsia, Stein-Leventhal syndrome, threatened abortion, toxemia of pregnancy, Turner's syndrome, and primary and secondary hypogonadism. Drugs include ampicillin, ethinyl estradiol.

Description. Progesterone is a steroid sex hormone secreted by the corpus luteum during the latter half of the menstrual cycle in nonpregnant women, by the placenta in large amounts in pregnant women, and by the adrenal cortex in men. Progesterone causes secretory changes in the mucosa of the fallopian tubes and assists in nourishing the fertilized ovum as it travels through the tubes to the uterus. It prepares the endometrium for implantation of the fertilized ovum, stimulates growth of the breasts and proliferation of the vaginal epithelium, and decreases myometrial excitability and uterine contractions.

Professional Considerations
Consent form NOT required.

Preparation
1. Tube: Red topped or green topped.
2. Specimens MAY be drawn during hemodialysis.

Procedure

1. Draw a 7-mL blood sample.

Postprocedure Care

1. Record the first day of the last menstrual cycle or the week of gestation on the laboratory requisition.

Client and Family Teaching

1. Results are normally available within 24 hours.

Factors That Affect Results

1. The sample may be refrigerated for 4 days or frozen up to 1 year and is stable at room temperature for 7 days.

Other Data

1. Serial testing is recommended.
2. For diagnosis of a short luteal phase, correlation with endometrial biopsy is recommended.
3. Topical progesterone was shown in one study to increase salivary progesterone levels, but not serum levels.
4. IVF patients with serum progesterone levels ≤1.5 ng/mL had higher ongoing pregnancy rates.
5. Avoid false negative breast MRIs by having patient scheduled for MRI 5 days after menstruation (Ganau et al, 2010).

Progesterone Receptor Assay—Specimen

Norm. Negative.

	Percent of Nuclei Staining		SI Units
Negative	<5	<5 fmol/mg protein	<5 nmol/kg protein
Borderline	5-19		
Positive	≥20	>10 fmol/mg protein	>10 nmol/kg protein

Usage. Determination of the likelihood of carcinoma to respond to hormone or antihormone therapy, monitoring the responsiveness of tumors to hormone or antihormone therapy, and determination of the need for oophorectomy.

Positive. Breast cancer (including invasive lobular), hormonal therapy, meningioma, and metastasis.

Negative. Normal finding. Normal results may be obtained in the presence of a benign and nonresponsive tumor.

Description. Progesterone receptors are located primarily in mammary gland tissue but are also present in the corpus luteum, prostate, uterus, vaginal epithelium, and placenta. Progesterone receptors transfer and bind steroid molecules into cell nuclei to exert hormonal function. This test is usually performed with an estrogen receptor assay and involves testing an excised or biopsied tumor for the degree of responsiveness (positivity) of the progesterone receptors in the tissue. In some clients with carcinoma, the degree of progesterone receptor positivity correlates to the amount of cellular subtype differentiation and is a measure of potential tumor responsiveness to hormonal

or antihormonal therapy. Clients with positive tests are more likely to respond to these types of therapy than those with negative results. In monitoring tumor response to therapy, the best prognosis can be expected in clients whose progesterone receptor assay results remain positive. In clients who have negative tests after positive initial tests, the prognosis is poor. Clients who remain negative have the poorest outcome.

Professional Considerations

Consent form NOT required for this test but IS required for the procedure used to obtain the specimen tested. See individual procedure for risks and contraindications.

Preparation

1. The client is prepared for a surgical biopsy or resection.
2. Arrange for a person to be standing by to transport the iced specimen to the pathology laboratory immediately after excision.
3. Obtain a waxed cardboard specimen container without preservatives. Do not place it into formalin.

Procedure

1. A fresh tissue specimen of at least 150 mg and preferably 1 g (1 mL) is obtained by

means of needle biopsy or resection and placed into a container free of formalin.

2. The specimen is transported to the pathology laboratory immediately.

Postprocedure Care

1. Apply a dry, sterile dressing to the biopsy or operative site.

2. Specimens must be stored at temperatures lower than −70 degrees C.

3. Specimens transported to another institution must be packed in dry ice.

Client and Family Teaching

1. Results of the test may dictate the type of anticipated therapy.

Factors That Affect Results

1. Reject specimens not stored at temperatures lower than −70 degrees C or those contaminated with formalin.

2. Reject specimens not transported to the pathology laboratory immediately because a delay of even 15 minutes results in degradation of receptor sites.

3. The presence of massive tumor necrosis or tumors with low cellular composition lowers the assay result.

Other Data

1. The estrogen receptor assay should also be performed on all specimens.

2. Progesterone receptors are found in up to 75% of estrogen receptor-positive mammary cancers.

3. Estrogen- and progesterone-positive tumors have a 75% response rate to endocrine therapy, whereas estrogen- and progesterone-negative tumors have a 5%-10% response rate.

Prolactin (Human Prolactin, HPRL)—Serum

Norm. Prolactin levels do not differ between males and females before the onset of puberty.

		SI Units
Adult female, nonlactating	<23 ng/mL	<23 ng/dL
Follicular phase	<28 ng/mL	<28 ng/dL
Luteal phase	5-40 ng/mL	5-40 ng/dL
Postmenopause	<12 ng/mL	<12 ng/dL
Pregnancy		
Trimester 1	<80 ng/mL	<80 ng/dL
Trimester 2	<160 ng/mL	<160 ng/dL
Trimester 3	<400 ng/mL	<400 ng/dL
Adult male	<20 ng/mL	<20 ng/dL
Children 1-9 years	2.7-17.7 ng/mL	2.7-17.7 ng/dL
Newborn	>10 times adult levels	>10 times adult levels
Pituitary tumor	>100 ng/mL	>100 ng/dL

Prolactin Levels in Response to TRH Stimulation Test (Used for Differentiation of Prolactinoma from Other Causes of Hyperprolactinemia)

	Baseline Value	Peak after Injection of 400 mg of TRH Intravenously
Adult female	4.0-25 μg/L	Relative increase: >250%
	Median: 10.0 μg/L	Median: 51 μg/L
Adult male	0.5-19.0 μg/L	Relative increase: >250%
	Median: 8.5 μg/L	Median: 41 μg/L

Increased. Serum level >300 ng/mL is assumed to be pathognomonic of a pituitary tumor.

Other conditions in which increases may be found: Acromegaly, Addison's disease, amenorrhea, anorexia nervosa, breast stimulation, bronchogenic carcinoma, Chiari-Frommel syndrome, chromium exposure, coitus, del Castillo's syndrome, diabetes mellitus, ectopic tumors, endometriosis, erectile dysfunction, exercise (prolonged exhaustive), Forbes-Albright syndrome, galactorrhea, HIV infection (20% of males with stable HIV), hyperestrogen states, hyperpituitarism, hypothalamic disorders, hypothyroidism (primary), hysterectomy, idiopathic causes (such as early microadenomas that are undetectable by radiology), impotence, lactation, multiple myeloma (advanced), Nelson's syndrome, neurogenic causes, pemphigus vulgaris, pituitary tumors, polycystic ovaries, postmenopausal hypertension, pregnancy, renal failure (chronic), schizophrenia, seizures (values return to normal within 1 hour), sleep, smokers, stress, systemic lupus erythematosus, uterine fibroids and venous thrombosis. Drugs include amitriptyline, amoxapine, amphetamines, benzamides, chlorprothixene, desipramine, doxepin, droperidol, estrogens, gamma-hydroxybutyrate (GHB), haloperidol, imipramine, isoniazid, maprotiline, meprobamate, methamphetamine use/abuse, methyldopa, metoclopramide, nortriptyline, opiates, oral contraceptives, paliperidone, phenothiazines, procainamide hydrochloride, protriptyline, reserpine, risperidone, thioridazine, thiothixene, thyrotropin, Triavil (perphenazine and amitriptyline HCl), and trimipramine maleate.

Decreased. CPAP use, gynecomastia, heavy metals (arsenic, cadmium, copper, lead, manganese, molybdenum, zinc), hirsutism, osteoporosis, and pituitary necrosis or infarction. Drugs include apomorphine hydrochloride, bromocriptine mesylate, clonidine, dihydroergotamine mesylate, dopamine, ergoloid mesylate, ergonovine maleate, ergotamine tartrate, lergotrile, levodopa, lisuride hydrogen maleate, olanzapine, and quetiapine. Herbal or natural remedies include licorice and St. John's wort. In addition, chaste tree (*Vitex agnus-castus*) berry has been shown to reduce prolactin

levels in a study of women with hyperprolactinemia.

Description. Prolactin is a peptide hormone produced by the anterior pituitary gland that promotes growth of breast tissue and is essential for the initiation and maintenance of milk production. Also called the lactogenic hormone, luteotropic hormone, LTH, and mammotropin. It is identical to luteotropin.

Professional Considerations
Consent form NOT required.

Preparation
1. Tube: Red topped, red/gray topped, or gold topped.
2. Specimens MAY be drawn during hemodialysis.
3. Screen client for the use of herbal preparations or natural remedies.
4. See Client and Family Teaching.

Procedure
1. Draw a 5-mL blood sample without trauma.
2. Samples should be drawn in the morning.

Postprocedure Care
1. Samples remain stable for 4 days at room temperature and then must be frozen if analysis is delayed.

Client and Family Teaching
1. Fast for 12 hours before testing.

Factors That Affect Results
1. Hemolysis of the specimen invalidates the results.

Other Data
1. Differentiation between a pituitary tumor and other prolactin disorders can be done by means of the thyrotropin-releasing hormone (TRH) stimulation test. Prolactin levels in clients with pituitary tumors do not increase.
2. Men with elevated prolactin levels generally have low serum testosterone. Symptoms will not reverse unless prolactin is reduced.
3. High levels of serum prolactin protect against diabetic retinopathy.

Propoxyphene Hydrochloride (Darvocet-N 100)—Blood

NOTE: This medication was banned from the United States in November 2010 based on cardiotoxicity in healthy subjects, including prolongation of QT interval, prolonged PR interval, and widening of QRS complex on ECG.

Propranolol—Blood

Norm. Negative.

Propranolol Therapy		SI Units
Therapeutic level	50-100 ng/mL	193-386 nmol/L
Panic level	>500 ng/mL; 0.53 m/m/L	>1930 nmol/L

Increased. Propranolol overdosage. Drugs include flecainide, methimazole, and propylthiouracil.

Description. Propranolol hydrochloride is a beta-adrenergic blocking drug classified as a type II cardiac antidysrhythmic. It competes with epinephrine and norepinephrine for beta-adrenergic receptors, resulting in inhibition of myocardial beta-adrenergic stimulation. Cardiac effects include reduced irritability and heart rate because the automaticity of the SA node, AV node, and intraventricular conduction velocity is depressed. Large doses depress cardiac function. Brugada syndrome may be present on ECG noted by RBBB, coved ST segment elevation in precordial leads V1 to V3 and this increases the risk for cardiac death. Propranolol may also cause hypoglycemia without warning in diabetic clients. Propranolol is bound to plasma proteins, metabolized in the liver, and excreted in the urine, with a half-life of 2-6 hours. Steady-state levels are reached after 10-30 hours.

Professional Considerations
Consent form NOT required.

Preparation
1. Tube: Red topped, red/gray topped, or gold topped.
2. Specimens MAY be drawn during hemodialysis.

Procedure
1. Draw a 7-mL blood sample in a syringe.
2. After removing the stopper, inject the specimen promptly into the tube (plasma propranolol binding is reduced when blood passes through the stopper of a vacuum tube).
3. Replace the stopper.
4. Collect the specimen before the next dose (trough) if drawing to evaluate therapeutic value.

Postprocedure Care
1. Monitor the client for evidence of increasing congestive heart failure.

Client and Family Teaching
1. Take mediation as prescribed to prevent overdose.
2. Report any side effects to the physician.
3. Record your pulse rate daily and notify the physician if it falls below the level your physician specifies.
4. For intentional overdose, refer client and family for crisis intervention.

Factors That Affect Results
1. Smoking decreases plasma concentration of propranolol.
2. Peak propranolol levels occur 1-2 hours after oral administration.
3. Propranolol metabolism and excretion are delayed with hepatic and renal dysfunction.

Other Data
1. When you are obtaining serial levels, the same time interval between drug dosing and specimen collection should be maintained.
2. Overdose treatment includes oxygen treatment, IV fluids, use of 20% Intralipid™.
3. Animal research (pigs) shows IV levosimendan may successfully treat propranolol overdose in humans.

Prostate Ultrasonography (Prostate Echogram, Prostate Ultrasound)—Diagnostic

Norm. The prostate gland is round and about 3 cm in diameter. Prostatic tissue is homogeneous and causes only a slight bladder wall indentation.

Usage. Adjunct to digital examination of the prostate, diagnosis and staging of and screening for prostate cancer, evaluation of the size and shape of the prostate gland, monitoring response to treatment in prostate disease (e.g., acute prostatitis, benign enlargement, cancer), and providing guidance for transrectal biopsy of the prostate gland or for positioning of clients for radiation of the prostate gland.

Description. Evaluation of the prostate gland by the creation of an oscilloscopic picture from the echoes of high-frequency sound waves passing through the anterior rectal wall or through the urethra over the pelvic area (acoustic imaging, endosonography). The time required for the ultrasonic beam to be reflected back to the transducer from differing densities of tissue is converted by a computer to an electrical impulse displayed on an oscilloscopic screen to create a three-dimensional picture of the pelvic contents. Because of the risk of sepsis and trauma from transurethral ultrasonography, the transrectal route is preferred. For staging prostate cancer, transrectal ultrasonography costs less than magnetic resonance imaging, with comparable or superior accuracy. This technique may help detect prostate lesions before they become large enough to palpate. Ultrasound techniques are still inferior to prostate biopsy in sensitivity for diagnosing prostate cancer.

Professional Considerations

Consent form IS required.

Risks

Transurethral route: Sepsis and trauma.
Transrectal route: Hematuria, infection, urinary retention.
NOTE: Complications are more frequent in clients who receive a preprocedural enema.

Contraindications

Nonprostate disease.
Transurethral route: Bleeding disorders, thrombocytopenia.

Preparation

1. This test should be performed before intestinal barium tests or after the barium is cleared from the system.
2. Obtain ultrasonic gel or paste.
3. For transrectal ultrasonography, a hypertonic enema of sodium phosphate or a bisacodyl suppository may be prescribed.
4. The client must disrobe below the waist or wear a gown.
5. See Client and Family Teaching.
6. Just before beginning the procedure, take a "time out" to verify the correct client, procedure, and site.

Procedure

1. An injection of lidocaine or inhalation of a nitrous oxide/air mixture may be used to manage procedure-associated pain.
2. The client is positioned supine, and a short transabdominal ultrasonogram may be performed to evaluate for kidney distention.
3. A suprapubic examination of the prostate is performed, and the rectum is examined digitally for obstruction.
4. The client is assisted to a knee-elbow, lateral decubitus, or rising position.
5. The probe is covered with an air-free, sterile, transparent cover or condom. The condom is then coated with sterile lubricant, and the probe is slowly inserted into the rectum.
6. After the probe is inserted into the rectum, the condom may be inflated with 20-60 mL of deaerated water, depending on the practitioner's preference.
7. The probe is angled anteriorly, and ultrasonography of the prostate is performed.
8. Photographs of the oscilloscopic display are taken. Doppler ultrasonography may be used to further define abnormalities in vascular supply and differentiate vascular differences in the prostate tissue.
9. A biopsy of the prostate lesions may be performed during ultrasonography.

Postprocedure Care

1. Remove the gel from the skin.
2. Sterilize the endosonography probes by soaking them in glutaraldehyde solution for 10 minutes.

Client and Family Teaching

1. An enema may be prescribed before the procedure.
2. Drink normal amounts of fluids for 24 hours before the procedure.
3. Clients under age 60 experience more discomfort than older men during the procedure. Both local and topical anesthesia may be used to reduce discomfort.

Factors That Affect Results

1. Dehydration interferes with adequate contrast between organs and body fluids.
2. Lower intestinal barium obscures results by preventing proper transmission and deflection of the high-frequency sound waves.

Other Data

1. Allow at least 6 weeks between procedures if biopsies are taken.
2. Ultrasound approach for lymphoscintigraphy and sentinel node identification is a valuable tool in the staging of localized prostate cancer.

Prostate-Specific Antigen (PSA)—Serum

Norm.

Free PSA		Total PSA*	Complexed (Bound to Alpha-chymotrypsin)	PSA Density
Male (Normal levels increase with age, secondary to increasing prostate size)				
0-49 years	<0.5 ng/mL	<2.5 ng/mL or µg/L	<3.75 µg/mL	<0.15
African-American		<2.0 ng/mL or µg/L		
Asian		<2.0 ng/mL or µg/L		
Caucasian		<2.5 ng/mL or µg/L		
50-59 years	<0.7 ng/mL	<3.5 ng/mL or µg/L	<3.75 µg/mL	<0.15
African-American		<4.0 ng/mL or µg/L		
Asian		<3.0 ng/mL or µg/L		
Caucasian		<3.5 ng/mL or µg/L		
60-69 years	<1.0 ng/mL	<5.5 ng/mL or µg/L	<3.75 µg/mL	<0.15
African-American		<4.5 ng/mL or µg/L		
Asian		<4.0 ng/mL or µg/L		
Caucasian		<4.6 ng/mL or µg/L		
>69 years	<1.2 ng/mL	<6.5 ng/mL or µg/L	<3.75 µg/mL	<0.15
African-American		<5.5 ng/mL or µg/L		
Asian		<5.0 ng/mL or µg/L		
Caucasian		<6.5 ng/mL or µg/L		
Female		<0.5 ng/mL or µg/L		

*Data from Vashi, 1997.

Probability of Prostate Cancer*

PSA	
0-2 ng/mL	1%
2-4 ng/mL	15%
4-10 ng/mL	25%
>10 ng/mL	50%-70%
>20 ng/mL	91%
% Free: Total PSA Ratio = (Free PSA/Total PSA) × 100	
0%-10%	56%
10%-15%	28%
15%-20%	20%
20%-25%	16%
>25%	8%

*Findings in combination with a negative digital rectal examination.

Usage. Assists in the identification, differentiation, classification, staging, and localization of prostate tumor in men beginning at age 40 years; monitoring preoperatively, postoperative therapeutic interventions or cytotoxic drug therapy; and assists in assessment of tumor response to treatment protocols. Can serve as a marker for the success of total prostatectomy for prostate cancer.

Increased. Benign prostatic hypertrophy (levels up to 10 ng/mL), cirrhosis, impotence, osteoporosis, prostate cancer or infarct, prostatic needle biopsy, prostatitis, pulmonary embolism, renal osteopathy, transurethral resection (TUR), urethral instrumentation, and urinary retention.

Herbal or natural remedies include *Dendranthema morifolium Tzvel, Ganoderma lucidum Karst, Isatis indigotica Fort, Panax pseudo-ginseng,* and *Rabdosia rubescens Hara.*

Decreased. Drugs include finasteride (decreases levels by 50%). Herbal or natural remedies include *Glycyrrhiza uralensis Fisch, Scutellaria baicalensis Georgi,* and *Serenoa repens.*

Description. Prostate-specific antigen (PSA) is a glycoprotein produced by the prostate gland that liquefies clotted semen. PSA was previously believed to be exclusive to the prostate epithelium, but is now known to exist in normal and cancerous breast tissue, as well as some female body fluids. *Total* PSA is comprised of free and complexed PSA. The percent of free PSA is lower in men with prostate cancer than in men free of the disease because tumor catabolic activity and accelerated metabolic rate in prostate carcinoma elevate the serum value of PSA without proportionately elevating the free PSA level. The *free* PSA test includes measuring both free and total PSA and then calculating the ratio; this test has been recommended in men with a negative digital rectal exam accompanied by an elevated total PSA level. It can help provide guidance to select those that need prostate biopsies, particularly when PSA levels are between 4 and 10 ng/mL.

More recently, testing for *complexed* PSA alone has been found in one large study to be more sensitive than free or total PSA in detecting prostate cancer. However, subsequent studies have not reproduced the same findings. Currently being investigated is PSA *fractionation*, in which subforms of PSA, called "Intact" PSA and "Nicked" PSA, have been identified; PSA fractionation may be helpful in more specifically differentiating between benign and malignant disease of the prostate. In one study, the ratio of intact to free PSA was higher in malignant than in benign cancer. PSA *density* is a division of the total PSA level by the prostate size in cubic centimeters and provides insight into whether the amount of PSA produced is out of proportion to the size of the prostate gland. PSA velocity (PSAV) is a term used by some to describe changes over time in the PSA levels. Overall, PSA is a reliable

immunocytochemical marker used in the detection of prostate cancer. The majority of PSA elevation is attributed to benign prostatic hypertrophy, which normally raises PSA no higher than 10 ng/mL and also produces higher free-to-total ratios. Although 70% of those men with elevated values are free of prostate cancer, when values are higher than 50 ng/mL, PSA is 98.5% accurate in predicting that a prostate biopsy will be positive for cancer. Only about 45% of clients with prostate cancer have PSA values >10 ng/mL. PSA is smaller than the prostatic acid phosphatase molecule, more stable, and does not demonstrate diurnal variations. It is measured using an immunoreactive antibody assay. Genome associations between PSA levels and single-nucleotide polymorphisms (SNPs) include SNPs 10q26, 12q24, 10q11, 5p15.33, 17q11 and 19q13.33. Incorporating genetics, molecular markers, PSA velocity, age, ethnicity, and family history can strengthen the predictive value of the serum PSA.

Professional Considerations
Consent form NOT required.

Preparation
1. Draw sample BEFORE performing digital rectal examination.
2. Tube: Red topped, red/gray topped, or gold topped.
3. Specimens MAY be drawn during hemodialysis.
4. See Client and Family Teaching.

Procedure
1. Draw a 4-mL blood sample.

Postprocedure Care
1. The sample is stable at room temperature for 24 hours and may be refrigerated.

Client and Family Teaching
1. Fast for 8 hours.
2. Do not have the test drawn less than 24 hours after a rectal or prostate examination.

Factors That Affect Results
1. Falsely elevated results may be associated with blood drawn 1 to 24 hours after a rectal examination.
2. Levels can rise and remain elevated up to 50 times higher than baseline values for several weeks after prostate procedures, such as transurethral resection of prostate needle biopsy.

3. This test is nonspecific for prostate cancer when levels are mildly elevated. Approximately 25% of men with benign prostatic hypertrophy have an elevated PSA. Up to one third of clients with localized prostate cancer have false-negative values.
4. Levels can normally vary 20% from one day to the next.

Other Data

1. Although this test aids in the diagnosis of malignant states, some benign diseases can also demonstrate antigen marker abnormalities.
2. Adult levels are reached at approximately 15 years.
3. In 2011, the United States Preventive Services Task Force withdrew its recommendation for routine PSA screening of males. The change in recommendation was made after examining the risks and benefits of treatment and mortality rates.
4. PSA above 1.5 ng/mL between ages 45-49 for males predicts long-term risk for prostate cancer.
5. In a study of women with breast cancer, one study found a 30% decrease in the risk of relapse or of death in clients with PSA-positive disease as compared to those with disease that was PSA-negative.
6. If serum PSA is undetectable 3 months post radical cystoprostatectomy with benign prostate pathology, there is no need for continued PSA monitoring. With prostate pathology, undetectable levels at 10 years after radical prostatectomy indicate no further testing is needed.

Prostatic Acid Phosphatase (PAP)—Blood

Norm. Values are dependent on laboratory method.

		SI Units
Fishman-Lerner	0-0.7 U/dL	
Bessey, Lowry, and Brock (BLB)		
Female	0.02-0.55 U at 37 degrees C	0.3-9.2 U/L
Male	0.15-0.65 U at 37 degrees C	2.5-10.8 U/L
Bodansky	0-3 U/dL	0-16.1 U/L
King-Armstrong	0-3 U/dL	0-5.3 U/L
RIA	2.5-3.7 ng/mL	

Increased. Hyperparathyroidism, metastatic bone cancer (elevated in 75%-80%), metastatic prostatic carcinoma (elevated in 50%-75%), multiple myeloma, nonmetastatic prostatic carcinoma (10%-25%), osteogenesis imperfecta, Paget's disease, and prostatic infarct.

Decreased. Down syndrome. Drugs include estrogen therapy for prostatic carcinoma and ethyl alcohol (ethanol).

Description. Prostatic acid phosphatase, an isoenzyme of acid phosphatase, is a lysosomal enzyme that hydrolyzes phosphate esters. It is found in the prostate, erythrocytes, kidneys, liver, and spleen. Prostatic acid phosphatase is a prostate-specific epithelium differentiation antigen that regulates the growth of the prostate; thus prostate tissue has a concentration of acid phosphatase 100 times higher than that of other tissues. Serum activity of the prostatic isoenzyme is greatly increased in metastatic cancer of the prostate in which the tumor has extended beyond the capsule surrounding the prostate gland. Therefore this test is used as both a marker for and a monitor of the disease course.

Professional Considerations

Consent form NOT required.

Preparation

1. Draw sample BEFORE performing digital rectal examination.
2. Tube: Red topped, red/gray topped, or gold topped or lavender topped.
3. Specimens MAY be drawn during hemodialysis.

Procedure

1. Draw an early-morning, 5-mL blood sample.

Postprocedure Care

1. Transport the specimen to the laboratory immediately. Serum specimens deteriorate rapidly at room temperature.

Client and Family Teaching

1. Wait at least 24 hours after prostatic massage, extensive prostate palpation, or a transurethral resection before the blood test.
2. This test may be drawn in conjunction with the prostate-specific antigen test.

Factors That Affect Results

1. PAP levels exhibit a diurnal variation, with the highest levels occurring during the early morning.
2. Recent administration of clofibrate invalidates the results.

3. Falsely elevated results may be associated with blood drawn 1 to 24 hours after a rectal examination.
4. False-positive results have been reported in hemolyzed serum samples.
5. False-negative results have been reported in serum specimens contaminated with fluoride, oxalate, or phosphate.

Other Data

1. Refrigerated specimens or specimens frozen with 0.01 mL of 20% acetic acid per milliliter of serum can remain stable for up to 1 week.
2. With the increased reliability of prostate-specific antigen (PSA), screening, serum PAP testing may become more limited in value for prostate carcinoma.

Protein, Cerebrospinal Fluid

See Cerebrospinal Fluid, Heparin-Binding Protein, Myelin Basic Protein, Oligoclonal Bands, Protein, and Protein Electrophoresis—Specimen

Protein Electrophoresis, Cerebrospinal Fluid

See Cerebrospinal Fluid, Heparin-Binding Protein, Myelin Basic Protein, Oligoclonal Bands, Protein, and Protein Electrophoresis—Specimen.

Protein Electrophoresis—Serum

Norm. Norms are dependent on laboratory procedure. Percentage values represent the percentage of total protein for the agarose method:

		SI Units
Adult percentage		
Total protein	100%	5.90-8.00
Albumin	58%-74%	0.58-0.74
Alpha$_1$ globulin	2.0%-3.5%	0.02-0.04
Alpha$_2$ globulin	5.4%-10.6%	0.05-0.11
Beta globulin	7.0%-14.0%	0.07-0.14
Gamma globulin	8.0%-18.0%	0.08-0.18
Adult quantitative		
Total protein	6.0-8.0 g/dL	60-80 g/L
Albumin	3.3-5.0 g/dL	35-50 g/L
Alpha$_1$ globulin	0.1-0.4 g/dL	1-4 g/L
Alpha$_2$ globulin	0.5-1.0 g/dL	5-10 g/L
Beta globulin	0.7-1.2 g/dL	7-12 g/L
Gamma globulin	0.8-1.6 g/dL	8-16 g/L
Premature infant		
Total protein	4.4-6.3 g/dL	44-63 g/L
Albumin	3.0-4.2 g/dL	30-42 g/L

Continued

		SI Units
Alpha$_1$ globulin	0.11-0.5 g/dL	1.1-5 g/L
Alpha$_2$ globulin	0.3-0.7 g/dL	3-7 g/L
Beta globulin	0.3-1.2 g/dL	3-12 g/L
Gamma globulin	0.3-1.4 g/dL	3-14 g/L
Newborn		
Total protein	4.6-7.4 g/dL	46-74 g/L
Albumin	3.5-5.4 g/dL	35-54 g/L
Alpha$_1$ globulin	0.1-0.3 g/dL	1-3 g/L
Alpha$_2$ globulin	0.3-0.5 g/dL	3-5 g/L
Beta globulin	0.2-0.6 g/dL	2-6 g/L
Gamma globulin	0.2-1.2 g/dL	2-12 g/L
Infant		
Total protein	6.0-6.7 g/dL	60-67 g/L
Albumin	4.4-5.4 g/dL	44-54 g/L
Alpha$_1$ globulin	0.2-0.4 g/dL	2-4 g/L
Alpha$_2$ globulin	0.5-0.8 g/dL	5-8 g/L
Beta globulin	0.5-0.9 g/dL	5-9 g/L
Gamma globulin	0.3-0.8 g/dL	3-8 g/L
Child		
Total protein	6.2-8.0 g/dL	62-80 g/L
Albumin	4.0-5.8 g/dL	40-58 g/L
Alpha$_1$ globulin	0.1-0.4 g/dL	1-4 g/L
Alpha$_2$ globulin	0.4-1.0 g/dL	4-10 g/L
Beta globulin	0.5-1.0 g/dL	5-10 g/L
Gamma globulin	0.3-1.0 g/dL	3-10 g/L

Usage. Assists in the diagnosis of amyloidosis, B-cell non-Hodgkin's lymphoma, blood dyscrasias, dysproteinemias, gastrointestinal disorders, hepatic disease, hypergammaglobulinemias, hypogammaglobulinemias, inflammatory states, multiple myeloma, plasma cell leukemia, neoplasms, renal disease, and Waldenström's macroglobulinemia.

Increased Total Protein. Macroglobulinemia, multiple myeloma, and sarcoidosis.

Increased Prealbumin Zone Intensity. Alcoholism.

Increased Albumin Zone Mobility. Acute pancreatitis. Drugs include aspirin and penicillins.

Increased Albumin-Alpha$_1$ Globulin Interzone Intensity. Alcoholism (chronic), females during puberty, and pregnancy.

Increased Alpha Globulin Zone Intensity. Acute-phase response in inflammation (alpha$_1$, alpha haptoglobin), acute rheumatic fever (alpha$_2$), aged (alpha$_2$), analbuminemia (alpha$_2$), chronic glomerulonephritis (alpha$_2$), cirrhosis (increased alpha$_1$ with normal or only slightly elevated alpha$_2$), diabetes mellitus (alpha$_2$), dysproteinemia (familial idiopathic), glomerular protein loss (alpha$_2$-macroglobulin), hepatic damage, hepatic metastasis (increased alpha$_1$ with normal alpha$_2$), Hodgkin's disease (alpha$_1$, alpha$_2$), hypoalbuminemia, infancy (alpha$_2$ zone dominated by macroglobulin), infection (acute), meningitis (alpha$_2$), metastatic carcinomatosis (alpha$_1$, alpha$_2$), myocardial infarction, myxedema, nephrosis (alpha$_2$), nephrotic syndrome (alpha$_2$), osteomyelitis (alpha$_2$), peptic ulcer disease (alpha$_1$, alpha$_2$), pneumonia (alpha$_2$), polyarteritis nodosa (alpha$_2$), pregnancy (increased alpha$_1$, with normal alpha$_2$), protein-losing enteropathy (alpha$_1$, alpha$_2$), rheumatoid arthritis (alpha$_2$), sarcoidosis (alpha$_2$), stress (alpha$_1$, alpha$_2$), systemic lupus erythematosus (alpha$_2$), and ulcerative colitis (alpha$_1$, alpha$_2$). Drugs that increase alpha$_1$ with little change in alpha$_2$ include estrogens.

Increased Alpha$_2$-Beta$_1$ Interzone Intensity. Hypercholesterolemia (type II), nephrotic syndrome, and pregnancy.

Increased Beta Globulin Zone Intensity.

Acute-phase response (beta$_2$), analbuminemia, diabetes mellitus (poorly controlled), dysproteinemia (familial idiopathic), glomerular protein loss, hepatitis (viral), hypercholesterolemia, hyperlipemia, iron-deficiency anemia (beta$_1$), jaundice (obstructive), macroglobulinemia, nephrotic syndrome, pregnancy (beta$_1$), rheumatoid arthritis, and sarcoidosis. Drugs that increase beta$_1$ globulin include estrogens and oral contraceptives.

Increased Gamma Globulin Zone Intensity.

Acute viral hepatitis (sometimes), amyloidosis, analbuminemia, carcinoma (advanced), chronic aggressive hepatitis (appearance of oligoclonal bands), chronic hepatic disease (IgM), chronic lymphatic leukemia (IgM paraprotein), chronic viral infections (appearance of oligoclonal bands), cirrhosis (IgA), cryoglobulinemia, cystic fibrosis (IgG, IgA), Hashimoto's disease, hepatic disease, Hodgkin's disease, hypergammaglobulinemia, hypersensitivity reaction, infection (severe), juvenile rheumatoid arthritis (IgG, IgA, IgM), Laënnec's cirrhosis, leukemia (myelogenous, monocytic), lymphosarcoma (IgM paraprotein), macroglobulinemia, multiple myeloma, respiratory tract infection (IgA), rheumatoid arthritis (IgA, IgM), sarcoidosis, scleroderma (sometimes), skin disease (IgA), Sjögren's syndrome (IgG), systemic lupus erythematosus (active) (IgM), and Waldenström's macroglobulinemia (IgM paraprotein).

Decreased Total Protein.

Analbuminemia, cholecystitis (acute), chronic glomerulonephritis, Hodgkin's disease, hypertension (essential with congestive heart failure), hypogammaglobulinemia, leukemia (myelogenous, monocytic), nephrosis, peptic ulcer disease, and ulcerative colitis.

Decreased Prealbumin Zone Intensity.

Acute-phase response (day 1) and cirrhosis.

Decreased Albumin Zone Intensity.

Acute rheumatic fever, analbuminemia, carcinomatosis (metastatic), cholecystitis (acute), diabetes mellitus, gastrointestinal protein loss (inflammatory or neoplastic disease), glomerular protein loss, glomerulonephritis (chronic), hepatic disease, hepatitis (acute viral), Hodgkin's disease, hyperthyroidism, hypertension (essential with congestive heart failure), Laënnec's cirrhosis, leukemia (lymphatic, myelogenous, monocytic), lymphoma, macroglobulinemia, malnutrition, meningitis, multiple myeloma, nephrosis, nephrotic syndrome, osteomyelitis, peptic ulcer disease, pneumonia, polyarteritis nodosa, protein-losing enteropathy, pyrexia, rheumatoid arthritis, sarcoidosis, stress, systemic lupus erythematosus, and ulcerative colitis. Drugs include corticosteroids.

Decreased Albumin-Alpha$_1$ Interzone Intensity.

Cirrhosis, hepatitis (acute), and inflammation (severe).

Decreased Alpha Globulin Zone Intensity.

Acute viral hepatitis (alpha$_1$, alpha$_2$), congenital hypohaptoglobinemia (alpha$_2$ haptoglobin), hepatic disease, intravascular hemolysis (hemolytic anemia, hepatic metastases, cirrhosis, and splenomegaly cause decreased alpha$_2$ haptoglobin), malabsorption, pulmonary emphysema (alpha$_1$), scleroderma, starvation, and steatorrhea.

Decreased Alpha$_2$-Beta$_1$ Interzone Intensity.

Diabetes mellitus, inflammation, and pancreatitis.

Decreased Beta Globulin Zone Intensity.

Autoimmune disease, carcinomatosis (metastatic), hepatic disease (beta$_1$), immune complex disease (beta$_2$), leukemia (lymphatic, monocytic, myelogenous), lymphoma, malabsorption, malnutrition (beta$_1$), nephrosis, scleroderma, starvation, steatorrhea, systemic lupus erythematosus, and ulcerative colitis.

Decreased Gamma Globulin Zone Intensity.

Acute viral hepatitis (sometimes), agammaglobulinemia, glomerular protein loss, hypogammaglobulinemia, leukemia (lymphatic), lymphoma, nephrosis, nephrotic syndrome, malabsorption, protein-losing enteropathy, scleroderma (sometimes), starvation, steatorrhea, and ulcerative colitis. Drugs include imatinib.

Description.

Protein electrophoresis is the most frequent measurement of the primary blood proteins: albumin and globulins (alpha$_1$, alpha$_2$, beta, and gamma). Under the influence of an electrical field, at a pH of 8.6, the proteins separate by electrical charge, molecular size, and shape. Plotted on treated paper, the serum proteins form five homogeneous bands of the relative protein values in percentages. These percentages, when multiplied by the total protein concentration, reflect the absolute value of each protein. High-resolution electrophoresis allows the detection of additional bands or zones. Immunoelectrophoresis may be performed to identify the nature of suspicious bands or to monitor the progress of gammopathies, disturbances in immunoglobulin synthesis. The most rapid form of unknown band identification combines high-resolution electrophoresis with immunoprecipitation. Certain protein electrophoresis band patterns are characteristic of specific disease states.

Professional Considerations
Consent form NOT required.

Preparation
1. Tube: Red topped, red/gray topped, or gold topped.
2. Specimens MAY be drawn during hemodialysis.

Procedure
1. Draw a 4-mL blood sample, without trauma.

Postprocedure Care
1. None.

Client and Family Teaching
1. Immunoelectrophoresis may take up to 3 days for results.
2. Medications that interfere with serum protein levels may be prescribed to be withheld.

Factors That Affect Results
1. Falsely elevated total protein levels may occur with the use of contrast dyes.
2. Hemolysis of the specimen invalidates the results.
3. Electrophoresis may be performed on plasma or serum. The alpha-beta interzone is absent in heparinized plasma.
4. At least a 30% drop in albumin level is required before changes can be detected by electrophoresis.
5. Aged serum samples may cause decreased beta globulin and increased beta globulin density.
6. Protein electrophoresis is unreliable for diagnosis of IgA deficiency.
7. Recent dialysis distorts protein values.

Other Data
1. Multiple myeloma patients present with serum M protein 82% of the time and 40% have an M protein level <3 g/dL.

Protein Electrophoresis—Urine

Norm. Interpretation of urine electrophoretic patterns is required. Normal urine electrophoretograms show individual variance and a globulin pattern that is generally diffuse. Distinct bands may not be identifiable. The dominant protein, albumin, rapidly migrates to the anode, producing a spike in the pattern. Normally there is only a trace amount of alpha$_1$ globulin and alpha$_2$ globulin. The beta globulin and gamma globulins are negligible to absent. In contrast to serum electrophoresis, urine electrophoresis does not contain beta lipoproteins and beta globulin.

	Total Protein	SI Units
Albumin	37.9%	0.379
Alpha$_1$ globulin	27.3%	0.273
Alpha$_2$ globulin	19.5%	0.195
Beta globulin	8.8%	0.088
Gamma globulin	3.3%	0.033

Usage. Detection of albumin, Bence Jones proteins, hemoglobin, myoclonal gammopathies, myoglobin, renal disease, and systemic lupus erythematosus.

Interpretation of Abnormals. Proteinuria associated with increased glomerular permeability exhibits an electrophoretic pattern that is dominated by albumin, with moderate beta globulin, some alpha globulin, trace alpha$_1$ globulin, and trace gamma$_1$ globulin. Basement-membrane glomerular capillary damage occurs with amyloidosis, congestive heart failure, glomerulosclerosis (diabetic), increased venous pressure, inflammation, nonrenal infectious disease, or renal vein thrombosis. Glomerular dysfunction may occur with idiopathic nephrotic syndrome, membranous glomerulonephritis, immune complex disorders such as poststreptococcal glomerulonephritis, and systemic lupus erythematosus. These conditions produce proteinuria. Proteinuria can result from chyluria, increased circulating proteins, increased glomerular permeability, or renal tubular dysfunction.

Prerenal conditions include hemoglobinuria, inflammatory syndrome, monocytic leukemia, myoglobinuria, and paraproteinemias. Prerenal electrophoretic patterns vary, based on the specific low-molecular-weight excess protein present in serum. These circulating proteins may be normal or abnormal. Their excess results in the excretion of proteins in the presence of normal glomerular function.

Hemoglobinuria or intravascular hemolysis produces an electrophoretic pattern that is dominated by beta globulin, with some albumin, trace alpha$_1$ globulin, trace alpha$_2$ globulin, and negligible to absent gamma$_1$ globulin.

Inflammatory syndromes include acute infection, burns, cancer, collagen diseases, hyperthyroidism, and pregnancy. This electrophoretic pattern consists of moderate alpha$_1$ globulin, some albumin, some alpha$_2$ globulin, and negligible to absent beta$_1$ globulin and gamma$_1$ globulin.

Monocytic and monomyelocytic leukemia result in a cationic peak or dominant migration to the cathode, moderate albumin, trace alpha$_1$ globulin, trace alpha$_2$ globulin, and negligible to absent beta$_1$ globulin and gamma$_1$ globulin.

Myoglobinuria associated with crushing injuries or electrocution demonstrates a pattern of dominant to absent gamma$_1$ globulin, some albumin, trace alpha$_1$ globulin, trace alpha$_2$ globulin, and negligible to absent beta$_1$ globulin.

Paraproteinemias such as multiple myeloma with Bence Jones proteinuria produce moderate to absent beta$_1$ globulin and gamma$_1$ globulin, with some albumin, trace alpha$_1$ globulin, and alpha$_2$ globulin.

Inflammatory conditions (such as chronic osteomyelitis), increased glomerular permeability, and tubular dysfunction (such as chronic renal failure) produce a pattern that is dominated by albumin, with moderate alpha$_1$ globulin elevation, some alpha$_2$ globulin, trace beta$_1$ globulin, and negligible to absent gamma$_1$ globulin.

Renal tubular disorders include acute renal tubular failure, Balkan neuropathy, cadmium poisoning (chronic), cystinosis, Fanconi syndrome, galactosemia, hypokalemia (chronic, severe), intoxication (phenacetin or vitamin D), medullary cystic disease, monoclonal gammopathy, oculocerebral renal syndrome, polycystic kidney disease, pyelonephritis (chronic), renal transplantation, renal tubular acidosis, sarcoidosis, and Wilson's disease. The electrophoretic pattern is dominated by beta$_1$ globulin, with some alpha$_2$ globulin, some gamma$_1$ globulin, trace albumin, trace alpha$_1$ globulin, and a trace cationic migration or peak.

Retroperitoneal lymphatic injury from inflammation, obstruction, or trauma can result in aberrant communication of the retroperitoneal lymph vessels, chyle ducts of the intestine, and urinary tract. This condition causes chyluria. The electrophoretic pattern noted in chyluria is one dominated by albumin, with moderate gamma$_1$ globulin, some alpha$_2$ globulin, some beta$_1$ globulins, and trace alpha$_1$ globulin.

Upright or orthostatic position–dependent proteinuria is characterized by dominant albumin, moderate beta$_1$ globulin, some alpha$_1$ globulin, trace alpha$_2$ globulin, and trace gamma$_1$ globulin. The recumbent position reflects a normal electrophoretic pattern. Activity-related proteinuria demonstrates a pattern that is more accentuated than normal but not so elevated as orthostatic proteinuria. An exercise pattern produces moderate albumin, some alpha$_1$ globulin and alpha$_2$ globulin, trace beta$_1$ globulin, and trace gamma$_1$ globulin.

Description. Normally the urine is free of protein or contains only trace amounts of albumin and globulin because the glomeruli prevent the passage of proteins from the plasma to the glomerular filtrate. Protein electrophoresis is a quantitative measurement of proteins, which under the influence of an electrical field, at a pH of 8.6, separate by charge, size, and shape. The separation produces homogeneous bands that are plotted on treated paper. Protein electrophoresis detects the presence of free light chains and other proteins associated with myoclonal gammopathies. The normally round and broad curves form a "church spire," or sharp peak. The immunoelectrophoretic technique is able to demonstrate a large number of components that are identical to the serum electrophoretic patterns. It is used to identify light-chain, Bence Jones, and kappa-, lambda-, and heavy-chain proteins. The test helps detect specific abnormalities by identifying patterns of protein characteristic of different disease states. The meaning of the results of urine electrophoresis is best interpreted when the test is run simultaneously with a serum sample for electrophoresis.

Professional Considerations
Consent form NOT required.

Preparation
1. Obtain a clean 50-mL container for a random urine collection or a 3-L container without preservatives or to which toluene or acetic acid has been added. For pediatric/infant specimen collection, also obtain a pediatric urine collection device/bag and tape.
2. Write the beginning time of the 24-hour collection on the laboratory requisition.
3. See Client and Family Teaching.

Procedure
1. *Random sample*: Obtain a 25-mL fresh, first morning-voided urine sample in a clean container. A fresh specimen may be taken from a urinary drainage bag.
2. *24-Hour sample*: Discard the first morning urine specimen. Save all urine voided for 24 hours in a refrigerated, clean 3-L container without preservatives or to which toluene or acetic acid preservative has been added. Document the quantity of urine output during the specimen collection period. Include the urine voided at the end of the 24-hour period. For catheterized clients, keep entire drainage bag on ice and empty the urine into the collection container hourly.
3. *Pediatric/infant specimen collection*: Empty the urine into the refrigerated collection container after each void.
   a. The child is placed in a supine position with the knees flexed and the hips externally rotated and abducted.
   b. Cleanse, rinse, and thoroughly dry the perineal area.
   c. To prevent the child from removing the collection device/bag, a diaper may be placed over the genital area.
   d. *Females*: Tape the pediatric collection device/bag to the perineum. Starting at the area between the anus and vagina, apply the device/bag in an anterior direction.
   e. *Males*: Place the pediatric collection device/bag over the penis and scrotum and tape it to the perineal area.

Postprocedure Care
1. Compare the urine quantity in the specimen container with the urinary output record for the test. If the specimen contains less urine than what was recorded as output, some of the sample may have been discarded, invalidating the test.
2. Document the urine quantity on the laboratory requisition.

Client and Family Teaching
1. For 24-hour urine collection for home collection: Save all urine voided in the 24-hour period and urinate before defecating to avoid loss of urine. If any urine is accidentally discarded, discard the entire specimen and restart the collection the next day.
2. Avoid drugs that may cause proteinuria (listed below) for specific lengths of time before the test as specified by the physician.

Factors That Affect Results
1. Contamination of the specimen with stool invalidates the results. The test must be repeated or restarted.
2. Drugs that cause proteinuria include amikacin sulfate, amphotericin B, aurothioglucose, bacitracin, gentamicin sulfate, gold sodium thiomalate, kanamycin, neomycin sulfate, netilmycin sulfate, penicillins, phenylbutazone, polymyxin B, streptomycin sulfate, sulfonamides, tobramycin sulfate, and trimethadione.

Other Data
1. Urine protein electrophoresis results should be evaluated with consideration given to serum protein electrophoresis patterns.
2. Multiple myeloma patients present with urine M protein 75% of the time.

Protein, Quantitative

See **Protein—Urine.**

Protein, Semiquantitative

See **Protein**—Urine.

Protein, Total—Serum

Norm.

		SI Units
Adults	6.0-8.0 g/dL	60-80 g/L
Children	4.3-7.6 g/dL	43-76 g/L
Premature	4.6-7.4 g/dL	46-74 g/L
Newborn	6.0-6.7 g/dL	60-67 g/L
Infant	6.2-8.0 g/dL	62-80 g/L

Increased. Addison's disease, amyloidosis, autoimmune collagen disorders, chronic infection, Crohn's disease, dehydration (relative increase), diarrhea, Franklin's disease, hemolysis, liver disease, macroglobulinemia, multiple myeloma, protozoal diseases (kala-azar), renal disease, sarcoidosis, vomiting, and wound drainage. Drugs include clofibrate, corticosteroids, corticotropin, dextran, growth hormone, heparin calcium, heparin sodium, insulin, levothyroxine sodium/T, radiographic contrast dye, somatotropin, sulfobromophthalein (Bromsulphalein), thyrotropin, and tolbutamide.

Decreased. Acute cholecystitis, analbuminemia, burns, chronic glomerulonephritis, cirrhosis, congestive heart failure, Crohn's disease, diarrhea, edema, essential hypertension, exfoliative dermatitis, frequent plasma donation, hemorrhage, hepatic disease (severe), Hodgkin's disease, hyperalimentation, hyperthyroidism, hypoalbuminemia, hypogammaglobulinemia, infectious hepatitis, kwashiorkor, leukemia (monocytic, myelogenous), malabsorption, malnutrition, nephrosis, nephrotic syndrome, peptic ulcer, pregnancy, protein-losing enteropathies, sprue, ulcerative colitis, and water intoxication. Drugs include ammonium ion, dextran, excessive intravenous fluids containing glucose, oral contraceptives, pyrazinamide, and salicylates.

Description. Total serum protein reflects the total amount of albumin and globulins in the serum. The serum proteins that are synthesized in the liver and reticuloendothelial system constitute more than 100 different substances and are grouped as albumin and globulins. Serum proteins are essential to the regulation of colloid osmotic pressure, and comprise coagulation factors for hemostasis, enzymes, hormones, tissue growth and repair, and pH buffers. They produce antibodies, transport blood components (bilirubin, calcium, lipids, metals, oxygen, steroids, thyroid hormones, and vitamins), and are the preservers of chromosomes.

Professional Considerations

Consent form NOT required.

Preparation

1. Tube: Red topped, red/gray topped, or gold topped.
2. Medications that interfere with serum protein levels may be withheld.
3. Do NOT draw specimens during hemodialysis.
4. See Client and Family Teaching.

Procedure

1. Draw a 4-mL blood sample without trauma.
2. Avoid prolonged application of a tourniquet, which can cause an increase in protein concentrations.
3. Obtain the sample away from IV solution, which can lower protein levels through local dilution.

Postprocedure Care

1. Samples may be refrigerated for up to 1 week.

Client and Family Teaching

1. Do not ingest a high-fat diet for 8 hours before the test.
2. Medications that interfere with serum protein levels may be prescribed to be withheld before the test.

Factors That Affect Results

1. Reject hemolyzed or lipemic specimens.
2. Falsely elevated total protein levels occur for up to 48 hours after the use of sulfobromophthalein contrast dye.

3. Recent dialysis distorts protein values.
4. Hyperglycemia may cause total protein concentration to appear to be greater than actual.
5. Serum total protein levels for bedridden clients is lower by approximately 0.3 g/dL than expected for the same age.

Other Data

1. See also Protein electrophoresis—Serum.
2. The significance of the total protein is difficult to interpret without knowledge of the level of the individual fractions (albumin/globulin) obtained through electrophoresis.

Protein—Urine

Norm. Negative; no detectable protein.

Semiquantitative Norms		SI Units
Normal	<20 mg/%	<0.2 g/L
Reagent Strip/Stick		
Negative	0-5 mg/dL	0-0.05 g/L
Trace	5-20 mg/dL	0.05-0.2 g/L
1+	30 mg/dL	0.3 g/L
2+	100 mg/dL	1.0 g/L
3+	300 mg/dL	3.0 g/L
4+	1000 mg/dL	10.0 g/L

Quantitative Norms		SI Units
Adults	30-150 mg/24 hours	0.03-0.15 g/day
Children <10 years	<100 mg/24 hours	<0.10 g/day
Newborn: Increased protein in urine for 3 days after delivery		

Increased or Positive

Nonrenal Disease. Abdominal tumor, aging, anemia (severe), ascites, bacterial toxins (acute streptococcal, diphtheria, pneumonia, scarlet and typhoid fever), cardiac disease, central nervous system lesion, convulsive disorders, fever, hepatic disease (jaundice), hypersensitivity reaction, hyperthyroidism, infection (acute), ingestion of or overexposure to certain substances (arsenic, carbon tetrachloride, ether, lead, mercury, mustard, opiates, phenol, propylene glycol, sulfosalicylic acid, turpentine), intestinal obstruction, leukemia (chronic lymphocytic), subacute bacterial endocarditis, toxemia, and trauma.

Transient Proteinuria. Dehydration, diet (excessive protein), emotional stress, exposure to cold, exercise (strenuous), fever, orthostatic hypotension, proteinuria, posthemorrhage, and sodium depletion. Drugs include epinephrine bitartrate, epinephrine borate, epinephrine hydrochloride, and levarterenol bitartrate.

Prerenal Disease. Amyloidosis, Bence Jones proteinuria associated with myeloma, congestive heart failure, convulsions, exercise, leukemia (myelocytic), orthostatic hypotension, proteinuria, and Waldenström's macroglobulinemia.

Renal Disease. Collagen diseases, cryoglobulinemia, Henoch-Schönlein purpura, hypertension (malignant, renovascular), and thrombotic thrombocytopenic purpura.

Glomerular Disease. Amyloidosis, diabetic glomerulosclerosis and nephropathy, glomerulonephritis and lesion, Goodpasture's syndrome, high-molecular-weight proteinuria, membranous nephropathy, polycystic disease, pyelonephritis (chronic), renal vein thrombosis, and systemic lupus erythematosus.

Interstitial Disease. Bacterial pyelonephritis; deposition of calcium, uric acid, or urate; and idiosyncratic pharmacologic reactions to the following drugs: methicillin sodium, phenindione, phenytoin, phenytoin sodium, and sulfonamides.

Tubular Disease. Acute tubular necrosis, Bartter syndrome, beta-microglobulinemia, Bright's disease, Butler-Albright syndrome, Fanconi syndrome, galactosemia, heavy-metal poisoning (cadmium, lead, mercury),

P

Kimmelstiel-Wilson syndrome, nephrotic syndrome, and renal tubular acidosis.

Postrenal Disease. Cystitis (severe), tumor metastasis of the bone, and tumor (urinary bladder, renal pelvis). Drugs that cause proteinuria include amikacin sulfate, amphotericin B, aurothioglucose, bacitracin, gentamicin sulfate, gold sodium thiomalate, netilmicin sulfate, neomycin sulfate, penicillins, phenylbutazone, polymyxin B, streptomycin sulfate, sulfonamides, and trimethadione.

Decreased. Not applicable.

Description. The semiquantitative urine test is a random screening test for urinary protein and is part of the routine urinalysis. The reagent-strip color indicators and use of sulfosalicylic acid in the laboratory are two methods used to confirm the presence of urinary protein. A small amount of protein in the urine is regarded as normal and consists of albumin and low-molecular-weight plasma proteins (beta microglobulin, globulins, haptoglobulin, light chains, and Tamm-Horsfall glycoprotein). Protein in the urine is a key indicator of renal disorder.

Quantitation of urinary protein is indicated when a random urine sample is positive for more than a trace of protein. Normally, only low-molecular-weight proteins are small enough to pass through the glomerular membrane into the glomerular filtrate, and most of these are reabsorbed by the renal tubules. Proteinuria is a key indicator of renal disorder and can result from glomerular leakage, tubular impairment, breakdown of renal tissue, or excessive concentrations of low-molecular-weight proteins. Transient proteinuria may result from nonpathologic states such as physical or emotional stress and body position. Protein substances are excreted at different rates and at varying times in a 24-hour period; thus the 24-hour timed quantitative urine test for protein provides the most accurate reflection of kidney function.

Professional Considerations
Consent form NOT required.

Preparation
1. Semiquantitative test:
   a. Obtain a clean, dry plastic container or a pediatric urine-collection device and a container of reagent strips.

2. Quantitative test:
   a. Obtain a clean, 3-L container that is free of preservative. For pediatric/infant collections, also obtain tape and a pediatric urine-collection device/bag.
   b. Write the beginning time of the 24-hour collection on the laboratory requisition.

Procedure
1. *Semiquantitative test:*
   a. An early morning specimen or the first-voided specimen of the day after the client stands upright is preferred.
   b. Instruct the client to void into a clean, dry container. The specimen may be transferred to a plastic container.
   c. Specimens may be tested immediately or sent to the laboratory for testing.
   d. To test the sample immediately, dip the reagent strip into the urine and remove any excess urine by gently tapping the strip on the side of the collection container. The strip should then be held at a horizontal plane to prevent mixing of any other chemicals on the strip. Immediately and carefully compare the color of the test pad on the reagent strip to the color chart provided on the container from which it was taken. Record the result according to the negative to 4++ range of approximate milligrams per deciliter (mg/dL) of protein.

2. *Quantitative test:*
   a. Early morning is the preferred time to begin a 24-hour collection.
   b. Discard the first morning urine specimen.
   c. Save all the urine voided for 24 hours in a refrigerated, clean, 3-L container that is free of preservatives. Document the quantity of urine output during the specimen collection period. Include the urine voided at the end of the 24-hour period. For catheterized clients, keep the drainage bag on ice and empty the urine into the refrigerated collection container hourly.
   d. Pediatric/infant specimen collection:
      i. Empty the collection bag into the refrigerated collection container after each void.

ii. The child is placed in a supine position with the knees flexed and the hips externally rotated and abducted.

iii. Cleanse, rinse, and thoroughly dry the perineal area.

iv. To prevent the child from removing the collection device/bag, a diaper may be placed over the genital area.

v. *Females*: Tape the pediatric collection device/bag to the perineum. Starting at the area between the anus and vagina, apply the device/bag in an anterior direction.

vi. *Males*: Place the pediatric collection device/bag over the penis and scrotum and tape it to the perineal area.

Postprocedure Care

1. *Semiquantitative test:*
   a. To be most accurate, specimens sent to the laboratory must be transported within 2 hours of the collection of the sulfosalicylic acid precipitation of the protein. Specimens must be refrigerated.
2. *Quantitative test:*
   a. Compare the urine quantity in the specimen container with the urinary output record for the test. If the specimen contains less urine than what was recorded as output, some of the sample may have been discarded, thus invalidating the test.
   b. Document the urine quantity and ending time on the laboratory requisition.

Client and Family Teaching

1. Save all the urine voided in a 24-hour period; urinate before defecating to avoid loss of urine; and avoid contamination of the specimen with stool, toilet tissue, or prostatic or vaginal secretions. If any urine is accidentally discarded, discard the entire specimen and restart the collection the next day.
2. Parents may be taught a pediatric collection technique for specimens collected on infants at home.

Factors That Affect Results

1. Drugs that may cause false-positive semiquantitative results include acetazolamide, aminosalicylic acid, cephaloridine, chlorpromazine, penicillins, phenazopyridine, promazine hydrochloride, radiographic contrast media, sodium bicarbonate, sulfisoxazole, sulfonamides, thymol, and tolbutamide.

2. Drugs that may cause falsely elevated quantitative results include acetazolamide, aminosalicylic acid, aspirin, barbiturates, cephalosporins, corticosteroids, iodine, iodine contrast medium, mercurial diuretics, penicillins, sodium bicarbonate, sulfonamides, tolbutamide, and tolmetin sodium.

3. First-voided urine samples are the most accurate for semiquantitative measurement because they are the most uniformly concentrated, are the most acidic pH, and are most likely to exhibit abnormalities.

4. False-positive semiquantitative results can occur with incorrect matching of the reagent strip to the color chart and with prolonged exposure of the strip or stick to the urine.

5. False-positive results have been reported with gross hematuria.

6. Reject specimens contaminated with blood, heavy mucus, purulent drainage, stool, prostatic or vaginal secretions, or toilet tissue.

7. The presence of many white blood cells can alter the results.

8. False-negative results have been reported with very dilute urine, highly buffered alkaline urine, urine high in sodium, and urea-splitting infectious organisms of the urinary tract.

9. Reject quantitative specimens in which the last void before the testing period was not discarded.

10. All urine voided for the 24-hour period must be included to avoid a falsely low quantitative result.

11. Increased protein concentrations are found during the daytime and after exercise.

12. The reagent strip is most sensitive to albumin and less sensitive to globulins.

13. The reagent strip method will not detect Bence Jones protein, globulins, mucoproteins, or myeloma protein.

14. Semiquantitative testing with a reagent strip will show a trace positive reaction at a protein concentration of 100-200 mg/L.

Other Data

1. The creatinine clearance test is often prescribed with the quantitative urine protein test.
2. Bence Jones protein may be present if the reagent strip method is negative and the sulfosalicylic acid test is positive. An electrophoresis and immunoelectrophoresis search for light chains is indicated because Bence Jones proteins are associated with amyloidosis, chronic lymphocytic leukemia, hyperparathyroidism, macroglobulinemia, malignant lymphoma, metastatic bone tumor, multiple myeloma, and osteomalacia.
3. See also Protein electrophoresis—Urine.

Protein C (Autoprothrombin IIA)—Blood

Norm.

Protein C	Range
Critical value	<50%
Heterozygous protein C	20%-74% deficiency
Homozygous protein C	As low as 0% deficiency

Functional Protein C	
Adults	77%-173%
Children	
1-4 days	17%-53%
5-29 days	20%-64%
1-3 months	21%-65%
3-6 months	28%-80%
6-12 months	37%-81%
1-6 years	40%-92%
7-9 years	56%-144%
10-11 years	59%-143%
12-13 years	57%-142%
14-15 years	56%-162%
16-17 years	68%-154%

Total Antigen Protein C	
1-4 days	17%-53%
5-29 days	20%-64%
1-3 months	21%-65%
3-6 months	28%-80%
6-12 months	37%-81%
1-6 years	40%-92%
6-10 years	45%-93%
11 years and older	65%-153%

Activated Protein C Resistance Test	
APC-APTT: APTT	>2.0
Resistance to activated protein C	≤2.0 with confirmatory DNA testing to identify factor V Leiden mutation

Usage. Helps diagnose cause of thrombosis. Protein C/protein S ratio is helpful in identifying carriers of congenital protein C deficiency.

Increased. Diabetes, nephrotic syndrome, pregnancy. Drugs include oral contraceptives.

Decreased. Congenital protein C deficiency. Acquired protein C deficiency conditions such as disseminated intravascular coagulation, hepatic disease, vitamin K deficiency.

Description. Activated protein C is a plasma, vitamin K–dependent glycoprotein anticoagulant that inhibits factors V and XIII. Protein C was first identified in the early 1980s. Sixty percent of protein C is bound to complement protein, and it is converted to an activated functional form by active serine protease and its activity is enhanced by cofactor protein S. Protein C deficiency may be congenital or acquired. *Congenital protein C deficiency* is an inherited, autosomal dominant thrombophilia present in 3%-5% of clients with venous thrombosis. Congenital deficiency may be exhibited either as reduced protein C levels or as resistance to protein C despite normal levels. Clients with homozygous deficiencies usually die as a result of thrombosis during their first year of life, which is often preceded by neonatal purpura fulminans. Those with heterozygous deficiency often have venous thromboembolisms, such as deep vein thrombosis or pulmonary embolism, at a young age. *Acquired protein C deficiency* is seen in acute respiratory distress syndrome, disseminated intravascular coagulation, hemolytic uremic syndrome, hepatic disease, infection, postoperative states, vitamin K deficiency, and clients receiving warfarin sodium (Coumadin). Protein C deficiency is responsible for a much greater proportion of venous thromboses than arterial thromboses. *The factor V Leiden mutation, newly identified in the 1990s, is a* thrombotic molecular defect in factor V making it resistant to anticoagulant activation by protein C. It is a significant cause of deep vein thrombosis, as the mutation is thought to be present in 5% of the population. The Leiden mutation is identified by performing an activated protein C resistance test (APTT with and without commercially available activated protein C) and confirming an abnormal result with DNA evaluation for the Leiden mutation.

Professional Considerations

Consent form NOT required.

Preparation

1. Tube: 4.5-mL blue topped. Also obtain ice.
2. Indicate on the laboratory requisition if the activated protein C resistance testing is needed.
3. For recurrent venous thrombosis, perform test at least 2 months after the last event, and with anticoagulants held.

Procedure

1. Withdraw 2 mL of blood into a syringe or vacuum tube. Remove the syringe or tube, leaving the needle in place. Attach a second syringe, and draw a 2.4-mL sample in a 2.7-mL tube or a 4.0-mL sample in a 4.5-mL tube. Place the specimens immediately into a container of ice.
2. Gently tilt the tube five or six times to mix.

Postprocedure Care

1. Place the specimens on ice immediately.
2. For clients with coagulopathy, hold pressure over the sampling site for at least 5 minutes and observe the site closely for development of a hematoma.
3. Write the collection time on the laboratory requisition.
4. Transport the specimens to the laboratory immediately, discard the ice, and refrigerate the specimens.

Client and Family Teaching

1. For results showing congenital deficiency, refer client or parents for genetic counseling as appropriate.

Factors That Affect Results

1. Reject hemolyzed or clotted specimens, specimens not completely mixed, tubes partially filled with blood, specimens not refrigerated, specimens diluted or contaminated with heparin, or specimens received more than 2 hours after collection.
2. Specimen results are invalidated if client is receiving a recently adjusted (within previous week) dose of warfarin. Oral anticoagulants decrease functional protein C values.
3. Falsely decreased functional protein C values occur in clients with abnormally high levels of factor VIII.
4. Falsely increased functional protein C values occur in clients receiving heparin.

Other Data

1. Protein C deficiency is treated with ongoing anticoagulation with or without protein C or factor IX concentrates. There is no treatment for factor V Leiden mutation.
2. Decreased protein C may contribute to coronary heart disease (He et al, 2008).

Protein S, Total and Free—Blood

Norm.

	Total	Free	% Free as Percentage of Healthy Control
Protein S	74-112 U/dL	27-63 U/dL	68-140
Critical low			<50

Functional Protein S	Female	Male
Adults	57%-131%	77%-173%
Children		
1 days-3 months	15%-55%	15%-55%
3-6 months	35%-92%	35%-92%
6-12 months	45%-115%	45%-115%

Functional Protein S	Female	Male
1-6 years	62%-120%	62%-120%
7-9 years	58%-154%	64%-141%
10-11 years	68%-140%	68%-180%
12-13 years	60%-150%	65%-143%
14-15 years	53%-147%	66%-149%
16-17 years	51%-150%	75%-157%

Total Antigen Protein S	
1-4 days	12%-60%
5-29 days	22%-78%
1-3 months	33%-93%
3-6 months	54%-118%
6-12 months	55%-119%
1-5 years	54%-118%
6-10 years	41%-114%
11 years and older	58%-146%

Usage. Helps diagnose cause of thrombosis. Protein C/Protein S ratio is helpful in identifying carriers of congenital protein C deficiency. Useful in clients with recurrent arterial thrombosis. Decreased in acute hepatitis, chronic kidney disease, chronic viral hepatitis, cirrhosis, hepatitis B carriers, hepatocellular carcinoma, protein S deficiency, acquired protein S deficiency (may be caused by hepatic disease, pregnancy, nephrotic syndrome, and use of estrogen).

Description. Protein S is a plasma, vitamin K–dependent glycoprotein manufactured in the liver that functions in the coagulation pathway. It exists in free form (active) and bound to a complement protein (inactive). Protein S functions as a cofactor to protein C, which inactivates factors Va and VIIIa. Deficiencies of protein S may be of two types. *Congenital protein S deficiency* is an autosomal dominant disorder responsible for about 5% of thromboses, in which the client has a higher-than-normal risk of thrombosis at a young age. *Acquired protein S deficiencies* are seen in pregnancy, disseminated intravascular coagulation, hepatic disease, and clients receiving warfarin. Protein S deficiency is responsible for a much greater proportion of venous thromboses than arterial thromboses.

Professional Considerations
Consent form NOT required.

Preparation
1. Tube: 4.5-mL blue topped. Also obtain ice.
2. For clients with recurrent arterial thrombosis, perform test at least 2 months after an event, and with anticoagulants held.

Procedure
1. Withdraw 3 mL of blood into a syringe or vacuum tube. Remove the syringe or tube, leaving the needle in place. Attach a second syringe, and draw a 2.4-mL sample in a 2.7-mL tube or a 4.0-mL sample in a 4.5-mL tube. Place the specimens immediately into a container of ice.
2. Gently tilt the tube five or six times to mix.

Postprocedure Care
1. Place the specimens on ice immediately.
2. For clients with coagulopathy, hold pressure over the sampling site for at least 5 minutes and observe the site closely for development of a hematoma.
3. Write the collection time on the laboratory requisition.
4. Transport the specimens to the laboratory immediately, discard the ice, and refrigerate the specimens.

Client and Family Teaching
1. For results showing congenital deficiency, refer client or parents for genetic counseling as appropriate.

Factors That Affect Results
1. Reject hemolyzed or clotted specimens, specimens not completely mixed, tubes partially filled with blood, specimens not refrigerated, specimens diluted or contaminated with heparin, or specimens received more than 2 hours after collection.
2. Specimen results are invalidated if client has recently received (within previous

week) a dose of warfarin. Oral anticoagulants decrease functional protein S values.

3. Falsely decreased functional protein S values occur in clients with abnormally high levels of factor VIII.

4. Falsely increased functional protein S values occur in clients receiving heparin.

Other Data

1. Once discovered, protein S deficiency is treated with ongoing anticoagulation.

Prothrombin Time (PT) and International Normalized Ratio (INR)—Blood

Normal PT. Each laboratory establishes a normal value, or control, based on the method and reagents used to perform the test. A value within ±2 seconds of the control set by each laboratory is considered within a normal range.

	Prothrombin Time
Adult	8.7-11.5 seconds
Newborn	<17 seconds
Child	11-14 seconds
Panic value	>40 seconds
Nonanticoagulated condition	>20 seconds
Anticoagulated condition	>3 times the control

Normal International Normalized Ratio (INR). Norm = 0.8-1.2, Routine therapy 2.0-3.0, Recurrent MI or mechanical valve prosthetic 2.5-3.5.

Coumadin therapy. There are, in general, two therapeutic ranges for clients receiving warfarin sodium (Coumadin). NOTE: Guidelines are updated periodically, and values below may not be the most current recommendations. Check the National Guideline Clearinghouse at http://www.guideline.gov for the most current recommendations.

Standard (Low-Intensity) Therapy	High-Dose (High-Intensity) Therapy
≤2.5 INR is recommended to minimize risk of bleeding during endoscopic procedures. 2.0 INR (range 1.6-2.5) is recommended for stroke prevention in clients over 75 years of age who have atrial fibrillation. 2.5 INR (range 2.0-3.0) is appropriate for stroke prevention in clients age 75 years or younger who have atrial fibrillation. 2.0-3.0 INR is appropriate for management of deep vein thrombosis, for prevention of systemic embolism, for clients with mitral or aortic prosthetic tissue valves, and for post myocardial infarction with concomitant aspirin therapy. 1.5 INR is recommended for those with moderate risk for a coronary event.	3.0-4.0 INR (target 3.5 INR post myocardial infarction if concomitant aspirin therapy is not used) is appropriate. 2.5-3.5 INR is appropriate for management of client's status after recent acute myocardial infarction, for management of clients with bi-leaflet or tilting-disk mechanical heart valves, or for evaluation of client's status after left-sided prosthetic valve thrombosis and recurrent systemic embolism; also used for prophylaxis in high-risk surgery.

Panic Level Symptoms and Treatment
Symptoms. Bleeding from venipuncture, arterial, or intravenous catheter sites; ecchymosis; hematoma; hematuria; blood in stool; or hallmark signs of intracerebral, gastrointestinal, or retroperitoneal bleeding.

Treatment

NOTE: Treatment choice(s) depend(s) on client's history and condition and episode history.

1. Discontinue or reduce rate of IV anticoagulant.
2. Maintain patent airway.
3. Apply pressure for 10 minutes or more to bleeding line or venipuncture sites.
4. Observe and intervene for hemodynamic stability.
5. For active bleeding, consider administration of whole blood, fresh frozen plasma, or prothrombin complex concentrate.
6. Administer vitamin K. Crowther et al (2002) found that the oral route of administration is faster than the subcutaneous route in reducing the INR.

Route	Coagulation Factors Increase	Bleeding Control Occurs	INR Becomes Normal	Risks
IV (Aqua-MEPHYTON) (route not recommended unless other routes are not feasible)	1-2 hours	3-8 hours	12-14 hours	Anaphylaxis
Subcutaneous (Aqua-MEPHYTON)	Progressive length ↓	Progressive length ↓	24-48 hours	Hemorrhage at injection site
Intramuscular (Aqua-MEPHYTON)			24-48 hours	Hemorrhage at injection site
Oral (Mephyton)	6-12 hours		24-48 hours	Considered safest and preferred method of administration

Increased PT. Afibrinogenemia, alcoholism, biliary obstruction, cancer, celiac disease, circulating anticoagulants, cirrhosis, colitis, collagen disease, congestive heart failure, diarrhea (chronic), disseminated intravascular coagulation (DIC), dysfibrinogenemia, factor deficiency (I, II, V, VII, X), fever, fibrinogen degradation products (FDPs), fistula, hemorrhagic disease of the newborn, hepatic disease (abscess, biopsy, failure, jaundice, infectious hepatitis), hypernephroma of kidney, hyperthyroidism, hypervitaminosis A, hypofibrinogenemia (<100 mg/dL), idiopathic familial hypoprothrombinemia, idiopathic myelofibrosis, increased fibrinolytic activity, jaundice (hemolytic, hepatocellular, obstructive), leukemia (acute), malabsorption, malnutrition, obstetric complications, pancreatic carcinoma, pancreatitis (chronic), polycythemia vera, premature infants, prolonged hot weather, prothrombin deficiency, Reye's syndrome, snakebite, sprue, steatorrhea, toxic shock syndrome, vitamin K deficiency, and vomiting. Drugs include acenocoumarol, alcohol, allopurinol, aminosalicylic acid, amiodarone hydrochloride, anabolic steroids, antibiotics, bromelains, chenodiol, chloral hydrate, chlorpropamide, chymotrypsin, cimetidine, clofibrate, dextran, dextrothyroxine, diazoxide, diflunisal, disulfiram, diuretics, ethacrynic acid, fenoprofen, fluoroquinolone antibiotics, fluoxetine, glucagon, hepatotoxic drugs, ibuprofen, indomethacin, influenza virus vaccine, mefenamic acid, methyldopa, methylphenidate, metronidazole, miconazole, monoamine oxidase inhibitors, nalidixic acid, naproxen, narcotics (prolonged), pentoxifylline, phenylbutazone, phenytoin sodium, propafenone, pyrazolones, quinidine, quinine, ranitidine, rivaroxaban, salicylates, sulfinpyrazone, sulfonamides (long-acting), sulindac, tamoxifen, thyroid drugs, tolbutamide, trimethoprim-sulfamethoxazole, and warfarin sodium (under dosage).

Increased INR. Excess oral anticoagulant. INR is also increased by conditions that increase PT. Concomitant administration of warfarin and erlotinib. Herbs or natural remedies include *dan shen* ('red-ginseng,' *Salvia miltiorrhiza*), *dang gui* (variants: *tangkuei*, *dong quai, Angelica sinensis*) (in clients receiving warfarin concurrently), feverfew, garlic, *Ginkgo biloba*, ginseng, and ginger. See warfarin interactions with herbals under Factors That Affect Results, below.

Decreased PT. Arterial occlusion, deep vein thrombosis, edema, hereditary coumarin resistance, hyperlipemia, hyperthyroidism, hypothyroidism, multiple myeloma, myocardial infarction, peripheral vascular disease, pulmonary embolism, spinal cord injury, thromboembolism (acute), and transplant rejection. Drugs include adrenocortical steroids, alcohol, aminoglutethimide, antacids, antihistamines, barbiturates, carbamazepine, chloral hydrate, chlordiazepoxide, cholestyramine, diuretics, ethchlorvynol, glutethimide, griseofulvin, haloperidol, meprobamate, nafcillin, oral contraceptives, paraldehyde, primidone, ranitidine, rifampin, sucralfate, trazodone, vitamin C, and warfarin sodium (underdosage).

Decreased INR. Insufficient oral anticoagulant. INR is also decreased by conditions and drugs that decrease PT.

Description. Prothrombin is a vitamin K–dependent glycoprotein produced by the liver that is necessary for firm fibrin clot formation. It converts to thrombin in the clotting-cascade process and should not appear in the serum after clot formation. Prothrombin time (PT) measures the amount of time taken for clot formation after reagent tissue thromboplastin (brain tissue extract) and calcium are added to citrated plasma. PT is used to monitor response to warfarin therapy or to screen for dysfunction involving the extrinsic system resulting from liver disease, vitamin

K deficiency, factor deficiency, or DIC. The most accurate PT values are reported as the number of seconds taken for the client's plasma to form a clot along with the number of seconds taken for a laboratory control sample to clot. Very small PT fluctuations can have profound physiologic effects. The PT is usually not prolonged until factors (II, V, VII, X) are decreased or less than 50% of normal or the fibrinogen is decreased to less than 80-100 mg/dL.

Because individual responses to same-dose warfarin anticoagulant therapy vary, the efficacy and safety of management are dependent on maintaining the anticoagulant effect within a defined therapeutic range. The INR improves the usability of the PT test in monitoring response to anticoagulation therapy. Since 1977 the World Health Organization (WHO) has advocated that all PT results be reported as an INR, which is the PT ratio that would result if the sample was tested with WHO international standard reference thromboplastin reagent. The standardization guidelines of the WHO state that freshly prepared specimens from 20 normal individuals and 60 clients receiving coumarin must be used to calibrate the International Sensitivity Index (ISI). An ISI number is assigned to each thromboplastin reagent that is used in mathematically calculating the INR to correct for varying thromboplastin sensitivities: The INR is calculated when the observed PT ratio is raised to the power of the ISI specific to the particular thromboplastin reagent used, or:

$$INR = (Client's\ PT\ in\ seconds)^{ISI} / (Mean\ normal\ PT\ in\ seconds)$$

Circumstances	Recommended INR Frequency
5-mg loading dose* of Coumadin	Baseline prior After 24 hours of therapy, then 2-4 times per week until steady levels are obtained.
Ongoing Coumadin therapy	Every 4-6 weeks. Lidstone et al (2000) found it safe to extend intervals between INR testing to 14 weeks in clients with a wide INR target range of 3-4.5.

*The literature contains several studies that demonstrate that using 5-mg instead of 10-mg loading doses of Coumadin is as effective in reaching a therapeutic INR between 2.0 and 3.0 by day 4-5, but poses less incidence of over-anticoagulation.

Professional Considerations

Consent form NOT required.

Preparation

1. Baseline PT should be drawn before anti-coagulant therapy is started.
2. Tube: 2.7-mL or 4.5-mL blue topped tube, a control tube, and a waste tube or syringe.
3. Do NOT draw specimens during hemodialysis.
4. Screen client for the use of herbal preparations or medicines or natural remedies. See #6 under Factors That Affect Results, below.
5. See Client and Family Teaching.

Procedure

1. Perform venipuncture (do not leave tourniquet on >1 minute, avoid traumatic stick) and withdraw 2 mL of blood into a syringe or vacuum tube. Remove the syringe or tube, leaving the needle in place.
2. Attach a second syringe and completely fill a blue topped tube with a blood sample collected without trauma. The sample quantity should be 2.4 mL for a 2.7-mL tube and 4.0 mL for a 4.5-mL tube.
3. A 9:1 ratio of blood to citrate is critical.
4. Gently tilt the tube several times to thoroughly mix the specimen.

Postprocedure Care

1. Write the specimen collection time on the laboratory requisition.
2. Send the specimen to the laboratory immediately. Results take about 1 hour, if the test is performed immediately.
3. The specimen should be refrigerated until testing. Testing should be performed within 12-18 hours.
4. In the presence of a coagulation defect, the venipuncture site should have digital direct pressure to the site for 3-5 minutes after the needle is removed. The venipuncture site should be observed for bleeding or excessive ecchymosis.

Client and Family Teaching

1. Abstain from coffee and alcohol for 24 hours before the test.
2. Follow normal dietary patterns for vitamin K–containing foods during the 24 hours before the test.
3. Oral anticoagulant medication should be taken at the same time daily. Regular PT checks may be required for clients on long-term anticoagulant medication.
4. Report any unusual bleeding.
5. Women of childbearing age should be advised to avoid pregnancy when oral anticoagulation is being used, because warfarin is teratogenic and can cause fetal death. Heparin, which does not cross the placenta, should be used if pregnancy is desired.
6. Warfarin enters breast milk. Women should not breast-feed when taking warfarin.
7. Many herbs can interfere with Coumadin's effects. For this reason, do not take any herbal preparations or natural remedies without receiving your doctor's approval.
8. It is important to keep taking the same brand of warfarin, if prescribed, because changing brands can alter the anticoagulation effect and INR.

Factors That Affect Results

1. Reject specimens if:
   a. Hemolyzed.
   b. Lipemic.
   c. Received more than 3 hours after collection.
   d. Collection tubes are incompletely filled.
   e. Not promptly transported to the laboratory.
   f. Not refrigerated.
2. Concurrent therapy with heparin can lengthen PT for up to 5 hours after dosing. To minimize this influence, blood for PT determinations should be drawn 5 hours after IV heparin and 24 hours after subcutaneous heparin injection. Concurrent therapy with warfarin and fluoxetine can cause a slightly increased PT and delayed normalization.
3. The problem of loss of accuracy of the INR system can be resolved by the use of sensitive thromboplastins with ISI values close to 1.0 (WHO reagent ISI = 1.0). However, even without this sensitivity, the INR system has been shown to be more accurate than reporting the results as a PT ratio.

4. The use of automated clot detectors requires the use of sensitive thromboplastins or calibration of each new batch of thromboplastins with lyophilized plasmas with certified INR values obtained by the manual method to obtain valid and reliable results. ("True" INR values were obtained by the manual method.)

5. It is recommended that reagents insensitive to heparin be used to avoid obtaining falsely elevated INRs when a client is receiving heparin and Coumadin concurrently. Innovin and Thromboplastin C Plus meet this criterion.

6. Herbs or natural remedies that have a synergistic effect with warfarin to prolong bleeding include *dan shen* (*Salvia miltiorrhiza*), *dang gui* (variants: *tangkuei, dong quai, Angelica sinensis*), *chuan xiong* (*ch'uanhsiung, Ligusticum chuanxiong* or *L. wallichii, Cnidium,* or *Conioselinum universatutum*), papaya (*Carica papaya*), *tao ren* (*Prunus persica* and *P. davidiana,* Semen Persicae, peach seed), *hong hua* (safflower, *Carthamus tinctorius*), and *shui zhi* (leech, *Hirudo* and *Whitmania*).

7. Antibiotic therapy, mineral oil, and clofibrate can affect the PT.

8. Diets excessively high in green, leafy vegetables can increase the absorption of vitamin K, which shortens the PT.

9. Intake of alcohol within 48 hours before the test can falsely decrease the INR.

10. Intake of the herb coffee (*Coffea*) within 48 hours before the test can falsely decrease the INR.

11. A minimum of 100 g/dL of fibrinogen must be present for the PT to be accurate.

12. The PT is affected by many pharmacologic agents, including those that alter protein-binding patterns, those that inhibit the formation of intestinal microorganisms, and those that are precursors of enzyme production.

13. Contamination of the specimen with tissue thromboplastin may alter the results. This is the reason for the double-draw technique.

14. 33% of INR values are falsely elevated due to poor blood drawing techniques (Froom and Barak, 2010).

Other Data

1. PT/INR should be measured frequently: daily × 5 when treatment is initiated, twice a week the following 1-2 weeks, once a week for the next 1-2 months, and every 2-4 weeks thereafter. Also, PT/INR should be performed whenever a drug that interacts with warfarin is added to or deleted from the regimen.

2. The INR system is invalid in clients with liver disease (different reagents do not give the same INR for the same sample) but is no less valid than the PT in this client population.

3. The PT should be evaluated daily and used as a basis for dose adjustments during initial anticoagulation therapy.

4. A time interval of 16-48 hours may occur before warfarin affects the PT value.

5. A PT >30 seconds places the client at risk for hemorrhage.

6. Home testing kits are now available for clients on warfarin therapy.

7. Portable bedside INR testing is not recommended for anticoagulated clients.

8. The American Society of Regional Anesthesia and Pain Medicine recommend that epidural catheters be removed with INR ≤1.4.

9. Dabigatran etexilate (Pradax, Pradaxa, Prazaxa) is an oral capsule blood thinner (direct thrombin inhibitor with predictable pharmacokinetics) that replaces Coumadin (FDA approved 2010). Half-life is 12-17 hours and largely eliminated in the urine. Usual dose is 150 mg twice daily or 75 mg BID if creatine clearance 15-30 mL/min. It is more effective, easier to use but should be used in caution on person taking Amiodarone, quinidine, rifampin or verapamil. Uses include stroke prevention for clients with atrial fibrillation; ACS, chronic thromboembolic pulmonary hypertension, mechanical heart valve recipients, recurrent DVT, and venous thromboembolic disease. It has lower rates of DVT and also lower rates of stroke compared to use of warfarin in patients with a-fib. PT/INR is NOT sensitive to dabigatran and these tests should not be used in patients on this medication.

10. Rivaroxaban (Xarelto® by J&J) is an oral tablet (FDA approved 2011) that reduces blood clots by blocking factor Xa in

patients undergoing knee and hip surgery and fore prevention of DVT. No routine monitoring of PT, PTT, or INR required. Drug interactions include amiodarone, aspirin, clopidogrel, quinidine, NSAIDS, verapamil.

Protoporphyrin, Free Erythrocyte—Blood
Norm.

		SI Units
Piomelli Method		
Adult female	19-52 mg/dL	0.34-0.92 µmol/L
Adult male	11-45 mg/dL	0.20-0.80 µmol/L
Hematofluorometer		
Adult female	<40 mg/dL	0.71 µmol/L
Adult male	<30 mg/dL	0.53 µmol/L
Panic level	>190 mg/dL	>3.38 µmol/L
Erythrocyte Precursor		
Protoporphyrin	4-52 mg/dL	0.07-0.92 µmol/L

Increased. Cancer, diabetes mellitus, erythropoiesis, erythropoietic protoporphyria (>2200 mg/dL), hemolytic anemia (>50 mg/dL), infection (>50 mg/dL), iron deficiency (>200 mg/dL), lead poisoning (>200 mg/dL), protoporphyria, psoriasis, sideroachrestic anemia (acquired) (>50 mg/dL), and thalassemia.

Decreased. Megaloblastic anemia (<30 mg/dL).

Description. Protoporphyrin is a derivative of porphin that combines with iron to form the heme portion of hemoglobin and constitutes the predominant porphyrin in red blood cells (RBCs). After hemoglobin breakdown, protoporphyrin is converted into bilirubin, combines with albumin, and remains unconjugated in the circulation.

In conditions interfering with heme synthesis, increased amounts of protoporphyrin can be detected in erythrocytes, urine, and stool. Protoporphyria is an autosomal dominant disorder in which increased amounts of protoporphyrin are secreted and excreted. It is believed to be caused by an enzyme deficiency and is detected by the identification of increased concentrations of protoporphyrin in RBCs. Protoporphyria causes photosensitivity and may lead to cirrhosis and cholelithiasis because of protoporphyrin deposition. The free erythrocyte protoporphyrin (FEP) test measures the concentration of protoporphyrin in RBCs.

Professional Considerations
Consent form NOT required.

Preparation
1. Write the current hematocrit value on the laboratory requisition.
2. If this test is being used for evaluation of lead intoxication, a blood sample for lead measurement should also be obtained.
3. Tube: Green topped, lavender topped, or black topped.
4. Do NOT draw specimens during hemodialysis.

Procedure
1. Draw a 3-mL blood sample, without hemolysis.
2. Capillary tube samples from pediatric heelsticks are acceptable. (See notation regarding infant testing in #2 under Factors That Affect Results.)

Postprocedure Care
1. Protect specimens from light.

Client and Family Teaching
1. Because protoporphyria is a hereditary disease, genetic counseling may be advised.
2. Inform the client of lead poisoning detection and prevention.

Factors That Affect Results
1. Hemolysis of the specimen invalidates the results.
2. This test is considered to be unreliable in infants less than 6 months of age.

Other Data

1. This test can be used to screen for elevated lead in children after iron deficiency is ruled out.

2. See also Porphyrins, Quantitative—Blood; Coproporphyrin—Urine.

Protriptyline

See Tricyclic Antidepressants—Plasma or Serum.

PSA

See Prostate-Specific Antigen—Serum.

PSA Density

See Prostate-Specific Antigen—Serum.

PSA Fractionation

See Prostate-Specific Antigen—Serum.

PSA Velocity

See Prostate-Specific Antigen—Serum.

PSAV

See Prostate-Specific Antigen—Serum.

P-Selectin—Plasma

Norm. sP-selectin: 0.6-10 ng/mL.

Usage. Being developed for use in helping to identify a myocardial origin of chest pain symptoms earlier than other markers available. Also being tested for its use as a first trimester marker for risk for preeclampsia.

Increased. Acute coronary syndromes, acute lung injury, acute myocardial infarction (AMI), acute respiratory distress syndrome (ARDS) with potential for DIC, angina, arthritis (rheumatoid), connective tissue diseases, coronary spasm, diabetes mellitus, Graves' disease, *H. pylori*, inflammatory bowel disease (active), metabolic syndrome, polycystic ovary syndrome (PCOS), postsplenectomy associated with splenic portal vein thrombosis, posttraumatic stress disorder (PTSD), preeclampsia (severe), psoriasis, stent thrombosis predictor post PCI day 10, surgical trauma, thrombosis (arterial).

Description. P-selectin is a glycoprotein that exists in two forms—a soluble protein (sP-selectin) and bound to platelets and endothelial cells—and is thought to help modulate platelet-leukocyte-endothelial activity during acute coronary syndromes and during inflammatory activity. P-selectin is thought to be a marker for platelet activation because it exists only on platelets that have undergone the release action and is involved with leukocytes on endothelial tissue, and levels increase within minutes of triggers. Levels of both the soluble and bound forms of P-selectin have been found to be elevated in clients with acute coronary syndromes, and so it is possible that P-selectin levels may serve as a coronary marker. The P-selectin profile measures both soluble and bound forms of the glycoprotein via enzyme immunoassay. While the sensitivity of this test is more than 90%, the specificity for chest pain is currently only about 55%. This is because many other noncardiac causes of chest pain also involve inflammatory processes that trigger increases in P-selectin level.

Professional Considerations
Consent form NOT required.

Preparation
1. Tube: 2.7-mL or 4.5-mL blue topped tube, a control tube, and a waste tube or syringe.
2. Do NOT draw specimens during hemodialysis.

Procedure
1. Perform venipuncture and withdraw 2 mL of blood into a syringe or vacuum tube. Remove the syringe or tube, leaving the needle in place.
2. Attach a second syringe and completely fill a blue topped tube with a blood sample collected without trauma. The sample quantity should be 2.4 mL for a 2.7-mL tube and 4.0 mL for a 4.5-mL tube.
3. A 9:1 ratio of blood to citrate is critical.
4. Gently tilt the tube several times to thoroughly mix the specimen.

Postprocedure Care
1. Write the specimen collection time on the laboratory requisition.
2. Send the specimen to the laboratory immediately.

Client and Family Teaching
1. None.

Factors That Affect Results
1. Lower levels on serial measurements may indicate depletion.
2. Aspirin has been found experimentally to decrease levels more than warfarin.
3. One study found that drinking five cups of black tea per day lowered levels of plasma P-selectin.

Other Data
1. Heparin does not affect P-selectin levels.

Pseudocholinesterase (Cholinesterase, Cholinesterase II, CHS, PCHE)—Plasma

Norm. Norms vary, depending on the laboratory substrate test method.

		SI Units
RID method	0.5-1.5 mg/dL	5-15 mg/L
DuPont ACA method	7-19 U/mL	7-19 kU/L
Other methods	3.0-8.0 U/mL	
	8-18 IU/L	3200-6600 IU/L
	0.5-1.3 pH U/hour	
	2900-7100 U/L	
Female	204-500 IU/dL	
Male	274-532 IU/dL	
Dibucaine inhibition	81%-87%	0.81-0.87
	2900-7100 U/L	
Fluoride inhibition	44%-54%	0.44-0.54

Increased. Diabetes mellitus, hyperthyroidism, insecticide exposure of organic phosphates, leprosy, nephrotic syndrome, and radiation therapy.

Decreased. Acute burns, anemia (severe pernicious, aplastic), burns, carcinomatosis, cardiopulmonary bypass, cirrhosis, congenital deficiency, congestive heart failure (causing liver disease), dermatomyositis, HELLP syndrome, hepatic carcinoma (metastatic), hepatitis (infectious), hypoproteinemia, infections (acute), infectious mononucleosis, insecticide exposure (carbamate, organophosphate), jaundice (obstructive), malignancy, malnutrition, metastasis, muscular dystrophy, myocardial infarction, organophosphate insecticide poisoning

(DFP, parathion, sarin, tricresyl phosphate), parenchymatous liver disease, pregnancy, pseudocholinesterase deficiency, recent plasmapheresis, renal disease, shock, skin diseases, succinylcholine hypersensitivity, tuberculosis, and uremia. Drugs include aspirin, cocaine, cyclophosphamide, echothiophate eyedrops, estrogens, MAOIs, metoclopramide, morphine sulfate, neostigmine bromide, neostigmine methylsulfate, oral contraceptives, phospholine iodine, physostigmine salicylate, physostigmine sulfate, and pyridostigmine bromide.

Description. Pseudocholinesterase (PCHE) is a nonspecific cholinesterase that hydrolyzes noncholine esters as well as acetylcholine. It exists in several forms and serves to inactivate acetylcholine. PCHE is synthesized by the liver and found in plasma and is well distributed throughout the body though not found in RBCs. This enzyme's activity is inhibited reversibly by carbamate insecticides and irreversibly by organophosphate insecticides. Clients with an inherited PCHE deficiency exhibit an increased sensitivity to the effects of succinylcholine, which is normally inactivated by PCHE. There is no cure for pseudocholinesterase deficiency. Inherited deficiencies can be detected by the identification of abnormal genotypes of PCHE through dibucaine and fluoride inhibition tests. Although normal forms of PCHE are inhibited by these substances, the abnormal forms are not. Inherited type is an autosomal recessive trait located on BChE gene of long arm 3 at 3q26.1-26.2. There are also 65 inherited variants resulting in apnea to paralysis.

Professional Considerations
Consent form NOT required.

Preparation
1. Tube: Red topped or green topped.
2. Specimens MAY be drawn during hemodialysis.
3. See Client and Family Teaching.

Procedure
1. Draw a 5-mL blood sample without trauma.

Postprocedure Care
1. If the test purpose is to screen for organophosphate insecticide poisoning, the sample should be transported to the laboratory for immediate spinning and refrigeration. For other purposes, serum samples remain stable at room temperature for up to 1 week, refrigerated for 2 weeks, and frozen for up to 3 months.

Client and Family Teaching
1. Ten percent of the population may carry the gene for an uncommon form of PCHE.
2. Elevated results may indicate exposure to organophosphates, and the source would need to be identified.
3. If the test is inhibition by dibucaine with fluoride, the client should not have taken muscle relaxants or anticholinergic drugs within 24 hours.

Factors That Affect Results
1. Hemolysis of the specimen causes falsely elevated results.
2. Pregnancy decreases values by 30%.
3. Exposure of the sample to chemicals such as fluoride, citrate, and borate will cause falsely decreased results.

Other Data
1. A 20% drop in PCHE activity between baseline value and subsequent samples indicates overexposure to organophosphate insecticides.
2. PCHE (pseudocholinesterase) is not to be confused with acetylcholinesterase (true cholinesterase, cholinesterase I, AcCHS).
3. PCHE levels are an earlier indicator of organophosphate exposure than acetylcholinesterase levels.
4. Normal level means no detectable cancer and is a prognostic biomarker.

Psittacosis Titer—Blood
See **Chlamydia Culture and Group Titer**—Specimen.

PTH
See *Parathyroid* Hormone—Blood.

PTT

See Activated Partial Thromboplastin Time and Partial Thromboplastin Time—Plasma.

Pulmonary Angiogram (Pulmonary Angiography, Pulmonary Arteriography)—Diagnostic

Norm. Radiopaque iodine contrast material should circulate symmetrically and without interruption through the pulmonary circulatory system.

Usage. Visualization of the size and shape of the pulmonary artery, its branches, and the pulmonary vascular bed; measurements of pressures within these structures, cardiac output, and pulmonary vascular resistance; assessment of pulmonary vascular perfusion defects, including aneurysms, blood vessel displacement, stenosis, thrombi, and vascular filling defects; definitive diagnostic test for pulmonary thromboembolism, in the symptomatic client and in clients at risk on anticoagulation therapy and when lung scans are normal or inconclusive; definitive test for lung torsion; and evaluation of the pulmonary circulatory system preoperatively in clients with congenital heart disease and for evaluation of snoring associated with obstructive sleep apnea.

Description. Pulmonary angiography is an invasive roentgenographic, fluoroscopic procedure after injection of iodine radiopaque contrast material via a catheter inserted through an antecubital or femoral vein into the pulmonary artery or one of its branches. Recurrence rates of pulmonary embolism are low if a normal result is found.

Professional Considerations

Consent form IS required.

Risks

Acute pulmonary hypertension, acute renal failure (related to the presence of contrast material), arterial occlusion, dysrhythmias, embolism, hemorrhage, infection, allergic reaction to dye (itching, hives, rash, tight feeling in the throat, shortness of breath, bronchospasm, anaphylaxis, death), perforation of pulmonary artery or myocardium, renal toxicity from contrast medium, venous occlusion, ventricular dysrhythmias.

Contraindications

Previous allergy to iodine, radiographic dye, or shellfish; pregnancy (because of radioactive iodine crossing the blood-placental barrier); renal insufficiency. Sedatives are contraindicated in clients with central nervous system depression.

Preparation

1. Recent coagulation times, platelet count, and renal function should be noted.
2. A mild sedative may be prescribed.
3. Establish intravenous access for use in the event of a hypersensitivity or dysrhythmic complication.
4. Obtain electrocardiographic patches, surgical scrub solution, povidone-iodine solution, sterile drapes, 1%-2% lidocaine (Xylocaine), radiopaque contrast material, a pulmonary artery catheter, and a pulmonary angiography tray. The amount of contrast dye used is based on the client's body weight.
5. Have an emergency cart readily available.
6. See Client and Family Teaching.
7. Just before beginning the procedure, take a "time out" to verify the correct client, procedure, and site.

Procedure

1. The client is placed in the supine position. Electrodes are connected to a cardiac monitor.
2. The femoral or antecubital vein site is cleansed with surgical scrub solution followed by povidone-iodine solution, and the area is then covered with sterile drapes.
3. After a local anesthetic is injected over the site, a needle puncture is made into the vein, a guidewire is placed through the needle, and a long catheter is introduced over the wire through the antecubital or femoral vein and advanced into the pulmonary vasculature. Pressures are measured as the catheter passes through the

right atrium, right ventricle, and into the pulmonary artery.

4. As the contrast material (e.g., 150 mg iodine/mL) is injected, rapid, serial roentgenographic images or films record the circulation of the dye through the pulmonary vasculature.

5. Monitor the client throughout the procedure for cardiac dysrhythmias or a hypersensitivity reaction to the contrast material.

6. The catheter is removed, and a pressure dressing is applied over the insertion site.

Postprocedure Care

1. Monitor the catheter insertion site for bleeding, inflammation, or hematoma formation.

2. Assess vital signs according to institutional protocol (usually every 15 minutes × 4 and then every 4 hours × 4).

3. Although hypersensitivity reactions usually occur during the first 30 minutes after injection of radiopaque iodine, a delayed reaction is possible.

4. Resume previous diet.

5. No blood pressures should be taken from the extremity used for injection for 24 hours.

Client and Family Teaching

1. Fast for 8 hours before the procedure.

2. For 5 minutes after the injection of the contrast material, an urge to cough, flushing, nausea, or salty taste may occur.

3. The client must lie motionless during the procedure.

Factors That Affect Results

1. The client must be able to lie motionless during the procedure.

Other Data

1. Small peripheral emboli may not be visible with angiography, but these rarely produce symptoms or result in the usual outcomes of embolism.

2. Pulmonary embolism is best diagnosed with computed tomographic angiogram (CTA).

3. Right ventricular dilatation of CT pulmonary angiogram is a predictor of 30-day mortality in acute pulmonary embolism.

Pulmonary Arteriography

See **Pulmonary Angiogram**—Diagnostic.

Pulmonary Artery Catheterization—Diagnostic

Norm.

Adult Pressures	
Right atrial (RA) pressure	3-11 mm Hg
Central venous pressure (CVP)	2-6 mm Hg (2.7-12 cm H_2O)
Right ventricular systolic pressure (RVSP)	20-30 mm Hg
Right ventricular end-diastolic pressure (RVEDP)	<5 mm Hg
Pulmonary artery systolic (PAS) pressure	20-30 mm Hg
Pulmonary artery end-diastolic pressure (PAEDP)	8-15 mm Hg
Pulmonary artery mean (PAM) pressure	<20 mm Hg
Pulmonary artery wedge pressure (PAWP) or pulmonary capillary wedge pressure (PCWP)	4-12 mm Hg
Cardiac output (CO)	5-8 L/minute
Cardiac index	2.5-3.5 L/minute/m²
Pulmonary vascular resistance	80-240 dyne/second/cm⁻⁵
Systemic vascular resistance	800-1300 dyne/second/cm⁻⁵

Usage. Assessment, diagnosis, and evaluation of the effects of therapy on right and left ventricular function; measurement of cardiac output and cardiac and pulmonary pressures; access to central venous blood and mixed venous blood samples; monitoring of mixed venous oxygen saturation (SvO_2); temporary atrial, ventricular, or atrioventricular sequential pacing by means of a thermodilution pulmonary arterial pacing catheter; and preoperative, intraoperative, and postoperative uses, including monitoring of high-risk clients (those with a history of angina, cardiopulmonary disease, or potential fluid shifts during surgery), elderly clients, and high or low cardiac output states, and in situations when hypotensive anesthesia is used. Indications for pulmonary artery catheterization include acute myocardial infarction, angina (severe), burns (severe), cardiomyopathy, congestive heart failure, cardiac tamponade, intraoperative cardiac collapse, failure to respond to appropriate resuscitative measures, fluid-related hypotension and hypovolemia, intravascular control problems, noncardiogenic pulmonary edema, pulmonary congestive states, pulmonary edema, pulmonary failure, pulmonary hypertension, renal disease, right and left ventricular failure, shock states (cardiogenic, hypovolemic, septic, traumatic with concomitant heart failure), tissue perfusion (altered), and titration of chronotropic, inotropic, or vasoactive pharmacologic agents.

Description. Pulmonary artery (PA) catheterization is an invasive procedure using a radiopaque polyvinyl chloride, flow-directed, balloon-tipped catheter containing fluid-filled proximal, distal, and thermistor lumens and a balloon inflation lumen with a valve. Proper placement of the catheter in the PA, in the lower one third of the lung (zone 3), where venous pressures are greater than alveolar pressure, allows for measurement of CVP, PAS, PAEDP, PAM, and PAWP pressures. Intermittent occlusion of the PA branch by inflation of the balloon tip with air or carbon dioxide (never fluid) temporarily impedes blood flow from the right side of the heart to the lungs. The mitral valve opens during diastole, permitting the distal part of the catheter to record pressure that is reflected backward through the left atrium and pulmonary capillary bed. Identical pressures in the left ventricle, left atrium, and pulmonary vasculature momentarily occur during diastole and are captured as the PAWP when the balloon is inflated.

Professional Considerations

Consent form MAY be required.

Preparation

1. Cardiac assessment for history of complete left bundle branch block is indicated before insertion of a PA catheter because there is slight risk for developing a right bundle branch block during catheter insertion, resulting in complete heart block. Standby external transcutaneous pacemaker, insertion of temporary pacemaker, or use of a pacing thermodilution PA catheter can be used for those at risk for this complication.

2. Assemble and prepare monitoring equipment according to institutional protocol. This includes the following:
   a. Program the monitor for PA pressure display.
   b. Prepare a transducer with high-pressure tubing for hemodynamic monitoring and a pressure bag of normal saline or heparin flush solution according to institutional protocol.
   c. Balance the transducer at the phlebostatic axis (the level of the client's right atrium, the fourth intercostal space at the midaxillary line).

3. Have an emergency cart on standby. Have lidocaine (100 mg) for intravenous use at the bedside in the event of sustained ventricular tachycardia caused by catheter irritation of the right ventricle.

4. Obtain povidone-iodine solution, sterile drapes, 1%-2% lidocaine (Xylocaine), introducer (sheath, Cordis) trays, a pulmonary artery catheter tray, and 0.9% saline or heparin flush solution.

5. The physician(s) performing the procedure should wear the following: a sterile gown, a sterile mask, a cap, and sterile gloves.

6. The procedure may be performed at the bedside or under fluoroscopy.

Procedure

1. The PA catheter may be inserted percutaneously into the external or internal jugular veins, femoral or subclavian veins, and the antecubital fossa veins by venous cutdown.

2. The client is placed in the supine position. For subclavian or internal jugular insertions, the head of the bed is lowered slightly into a shallow Trendelenburg position. The flat supine position is preferred; however, if not tolerated by the

client, a low semi-Fowler's position is acceptable, provided that the same position is maintained throughout the procedure.

3. Electrocardiographic monitoring is performed throughout the procedure.

4. After the site is cleansed with povidone-iodine solution and allowed to dry, it is covered with sterile drapes.

5. A protective sleeve is placed over the PA catheter, and the catheter is flushed with sterile 0.9% saline or heparin flush solution (heparin 100 U/mL of 0.9% saline). The balloon at the distal end of the PA catheter is tested for proper inflation and integrity by injection of 1-1.5 cc of air into the PA distal injection port.

6. The PA distal port is connected to the transducer tubing and a paper printout of the PA tracing is started and run continuously throughout the catheter insertion.

7. The site is anesthetized with 1%-2% lidocaine. For subclavian or internal jugular (IJ) insertions, the Seldinger technique is used as follows: The vessel is cannulated with a 22- or 25-gauge needle (IJ insertions only; subclavian insertions omit this step). A large-bore needle is inserted over the small needle, and the small needle is removed. A guidewire is inserted through the large-bore needle, and that needle is removed. The introducer is then inserted over the guidewire, and the guidewire is removed. The introducer is then secured into place.

8. The PA catheter is inserted through the introducer and directed into the right atrium and through the tricuspid valve into the right ventricle. As the catheter traverses the right ventricle, the balloon at the distal portion of the catheter is inflated to permit normal cardiac blood flow to carry (float) the catheter through the pulmonic valve into the PA. Inflation of the balloon and flow-direction minimize the potential of catheter-induced ventricular dysrhythmias and irritability. However, the risk for ventricular tachycardia is greatest while the PA catheter tip is passing through the right ventricle. If ventricular tachycardia occurs, the catheter should be either advanced through the pulmonary valve or withdrawn into the right atrium. Lidocaine and emergency measures are seldom needed because the removal of the catheter as a ventricular irritant is usually sufficient to stop the tachycardia.

9. As the catheter is slowly inserted, placement and progress are assessed by observation of the monitor for the waveform and pressure changes characteristic of the different chambers and vessels of the cardiac and pulmonary anatomy. When the waveform changes from a PA waveform to a PAWP waveform, the balloon is allowed to deflate, and the catheter is secured into this position. The syringes of flush solution are removed, and the ports are either connected to a continuous flush solution or capped, according to the policy of the institution.

Postprocedure Care

1. Apply an occlusive sterile dressing to the PA catheter insertion site.

2. Obtain a chest radiograph for verification of the catheter placement if fluoroscopy has not been used.

3. PA pressures should be monitored continuously. The waveform should be frequently observed for progression of the catheter tip into a wedge position.

Client and Family Teaching

1. If the access is subclavian or jugular, the head will be covered with a sterile drape during the procedure.

2. Activity may be limited during the time a PA catheter is in place.

Factors That Affect Results

1. The mechanical factors that invalidate pressure measurements include the following:

   a. *Air bubbles* in pressure tubing system or transducer cause dampening of the waveform.

   b. *Kinking of pressure tubing* causes dampening of the waveform.

   c. Improper tubing length: Tubing should not exceed 48 inches in length from the client to the transducer.

   d. *Loose connections* interfere with the high-pressure pathway along the tubing and may cause waveform artifact and false readings.

   e. *Stopcocks* between the transducer and the PA distal port distort PA pressures slightly, but effects increase with an increased number of stopcocks. For this reason, use no more than one stopcock for ports through which pressures are monitored.

f. *Blood return* in the transducer tubing. The continual flush–counteracting pressure should be maintained at 300 mm Hg.

g. *Catheter artifact* (catheter whip, catheter fling) results from excessive catheter movement during cardiac contraction when the distal tip of the catheter is too close to the pulmonary valve.

h. *Catheter displacement* may result from backward recoil into the right ventricle as evidenced by large RV waveforms. It may also result from forward migration into a wedged position.

i. *Migration of the catheter against the vessel wall* may cause a dampened waveform and affect pressure readings. Repositioning the client or asking the client to cough may help to return the tip to a floating position. The catheter should never be flushed if a spontaneous wedge position is suspected.

j. *Flush solution rate* affects pressure readings. Clot formation near the distal port as a result of too slow a flush rate dampens the waveform and causes falsely low readings. Falsely high readings may result from a flush rate >3-6 mL/hour.

k. *Incorrect transducer position* below the phlebostatic axis causes falsely low pressure readings. A transducer higher than the phlebostatic axis causes falsely high pressure readings. Each 1-cm difference alters the reading by 1 mm Hg.

l. *Malfunction of equipment*, which may include the amplifier, the oscilloscope, the recording devices, or the transducer.

m. *Positive-pressure mechanical ventilation* (PEEP) elevates pressures slightly. Formulas are available to compensate for this effect. PEEP should never be discontinued to obtain pressure readings because the discontinuation has been shown to be deleterious to the client's condition.

n. *Overinflation of the balloon* results in inflation larger than what is necessary for the vessel size, recognized by a drifting up or down of the PAWP waveform. Overinflation may cause rupture of the pulmonary capillary. Air should be injected into the balloon very slowly while one continuously watches for a waveform change to a wedge position. Proper placement of the PA catheter is indicated when a PAWP waveform is obtained with 0.8-1.2 cc of air. At no time should more than 1.5 cc of air be injected into the balloon. Assessment or adjustment of PA catheter placement by a physician is indicated if a PAWP waveform cannot be obtained with ≥1.5 cc of air.

o. *A ruptured balloon* is indicated when one feels no resistance to air injection into the balloon port, along with an absence of a PAWP waveform, or by the presence of blood in the PA distal (balloon) port. Balloon rupture may result from a manufacturing defect or from balloon weakening after many inflations. Manual deflation may accelerate balloon weakening. If a ruptured balloon is suspected, no more air should be injected, and a physician should immediately assess the client.

p. *Respiratory variation* as a result of inspiration and expiration cannot be accounted for by digital averaging. The most accurate readings of pressures are calculated manually from paper recordings of the waveforms at end expiration.

q. *Retrograde injection* during cardiac output measurement is indicated when a backflow of blood or fluid is detected in the introducer or protective sleeve of the catheter. This is an indication that the catheter injectate opening is located within the lumen of the introducer, rather than in the right atrium. Retrograde injection results in inadequate thermodilution and falsely high cardiac output values.

2. Physiologic conditions that alter pressure measurements of the different chambers and vessels include the following:

a. *RA/CVP*: Cardiac tamponade, fluid overload, pulmonary disease, pulmonary hypertension, right heart failure, tricuspid regurgitation, and tricuspid stenosis.

b. *RV*: Chronic congestive heart failure, constrictive pericarditis, pericardial effusion, pulmonary hypertension, pulmonary valvular stenosis, right ventricular failure, and ventricular septal defects.

c. *PAS/PAD*: Chronic obstructive pulmonary disease, increased pulmonary blood flow, left-to-right shunts secondary to atrial or ventricular septal defects, mitral stenosis, pulmonary edema, pulmonary embolus, and pulmonary hypertension.

d. *PAWP/PCWP*: Cardiac insufficiency, cardiac tamponade, left ventricular failure, mitral regurgitation, and mitral stenosis.

Other Data

1. Transducers should be balanced every 2-4 hours with position and ventilator changes and before each measurement of PA catheter parameters.

2. PA catheter balloons should never be manually deflated. The air should be allowed to flow back into the syringe spontaneously.

3. The flexible PA catheter includes two-lumen, three-lumen, four-lumen thermo dilutional, and five-lumen catheters of varying lengths. Sizes include 5, 6, 7, and 7.5 Fr, with markings at 10-cm increments along the outer surface.

4. Although the information obtained from the pulmonary artery catheter can help diagnose certain conditions, a meta-analysis routine perioperative use in vascular surgery and a study of use of continuous SvO_2 monitoring during cardiac surgery have not consistently been shown to reduce morbidity and mortality.

5. Later generations of catheter development include the capability for atrial, ventricular, or AV sequential pacing; continuous mixed venous oxygen saturation (SvO_2); continuous cardiac output; using fiberoptic oximetry; and additional lumens or ports for fluid infusions.

Pulmonary Function Tests (PFT)—Diagnostic

Norm. The observed values are reported as percentages of normal with use of prediction equations calculated according to age, height, sex, race, and weight. Results are considered abnormal if they are less than predicted 80% of the calculated values. For spirometry measurement, forced vital capacity, forced expiratory volumes, and peak expiratory flow rates are at predicted value for age, race, sex, and height.

Volume	Average Results for Adults
Tidal volume (V_T)	500 cc
Expiratory reserve volume (ERV)	1500 cc
Residual volume (RV)	1500 cc
Inspiratory reserve volume (IRV)	2000 cc
Diffusion capacity carbon monoxide	25 mL/min/mm Hg
Spirometry Norms	
Forced vital capacity (FVC)	>80% of predicted volume
Forced expiratory volume (FEV_1)	>80% of predicted volume
FEV_1/FVC ratio	>80%
Elderly clients	70%-80%
Forced expiratory flow (FEF) 25-75	>50%

Usage. Diagnosis and monitor the progress of pulmonary dysfunction (asthma, bronchitis, bronchiolitis obliterans, emphysema, and myasthenia gravis); quantify the severity of known lung disease; evaluate the effectiveness of medications (bronchodilators); determination of whether a functional abnormality is obstructive or restrictive;

identification of clients at high risk for post-operative pulmonary complications; evaluation of the risk of pulmonary resection; used in conjunction with a cardiopulmonary exercise stress test for evaluation of functional ability; serial measurements used to evaluate response to treatment in cardiopulmonary vascular disease.

Measurement	Increased	Decreased
Total Lung Capacity (TLC) = (V_T + ERV + RV + IRV) (Total volume of lungs when maximally inflated is divided into four volumes)	Overdistention of the lungs associated with obstructive disease	Restrictive disease
Tidal Volume (V_T) (Volume of air inhaled and exhaled in normal quiet breathing)	May indicate bronchiolar obstruction with hyperinflation or emphysema	May indicate fatigue, restrictive parenchymal lung disease, atelectasis, cancer, edema, pulmonary congestion, pneumothorax or thoracic tumor; decreased V_T necessitates further testing
Inspiratory Reserve Volume (IRV) (Maximum volume that can be inhaled after a normal quiet inhalation)	n/a	Decreased IRV as an isolated value does not indicate disease
Expiratory Reserve Volume (ERV) (Maximum volume that can be exhaled after a normal quiet exhalation)	n/a	May occur with obesity, pregnancy, or thoracoplasty
Residual Volume (RV) (Volume remaining in lungs after maximal exhalation)	Increased RV above 35% of the TLC indicates obstructive disease; RV is also increased with aging	n/a
Forced Expiratory Volume (FEV) (Volume expired during specified time intervals [0.5 and 1 second])	Restrictive disease	Decreased FEV_1 after administration of beta-blockers may indicate presence of bronchospasm and contraindicate continued use of specific pharmacologic therapy involved
Forced Expiratory Volume 1 (FEV_1) (Air volume forcefully exhaled in 1 second)	Restrictive disease	Decreased FEV_1 as percentage of vital capacity (FEV_1/FVC) indicates obstructive disease: 65%-80% of predicted = mild disease 50%-65% of predicted = moderate disease <50% of predicted = severe disease

Continued

Measurement	Increased	Decreased
Functional Residual Capacity (FRC) = (ERV + RV) (Amount of volume in lungs after normal exhalation)	Overdistention of lungs associated with chronic obstructive pulmonary disease Pulmonary cysts	Acute respiratory distress syndrome (ARDS) Heart failure Kyphoscoliosis Muscular weakness Pulmonary granulomatosis Restrictive diseases and mixed obstructive and restrictive diseases
Inspiratory Capacity (IC) = (IRV + V_T) (Maximum volume that can be inhaled after a normal quiet exhalation; useful in evaluating timeliness of weaning from mechanical ventilation)	n/a	Restrictive disease
Vital Capacity (VC) = (IRV + V_T + ERV) (Total volume that can be exhaled after maximum inspiration)	Increased or normal VC and FVC with decreased flow rates indicates obstructive defect (airway diseases)	Decreased VC with normal or increased flow rates indicates restrictive defect (diaphragmatic impairment, drug overdose, head injury, limited thoracic expansion, and neuromuscular disease)
Forced Vital Capacity (FVC) (Total volume exhaled forcefully and rapidly after maximum inhalation)	Increased or normal VC and FVC with decreased rates indicates obstructive defect (airway diseases)	With concurrent heart disease, may indicate pulmonary congestion, pleural effusion, cardiomegaly, or muscular weakness
Thoracic Gas Volume (TGV) (Total volume of lungs, including nonventilated and ventilated airways)	Indicates air trapping caused by obstructive disease and requires special equipment to monitor	n/a
Minute Volume (MV) = (Respiratory Rate × V_T) (Total amount of gas breathed during 1 minute)	Air embolism Bronchospasm Burns Hyperthyroidism Hypovolemia Metabolic or respiratory acidosis PEEP causing increased intrathoracic pressure Pulmonary embolism Pulmonary parenchymal disease Sepsis Shallow breathing Shock	n/a

Continued

Measurement	Increased	Decreased
Maximum Voluntary Ventilation (MVV) (Maximum volume of gas breathed during rapid, forced breathing in 1 minute under testing conditions)	n/a	Obstructive disease
Maximum Breathing Capacity (MBC) (Largest volume of air that can be inhaled and exhaled in 1 minute)	n/a	Obstructive disease
Peak Expiratory Flow Rate (PEFR) (Peak flow rate during expiration)	n/a	Asthma
FEV$_1$/FVC (Ratio of FEV$_1$ to FVC, expressed as a percentage)	n/a	Obstructive airway disease Obstruction
Forced Expiratory Flow (FEF 25-75) (Average forced expiratory flow during midportion [25%-75%] of forced vital capacity; useful in clients with small airways, such as children)	n/a	Obstructive airway disease

Description. Pulmonary function tests (PFTs) are several different tests used to evaluate lung mechanics, gas exchange, and acid-base disturbance through spirometric measurements, lung volumes, and arterial blood gases. Spirometry testing is included in pulmonary function testing. A spirometer is an instrument that measures lung capacity, volume, and flow rates. The instrument consists of a bell suspended in a container of water. The bell rises and falls in response to the client's breathing. The movement of the bell is recorded on a kymograph or electrical potentiometer. The pattern of the air flow on the graph must be interpreted to identify artifact and abnormalities, such as cough and upper airway obstruction. Full PFTs include measuring the amount of air that can be maximally exhaled after a maximum inspiration and the time required for that expiration and determining the ability of the alveolar capillary membrane to transport oxygen into the blood and carbon dioxide from the blood into the expired air.

Professional Considerations
Consent form NOT required.

Risk
Pneumothorax, increased intracranial or intraocular pressure, syncope, dizziness, chest pain, paroxysmal coughing, bronchospasm, oxygen desaturation, hypertension, strain on recent abdominal or thoracic incisions, aneurysm rupture.

Contraindications
Relative contraindications include hemoptysis of unknown origin, pneumothorax, unstable cardiovascular status, recent cardiac event or pulmonary embolus, recent eye surgery, concurrent nausea or vomiting, recent thoracic or abdominal surgery, or thoracic, abdominal, or cerebral aneurysm.

Preparation

1. Assess medication record for recent analgesic that may depress respiratory function.
2. Bronchodilators and intermittent positive-pressure breathing therapy may be withheld before the tests.
3. The client should void and then loosen any restrictive clothing.
4. Record the client's age, sex, and race on the test requisition.
5. Carefully measure and record weight and height.
6. Assess baseline vital signs.
7. See Client and Family Teaching.

Procedure

1. Position the client sitting with both feet flat on the floor or standing with something to lean on and a chair behind him or her for use if dizziness occurs.
2. Connect the mouthpiece to the spirometer (even in the handled version) and place mouthpiece in the client's mouth.
3. Place the clip over the nose so that only breathing through the mouth is possible.
4. Instruct the client to breathe through a mouthpiece. Up to eight efforts per measurement period may be needed to obtain results that are reproducible three times.
5. Criteria for acceptable test:
   a. Extrapolated volume of 95% of the FVC or 150 cc, whichever is greater.
   b. No false starts.
   c. Rapid start-to-rise time.
   d. No cough.
   e. Exhalation time of at least 6 seconds.
   f. The two largest FEV and FEV_1 values vary by no more than 0.200 L.
   g. MVV 12-15 seconds.
6. The two highest MVVs are within 10% of each other.
7. If the test is ordered to include a bronchodilator, administer bronchodilator and wait 15 minutes before repeating the procedure.

Postprocedure Care

1. Assess vital signs every 5 minutes until they return to baseline values.
2. Resume normal diet and any bronchodilators or intermittent positive-pressure breathing therapy.
3. Results are normally available within 30 minutes. Consideration of client's clinical condition is necessary when one is interpreting results.
4. Flush out air at least five times in a volume-displacement spirometer to reduce risk of airborne spread of infection to future clients.
5. Dispose of or disinfect any portions of the test equipment that come into contact with the client.

Client and Family Teaching

1. Withhold short-acting bronchodilator medication for 5 hours before the test or as ordered by physician. Long-acting bronchodilators will be withheld for a longer period of time. If you experience difficult breathing, you should use your bronchodilator.
2. Refrain from smoking or eating a heavy meal for 4-6 hours.
3. Dentures should not be removed.
4. Take a maximal inhalation, hold it, and then maximally and forcibly exhale. A modified technique with an initial forced exhalation followed by a relaxed exhalation continued for as long as possible may be used.
5. After a short rest period, the procedure is repeated two more times.
6. The procedure takes about 20 minutes.

Factors That Affect Results

1. The client's ability to voluntarily and actively participate is essential to complete the indicated tests.
2. An inadequate seal around the mouthpiece invalidates the results.
3. An ineffective nose clip causes unreliable results.
4. Gastric distention, hypoxia, metabolic disturbances, narcotic analgesia, pregnancy, and sedatives may alter the results. Fatigue as a result of repeated efforts may also alter the results.
5. Daily monitoring and calibration are required to ensure accuracy and reproducibility of spirometry results.
6. In one study, obstruction of PFTs included use of tobacco, history of hay fever, age, and male sex.
7. Bronchodilators administered before the tests may obscure true pulmonary function.
8. Herbs or natural remedy effects: In one study, people who received 200 mg of ginseng twice each day for 3 months

demonstrated improved FVC, FEV₁, and PEFR as well as arterial blood oxygen levels and walking distance.

2. See also Lung scan, Perfusion and ventilation—Diagnostic; Diffusing capacity for carbon monoxide—Diagnostic.

Other Data

1. Pulmonary function tests are normally performed in a pulmonary laboratory.

Pulmonary Scintiphotography

See Lung Scan, Perfusion and Ventilation—Diagnostic.

Pulsatility Index Ratio

See Pulse Volume Recorder Testing of Peripheral Vasculature—Diagnostic.

Pulse Oximetry

See Oximetry—Diagnostic.

Pulse Volume Recorder Testing of Peripheral Vasculature—Diagnostic

Norm. The waveform recording demonstrates rapid upstroke or an anacrotic limb, a sharp peak, a brisk decline or catacrotic limb, and a clearly discernible visual diastolic wave. Bilateral consistent augmentation of the pulse amplitude from proximal-to-distal measurement sites is present throughout the waveform recordings.

Usage. Assists in the diagnosis, location, and monitoring of the progression of arterial vascular lesions and arterial narrowing; used for preoperative, intraoperative, and postoperative evaluations; aids in the determination of the need for arterial angiography; aids in differentiation of aortoiliac and superficial femoral artery occlusion and neuropathies; assists in the evaluation of the severity of arterial occlusions and the detection of arterial pressure changes in distal extremity vessels that cannot be measured by a Doppler probe; measures peripheral vascular status in persons with diabetes mellitus and can be used in patients with edema; helps evaluate penile blood flow and intercavernous pressure; TFI method used to monitor venous grafts at risk for failing.

Description. *Pulse volume recording* measures pressure changes of arterial vessels and displays the pressure changes as waveforms.

Pressure changes are recorded by a transducer during blood pressure cuff inflation and deflation. Segmental air plethysmography records the pulse waveform tracings onto graph paper. These pressure recordings supplement segmental limb pressure studies and are a sensitive indicator of arterial vascular occlusive disease of the distal vessels of the feet and toes. Recordings may be taken before or after segmental limb-pressure measurements. Arterial narrowing distal to a vascular lesion produces a loss of the diastolic wave, a prolonged catacrotic limb (prolonged downstroke tracing), rounding of the normally sharp peak, and a decrease in the slope of the anacrotic limb (vertical ascending limb). Progression of arterial occlusive disease results in a broadened, flattened, lengthened, and dampened waveform with depression in the amplitude of the diastolic wave. A *transfer function index* (TFI) or *pulsatility index ratio* (PIR) may be generated by the equipment to demonstrate abnormalities in perfusion via color coding. A variation of the pulse volume recording procedure is *pulse volume plethysmography,* in which a water-filled cuff is placed around the penis and an assessment of continuous blood flow and intercavernous pressure is taken.

Professional Considerations
Consent form NOT required.

Preparation
1. Remove clothing from each extremity.

Procedure
1. *Traditional pulse volume recording:*
   a. The client is placed in the prone position.
   b. Blood pressure cuffs that have a length of 80% of the limb circumference and a width of 40% of the limb circumference and a pneumatic inflatable bladder that is 20% wider than the limb diameter are selected.
   c. The pressure cuffs are placed bilaterally 2.5 cm above the antecubital crease of the arm, just above the wrist, as high as possible on the thigh, just below the knee, and just above the malleolus of the ankle.
   d. Transmetatarsal and penile pressure recordings may be obtained.
   e. Pulse volume recordings are measured at brachial, radial, ulnar, femoral, popliteal, dorsalis pedis, and posterior tibial levels of each resting extremity.
   f. Pressure changes are recorded by a transducer during cuff inflation and deflation.
   g. Cuff inflation is measured by standard mercury-gravity or aneroid manometer
   h. Cuff deflation is measured by stethoscope, plethysmography, or the Doppler velocity detector, which is the most convenient and sensitive measurement device.
   i. A segmental air plethysmography records the pulse-waveform tracings onto graph paper.
   j. The same procedure is used for pediatrics.
2. *Pulse volume plethysmography of penile blood flow:*
   a. The procedure may be performed to measure natural variations in blood flow while the client sleeps, or during visual sexual stimulation or during artificial erection.
   b. A cuff filled with water is placed around the penis and connected to a three-way tap. One of the taps is covered with a latex membrane, which displaces in response to penile blood flow. Another tap is connected to a pressure bag positioned 30 cm above the penis. A second cuff is placed around the base of the penis.
   c. As variations in blood flow occur, the displacement of the latex membrane is recorded by a photoplethysmograph. Artificial variations in blood flow may be induced by compression of the penis artery via the base cuff.
   d. Findings are used by the equipment to determine a *pulsatility index ratio* (PIR), which is a ratio of total vascular resistance in the penis divided by functional impedance at the current heart rate. The PIR along with the transfer function index display a color-coded screen that represents differing perfusion between adjacent cuff segments.

Postprocedure Care
1. Remove cuffs.

Client and Family Teaching
1. The procedure takes 30 minutes, unless performed during sleep.
2. Results are available immediately.

Factors That Affect Results
1. Improper size, inflation, or loose cuff application causes inaccurate results.
2. False-negative results have been reported in clients with a short segmental occlusion of the superficial femoral artery in which they have developed large femoral collateral circulation. The pulse-volume recording produced a very depressed thigh tracing without discernible augmentation over the occluded site while circulation to the extremity was maintained.

Other Data
1. Pulse-volume recording of peripheral vascular pulses reports 97% accuracy for detecting superficial femoral artery occlusion.

Pure Tone Audiometry
See **Audiometry Test—Diagnostic.**

Pyelography, Antegrade
See **Antegrade Pyelography**—Diagnostic.

Pyelography, Retrograde
See **Retrograde Pyelography**—Diagnostic.

PYP Scan
See **Heart Scan**—Diagnostic.

Pyridoxal
See **Vitamin B₆**—Plasma.

Pyridoxamine
See **Vitamin B₆**—Plasma.

4-Pyridoxic Acid
See **Vitamin B₆**—Urine.

Pyridoxine
See **Vitamin B₆**—Plasma.

QFT
See **RD1-Interferon Tests for Tuberculosis**—Blood.

QuantiFERON-TB Gold
See **RD1-Interferon Tests for Tuberculosis**—Blood.

Quinidine—Serum

Norm. NOTE: Quinidine takes 2 days to reach steady-state.

	Trough	SI Units
Therapeutic level	2-5 µg/mL	6.16-15.41 µmol/L
Toxic level	>6 µg/mL	>18.49 µmol/L
Lethal level	>30 µg/mL	>92.46 µmol/L

Panic Level Symptoms and Treatment
65% of people with levels >14 µg/mL (for the double extraction test methodology) have toxic symptoms.

Symptoms. Asthmatic or angioneurotic phenomena, ataxia, cinchonism (headache, dizziness, hearing loss, ringing in the ears), respiratory depression, vomiting, diarrhea, severe hypotension, syncope, anuria, cardiac dysrhythmia (asystole, heart block, widening of QRS and Q-T interval, sodium-channel blockade manifesting as early prolonged QRS interval, rightward axis of 40 msec, presence of an R wave in the aV_R lead and an S wave in leads I and aV_L, paradoxical tachycardia, ventricular tachycardia), embolism, hallucinations, paresthesia, irritability.

Treatment
NOTE: Treatment choice(s) depend(s) on client's history and condition and episode history.
1. Maintain airway and hemodynamic stability.
2. Provide transcutaneous or transvenous temporary pacemaker.
3. Acidify urine.
4. Perform gastric lavage.
5. Implement forced emesis.
6. Administer infusion of a sodium molar lactate.
7. Treat respiratory depression with caffeine, ephedrine, oxygen, or mechanical ventilation.
8. Administer epinephrine and/or anti-asthmatics for angioneurotic or asthmatic symptoms' phenomena.
9. Consider administration of nitrates and methacholine for toxic amaurosis (residual visual impairment).
10. Provide transfusion, if warranted because of severe hemoglobinuria.
11. Hemodialysis and peritoneal dialysis will NOT remove quinidine. Hemoperfusion WILL remove quinidine.

Increased. Impaired hepatic function, impaired renal function, and urine alkalinity. Drugs include acetazolamide, amiodarone, antacids, carbonic anhydrase inhibitors, cimetidine, magnesium hydroxide, nifedipine, propranolol, sodium bicarbonate, thiazide diuretics, and verapamil.

Decreased. Urine acidity. Drugs include ascorbic acid, barbiturates, nifedipine, phenobarbital, phenytoin, phenytoin sodium, primidone, and rifampin.

Description. Quinidine is a class 1A antidysrhythmic that exerts a depressant effect on myocardial excitability, conduction velocity, and contractility. It causes decreased sodium, potassium, and calcium influx across the cell membrane, resulting in a prolongation of the myocardial refractory period. In larger doses, the ventricular response rate is increased through anticholinergic inhibition of vagal stimulation of the AV node. Quinidine is metabolized by the liver and excreted unchanged in the urine, with a half-life of 4-10 hours. Steady-state levels are reached after 20-35 hours. Toxicity may result in prolongation of the QRS complex >25% from baseline value, hypotension, and cardiac standstill. Because 70%-80% of quinidine is bound to plasma protein and plasma binding varies among individuals, it is recommended that the unbound portion of quinidine be measured and doses be adjusted in conjunction with serial measurements. This is of particular importance during pregnancy, when changes in protein binding occur.

Professional Considerations
Consent form NOT required.

Preparation
1. Tube: Royal blue topped. Do NOT use a serum separator tube.
2. Do NOT draw specimens during hemodialysis.

Procedure
1. Draw a 3-mL TROUGH blood sample. Obtain serial measurements at the same time each day.

Postprocedure Care
1. None.

Client and Family Teaching
1. Take medication as prescribed.
2. Report any side effects, such as nausea, vomiting, and dizziness.
3. Check pulse rate every day when taking quinidine. The client should notify the physician when panic level symptoms are noted.
4. Toxicity in children occurs after ingestion of more than two pills having cardiovascular and neurological effects including death.

Factors That Affect Results
1. When obtaining serial samples, the same time interval between drug dosing and sample collection should be observed.
2. Peak quinidine levels occur 1.5-2 hours after oral administration.

3. Acidification of the urine increases excretion of quinidine. Alkalinization of the urine decreases excretion of this drug.
4. If the radioimmunoassay is used for testing, instead of high-performance liquid chromatography (HPLC), values may be overestimated because of the cross-reactivity of dihydroquinone, an impurity present in up to 15% of quinidine preparations.

Other Data
1. Coadministration of quinidine with digoxin increases the risk of digoxin toxicity.
2. Quinidine may cause an increase in bleeding tendencies secondary to inhibition of hepatic production of vitamin K–dependent clotting factors.
3. Ingestion of more than two tablets causes toxicity in toddlers.

Rabies

See Fluorescent Rabies Antibody—Specimen.

Radioallergosorbent Test

See Allergen-Specific IgE Antibody—Serum.

Radiographic Absorptiometry

See Bone Densitometry—Diagnostic.

Radiography

See Bone Radiography—Diagnostic; Chest Radiography—Diagnostic; Esophageal Radiography—Diagnostic; Esophageal Radiography—Diagnostic; Flat-Plate Radiography of Abdomen—Diagnostic; Radiography of Skull, Chest, and Cervical Spine—Diagnostic; Sinus Radiography—Diagnostic.

Radiography of Skull, Chest, and Cervical Spine—Diagnostic

Norm. Negative for fracture or dislocation.

Usage. Trauma and determination of location and extent of suspected skull fracture or cervical spine damage. Detection of Kimura disease, neonatal acute gastric volvulus, and pituitary macro adenoma.

Description. This procedure involves radiographic examination of the skull, chest, and cervical spine to detect skull and spinal injuries resulting from accidents or physically induced. Fractures of the skull are classified by location and type. Types of skull fractures may be penetrating, depressed, bending, linear, or diastatic (involving the skull suture area or areas). The orbits are examined for the presence of free air, which indicates a fractured sinus area. Radiography of the chest and cervical spine identifies the seven cervical spine segments as

well as the C7-T1 area and relationship. Definite indications for cervical spine radiographs include neck pain or a tender cervical area. Other indications may include decreased level of consciousness, paresthesias, decreased sensation, weakness, muscle spasm near the cervical area, or decreased anal tone.

Professional Considerations
Consent form NOT required.

Precautions
During pregnancy, risks of cumulative radiation exposure to the fetus from this and other previous or future imaging studies must be weighed against the benefits of the procedure. Although formal limits for client exposure are relative to this risk:benefit comparison, the United States

Nuclear Regulatory Commission requires that the cumulative dose equivalent to an embryo/fetus from occupational exposure not exceed 0.5 rem (5 mSv). Radiation dosage to the fetus is proportional to the distance of the anatomy studied from the abdomen and decreases as pregnancy progresses. For pregnant clients, consult the radiologist/radiology department to obtain estimated fetal radiation exposure from this procedure.

Preparation

1. Move the client only the minimal amount necessary to obtain the different radiographic views.
2. Maintain strict body alignment throughout transport and transfer of the client. If uncooperative or combative, the client may need to be intubated, paralyzed, and mechanically ventilated to maintain alignment.

Procedure

1. *Skull radiography*: Conventional plain-film radiography of the skull is performed, including the following views: posteroanterior, anteroposterior in Towne's projection, two lateral views, posteroanterior Waters, and lateral views designed to highlight the facial area.
2. *Chest and cervical spine radiography*: Conventional plain-film radiography of the cervical spine is performed, including the following views: anteroposterior, lateral, both obliques, and one that shows the odontoid process. Risks versus benefits must be considered before flexion and extension views are taken.

Postprocedure Care

1. Maintain strict body alignment until radiograph results are known.
2. Perform post-sedation or paralytic monitoring per institutional protocol if either was used.

Client and Family Teaching

1. Results are normally available within 24 hours or immediately in case of emergency.
2. Body alignment should be maintained until results are known.

Factors That Affect Results

1. Linear skull fractures may not be detected if their location is not on the side of the skull closest to the film. They must be distinguished from vascular grooves of the skull.
2. Skull suture area (diastatic) fractures are difficult to detect without a great deal of experience in radiographic interpretation.
3. Skull radiograph interpretation should take into consideration clinical findings from scalp and soft-tissue examination.

Other Data

1. Nuclear medicine studies can help pinpoint fractures near the base of the skull that are not demonstrable by conventional radiography.
2. Computed tomography of the spine may be needed to detect spinal fractures not demonstrable by conventional radiography.
3. Because as many as half of spinal injuries occur below the cervical area, radiographs of the lower spine should also be taken.

Radionuclide Breast Imaging

See **Scintimammography**—Diagnostic.

Radionuclide Venography

See **Venography**—Diagnostic.

Raji Cell Immune Complex Assay—Blood

Norm.

Normal	<13 µg AHG Eq/mL
Borderline	13-25 µg AHG Eq/mL
Abnormal	≥26 µg AHG Eq/mL

Usage. Detection of immune complexes in the following: autoimmune disorders, celiac disease, cirrhosis, Crohn's disease, cryoglobulinemia, dermatitis herpetiformis, disseminated malignancy, drug reactions, infections (microbial, parasitic, viral), rheumatoid arthritis, sickle cell anemia, and systemic lupus erythematosus. Assists in staging immunological disorders such as RA and SLE.

Description. Complement receptors for IgG are found on the Raji cells, which are lymphoblastoid cells that contain receptors for complement, particularly C3b. Raji cells are derived from Burkitt's lymphoma and are used to recognize and bind protein-bound immune complexes that contain C3b. Results are reported as the quantity of precipitated immune complexes. Detection of circulating immune complexes is used to help determine the mechanisms of autoimmune diseases.

Professional Considerations

Consent form NOT required.

Preparation

1. Preschedule this test with the laboratory.
2. Tube: Chilled green topped.

3. Specimens MAY be drawn during hemodialysis.

Procedure

1. Draw a 5-mL blood sample.
2. Heelstick is acceptable, collected in a Microtainer.
3. Place the tube in a container of ice and water.

Postprocedure Care

1. Transport the specimen to the laboratory immediately.

Client and Family Teaching

1. The test is used to help diagnose autoimmune diseases.

Factors That Affect Results

1. Results may be unreliable if the client has undergone a recent scan involving the injection of radioactive dye.

Other Data

1. AHG measurement is defined as aggregated human gamma globulin equivalents.
2. See also Immune complex assay—Blood.

Rapid HIV Test

See OraQuick Rapid HIV Tests—Specimen.

Rapid Plasma Reagin (RPR) Test—Blood

Norm. Negative, nonreactive sample. *Treponema pallidum titer* <1:2. NOTE: Titers are indicated when samples are weakly positive or positive.

Positive. Borderline, reactive, and weakly reactive are considered positive results for the syphilis antibody. A reactive result is suggestive of contraction of syphilis, but diagnosis must be confirmed by medical examination and history. Hidradenitis suppurative of groin and axilla, Jarisch-Herxheimer reaction (incidence 31.5%) in HIV infected persons receiving penicillin therapy for syphilis.

Negative. RPR nonreactive results may be reported in clients who are treated before the appearance of the primary chancre (in the primary phase), those treated after the appearance of the primary chancre but

before the appearance of the reagin, and those treated in the secondary phase of the disease. Seronegative results occur with alcohol ingestion before the test and during inactive or latent-phase syphilis.

Description. Syphilis is a complex sexually transmitted disease characterized by a wide range of symptoms that imitate other diseases. It is caused by the organism *Treponema pallidum*. The RPR test is a macroscopic agglutination screening test for the presence of reagin, the antibody specific for the treponemal spirochete. In this test, an antigen (cardiolipin phospholipid derived from beef heart) to reagin is used to detect an agglutination reaction, indicating a positive test result. The RPR test is most useful during the secondary stage of syphilis, at the peak of reagin antibody presence in the blood. This test is more sensitive than and can be substituted for the Venereal Disease Research Laboratory (VDRL) test. This test is inexpensive and widely used for mass testing for syphilis. However, its sensitivity in primary syphilis is fairly poor, and many biologic false-positive results are possible. Positive results should be confirmed with the fluorescent treponemal antibody-absorbed double-stain test (see Fluorescent treponemal antibody-absorbed double-stain test—Serum).

Professional Considerations
Consent form NOT required.

Preparation
1. Tube: Red topped, red/gray topped, or gold topped.
2. See Client and Family Teaching.
3. Specimens MAY be drawn during hemodialysis.

Procedure
1. Draw a 4-mL blood sample.
2. Heelstick is acceptable, collected in a Microtainer.

Postprocedure Care
1. State law may require completion of a confidential department of health form when a specimen is reported as reactive.

Client and Family Teaching
1. Do not drink alcohol for 24 hours before the test.
2. Assess the client's understanding of safe sexual practices.
3. If testing is positive and a syphilis diagnosis is confirmed:
   a. Notify all sexual contacts from the last 90 days (if early stage) to be tested for syphilis.
   b. Syphilis can be cured with antibiotics. These may worsen the symptoms for the first 24 hours.
   c. Do not have sex for 2 months and until after repeat testing has confirmed that the syphilis is cured. Use condoms after that for 2 years. Return for repeat testing every 3-4 months for the next 2 years to make sure the disease is cured.
   d. Do not become pregnant for 2 years because syphilis can be transmitted to the fetus.
   e. If left untreated, syphilis can damage many body organs, including the brain, over several years.

Factors That Affect Results
1. Alcohol ingestion within the previous 24 hours produces transient nonreactive results.
2. Hemolysis of the specimen invalidates the results.
3. Serum samples should be drawn before meals because chyme alters the reaction.
4. Refrigeration destroys *Treponema* spirochetes in 72 hours.
5. Conditions that may cause false-positive results include active immunization in children, antinuclear antibodies, antiphospholipid antibody syndromes, blood loss (with multiple transfusions), chancroid, chickenpox, cirrhosis, the common cold, diabetes mellitus, fever (relapsing), hepatitis (infectious), HIV, hypergammaglobulinemia, leprosy, leptospirosis (Weil's disease), Lyme disease, lymphogranuloma venereum, lymphoma, infection (chronic), malaria, measles, mononucleosis (infectious), *Mycoplasma* pneumonia, non-syphilitic treponemal diseases (bejel, pinta, yaws), periarteritis nodosa, pneumococcal pneumonia, pneumonia, pregnancy, rat-bite fever, rheumatic fever, rheumatic heart disease, rheumatoid arthritis, scarlet fever, scleroderma, senescence, subacute bacterial endocarditis, systemic lupus erythematosus, tuberculosis (advanced pulmonary), treponematosis, trypanosomiasis, tuberculosis, typhus fever, and vaccinia.

Other Data
1. Results may be nonreactive while infectious organisms are present in the bloodstream because immunologic response is not detectable for 14-21 days after contraction of the spirochetes.
2. The greatest risk for transmission of syphilis occurs in freshly drawn blood products that must be administered immediately (platelets) or those not refrigerated for 72 hours before infusion.
3. Negative results in the presence of definite clinical signs of syphilis or suspected biologic false-positive tests necessitate the *fluorescent treponemal antibody absorption test.*
4. This test has been found to be highly sensitive and specific, even if antigen is

improperly stored at a temperature of 36 degrees C.

5. A newer test, the *Treponema pallidum* enzyme-linked immunosorbent assay (ELISA), is being studied for possible replacement of this test for large-scale screening for syphilis.

6. Azithromycin and penicillin resistance is common.

Rapid Streptococcal Antigen Testing

See Throat Culture for Group A Beta-Hemolytic Streptococci—Culture.

RAST Test

See Allergen-Specific IgE Antibody—Serum.

Raynaud's Cold Stimulation Test—Diagnostic

Norm. Within 15 minutes, digital temperature returns to prebath temperature. Recovery time >20 minutes indicates Raynaud's syndrome.

Usage. Detection of Raynaud's syndrome or hand arm vibration syndrome (HAVS) after occlusive disease of the peripheral arteries is ruled out.

Description. This test records digital temperature changes after submersion of the digits in an ice-water bath. Raynaud's syndrome is an idiopathic, vasospastic disorder of small cutaneous arteries and arterioles of the extremities characterized by intense paroxysmal bilateral pallor and cyanosis of the fingers or toes with or without local gangrene. The attacks may occur in response to exposure of the affected extremities to cold temperature. Idiopathic or primary occurrence of this syndrome is referred to as "Raynaud's disease." "Raynaud's phenomenon" is the term used when accompanied by paresthesia and caused by underlying disease processes such as connective tissue disorders.

Professional Considerations
Consent form NOT required.

Risks
Increased infection in open wounds on fingers.

Contraindications
Gangrenous digits, or open or infected wounds on the hands.

Preparation
1. All jewelry should be removed from the fingers and wrists.

Procedure
1. Digital temperatures are measured by thermistors attached to each digit.
2. The hands are then submerged in an ice-water bath for 20 seconds.
3. Serial temperature recordings are taken beginning immediately after the hands are removed from the bath and continue every 5 minutes for 20 minutes.

Postprocedure Care
1. None.

Client and Family Teaching
1. Avoid exposing the hands to extreme cold.
2. Smoking greatly increases difficulties in clients with peripheral circulatory problems.

Factors That Affect Results
1. Excessively cold or warm ambient temperature can alter the physiologic response.

Other Data
1. Laser Doppler flowmetry is being studied for its usefulness as an adjunctive diagnostic tool for Raynaud's conditions.

RBC

See **Red Blood Cell**—Blood.

RD1-Interferon Tests for Tuberculosis (QuantiFERON-TB Gold (QFT-G), QuantiFERON-TB Gold In-Tube test (QFT-GIT), Interferon Gamma Release Assays, IFN-Gamma Assay, T-SPOT®.TB)—Blood

Norm. Negative.

Usage. Helps diagnose *M. tuberculosis* infection; may be used for surveillance or to identify persons likely to benefit from treatment. Preferred over skin testing for detecting latent tuberculosis infections in which clients have previously been vaccinated with BCG or received BCG cancer therapy. Useful for screening clients at high risk for latent tuberculosis, such as recent immigrants from high-prevalence countries, health care workers, and those persons working or living in prisons. This test is preferred over the tuberculin skin test in persons who are unlikely to return to have the skin test read. May be used to increase diagnostic sensitivity as an adjunct to the tuberculin skin test in children under 5 years of age. Not for use in those with a low risk for infection.

Description. These enzyme-linked immunoassays measure cell-mediated immune response by quantifying interferon (IFN)-gamma released by T cells in response to stimulation by *Mycobacterium tuberculosis*. The IFN-gamma is specific to *M. tuberculosis* and not to the BCG vaccine strain.

Thus this test has particular value in detecting latent tuberculosis in clients who previously received BCG vaccination because it does not produce false-positive results as does tuberculin skin testing. Because it does not require two visits, as does the Mantoux skin test, the interferon tests are valuable for use in areas such as emerging countries where client follow-up is unreliable. In addition, because this test is an assay, it is not subject to reader error, as is the Mantoux test. The QuantiFERON-TB Gold (produced by Cellestis Ltd., Carnegie, Victoria, Australia) is included in the 2005 U.S. CDC guidelines for screening of health care workers.

Professional Considerations
Consent form NOT required.

Risks
None.

Contraindications
This test is not recommended for use in clients with suspected active tuberculosis, which is associated with suppressed interferon response. Also not recommended for contact screening, screening of those under age 17, during client pregnancy, or in clients with HIV infection.

Preparation
1. Tube: Heparinized.

Procedure
1. Obtain a 5-mL blood sample.
2. Notify receiving laboratory that test is needed, to assure that testing will be completed in the required time frames.

Postprocedure Care
1. Transport specimen to the laboratory promptly.

Client and Family Teaching
1. Tuberculosis is treatable in most clients. It is important to follow up with your physician to learn the results of this test and plan further treatment, if necessary.

Factors That Affect Results
1. Results are invalidated if the specimen is not incubated with the test antigen within 12 hours of collection.

Other Data
1. Not useful for confirmation of Mantoux skin testing results because PPD injection skews results of this test. Test may be used at least 12 months after the last Mantoux skin test. Also not used for diagnosis of *M. avium* disease.
2. Mantoux test is preferred in children.
3. t IGRAs (tuberculosis interferon-gamma release assays) have a similar sensitivity but a greater specificity in diagnosing tuberculosis than the tuberculin skin test.

RDI

See Polysomnography—Diagnostic.

Recombigen Latex Agglutination Assay

See Acquired Immune Deficiency Syndrome Evaluation Battery—Diagnostic.

Rectal Culture, Swab—Diagnostic

Norm. Negative for pathogenic organisms.

Usage. Screening for prenatal group B streptococci, vancomycin resistant enterococci (VRE) that has been found in 38% of acute hospitalized patients, and causes of bacterial diarrhea such as *Campylobacter, Chlamydia, Neisseria gonorrhoeae, Salmonella* (e.g., detection of *Salmonella* Urbana in infected child from turtle tank water), and *Shigella*; detection of aerobic and anaerobic intestinal flora (e.g., before TRUS-guided prostate biopsies), and detection of cholera, and norovirus, rotavirus, and adenovirus in gastroenteritis.

Description. The rectal swab culture is a screening test for pathogenic organisms of the rectum.

Professional Considerations

Consent form NOT required.

Preparation

1. Obtain a sterile culture swab, a closed sterile container, and drapes.
2. The client should disrobe below the waist.

Procedure

1. Drape the client in the left lateral position with the knees and hips flexed.
2. Gently insert a sterile, cotton-tipped swab at least 2.5-3 cm into the rectum. Rotate the swab from side to side and leave it in place for a few seconds to allow absorption of rectal flora.
3. If the swab is being obtained for *N. gonorrhoeae* culture, the swab must be discarded and the procedure repeated if fecal material contaminates the swab.
4. Place the swab in a sterile container and cover it tightly. If a Culturette is used, insert the swab into the medium compartment of the culture tube and crush the distal end to release the ampule of medium.

Postprocedure Care

1. Label the specimen with the site and collection time.

Client and Family Teaching

1. The test is used to determine the potential bacterial cause of diarrhea.

Factors That Affect Results

1. Swabs should be sent to the laboratory immediately.
2. Refrigerate specimens not tested immediately.
3. There is a high false-negative rate when testing for vancomycin-resistant enterococcus (VRE) in stool.

Other Data

1. The rectal culture is not used to determine carrier state.

Rectal Manometry

See Rectal Motility Test—Diagnostic.

Rectal Motility Test (Rectal Manometry)—Diagnostic

Norm. *Adult:* 40-120 mm Hg. Distention of the rectum produces relaxation of the internal sphincter and contraction of the external sphincter.

Usage. Assists in the diagnosis of colonic dilation, constipation, diarrhea, external sphincter disorders (hypothyroidism, myasthenia gravis, myotonic dystrophy, polymyositis), Hirschsprung's disease, incontinence from rectum, and internal sphincter disorders (scleroderma); detection of anal achalasia; and evaluation of children with nonneuropathic overactive bladder and persons with intrinsic ganglionic innervation of the internal sphincter of the rectum.

Increased. Crohn's disease. Decreased anal squeeze pressure and/or rectal motility and/or rectal sensation: hyperglycemia, irritable bowel syndrome, post-anorectal repair or microscopic surgery, post-irradiation of the prostate, multiple sclerosis, proctalgia fugax, severe idiopathic chronic constipation, and ulcerative colitis.

Description. This test measures the pressures within the rectum and provides an evaluation of the strength and function of the internal and external anal sphincters. The anal canal length is 5 cm, with a functional length of 3-5 cm. Functional length is determined by the extent of pressure generated by the involuntary internal and voluntary external anal sphincter muscles within the anal canal. Increasing rectal distention from filling produces progressive increasing electromechanical activity in the surrounding tissue accompanied by increasing proximal pressure and decreasing distal pressure along the rectal canal until the contents are expelled. This test is a more sensitive indicator of short segments of anal achalasia than barium enema. A small, thin, flexible balloon catheter with four sensing ports is introduced into the proximal portion of the rectum. The catheter is connected to three pressure transducers. Pressure readings of the rectum and sphincter are measured and recorded onto a graph or computer.

Professional Considerations
Consent form NOT required.

Preparation
1. The client should disrobe below the waist.
2. If a large amount of stool is present, a Fleet enema is given, and the examination is performed 1 hour after rectal evacuation.

Procedure
1. *Adults:*
   a. The client is placed in the left lateral position.
   b. A small, thin, flexible balloon catheter with four sensing ports is introduced into the proximal portion of the rectum.
   c. The catheter is inserted 8-10 cm above the mucocutaneous level, with the balloon portion in the proximal portion of the rectum and the sensing ports in the anal canal.
   d. The catheter is connected to three pressure transducers.
   e. The rectum is distended with an inflated balloon for 7-12 seconds until resistance to balloon distention is demonstrated by passive movement of a syringe. Usually 30-50 mL of air is required and is dependent on the client's age, the balloon size, and rectal dilation capacity.
   f. The amount of air required for the client to feel resistance is recorded as the internal anal sphincter response.
   g. Air is withdrawn in 5- to 10-mL amounts until distention is no longer felt. This smallest volume reflects the threshold of rectal sensation. Most people have relaxation of the internal sphincter with a distention volume of 15 mL.
   h. The client is asked to squeeze the external sphincter tightly for 2 seconds and then relax.
   i. Anal canal pressures are measured at eight points, in 0.5- to 1.0-cm increments, with the highest resting and voluntary squeeze pressures recorded at each point.
   j. Pressure readings of the rectum and sphincters are recorded onto graph paper, or images are configured on a computer.
   k. The catheter is removed.
2. *Children:*
   a. The same procedure as that described previously for adults is used with the following changes: The catheter is inserted 5 cm above the mucocutaneous level, and the child may be sedated to prevent unnecessary movements and crying.
3. *Infants:* A cleansing enema is not given.

Postprocedure Care
1. Cleanse the anal area.

Client and Family Teaching
1. Once home, call your doctor if rectal bleeding or discharge occurs.

Factors That Affect Results

1. Rectal stool decreases pressure readings.
2. Insufficient rectal distention results in decreased pressure readings.
3. Improper placement of the anal balloon or equipment malfunction.

Other Data

1. Rectal manometry has not been demonstrated to be reliable in the newborn.
2. To avoid bacterial growth, store the equipment tubing dry. To detect bacterial growth, perform regular water quality testing.

Rectosphincteric Manometry

See Rectal Motility Test—Diagnostic.

Red Blood Cell (RBC)—Blood

Norm.

		SI Units
Adult female	4-5.5 million/μL	4-5.5 × 10^{12}/L
Pregnant	3-5.0 million/μL	3-5.0 × 10^{12}/L
Adult male	4.5-6.2 million/μL	4.5-6.2 × 10^{12}/L
Infant	3.8-6.1 million/μL	3.8-6.1 × 10^{12}/L
1-2 years	3.6-5.5 million/μL	3.6-5.5 × 10^{12}/L
6-15 years	4.7-4.8 million/μL	4.7-4.8 × 10^{12}/L

Increased. Anoxia, burns (severe), cardiovascular disease, cerebellar hemangioblastoma, Cushing's disease, dehydration (severe), diarrhea, erythema, erythropoietin production increase, hemoconcentration (exercise, fright, stress), hemorrhage, hepatic carcinoma, hereditary spherocytosis, high-oxygen-affinity hemoglobinopathy, hypernephroma, poisoning, polycythemia vera, pulmonary disease and fibrosis, renal cyst, shock, sickle cell disease, surgery, thalassemia, and trauma. Drugs include gentamicin sulfate, methyldopa, and methyldopate hydrochloride.

Decreased. Addison's disease, anemias (aplastic, hemolytic, hemorrhagic, iron deficiency, pernicious, pure red cell), bone marrow suppression, cirrhosis, fatty liver, fluid overload, Gaucher disease, hemodilution, hemolysis, hemorrhage, Hodgkin's disease, hydremia in pregnancy, hypothyroidism, idiopathic steatorrhea, infection (chronic), leukemia (chronic myelogenous), malaria, multiple myeloma, myxoma of left atrium of the heart, rheumatic fever, smokers, subacute bacterial endocarditis, systemic lupus erythematosus, and vitamin deficiency (B_6, B_{12}, folic acid). Drugs include acetaminophen, aminosalicylic acid, ampicillin, antineoplastics, carbamazepine, chloramphenicol, chloroquine hydrochloride or phosphate, haloperidol, hydralazine hydrochloride, hydroxychloroquine sulfate, indomethacin, isoniazid, lithium, mefenamic acid, methsuximide, methyldopa, methyldopate hydrochloride, nitrofurantoin, novobiocin sodium, penicillamine, phenobarbital, phenylbutazone, phenytoin, phytonadione, rifampin, spectinomycin hydrochloride, tetracyclines, thiazide diuretics, thiocyanates, tolbutamide, tripelennamine hydrochloride, valproic acid, and vitamin A. Herbs or natural remedies that potentiate anemia include American mandrake or mayapple (*Podophyllum peltatum*), European mistletoe (*Viscum album*), pennyroyal (*Hedeoma pulegioides*), *Rauwolfia serpentina*, Indian squill (*Urginea indica*), and squill (*Urginea maritima*).

Description. Red blood cells constitute the majority of peripheral blood cells. They are formed by red bone marrow, have a life span of about 120 days, and are removed from the blood by the liver, spleen, and bone marrow. Red blood cells function in hemoglobin transport, which results in delivery of oxygen to the body tissues. Red blood cell development is characterized by passage through several characteristic stages, beginning with erythroblasts, which are immature, nucleated red blood cells.

Professional Considerations
Consent form NOT required.

Preparation
1. Tube: Lavender topped.
2. Draw the sample from an extremity that does not have intravenous fluids infusing.
3. Do NOT draw specimens during hemodialysis.

Procedure
1. Draw a 4-mL blood sample.
2. Heelstick is acceptable, collected in a Microtainer.

Postprocedure Care
1. Invert the tube 10 times to mix the contents.
2. The sample is stable at room temperature for 10 hours and refrigerated for 18 hours.

Overnight hold before processing has no deleterious effects.

Client and Family Teaching
1. This test evaluates the body's ability to produce red blood cells in sufficient numbers.

Factors That Affect Results
1. False low values occur in the presence of cold agglutinins.
2. Traumatic venipuncture and hemolysis invalidate the results.
3. Diltiazem can cause hemolysis of RBCs.

Other Data
1. Red blood cell indices are useful in further differentiating conditions. See Blood indices—Blood.
2. Ringer's lactate is compatible with saline-adenine-glucose-mannitol (SAGM) preserved packed red blood cells for infusions <60 minutes.

Red Blood Cell Count
See **Red Blood Cell**—Blood.

Red Blood Cell Mass—Blood

Norm. *Female*: 24.24 ± 2.59 mL/kg (standard deviation).
Male: 28.27 ± 4.11 mL/kg (standard deviation).

Increased. Addison's disease, burns, carboxyhemoglobinemia, cerebellar hemangioblastoma, Cushing's disease, dehydration, emphysema, Gilbert's syndrome, hepatoma, high altitude, idiopathic erythrocytosis, increased erythropoietin production, left-to-right shunt (because of cardiovascular disease), lung disease (producing hypoxia), methemoglobinemia, myeloproliferative syndrome, Philadelphia-negative chronic myeloproliferative disorders (CMPD), pickwickian syndrome, polycythemia vera, renal cell adenocarcinoma, renal cyst, secondary polycythemia, smokers, stress states, and uterine myoma. Drugs include epogen.

Decreased. Addison's disease, anemias, blood loss (acute), carcinoma, edema (severe), hemorrhage, hypothyroidism, infection (chronic), inflammation (chronic), myxedema, panhypopituitarism, radiation, renal failure (chronic), and starvation.

Description. Red blood cell mass is a direct measurement of the total number of red blood cells in the systemic circulation and is expressed in relation to body weight as milliliters per kilogram (mL/kg). Red blood cell mass reflects the equilibrium between the rate that the bone marrow produces and releases erythrocytes and the rate of peripheral erythrocyte destruction. This test assists in differential diagnosis of absolute and relative polycythemia, anemia, erythrocytosis, and Gaisböck's disease.

Professional Considerations
Consent form NOT required.

Preparation
1. Tube: Two green topped.
2. Do NOT draw specimen during hemodialysis.

R

Procedure
1. Draw an 8-mL blood sample.
2. The sample is mixed with a radioactive isotope (^{51}Cr-, ^{131}I-, or ^{125}I-labeled albumin) and is reinjected into the client after 15 minutes.
3. Draw an 8-mL blood sample 15 minutes after reinjection.

Postprocedure Care
1. Observe the client carefully for up to 60 minutes after the study for a possible (anaphylactic) reaction to the radionuclide.
2. When urine is being discarded, rubber gloves should be worn for 24 hours after the procedure. Wash the gloved hands with soap and water before removing the gloves. Wash the ungloved hands after gloves are removed.

Client and Family Teaching
1. This test is a measurement of the body's ability to produce RBCs.

2. Instruct the client to meticulously wash the hands with soap and water after each void for 24 hours.

Factors That Affect Results
1. Active bleeding, edematous extremities, or intravenous infusions during measurement may alter the results.
2. Recent scans involving the administration of radioactive isotopes will obscure the results.

Other Data
1. Total blood volume and plasma volume are obtained at the time of this test.
2. Health care professionals working in a nuclear medicine area must follow federal standards set by the Nuclear Regulatory Commission. These standards include precautions for handling the radioactive material and monitoring of potential radiation exposure.
3. Iodine-131 half-life is 8 days. Iodine-125 half-life is 60 days. Chromium-51 half-life is 27.8 days.

Red Blood Cell Morphology—Blood

Norm. Microscopic interpretation is required.

Color	Uniformly normochromic	Acanthocytes	Absent
Size	6-8 μm, only slight size variation	Crescent bodies	Absent
		Drepanocytes	Absent
Shape	Round, biconcave disk	Echinocytes	Absent
Stained appearance	Mature erythrocytes stain uniformly and contain a normal concentration of hemoglobin with an area of central pallor	Leptocytes	Absent
		Poikilocytes	Absent
		Schizocytes	Absent
		Spherocytes	Absent
		Stomatocytes	Absent
Nucleus	Absent	Cabot rings	Absent
Nuclear remnants	Absent	Heinz bodies	Absent
		Siderocytes	Absent
Cellular inclusions	Absent		

Classification of Variation from Normal

Abnormal RBCS/HPF	Score	Interpretation
3-6	1+	Slight
7-10	2+	Moderate
11-20	3+	Significant
>20	4+	Pronounced

Usage. Detection of blood dyscrasias; differentiation of anemias, leukemia, and thalassemia.

Description of Abnormalities of RBC Color	Possible Causes of Abnormal RBC Color
Anisochromia is demonstrated by variable staining intensities, indicating unequal hemoglobin content because of multiple populations of red blood cells (RBCs).	*Anisochromatism*: Iron-deficiency anemia treated with transfused blood
Hyperchromia is demonstrated by the presence of cells having a smaller-than-normal area of central pallor, causing the cells to absorb excessive stain and demonstrate higher-than-normal pigmentation. Increased amounts of these cells are called "hyperchromatism."	*Hyperchromatism*: Dehydration, increased bone marrow iron stores, inflammation (chronic), and in the presence of spherocytes that have increased cell wall thickness
Hypochromia is demonstrated by the presence of cells having a larger-than-normal area of central pallor, causing the cells to stain weakly and appear to have less-than-normal pigmentation. Increased amounts of these cells are called "hypochromatism."	*Hypochromatism*: Anemia (iron deficiency), HIV/AIDS, and decreased hemoglobin concentration
Polychromatophils are cells that are stainable with many types of stains, such as stains with both an acid and a base component. They are demonstrated by a bluish pink tinge caused by the presence of both hemoglobin stained by acid and cytoplasmic ribonucleic acid (cRNA) stained by the basic component. Both the larger-than-normal cell size and the presence of cytoplasmic RNA indicate that polychromatophils are reticulocytes (newly made red blood cells). Increased amounts of polychromatophils are called "polychromatosis" and occur in accelerated RBC production.	*Polychromatosis*: Hemorrhage, hemolysis, reticulocytosis, and therapy for iron-deficiency anemia or pernicious anemia
Acanthocytes are cells with irregular, thorny, spiculated membrane surface projections containing bulbous, rounded ends. They result from an irreversible defect in the lipid content of the RBC membrane. The presence of acanthocytes is called "acanthocytosis."	*Acanthocytosis*: Abetalipoproteinemia (most common cause), alcoholic cirrhosis, hemolytic anemia (induced by pyruvate kinase deficiency), hepatic disease, status after splenectomy, and retinitis pigmentosa; drugs include heparin calcium and heparin sodium

Description of Abnormalities of RBC Shape	Possible Causes of Abnormal RBC Shape
Crescent bodies (achromocytes) are cells with a faint quarter-moon shape caused by RBC rupture.	*Achromocytosis*: Condition that increases the fragility of red blood cells (that is, sickle cell anemia, reduced oxygen supply)
Drepanocytes, or sickle cells, are cells formed in the shape of a sickle with a point at one end. The presence of these cells is called "drepanocytosis."	*Drepanocytosis*: Anemia (hemolytic, sickle cell) and hemoglobin SC disease

Description of Abnormalities of RBC Shape	Possible Causes of Abnormal RBC Shape
Echinocytes, burr cells, or *crenated RBCs* have a cell surface with 10-30 uniformly distributed, blunt spicules. Echinocytes may be commonly attributable to pH changes caused by faulty drying during smear preparation, but certain physiologic conditions, including a reversible defect in the lipid content of the RBC membrane, have been associated with their presence. The presence of these cells is called "echinocytosis."	*Echinocytosis*: Bile acid abnormalities, blood loss (acute), burns (extensive), carcinoma of the stomach, disseminated intravascular coagulation (DID), gastric ulcers (bleeding), increased free fatty acids, microangiopathic hemolytic anemia, pyruvate kinase deficiency, renal failure, thrombotic thrombocytopenic purpura, and uremia; drugs include barbiturates, heparin calcium, heparin sodium, and salicylates
Elliptocytes, or *ovalocytes,* have a cigar shape, which distinguishes them from the more oval shape of the ovalocytes. They are normal constituents of mature RBCs. Higher-than-normal amounts of these cells are called "elliptocytosis."	*Elliptocytosis*: Anemias (iron deficiency, pernicious, sickle cell), hereditary elliptocytosis, leukemia, megaloblastic hematopoiesis, and thalassemia
Leptocytes, or *target cells,* have an increased ratio of surface to volume, often because of a shape that looks like a cup, bell, or hat. They have a colorless center and are thinner and lighter staining than normal RBCs because of abnormally low amounts of hemoglobin. When they are stained, the depth of the "cup" collapses, causing a bull's-eye appearance. The presence of leptocytes is termed "leptocytosis."	*Leptocytosis*: Anemia (iron deficiency, sickle cell), cellular dehydration, cirrhosis, hemoglobin C disease, hemoglobin SC disease, hepatitis, jaundice (obstructive), status after splenectomy, and thalassemia
Poikilocytes occur in varying shapes, ranging from slightly irregular to dumbbell-like, pear shaped, or teardrop shaped. Defective bone marrow production causes poikilocytosis, a general term used to describe the presence of cells demonstrating variation from the normal shape of the RBC.	*Poikilocytosis*: Anemia (iron deficiency, hemolytic, megaloblastic, pernicious), myelofibrosis, and thalassemia myeloid metaplasia
Schizocytes, or *schistocytes,* are RBCs with adhesions of spiral and triangular red blood cell fragments because of hemolysis, hemoglobinopathies, or erythrocytic mechanical damage from fibrin strands. The presence of these cells is called "schizocytosis."	*Schizocytosis* or *schistocytosis*: Anemia (acute hemolytic, microangiopathic hemolytic), burns (severe), disseminated intravascular coagulation (DIC), prosthetic heart valves, pyruvate kinase deficiency, renal graft rejection, uremic hemolytic syndrome, valve prosthesis, and valvular stenosis
Spherocytes are cells that are globelike rather than biconcave, with an abnormally small dimple. They are thicker than normal, with many fine needlelike projections. Spherocytes lack an area of central pallor (as a result of an increased mean corpuscular hemoglobin concentration) and have a smaller surface area relative to their size. Spherocytes are caused by mechanical fibrin strand damage to circulating RBCs. The presence of spherocytes is called "spherocytosis."	*Spherocytosis*: ABO hemolytic disease of the newborn, accelerated reticuloendothelial red blood cell destruction, anemia (hemolytic), status after blood transfusion, hereditary spherocytosis, and thermal injury of the cell membrane

Continued

R

Description of Abnormalities of RBC Shape	Possible Causes of Abnormal RBC Shape
Stomatocytes are cup-shaped RBCs with an abnormal area of central pallor that may be oval or rectangular, elongated, or slitlike. These cells are produced by antibodies or hydrocytosis. The presence of these is called "stomatocytosis."	*Stomatocytosis*: Alcoholism, cirrhosis, erythrocyte sodium pump defect, hepatic disease (obstructive), hereditary spherocytosis, hereditary stomatocytosis, and Rh_{null} (Rh_0) cells

Description of Abnormalities of RBC Size	Possible Causes of Abnormalities of RBC Size
Anisocytosis is a general term that describes any variation in the size of the RBC.	*Anisocytosis*: Anemias (iron deficiency, pernicious), folic acid deficiency, status after blood transfusion of normal cells into an abnormal red blood cell population, leukemia, newborns, and reticulocytosis
Macrocytes are large erythrocytes having a diameter >8 μm, a mean corpuscular volume >95 μm³, and higher-than-normal hemoglobin content. They are usually increased because of stress erythropoiesis. Increased amounts of macrocytes are called "macrocytosis."	*Macrocytosis*: Alcoholic liver disease, anemia (hemolytic, pernicious), folic acid deficiency, hepatic disease, hyperthyroidism, idiopathic steatorrhea, newborns, reticulocytosis, status after hemorrhagic states, and thalassemia
Microcytes have a RBC diameter <6 μm, a mean corpuscular volume <80 μm³, and a mean corpuscular hemoglobin <27%. Increased amounts of microcytes are called "microcytosis."	*Microcytosis*: AIDS, anemia (from chronic hemorrhage, iron deficiency), hemoglobinopathies, hereditary concentration spherocytosis, HIV, and thalassemia

Description of Abnormalities of RBC Content or Structure	Possible Causes of Abnormal RBC Content or Structure
Agglutination: Clumping together of RBCs is an immune mechanism caused by antibody formation.	*Agglutination*: Invading antigen(s)
Basophilic stippling is demonstrated by the presence of minute basophilic granules that cause a bluish-to-purple color when reticulocytes are stained. They are caused by ribosomal aggregation that occurs as smears are prepared. Small amounts of basophilic stippling normally occur as the smears are dried. Increased amounts occur in conditions in which RNA has aggregated in the cells.	*Increased basophilic stippling*: Alcoholism, anemia (megaloblastic, sickle cell), heavy-metal intoxication (bismuth, lead, mercury, and silver), hemorrhage (gastrointestinal), leukemia, and thalassemia
Cabot's rings are cells containing mitotic spindle remnants appearing as fine, threadlike filaments of bluish purple color in the shape of a single ring or a double ring (figure-eight shape).	*Presence of Cabot's rings*: Anemia (severe, pernicious), lead poisoning, myelofibrosis, and myeloid metaplasia

Description of Abnormalities of RBC Content or Structure	Possible Causes of Abnormal RBC Content or Structure
Heinz bodies are denatured particles of hemoglobin attached to the RBC membrane that appear when stained with cresyl blue or new methylene blue. Heinz bodies usually indicate abnormal erythrocyte stability because of hemolytic conditions or hemoglobinopathies.	*Presence of Heinz bodies:* Alpha-thalassemia, anemia (hemolytic), glucose-6-phosphate dehydrogenase deficiency, hemoglobinopathies, methemoglobinemia, and status after splenectomy; drugs include analgesics, antipyretics, chlorates, phenacetin, phenothiazines, phenylacetamide, phenylamine, phenylhydrazine, primaquine phosphate, resorcinol, and sulfapyridine
Howell-Jolly bodies are nuclear fragments contained in red cells that stain purple or violet. They are normally present in immature RBCs and in mature erythrocytes before they pass through the splenic circulation. In conditions causing increased RBC production, erythrocytes contain higher-than-normal amounts of these bodies.	*Presence of Howell-Jolly bodies:* Anemia (hemolytic, megaloblastic), leukemia, splenic absence (congenital or surgical removal), and splenic atrophy
Platelets on red blood cells appear as a halo that resists staining and can easily be confused with RBC inclusion bodies.	n/a
Rouleaux formation is demonstrated by a cellular configuration in stacks or rolls. Increased rouleaux formation may be caused by increased fibrinogen or globulins in the blood. Rouleaux formation is decreased by the presence of abnormally shaped RBCs, which inhibit adherence of the cells in a stacked shape. Rouleaux formation may also result from a delay in slide preparation.	*Increased rouleaux formation:* Hyperfibrinogenemia, macroglobulinemia, and multiple myeloma *Decreased rouleaux formation:* Hereditary spherocytosis
Siderocytes or *Pappenheimer bodies* are cells with mitochondrial concentrations of ferritin (non-hemoglobin iron) deposits. These cells stain as purple bluish granules only in the presence of iron stains such as Prussian-blue reactions. Pappenheimer bodies are non-iron basophilic granules contained in the iron-protein matrix and stain positive for iron in the presence of non-iron stains. Ferritin is normally absent in RBCs. During hemoglobin formation in the premature infant and newborn, siderocyte free-iron granules commonly occur in developing normoblasts and reticulocytes. The presence of siderocytes is called "siderocytosis."	*Siderocytosis* or *Pappenheimer* bodies: Anemia (chronic hemolytic, congenital spherocytic, dyserythropoietic, megaloblastic, pernicious, refractory, sideroblastic), burns (severe), hemochromatosis, infection, lead poisoning, status post splenectomy, and thalassemia

R

Description. Red blood cells (RBCs) constitute the majority of peripheral blood cells and function in hemoglobin transport, which results in delivery of oxygen to the body tissues. RBC development is characterized by passage through several characteristic stages, beginning with erythroblasts, which are immature, nucleated RBCs. RBC morphology is the examination of red blood cells under a microscope, comparing the actual appearance with calculated values for each index of color, size, shape, developmental stage, and structure or content.

Professional Considerations
Consent form NOT required.

Preparation
1. Tube: Lavender topped.
2. Specimens MAY be drawn during hemodialysis.

Procedure
1. Draw a 7-mL blood sample.
2. Heelstick is acceptable, collected in a Microtainer.

Postprocedure Care
1. None.

Client and Family Teaching
1. This test evaluates the structure of the RBCs.

Factors That Affect Results
1. Automated methods of counting and sizing of the RBCs should not be used in the presence of red cell agglutination. Instead, hand counts must be performed.

Other Data
1. RBC morphology stained smear is usually carried out at the same time as the differential white blood cell count.

Red Blood Cell Size Distribution Width (RDW)—Blood

Norm. 12.8%-14.6%. Microscopic electronic interpretation is required.

Increased. Alcoholic liver disease, celiac disease, coronary heart disease, Crohn's disease, Harris platelet syndrome (HPS), inflammatory bowel disease, iron deficiency, stroke and ulcerative colitis. See Red blood cell—Blood; Red blood cell morphology—Blood.

Decreased. Defects in iron reutilization, renal failure See Red blood cell—Blood; Red blood cell morphology—Blood.

Description. Red blood cell volume distribution width, or RDW, is a coefficient of variation (CV) in red blood cell volume. This is derived from anisocytosis. RDW becomes abnormal earlier in iron deficiency than in any other blood cell parameters. RDW may be a useful tool in differential diagnosis of microcytic and macrocytic anemias. It may also be used in monitoring for improved absorption of nutrients in response to a gluten-free diet in celiac disease. It should be remembered that RDW is a CV, and it should be correlated with other erythrocytic indices for the most accurate diagnoses (see Red blood cell morphology—Blood).

Professional Considerations
Consent form NOT required.

Preparation
1. Tube: Lavender topped.
2. Specimens MAY be drawn during hemodialysis.

Procedure
1. Draw a 5-mL blood sample.

Postprocedure Care
1. None.

Client and Family Teaching
1. This test will evaluate iron intake and utilization in the body.

Factors That Affect Results
1. RDW is obtained by electronic evaluation (anisocytosis).
2. See Reticulocyte count—Blood; Hematocrit—Blood.

Other Data
1. RDW values affect left ventricular ejection fraction in acute coronary syndrome patients (Zhang, Zhang, Zhao et al, 2010).
2. Elevated RDW is a strong independent predictor of all-cause mortality in males referred for coronary angiography, persons post AMI, in patients undergoing PCI who were not anemic at baseline,

post stroke, and in older persons living in community dwellings.

3. See Reticulocyte count—Blood; Hematocrit—Blood.

Red Blood Cell Survival

See ^{51}Cr-Red Cell Survival—Blood.

Reducing Substances—Stool

Norm.

Normal	<2 mg/g of stool
Borderline	2-5 mg/g of stool
Abnormal	>5 mg/g of stool

Increased. Disaccharidase deficiencies, infant diarrhea (some forms), intestinal mucosal defects, metabolic disorders, and rotavirus.

Decreased. Beta-lipoprotein deficiency, blind loop syndrome, celiac disease, cystic fibrosis of the pancreas, *Giardia* infestation, lactose intolerance, and malnutrition (severe). Drugs include colchicine, neomycin sulfate, and oral contraceptives.

Description. The presence of reducing substances in the stool demonstrates the inability of intestinal border enzymes to absorb disaccharide carbohydrates, especially sucrose and lactose. These unabsorbed sugars are reduced by metal ions, such as copper contained in the frequently used Clinitest reduction tablet.

Professional Considerations
Consent form NOT required.

Preparation
1. Obtain a clean, dry, plastic specimen container.

Procedure
1. Collect at least 1 g of stool in a clean, dry, plastic specimen container with a lid.

Postprocedure Care
1. Send the specimen to the laboratory immediately.
2. Freeze the specimen if not tested immediately.

Client and Family Teaching
1. This test measures the digestive tract's ability to absorb disaccharides.
2. Urinate before defecating to avoid contaminating the stool sample with urine.

Factors That Affect Results
1. False-low results because of bacterial fermentation may occur when analysis is delayed in nonfrozen specimens.
2. Reject specimens that have been placed on an absorbent surface (diaper, cardboard).

Other Data
1. The weight and pH of the specimen are usually obtained and included in the results.

Renal Angiogram (Renal Arteriogram)—Diagnostic

Norm. Radiopaque iodine contrast material should circulate symmetrically and without interruption through the renal parenchyma and renal vasculature.

Usage. Visualization of the renal parenchyma and renal vasculature; assists in differentiation of renal masses; identification of extravasation, renovascular abnormalities such as abscesses, aneurysms, arteriovenous fistula, emboli, fibrosis, hypervascularity, hypovascularity, infarction, intrarenal hematoma, parenchymal laceration, polyarteritis nodosa, renal artery dysplasia, stenosis, thrombolic occlusions, and accidental injury; and evaluation of chronic renal disease, renal failure, and transplant donors and recipients as well as posttransplantation evaluation of vascular flow and rejection of the donor organ.

Description. Renal angiogram is an invasive radiographic procedure involving injection of iodine radiopaque contrast material through a catheter inserted into the aorta near the bifurcation of the renal arteries or directly into the renal arteries. For clients with preexisting renal impairment, gadolinium-enhanced magnetic resonance angiography or magnetic resonance urography is a better choice than this procedure, because it is nonnephrotoxic.

Professional Considerations
Consent form IS required.

Risks
Embolus, hematoma, hemorrhage, infection, allergic reaction to contrast material (itching, hives, rash, tight feeling in the throat, shortness of breath, bronchospasm, anaphylaxis, death), renal toxicity from contrast medium.

Contraindications
Previous allergy to iodine, shellfish, or radiographic dye; renal insufficiency. The procedure may be contraindicated during pregnancy if iodinated contrast medium is used, because of the radioactive iodine crossing the blood-placental barrier. Caution should be taken with clients who have bleeding tendencies and those with renal failure because of end-stage renal disease. Sedatives are contraindicated in clients with central nervous system depression.

Preparation
1. Establish intravenous access.
2. A narcotic or sedative may be prescribed.
3. The client should void and remove all jewelry and metal objects.
4. Have an emergency cart readily available.
5. Obtain local anesthetic, povidone-iodine solution, intravenous fluid, contrast material, guidewire, vascular and renal catheters, and sterile gloves.
6. See Client and Family Teaching.
7. Just before beginning the procedure, take a "time out" to verify the correct client, procedure, and site.

Procedure
1. The client is positioned supine.
2. A peripheral intravenous infusion is started.
3. The arterial site is cleansed and anesthetized.
4. A catheter is introduced in accordance with the Seldinger technique into the femoral artery or into the transaxillary, transbrachial, or translumbar vessels, and advanced under fluoroscopy to the aorta. Test aortograms with a small amount of contrast material are completed.
5. The catheter is then replaced with a renal catheter, and larger amounts of radiopaque contrast material are injected through the catheter directly into the aorta near the bifurcation of the renal arteries or directly into the renal arteries.
6. Rapid, serial radiographic films are then taken to record circulation of the contrast material through the renal parenchyma and vasculature.
7. The catheter is removed, and a pressure dressing is applied over the insertion site.

Postprocedure Care
1. If sedation was used, continue assessment of respiratory status. If deep sedation was used, follow institutional protocol for post-sedation monitoring. Typical monitoring includes continuous ECG monitoring and pulse oximetry, with continual assessments (every 5-15 minutes) of airway, vital signs, and neurologic status until the client is lying quietly awake, is breathing independently, and responds to commands spoken in a normal tone.
2. Monitor the catheter insertion site for bleeding, inflammation, or hematoma formation.

Client and Family Teaching
1. This test determines the adequacy of blood flow through both renal arteries.
2. Fast for 8 hours before the procedure.
3. For 5 minutes after injection of the contrast material, an urge to cough, a flushed sensation, nausea, or a salty taste may occur.
4. It is important to lie motionless throughout the procedure. Sedation may be used to help you relax.

Factors That Affect Results
1. Interpretation of the results may be impaired by the presence of gas, feces, or

contrast material such as barium in the gastrointestinal tract.

2. Movement of the client during the procedure obscures the radiography.

3. Calcium antagonists can cause false-positive captopril renograms.

4. False negative results can be decreased by use of adjunctive catheter-based techniques (Pratap et al, 2008).

Other Data

1. None.

Renal Arteriogram

See **Renal Angiogram**—Diagnostic.

Renal Echogram

See **Kidney Ultrasonography**—Diagnostic.

Renal Failure Index

See **Sodium, Plasma**—Serum or Urine.

Renal Function Tests—Diagnostic

See **Concentration Test**—Urine; **Creatinine Clearance**—Serum and Urine; **Renal Indices**—Diagnostic.

Description. The renal function test may consist of up to four tests: the urine concentration test, the creatinine clearance test, calculation of the renal indices, and the inulin clearance test. These tests reflect glomerular filtration, tubular reabsorption, renal blood flow, and tubular secretion. Measurement of these separate kidney functions assists in the determination of the origin and degree of renal dysfunction and renal tissue destruction. These tests are limited in their scope to detect early or mild renal disorders. (See individual test listings for more information.)

Renal Indices (FE$_{Na}$, RFI)—Diagnostic

Norm. Norm not applicable. Indices are used only for clients experiencing or suspected of experiencing renal failure.

Renal Indices: Differentiating Categories of Renal Failure

	Fractional Excretion of Sodium in Urine (Urine NA$^+$ × Serum Creatinine × 100)/(Serum NA$^+$ × Urine Creatinine)	Urine Sodium	Renal Failure Index: Urine NA$^+$ × (Plasma Creatinine/ Urine Creatinine)
Prerenal and volume depletion	<1%	<20 mmol/L	<1%
Renal (acute tubular necrosis)	>1%	>40 mmol/L	>1%
Postrenal	>4%		

Usage. Determination of the category of renal failure; ongoing monitoring during recovery from acute tubular necrosis and development of lupus nephritis.

Description. Both renal indices are mathematically calculated values of renal sodium handling, using laboratory measurement results. Urinary sodium levels are used in conjunction with urine and plasma or serum creatinine levels in two formulas that help narrow down the source of renal failure into prerenal, renal, and postrenal causes. Both the *fractional excretion of sodium in urine (FE_{Na})* and the *renal failure index (RFI)* determine how well the kidneys are able to remove urine from the blood into the urine. They are expressed as the percentage of serum sodium that is excreted in the urine.

Professional Considerations
Consent form NOT required.

Preparation
1. Obtain a clean-catch urine container, towelettes, and a red topped tube. For pediatric/infant collections, also obtain tape and a pediatric urine collection device/bag.

Procedure
1. Obtain a clean-catch urine sample and a 3-mL blood sample.
2. Pediatric/infant specimen collection:
   a. The child is placed in a supine position with the knees flexed and the hips externally rotated and abducted.
   b. Cleanse, rinse, and thoroughly dry the perineal area.
   c. To prevent the child from removing the collection device/bag, a diaper may be placed over the genital area.
   d. *Females*: Tape the pediatric collection device/bag to the perineum. Starting at the area between the anus and vagina, apply the device/bag in an anterior direction.
   e. *Males*: Place the pediatric collection device/bag over the penis and scrotum and tape it to the perineal area.
   f. Empty the collection bag into the refrigerated collection container after the infant or child voids.

Postprocedure Care
1. Remove the collection device/bag by gently peeling it away from the skin.

Client and Family Teaching
1. Caffeine consumption does not act chronically as a diuretic.

Factors That Affect Results
1. Both tests are most useful when urine output is oliguric.

Other Data
1. Tacrolimus has been known to cause hemolytic uremic syndrome following lung transplantation.
2. Terlipressin improved renal indices in children with extremely low cardiac output after open heart surgery.
3. Urocortin 2 with captopril treatment in heart failure patients improves renal function.

Renal Scan
See **Renocystogram**—Diagnostic.

Renal Ultrasonography
See **Kidney Ultrasonography**—Diagnostic.

Renin Activity (Plasma Renin Activity, PRA)—Plasma

Norm. Norms are dependent on age, diet, position, and vein site.

		SI Units
Normal-Sodium Diet, Upright, and from Peripheral Vein		
Age 20-39	0.6-4.3 ng/mL/hour	0.6-4.3 µg/L/hour
Mean	1.9 ng/mL/hour	1.9 µg/L/hour
Age ≥40	0.6-3.0 ng/mL/hour	0.6-3.0 µg/L/hour
Mean	1.0 ng/mL/hour	1.0 µg/L/hour

		SI Units
Low-Sodium Diet, Upright, and from Peripheral Vein		
Age 20-39	2.9-24 ng/mL/hour	2.9-24 µg/L/hour
Mean	10.8 ng/mL/hour	10.8 µg/L/hour
Age ≥40	2.9-10.8 ng/mL/hour	2.9-10.8 µg/L/hour
Mean	5.9 ng/mL/hour	5.9 µg/L/hour

Renal venous renin ratio: <15:2.
Unilateral renal stenosis: normal kidney/affected kidney renin level ratio >1:1.4.

	Renin Activity	Aldosterone
Primary hyperaldosteronism	Decreased	Increased
Secondary hyperaldosteronism	Increased	Increased

NOTE: Samples obtained during renal vein catheterization are compared with levels obtained in the inferior vena cava to obtain the renal venous renin ratio.

Usage. Helps differentiate cause of hypertension (hyperaldosteronism versus renal vascular disease).

Increased. Addison's disease, aldosteronism (secondary), ambulatory clients (compared to clients prescribed bed rest), Bartter syndrome, chronic renal failure, cirrhosis, Conn's syndrome, erect posture for 4 hours (twofold increase), essential hypertension (rare), hypokalemia, hypovolemia (hemorrhage-induced), last half of menstrual cycle (twofold increase), low-sodium diet, nephropathy (sodium-losing), normal pregnancy, oxonic acid diet (rat study), pheochromocytoma, renal hypertension, renin-producing renal tumors, and transplant rejection. Drugs include antihypertensives, diazoxide, estrogens, furosemide, guanethidine sulfate, hydralazine hydrochloride, minoxidil, nitroprusside sodium, saralasin, spironolactone, telmisartan, and thiazides.

Description. Renin is a proteolytic enzyme that is synthesized, stored, and secreted by the juxtaglomerular cells of the kidneys and is a primary catalyst in regulation of blood pressure, potassium level, and fluid volume balance. Hydrolytic activity of the renin-angiotensin-aldosterone cycle results in the production of angiotensin II, a potent vasoconstrictor that stimulates the production of aldosterone in the adrenal cortex. Decreased renal blood flow stimulates renin secretion and an increased secretion of aldosterone. Blood loss and sodium depletion stimulate the release of renin. For this reason, the test may be preceded by the intake of a low-sodium diet for a several days. Hypertensive states with low plasma renin activity are suggestive of body fluid expansion imbalance. The test is an indirect measurement of the activity of renin through measurement of the rate of production of angiotensin I, which increases as a result of renin stimulation. Aldosterone levels are usually measured at the same time. High plasma renin activity suggests hypertension from the vasoconstrictive effects of angiotensin. The sample may be drawn peripherally or directly from the renal vein during a renal vein catheterization.

Professional Considerations

Consent form IS required for the renal artery catheterization procedure if it will be done in conjunction with sample collection for renin determination.

Preparation

1. Preparation and cooperation of the client are critical for accurate results.
2. The client must be assessed for medications that affect the results (estrogens can affect results for up to 6 months), and certain medications may be withheld for 2-4 hours before the test.
3. See Client and Family Teaching.
4. Preschedule this test with the laboratory.
5. Tube: Lavender topped, ice-cold. Also obtain a container of ice.
6. A local anesthetic may be administered before renal vein catheterization.
7. Just before beginning the procedure, take a "time out" to verify the correct client, procedure, and site.

Procedure

1. The test should be performed in the morning because renin levels exhibit a diurnal variation.
2. Completely fill an ice-cold lavender topped tube with blood. Avoid prolonged tourniquet use to avoid causing a drop in renin level.
3. Gently tilt the tube several times to mix the sample.
4. The same procedure is used in handling blood samples obtained during renal vein catheterization.

Postprocedure Care

1. Place the specimen immediately on ice.
2. Send the specimen to the laboratory immediately.
3. If a renal artery catheterization was performed, monitor vital signs, catheterization site, and distal pulses every 15 minutes × 2, then every 30 minutes × 2.

Client and Family Teaching

1. This test measures one of the fluid balance controls in the body.
2. Follow a 3 g/day sodium diet for 3-14 days before the test. Do not eat licorice before the test.
3. If the sodium depletion renin level will be measured, follow a low-sodium diet for 3 days before the test. Diuretics may also be prescribed before the test.

4. Fast for 8 hours before the test.
5. The recumbent position test requires that you be able to lie on your back for at least 1 hour. The upright position test requires that you be able to stand or sit upright for 2 hours.

Factors That Affect Results

1. Improper position of the client provides unreliable results. Levels are highest when drawn with the client in an upright position.
2. Failure to follow the dietary restrictions or failure to withhold appropriate medications before the test invalidates the results.
3. Results are invalid if the collection tube was not chilled before venipuncture or if the specimen was not placed on ice after collection.
4. Reject tubes incompletely filled or specimens not well mixed.
5. Total paracentesis with albumin infusion immediately suppresses plasma renin activity in patients with liver cirrhosis.

Other Data

1. Renin is very unstable and samples must be handled properly.
2. The 24-hour urine sample for sodium should be indexed against renin levels.
3. A second nonfasting blood sample, with exercise, may also be prescribed.

Renocystogram (Renogram Scan, Renal Scan)—Diagnostic

Norm. Radionuclide contrast material should circulate bilaterally, symmetrically, and without interruption through the renal parenchyma, ureters, and urinary bladder; 50% of radionuclide should be excreted within the first 10 minutes. The initial uptake or vascular phase occurs within 30-45 seconds after administration of the radionuclide. The transit or tubular phase follows over the next 2-5 minutes, and drainage of the radionuclide from the kidneys occurs during the excretory phase.

Captopril Radiography Method. Renovascular hypertension: GFR decreases more than 20%, with a 10% difference between the left and right kidneys.

Renal Artery Stenosis The kidney shows a disproportionate reduction in perfusion after administration of captopril.

Usage. Azotemia, excretory defects, nephroureteral dilation, renal ischemia (acute tubular necrosis), renal obstruction or mass, renal parenchymal disease, renovascular hypertension, unilateral kidney disease, and upper urinary tract obstruction; assessment of renal perfusion and status before transplantation and after transplantation (to differentiate between acute tubular necrosis and transplant rejection); evaluation of hydroureteronephrosis and urinary tract patency; also used for clients hypersensitive to iodine-based contrast material used with intravenous pyelography or those in whom urethral catheterization is contraindicated. This study records the activity of the entire kidney but does not distinguish between specific areas of disease within the kidneys.

Description. The renocystogram is a dynamic nuclear medicine study of the kidneys and ureters in which the dispersion, clearance, and excretion of a radionuclide are recorded by means of a gamma radiographic scan. Radionuclide uptake, transit, and excretion times are computed, and renogram curves are plotted on a graph for each kidney and ureter. Quantitative evaluation of renal function occurs as the external radiation detectors record vascular supply, perfusion, tubular filtration, and excretory phases. A renogram curve is produced as the radionuclide dispersion is plotted on a graph or computed. Comparisons of the right and left kidneys, curve shapes, and relative functions are calculated. Curve shapes are characteristic of certain disorders. This scan uses less radiation than an IVP or CT scan. However, IVP is better for anatomic definition, and arteriography is better for assessment of renal arterial anatomy. Renocystogram is superior to magnetic resonance imaging for medullary renogram evaluation (which must derive medullary information from a mixed study renogram), but equivalent in use for cortical renograms. When the evaluation is being done to identify the presence of renal vascularization abnormalities in hypertension and suspected renal artery stenosis, captopril radiography may be used. For suspected renal artery stenosis only, duplex ultrasound is less costly and invasive and provides similar diagnostic accuracy to captopril radiography.

Professional Considerations
Consent form IS required.

Risks
Allergic reaction, bleeding, infection, urinary tract obstruction.

Contraindications
During pregnancy, this test is performed only when imperative. It is contraindicated during breast-feeding, with congenital renal abnormality, clients with open flank wounds present, or with previous allergic reaction to the same radionuclide.

Preparation
1. Obtain the client's current weight.
2. The client should empty the bladder. Insert an indwelling urinary catheter for pediatric clients.
3. Establish intravenous access and infuse 500 mL of IV fluids (unless contraindicated). Unless contraindicated, the client should be well hydrated with 10 mL of water per kilogram of body weight.
4. Have emergency equipment readily available.
5. Just before beginning the procedure, take a "time out" to verify the correct client, procedure, and site.

Procedure
1. The client is positioned upright.
2. After placement of external posterior radiation detectors over both kidneys, an intravenous injection of radionuclide ^{99m}Tc-DTPA (technetium with the chelating agent diethylenetriaminepentaacetic acid) or ^{131}I-ortho-iodohippurate (radioiodine hippuran) is administered. Detectors record the uptake and excretion radiation counts when gamma scanning of both kidneys is completed.
3. The scan takes about 45 minutes.
4. If captopril renography will be done, captopril is administered and the scan is repeated 1 hour later. Monitor blood pressure every 15 minutes throughout the procedure.

Postprocedure Care
1. Urine or serum blood samples may be obtained.
2. Assess the injection site for infiltration of radionuclide analog.
3. Observe the client carefully for up to 60 minutes after the study for a possible (anaphylactic) reaction to the radionuclide.
4. When urine is being discarded, rubber gloves should be worn for 24 hours after the procedure. Wash the gloved hands with soap and water before removing the gloves. Wash the ungloved hands after gloves are removed.
5. If captopril was administered, continue blood pressure measurements every 30 minutes until the client meets discharge criteria. Assess for orthostatic hypotension.

Client and Family Teaching

1. This is a screening test used when it is suspected that renal blood flow is reduced.
2. This examination takes approximately 45 minutes and involves receiving an IV line to administer the test material and some fluids.
3. Immediately flush the toilet after each voiding after the procedure, and meticulously wash your hands with soap and water after each void for 24 hours after the procedure.
4. There will be a small amount of radiation exposure during testing.
5. For captopril renography, eat and drink only liquids beginning midnight before the test. Do not ingest any milk products.
6. For captopril renography, you will be given a glass of water to drink.
7. For captopril renography, you will need to slowly change from a lying or sitting position to a standing position in case you experience dizziness.
8. If you are breast-feeding, substitute formula for breast milk for 1 or more days after the procedure.

Factors That Affect Results

1. The presence of contrast material from prior diagnostic testing within 7 days interferes with accuracy.
2. Abnormalities may be accentuated in the presence of dehydration or masked in the presence of overhydration.
3. Injection of radiographic contrast material within 24 hours before the test invalidates the results.

Other Data

1. Health care professionals working in a nuclear medicine area must follow the federal standards set by the Nuclear Regulatory Commission. These standards include precautions for handling the radioactive material and monitoring of potential radiation exposure.
2. Technetium half-life is 6 hours.

Renogram Scan

See **Renocystogram**—Diagnostic.

Reptilase Time—Serum

Norm. 18-20 seconds or ±2 seconds of normal control.

Increased. Congenital afibrinogenemia, acquired dysfibrinogenemia (from liver or biliary disease), inherited dysfibrinogenemia (gene AalphaR16C), elevated fibrinogen during an acute phase reaction multiple myeloma (IgG kappa). Drugs include interferon therapy.

Decreased. Not clinically significant.

Description. Reptilase is an enzyme from Russell's viper (*Vipera russellii*, syn. *Daboia russelli*) venom used to determine blood coagulation time. Reptilase is one of a group of nine known snake venom thrombin-like enzymes (SVTLEs) that are similar to thrombin in their structure and function. It is a variation of the thrombin time used to detect the presence of adequate fibrinogen levels without interference from heparin, fibrin-fibrinogen degradation products, or increased concentrations of plasmin. Prolonged thrombin time in the presence of a normal reptilase time is confirmation that heparin, rather than low fibrinogen levels, is the cause of the coagulation defect.

Professional Considerations
Consent form NOT required.

Preparation
1. Tube: 2.7-mL or 4.5-mL blue topped.
2. Specimens MAY be drawn during hemodialysis.

Procedure
1. Draw a 3-mL blood sample and discard, leaving the needle in place.
2. Withdraw 2 mL of blood into a syringe or vacuum tube. Remove the syringe or tube,

leaving the needle in place. Attach a second syringe, and draw a blood sample quantity of 2.4 mL for a 2.7-mL tube and 4.0 mL for a 4.5-mL tube.

Postprocedure Care
1. None.

Client and Family Teaching
1. The test will measure your blood's ability to clot properly.
2. Results are normally available within 24 hours.

Factors That Affect Results
1. Send specimens to the laboratory immediately.
2. Contamination of the sample with tissue thromboplastin causes falsely elevated results. This is the reason for the double-draw technique.

Other Data
1. The reptilase time may be used in place of the thrombin time in fibrinogen evaluation in clients anticoagulated with heparin.

Reserpine—Plasma or Serum

Norm. Negative. *Serum therapeutic level:* 20 ng/mL.

Overdose Symptoms and Treatment
Symptoms. Lethargy, drowsiness, hypotension, respiratory depression.

Treatment
NOTE: Treatment choice(s) depend(s) on client's history and condition and episode history.
1. Protect airway.
2. Support blood pressure with vasopressors.
3. Monitor neurologic checks every hour.
4. Hemodialysis and peritoneal dialysis will NOT remove reserpine.

Increased. Parkinson's disease, reserpine-induced gastric mucosal lesions.

Description. Reserpine, an alkaloid of the *Rauwolfia serpentina* and *Rauwolfia vomitoria* plants, is used primarily as an anti-hypertensive (reduces SBP), sedative, or tranquilizer. It acts at adrenergic receptor sites, primarily of the central and peripheral nervous systems and heart, by interfering with the binding of serotonin. Reserpine is metabolized in the liver and excreted as an inactive metabolite in small amounts in the urine and stool. Reserpine has a very slow onset of peak action (2-3 weeks) with a prolonged effect (4-6 weeks); thus alterations in dosage occur in small increments and at 7- to 14-day intervals. Half-life is 4.5 hours and duration 45-168 hours.

Professional Considerations
Consent form NOT required.

Preparation
1. Tube: Lavender topped.
2. Specimens MAY be drawn during hemodialysis.

Procedure
1. Draw a 7-mL blood sample.
2. Heelstick is acceptable, collected in a Microtainer.

Postprocedure Care
1. None.

Client and Family Teaching
1. This test measures the level of reserpine in your body.
2. Results are normally available within 24 hours.
3. Know and understand the side effects of this drug and recognize the signs of overdose.
4. For intentional overdose, refer the client and family for crisis intervention.

Factors That Affect Results
1. Specimens collected in heparin invalidate results.

Other Data
1. *Rauwolfia* alkaloids lower seizure threshold. Clients with convulsive disorders should be observed closely.
2. Green tea extract was shown to reverse hepatic damage in reserpine toxicity (rat study).

Respiratory Antigen Panel (Antigen Detection Test, ADT, Respiratory Virus Immunofluorescence, Respiratory Virus Direct Stain Panel)—Specimen

Norm. Negative for adenovirus; influenza viruses A and B; parainfluenza viruses 1, 2, and 3; and respiratory syncytial virus (RSV).

Usage. Enables early and direct detection of seven common respiratory viruses so that treatment can begin while one is awaiting confirmatory cultures.

Description. The respiratory antigen panel allows for direct immunofluorescence detection of respiratory viral antigens from nasopharyngeal secretions and sputum, with specificity of 97%-99% and varying sensitivities. The seven viruses that are responsible for common and severe respiratory illness are included in the panel: respiratory syncytial virus, respiratory adenovirus, influenza viruses A and B, and parainfluenza viruses 1, 2, 3. After the virus is identified, antibodies are added, and the sample is incubated. Antigen-antibody complexes are observed under direct immunofluorescence after IgG is added to the specimen. Sensitivity for RSV is 95%-99%. Thus confirmatory culture is not needed. For all other organisms, sensitivity ranges from only 20%-50%; therefore confirmatory culture is recommended.

Professional Considerations
Consent form NOT required.

Preparation
1. Obtain viral transport media.

Procedure
1. Collect a 4-mL nasal aspirate, sputum, or a throat swab. Place immediately in viral transport media.

Postprocedure Care
1. Document source of specimen on the laboratory requisition and send specimen to the laboratory.
2. Specimen is viable for 2 hours at room temperature or for 3 days when refrigerated.

Client and Family Teaching
1. Teach client the proper method to produce a deep cough specimen.

Factors That Affect Results
1. Results are invalidated if swab or specimen was allowed to dry.
2. False-positive reactions for group A streptococcus have been found in the presence of *S. milleri.*
3. Interpretation may be inaccurate if smear is contaminated with red blood cells.

Other Data
1. Houben et al (2011) found that children had a 10 times higher risk of RSV lower respiratory tract infection if they had a birth weight more than 4 kilograms or were born during April through September, or had attended day care, or had siblings, as compared to children with none of these characteristics.

Respiratory Distress Index
See **Polysomnography**—Diagnostic.

Respiratory Syncytial Virus (RSV)—Culture

Norm. Negative for respiratory syncytial virus (RSV).

Usage. Detection of the presence of RSV in obtained medium.

Description. RSV is an important cause of lower respiratory tract infections in infants, especially <33 weeks gestational age. This virus, originally isolated in 1956, has become a major pathogen in children worldwide. It typically occurs seasonally during the winter months (November-April), afflicts almost all infants by 2 years of age, and can be very severe causing pneumonia and bronchiolitis and even fatal in the immunocompromised (e.g., bronchiolitis obliterans in lung transplant recipients). Symptoms are most pronounced in those infants with the lowest cellular and humoral immunity. Thus those with prematurity, congenital heart disease, neuromuscular disease, immunodeficiencies and cystic fibrosis or other underlying respiratory problems are at greatest risk of having RSV. RSV risk is also increased in those infants in day care, living in crowded conditions, or exposed to passive smoke. In adults, RSV manifests itself as an upper respiratory tract infection. Currently, there is no antiviral medication available that will treat RSV though a vaccine is in development (2011); thus treatment is primarily supportive and includes oxygenation, hydration, nasal suctioning, and nutritional interventions.

Professional Considerations
Consent form NOT required.

Preparation
1. Obtain a chilled viral transport medium and a sterile wire swab in a pack.
2. Open the transport medium, and place it in ice.
3. Obtain assistance for restraint of the client if necessary.

Procedure
1. Explain the procedure to the client and offer reassurance.
2. Bend the wire swab; open the pack.
3. Restrain the client if necessary, pass the wire through one naris and into the nasopharynx, and rotate the swab quickly.
4. Remove the swab, place it into the medium, and close.
5. Transport to the laboratory immediately.

Postprocedure Care
1. None.

Client and Family Teaching
1. This test is performed to try to isolate the pathogen causing the illness.
2. Results are normally available within 48-72 hours.
3. Having child wash his/her hands often can lower risk of spreading the disease.
4. Mean range of hospital length of stay is 1.4-6.65 days.
5. Websites for more information include http://www.cdc.gov/rsv/ and http://familydoctor.org/020.xml

Factors That Affect Results
1. Specimens must remain cold and do not tolerate freezing and thawing well.
2. Inaccurate swabbing or swabbing of the wrong location.

Other Data
1. Serologic isolation should also be considered.
2. Many efforts are underway to develop vaccines, monoclonal antibodies, and other prophylactic measures for RSV. RSV intravenous immune globulin and palivizumab are two products now available for immunoprophylaxis and are recommended as described below:
   a. Palivizumab monoclonal immune globulin (12% death rate in patients with upper respiratory infections):
      • Prophylaxis in children <2 years with respiratory disease requiring continuous oxygen or inhalation or steroid treatment for at least 6 months.
      • Premature infants (born before week 26 of gestation).
   b. Ribavirin inhalation:
      • High-risk infants with severe RSV infection.
   c. Ribavirin plus intravenous polyclonal immunoglobulin:
      • Clients (any age) after allogeneic stem cell or organ transplant.
      • Accompanied by more than one course of treatment for transplant rejection.
      • Accompanied by RSV pneumonia.
3. Aerosolized ALN-RSV01 (0.6 mg/kg) daily may have beneficial effects on long-term allograft function in lung transplant patients infected with RSV.
4. There is some evidence showing later development of reactive airways disease in those who had active RSV illness at an early age.
5. Development of bronchiolitis in infants associated with RSV genotypes GA2 and BA.
6. Breast milk can protect against respiratory viruses.

Respiratory Virus Direct Stain Panel

See **Respiratory Antigen Panel**—Specimen.

Respiratory Virus Immunofluorescence

See **Respiratory Antigen Panel**—Specimen.

Reticulocyte Count—Blood

Norm. Constitutes 1%-2% of the total RBC count.

		SI Units
Adult females	0.5%-2.5%	$0.005\text{-}0.025 \times 10^{-3}$
Adult males	0.5%-1.5%	$0.005\text{-}0.015 \times 10^{-3}$
Cord blood	3.0%-7.0%	$0.030\text{-}0.070 \times 10^{-3}$
Newborn	1.1%-4.5%	$0.011\text{-}0.045 \times 10^{-3}$
Neonates	0.1%-1.5%	$0.001\text{-}0.015 \times 10^{-3}$
Infants	0.5%-3.1%	$0.005\text{-}0.031 \times 10^{-3}$
Children >6 months	0.5%-4.0%	$0.005\text{-}0.040 \times 10^{-3}$
Immature reticulocyte fraction (IRF)	0.13%-0.31%	$0.001\text{-}0.004 \times 10^{-3}$

Increased Total Reticulocyte Count. Acquired autoimmune hemolytic anemia, Di Guglielmo's disease, erythremic myelosis (chronic), erythroblastosis fetalis, hemoglobin C disease, hemolytic anemias, hemorrhage (chronic), hereditary spherocytosis, infants, leukemia, malaria, metastatic carcinoma, myxoma of left heart atrium, paroxysmal nocturnal hemoglobinuria, polycythemia, posthemorrhagic anemia (acute), pregnancy, sickle cell disease, thalassemia major, thrombotic thrombocytopenic purpura, transfusion therapy, treatment of iron-deficiency anemia, vitamin B_{12} deficiency, or folic acid deficiency.

Increased Immature Reticulocyte Fraction. Anemia (hemolytic), blood loss, bone marrow regeneration, folic acid/folate deficiency, iron deficiency, myelodysplasia, and thalassemia.

Decreased Total Reticulocyte Count. Alcoholism, anemia (aplastic, hemolytic [aplastic crisis], iron deficiency, megaloblastic, pernicious, pure red cell), anoxia, aregenerative crisis, blood loss, bone marrow regeneration, chronic infection, myxedema, and radiation therapy. Drugs include carbamazepine and chloramphenicol.

Children <6 months old who were born before gestational week 26. Ribavirin inhalation treatment may be considered in high-risk infants with clinical symptoms indicating a serious course of an RSV infection. Treatment with ribavirin in combination with intravenous polyclonal immunoglobulin should be considered in clients who have received an allogeneic stem cell transplantation or organ transplantation with >1 episode of rejection treatment and who have mild or moderate RSV pneumonia. Evidence-based documentation for treatment of other groups of clients is lacking.

Description. Reticulocytes are nonnucleated red blood cells containing a basophilic network of granules or filaments characteristic of an immature cell of the erythrocyte class. Formed in the bone marrow, reticulocytes reach maturity after 1 day in the circulating blood and are an index of bone marrow function. The reticulocyte count is the number of reticulocytes per 1000 erythrocytes and is significant only when reported as a percentage of the total number of erythrocytes. This test helps differentiate bone marrow depression from anemias, hemorrhage, hemolysis, or radiation, and helps evaluate bone marrow activity and response to therapeutic interventions. Some test results include an immature reticulocyte fraction (IRF), determined by the staining abilities of the reticulocytes. Young reticulocytes have a higher degree of RNA staining. Higher than normal amounts of immature reticulocytes can indicate conditions in which there is more red blood cell production, such as after erythropoietin administration. The IRF is also useful in detecting new or increasing erythropoiesis after bone marrow or stem cell transplant.

Professional Considerations
Consent form NOT required.

Preparation
1. Obtain venipuncture supplies and a lavender topped tube or white blood cell pipette and supravital dye (such as brilliant cresyl blue or new methylene blue).
2. Do NOT draw specimens during hemodialysis.

Procedure
1. Adult:
   a. Leave the tourniquet on no more than 1 minute, draw a 4-mL blood sample without trauma.
   b. Gently tilt or roll the specimen six to eight times to mix the anticoagulant and the blood.
2. Infant:
   a. Draw a fresh drop of capillary blood into a white blood cell pipette and mix with an equal volume of a supravital dye.

Postprocedure Care
1. None.

Client and Family Teaching
1. This test measures your body's ability to make adequate numbers of red blood cells.
2. Results are normally available within 4 hours.
3. Visual counting is a reliable tool for estimating reticulocytes in resource-strained countries.

Factors That Affect Results
1. Reject hemolyzed specimens or specimens not thoroughly mixed with EDTA anticoagulant.
2. Hemodilution of the sample may occur if the specimen is drawn from an extremity that is being infused with intravenous solution.
3. False-positive results have been reported with laboratory handling of the specimen that included drying of the coverslip preparation; incorrect concentration of sodium metabisulfite; and mixture with fibrinogen, gelatin, or thrombin on the slide.
4. After transfusion with blood containing the sickle cell trait, cells with the sickle cell trait are present for 4 months.
5. False low results may occur when the sample is drawn soon after a blood transfusion.
6. Drugs that may cause false-positive results include antipyretics, chloroquine hydrochloride, chloroquine phosphate, corticotropin, furazolidone (in infants), hydroxychloroquine sulfate, levodopa, primaquine phosphate, pyrimethamine, quinacrine hydrochloride, quinine sulfate, and sulfonamides.
7. Drugs that may cause false-negative results include azathioprine, chloramphenicol, dactinomycin, methotrexate sodium, and sulfonamides.

Other Data
1. Reticulocyte count corrected for abnormal hematocrit (Hct) only = Reticulocyte % × (Hct/45).
2. The immature reticulocyte fraction (IRF) was formerly called the reticulocyte maturity index (RIM).

Reticulocyte Production Index (RPI)—Diagnostic

Norm. Index of 1.

Increased. Accelerated red blood cell production, preeclamptic mothers. Drugs include epogen and Vitamin A.

Decreased. Alcoholism; anemia (aplastic, iron deficiency, megaloblastic, pernicious, pure red cell); aplastic crisis of hemolytic anemia; aregenerative crisis; chronic infection; iron deficiency, myxedema; and radiation therapy.

Description. The reticulocyte production index (RPI) is a calculated measurement of the number of circulating reticulocytes in the packed cell volume of hematocrit. The raw reticulocyte count is expressed as a percentage of erythrocytes. In anemia, a 1%-2% reticulocyte count is not really normal because it is based on a lower-than-normal amount of erythrocytes. Also, the normal life span of reticulocytes is 2 days, but in the presence of accelerated red blood cell production, reticulocytes are released prematurely and circulate for up to 4 days. The RPI normalizes the reticulocyte count by multiplying it by the hematocrit divided by 45 and by correcting for the increased life span of reticulocytes (based on the degree of anemia) to give a more accurate portrayal of the rate of reticulocyte production. This index is used to calculate the degree of increased erythropoietic activity associated with the premature release of reticulocytes (shift) from the bone marrow in anemia.

Professional Considerations
Consent form NOT required.

Preparation
1. See Reticulocyte count—Blood; Hematocrit—Blood.
2. Do NOT draw specimens during hemodialysis.

Procedure
1. Obtain samples for reticulocyte count and for VPRC (volume of packed red cells, hematocrit). See Reticulocyte count—Blood; Hematocrit—Blood.
2. Calculation: Reticulocyte maturation time in the circulating blood changes as follows:

Hematocrit	Reticulocyte Maturation Time
35	1.5 days
30	1.75 days
25	2.0 days
20	2.25 days
15	2.5 days

The RPI is calculated as:

$$RPI = \frac{\text{Reticulocyte percentage}}{\text{Reticulocyte maturation time (days)}} \times \frac{\text{Client's VPRC (1)}}{0.45}$$

Postprocedure Care
1. See Reticulocyte count—Blood; Hematocrit—Blood.

Client and Family Teaching
1. This test measures the number of immature red blood cells in your bloodstream.
2. Results are normally available within 24 hours.

Factors That Affect Results
1. See Reticulocyte count—Blood; Hematocrit—Blood.

Other Data
1. See Reticulocyte count—Blood; Hematocrit—Blood.

Retinoblastoma Chromosome Abnormalities—Diagnostic

Norm.

Female	44 autosomes + 2X chromosomes
Karyotype	46,XX
Male	44 autosomes + 1X and 1Y chromosome
Karyotype	46,XY

NOTE: Retinoblastoma chromosomal defect is identified as female, 46,XX,13q–; male, 46,XY,13q–.

Usage.
Screening for retinoblastoma, identification of numerical chromosomal defects, and genetic counseling.

Description.
Retinoblastoma is an inherited type of cancer caused by mutations of the RB1 gene and associated with the MDM2 309G allele. It is the most frequently occurring congenital ocular tumor in children, occurring in 1 in 20,000 births. Tumor occurrence is unilateral in 60% of cases and is usually nonmetastatic and may occur up to several years later in the second eye. The risk for metastasis of retinoblastoma is elevated when diagnosis is delayed, when both eyes are involved, and when there is invasion to the uvea, orbit, and optic nerve. Clinical symptoms include leukocoria (57%), strabismus, impaired vision, and the appearance of white to yellow reflex from the pupil, referred to as "cat's-eye." Left untreated, this tumor is fatal because optic nerve, subarachnoid space, and cerebral tissue invasion occurs. If caught early enough, retinoblastoma is considered curable with years of chemotherapy treatment. Leukocyte screening of peripheral blood is the most common technique for chromosomal abnormality detection and analysis. Tissue cultures are cultivated from the blood sample, fixed, and stained. The chromosomes are then counted and photographed, and the karyotype is arranged according to the Denver nomenclature from cut photographs. Diagnosis is

confirmed by computed tomography with or without magnetic resonance imaging, and radiotherapy is a common approach to treatment. Prognosis is dependent on location, size, and the amount of ocular and extraocular involvement. Retinoblastoma patients have a strong increased risk of second (sarcomas, melanomas, lipomas, leukemia, lymphoma) and third subsequent malignancies.

Professional Considerations
Informed consent is recommended for genetic testing.

Preparation
1. See Client and Family Teaching.
2. Tube: Green topped.
3. Specimens MAY be drawn during hemodialysis.

Procedure
1. A morning sample is preferred. Draw a 10-mL blood sample.

Postprocedure Care
1. None.

Client and Family Teaching
1. This test is a genetic screen. Refer Appendix B, "Informed Consent for Genetic Testing."
2. Fast for 3 hours before the blood is drawn.
3. Refer the client with abnormal results for genetic counseling.

Factors That Affect Results
1. Insufficient number of cells in sample.

Other Data
1. Retinoblastoma is also associated with elevated plasma somatostatin levels.
2. The Genetic Information Nondiscrimination Act of 2008 prohibits health plans from using genetic family history or genetic test results from influencing eligibility or premiums for health insurance. It also prohibits employers from using this information to influence decisions about hiring, terminating employment, or employment pay, promotions, or privileges.

Retrograde Pyelography—Diagnostic

Norm. Bilateral, symmetric, and uniform opacification of ureters, renal calyces, and renal pelvis. Normal size and architecture of these structures. Superimposed films on inspiration and expiration normally show two outlines of the renal pelvis 2 cm apart.

Usage. Assessment of displacement, drainage, enlargement, or fixation of the structures of the renal collecting system; detection of complete or partial obstruction as a result of blood clot, calculus, inflammation, perinephric abscess, stricture, or tumor formation; assessment for integrity of the renal pelvis and ureters after blunt trauma to the ureteropelvic junction. Also used in clients with bladder tumor, severe renal insufficiency, or hypersensitivity to iodine-based contrast material, and when visualization of the renal collecting system with excretory urography is inadequate. Detection of hematuria, lymphoma, plasmacytoma of bladder, renal cyst, transitional cell carcinoma of renal pelvis, ureteral diverticulosis, urethral obstruction from endometriosis, urinary fistula, urinary leaks post op, and urothelial tumors.

Description. Retrograde pyelography is an invasive radiographic (fluoroscopic) examination of the kidneys from a distal direction via the ureters. During cystoscopy, catheters are passed into the ureters, and radiopaque contrast material is injected. The mucous membrane absorbs minimal amounts of the iodine radiopaque contrast material. Thus the complications of hypersensitivity reactions or delayed excretion of the dye in renal impairment that are associated with intravenous dye injections are avoided.

Professional Considerations
Consent form IS required.

Risks
Bladder perforation, hemorrhage, nausea, vomiting, urinary tract infection, vasovagal response.

Contraindications
Pregnancy (because of the radioactive iodine crossing the blood-placental barrier); severe dehydration. Sedatives are contraindicated in clients with central nervous system depression.

R

Preparation

1. See Client and Family Teaching.
2. The client should disrobe below the waist.
3. Just before beginning the procedure, take a "time out" to verify the correct client, procedure, and site.

Procedure

1. If deep sedation or anesthesia is used, monitor respiratory status and ECG continuously throughout the procedure.
2. The client is placed in a dorsal lithotomy position, and a cystoscopic examination is performed (see Cystoscopy—Diagnostic).
3. A catheter is then advanced through the ureter(s) into the renal pelvis. After drainage of the renal pelvis, iodine radiopaque contrast material is injected through the catheter(s) into the kidney(s), and anterior, posterior, lateral, and oblique radiographic films are obtained. A small amount of contrast material may be injected into the ureters as the catheter is removed, and radiographs of the ureters may then be taken.
4. The procedure may also be performed without cystoscopy by injection of the radiopaque contrast material into the lower ureter after wedging a bulb catheter at the distal end of the ureter.

Postprocedure Care

1. A ureteral or Foley catheter may be left in place after the examination.
2. Continue assessment of respiratory status. If deep sedation or anesthesia was used, follow institutional protocol for post-sedation monitoring. Typical monitoring includes continuous ECG monitoring and pulse oximetry, with continual assessments (every 5-15 minutes) of airway, vital signs, and neurologic status until the client is lying quietly awake, is breathing independently, and responds to commands spoken in a normal tone.

3. Monitor vital signs at the end of the procedure and then every 4 hours for 24 hours.
4. Observe for signs of allergic reaction to the dye for 24 hours.
5. Encourage the oral intake of fluids when not contraindicated. Monitor urinary output for quantity and hematuria for 24 hours. Notify physician for bladder distention, anuria, oliguria, or hematuria. Gross hematuria or persistent hematuria after the third voiding is abnormal.
6. Notify the physician if there are symptoms of infection (fever, tachycardia, hypotension, chills, dysuria, flank pain).
7. Resume previous diet.
8. Administer analgesics as prescribed.

Client and Family Teaching

1. This test helps to evaluate kidney structure.
2. Fast for 8 hours before the procedure if general anesthesia is to be administered.
3. A laxative may be prescribed the evening before the procedure. A cleansing enema may be prescribed to be given the morning of the procedure.
4. A sedative may be prescribed to be given just before the procedure.
5. After the procedure is over, save all the urine voided and report chills or pain with urination. Notify the physician if there are symptoms of infection (see #6 under Postprocedure Care).

Factors That Affect Results

1. Views are obscured by the presence of feces, gas, or barium in the bowel.

Other Data

1. Impaired renal function does not affect test results.
2. If the renal pelves are not visualized by this exam, ureteral obstruction may be present and may be localized by antegrade pyelography (see separate test listing).

Reverse Giemsa

See Banding in Genetic Disorders—Diagnostic.

Review of Peripheral Blood Smear: Red Blood Cell Morphology

See Red Blood Cell Morphology—Blood.

RFI

See **Renal Indices**—Diagnostic.

Rh Type

See **ABO Group and Rh Type**—Blood.

Rheumatoid Factor (RF)—Blood

Norm.

Qualitative	Negative
Quantitative	
Normal	<1:20
Chronic inflammatory disease	<1:40
Rheumatoid arthritis	1:40-1:60
	>300 IU/mL
Advanced rheumatoid arthritis	>1:60
Sjögren's syndrome	>300 IU/mL

Increased. Allografts (skin, renal), ankylosing rheumatoid spondylitis, cancer, cirrhosis, dermatomyositis, diabetes mellitus, diseases (of the kidney, liver, or lung), endocarditis, healthy clients more than 60 years of age, hepatic neoplasms, hepatitis, hypertension, infectious mononucleosis, juvenile rheumatoid arthritis, kala-azar, leishmaniasis, leprosy, lymphomas, macroglobulinemia, malaria, mixed connective tissue disease, neuropathy, osteoarthritis, paraproteinemia, polyarteritis nodosa, pulmonary interstitial fibrosis, rheumatoid arthritis, sarcoidosis, schistosomiasis, scleroderma, Sjögren's syndrome, smokers, splenomegaly, subacute bacterial endocarditis, syphilis, systemic lupus erythematosus, transfusions (multiple), tuberculosis, vaccinations (multiple), vasculitis, viral infections, and yaws.

Decreased After Previous Elevations. Gold salt therapy.

Description. Rheumatoid factor is an immunoglobulin present in the serum of approximately 65% of adults with rheumatoid arthritis (RA). It appears in the serum and synovial fluid several months after the onset of rheumatoid arthritis and is present for up to years after therapy. The antibody of the macroglobulin type produced in the synovium appears in the presence of autoimmunity, chronic infections, or connective tissue defects. This factor, though not specific for rheumatoid arthritis, is very helpful in diagnosis because high titers correlate with severe disease as compared to titers with other diseases. Analgesia and antiinflammatory pharmacologic preparations do not affect the presence of rheumatoid factor.

Professional Considerations

Consent form NOT required.

Preparation

1. Tube: Red topped, red/gray topped, or gold topped.
2. Specimens MAY be drawn during hemodialysis.

Procedure

1. Draw a 2-mL blood sample.

Postprocedure Care

1. None.

Client and Family Teaching

1. This is a screening test for many different disorders.
2. Results are normally available within 24 hours.
3. 50% of the risk for developing rheumatoid arthritis is attributable to genetic factors. Smoking is the main environmental risk.

Factors That Affect Results

1. Anticoagulant in the specimen tube invalidates the results.

Other Data

1. Clients who have rheumatoid factor identified early in the course of their rheumatoid arthritis have a greater risk of developing articular destruction than those identified later.

2. In general population, RF was associated with increased all-cause mortality and cardiovascular mortality.

3. Higher serum RF titers at baseline might predict better patient response to infliximab (Nozaki et al, 2010).

Rinne Test

See Tuning Fork Test, of Weber, Rinne, and Schwabach Tests—Diagnostic.

Rivaroxaban (Xarelto®)

See Prothrombin Time and International Normalized Ratio—Blood.

Rochalimaea henselae Antibody—Serum

Norm. Titer <1:64.

Increased. Titer >1:64 or a fourfold rise in titer between acute and convalescent sera: cat-scratch disease.

Description. A serologic test to identify antibodies to *Rochalimaea henselae* (*Bartonella* species), an organism implicated in 1992 as the causative agent of cat-scratch disease in humans who have been bitten or scratched by an infected cat as well as the cause of endocarditis and peliosis hepatis. The disease is characterized by unexplained regional lymphadenopathy, fever, malaise, and skin lesion at the site of injury. Although the cause of cat-scratch disease is not firmly established, *R. henselae* has been found in significantly higher levels in cats owned by clients infected with the disease who have recently been wounded by the cat. *R. henselae* is believed to be transmitted through the saliva or other body fluids of the sick cat when biting or scratching a human. In this indirect fluorescent antibody test, a sample of the client's serum with the *R. henselae* antigen and titers of antibodies to the antigen are measured. This test is more sensitive and specific than the skin test for *Bartonella* species.

Professional Considerations
Consent form NOT required.

Preparation
1. Tube: Red topped, red/gray topped, or gold topped.
2. Specimens MAY be drawn during hemodialysis.

Procedure
1. Draw a 2-mL blood sample.

Postprocedure Care
1. None.

Client and Family Teaching
1. Avoid traumatic contact, such as rough playing, with kittens and cats because this disease may be transmitted through bites and scratches from the animals.
2. Results are normally available within 24 hours.

Factors That Affect Results
1. None found.

Other Data
1. Fleas have also been suspected as transmission sources for this disease.
2. Most cases resolve spontaneously. Many antibiotics, such as gentamicin, are not effective against *R. henselae* infections. Aminoglycosides have been found to be bactericidal against the organism. Minocycline and macrolides antibiotics show high susceptibility and are currently the primary treatment for cat-scratch disease.

Rocky Mountain Spotted Fever (RMSF, *Rickettsia rickettsii* Antibodies) Serology—Serum

Norm. Negative.
Indirect fluorescent antibody assay (most sensitive): Diagnostically significant: titer >128 in a single specimen, or fourfold rise in paired serum titers, or any positive titer for IgM.

Latex agglutination test: Active Rocky Mountain spotted fever: titer >128.

Complement fixation for rickettsial infection: >1:160 or fourfold increase in paired samples within 7 days.

Weil-Felix agglutination reaction for rickettsial disease (least sensitive test): Strong agglutination response to *Proteus* Ox-19++++ is suggestive of rickettsial disease.

Enzyme-Linked Immunosorbent Assay

	IgG	IgM
<0.8 IV	Negative	Negative
0.9-1.1 IV	Equivocal	Equivocal
	Repeat testing in 2 weeks	Repeat testing in 2 weeks
1.2-2.3 IV	Positive	Low positive
		Repeat testing in 2 weeks
>2.3 IV	Positive	Positive
	Suggests current or past infection	Suggests current or recent infection

Positive. High titers occur with continuous exposure to bacterial, *Proteus*, or rickettsial infection and recent vaccinations.

Negative. Normal finding. Low titers occur with antibiotic therapy (early in the disease course) and in symptomatic clients who are unable to produce antibodies during active infection (immune deficiency disorders).

Description. Rocky Mountain spotted fever (RMSF) is an infectious disease caused by the parasite *Rickettsia rickettsii* transmitted to humans by the bite of an infected tick (usually the wood tick, *Dermacentor andersoni*; the dog tick, *Dermacentor variabilis*; and occasionally the Lone Star tick, *Amblyomma americanum*). Although believed to exist in the Western Hemisphere, this disease can occur anywhere that the vector is present. Symptoms include the sudden onset of fever lasting 2-3 weeks and the appearance of a rash spreading from the palms of the hands and soles of the feet to the entire body. Other symptoms include headache and abdominal pain. Myocarditis and death may occur if RMSF diagnosis is delayed or the disease is left untreated (death occurs 8 days after onset of symptoms) or treated only with chloramphenicol and not tetracycline or doxycycline (treatment of choice in adults and children). Other factors placing the client at higher risk of death include elderly age, absence of classic symptoms, and lack of noted tick bite. This test measures IgG and IgM antibodies to *R. rickettsii*.

Professional Considerations

Consent form NOT required.

Preparation

1. Tube: Red topped, red/gray topped, or gold topped.
2. Specimens MAY be drawn during hemodialysis.

Procedure

1. Draw a 5-mL blood sample, without trauma.
2. An acute sample should be drawn with the onset of symptoms.
3. Draw a convalescent sample 7 days later.

Postprocedure Care

1. Send specimens to the laboratory immediately.

Client and Family Teaching

1. This is a screening test to determine exposure to certain bacteria, including *Rickettsia*.
2. Return in 1 week to have a convalescent sample drawn. This will help determine if the disease is responding to treatment.

Factors That Affect Results

1. Weil-Felix false-positive reactions have been reported in *Borrelia* infection, *Proteus* infection, endemic typhus, leptospirosis, and liver disease (severe) and in clients who have been recently vaccinated.
2. Weil-Felix false-negative reactions have been reported when antibiotic therapy is started before the first specimen is drawn.
3. The latex agglutination test is useful only during active infection.
4. Low levels of IgM antibodies may persist for up to a year after an active infection.

Other Data

1. The Weil-Felix test is able to establish titers but does not use the causal agent as the reactive antigen. It is useful in screening for rickettsial infections but is unable to distinguish murine typhus from spotted fever. Indirect fluorescent antibody testing can be used for specific identification of RMSF.
2. If the Weil-Felix agglutination test is positive, the possibility of a *Proteus* urinary tract infection should be considered.

Roentgenography

See **Bone Radiography**—Diagnostic; **Chest Radiography**—Diagnostic; **Esophageal Radiography**—Diagnostic; **Esophageal Radiography**—Diagnostic; **Flat-Plate Radiography of Abdomen**—Diagnostic; **Radiography of Skull, Chest, and Cervical Spine**—Diagnostic; **Sinus Radiography**—Diagnostic.

Rotavirus Antigen—Blood

Norm. Negative antigen screen.

Positive. Presence of rotavirus antibodies and postviral lactase deficiency.

Negative. Normal finding. Also disaccharidase deficiencies.

Description. Rotavirus is a sporadic, acute, infectious, diarrheal disease of the Reoviridae viral class in which five serigraphs have been identified. It replicates exclusively in the epithelial cells of the small intestine during the winter or cooler months. This virus is the major cause of sporadic acute enteritis in infants and of epidemic acute gastroenteritis in small children. Occurrence in the young is presumed to be caused by the absence of a well-developed immune system. Rotavirus is presumed to be transmitted by the fecal-oral route and is detectable only during the first 7-8 days of illness. Symptoms in children start with vomiting and progress to fever, diarrhea, and abdominal cramping. Radioimmunoassay and complement-fixing antibody titers are used for rotavirus detection. Dominant genotypes include G1P (49%) and G2P (21%).

Professional Considerations

Consent form NOT required.

Preparation

1. Tube: Red topped, red/gray topped, or gold topped.
2. Specimens MAY be drawn during hemodialysis.

Procedure

1. Draw a 5-mL blood sample without trauma.
2. Heelstick is acceptable, collected in a Microtainer.

Postprocedure Care

1. None.

Client and Family Teaching

1. These clients are most often children; therefore emotional support and comfort measures should be offered during blood draws.
2. Results are normally available within 24 hours.
3. Parents should maintain enteric precautions during the client's diarrheal symptoms.
4. A live, attenuated rotavirus vaccine, RotaTeq, was approved in 2006 in the United States for immunization of infants.

Factors That Affect Results

1. Hemolysis of the specimen invalidates the results.

Other Data

1. Clients with the rotavirus may be free of symptomatic illness.
2. There is no specific treatment for rotavirus. Fluid and electrolyte balance should be supported to prevent severe dehydration.
3. Rectal swabs and stool samples should be examined for the presence of rotavirus antigen (see Rotavirus antigen—Stool).
4. Rotavirus should be suspected when the symptoms of diarrhea, vomiting, and fever occur together in children.
5. In 1998 a vaccine for rotavirus was made available, and subsequently recalled by the FDA because of an increase in

incidence of intestinal intussusception. Although the risk of intussusception was subsequently estimated to be between 1:10,000 and 1:32,000, the manufacturer is not planning a reintroduction of the vaccine. However, one new vaccine (Rotarix) has been used in Mexico since 2004, and another (RotaShield) is undergoing clinical trials. There is some expectation in the literature that they are safer vaccines and that one or both will become approved for use in 2006 or later.

Rotavirus Antigen—Stool

Norm. Negative. The presence of rotavirus in neonates less than 2 weeks of age is inconclusive.

Usage. Directly detects the rotavirus antigen that is shed in large amounts in the stool.

Description. Rotavirus illness, first discovered in 1970, is a diarrheal disease of the Reoviridae viral family in which five serogroups have been identified. It replicates exclusively in the epithelial cells of the small intestine and is pathogenic primarily in infants and children during the winter or cooler months. Rotavirus is presumed to be transmitted by the fecal-oral route. Rotavirus antigen in the stool is detected by direct visualization with electron microscopy or by the more common enzyme-linked immunosorbent assay (ELISA) screen. See also Rotavirus antigen—Blood.

Professional Considerations

Consent form NOT required.

Preparation

1. Obtain a clean, dry, preservative-free, covered cardboard specimen container or a tube with a screw topped cap, and a larger container of ice; or obtain a sterile culture swab and a closed, sterile container.
2. The client should disrobe below the waist for rectal swab collection.

Procedure

1. *Stool collection:*
   a. Obtain 5 mL or 5 g of liquid stool in a closed container or soiled diaper as soon as possible after evacuation from the bowel.
2. *Rectal swab collection:*
   a. Place the client in the left lateral position with knees and hips flexed and draped.
   b. Gently insert a sterile cotton-tipped swab at least 2.5-3.0 cm into the rectum. Rotate the swab from side to side and leave it in place for a few seconds to allow absorption of rectal flora.
   c. Place the swab into a sterile container without preservatives and cover tightly.

Postprocedure Care

1. The stool container should be placed on ice and transported promptly to the laboratory.
2. The rectal swab container should be labeled with the site and time of collection, packed in ice, and sent promptly to the laboratory.

Client and Family Teaching

1. These clients are most often children; therefore supportive measures should be offered if collection occurs by rectal swabbing.
2. Results are normally available within 24 hours.
3. Parents should maintain enteric precautions during the client's diarrheal symptoms.

Factors That Affect Results

1. Reject specimens placed in preservatives or those not placed on ice.
2. Prolonged rotaviral shedding has been found in clients with immunosuppression.

Other Data

1. Clients with the rotavirus may be free of symptomatic illness.
2. See Rotavirus antigen—Blood for information about the status of vaccines for rotavirus infections.

RPR

See Rapid Plasma Reagin Test—Diagnostic.

Rubella Serology—Serum and Specimen

Norm. Negative titer. A fourfold rise in titer of paired titer or a sample positive for rubella-specific IgG or IgM is diagnostic of exposure to rubella.

Hemagglutination Inhibition Test

Susceptibility to rubella infection	<1:8
Immunity uncertain	1:8
Immunity from prior infection or vaccination	>1:8
Resistance to rubella infection	>1:64

Fluorescent Antibody Test

Susceptibility to rubella infection	<1+
Positive for rubella antibodies	>1+

Time-Resolved Fluorometric Immunoassay for Rubella Antibody

Low levels of antibody	15 IU/mL

Chemilucent Immunoassay

IgG (IU/ML)		IgM Index Value (IV)	
<5	Negative	≤0.89	Negative
5-9	Equivocal		Equivocal
	Repeat testing in 2 weeks	0.90-1.09	Repeat testing in 2 weeks
>9	Positive	≥1.10	Positive
	Suggests current or past exposure to or immunization for rubella		Suggests current or recent infection or immunization

Usage. Determination of rubella immune status. Differentiation of rubella, measles, scarlet fever, erythema infectiosum, and exanthema subitum during pregnancy.

Description. Rubella, also known as "German measles," is an acute viral communicable disease of children and young adults. This infection is caused by the togavirus and produces a discrete red or pink macular rash that desquamates and vanishes in 2-3 days. It is transmitted client to client by direct contact with the discharges of infected clients or droplet-spray inhalation. Symptoms include rash, arthritis, and mild fever. Rubella is most common in underdeveloped countries, but outbreaks have occurred in well-developed countries secondary to suboptimal uptake of the vaccine. This test is useful when a pregnant woman is exposed to the rubella virus or an illness similar to rubella. Apparent or nonapparent transplacental fetal infection during the first trimester of pregnancy can result in spontaneous abortion or fetal congenital defects such as cardiac lesions, cataracts, congenital heart defects, deafness, encephalitis, growth and mental retardation, hepatitis, microcephaly, ocular lesions, pulmonary stenosis, radiolucencies of long bones, or retinopathy. This test measures IgG and IgM rubella antibody levels to determine the existence of active disease or active immunity. The oral fluid test measures rubella antibodies from fluid taken from around the gum line. IgM antibody levels are detectable a few days after the onset of symptoms, then peak in 7-10 days, and decrease to the undetectable level over the next 28-35 days.

Professional Considerations

Consent form NOT required.

Preparation

1. Tube: Red topped, red/gray topped, or gold topped. For oral fluid specimens, obtain a sponge oral fluid collection device.
2. Specimens MAY be drawn during hemodialysis.

Procedure

1. Draw a 3-mL blood or umbilical cord blood sample. Heelstick is acceptable, collected in a Microtainer.

2. Collect oral fluid by saturating well the sponge device around the gum line.
3. An acute sample should be drawn as soon as possible after symptoms appear.
4. The convalescent sample should be drawn at least 7-14 days after the acute sample and preferably 14-21 days after the onset of symptoms.

Postprocedure Care
1. Label specimen as acute or convalescent.

Client and Family Teaching
1. This test will show exposure to togavirus, the causative virus of rubella.
2. If pregnant, avoid anyone known to have rubella.
3. Return in 7-14 days for repeat testing.
4. A negative test result in the mother rules out infection in the fetus.
5. Rubella is highly communicable from adults for a week before and 4 days after the appearance of rash. Infants may transmit the virus in feces for up to 6 months.

Factors That Affect Results
1. Rubella antibodies remain present and static for many years.
2. The antibody levels decline with age.
3. The incidence of false-negative tests increases with age.

Other Data
1. The presence of rubella IgM in a newborn's sample indicates congenital infection. Confirmation of congenital infection requires that samples be drawn from the mother and the infant.
2. The MMR vaccination is recommended to be done twice, first between 12 and 15 months of age, and repeated between 4 and 6 years of age. It should NOT be given during pregnancy or within 28 days before becoming pregnant.

Rubeola Serology (Measles Antibodies)—Serum

Norm. Negative. The presence of antibodies 1 week after the onset of symptoms is indicative of susceptibility to rubeola infection. Recent exposure to the virus shows a fourfold or greater increase in antibody titers in two consecutive samples (acute and convalescent) drawn 1-4 weeks apart with use of hemagglutination inhibition or complement fixation methods.

Chemilucent Immunoassay

IgG Index Value (IV)		IgM Arbitrary Units (AU)	
<0.89	Negative	<0.89	Negative
0.9-1.09	Equivocal	0.90-1.10	Equivocal
	Repeat testing in 2 weeks		Repeat testing in 2 weeks
≥1.10	Positive	≥1.11	Positive
	Suggests current or past exposure to or immunization for rubeola		Suggests current or recent infection or immunization
	Indicates immunity if no symptoms are present		

Usage. Diagnosis of measles.

Description. Rubeola is an acute, highly contagious, viral, communicable disease caused by the measles virus of the Paramyxoviridae family. It is transmitted by direct contact with or inhalation of the infected oral or nasal secretions of infected clients. Rubeola is characterized by the appearance of a blotchy red facial rash appearing 3 days after a fever, with progression to a generalized rash lasting about 1 week. Other symptoms include Koplik's spots in the mouth, rose-colored maculopapular skin eruptions, photosensitivity, and catarrhal symptoms. Uncomplicated cases are usually self-limiting, but death may occur from complications and in undernourished children.

Professional Considerations
Consent form NOT required.

Preparation

1. Tube: Red topped, red/gray topped, or gold topped.
2. Specimens MAY be drawn during hemodialysis.

Procedure

1. Draw a 2-mL blood sample.
2. Heelstick is acceptable, collected in a Microtainer.

Postprocedure Care

1. Label specimen as acute or convalescent.

Client and Family Teaching

1. This test can show exposure to the Paramyxoviridae, which includes measles.

2. Results are normally available within 24 hours.

Factors That Affect Results

1. Hemolysis or contamination alters the results.

Other Data

1. ELISA assay is 20 times more sensitive than the complement fixation test and the hemagglutination inhibition test and is the assay of choice.
2. Measles deaths fell by 90% worldwide from 2000-2008 except in southern Asia.
3. Serum levels of sE-selectin were found to be significantly higher in children with measles versus healthy controls (Park et al, 2008).

Rubin's Test (Uterotubal Insufflation)—Diagnostic

Norm. Bilaterally patent fallopian tubes.

Normal patency: Pressure rises to 80-100 mm Hg and then decreases as carbon dioxide passes through the fallopian tubes.

Partial patency: Pressure rises to between 120 and 130 mm Hg.

Occlusion of tubes: Pressure rises above 200 mm Hg.

Usage. Diagnosis of obstruction, stenosis, or stricture of the fallopian tubes; and detection of spasm of the uterine end of the fallopian tubes.

Description. Rubin's test involves transuterine fallopian tube insufflation with carbon dioxide. A flowmeter and pressure gauge are attached to the source of the carbon dioxide. Changes in pressure are recorded on a kymograph. Displacement of adhesions and removal of debris from the tubes may occur during the procedure.

Professional Considerations

Consent form NOT required.

Risks

Air embolism, hemorrhage, infection, and referred shoulder pain.

Contraindications

Infections of the cervix, fallopian tubes, or vagina; in suspected pregnancy; and with uterine bleeding.

Preparation

1. See Client and Family Teaching.
2. An analgesic may be given 1 hour before the procedure to minimize tubal spasm from anxiety or discomfort.
3. Obtain povidone-iodine solution, a vaginal speculum, cervical swabs, and a cervical cannula.
4. The client should void.

Procedure

1. The client is placed in the dorsal lithotomy position, and the perineal area is cleansed with 1% povidone-iodine solution.
2. The physician introduces a vaginal speculum and exposes the cervix.
3. The cervix is swabbed.
4. A sterile cannula with a rubber tip is inserted into the cervical canal.
5. The cannula tip is pressed tightly against the cervical os to seal the opening and is secured with a tenaculum.
6. A rest period of approximately 2 minutes permits relaxation of the fallopian tubes.
7. 60 mL/minute of carbon dioxide (never air because of the risk of embolism) is administered into the uterus, and pressures are recorded by means of a kymograph.
8. During insufflation, a swishing sound may be heard with a stethoscope as the carbon dioxide passes through the tubes.

9. Shoulder pain caused by gas-induced subphrenic pneumoperitoneum is an indication of patency of at least one fallopian tube.

Postprocedure Care
1. Nausea, vomiting, cramping, dizziness, and pain associated with carbon dioxide gas absorption may be reduced by having the client rest for 2-3 hours with the pelvis elevated.

Client and Family Teaching
1. This test will determine the patency of the fallopian tubes.
2. Rubin's test takes approximately 30 minutes and is performed on an ambulatory care basis.
3. You may be prescribed a laxative to take the night before the examination or may be given a suppository or enema before the procedure.
4. Shoulder pain may be felt with insufflation.
5. You may rest with the pelvis elevated for several hours to reduce discomfort secondary to gas absorption.

Factors That Affect Results
1. Anxiety can cause fallopian tube spasm.

Other Data
1. This test is performed 4-5 days after the last day of menstruation.
2. Because Rubin's test can ensure only that at least one fallopian tube is patent, it is of limited value.
3. See also Hysterosalpingography—Diagnostic.

SAECG
See Signal-Averaged Electrocardiography—Diagnostic.

Sahara Clinical Bone Ultrasonometry
See Bone Ultrasonometry—Diagnostic.

Salicylate (Aspirin, Acetylsalicylic Acid)—Blood
Norm. Negative.

		SI Units
Analgesia therapeutic level	20-100 mg/L 20-100 µg/mL 2-10 mg/dL	0.14-0.72 mmol/L
Antiinflammatory therapeutic level	100-300 mg/L 100-300 µg/mL 10-30 mg/dL	1.09-2.17 mmol/L
Panic level	>50 µg/dL	3.62 mmol/L

Overdose Symptoms and Treatment
Symptoms. Acidemia, alkalosis, convulsions, dizziness, hyperactivity, hyperglycemia, hyperpnea, hyperthermia, ketosis, nausea, respiratory arrest, seizures, tinnitus, vomiting.

Treatment
NOTE: Treatment choice(s) depend(s) on client's history and condition and episode history.

1. Removing topical agents with soap and water and early emptying of the stomach is important.
2. Monitor salicylate levels with serial serum draws.
3. Position statements on the use of single-dose activated charcoal and on the use of multi-dose activated charcoal (Chyka, Erdman, Christianson et al, 2007) from the American Academy of Clinical

Toxicology indicate that data are insufficient to recommend the use of charcoal therapy for salicylate poisoning.

4. Maintain arterial pH at 7.4 and urine alkalinization to pH >7.5 with bicarbonate and fluids. Measure urine pH every hour. Potassium infusion may be necessary to achieve alkaline urine.
5. Fluid resuscitation may be necessary. This may be orally in mild cases, intravenously in severe cases.
6. A single dose of vitamin K may be given for the rare case of hypoprothrombinemia.
7. Diazepam is generally effective for seizures.
8. In the case of renal failure, dialysis is indicated. Both hemodialysis and peritoneal dialysis WILL remove acetylsalicylic acid.

Usage. Monitoring for salicylate toxicity during salicylate therapy or when overdose is suspected.

Description. Salicylates are a group of non-narcotic drugs with analgesic, antipyretic, antiinflammatory, and platelet aggregation–inhibiting (aspirin only) effects. Salicylates are absorbed in the gastrointestinal tract, metabolized in the liver, and excreted in the urine, with a half-life of 2-3 hours in short-term use and 15-30 hours in chronic use.

Professional Considerations
Consent form NOT required.

Preparation
1. Optimal sampling time for blood is 2-6 hours after salicylate ingestion.
2. Tube: Red topped, red/gray topped, or gold topped.
3. Do NOT draw specimens during hemodialysis.

Procedure
1. Draw a 4-mL blood sample.
2. Heelstick is acceptable, collected in a Microtainer.

Postprocedure Care
1. Assess for tinnitus and dizziness, signs of mild salicylate toxicity.

Client and Family Teaching
1. Watch for and seek medical attention for signs of toxicity, such as tinnitus and dizziness.
2. If activated charcoal was given for elevated levels, the client should drink 4-6 glasses of water each day for 2 days to prevent constipation. The activated charcoal will cause stools to be black for a few days.
3. For intentional overdose, refer client and family for crisis intervention.
4. Known causes include use of salicylate containing teething gel in infancy, inadequate mechanical ventilation (Stolbach et al, 2008), use of musculoskeletal preparations/rubs such as Ben-Gay (Pfizer) or oil of wintergreen (sweet birch oil). Note that even one lick of wintergreen oil can be fatal in children under 6 years old.

Factors That Affect Results
1. Negative result found in ketoacidosis.
2. Falsely elevated values have been found in infants with hyperbilirubinemia.
3. Sodium azide increases results.
4. An herbal or natural remedy that increases results is *Ginkgo biloba*.
5. Urine alkalinization (as by antacids) speeds renal excretion.
6. Lab error (false elevation) by not using a polymer-based lipid-clearing reagent prior to use of spectrometry in person with hyperlipidemia.

Other Data
1. Salicylate poisoning may include alkalemia, followed by acidemia, ketosis, and hyperglycemia. Treatment may include diuresis and dialysis.
2. Salicylate hepatitis can occur at blood concentrations of 20-25 mg/dL.

Salmonella Titer—Blood

Norm. Less than a fourfold rise in titer between acute and convalescent specimens.

Positive. Fever of undetermined origin and salmonellosis.

Description. *Salmonella* is a complex genus of gram-negative, non–spore-forming rods that are facultatively anaerobic. There are four subgenera of *Salmonella* (*S. typhi*, *S. choleraesuis*, *S. enteritidis*, and *S. arizonae*) as well as 1500 serotypes. *Salmonella* causes salmonellosis, typhoid fever, paratyphoid fever, septicemia, and sometimes inflammations of the joints and organs. The mode of transmission is through the fecal-oral route, most commonly by ingestion of food contaminated with the feces of infected clients or animals (e.g., reptiles). *Salmonella* organisms enhance their own uptake into the intestinal epithelium of the host. This test uses cellular (O) antigens and flagellar (H) antigens to detect the presence of *Salmonella* antibodies in a sample of serum.

Professional Considerations
Consent form NOT required.

Preparation
1. Specify for *Salmonella* antigens of groups A, B, C, or D on the laboratory requisition.
2. Tube: Red topped, red/gray topped, or gold topped.
3. Specimens MAY be drawn during hemodialysis.

Procedure
1. Draw a 7-mL blood sample. Label the specimen as the acute sample.
2. Repeat the test in 3-5 days and label the tube as the convalescent sample.
3. Heelstick is acceptable, collected in a Microtainer.

Postprocedure Care
1. None.

Client and Family Teaching
1. Thoroughly cook food, and avoid ingesting raw eggs or foods that have been sitting at room temperature for more than 2 hours.
2. 22.2% of all retail meat products were positive for *Salmonella* (Turkish study).
3. In addition to standard precautions, practice enteric precautions with the clothing and linen of infected clients.

Factors That Affect Results
1. Hemolysis or insufficient volume invalidates the results.
2. Titers on a single specimen are not diagnostically significant.
3. False-positive results may occur because of cross-reacting bacterial antibodies.
4. Antibiotic treatment may cause false-negative results.

Other Data
1. Stool culture is the definitive technique for diagnosing bacterial diarrhea.
2. The use of fluoroquinolones in animals has contributed to increasing emergence of strains of *Salmonella* resistant to these drugs. For this reason, this class of drugs is recommended to be restricted to use in humans only.
3. Antibiotic resistance has occurred with ampicillin, cephazolin, and amoxicillin-clavulanic acid.

SaO$_2$

See **Blood Gases, Arterial—Blood**.

SARS Test

See **Severe Acute Respiratory Syndrome—Associated Coronavirus Antibody and Reverse Transcriptase Polymerase Chain Reaction Tests**—Specimen.

SCA Gene Test—Diagnostic

Norm. Normal repeat numbers range from 15 to 29.

Cytosine Adenosine Guanine Repeat Range

	SCA1	SCA2	SCA3	SCA6	SCA7	SCA12
Normal	6-39	14-31	12-41	7-18	7-17	Not found
Pathologic	41-81	35-64	40-84	21-27	38-130	Not found

From Wilmot GR, Warren ST: A new mutational basis for disease: In Wells RD, Warren ST, eds.: *Genetic instabilities and hereditary neurological diseases*, San Diego, 1998, Academic Press.

Usage. Genetic testing determines diagnosis, course of disease, and likelihood of transmission of disease from generation to generation.

Description. SCA gene testing identifies autosomal dominant neurodegenerative spinocerebellar ataxia (SCA) genes found in Machado-Joseph disease (MJD) and other ataxias. SCA1, SCA2, SCA3, SCA6, SCA7, and SCA12 are members of a group known as "triplet repeat diseases" or "CAG repeat diseases" (cytosine, adenine, and guanine). In CAG repeat diseases, the trinucleotide sequence repeats abnormally within the gene coding sequence. At least 8 genes have been identified as causative for the cerebellar ataxias with a possible linkage to chromosome 15q. MJD, one of the most common ataxias, is characterized by abnormalities in the SCA3 gene. It includes symptoms of progressive weakness of the extremities, spasticity, dysphagia, exophthalmos, diplopia, and urinary frequency, and can occur in either mild or severe form, beginning at age 10 years. By identification of the intricate intracellular mechanisms by which SCA functions, treatments and cures for neurodegenerative diseases may eventually be found. This test involves isolating the DNA from the blood sample and then amplifying the CAG repetitions via polymerase chain reaction.

Professional Considerations

Informed consent is recommended for genetic testing.

Preparation

1. Tube: Lavender topped.

Procedure

1. Collect a 3.5-mL blood sample. Lavender topped tubes need 10-20 mL of whole blood.

Postprocedure Care

1. None.

Client and Family Teaching

1. Refer to Appendix B, "Informed Consent for Genetic Testing".
2. Persons with the disease had numbers from 35 to 59.
3. A repeat number in the low fifties for SCA2 probably represents a severe form of the disease.

Factors That Affect Results

1. Less than 3 mL in EDTA tube.
2. SCA diseases vary considerably across different ethnic groups and geographic regions.

Other Data

1. The Genetic Information Nondiscrimination Act of 2008 prohibits health plans from using genetic family history or genetic test results from influencing eligibility or premiums for health insurance. It also prohibits employers from using this information to influence decisions about hiring, terminating employment, or employment pay, promotions, or privileges.

SCC Antigen

See **Squamous Cell Carcinoma Antigen—Serum.**

Schick Test for Diphtheria—Diagnostic

Norm. Negative test.

Usage. Measurement of immunity to diphtheria. To eliminate the carrier state of strains during epidemics.

Description. The Schick test is an intracutaneous skin test to determine the immunity strain for diphtheria by detecting the presence of antitoxins in the blood to this respiratory disease. One performs the test by injecting $\frac{1}{50}$ of the minimum lethal dose of diphtheria toxin and then observing the site for a reaction, which would indicate lack of diphtheria immunity. A negative response indicates the presence of diphtheria antitoxin in the client's bloodstream. Immunity to diphtheria wanes over time; therefore a childhood vaccination does not guarantee immunity in adulthood.

Professional Considerations

Consent form NOT required.

Preparation

1. Obtain two intradermal needles with syringes, and two alcohol pads.

Procedure

1. Cleanse areas on the forearm with alcohol pads and allow the areas to dry.
2. Inject intracutaneously 0.1 mL of purified diphtheria toxin into one forearm and 0.1 mL of inactivated diphtheria toxoid into the other forearm.
3. Observe the sites for reaction 24-48 hours later (no longer than 120 hours). Absence of erythema, induration, and necrosis at the site is indicative of immunity to diphtheria.

Postprocedure Care

1. Leave the injection sites open to air.

2. For positive responses, inject $\frac{1}{13}$ U of diphtheria antitoxin to neutralize the toxin.

Client and Family Teaching

1. This test will indicate whether you are immune to diphtheria.
2. The recommended schedule for active immunization of children is 2 months, 4 months, 6 months, 18 months, and 4-6 years of age.

Factors That Affect Results

1. Expired toxin will cause false-negative results.

Other Data

1. If a client has been actively immunized but the Schick test is positive, the client is unable to produce antibodies.

Schilling Test—Diagnostic

Description. The Schilling test is a vitamin B_{12} (cyanocobalamin) absorption test that indicates if a client lacks intrinsic factor by measuring excretion of orally administered, radiolabeled cyanocobalamin (vitamin B_{12}) in a 24-hour urine sample. Vitamin B_{12} normally combines with intrinsic factor from the stomach and is absorbed in the terminal ileum. The test is based on the fact that, in normal clients, absorbed vitamin B_{12} in excess of the body's needs is excreted in the urine. Because parenteral nonradiolabeled cyanocobalamin is also administered to saturate the vitamin B_{12} binding sites, all the radiolabeled cyanocobalamin should eventually be excreted in the urine. Because this test requires the use of radioactive cobalt and the diagnosis of pernicious anemia can be made using other tests, the Schilling test is no longer performed and has not been available since 2003. See Pernicious Anemia in Part One for a full listing of tests used to diagnose pernicious anemia.

Schirmer Tearing Eye Test—Diagnostic

Norm. ≥10 mm of moisture from each eye after 5 minutes.

Absent tear production in Sjögren's syndrome.

Reduced tear production in meibomian gland dysfunction.

Usage. Aging that results in tearing, leukemia, lymphoma, Sjögren's syndrome, and rheumatoid arthritis.

Description. The Schirmer test differentiates "keratoconjunctivitis sicca" from abnormal or reduced tearing of the eyes. In normal eyes, both basic and reflex tearing keep the eyes moist. Basic tearing occurs throughout the day, supplying basic essential nutrients and lubricants to the eyes, and reflex tearing occurs in response to eye irritation. Either or both types of tearing capability may be absent or reduced in different disorders and lead to ocular surface damage. The Schirmer tearing eye test involves the simultaneous testing of the tearing ability of both eyes to assess the function of the lacrimal glands. The amount of moisture accumulating on filter paper held against the conjunctival sac is evaluated. Filter paper that remains dry for 15 minutes indicates insufficient tear formation.

Professional Considerations

Consent form NOT required.

Preparation

1. Two sterile strips of filter paper ruled in millimeters.
2. Topical anesthetic such as proparacaine.

Procedure

1. To measure the function of accessory lacrimal glands, instill one drop of topical anesthetic into each conjunctival sac before inserting the strips.
2. Position the client sitting upright with the head tilted back against a headrest.
3. Instruct the client to look upward and gently lower the inferior lids. Hook the folded ends of the filter paper strips over the inferior eyelids at the juncture between the middle and the lateral third.
4. After 5 minutes, remove the strips and measure the length of the moistened area in millimeters, starting from the folded ends of the strips.
5. The diagnosis of aqueous, tear-deficient dry eye is confirmed if 5 mm or less of tearing is evident on the filter paper.

Postprocedure Care

1. Assess for corneal abrasion caused by rubbing the eyes before the topical anesthetic has worn off.

Client and Family Teaching

1. This test assesses the tearing ability of the eyes.

2. After the test, do not rub your eyes until the topical anesthetic has worn off (usually about 30 minutes). Rubbing the eyes before this time can cause a corneal abrasion, which is painful and takes several days to heal.

Factors That Affect Results

1. Rubbing or squeezing the eyes increases tearing.

Other Data

1. The results of the Schirmer test are not consistently reproducible. The test also is not very sensitive for detecting dry eyes. Two additional tests being developed are the tear break-up time (TBUT) test and the fluorescein meniscus time (FMT) test. The TBUT test identifies unstable tears that contribute to dry eye, and the FMT test measures how long it takes for tears to form.
2. Drops containing sodium hyaluronidate are sometimes helpful in preventing ocular surface damage from dry eye. Punctal occlusion increases the amount of tears remaining on the eye surface by reducing the rate of tear outflow.
3. A modified version of this test is being used experimentally to test for dry mouth, or xerostomia.

Schlichter Test (MBD, Maximum Bactericidal Dilution, Serum Killing Test)—Specimen

Norm. Bactericidal activity >1:8 dilution.

Usage. Endocarditis and osteomyelitis.

Description. Determination of the maximum dilution necessary to be bactericidal for 99.9% of clients with an infecting organism. The maximum inhibitory dilution (MID) is the highest dilution of the client's serum that will inhibit the growth of the pathogen. The maximum bactericidal dilution (MBD) is the highest dilution of the serum that will eradicate the organism.

Professional Considerations

Consent form NOT required.

Preparation

1. Obtain venipuncture supplies and a red topped, red/gray topped, or gold topped tube, or a sterile tube and sterile aspiration set for body fluid testing.
2. Document recent antibiotics.
3. MAY be drawn during hemodialysis.

Procedure

1. Obtain both peak and trough levels: One before antibiotic treatment and the other 30-45 minutes after an antibiotic dose. Draw a 3-mL blood sample in the blood tube or a 2-mL body fluid sample by sterile aspiration.

Postprocedure Care

1. Transport to laboratory within 1 hour.

Client and Family Teaching

1. This test evaluates the success of antibiotic treatment.

Factors That Affect Results

1. Specimens more than 4 hours old invalidate the results.

Other Data

1. Results take 2-3 days.

S

Scintimammography (Miraluma, Sestamibi Breast Imaging, Radionuclide Breast Imaging)—Diagnostic

Normal or Negative. No uptake, or minimal symmetric, bilateral, uniform, diffuse uptake; equal to soft-tissue uptake.

Abnormal or Positive. Malignant lesions are noted by focal areas of increased uptake of the radioisotope. The results may be graded from 1 to 5, reflecting the progressive probability of a malignant lesion, or as equivocal, low, moderate, or high uptake of the isotope, with low, moderate, and high generally associated with malignant disease.

Usage. Follow-up or adjunct test to mammography in evaluating breast lesions in clients with an abnormal mammogram or palpable breast mass. Because the test depends on the molecular differences between cancer cells and normal cells and not on tissue density, it is useful in the further evaluation of breast lesions in women, especially if the woman has dense breast tissue (that is, fibrocystic disease, fatty tissue, or previous breast surgery, radiation therapy, chemotherapy, biopsy, breast implants, or silicone injections). It is not used for routine breast cancer screening, for confirming the presence or absence of breast cancer, or in place of biopsy. It helps the health care professional more accurately predict the chances of a breast lesion being cancerous. Research is being conducted to establish the effectiveness of the test in detecting axillary lymph node involvement in breast cancer and in the evaluation of breast tumor response to chemotherapy.

Description. A nuclear medicine planar scan in which a radioisotope, technetium-99m sestamibi (Miraluma, ^{99m}Tc-sestamibi, ^{99m}Tc-MIBI), is used to provide pictures of breast lesions. A "trace" amount of the radioisotope (producing a low dose of radiation) is injected intravenously and accumulates in areas of increased metabolic activity, such as that found in malignant cells. Images of each breast are taken by a gamma (Anger) camera to identify any areas of focal uptake of the isotope, indicating the possible presence of a cancerous lesion. A high-resolution method of this procedure has been shown to be more sensitive than a conventional camera for differentiating indeterminate breast lesions, but is still inferior to biopsy. However, this test has a high negative predictive value (93%) making it valuable in reducing the number of negative breast biopsies. Sensitivity is 87.8%, specificity 92.8% and positive predictive value 96.6%.

Professional Considerations

Consent form IS required.

Risks

Rare reports of severe hypersensitivity or seizures. Allergic reaction (itching, hives, rash, tight feeling in throat, shortness of breath, bronchospasm, anaphylaxis, death). Women of childbearing age should have minimal exposure because of the relatively high radiation dose to the ovaries.

Pregnant females: No studies have been done in pregnant females; the test should be administered only if clearly needed.

Nursing mothers: Components of ^{99m}Tc-sestamibi are excreted in breast milk; therefore formula feedings should be substituted for breast feedings.

Pediatric population: Safety has not been established.

Contraindications

Previous allergic reaction to Cardiolite or Miraluma (which are the same drug) or other radioactive dyes.

Preparation

1. Have emergency equipment readily available.
2. Assess for hypersensitivity to radioactive dyes.
3. Ask if the female client is pregnant or nursing.

4. Ask the client if there are any known breast lumps or other problems with the breast, a surgery or injury to the breasts, breast implants, or injections. The test should be performed before or at least 7-10 days after fine-needle aspiration, 4-6 weeks after a breast biopsy, and at least 2-3 months after breast surgery or radiotherapy. (This decreases the risk of nonspecific uptake of ^{99m}Tc-sestamibi.)

5. No fasting is necessary. The client may eat, drink, and take prescribed medications as usual before the test.

6. Have client remove all clothing and jewelry above the waist and provide hospital gown.

7. Establish intravenous access in the arm opposite from the breast with the suspected lesion.

8. At this time there are no definite guidelines regarding the timing of the test with a specific phase of the menstrual cycle.

9. Just before beginning the procedure, take a "time out" to verify the correct client, procedure, and site.

Procedure

1. The radioisotope (20-30 mCi of ^{99m}Tc-sestamibi) is injected intravenously in the arm opposite that of the breast in question. (This minimizes false uptake of the isotope in the ipsilateral axillary lymph nodes.) The dorsal pedal vein may be used if bilateral lesions are suspected or the client has had a mastectomy.

2. The client is positioned in a prone position on an imaging table that has an overlay with "cutouts" that allow the breasts to hang free. Five minutes after the injection of isotope, the camera will be positioned to take a lateral view of each breast, beginning with the breast with the abnormality and followed by the contralateral breast. The client may be asked to lie supine or to sit up with hands clasped behind head to obtain additional images of each breast. Each view takes about 10 minutes. The total test time is about 45 minutes to 1 hour.

Postprocedure Care

1. Encourage the intake of fluids to aid excretion of the radioactive medium from the body.

Client and Family Teaching

1. You may be asked to bring previous mammograms or other test results for the doctor to compare with scintimammograms.

2. You will be asked to remove all clothing and jewelry above your waist.

3. A venous access line will be necessary.

4. You may experience a slight metallic taste after the injection of the isotope.

5. You should remain still and breathe normally while the images are being taken by the camera.

6. There is no compression of the breasts during the procedure.

7. You should allow 60-90 minutes for the test.

8. Most of the radioactive material will be excreted from the body through urine and feces within 48 hours and is not harmful to other persons nearby.

9. The nuclear medicine physician will interpret the test and report the results to your doctor within several days.

Factors That Affect Results

1. The sensitivity of scintimammography is decreased in lesions that are less than 1.0 cm at the largest dimension.

2. False-positive results have been found with fibroadenomas, sclerosing adenomas, and juvenile adenomas.

3. The uptake of ^{99m}Tc-sestamibi by the myocardium and the liver may mask overlying breast activity in certain client positions.

4. Ibuprofen induces significant uptake reduction of the radiotracer ^{99m}Tc-(V) DMSA.

Other Data

1. Other radioisotopes being evaluated for use in scintimammography include ^{99m}Tc-tetrofosmin (Myoview) and ^{99m}Tc-MDP (methylene diphosphate).

2. Health care professionals working in a nuclear medicine area must follow federal standards set by the Nuclear Regulatory Commission. These standards include precautions for handling the reactive material and monitoring of potential radiation exposure.

3. Scintimammography and ultrasonography together have a 100% sensitivity, 77% specificity and 93% accuracy in breast cancer recurrence.

Scleroderma Antibody—Blood

Norm. Negative.

Positive. CREST (calcinosis, Raynaud's, esophageal dysfunction, sclerodactyly, telangiectasia) syndrome, and scleroderma.

Description. Scleroderma antibody (Scl-70) is found in the blood of clients with progressive systemic sclerosis.

Professional Considerations
Consent form NOT required.

Preparation
1. Tube: Red topped, red/gray topped, or gold topped.
2. Specimens MAY be drawn during hemodialysis.

Procedure
1. Draw a 5-mL blood sample.

Postprocedure Care
1. Refrigerate separated serum.

Client and Family Teaching
1. This test evaluates you for possible systemic sclerosis.
2. Results are normally available within 24 hours.

Factors That Affect Results
1. False-positive results may be created by aminosalicylic acid, diphenylhydantoin, ethosuximide, isoniazid, methyldopa, penicillin, propylthiouracil, streptomycin sulfate, tetracycline, and trimethadione.

Other Data
1. Absence of scleroderma antibody does not exclude diagnosis.
2. There is an increase in liver autoantibodies in patients with scleroderma.

Scout Film

See Flat-Plate Radiography of Abdomen—Diagnostic.

Screen Film Mammography

See Mammography—Diagnostic.

Scrotum and Testicular Ultrasonography—Diagnostic

Norm. Normal size, shape, and position of scrotum and testicles; negative for cyst, foreign body, stones, or tumor.

Usage. Evaluation of the size, shape, and position of the scrotum and testicles; differentiation of extratesticular from intratesticular mass. Color Doppler method used for detection of testicular torsion. Evaluate scrotal pain. Detection of inguinal hernia, varicocele, tumor, trauma to the scrotum.

Description. Scrotum and testicular high-resolution ultrasonography (ultrasound) is the evaluation of the pelvic structures by the creation of an oscilloscopic picture from the echoes of high-frequency sound waves passing over the pelvic area (acoustic imaging). The time required for the ultrasonic beam to be reflected back to the transducer from differing densities of tissue is converted by a computer to an electrical impulse displayed on an oscilloscopic screen to create a three-dimensional picture of the pelvic contents.

Professional Considerations
Consent form NOT required.

Preparation
1. The client should disrobe below the waist or wear a gown.
2. Obtain ultrasonic gel.
3. See Client and Family Teaching.

Procedure
1. The client is positioned supine in bed or on a procedure table.
2. The scrotum is covered with ultrasonic gel, and a lubricated transducer is passed slowly and firmly over the exterior

scrotum at a variety of angles and at 1- to 2-cm intervals.

3. Photographs are taken of the oscilloscopic pictures.

4. The procedure takes less than 30 minutes.

Postprocedure Care

1. Remove the lubricant from the skin.

2. Disinfect the transducer probe by soaking in glutaraldehyde solution for 10 minutes.

Client and Family Teaching

1. The procedure is painless and carries no risks.

Factors That Affect Results

1. Dehydration interferes with adequate contrast between organs and body fluids.

Other Data

1. Further studies may include tomography or other radiographic imaging.

Secretin Provocation Test

See Secretin Stimulation for Zollinger-Ellison Syndrome—Diagnostic.

Secretin Stimulation for Zollinger-Ellison Syndrome (Secretin Provocation Test)—Diagnostic

Norm. Serum gastrin: ≤200 pg/mL with no increase in production.

Increased. Gastrinoma (gastrin levels increase <100 pg/mL) and Zollinger-Ellison (ZE) syndrome (gastrin levels increase ≥110 pg/mL within 10 minutes). Drugs include amino acids, calcium, catecholamines, and insulin. Herbal or natural remedies include coffee (*Coffea*).

Decreased. Duodenal ulcer, G-cell hyperplasia (astral), and pancreatic dysfunction. Drugs include atropine.

Description. A stimulation test to assess for gastrinomas that can be correlated with chemical findings for diagnostic purposes. Secretin is a polypeptide secreted by the duodenal mucosa and the upper jejunum in response to gastric acidity. It acts to stimulate gastric pepsinogen, hepatic duct bicarbonate and water, pancreatic juice, bile, and intestinal fluid secretion and to inhibit gastric acid and gastrin secretion and intestinal smooth muscle contraction. ZE syndrome is a gastrointestinal disease in which elevated gastrin is formed, and pancreatic gastrinomas are present. In clients with ZE syndrome, the intravenous administration of secretin produces a paradoxical increase in serum gastrin levels. This test aids diagnosis of ZE syndrome for clients with baseline gastrin levels of 100-500 pg/mL (equivocal levels).

Professional Considerations

Consent form NOT required.

Risks

Allergic reaction to secretin.

Contraindications

Positive reaction to secretin skin testing.

Preparation

1. See Client and Family Teaching.

2. Establish intravenous access.

3. Obtain secretin for intravenous administration, a tourniquet, and 7 each of alcohol wipes, needles, syringes, and red topped tubes. Number the tubes sequentially.

4. Perform secretin skin testing to assess for allergy to the foreign protein. Inject 0.1 mL intradermally and observe 30 minutes for development of a wheal at the injection site.

Procedure

1. Draw a 5-mL blood sample for the gastrin level.

2. Inject intravenously 2-3 U/kg of body weight of secretin over 30 seconds. Repeat step 1 above every 5 minutes × 6 for a total of 30 minutes after injection, using the tubes in sequential order.

3. An alternative procedure is to infuse secretin 9 U/kg of body weight over 1 hour and draw blood specimens every 15

minutes. In ZE syndrome, gastrin levels peak after 45-90 minutes.

4. A 0.26 microg/kg secretin stimulation test has the best diagnostic efficacy for ZE syndrome.

Postprocedure Care

1. Label all the tubes and laboratory requisitions with the time the specimens were collected.

Client and Family Teaching

1. This test helps diagnose ZE syndrome.

2. Fast from food and fluids from midnight before the test.

Factors That Affect Results

1. None.

Other Data

1. Gastrin secretion may increase by 100-200 pg/mL (ng/L) every 5 minutes after secretin injection when gastrinoma is present.

2. Calcium provocation tests are also sometimes performed to aid in the diagnosis of ZE syndrome.

Secretin Test for Pancreatic Function—Diagnostic

Norm.

Duodenal Fluid		SI Units
Volume	95-235 mL/hour	
Bicarbonate	74-121 mEq/L	74-121 mmol/L
Amylase	87,000-267,000 mg	
Lipase	<1.5 U/mL	<415 IU/L

Usage. Assessment of exocrine secretory ability of the pancreas for carcinoma, ductal obstruction, or chronic pancreatitis.

Description. Secretin is a polypeptide secreted by the duodenal mucosa and the upper jejunum in response to gastric acidity. Some of its actions are to stimulate pancreatic enzyme secretion and bicarbonate pancreatic juice production. This test allows an assessment of pancreatic endocrine function by assessing duodenal contents for volume and bicarbonate, amylase, lipase, and trypsin levels before and after pancreatic stimulation by secretin. In chronic pancreatitis and cystic fibrosis, all values are low because of pancreatic tissue destruction. In early stages of obstructive pancreatic cancer, volume may be low, with other values normal. In pancreatic pseudocyst, bicarbonate level may be decreased, with other values normal. This test is usually followed by magnetic resonance cholangiopancreatography (MRCP), endoscopic ultrasound (EUS), or spiral computed tomography (spiral CT) and is replacing endoscopic retrograde cholangiopancreatography for confirming diagnosis of chronic pancreatitis.

Professional Considerations

Consent form IS required.

Risks
Allergic reaction to secretin. Complications of nasogastric tube insertion include bleeding, dysrhythmias, esophageal perforation, laryngospasm, and decreased mean po_2.

Contraindications
Positive reaction to secretin skin testing.

Preparation

1. Obtain a double-lumen orogastric tube, pH paper, secretin, and two aspiration syringes or mechanical suction.

2. Perform secretin skin testing to assess for allergy to the foreign protein. Inject 0.1 mL intradermally and observe 30 minutes for development of a wheal at the injection site.

3. Establish intravenous access.

4. See Client and Family Teaching.

5. Just before beginning the procedure, take a "time out" to verify the correct client, procedure, and site.

Procedure

1. An orogastric tube is passed into the duodenum to the ligament of Treitz. Placement is assessed by analysis of the pH of secretions. Gastric pH is acidic, whereas duodenal secretions are alkaline.

S

2. The gastric (proximal) lumen is continuously aspirated to prevent acidic gastric secretions from contaminating duodenal contents.
3. All the duodenal fluid is aspirated from the distal portion of the lumen and placed into a sterile container. The container is labeled with the date, time, and specimen source and sent to the laboratory for baseline volume and bicarbonate and amylase measurement.
4. Secretin, 1-2 U/kg of body weight, is administered intravenously.
5. All fluid is aspirated from the distal lumen every 20 minutes and analyzed for volume and bicarbonate, amylase, and lipase levels, as for the baseline sample.
6. Test may be followed by MRCP, EUS, or spiral CT.

Postprocedure Care
1. Remove the orogastric tube.

Client and Family Teaching
1. This test is one of several used to screen for pancreatic cancer or pancreatitis.

2. A nasogastric tube will be inserted through your nose into your stomach. Insertion may be uncomfortable and cause a pressurelike feeling or cause you to gag and cough. You will be asked to take sips of water and swallow to make tube insertion easier.

Factors That Affect Results
1. Failure to insert the tube fully into the duodenum causes unreliable results.

Other Data
1. There is a 5.1% chance of false-positive results and a 5.2% chance of false-negative results.
2. This test is somewhat out of favor because duodenal intubation is unpopular, and pancreatic disease is usually far advanced before exocrine function is appreciably reduced.
3. This test is of little help in distinguishing chronic pancreatitis from advanced pancreatic cancer.
4. Pancreozymin may be used in place of secretin for pancreatic stimulation, but it is more expensive.

Sedimentation Rate, Erythrocyte (ESR, Zeta Sedimentation Ratio)—Blood

Norm.

Age	Females	Males
Westergren, Modified Westergren Methods		
Pregnancy weeks 1-20	18-48 mm/hour	
Pregnancy weeks 21-40	30-70 mm/hour	
<50 years	0-20 mm/hour	0-15 mm/hour
50-85 years	0-30 mm/hour	0-20 mm/hour
>85 years	0-42 mm/hour	0-30 mm/hour
Children	0-10 mm/hour	0-10 mm/hour
Wintrobe Method	0.36-0.45	0.41-0.51
Zeta Sedimentation Ratio: 41%-54% (41-54 arbitrary units, SI units)		

Increased. Abscesses, acute pancreatitis (>60 mm/hour), anemia, ankylosing spondylitis, arteritis (temporal), arthritis (rheumatoid), autoimmune diseases, cat-scratch disease, cholesterol, coccidioidomycosis, colon cancer, Crohn's disease, dental decay, dermatomyositis, endocarditis, fever of undetermined origin, fibrinogen elevation, giant cell arteritis with severe ocular complications, hemolytic anemia, HIV, hyperfibrinogenemias, industry-related diseases, infection, inflammation, lymphoma, macroglobulinemia, malignancy, multiple myeloma, obstructive hepatic disease, osteomyelitis, pain (acute, chronic, abdominal, pelvic), paraproteinemia, pelvic inflammatory disease, pericarditis, peritonitis, polyclonal hyperglobulinemias, polymyalgia rheumatica, pregnancy, pulmonary embolism, renal disease, rheumatoid arthritis (65%-75% of clients), sepsis of unknown origin, sickle cell disease, sinusitis, Sjögren's syndrome, subacute bacterial endocarditis, systemic lupus erythematosus, tissue destruction, trauma, tuberculosis, and UTI. Drugs include angiotensin receptor blockers, dextran, fat emulsion, oral contraceptives, and vitamin A.

Decreased. Congestive heart failure and poikilocytosis. Drugs include albumin, corticotropin, cortisone, and lecithin.

Description. The erythrocyte sedimentation rate (ESR) is the most widely used lab test to monitor the course of inflammatory disease, as well as infections. When a tube of well-mixed venous blood is positioned vertically, the red blood cells will tend to fall to the bottom. The rate at which they fall is the ESR. The ESR is a reflection of acute-phase reaction in inflammation and infection. A limitation of this test is that it lacks sensitivity and specificity for disease processes. In addition, ESR cannot detect inflammation as quickly or early as can the C-reactive protein test. Thus C-reactive protein is sometimes used preferentially over ESR as a marker of inflammation (see C-reactive protein—Plasma or serum). Various methods are used to measure the ESR. The Westergren method is used most often because of the simplicity of the procedure. The Wintrobe method is more accurate for borderline elevations in the ESR. The zeta sedimentation ratio is a sedimentation rate calculation that provides more accurate data than the ESR in clients with anemia, requires the smallest amount of blood for testing, and provides the fastest results.

Professional Considerations
Consent form NOT required.

Preparation
1. Specimens MAY be drawn during hemodialysis.
2. *Westergren method:*
   a. Obtain venipuncture supplies and a blue topped tube, a 30-cm-long pipette with a 2.5-mm internal diameter and calibrated 0-200 mm, and a Westergren rack.
   b. For the modified Westergren method, substitute a lavender topped tube for the blue topped tube.
3. *Wintrobe method:*
   a. Obtain venipuncture supplies, a lavender topped tube, and a Wintrobe hematocrit tube.

4. *Zeta sedimentation ratio:*
   a. Obtain venipuncture supplies, a lavender topped tube, and a capillary tube.
5. Screen client for the use of herbal preparations or medicines or natural remedies.

Procedure
1. *Westergren method:*
   a. Draw a 4-mL blood sample in a blue topped tube. Gently roll the tube to mix the sample.
   b. Fill a pipette to the 0 mark with the blood sample.
   c. Place the filled pipette vertically in the Westergren rack at room temperature.
   d. After exactly 60 minutes, measure and record the distance to the top of the column of cells. Note that current research shows that a 30-minute estimation is applicable to hospitalized patients (Shteinshnaider et al, 2010). The 60 minute estimate = 10.7+1.2X where X = ESR at 30 minutes.
2. *Modified Westergren method:*
   a. Draw a 2-mL blood sample in a lavender topped tube.
   b. Add 0.5 mL of 3.8% sodium citrate or 0.85% sodium chloride to the sample, and follow the steps as for the Westergren method above.
3. *Wintrobe method:*
   a. Draw a 7-mL blood sample in a lavender topped tube.
   b. Fill a 7-cm-long Wintrobe capillary hematocrit tube with the blood sample, and then place the cap on the tube.
   c. Spin the tube for 5 minutes.
4. *Zeta sedimentation ratio:*
   a. Draw a 7-mL blood sample. Gently roll the tube to mix the sample.
   b. Heelstick is acceptable, collected in a Microtainer.
   c. Fill a capillary tube with 100 mL of the blood sample.
   d. Place the capillary tube vertically into a centrifuge.
   e. Spin for cycles of 45 seconds.
   f. Read the capillary tube like a standard hematocrit tube. The results are called the "zetacrit."
   g. Divide the true hematocrit by the zetacrit and express the result as a percentage.

Postprocedure Care

1. Perform the Westergren method within 2 hours, the modified Westergren method within 12 hours, the Wintrobe method within 4 hours, and the zeta method within 4 hours of collection.

Client and Family Teaching

1. This test is used in situations in which acute infection or inflammation is suspected. It is a screening test only.
2. Results are normally available within 4 hours.

Factors That Affect Results

1. *All methods:*
   a. Conditions that counteract accelerated ESR in the conditions listed under Increased include hypofibrinogenemia, polycythemia vera, sickle cell anemia, and spherocytosis.
   b. Results are elevated in the presence of anemia during pregnancy.
   c. Purified polysaccharides taken from cultures of the herb *Echinacea purpura* have been shown to slightly increase the ESR.
   d. Hemolysis or clotting invalidates the results.
2. *Westergren or modified Westergren method:*
   a. Heparin falsely increases the results.
   b. Bubbles in the pipette decrease the results.
   c. Tilting the pipette more than 3 degrees from vertical can increase the results by as much as 30%.
3. *Wintrobe method:*
   a. Inadequate duration or speed of the centrifuge or specimens overdiluted with EDTA cause unreliable results.
4. ESR results will be higher for the same client when plastic pipettes instead of glass tubes are used for the test.

Other Data

1. ESR is often normal in clients with connective tissue disease or neoplasms.

Segmented Neutrophils

See **Differential Leukocyte Count**—Peripheral Blood.

Selective Serotonin Reuptake Inhibitors (SSRIs)—Blood

Norm.

	Therapeutic Levels	Panic Level
Citalopram	25-550 ng/mL	Not established
Desmethylcitalopram	25-750 ng/mL	Not established
Didesmethylcitalopram	25-800 ng/mL	Not established
Desmethylvenlafaxine	200-400 ng/mL	Not established
Fluoxetine	50-480 ng/mL	>2000 ng/mL
Fluvoxamine	50-1000 ng/mL	Not established
Milnacipran	25-650 ng/mL	Not established
Norfluoxetine	25-500 ng/mL	>2000 ng/mL
Paroxetine	20-500 ng/mL	Not established
Sertraline	50-500 ng/mL	>500 ng/mL
Venlafaxine	25-500 ng/mL	Not established

Usage. Monitoring for therapeutic levels during drug therapy with selective serotonin reuptake inhibitors (SSRIs).

Description. SSRIs are a group of drugs that act by reducing serotonin reentry into the neurons of the brain. This leads to higher levels of serotonin and an improved mood in some clients. SSRIs are used to treat depression, with similar efficacy to the 50%-60% improvement rate achieved by tricyclic antidepressants. SSRIs are most effective in mild depression or when taken early in a course of depression.

Professional Considerations

Consent form NOT required.

Preparation

1. Tube: Red, gray/green/lavender, or pink topped.

Procedure

1. Draw a TROUGH 5-mL blood sample.

Postprocedure Care

1. None.

Client and Family Teaching

1. Specific to the medication; however, methylene blue is contraindicated in patients on SSRIs.

Factors That Affect Results

1. SSRI toxicity may occur with concomitant alcohol intake.
2. Trough levels are most consistently reproducible.
3. Increases and decreases (see following table):

	Drugs That May Cause Increased Levels	Drugs That May Cause Decreased Levels
Citalopram	Azole antifungals	Carbamazepine
	Cimetidine	Omeprazole
	Cyproheptadine (Periactin)	
	Erythromycin	
Fluoxetine	Benzodiazepines	
Paroxetine	Cimetidine	
Sertraline	Benzodiazepines	

Other Data

1. SSRIs are protein bound, so assess client serum albumin levels.
2. Fluoxetine has antiproliferative effect against Burkitt's lymphoma. If used in early pregnancy may be associated with a small increased risk for cardiovascular malformations (Ellfolk & Malm, 2010).
3. Citalopram can cause tachycardia, drowsiness, hypertension, severe hypoglycemia, vomiting, seizures, dysrhythmias, QTc prolongation, and metabolic acidosis in overdoses.
4. Paroxetine (Paxil), fluoxetine (Prozac) and bupropion (Wellbutrin) interfere with tamoxifen treatment in breast cancer.
5. Venlafaxine overdose associated with takotsubo cardiomyopathy.
6. Duloxetine is both a SSRI and norepinephrine reuptake inhibitor. Therapeutic serum levels are between 20-80 ng/mL.

Semen Analysis—Specimen

Norm per 1.5 mL

Appearance of semen	Highly viscid, opaque, white, or gray-white
Count (total spermatozoa)	39×10^6 spermatozoa/ejaculate or more
Liquefaction time of semen	20-30 minutes after collection
Odor of semen	Musty or acrid odor
pH of semen	7.2-8.0
Concentration of spermatozoa	$>15 \times 10^6$ spermatozoa/mL or more
Morphology of spermatozoa	>70% are of normal shape
	15% or more with normal forms
	85% or less with abnormal forms
Defective heads	<35
Defective mid pieces	≤20
Defective tails	≤20
Immature	<4
Motility of spermatozoa	>40% or progressive motility score of 3-4

Continued

Motility is graded as	60%-80% are motile
0 = none	50% or more with forward progression or
1 = poor	25% or more with rapid progression within
	60 minutes of ejaculation
2 = moderate	
3 = good	
4 = excellent	
Volume of semen	2-6 mL (0.002-0.006 L, SI units)
Vitality of spermatozoa	58% or more live
White blood cells	$<1 \times 10^6$/mL

Increased. Not applicable.

Decreased . Number. Cryptorchidism, hyperpyrexia, infertility, Klinefelter's syndrome, testicular irradiation. Drugs include heavy tobacco smoking and heavy consumption of the herb coffee (*Coffea*), which may decrease the number of motile spermatozoa.

Decreased Motility. Drugs include chemotherapeutics, cimetidine, and ketoconazole. Herbs include St. John's wort at highly concentrated doses of 0.6 mg/mL.

Description. Semen consists of spermatozoa in seminal plasma, which provides a nutritive medium for conveying the sperm to the endocervical mucus. The components of semen are obtained from the testes, seminal vesicles, prostate, epididymis, vas deferens, bulbourethral glands, and urethral glands. Because the interpretation is derived from microscopic visualization, the literature discusses common problems with interoperator reliability in interpretation of the results. Some computerized systems are being tested for semen analysis.

Professional Considerations
Consent form NOT required.

Preparation
1. Obtain a clean glass container.
2. Verify that the client's last ejaculation was between 7 days and 48 hours before collection.
3. Screen client for the use of herbal preparations or medicines or natural remedies.
4. If the semen is to be collected on-site, provide privacy for the male client.
5. See Client and Family Teaching.

Procedure
1. Collect a fresh specimen in a clean glass jar. The client may obtain the specimen at home if he is unable to masturbate or is uncomfortable with masturbation.

Postprocedure Care
1. Document specimen collection time. Specimens must be received within 1 hour and examined within 3 hours.
2. Reject semen specimens over 2 hours old.
3. Heavy tobacco smoking and heavy coffee consumption may decrease the number of motile spermatozoa. However, one recent study found that sperm motility increased significantly with coffee drinking and with smoking when evaluated in infertile couples.
4. Coital lubricants reduce sperm motility.
5. The presence of antisperm antibodies has been shown to affect sperm linearity, but not sperm motility.

Client and Family Teaching
1. This test is used to estimate the number of sperm and evaluate fertility.
2. Do not have intercourse or masturbate for 48 hours before specimen collection. Make sure to ejaculate at least once between 48 hours and 7 days before collection.
3. Collect a fresh semen specimen in a plastic cup without using a condom or lubricants other than saliva. The specimen should be collected by masturbation at the institution or at home.
4. Keep track of the time the semen was collected.
5. For home collection: After collecting the specimen, keep the container of semen warm by putting it in a pocket next to the human's body.
6. If the specimen is collected at home, it must be delivered to the laboratory within 1 hour.

7. Consult with your physician before using natural or herbal remedies or medicines because some have been shown to impair the activity of or damage sperm as well as oocytes.

Factors That Affect Results
1. Temperature extremes decrease the sperm count.
2. Reject semen specimens more than 1 hour old.
3. Males with infertility tend to have increased semen volume, which is associated with diminished sperm count.

4. *Herbal effects:* Several studies have shown that St. John's wort is mutagenic to sperm cells and saw palmetto induces metabolic changes in sperm. High doses of *Echinacea purpura* have been found to interfere with sperm enzyme activity.
5. An herbal or natural remedy that has been shown to increase sperm motility in vitro is *Astragalus membranaceus.*

Other Data
1. Repeat testing may be necessary because results vary with samples.
2. See also Infertility screen—Specimen.

Sensitive TSH Assay

See Thyroid-Stimulating Hormone, Sensitive Assay—Blood.

Sentinel Lymph Node Biopsy (SLNB)—Diagnostic

Norm. A sentinel lymph node is defined as a lymph node that stains blue or is radioactive.

Usage. Helps avoid total axillary node dissection during early breast cancer; provides staging information for operable invasive breast cancer; identifies location of sentinel node for subsequent tumor resection. Also used to help diagnose malignant melanoma, skin cancer, and head and neck cancer. SLNB is being studied for its usefulness in evaluating other types of solid tumors.

Description. Metastasis to lymph nodes can be determined by identifying lymph flow from the tumor site to the primary lymph node via radio-guided biopsy. The sentinel lymph node is the first lymph node in the lymphatic basin to receive lymph flow from a primary tumor. Thus it will be the first node to contain metastasis and can be identified on lymphoscintigraphy by following the blue dye to the most proximal node. SLNB is a standard of care for breast cancer.

Professional Considerations
Consent form IS required for the biopsy portion of this procedure.

Risks
Bleeding; infection; reaction to the dye, more so when isosulfan blue is used than when methylene blue is used.

Contraindications
Sentinel lymph node biopsy for work-up of breast cancer is contraindicated in clients who have had previous breast surgery or radiation to the breast, as well as in clients who have clinically palpable nodes, locally advanced breast disease, tumors in more than one location in the breast, lymphatic problems, burns, breast reduction surgery, or breast implants.

Preparation
1. 3-5 mL of isosulfan blue radioactive tracer is injected subdermally around the circumference of the tumor (for palpable masses) or peritumorally or intratumorally under the guidance of ultrasound. Alternatively, methylene blue dye has been used and has less incidence of allergic reaction.
2. The site is then massaged for 5 minutes to promote migration of the tracer.
3. Just before beginning the procedure, take a "time out" to verify the correct client, procedure, and site.

Procedure
1. 2-6 hours after tracer injection, the area of the tumor site is scanned via lymphoscintigraphy to identify the "hot spot," which is marked on the skin and later used for localization of tumor for excision. The remainder of the lymph

node basin is examined for residual radioactivity.

Postprocedure Care

1. A dry, sterile dressing is required.
2. Assess vital signs and the site for bleeding.

Client and Family Teaching

1. Consume only clear liquids after midnight and before the biopsy.
2. A lumpectomy is usually performed immediately after the sentinel node biopsy.
3. Do not lift more than 10 pounds for 48 hours after the procedure.
4. Final results may take up to 1 week.
5. Observe for signs of infection and report to the physician: increasing pain, redness, swelling, drainage, or temperature >101 degrees F (38.3 degrees C).

Factors That Affect Results

1. Surgeon's skill and frequency of performing procedure.

2. The shine-through effect of radiocolloid from the primary site may affect localization of the sentinel node.
3. If results are negative further immunohistochemical testing of the specimen is not clinically warranted (Giuliano et al, 2011).
4. Sensitivity is low when used for assessing nodal status in clients with colorectal cancer.
5. Rhodes (2011) found that for clients with melanoma, this test can be useful in determining prognosis when the tumor thickness is 1-4mm (intermediate classification) and is not helpful for tumors classified as "thin" or "thick".

Other Data

1. In one study (Izawa et al, 2005), SLNB was found not to be useful for evaluation of penile cancer.

Serotonin (5-Hydroxytryptamine)—Serum or Blood

Norm.

	Adults	SI Units
Whole blood, high-performance liquid chromatography(HPLC)	50-200 ng/mL or µg/L	0.28-1.13 µmol/L
Serum, HPLC	50-220 ng/mL or µg/L	0.28-1.24 µmol/L

Increased. Carcinoid syndrome, cystic fibrosis, Duchenne's muscular dystrophy, dumping syndrome, endocarditis, essential hypertension, Huntington's disease, metastasis, migraine, myocardial infarction, nontropical sprue, oat cell carcinoma of the lung (causing ectopic production), pain (chronic), pancreatic islet cell tumor (causing ectopic production), primary pulmonary hypertension, schizophrenia, and thyroid medullary carcinoma (causing ectopic production). Drugs include imipramine, methyldopa, monoamine oxidase (MAO) inhibitors, reserpine, selective serotonin reuptake inhibitors (SSRIs) (citalopram, desmethylcitalopram, didesmethylcitalopram, fluoxetine, milnacipran, norfluoxetine, paroxetine, sertraline, venlafaxine), and tramadol (decreasing the serotonin reuptake).

Decreased. Depression, Down syndrome, Parkinson's disease, phenylketonuria, renal insufficiency, and teratomas (benign cystic).

Description. Serotonin is an indolamine synthesized from L-tryptophan, an essential amino acid, by the argentaffin cells of the intestinal mucosa. Serotonin is stored in and transported by platelets, but it is also found in many body tissues, including the central nervous system and gastrointestinal tract. Serotonin mediates cardiovascular integrity, neurotransmission, smooth muscle contraction (gastrointestinal motility), prolactin release, and growth hormone release and functions in hemocoagulation. This broad array of actions occurs as a result of the location of serotonin receptors throughout the body. This test is used to confirm the diagnosis of carcinoid tumors, in which the highest increases in levels are found.

Professional Considerations
Consent form NOT required.

Preparation
1. Preschedule this test with the laboratory. Clarify whether the client must follow a low-indole diet for a period of time before testing.
2. MAO inhibitor drugs should be discontinued 1 week before the test.
3. Avoid radionuclide scans for 7 days before the test.
4. Tube: Chilled lavender topped, and a container of ice.
5. Specimens MAY be drawn during hemodialysis.

Procedure
1. Draw a 7-mL blood sample. Place the specimen on ice.
2. Heelstick is acceptable, collected in a Microtainer.

Postprocedure Care
1. Send specimens to the laboratory promptly. Specimens must be transferred to a plastic container of 10 mg of EDTA and 75 mg of ascorbic acid and frozen within 4 hours of collection.

Client and Family Teaching
1. This test is used to screen for carcinoid tumors.
2. Results are normally available within 48 hours.

Factors That Affect Results
1. Lithium either increases or decreases the level of serotonin in the brain.
2. A radioactive scan within 7 days before this test invalidates the results of the radioimmunoassay method.

Other Data
1. Because blood serotonin samples are unstable, urine measurements of 5-hydroxyindoleacetic acid are more commonly measured.

Sertraline
See **Selective Serotonin Reuptake Inhibitors**—Blood.

Serum Glutamic-Oxaloacetic Transaminase (SGOT)
See **Aspartate Aminotransferase**—Serum.

Serum Glutamic-Pyruvic Transaminase (SGPT)
See **Alanine Aminotransferase**—Serum.

Serum Killing Test
See **Schlichter Test**—Specimen.

Sestamibi Breast Imaging
See **Scintimammography**—Diagnostic.

Sestamibi-Dipyridamole Stress Test and Scan
See **Heart Scan**—Diagnostic.

Sestamibi Exercise Testing and Scan
See **Heart Scan**—Diagnostic.

Severe Acute Respiratory Syndrome (SARS)–Associated Coronavirus (CoV) Antibody and Reverse Transcriptase Polymerase Chain Reaction (RT-PCR) Tests—Specimen

Norm. Negative.

Positive. Any one of the following: Detection of SARS covalent RNA in two specimens from different sites, or from two same-site specimens collected on different days; isolation in culture of SARS coronavirus; detection of SARS-CoV antibody in a single serum sample; a fourfold increase in titer between acute and convalescent serum specimens.

Description. Helps rapidly identify persons with severe acute respiratory syndrome (SARS). SARS, thought to be caused by a human coronavirus, first appeared in late 2002. It causes mild respiratory symptoms of cough and fever and may progress to severe pneumonia and possibly death. SARS is thought to be transmitted by direct contact with infected droplets, but airborne transmission is also being considered. Selection of sites for specimens are determined by the timing of collection. Nasopharyngeal swab, oropharyngeal specimen, and serum are recommended if collection is done within 1 week of illness onset. Nasopharyngeal swab, oropharyngeal specimen, and stool specimens are recommended if collection is done later than 1 week after illness onset.

Professional Considerations

Consent form IS recommended by the Centers for Disease Control and Prevention (CDC). Consent to have the leftover specimen stored at the CDC should also be obtained.

Preparation

1. For aspirates, obtain NON bacteriostatic saline, a plastic catheter, and a sterile vial containing viral transport medium.
2. For swabs, obtain sterile swabs made of Dacron or rayon with plastic shafts and vials of viral transport medium.
3. For blood sample, obtain a red topped or lavender topped tube with external caps and internal O-ring seals.
4. For stool, obtain a clean container and paraffin for sealing.

Procedure

1. Collect acute specimens as soon as possible after illness is suspected. Collect convalescent specimens 22 days after the onset of symptoms.
2. *Nasopharyngeal wash/aspirate* (specimen of choice): Flush catheter with nonbacteriostatic saline. After instilling 1.5 mL of nonbacteriostatic saline into the nostril, aspirate from the nasopharynx. Repeat procedure through the other nostril.
3. *Nasopharyngeal swab*: Insert swab into the nostril, pressing lightly against the nasopharynx for a few seconds. Repeat in other nostril with another swab.
4. *Oropharyngeal swab*: Insert swab through the mouth, using care to avoid the tongue. Press lightly against the posterior pharynx and tonsillar area. Insert swab into vial containing viral transport medium.
5. *Lower respiratory tract*: Obtain bronchoalveolar lavage fluid. Place half of the fluid into sterile vials with external caps and internal O-ring seals. Spin the remaining fluid and fix the cell-pellet in formalin. For sputum, client should rinse mouth with water; then use stacked inhalations to produce expectorate of sputum into a sterile container.
6. *Blood*: Collect a 5-mL blood sample in a red- or purple topped tube. 1 mL is acceptable for pediatric collections. Both acute and convalescent specimens (at 4 weeks) should be obtained.
7. *Stool*: Collect 10-50 mL in a clean container. Seal the lid with paraffin and place in a bag.

Postprocedure Care

1. Label specimens with collection date, collection site, and identification numbers. Store at 4 degrees C and ship to CDC-approved testing laboratory.
2. If consent has been obtained for long-term storage, forward remaining specimen and client-identifying information to the CDC.

Client and Family Teaching

1. Prepare client for the possibility of false-positive and false-negative results.

2. Prepare client for the possibility of quarantine, even with negative test results.

Factors That Affect Results

1. Sensitivity and specificity of these tests are not yet known. Specimens stored with the CDC may be repeat-tested, as test methods improve.
2. False-negative RT-PCR may occur if viral RNA is not present in the specimen at the time of collection.
3. False-negative CoV antibody results may occur if specimen is collected earlier than 21 days or longer after the onset of illness.
4. Use of calcium alginate swabs or swabs with wooden shafts may cause false-negative results as a result of viral inactivation or inhibition of PCR.
5. The chances of positive findings are increased when specimens from multiple sites are collected.

Other Data

1. It is not known yet if there are other causative agents for SARS.

Sex Hormone Binding Globulin

See Testosterone, Free and Total—Blood.

SFM

See Mammography—Diagnostic.

SFMC

See Soluble Fibrin Monomer Complex—Serum.

SGNFD

See Sweat Gland Nerve Fiber Density Test—Specimen.

SGOT

See Aspartate Aminotransferase—Serum.

SGPT

See Alanine Aminotransferase—Serum.

Shake Test

See Foam Stability Index—Amniotic Fluid.

SHBG

See Testosterone, Free and Total—Blood.

S

Sickle Cell Test—Blood

Norm. *Sickling test*: negative, no sickled red blood cells seen, no hemoglobin S.
Solubility test: negative.

Positive. Pain (chronic) and sickle cell anemia.

Negative. Drugs include phenothiazines at concentrations >128 mg/mL.

Description. Sickle cell disease is an inherited disease characterized by chronic hemolytic anemia and painful episodes of "sickle cell crises," which usually require high doses of narcotics for relief. It is common in the African-American population, affecting 3 of every 1000 persons. Those inheriting the disease are at a higher risk for mortality and morbidity. Sickle cell disease causes pain crises, hemolytic anemia, splenic malfunction, and infections. The prevalence of asthma is higher in person with sickle cell trait. The sickle cell test is a screening test used to demonstrate the presence of hemoglobin S, which causes red blood cells to assume a sickle shape or crescent shape under reduced oxygen supply. The sickling test is positive in sickle cell anemia or sickle cell trait or in combinations of other hemoglobin S abnormalities.

Professional Considerations

Informed consent is recommended for genetic testing.

Preparation

1. Tube: Lavender topped, pink topped, green topped, or black topped.
2. Note whether the client received a blood transfusion within the previous 4 months because this may produce false-negative results.
3. Specimens MAY be drawn during hemodialysis.

Procedure

1. Draw a 3-mL blood sample. Gently roll the tube to mix the specimen.

Postprocedure Care

1. Observe for signs of sickle cell disease: fatigue, dyspnea, bone pain, joint swelling, and chest pain.

Client and Family Teaching

1. This test is used in screening for sickle cell disease. Refer to Appendix B, "Informed Consent for Genetic Testing".
2. Clients with sickle cell disease should avoid hypoxic situations such as high altitudes, strenuous activity, extreme cold, and traveling in an unpressurized aircraft.
3. Refer clients with sickle cell disease for genetic counseling.

Factors That Affect Results

1. If hemoglobin S concentration is <25%, erythrocytes will not sickle.
2. False-positive results may be caused by polycythemia, hemoglobin abnormalities, or high blood protein levels (such as systemic lupus erythematosus, multiple myeloma).
3. Collection of more than 7 mL of blood may cause false-positive results.
4. False-negative results may be caused by anemia in combination with less than 7 mL of blood drawn, blood transfusion of normal hemoglobin within the previous 4 months, phenothiazine drug therapy, concurrent iron deficiency or thalassemia, elevated hemoglobin F levels, and in infants less than 6 months of age.
5. Hemolysis, clotting, or lipemia of the specimen invalidates the results.

Other Data

1. This test cannot reliably differentiate the homozygous sickle cell state from the heterozygous trait.
2. The Sickledex is a trade name for the sickle cell test.
3. Treatment may include bone marrow transplantation.
4. The Genetic Information Nondiscrimination Act of 2008 prohibits health plans from using genetic family history or genetic test results from influencing eligibility or premiums for health insurance. It also prohibits employers from using this information to influence decisions about hiring, terminating employment, or employment pay, promotions, or privileges.

Sickledex Test

See **Sickle Cell Test**—Blood.

Siderophilin

See Transferrin—Serum.

Sigmoidoscopy—Diagnostic

Norm. Negative.

Usage. Identify bowel obstruction, carcinoma of sigmoid colon, celiac sprue, colitis, Crohn's disease, diverticulitis, diverticulosis; help diagnose causes of malabsorption.

Description. Sigmoidoscopy is the endoscopic visualization of the interior space and walls of the sigmoid colon, using a sigmoidoscope. A sigmoidoscope is a 50-cm fiberoptic tube with a lighted mirror lens system that illuminates the sigmoid colon for visualization. A rigid sigmoidoscope is rarely used, because of the degree of discomfort it causes. The most common method for this procedure is a flexible sigmoidoscopy, in which a short, flexible tube with a light source is inserted through the rectum and advanced to the sigmoid colon. Because flexible sigmoidoscopy examines only the lower one third of the colon, it cannot completely rule out colon cancer. However, it has been shown to identify 50%-70% of advanced colorectal neoplasms and thus is considered a cost-effective test for screening. The American Cancer Society recommends screening sigmoidoscopy every 5 years for all adults >50 years, followed by a colonoscopy in those with positive results.

Professional Considerations

Consent form IS required.

Risks

Air embolism (rare), bowel perforation (0.15%), hemorrhage, peritonitis, pneumatic perforation of cecum vasovagal reaction.

Contraindications

Anorectal fistula, diverticulitis, paralytic ileus, third-trimester pregnancy. Sedatives are contraindicated in clients with central nervous system depression.

Preparation

1. See Client and Family Teaching.
2. Obtain sterile specimen containers if a biopsy is planned.
3. The client should disrobe below the waist or wear a gown.

4. Just before beginning the procedure, take a "time out" to verify the correct client, procedure, and site.

Procedure

1. The client is placed in the left lateral position.
2. Monitor blood pressure, heart rate, and oxygen saturation rate by pulse oximeter before analgesic and sedative are given and then every 5 minutes during the procedure.
3. An analgesic and/or a sedative may be administered. Monitor respiratory status continually after sedation.
4. The sigmoidoscope is lubricated and inserted into the anus and rectum and then slowly advanced into the sigmoid colon. Insufflation occurs to aid in visualization. However, insufflation of CO_2 rather than air reduces abdominal pain and bowel distention after colonoscopy.
5. During the procedure, biopsy specimens and photographs may be taken, and suction is used to remove excess secretions.

Postprocedure Care

1. Assess for side effects of the sedative: hypotension, depressed respirations, and bradycardia.
2. Continue the assessment of the respiratory status. If deep sedation was used, follow institutional protocol for post-sedation monitoring. Typical monitoring includes continuous ECG monitoring and pulse oximetry, with continual assessments (every 5-15 minutes) of airway, vital signs, and neurologic status until the client is lying quietly awake, is breathing independently, and responds to commands spoken in a normal tone.

Client and Family Teaching

1. This test is performed to evaluate the colon for several different disorders.
2. Consume a full liquid diet the evening before the test.

3. Laxatives may be prescribed to be administered the night before the test with or without an enema or suppository 1 hour before the test, except in pregnant women. Magnesium citrate and a Fleet enema also produce excellent results.
4. The urge to defecate as the sigmoidoscope is inserted into the rectum is normal.
5. The procedure takes approximately 30 minutes.
6. Resume normal activities and diet as soon as you feel ready.
7. Call a physician if your temperature is higher than 101 degrees F (38.3 degrees C), or if you have trouble breathing or experience stomach pain, nausea, or bright-red rectal bleeding.

Factors That Affect Results

1. Retained barium from previous studies makes visualization impossible.

2. Fixation of the bowel from previous radiation therapy or surgery may inhibit the passage of the sigmoidoscope.
3. Older clients and female clients have a higher incidence of incomplete exams and inadequate sigmoidoscopies, because of failure to achieve at least a depth of insertion of 40 cm. The rate of complete exams can be increased by use of sedation, analgesia, and/or distraction during the examination.

Other Data

1. Women more than men fail to comply with recommendations to have this procedure done for cancer screening. A major contributor to this decision is a low perceived risk of bowel cancer because of current health/symptom status, and lack of having a family history of colorectal cancer.

Signal-Averaged Electrocardiography (Signal-Averaged ECG, SAECG)—Diagnostic

Norm. No late potentials detected.

Usage. Main value is in identifying low-risk patients for acute myocardial infarction. Also used in determination of the risk for developing life-threatening dysrhythmias for the following high-risk conditions: myocardial infarction, clients with a history of reentrant dysrhythmias, survivors of sudden cardiac death, and syncope. Aids decision-making about the need for further evaluation and treatment, including electrophysiologic study, drug treatment, antitachycardia pacemaker, or coronary artery bypass grafting. Better at predicting risk of VT than VF.

Description. Signal-averaged electrocardiography (SAECG) is an inexpensive, non-invasive method for detection of late ventricular potentials (late potentials). Late potentials are low-amplitude electrical activity occurring in diastole during a normally isoelectric phase. Their presence signals slowed conduction velocity and is usually associated with disease, ischemia, or scarring of the heart muscle. The existence of late potentials is believed to indicate a potential for the development of reentrant dysrhythmias, which may lead to sudden cardiac death. Traditional electrocardiography is not sensitive enough to detect the very-low-amplitude electrical activity of late potentials. Signal averaging is an electrocardiographic method that amplifies and averages up to 10,000 samples of electrical activity per second from the electrocardiographic signals of 100-1000 cardiac cycles to reduce the effect of random noise and artifact, thus allowing the detection of late potentials. The procedure may take up to 20 minutes, depending on the number of cardiac cycles averaged and the amount of electrical interference present. The presence of late potentials in the SAECG is determined by examination of the duration of the QRS complex, the root mean square voltage of the last 40 msec of the QRS complex, and the duration of the terminal QRS complex that measures under 40 mV.

Professional Considerations

Consent form NOT required.

Preparation

1. Provide a private, comfortable, calm, warm environment to help the client relax skeletal muscles and avoid shivering.
2. To minimize artifact caused by electrical interference, turn off all nonessential electrical equipment in the area. For example, run IV pumps on battery, and

turn off the hypothermia machine, television, and radio. Plug the SAECG machine into an outlet different from that of essential equipment such as a ventilator or monitor.
3. Obtain electrodes, conduction gel, and an SAECG machine.

Procedure
1. Position the client supine or with the head of the bed slightly elevated.
2. For electrode placement, clip hair from the sites, then cleanse the sites with an alcohol wipe, and scrape sites lightly with the edge of an electrode.
3. Lead placement varies by institutional protocol and SAECG machine manufacturer recommendations but generally involves the placement of bipolar lead sets on the anterior and posterior areas of the torso. Apply leads according to institutional protocol.
4. Follow the manufacturer's recommendations for obtaining the SAECG. This generally involves activating the SAECG machine, which runs an electrocardiographic template of the client's common cardiac cycle and then compares it to the template, amplifies it, and averages the electrical signals from a set number of subsequent cardiac cycles.

Postprocedure Care
1. Remove the electrodes and cleanse the skin of conductive gel.

Client and Family Teaching
1. This test is performed to determine the risk of developing life-threatening dysrhythmias in high-risk conditions.

This is a special kind of electrocardiogram that takes longer than a normal electrocardiogram.
2. It is important to lie motionless and try to relax the muscles as much as possible throughout the procedure.

Factors That Affect Results
1. Because a specific number of cardiac cycles will be averaged, the procedure will take longer than normal for clients with bradycardia and less time than normal for clients with tachycardia.
2. Ectopic beats are not included in the averaging. Thus the procedure time increases for clients demonstrating a great deal of ectopy.
3. Artifact is not included in the averaging. Thus movement or shivering of the client as well as electrical interference by nearby equipment will increase the procedure time.
4. Use of androgenic anabolic steroids includes a higher incidence of abnormal SAECG measurements immediately post exercise making them at greater risk for sudden death.
5. Hypoglycemia related to increased QT interval on SAECG.

Other Data
1. SAECG has not been found useful for atrial dysrhythmias, continuously irregular rhythms, or rhythms with wide QRS complexes.
2. Low dose bepridil reduces frequency of ventricular fibrillation in patients with Brugada syndrome with an SCN5A gene mutation.

Sims-Huhner Test—Diagnostic

Norm. *Mucus tenacity*: stretches ≥10 cm. *Number of motile sperm*: ≥6-20/HPF.

Usage. Infertility testing; rape trauma.

Description. Examination of the postcoital endocervical mucus to detect its quality and the ability of the spermatozoa to penetrate the mucus. It is believed that the presence of anti-sperm antibodies in cervical mucus may, in part, explain why sperm cannot penetrate normally. This test is included in infertility work-ups when prior semen analysis results are normal.

Professional Considerations
Consent form NOT required, unless the specimen is being collected for medicolegal purposes.

Preparation
1. The test should be timed to coincide with mid-ovulation. The male should abstain from ejaculation for 3 days before this test. Intercourse should be performed without using a lubricant. The woman should lie recumbent for 15-30 minutes after intercourse in which male

ejaculation has occurred and then arrive for testing within 1-5 hours.

2. Obtain a glass cannula with a rubber tube, a syringe, a Petri dish, slides, and a ruler.
3. The client should disrobe below the waist or wear a gown.
4. Obtain a speculum and a glass slide.

Procedure

1. Specimen collection must be witnessed if used for medicolegal purposes.
2. The client is placed in the dorsal lithotomy position and draped for privacy and comfort.
3. The external cervical os is wiped clear of mucus.
4. An endocervical mucus sample is obtained by aspiration in a glass cannula attached by a rubber tube to a syringe.

Postprocedure Care

1. For medicolegal specimens, place the specimen in a sealed plastic bag and label it as legal evidence. All persons handling the specimen must sign a record with the date and time received.
2. Deliver the specimen in a syringe to the laboratory, where the following occurs:

a. After the mucus volume is measured, the specimen is placed in a Petri dish, and color and viscosity are noted.
b. One measures the tenacity of the mucus (spinnbarkeit) by grasping a portion of the mucus and noting the distance it can be drawn before it breaks.
c. Next, a drop of mucus is placed on a microscope slide and covered with a coverslip, and the number of motile sperm are counted.

Client and Family Teaching

1. This test is performed to evaluate endocervical mucus as part of a fertility work-up when sperm counts have been normal.

Factors That Affect Results

1. Specimens collected more than 6 hours after coitus yield unreliable results.
2. An herb that has been found to decrease sperm motility and viability is St. John's wort.

Other Data

1. Mucus can also be microscopically examined for leukocytes, erythrocytes, and trichomonads.
2. See also Infertility screen—Specimen.

Single-Photon Emission Computed Tomography (SPECT Scan), Brain—Diagnostic

Norm. Normal brain and structures.

Usage. Evaluate AIDS, Alzheimer's disease, anoxia, brain death diagnosis, cerebrovascular accident, head trauma, mild brain injury, Parkinson's disease, transient ischemic attack; helps differentiate type of dementia (Alzheimer's, focal, multi-infarct, diffuse) by allowing identification of pattern of cerebral ischemia; helps differentiate Parkinson's disease from dopa-responsive dystonia; allows identification of the focus of seizure activity. Used to scan for ectopic (nonpituitary) tumor when acromegaly is suspected. SPECT is used in forensic psychiatry and experimentally in psychiatry to identify patterns coinciding with individual disorders.

Description. SPECT scan is a nuclear medicine procedure that gives clinical information about organ function (versus CT and radiography, which give information about anatomy). In this scan, a radiopharmaceutical selected for its absorptive properties is injected intravenously, crosses the blood-brain barrier, decomposes, and remains for several hours in the brain tissue, where its qualitative and quantitative distribution can be detected with the SPECT camera. The camera sends images to a computer that can reproduce visual images, or "slices," of the brain along several planes. Advantages of SPECT imaging over older nuclear medicine scans are that it can identify patterns of dementia earlier in the process and allow for early intervention for potentially reversible types of dementia. This scan can be done in a three-dimensional format. In addition to imaging the brain, SPECT is used for many organs, with different radiopharmaceuticals selected, based on their absorptive properties for the organ being imaged. Newer equipment called "dual mode imaging" combines SPECT with structural imaging modalities such as Ultrafast CT or MRI for improved imaging results. See Dual modality imaging—Diagnostic.

Professional Considerations
Consent form IS required.

Risks
Allergic reaction to the radiopharmaceutical (itching, hives, rash, tight feeling in the throat, shortness of breath, anaphylaxis, death).

Contraindications
Inability to lie motionless during the scan; women who are breast-feeding; previous allergic reaction to the radiopharmaceutical agent.

Precautions
During pregnancy, risks of cumulative radiation exposure to the fetus from this and other previous or future imaging studies must be weighed against the benefits of the procedure. Although formal limits for client exposure are relative to this risk:benefit comparison, the United States Nuclear Regulatory Commission requires that the cumulative dose equivalent to an embryo/fetus from occupational exposure not exceed 0.5 rem (5 mSv). Radiation dosage to the fetus is proportional to the distance of the anatomy studied from the abdomen and decreases as pregnancy progresses. For pregnant clients, consult the radiologist/radiology department to obtain estimated fetal radiation exposure from this procedure.

Preparation
1. Remove all metal objects from the client's clothes, hair, and body.
2. See Client and Family Teaching.

Procedure
1. The client is transported to the nuclear medicine department, positioned supine on the scanning table, and left to rest quietly for approximately 10 minutes to allow the brain to reach a basal activity level.
2. A radiopharmaceutical is injected intravenously and allowed to circulate and cross the blood-brain barrier.
3. The SPECT scan is then taken while the client lies motionless, with open eyes.

Postprocedure Care
1. See Client and Family Teaching.

Client and Family Teaching
1. Do not drink caffeine-containing beverages for 24 hours before the scan.
2. It is important to lie motionless during this scan. If the client is confused, a family member familiar to the client may remain in the room to reassure the client during the scan.
3. The scan takes about 30 minutes.
4. For about 24 hours after the scan, meticulously wash your hands after urination to remove any radioactivity from contaminated urine.

Factors That Affect Results
1. The presence of metal objects, such as metal eyeglasses, over the scanning area may block some views.
2. Movement of the client during imaging obscures the clarity of the images.

Other Data
1. The radiopharmaceutical half-life is about 6 hours.
2. Hybrid PET/CT scans are generally more precise than SPECT and take less time for the procedure, but are more expensive.

Single-Photon Emission Computed Tomography (SPECT Scan), Myocardial Perfusion—Diagnostic

Norm. Normal heart and structures.

Usage. Assessment of coronary artery disease (CAD). Women with an LVEF <52% are at increased risk for subsequent hard event (AMI, VF, death).

Description. A common test with high accuracy and incremental prognostic value for CAD. Limitations include suboptimal spatial resolution and significant radiation exposure. Ability to detect hemodynamic significance of lesions seen on multidetector CT angiogram (MDCTA) paves the path for a hybrid scan of SPECT/MDCTA (Berman, 2010). With the arrival of Tc-99m-labeled deoxyglucose to strengthen imaging it is anticipated that this will replace fluoride-18-labeled PET scan and glucose metabolism imaging agents.

Professional Considerations
Consent form IS required.

Risks
Allergic reaction to the radiopharmaceutical (itching, hives, rash, tight feeling in the throat, shortness of breath, anaphylaxis, death).

Contraindications
Inability to lie motionless during the scan; women who are breast-feeding; previous allergic reaction to the radiopharmaceutical agent.

Precautions
During pregnancy, risks of cumulative radiation exposure to the fetus from this and other previous or future imaging studies must be weighed against the benefits of the procedure. Although formal limits for client exposure are relative to this risk:benefit comparison, the United States Nuclear Regulatory Commission requires that the cumulative dose equivalent to an embryo/fetus from occupational exposure not exceed 0.5 rem (5 mSv). Radiation dosage to the fetus is proportional to the distance of the anatomy studied from the abdomen and decreases as pregnancy progresses. For pregnant clients, consult the radiologist/radiology department to obtain estimated fetal radiation exposure from this procedure.

Preparation
1. Remove all metal objects from the client's clothes, hair, and body.
2. See Client and Family Teaching.

Procedure
1. The client is transported to the nuclear medicine department, positioned supine on the scanning table, and left to rest quietly for approximately 10 minutes to allow the brain to reach a basal activity level.
2. A radiopharmaceutical is injected intravenously and allowed to circulate.
3. The SPECT scan is then taken while the client lies motionless.

Postprocedure Care
1. See Client and Family Teaching.

Client and Family Teaching
1. Do not drink caffeine-containing beverages for 24 hours before the scan.
2. It is important to lie motionless during this scan. If the client is confused, a family member familiar to the client may remain in the room to reassure the client during the scan.
3. The scan takes about 30 minutes.
4. For about 24 hours after the scan, meticulously wash your hands after urination to remove any radioactivity from contaminated urine.

Factors That Affect Results
1. The presence of metal objects, such as metal eyeglasses, over the scanning area may block some views.
2. Movement of the client during imaging obscures the clarity of the images.
3. A method to reduce attenuation resulting when the client has very large or very dense breasts includes using ^{99m}Tc-based agents.
4. Lung uptake of the radiopharmaceutical after stress and/or dilation of the left ventricle is likely due to ischemia and severe multivessel disease.

Other Data
1. The radiopharmaceutical half-life is about 6 hours.

Sinus Radiography—Diagnostic

Norm. Negative.

Usage. Cysts, postoperative nasal-sinus surgery, rhinitis, and sinusitis.

Description. Sinus x-rays (roentgen rays) are short electromagnetic waves that penetrate the soft sinus tissues to produce an image that is recorded on radiographic film. The sinuses are usually radiolucent because of the air content. Any deviation from total radiolucency indicates tumor or infection.

Professional Considerations
Consent form NOT required.

Precautions

During pregnancy, risks of cumulative radiation exposure to the fetus from this and other previous or future imaging studies must be weighed against the benefits of the procedure. Although formal limits for client exposure are relative to this risk:benefit comparison, the United States Nuclear Regulatory Commission requires that the cumulative dose equivalent to an embryo/fetus from occupational exposure not exceed 0.5 rem (5 mSv). Radiation dosage to the fetus is proportional to the distance of the anatomy studied from the abdomen and decreases as pregnancy progresses. For pregnant clients, consult the radiologist/radiology department to obtain estimated fetal radiation exposure from this procedure.

Preparation

1. Shield the pregnant uterus during x-ray exposure.

2. Remove earrings, glasses, hairpins, or other radiopaque objects from the head area.

Procedure

1. The head is placed in a fixed position.
2. Radiographs of sinuses are taken from several angles.
3. The exam takes 10-15 minutes.

Postprocedure Care

1. Remove the lead apron.

Client and Family Teaching

1. This test is performed to evaluate sinus cavities for signs of infection or growth.

Factors That Affect Results

1. Movement during radiography distorts the images.

Other Data

1. Anaerobic organisms are the predominant pathogens of chronic sinusitis.

Sjögren's Antibodies (SS-A [Ro] and SS-B [La])

See Anti-La/SS-B Test—Diagnostic; Anti-Ro/SS-A Test—Diagnostic.

Skeletal Muscle Antibody

See Striational Autoantibody—Specimen.

Skin, Fungus—Culture

Norm. Negative.

Usage. Dermatitis and fungal infections.

Description. Culture of skin scrapings, nails, scalp, hair, or debris under the nails is taken to isolate and identify fungi. A single negative culture does not rule out a fungal infection.

Professional Considerations

Consent form NOT required.

Preparation

1. Obtain a sterile scraper and a dermatophyte test medium or a sterile container.

Procedure

1. Place the skin or scalp scrapings, nail clippings, hair stubs, or nail debris scrapings into a dermatophyte medium or sterile container.

Postprocedure Care

1. Store the specimens at room temperature.

Client and Family Teaching

1. Culture results for *Candida* are usually available within 1 week and for dermatophytes within 2 weeks.
2. All negative cultures are final after 4 weeks.

Factors That Affect Results

1. Cotton-plugged tubes should not be used because they may cause the specimen to become trapped in the cotton and lost.

2. Closed rubber stopper tubes should not be used because they keep the specimen moist and aid in bacterial growth.

Other Data
1. None.

Skin, *Mycobacteria*—Culture

Norm. No growth.

Usage. Abscess, AIDS, amyloidosis, Buruli ulcers, granulomatous cutaneous lesions, and osteomyelitis.

Description. Isolation of mycobacteria on the skin as the cause of infection. Some of the common mycobacteria are *M. tuberculosis* and the nontubercular *M. avium-intracellulare, genavense,* and *marinum* found in clients with acquired immune deficiency syndrome (AIDS) or immunosuppression.

Professional Considerations
Consent form NOT required.

Preparation
1. Obtain a sterile scraper and a mycobacterial culture medium.

Procedure
1. Scrape the skin or lesion (do not use a swab) and place the specimen in the mycobacterial culture medium.

Postprocedure Care
1. Transport the specimen directly to the laboratory.

Client and Family Teaching
1. Negative cultures are reported after 9 weeks.

Factors That Affect Results
1. Specimens not incubated at 86 degrees F (30 degrees C) may not grow.

Other Data
1. The yield on cultures is proportional to the amount of specimen submitted.

Skin Culture

See **Culture, Skin**—Specimen.

Skin Test for Hypersensitivity—Diagnostic

Norm. Negative.

Positive. There is no agreement on a threshold value for a positive skin test result.

Usage. Allergies and cat-scratch disease.

Description. An intradermal test using allergen extracts to determine sensitivity to various drugs, materials, and pollens that a client may react to in an allergic manner, such reaction possibly resulting in anaphylaxis. The result is based on an immediate hypersensitivity reaction.

Professional Considerations
Consent form NOT required.

Preparation
1. Obtain an alcohol wipe, 0.1 mL of the test substance in question, and an intradermal 26- or 27-gauge needle.
2. Have emergency equipment and medications on hand for possible anaphylaxis.
3. See Client and Family Teaching.

Procedure
1. Wipe the skin with an alcohol wipe and let it air-dry.
2. Intradermally inject 0.1 mL of the test substance in question in the underpart of the forearm.

Postprocedure Care
1. Observe for redness and swelling (a wheal) at the site of the injection.
2. Results are read 15 minutes after injection. Assess the wheal size of the skin reaction by measuring the mean wheal diameter (MWD) or the mean of the largest wheal diameter and that perpendicular to it. MWDs of skin tests may be expressed in absolute values (millimeters), or they may be related to the size of a control. An MWD >7 mm has a higher diagnostic value for symptomatic allergies. An MWD greater than or equal to a histamine control also has a greater diagnostic value.

3. Assess for anaphylaxis symptoms for ½ hour.

Client and Family Teaching
1. Withhold allergy medications and antihistamines for 48 hours before the test.
2. Report drowsiness, skin rash or itching, difficulty breathing, and palpitations immediately.

Factors That Affect Results
1. A subcutaneous rather than an intradermal injection will produce a false-negative result.

Other Data
1. Most skin tests are available in prepackaged sterile kits.

Sleep Apnea Study

See **Polysomnography**—Diagnostic.

Sleep Oximetry

See **Polysomnography**—Diagnostic.

Sleep Study

See **Polysomnography**—Diagnostic.

Slit-Lamp Vision Test—Diagnostic

Norm. Normal.

Usage. Detection of conjunctivitis, corneal abrasions, glaucomatous damage, iritis, and opacities. Useful after bone-marrow transplantation to monitor clients for cataracts acquired secondary to chemotherapy and radiation therapy as well as to monitor for hemorrhage secondary to thrombocytopenia.

Description. The slit lamp is a special microscopic instrument with a lighting system that allows detailed visualization of the anterior segment of the eye. Slit-lamp vision testing involves visualization of the anterior chamber, conjunctiva, cornea, crystalline lens, eyelashes, eyelids, iris, sclera, tear film, and vitreous face and evaluation of ocular fluid and tissue size and shape by using a slit-lamp light source.

Professional Considerations
Consent form NOT required.

Risks
Allergic reaction to eye drops (itching, hives, rash, tight feeling in the throat, shortness of breath, anaphylaxis).
Contraindications
Allergy to mydriatic eye drops; narrow-angle glaucoma.

Preparation
1. Remove contact lenses and glasses.

Procedure
1. The client is positioned sitting upright with the chin resting on a chin rest and the forehead touching the forehead bar of the slit-lamp instrument.
2. The client is instructed to gaze into the eye of the microscope as the examiner examines the eye from the other side of the microscope.
3. Pupillary dilation drops may be needed, such as in iritis.

Postprocedure Care
1. See Client and Family Teaching.

Client and Family Teaching
1. If dilatory drops are used, vision will be blurred for up to 2 hours. The client should bring sunglasses to wear after the test. The client should not drive or operate machinery during this time.
2. The test takes 10 minutes and is painless.

Factors That Affect Results
1. Inability of the client to remain still during the examination prevents proper examination.

Other Data

1. Three other slit-lamp procedures may be used: fluorescein staining to detect scratches on the cornea or conjunctiva; Hruby lens to better visualize the posterior vitreous and retina; and gonioscopy, where a special contact lens eliminates the corneal curve so that glaucoma testing can be performed.

SLNB

See **Sentinel Lymph Node Biopsy**—Diagnostic.

SMA-6, -7, -12, -20 (CHEM-6, -7, -12, -20)—Blood

Norm. See individual test listings.

Increased or Decreased. See individual test listings.

Description. SMA is an acronym for the sequential multiple analyzer (SMA) automated system that analyzes multiple blood values from one tube of blood.

For the blood values of an SMA-6, see Carbon dioxide, Total content—Blood; Chloride—Serum; Creatinine—Serum; Potassium—Plasma or serum; Sodium, Plasma—Serum or urine; Urea nitrogen—Plasma or serum.

For the blood values of an SMA-7, see Carbon dioxide, Total content—Blood; Chloride—Serum; Creatinine—Serum; Glucose—Blood; Potassium—Plasma or serum; Sodium, Plasma—Serum or urine; Urea nitrogen—Plasma or serum.

For the blood values of an SMA-12, see Albumin—Serum, Urine, and 24-Hour urine; Alkaline phosphatase—Serum; Aspartate aminotransferase—Serum; Bilirubin—Serum; Calcium, Total—Serum; Cholesterol—Blood; Glucose—Blood; Lactate dehydrogenase—Blood; Phosphorus—Serum; Protein, Total—Serum; Urea nitrogen—Plasma or serum; Uric acid—Serum.

For the blood values of an SMA-20, see Alanine Aminotransferase—Serum; alkaline phosphatase—Serum; Aspartate aminotransferase—Serum; Bilirubin—Serum; Calcium, Total—Serum; Carbon dioxide, Total content—Blood; Chloride—Serum; Cholesterol—Blood; Creatine kinase—Serum; Creatinine—Serum; Gamma-glutamyltranspeptidase—Blood; Glucose—Blood; Lactate dehydrogenase—Blood; Phosphorus—Serum; Potassium—Plasma or serum; Protein, Total—Serum; Sodium, Plasma—Serum or urine; Triglycerides—Blood; Urea nitrogen—Plasma or serum; Uric acid—Serum. For further information, see individual test listings.

Professional Considerations

Consent form NOT required.

Preparation

1. Tube: Red topped, red/gray topped, or gold topped.
2. Do NOT draw specimens during hemodialysis.

Procedure

1. Draw a 5-mL blood sample.

Postprocedure Care

1. None.

Client and Family Teaching

1. See individual test listings.

Factors That Affect Results

1. See individual test listings.

Other Data

1. See individual test listings and also Basic metabolic panel—Blood; Comprehensive metabolic panel—Blood.

Small Bowel Series—Diagnostic

Norm. No abnormalities in the small bowel contour, position, or motility.

Usage. Cancer, Crohn's disease, diarrhea, enteritis, hematemesis, Hodgkin's disease, jejunal carcinoma, lymphosarcoma, malabsorption syndrome, melena, obscure GI bleeding, polyps, ulcers, and weight loss.

Description. Fluoroscopic examination of the small intestine after ingestion of barium sulfate. The barium enters the stomach and empties into the duodenal bulb. Circular folds appear as barium enters the duodenal loop. These folds deepen in the jejunum and then lessen in the ileum. The procedure takes 2-6 hours depending on barium transit time through the small bowel.

Professional Considerations
Consent form NOT required.

Risks
Aspiration of contrast material, bowel obstruction, constipation.

Contraindications
Obstruction or perforation of the small intestine because the barium may intensify the obstruction or cause seeping of the barium into the abdominal cavity.

Precautions
During pregnancy, risks of cumulative radiation exposure to the fetus from this and other previous or future imaging studies must be weighed against the benefits of the procedure. Although formal limits for client exposure are relative to this risk:benefit comparison, the United States Nuclear Regulatory Commission requires that the cumulative dose equivalent to an embryo/fetus from occupational exposure not exceed 0.5 rem (5 mSv). Radiation dosage to the fetus is proportional to the distance of the anatomy studied from the abdomen and decreases as pregnancy progresses. For pregnant clients, consult the radiologist/radiology department to obtain estimated fetal radiation exposure from this procedure.

Preparation
1. See Client and Family Teaching.

Procedure
1. Preliminary radiographs are taken in supine, erect, and lateral side positions.
2. The client is given 500 mL of flavored but chalky-tasting barium orally.
3. Radiographs are taken at 30- to 60-minute intervals with the client in supine, erect, and lateral side positions for 2-6 hours to track the barium passage through the small intestine.

Postprocedure Care
1. Encourage fluids (4-6 glasses of water per day for 2 days when not contraindicated) to promote the passage of the barium through the intestines.
2. A cathartic may be prescribed to prevent barium impaction.

Client and Family Teaching
1. Fast from food and fluids and refrain from smoking from midnight before the test.
2. A cathartic may be prescribed to be administered the evening before the test.
3. Bring reading material or other diversion to the test because the procedure is lengthy.
4. Stool will be barium colored for up to 72 hours.

Factors That Affect Results
1. Chronic narcotic use can cause delayed motility.

Other Data
1. Barium enema, gallbladder and biliary system ultrasound, and routine radiography should precede a small bowel series, since retained barium clouds details on the radiographs.

Smooth Muscle Antibody
See Anti–Smooth Muscle Antibody—Serum.

S Mucopolysaccharide Turnover—Diagnostic

Norm. Normal turnover.

Usage. Glucuronidase deficiency, Hurler's syndrome, Maroteaux-Lamy syndrome, mucopolysaccharidoses I-VII (except Morquio's syndrome), Sanfilippo's syndrome type A or B, and Scheie's syndrome.

Description. The mucopolysaccharidoses form a group of inherited disorders caused by the deficiency of enzymes required for the lysosomal degradation of glycosamino-glycans. Evaluation of the rate of turnover of ^{35}S-labeled mucopolysaccharidoses in cultures of the skin assists in their diagnosis. Skin containing fibroblasts that lack an enzyme necessary for the breakdown of mucopolysaccharides will accumulate polysaccharides.

Professional Considerations

Informed consent is recommended for genetic testing.

Preparation

1. Obtain a 4-mm punch biopsy instrument, sterile gauze, tape, and a sterile plastic container.

Procedure

1. Obtain a skin biopsy using a 4-mm punch biopsy instrument.
2. Place the specimen in the sterile plastic container.

Postprocedure Care

1. Transport the specimen to the laboratory immediately.

Client and Family Teaching

1. Genetic counseling is necessary for clients and families undergoing genetic testing. Refer to Appendix B, "Informed Consent for Genetic Testing".

Factors That Affect Results

1. An inadequate amount of biopsy tissue can cause false-negative results.

Other Data

1. The mucopolysaccharidoses, besides involving diseases of connective and vascular tissues, also secrete substantial amounts of chondroitin-6-sulfate, heparin sulfate, and keratin sulfate.
2. The Genetic Information Nondiscrimination Act of 2008 prohibits health plans from using genetic family history or genetic test results from influencing eligibility or premiums for health insurance. It also prohibits employers from using this information to influence decisions about hiring, terminating employment, or employment pay, promotions, or privileges.

Snellen Test

See Visual Acuity Tests—Diagnostic.

SO$_2$

See Blood Gases, Arterial—Blood.

Sodium, Plasma—Serum or Urine

Norm.

		SI Units
Plasma or serum		
Adult	136-145 mEq/L	136-145 mmol/L
Umbilical cord	116-166 mEq/L	116-166 mmol/L
Infant	139-146 mEq/L	139-146 mmol/L
Child	138-145 mEq/L	138-145 mmol/L
Panic level	≤110 mEq/L	≤110 mmol/L
Urine		
Adults	75-200 mEq/24 hours	75-200 mmol/day
Hypovolemia	<20 mmol/L	
Suggestive of SIADHS	>40 mmol/L	

		SI Units
Children		
Newborn	14-40 mEq/24 hours	14-40 mmol/day
6-10 years		
Female	20-69 mEq/24 hours	20-69 mmol/day
Male	41-115 mEq/24 hours	41-115 mmol/day
10-14 years		
Female	48-168 mEq/24 hours	48-168 mmol/day
Male	63-177 mEq/24 hours	63-177 mmol/day

Panic Level Symptoms and Treatment

Symptoms (Low Sodium). Impaired cognition, depressed level of consciousness, convulsions.

Treatment (Sodium ≤110 mEq/L, 110 mmol/L SI units)

NOTE: Treatment choice(s) depend(s) on client's history and condition and episode history.

1. Measure serum osmolality by blood test or by calculated means to determine if relative or true hyponatremia. Measure urine specific gravity.
2. Maintain a patent airway.
3. Monitor for convulsions caused by brain cell edema.
4. Monitor hourly neurologic checks.
5. The use of hypertonic saline is controversial because of its association with osmotic demyelinating syndrome. The literature demonstrates uncertainty over the cause of osmotic demyelinating syndrome, with the possible causes being rapid infusions of hypertonic saline, cerebral ischemia that occurs in severely hyponatremic clients, or some other unknown cause. However, most sources agree that slow infusions are indicated when levels reach the panic (low) level above. Give hypertonic saline (3%-5%) slowly and with extreme caution. Change to a less hypertonic infusion as soon as possible. Sodium should be replaced at about the amount of time over which the loss occurred.

Increased (Hypernatremia). Aldosteronism (primary), congestive heart failure, Cushing's disease, dehydration, diabetes insipidus, diaphoresis, diarrhea, hyperaldosteronism, hypertension, hypovolemia, insensible water loss, ostomies, salicylate toxicity, toxemia, vomiting, and Zollinger-Ellison syndrome with diarrhea. Drugs include ACTH, ampicillin, androgens, calcium, carbenicillin, carbenoxolone, clonidine, corticosteroids, diazoxide, estrogens, gamma-hydroxybutyrate (GHB), guanethidine, lactulose, mannitol, methoxyflurane, methyldopa, mineralocorticoids, oral contraceptives, oxyphenbutazone, phenylbutazone, rauwolfia alkaloids, reserpine, sildenafil, sodium bicarbonate, and tetracycline. Herbal or natural remedies include licorice.

Increased Urinary Sodium Concentration. Hyponatremia as a result of renal salt losses, osmotic diuresis, or renal failure with water retention. Also dehydration, fever, head trauma, hypernatremia, hyponatremia, kidney stone, nephrotic syndrome, salicylate toxicity, starvation, and syndrome of inappropriate antidiuretic hormone secretion (SIADHS). Drugs include caffeine, calcitonin, cisplatin, diuretics, dopamine, heparin, lithium, niacin, sulfates, tetracycline, and vincristine.

Decreased (Hyponatremia). Addison's disease, adrenal insufficiency, aminoglycoside toxicity, ascites in cardiac failure, bowel obstruction, burns, cerebral palsy, chronic renal failure, cirrhosis, congenital adrenal hyperplasia, diabetes mellitus, eating disorders (water loading, laxatives), emphysema, exercise (prolonged), glomerulonephritis, hyperglycemia, hyperosmolality, hyperthermia, hypophosphatemia, hypotension, hypothyroidism, hysterectomy, malabsorption, malnutrition, meningitis, metabolic acidosis, myxedema, nephrotic syndrome, ostomies, overhydration, pain (abdominal), paracentesis, paralytic ileus, psychogenic polydipsia, pyelonephritis (chronic), renal hypertension, sigmoidoscopy, sprue, syndrome of inappropriate antidiuretic hormone secretion (SIADHS), toxemia, toxic shock syndrome, and vomiting. Drugs include aminoglutethimide, ammonium chloride, amphotericin B, carbamazepine, clofibrate, chlorpropamide, cisplatin, clofibrate, chlorpropamide, cyclophosphamide, desmopressin, diuretics (loop, ethacrynic acid and furosemide; osmotic, mannitol; thiazide, hydrochlorothiazide), fosinopril, heparin, laxatives, miconazole, nonsteroidal anti-inflammatory agents (NSAIDs), oxytocin, risperidone, spironolactone, sulfonylureas, tolbutamide, tricyclic antidepressants, valproic acid, vasopressin, and vincristine.

Decreased Urinary Sodium Concentration. Hyponatremia associated with edema or with volume depletion from extrarenal causes. Also acute renal failure, diarrhea, emphysema, fluid retention, malabsorption, pyloric obstruction, and sprue. Drugs include corticosteroids, diazoxide, epinephrine, levarterenol, and propranolol.

Description. Sodium is the major cation of extracellular fluid. Its primary function is to maintain osmotic pressures and acid-base balance and to transmit nerve impulses. It is absorbed from the small intestine and excreted in the urine in amounts dependent on dietary intake. In normal clients, the sodium content of the body remains fairly constant despite wide variations in sodium intake.

Urinary sodium levels are used in conjunction with urine and plasma or serum creatinine levels in two formulas that help narrow down the source of renal failure into prerenal, renal, and postrenal causes. See Renal indices—Diagnostic for further explanation of the use of these formulas.

Professional Considerations
Consent form NOT required.

Preparation
1. *Plasma or serum:*
   a. Tube: Red topped, red/gray topped, or gold topped.
   b. Do NOT draw specimens during hemodialysis.
2. *Urine:*
   a. Obtain a clean, 3-L container without preservatives.
   b. Write the beginning time of collection on the laboratory requisition.

Procedure
1. *Serum:* Draw a 4-mL blood sample.
2. *Urine:*
   a. Discard the first morning urine specimen.

   b. Save all the urine voided for 24 hours in a refrigerated, clean 3-L container without preservatives. Document the quantity of urine output during the collection period. Include the urine voided at the end of the 24-hour period. For catheterized clients, keep the drainage bag on ice and empty the urine into the collection container hourly.

Postprocedure Care
1. Compare the urine quantity in the specimen container with the urinary output record for the test. If the specimen contains less urine than what was recorded as output, some of the sample may have been discarded, thus invalidating the test.
2. Document the quantity of urine output and the ending time for the collection period on the laboratory requisition.
3. Send the entire 24-hour urine specimen to the laboratory for testing.

Client and Family Teaching
1. Save all the urine voided in the 24-hour period and urinate before defecating to avoid loss of urine. If any urine is accidentally discarded, discard the entire specimen and restart the collection the next day.
2. Routine blood results are normally available within 2 hours.

Factors That Affect Results
1. Drawing blood samples proximal to intravenous infusion of sodium chloride will falsely elevate the results.
2. The herbal or natural remedy goldenseal (*Hydrastis canadensis*) causes increased renal water loss while sodium is spared. This will cause a relative increase in sodium value.

Other Data
1. An average dietary intake of 90-250 mEq/day will maintain sodium balance in adults.
2. Minimum daily requirement is 15 mEq.
3. The rate of sodium excretion during the night is one fifth the peak rate during the day.
4. Urinary excretion of sodium is highly dependent on dietary intake, state of hydration, and renal function.
5. Signs of hypernatremia include dry and sticky mucous membranes, fever, thirst, and rubbery skin turgor.

6. Signs of hyponatremia include abdominal cramping, apprehension, oliguria, and rapid, weak pulse.
7. Increased and decreased serum sodium levels in hospitalized patients are associated with in-hospital mortality (Silver, Farley, 2011).
8. The 2011 Third National Health and Nutrition Examination Survey (NHANES III), a prospective cohort study of 12,267 US adults, found that a dietary sodium/potassium ratio of <1 is protective in that it is associated with a decreased rate of mortality (Yang et al, 2011).

Soluble Fibrin Monomer Complex (SFMC)—Serum

Norm. Negative or <0.4 µg/mL.

Positive. Indicates low-grade or chronic intravascular coagulation.

Increased. Acute MI, acute thrombosis (including arterial, coronary, pulmonary, and deep vein), after cardiopulmonary bypass, before disseminated intravascular coagulation, disseminated intravascular coagulation, exacerbations of chronic relapsing pancreatitis, post hip fracture surgery.

Decreased. Elevation slows or stops with the administration of glycoprotein IIB/IIIA inhibitors.

Description. Fibrin monomers are intermediate products formed during the proteolysis of fibrinogen by thrombin. During the intravascular coagulation, low levels of thrombin are available in the blood, but the fibrin monomers formed are not in sufficient quantities to aggregate and form a clot. Instead, they associate themselves with fibrinogen or with fibrinogen degradation products to form soluble complexes. Demonstration of soluble fibrin monomer complex (SFMC) in plasma therefore indicates low-grade or chronic intravascular coagulation.

Professional Considerations
Consent form NOT required.

Preparation
1. Red topped tube, a buffered citrate collection tube.

Procedure
1. Draw a plain red topped tube to remove fluid contamination. Discard this tube.
2. Draw blood into a buffered citrate collection tube filled to the proper level (sodium citrate of 0.105 M should be used). Other anticoagulants may cause invalid results.
3. Gently invert tube six times to mix.

Postprocedure Care
1. Deliver specimen to lab immediately. If specimen is not processed immediately, it must be frozen at −94 degrees F (−70 degrees C) until testing takes place.
2. Assess the client for other signs or symptoms of thrombosis, emboli, or veno-occlusive disease.

Client and Family Teaching
1. Results are normally available within 24 hours.

Factors That Affect Results
1. Specimen is heat sensitive and deteriorates rapidly. Send the specimen to the lab immediately.

Other Data
1. Studies have suggested that fibrin monomer may play a role in tumor biology. Fibrin monomers may enhance platelet adhesion to circulating tumor cells and facilitate metastatic spread.
2. See also Fibrinopeptide A—Blood.

Soluble Transferrin Receptor Assay—Serum

Norm. Males: 2.2-4.5 mg/L.
Females: 1.8-4.6 mg/L.
Values are not affected by age or by inflammation.

NOTE: Reference ranges are not yet standardized. Results should be compared to the ranges on the individual test kit used for this test. No reference values have been established for pregnant females, and recent or frequent blood donors.

Increased. Tissue iron-deficiency states, with an increase proportional to the severity of the anemia; also hemolytic anemia, hereditary spherocytosis, megaloblastic anemia (caused by vitamin B_{12} and folate deficiency), myelodysplastic syndromes, polycythemia, and thalassemia.

Decreased. Aplastic anemia.

Parameter	Tests for Changes in	Iron-Deficiency Anemia	Anemia of Chronic Iron Disease	Deficiency and Anemia of Chronic Disease
Ferritin	Iron stores	Low	High	Normal or high
TIBC	Iron status	High	Low	Normal or high
Serum Fe	Iron status	Low	Low	Low
sTfR	Iron status	High	Normal	High

Usage. Helps distinguish between iron-deficiency anemia and anemia of chronic disease. Assessment of body iron status and tissue iron stores in conjunction with measured serum ferritin levels; helps detect and determine the cause of iron deficiency in inflammatory states and in the anemia of chronic disease because transferrin levels are not affected by the acute-phase response; may help evaluate erythropoiesis in clients receiving erythropoietin treatment; holds promise for usefulness in evaluating iron status during pregnancy because results are not affected by gestational changes. This test is NOT helpful in assessing iron status with coexisting conditions associated with greatly enhanced erythropoiesis (such as megaloblastic anemia, thalassemia.) This test is not as sensitive and specific as serum ferritin for differentiating iron-deficiency anemia from anemia of chronic disease in elderly clients with anemia.

Description. Transferrin is a beta globulin and a glycoprotein with a short (7-day) half-life. Formed in the liver, transferrin facilitates cellular iron uptake by transporting dietary iron from the intestinal mucosa to iron storage sites and hemoglobin synthesis sites in the body (bone, muscle, erythrocytes, lymphocytes). Transferrin enables iron storage by binding to two types of transferrin receptors (type 1 and type 2) at the iron storage sites. 80% of transferrin receptors are found in erythroid tissue (precursor cells of bone marrow), though these receptors are present in almost all body tissue. During transferrin receptor–mediated endocytosis in which iron is transported into the cells, a soluble form of transferrin receptor (sTfR) can be detected in serum and is closely related to erythroid transferrin receptor turnover. The major stimuli of the serum transferrin receptor concentration are cellular iron demands and erythroid proliferation rate. Therefore the serum transferrin receptor level can be a sensitive identifier of early tissue iron deficiency as long as hyperplastic erythropoiesis is not also present. Serum soluble transferrin receptor increases in iron deficiency and is usually unaffected by chronic disease states. In general, to increase sensitivity and specificity, the measurement of iron transferrin receptor should be performed in combination with other tests of iron status, including ferritin, TIBC, and serum iron (Fe). In this test, an enzyme-linked immunoassay measures serum transferrin receptors using monoclonal antibodies directed against the receptors.

Professional Considerations
Consent form NOT required.

Preparation
1. Tube: Lavender topped, green topped, or serum separator tube (SST). Also obtain ice.

Procedure
1. Draw a 5-mL (lavender topped tube), 7-mL (green topped tube), or 6-mL (SST) blood sample. Place tube immediately on ice.

Postprocedure Care
1. Document the date of last blood transfusion.
2. Separate cells from plasma within 30 minutes and freeze.

Client and Family Teaching
1. This test should be performed in combination with other tests.

Factors That Affect Results

1. Concentrations have been found to be higher in African-Americans.
2. Concentrations have been found to be higher in persons living at high altitudes than in persons living at sea level.

Other Data

1. The sTfR/ferritin index is used in research in an attempt to find predictive correlations with disease states. There is no official norm available for this index.

Somatomedin-C

See Insulin-Like Growth Factor-I—Blood.

Somatosensory Evoked Potential (SSEP)—Diagnostic

Norm. Results of the somatosensory evoked potential (SEP, SSEP) are interpreted by a physician trained in neurophysiology.

Usage. Aids in the diagnosis of demyelinating diseases, including multiple sclerosis; neurodegenerative diseases, including adrenoleukodystrophy, adrenomyeloneuropathy, and Friedreich's ataxia; and spinal cord lesions. May help predict recovery prognosis in coma, especially nontraumatic coma.

Description. SEP testing uses peripheral electrical nerve stimulation to examine the conduction velocity of impulses through the somatosensory pathway along peripheral nerves to the cortex of the brain in a fashion similar to that of the electroencephalogram (EEG). The test uses sophisticated signal averaging to filter out the effect of other brain activity during testing. Of significance are conduction time for the SEP to occur after stimulation (latency) and the amplitude of the SEP waveform.

Professional Considerations
Consent form NOT required.

Preparation

1. Obtain EEG electrodes, an EEG machine, and electroconductive gel.
2. Remove jewelry and metal objects from the client's head and limbs.

Procedure

1. Scalp electrodes are placed over the sensory cortex of the scalp on the side opposite that to be stimulated.
2. Small painless electrical stimuli are administered to large sensory fibers in the median or posterior tibial nerves.
3. The afferent volley is recorded as well as waves that reflect peripheral nerve trunk activity.

Postprocedure Care

1. Remove electrodes from the scalp and cleanse scalp of electroconductive gel.

Client and Family Teaching

1. The hair should be clean, dry, and free of hair spray or other hair fixatives.
2. Small, painless electrical stimuli are administered to peripheral nerves. The brain's response is recorded by means of scalp electrodes.

Factors That Affect Results

1. The client must be able to lie motionless during the test.
2. Results must be compared with the norms of the laboratory performing the test because different variations of the test will be performed, depending on the client's history and the purpose of the test.
3. Complete lesion of the spinal cord results in no SEP recording when nerves distal to the lesion are stimulated.
4. Lesions between the stimulated nerve and the thalamus increase the latency of the SEP.
5. Lesions of the somatosensory cortex reduce the amplitude of the SEP wave.
6. SEPs are a useful diagnostic tool for infants and children; however, growth and maturation of the nervous system complicate the technical application and interpretation of the results.
7. SEP examines a restricted anatomic pathway and does not reflect general brainstem or cerebral function.

Other Data

1. This test is unaffected by general anesthesia, medications (except ropivacaine), and metabolic abnormalities.

2. Patients receiving sevoflurane had faster suppression and faster recovery of SSEP amplitude compared to propofol. Hence propofol produces a better SSEP signal.

Somatostatin-Receptor Scintigraphy

See Octreotide Scan—Diagnostic.

Somatotropin

See Growth Hormone—Blood.

Sonometry

See Bone Ultrasonometry—Diagnostic.

Specific Gravity—Urine

Norm.

		SI Units
Adults	1.016-1.022	1.016-1.022
No fluids for 12 hours	1.007-1.030	1.007-1.030
No fluids for 24 hours	≥1.026 indicates normal renal concentrating ability	
Stress conditions	1.001-1.040	1.001-1.040
Newborns	1.012	1.012
Infants	1.002-1.006	1.002-1.006

Increased. Adrenal insufficiency, bacteriuria, congestive heart failure, diabetes mellitus, diarrhea, fever, fluid volume deficit, glomerulonephritis, obstruction uropathy, proteinuria, syndrome of inappropriate antidiuretic hormone secretion (SIADHS), toxemia of pregnancy, and vomiting. Drugs include dextran, radiographic contrast media, and sucrose.

Decreased. Chronic renal insufficiency, diabetes insipidus, fluid volume excess, hypothermia, intracranial pressure increase, and malignant hypertension. Drugs include aminoglycosides, carbenoxolone, lithium, and methoxyflurane.

Description. Specific gravity is the ratio of the density of urine compared to the density of an equal volume of water, which has a defined density of 1.000. Specific gravity is dependent on the number, size, and weight of urine solutes (chloride, creatinine, glucose, phosphates, protein, sodium, sulfates, urea, uric acid) dissolved in solvent.

Specific gravity evaluates the kidneys' ability to regulate fluid balance as well as the hydration status of the body.

Professional Considerations

Consent form NOT required.

Preparation

1. Obtain a calibrated hydrometer (urinometer) or a temperature-compensated refractometer and a random urine specimen.

Procedure

1. *Urinometer procedure:*
   a. The urinometer should be clean and dry before use.
   b. Place the urinometer on a level surface and fill it with 15 mL of urine.
   c. Insert a glass cylinder into the urinometer, using a spinning motion.
   d. When the spinning stops, read the base meniscus, avoiding surface bubbles.
   e. Subtract 0.001 from the reading for every 3 degrees C room temperature

S

below 20 degrees C to determine the specific gravity. Alternatively, add 0.001 to the reading for every 3 degrees C room temperature above 20 degrees C to determine the specific gravity.

f. For every 1 g/dL proteinuria, subtract 0.003 from the specific gravity.

g. For every 1 g/dL glucosuria, subtract 0.004 from the specific gravity.

2. *Refractometer procedure:*

a. Clean the cover and prism with a drop of distilled water and allow them to dry.

b. Close the cover.

c. Hold the instrument horizontally.

d. Apply a drop of urine at the notched bottom of the cover so that the drop flows over the prism surface.

e. Point the instrument toward a light.

f. Rotate the eyepiece until the scale is in focus.

g. Read the specific gravity between the sharp dividing line of the dark and light contrast.

Postprocedure Care

1. Cleanse the urinometer.

Client and Family Teaching

1. Give instructions about obtaining a urine specimen.

Factors That Affect Results

1. The reading is invalid if the glass cylinder touches the sides or bottom of the urinometer while the meniscus is being read.

2. The urine specimen must be at room temperature.

Other Data

1. The urinometer needs to be calibrated to produce accurate readings.

2. Dipstick methods of measuring urine specific gravity are unreliable.

SPECT Scan

See Single-Photon Emission Computed Tomography, Brain—Diagnostic.

SPECT/CT

See Dual Modality Imaging—Diagnostic.

Speech Audiometry

See Audiometry Test—Diagnostic.

Sperm Count

See Infertility Screen, Specimen and Semen Analysis—Specimen.

Sphingomyelinase—Diagnostic

Norm. 1.53-7.18 U/g.

Increased. Acute toxic hepatitis, *Clostridium perfringens* toxins, multiple sclerosis.

Decreased. Colitis (chronic), Niemann-Pick disease, types A and B.

Description. Sphingomyelinase is an enzyme that acts as a catalyst in the metabolism of sphingomyelin. Sphingomyelin is a phospholipid ubiquitously distributed in all membranes of mammalian cells and in serum lipoproteins. Niemann-Pick disease is an autosomal recessive lysosome storage disease caused by sphingomyelinase deficiency. Massive tissue accumulation of sphingomyelin results. Two types of Niemann-Pick disease have been identified: type A is a severe, neurodegenerative infantile form leading to death by 4 years of age; and type B is a chronic, nonneuronopathic form. A subacute form, similar to type B but with mild neuronal involvement (retinal storage, peripheral neuropathy, mild neurologic changes, or psychiatric disorders), has also been identified. In this test, a skin biopsy is used to perform fibroblast tissue culture and fibroblast assay for sphingomyelinase activity.

Professional Considerations
Informed consent is recommended for genetic testing.

Preparation
1. Obtain a skin punch biopsy setup and a sterile plastic cup.

Procedure
1. Cleanse the biopsy site with alcohol and allow it to air-dry.
2. Obtain a skin punch biopsy with a 4-mm punch.

Postprocedure Care
1. Place the biopsy specimen in a sterile cup.

Client and Family Teaching
1. A mild analgesic may be used for site tenderness.

2. Contact the physician for redness, swelling, increasing tenderness, purulent drainage, or slow healing noted at the site.
3. Genetic counseling must be provided for individuals and families undergoing genetic testing. Refer to Appendix B, "Informed Consent for Genetic Testing".
4. Results will be available in 10-14 days.

Factors That Affect Results
1. Inadequate punch biopsy specimen may cause false-negative results.

Other Data
1. The Genetic Information Nondiscrimination Act of 2008 prohibits health plans from using genetic family history or genetic test results from influencing eligibility or premiums for health insurance. It also prohibits employers from using this information to influence decisions about hiring, terminating employment, or employment pay, promotions, or privileges.

Spinal Puncture
See **Lumbar Puncture**—Diagnostic.

Spiral CT
See **Computed Tomography of the Body**—Diagnostic.

Spirometry
See **Pulmonary Function Tests**—Diagnostic.

Speech Recognition Threshold
See **Spondee Threshold Speech Test**—Diagnostic.

Spleen Echogram
See **Spleen Ultrasonography**—Diagnostic.

Spleen Scan—Diagnostic

Norm. Homogeneous distribution of the radiolabeled erythrocytes throughout the spleen.

Usage. Evaluation of the size, shape, and location of the spleen in suspected congenital anomalies, in cancer, or after trauma.

Description. The spleen scan is a nuclear medicine examination of the left upper quadrant of the abdomen after intravenous administration of either technetium-99m–labeled or chromium-51–labeled, heat-treated, red blood cells. Because erythrocytes are sequestered by the spleen, the radiolabeled cell accumulation in the spleen can be identified with the scinticounter.

Professional Considerations
Consent form IS required.

Risks
Hematoma, infection.
Contraindications
Inability to lie motionless during the scan; during pregnancy; or breast-feeding.

Preparation
1. Establish intravenous access.
2. Have emergency equipment available for potential anaphylaxis.
3. Just before beginning the procedure, take a "time out" to verify the correct client, procedure, and site.

Procedure
1. A 5-mL sample of the client's blood is removed with a heparinized syringe by means of venipuncture. It is heat-treated and labeled with the selected radionuclide in the nuclear medicine department.
2. The labeled blood is injected through the established intravenous access into the client.
3. After 1 hour, scintiscans are taken of the left upper quadrant of the abdomen from anterior, posterior, left lateral, and oblique views.
4. Scanning is repeated in 24 hours.

Postprocedure Care
1. Observe the individual for 1 hour after the study for possible anaphylactic reaction to the radionuclide.
2. General body-substance isolation precautions protect the health care professional from potential radiation exposure.

Client and Family Teaching
1. Technetium half-life is 6 hours. Chromium-51 half-life is 27.8 days.
2. General body-substance isolation precautions protect the client's family from potential radiation exposure.

Factors That Affect Results
1. Impaired hepatic function causes a greater-than-normal splenic uptake of the labeled cells.
2. Hematoma, infarct, abscess, or tumor causes decreased uptake.
3. Amyloidosis, sarcoidosis, or granulomas may cause many filling defects.

Other Data
1. This test may be performed with a liver scan.
2. Health care professionals working in a nuclear medicine area must follow federal standards set by the Nuclear Regulatory Commission. These standards include precautions for handling the radioactive material and monitoring of potential radiation exposure.

Spleen Ultrasonography (Spleen Echogram, Spleen Ultrasound)—Diagnostic

Norm. Proper size, shape, and position of the spleen. Negative for abscess, cyst, tumor, or splenomegaly. Spleen tissue stipples with fine, homogeneous, low-level echoes. Spleen is not visualized until the transducer reaches 9-11 cm above the umbilicus.

Usage. Assessment of status after trauma; detection or differentiation of splenic abnormalities such as abscess or cyst; ongoing monitoring of the spleen during medical therapy; guidance for splenic needle biopsy.

Description. Evaluation of the spleen's size, shape, and position by the creation of an oscilloscopic picture from the echoes of high-frequency sound waves passing over the abdominal area (acoustic imaging). The time required for the ultrasonic beam to be reflected back to the transducer from differing densities of tissue is converted by a computer to an electrical impulse displayed on an oscilloscopic screen to create a three-dimensional picture of the spleen. The echo-morphology of splenic lesions assists in the diagnosis of the lesion and can be described as isoechogenic, hyperechogenic, hypoechogenic, or complex in comparison to the normal spleen echogenicity. The differing tissue densities of specific lesions assists in the diagnosis of the lesion. However, spleen ultrasonography cannot definitively localize a splenic tumor because of close proximity of other organs in the area.

Professional Considerations
Consent form NOT required.

Preparation
1. This test should be performed before intestinal barium tests or after the barium is cleared from the system.
2. Obtain ultrasonic gel or paste.
3. See Client and Family Teaching.

Procedure
1. The client is positioned supine in a bed or on a procedure table.
2. The skin overlying the spleen is covered with ultrasonic gel, and a lubricated transducer is passed slowly and firmly over the left upper quadrant of the abdomen at various angles and at specific intervals 1-2 cm apart. The transducer is passed between rather than over the ribs. This may be performed with the client in several positions. The right lateral decubitus position provides the best information. Higher-frequency linear ultrasound probes are selected for clients who are thin.
3. Photographs are taken of the oscilloscopic display.

Postprocedure Care
1. Wipe the ultrasonic gel from the skin.

Client and Family Teaching
1. Fast from food and fluids overnight (when possible), and abstain from smoking for several hours before the test.
2. The procedure is painless and carries no risks.
3. The procedure takes less than 30 minutes.

Factors That Affect Results
1. Dehydration interferes with adequate contrast between organs and body fluids.
2. Intestinal barium, food, or gas (particularly in the supine position) obscures the results by preventing the proper transmission and deflection of the high-frequency sound waves.

Other Data
1. Further testing may include computed tomography or magnetic resonance imaging.

Spleen Ultrasound
See **Spleen Ultrasonography**—Diagnostic.

Splenoportography—Diagnostic

Norm. Splenic pulp pressure: 50-180 mm H_2O, or 3.5-13.5 mm Hg. Smooth flow of dye through the splenic venous system without obstruction or diversion. Timely flow of the dye through the hepatic portal system without evidence of collateral veins.

Usage. Cirrhosis, hepatocellular carcinoma, portal hypertension, and portal vein thrombosis.

Description. Splenoportography is the radiographic examination of the venous system of the spleen and portal system of the liver after injection of contrast medium directly into the splenic vein or splenic parenchyma. The measurement of splenic pulp pressure before dye injection helps detect portal hypertension.

Professional Considerations
Consent form IS required.

Risks
Allergic reaction to contrast media (itching, hives, rash, tight feeling in the throat, shortness of breath, anaphylaxis); renal toxicity from contrast medium; hemorrhage requiring blood transfusion or splenectomy, or both.

Contraindications
Previous allergy to iodine, shellfish, or radiographic contrast media; pregnancy (if

iodinated medium is used, because of the radioactive iodine crossing the blood-placental barrier); renal insufficiency; ascites; coagulation disorders; impaired hepatic or renal function; or splenic infection. Sedatives are contraindicated in clients with central nervous system depression.

Preparation

1. Establish intravenous access.
2. Assess platelet count, prothrombin time (PT), activated partial thromboplastin time (APTT), urea nitrogen, creatinine, and liver enzymes.
3. Administer a sedative and an analgesic, as prescribed, 30 minutes before the test.
4. Obtain antiseptic, sterile drapes, 1%-2% lidocaine (Xylocaine) local anesthetic, a percutaneous injection tray, a manometer, contrast medium, and material for a dry, sterile dressing.
5. See Client and Family Teaching.
6. Just before beginning the procedure, take a "time out" to verify the correct client, procedure, and site.

Procedure

1. The client is positioned supine with the left hand under the head.
2. The left sides of the thorax and abdomen are washed with an antiseptic.
3. The spleen is located by means of fluoroscopy.
4. The puncture site is marked, usually the ninth or tenth intercostal space at the mid- or post-axillary line.
5. After a local anesthetic is injected around the puncture site, a sheathed needle is inserted percutaneously into the spleen. The needle is removed, and the sheath is connected to a spinal manometer for splenic pulp pressure measurement.
6. After sheath placement is verified, radiographic contrast medium is injected through the splenic parenchyma into the splenic vein, and cineradiographic films are taken to record splenic venous system filling.
7. The needle is removed, and a dry, sterile dressing is applied to the puncture site.
8. The procedure takes less than 1 hour.

Postprocedure Care

1. Assess vital signs every 15 minutes × 4, then every 30 minutes × 4, then hourly × 4, and then every 4 hours until 24 hours after the procedure.
2. Observe for bleeding and swelling at the puncture site each time vital signs are taken.

Client and Family Teaching

1. Fast from food and fluids from midnight before the test.
2. A sensation of warmth or flushing after the dye injection is normal and will be transient.
3. Immediately report any left upper quadrant pain.
4. The client must assume a left side–lying position for 24 hours.
5. The client may resume previous diet after the procedure. Oral intake of fluids, where not contraindicated, is encouraged.

Factors That Affect Results

1. Cirrhosis causes delayed emptying of the intrahepatic radicles.
2. Portal hypertension causes elevated splenic pulp pressure and evidence of the development of collateral veins.

Other Data

1. The newer computed tomographic percutaneous transsplenic portography (CT-PTSP) utilizes thinner needles for splenic puncture and CT rather than cineradiography. The use of thinner needles decreases the amount of pain and the risk of hemorrhage associated with the procedure. CT has a high-contrast resolution and can thus detect a low dose of contrast dye. CT-PTSP thus decreases the length of time that the client must be monitored and be on bed rest after the procedure and allows the procedure to be performed on an outpatient basis.
2. A new technique of carbon dioxide wedged arterial splenoportography is useful for visualizing gastric varices associated with splenic vein occlusion.

SpO₂

See **Oximetry**—Diagnostic.

S

Spondee Threshold Speech Test—Diagnostic

Norm. 0-20 dB (decibels) in adults, 0-15 dB children.

Usage. Evaluates the ability to hear conversational speech and provides more specific evaluation after abnormal pure-tone audiometry results. Also used to determine proper gain when selecting a hearing aid for a client.

Description. Spondees are two-syllable words (such as "baseball," "airplane") presented to a client through earphones to measure the lowest level at which the client repeats 50% of the words. This test measures degree of hearing loss and is often performed after audiometric testing. The test is also used to validate the pure tone audiometry test, as there is a high correlation between the results of this test and the three-threshold (500 Hz, 1000 Hz, 2000 Hz) average.

Professional Considerations
Consent form NOT required.

Preparation
1. Obtain a speech audiometer, earphones, and a recorded spondee list.

Procedure
1. Explain to the client that a series of two-syllable words in decreasing loudness will be transmitted through the earphones. The client should repeat these words when he or she hears them to the best of his or her ability.

Postprocedure Care
1. A client with abnormal results should be referred to an audiologist.

Client and Family Teaching
1. The earphones are placed over the client's ears, and testing proceeds as described above, with only one ear tested at a time.

Factors That Affect Results
1. Unfamiliarity with the language or words used may make the results unreliable.
2. This test is unreliable in young children who do not yet have fully developed speech.

Other Data
1. See also Audiometry test—Diagnostic.

Sputum, Fungus—Culture

Norm. No growth.

Usage. Actinomycosis, AIDS, aspergillosis, candidiasis, coccidioidomycosis, fungal infections, histoplasmosis, neoplastic disease, and pneumonia.

Description. Fungi are slow-growing, eukaryotic organisms that can grow on living and nonliving organic materials and are subdivided into yeasts and molds. Only a few fungi species infect humans. Normal host defense mechanisms limit the damage these fungi cause superficially. When inhaled or inoculated deep into tissues or when acquired by an immunocompromised client, fungi can cause serious infections.

Professional Considerations
Consent form NOT required.

Preparation
1. A first morning specimen is preferred because it represents overnight secretions of the tracheobronchial tree.
2. Obtain a sterile plastic container or a sputum trap.

Procedure
1. Obtain 1-3 mL of sputum in a sterile container and cover it with a lid, or obtain a specimen in a sputum trap.

Postprocedure Care
1. Refrigerate the specimen or deliver it to the laboratory within 1 hour.
2. Preliminary reports will be available in 48-72 hours and negative reports after 4 weeks.

Client and Family Teaching
1. Cough deeply and expectorate 5-10 mL of sputum into a sterile plastic container and then cap it tightly. Deep coughs are necessary to produce sputum, rather than saliva. To produce the proper specimen, take several breaths in, without fully exhaling each, and then expel sputum with a "cascade cough."

Factors That Affect Results

1. A contaminated specimen cup invalidates the results.

Other Data

1. Pathogenic fungi include *Alternaria, Aspergillus, Blastomyces dermatitidis,* *Candida, Coccidioides immitis, Crypto-coccus, Histoplasma capsulatum, Monilia* (now called *Candida), Mucor, Penicillium, Rhizopus, Scopulariopsis,* and *Sporothrix schenckii.*

2. A single negative culture does not rule out a fungal infection.

Sputum, Gram Stain

See Gram Stain—Diagnostic.

Sputum, *Mycobacteria*—Culture and Smear

Norm. No growth.

Usage. Acquired immune deficiency syndrome, hemoptysis, mycobacteria, splenomegaly, and tuberculosis.

Description. Mycobacteria are rod-shaped, aerobic bacteria that resist decolorizing chemicals after staining, hence "acid fast." Many new species of nontuberculous mycobacteria (or new components of species complexes) as well as multiple drug-resistant isolates of *M. tuberculosis* have been recognized. *Mycobacterium* species are capable of producing human disease characterized by destructive granulomas that can necrose, ulcerate, and cavitate. *M. tuberculosis* is transmitted by the airborne route, most commonly to the lungs, where it survives well, causes areas of granulomatous inflammation, and, if not dormant, causes cough, fever, and hemoptysis. In this test, an acid-fast bacteria (AFB) culture and stain of sputum are performed to detect mycobacteria. The smear is followed by a confirmatory culture. Sputum culture for *M. tuberculosis* obtains a higher yield and is more cost-effective than blood culture. Newer methods of testing for tuberculosis include polymerase chain reaction and nucleic acid amplification (Palomino, 2006).

Professional Considerations

Consent form NOT required.

Preparation

1. A first morning specimen is preferred because it represents an accumulation of overnight secretions of the tracheobronchial tree.

2. Obtain a sterile plastic cup with a lid.

3. For clients who are inpatients, waiting until the morning after admission to obtain sputum samples produces a less false-negative result.

Procedure

1. Sputum may be induced by inhalation of hypertonic saline aerosol.

2. Laryngeal swabs and gastric isolates may also be useful in individuals unable to produce sputum or cooperate with induction procedures.

Postprocedure Care

1. Refrigerate the specimens if not delivered to the laboratory within an hour.

2. A preliminary report is available in 72 hours, the final report in 4-6 weeks.

Client and Family Teaching

1. Cough deeply and expectorate 5-10 mL of sputum into a sterile plastic container and then cap it tightly. Deep coughs are necessary to produce sputum, rather than saliva. To produce the proper specimen, take several breaths in, without fully exhaling each, and then expel sputum with a "cascade cough."

2. Repeat the procedure for three consecutive mornings.

Factors That Affect Results

1. Contamination of the specimen invalidates the results.

2. An insufficient sputum amount may cause false-negative results.

3. Repeated induction of sputum increases the yield via the polymerase chain reaction.

Other Data

1. Because 5-10 mL of sputum is required, the specimen may be collected over a 2-hour period. However, a 24-hour period is unacceptable.

2. Bronchial washings often do not contain enough sputum because they are diluted with anesthetics and irrigating fluid.

Sputum, Routine

See Culture, Routine.

Sputum Acid-Fast Bacteria

See Acid-Fast Bacteria—Culture and Stain.

Sputum Culture and Sensitivity

See Culture, Routine.

Sputum Cytology

See Cytologic Study of Respiratory Tract—Diagnostic.

Sputum for *Haemophilus* Species—Culture

Norm. No *Haemophilus* species isolated.

Positive. Chronic bronchitis, epiglottitis, *Haemophilus influenzae*, meningitis, otitis media, and pneumonia.

Negative. Viral pulmonary disease.

Description. The gram-negative *Haemophilus coccobacillus* is the leading cause of pediatric otitis, meningitis, epiglottitis, and adult pneumonia. The *Haemophilus* organisms usually live on the host and only cause disease when the immune system is disrupted or suppressed.

Professional Considerations
Consent form NOT required.

Preparation

1. A first morning specimen is preferred because it represents overnight secretions of the tracheobronchial tree.
2. Obtain a sterile plastic cup with a lid.

Procedure

1. Obtain 3-5 mL of sputum in a sterile container and cover it with a lid, or obtain a specimen in a sputum trap.

Postprocedure Care

1. Refrigerate the specimen within 2 hours of collection.
2. Results are normally available within 24 hours, the final report within 48 hours.

Client and Family Teaching

1. Cough deeply and expectorate 3-5 mL of sputum into a sterile plastic container and then cap it tightly.

Factors That Affect Results

1. Specimens more than 2 hours old and not refrigerated may cause false-negative results.

Other Data

1. 5%-15% of *H. influenzae* pathogens produce penicillinase and therefore are resistant to treatment with ampicillin.
2. *H. influenzae* meningitis has a high mortality. Therefore vaccination against this organism is recommended.

Sputum Hemosiderin Preparation—Specimen

Norm. Negative.

Usage. Blood in the alveolar space.

Description. Hemosiderins are iron-storage granules normally found in the liver cytoplasm, spleen, and bone marrow. Hemosiderin is also a by-product of macrophage degradation of erythrocytes. This test uses Prussian blue stain on a smear of sputum to detect the presence of hemosiderin in the lungs, representing previous alveolar hemorrhage (AH). AH has a variety of causes, including anti-basement-membrane–mediated diseases, pulmonary infection, and vasculitis. AH can also occur in immunocompromised clients with invasive fungal pneumonia and thrombocytopenia and in clients who have undergone heart transplantation for chronic congestive heart failure.

Professional Considerations
Consent form NOT required.

Preparation
1. Obtain a sterile plastic sputum cup, a sterile container with a lid, glass slides, and a cytologic sputum fixative.

Procedure
1. Obtain a sputum specimen in a sterile plastic container.

Postprocedure Care
1. Smear sputum on a glass slide and apply cytologic fixative. Place the slide in a sterile container and cap it tightly.

Client and Family Teaching
1. Cough deeply and expectorate 3-5 mL of sputum into a sterile plastic container. Deep coughs are necessary to produce sputum, rather than saliva. To produce the proper specimen, take several breaths in, without fully exhaling each, and then expel sputum with a "cascade cough."

Factors That Affect Results
1. Failure to "fix" the specimen invalidates the results.

Other Data
1. Results are available within hours but require interpretation with other clinical data.

Squamous Cell Carcinoma Antigen—Serum

Norm. Less than 2.2 ng/mL.

Usage. Levels correlate with certain squamous cell carcinoma (SCC) disease progression and response to treatment, and also as a prognostic indicator for the disease. After removal of SCC lesions, levels reach normal levels within about 4 days.

Increased. Squamous cell carcinomas (anal canal, cervix, esophagus, lungs, head, neck, penis, skin, uterus). Higher levels of SCC-antigen after treatment (especially ≥8 ng/mL) indicate progression of the carcinoma. Also may be elevated in up to 3% of healthy clients, and in acute respiratory distress syndrome, benign skin disease (eczema, pemphigus, psoriasis), endometriosis, hepatic disease (cirrhosis, hepatitis), pelvic inflammatory disease, pleural effusion, pneumonia, renal failure, sarcoidosis, and tuberculosis.

Decreased. Decreasing levels of previously elevated SCC-antigen are evident after irradiation.

Description. Squamous cell carcinoma antigen (SCC-antigen) is a glycoprotein contained in a neutral form inside normal epithelial tissues but is released in an acidic form when squamous cell carcinomas or nonmalignant lesions occur.

Professional Considerations
Consent form NOT required.

Preparation
1. Tube: Red topped or serum separator (red/gray or gold topped).

Procedure
1. Collect a 3-mL blood sample.
2. Refrigerate specimen.

Postprocedure Care
1. None.

Client and Family Teaching

1. This test is not used for early screening for squamous cell carcinomas.
2. This test is mainly used to evaluate the extent or prognosis of the disease and effectiveness of the treatments. Results may also indicate early recurrent disease after a period of time following initial treatment.
3. Results are normally available within 3-7 working days.

Factors That Affect Results

1. Levels are higher when the cancer is well differentiated than earlier in the disease course.

2. Levels increase as the tumor stage progresses.
3. Up to 3% of healthy clients have elevated SCC-antigen.

Other Data

1. This test is not widely available. An enzyme-linked immunosorbent assay test is available through ARUP laboratories.
2. Pretreatment levels of SCC-antigen >2.0 ng/mL and elevated urine poly-amines of >45 µmol/g of creatinine predict lymph node metastasis in early cervical carcinoma.

SSRI

See **Selective Serotonin Reuptake Inhibitors—**Blood.

St. Louis Encephalitis Virus Serology—Serum

Norm. A less than fourfold rise in titer between acute and convalescent samples.

Usage. Hemagglutination titer <1:10. Complement fixation titer <1:8. Indirect fluorescent IgG antibody <1:16.

Description. St. Louis encephalitis virus is a group B arbovirus, a member of Flaviviri-dae, that is transmitted to humans by the bite of infected mosquitoes, with the donor host being birds. This virus causes inflammation of the tissues of the central nervous system. Symptoms may range from mild headache and fever to encephalitis and death. This virus occurs in the western, central, and southern United States and in Jamaica, Panama, Brazil, and Trinidad.

Professional Considerations

Consent form NOT required.

Preparation

1. Tube: Red topped, red/gray topped, or gold topped.
2. Specimens MAY be drawn during hemodialysis.

Procedure

1. Draw a 7-mL blood sample as soon as possible after symptoms appear, and label it as the acute sample.

2. Repeat the test in 10-14 days, and label the tube as the convalescent sample.

Postprocedure Care

1. See Client and Family Teaching.

Client and Family Teaching

1. Return in 10-14 days to have a convalescent sample drawn, which is necessary to interpret the results of the acute sample.

Factors That Affect Results

1. Failure to collect a convalescent sample.
2. False-positive results may occur in clients recently vaccinated for yellow fever.

Other Data

1. 10%-15% of clients with St. Louis encephalitis do not develop complement fixation antibodies.
2. There is no specific treatment for this disease.
3. Standard precautions and vector-control practices are adequate to prevent spread of this disease.
4. Severe winter freezes enhance the virus amplification (Florida, U.S.A.).

Stable Factor

See **Factor VII**—Blood.

Stemline DNA Analysis

See **DNA Ploidy**—Specimen.

Stereotactic Breast Biopsy—Diagnostic

Negative. Benign.

Positive. Atypical or malignant cells.

Description. Stereotactic breast biopsy is a gold standard out-patient radiograph-guided method of localizing and sampling nonpalpable breast lesions that are discovered on mammography and considered to be suspicious for malignancy. The position of the lesion in the breast can be calculated relative to a fixed grid and usually an 11-gauge needle placed within the lesion with direct confirmation of its position on a stereotactic radiograph. The placement is accurate to within 2 mm. A lateral guidance device improves biopsy accuracy and can accurately sample lesions within thin breasts. Stereotactic breast biopsy can be performed by means of fine-needle aspiration cytology or core needle histology. Other abnormal findings where this test can be used include microcalcifications, distorted breast tissue, area of abnormal change or a new mass or microcalcification that formed since a previous breast surgery.

Professional Considerations

Consent form IS required.

Risks

Bruising, infection at needle aspiration site, vasovagal reaction.

Contraindications

Large, abnormal breast tissue area, breast augmentation with implants.

Precautions

During pregnancy, risks of cumulative radiation exposure to the fetus from this and other previous or future imaging studies must be weighed against the benefits of the procedure. Although formal limits for client exposure are relative to this risk:benefit comparison, the United States Nuclear Regulatory Commission requires that the cumulative dose equivalent to an embryo/fetus from occupational exposure not exceed 0.5 rem (5 mSv). Radiation dosage to the fetus is proportional to the distance of the anatomy studied from the abdomen and decreases as pregnancy progresses. For pregnant clients, consult the radiologist/radiology department to obtain estimated fetal radiation exposure from this procedure. In women who are breast-feeding, formula should be substituted for breast milk for 1 or more days after the procedure.

Preparation

1. This procedure is performed by a radiologist with mammographic experience.
2. Equipment is assembled according to the type of biopsy (fine-needle aspiration or core needle) and the radiologist's preference.
3. The client is assessed for any allergies, use of anticoagulants or antiplatelet agents, or bleeding disorders.
4. Just before beginning the procedure, take a "time out" to verify the correct client, procedure, and site.

Procedure

1. The client is positioned prone on the x-ray table with the breasts hanging down for the mammogram films and biopsy. An upright seated position with lateral arm support may also be used, but is associated with a higher incidence of vasovagal reactions.
2. The skin is prepared according to the radiologist's preference and institutional policy.
3. A local anesthetic is injected into the biopsy site.
4. A small incision is made at the site of needle insertion.

5. The needle (either a 14-gauge automated needle or an 11- to 14-gauge vacuum-assisted biopsy probe) is inserted percutaneously into the lesion with placement confirmed by radiography.

6. Three or more samples are taken from different positions in the lesion. At least 12 samples are required for best diagnostic accuracy. The first sample is usually taken from the core of the lesion, followed by samples taken from the periphery.

7. Metallic clips may be placed within the breast to mark the biopsy site for easy identification should later biopsy be needed.

8. The specimen obtained from core needle biopsy is placed in formalin and sent immediately to the laboratory.

9. The specimen obtained from fine-needle aspiration is fixed on cytology slides and sent immediately to the laboratory.

Postprocedure Care

1. Place Steri-Strips and a pressure dressing over the site.

2. If metal clips were placed, two orthogonal planes should be taken via mammogram to confirm clip location for later comparison.

Client and Family Teaching

1. The client may eat or drink as usual.

2. The procedure generally takes 45 minutes to 1 hour.

3. Most individuals are able to return to their usual routine, including driving or work, after the procedure.

4. The dressing may be removed the next day.

5. There may be some tenderness, swelling, bruising, or slight bleeding at the site. An ice pack or non-aspirin pain reliever will help to relieve these symptoms.

6. If the biopsy diagnosis is benign, routine mammograms should be continued.

Factors That Affect Results

1. Core needle biopsy yields better diagnostic results than does fine-needle aspiration. All specimens taken must be examined to avoid false-negative results.

2. Needle placement can be inaccurate and yield a false-negative result if the breast tissue is displaced during biopsy.

3. Physician experience with at least 5-14 prior biopsies of this type significantly improves the diagnostic accuracy of the procedure.

Other Data

1. If inadequate tissue was obtained or if a malignancy is suspected but not confirmed, an open surgical biopsy is recommended. Open surgical biopsy is also recommended if atypical cells are identified.

2. Although complications from this procedure may include infection and hematoma, the complication rate is low.

3. Results from either fine-needle aspiration or core needle biopsy are available within 24 hours.

4. A 1-year follow-up mammography is recommended for benign lesions.

Stool Culture, Routine—Stool

Norm. Negative for pathogens; no growth other than normal flora.

Usage. Coccidioidomycosis, dysentery, enteric fever, failure to thrive (fat, ova, and parasite), gastroenteritis, salmonellosis, typhoid with *Salmonella*, and ulcerative colitis.

Description. To screen for common pathogens such as *Helicobacter*, *Salmonella*, *Shigella*, *Campylobacter*, *Vibrio*, *Yersinia*, or *Clostridium difficile*. This test may be indicated in clients with persistent or bloody diarrhea accompanied by fever or recent out-of-country travel (to a third-world country), in clients with a history of recent antibiotic usage, or in clients known to be exposed to enteric pathogens.

Professional Considerations

Consent form NOT required.

Preparation

1. Obtain a bedpan or a plastic toilet-seat specimen hat, a wooden tongue blade, and a sterile container with a lid.

Procedure

1. Using a wooden tongue blade, place a fresh stool sample 1 inch in diameter in a sterile container and cap it tightly.

Postprocedure Care

1. Send the specimen to the laboratory immediately.
2. If there will be a 2- or 3-hour delay before testing, place the specimen in a transport medium such as buffered saline-glycol or alkaline peptone-water.

Client and Family Teaching

1. Defecate in a bedpan or toilet-seat specimen hat, and avoid contaminating the stool with urine, toilet tissue, soap, or water.

Factors That Affect Results

1. Refrigerate the specimens if they are not sent to the laboratory immediately.
2. Barium or mineral oil inhibits bacterial growth.
3. Keep the specimens free of toilet tissue, bismuth, soap, water, or urine, because these accelerate deterioration of ova.

Other Data

1. Rectal swabs can be used, but they are less likely to yield positive results.
2. *Vibrio parahaemolyticus*, a marine bacterium, causes gastrointestinal symptoms as a result of improperly refrigerated crab, lobster, or shrimp.
3. *Vibrio cholerae*, rice-watery in appearance with a fishy odor, causes both epidemic and environmental cholera.
4. *Helicobacter pylori* has been cultured from the diarrheal stools of infected individuals in developing countries. Immigration is responsible for the development of isolated areas of high prevalence in some Western countries.
5. The optimal specimen for the diagnosis of *C. difficile*–associated diarrhea is a watery or loose stool. However, stool culture is no longer widely used for *C. difficile* detection because of the lengthy turnaround time.
6. Results are normally available in 48-96 hours.

Streptodornase

See Antideoxyribonuclease B Antibody Titer—Serum.

Streptozyme—Blood

Norm. Titer <166 Todd units or <100 streptozyme units.

Positive. Bacterial endocarditis, glomerulonephritis, pharyngitis, reactive arthritis, recent streptococcal infection, rheumatic and connective tissue diseases, rheumatic fever, scarlet fever, and upper respiratory tract infections.

Negative. Hematuria.

Description. A nonspecific screening test for the detection of antibodies to multiple exoenzymes of various species of streptococci using a commercial reagent containing erythrocytes coated with streptococcal antigens (DNase, streptokinase, streptolysin O, and hyaluronidase). This test can determine current or recent streptococcal infection earlier than the ASO titer, but it cannot determine the location or type of streptococcal infection. In a positive test, antibodies begin increasing by week 3 after infection and decrease by week 10.

Professional Considerations

Consent form NOT required.

Preparation

1. Tube: Serum separator or lavender topped or gray topped.
2. Specimens MAY be drawn during hemodialysis.

Procedure

1. Draw a 4-mL blood sample as soon as possible after symptoms appear, and label it as the acute sample.

Postprocedure Care

1. Repeat testing in 10 days, and label the tube as the convalescent sample.
2. Subsequent samples, taken biweekly for the next 4-6 weeks, are recommended.

Client and Family Teaching

1. Serial testing is recommended.

Factors That Affect Results

1. Antibiotic therapy may cause decreased results.

Other Data

1. Serial testing over a period of weeks is more significant than a single determination.
2. This test is not as sensitive in children as it is in adults.
3. See also Antistreptolysin-O titer—Serum.

Stress/Exercise Test—Diagnostic

Norm. Negative.

Client reaches and maintains 85% of his/her target heart rate, without cardiac symptoms.

Test results usually include the following information:

ECG: baseline and during test, including the presence of changes

Estimate of exercise capacity

Any cardiac symptoms occurring during the test

Criteria used for ending the test: determination of whether the maximal heart rate was attained

Blood pressure and any arrhythmias occurring during the test

Usage. Coronary artery disease; evaluation of cardiopulmonary fitness and exercise tolerance; preoperative screening for clients at high risk for surgical cardiovascular compromise; assessment of the efficacy of interventions such as coronary artery bypass graft, coronary angioplasty, medications, and cardiac rehabilitation; dysrhythmias; and valvular competence.

Description. Stress testing measures the efficiency of the heart during a period of physical stress on a treadmill or on a stationary bicycle. The effects of exercise on cardiac output and myocardial oxygen consumption are evaluated by concurrent monitoring of electrocardiograms, blood pressure, and oxygen consumption. An advantage of exercise testing is that it can identify (in a safe environment) individuals prone to cardiac ischemia during activity, when resting electrocardiograms are normal.

Professional Considerations

Consent form IS required.

Risks

Cardiac ischemia, including myocardial infarction, dysrhythmias, hypotension, hypertension, dizziness.

Contraindications

Cardiac contraindications: Active unstable angina, aortic stenosis (hemodynamically significant), chest pain, cardiac inflammation (endocarditis, myocarditis, pericarditis), congestive heart failure (acute), coronary insufficiency syndrome, digitalis toxicity, electrolyte abnormalities (severe), heart blocks (2°, 3°), hypertension (SBP >200 mm Hg, or DBP >110 mm Hg), left bundle branch block or other uncontrolled dysrhythmias, left ventricular hypertrophy, myocardial infarction (recent), obesity (weight higher than capacity of equipment, usually 350 pounds), pacemaker (fixed-rate), recent significant changes in ECG, thromboembolic processes (active).

Other contraindications: Alcohol intoxication, asthma (severe) or chronic obstructive pulmonary disease, infection (acute), pulmonary embolism (recent), thrombophlebitis; also inability to walk on a treadmill or pedal a bicycle.

Preparation

1. Have emergency equipment readily available.
2. See Client and Family Teaching.

Procedure

1. The stress test is performed by specially trained (that is, ACLS-certified) nurses, exercise physiologists, and physical therapists. The American Association of Cardiovascular and Pulmonary Rehabilitation has recommended direct physician supervision of all initial stress tests and tests for individuals considered at high risk for complications.
2. Attach electrocardiogram leads and a blood pressure cuff.
3. While the client is on a treadmill, stationary bicycle, or stair stepper, computerized electrocardiographic recordings and blood pressure readings are obtained.

Oxygen consumption may be measured by having the client breathe through a special mouthpiece during exercise.

4. The client is stressed in stages by increases in miles per hour and the percentage grade of elevation of the treadmill.

5. The test is terminated when any of the following occurs:

   a. Signs of ischemia are present (ST-segment depression of ≤1-2 mm for a duration >0.06 second, or ST-segment elevation).

   b. Maximum effort has been achieved.

   c. A predetermined target has been achieved.

   d. Dyspnea or hypertension >250 mm Hg systolic blood pressure is achieved.

   e. Tachycardia >200 beats per minute minus the client's age is reached.

   f. New dysrhythmias, new conduction disturbances (that is, heart block), or increasing ectopy is seen.

   g. Chest pain with or without ECG changes is seen.

   h. Faintness, weakness, dizziness, or confusion is seen.

   i. Blood pressure fails to rise as body exercise stress increases.

   j. There is extreme fatigue or request by the client that the test be stopped.

Postprocedure Care

1. The client should be monitored at rest until the heart rate, blood pressure, and electrocardiogram are at baseline values.

2. Remove the electrodes and the blood pressure cuff.

Client and Family Teaching

1. Wear flat walking or tennis shoes and comfortable attire.

2. According to physician preference and instructions, gradually discontinue beta-blocker drugs before the test.

3. Fast from food and fluids and refrain from smoking and caffeine usage for 4 hours before the test.

4. Clients may take all their medications as usual.

5. During the test, immediately report to the technician any chest pain, dizziness, light-headedness, nausea, or discomfort you experience.

6. After the test, rest for a few hours at home.

Factors That Affect Results

1. False-positive electrocardiogram responses are caused by anemia, digitalis, diuretics, estrogen, hypertension, hypoxia, Lown-Ganong-Levine syndrome, syndrome X in women, or valvular heart disease.

2. False-positive results may be caused by the following baseline ECG abnormalities:

   a. 1 mm or more elevation or depression of the ST segment

   b. Right or left ventricular hypertrophy

   c. T-wave inversions in multiple leads from an old injury

   d. Abnormal conduction, such as increased Q-T interval, ST-T changes, and right or left bundle branch blocks

3. False-positive results occur more frequently in women than in men.

4. False-negative tests occur when individuals with known significant CAD fail to demonstrate exercise-induced ST-segment depression.

5. Conditions that may affect performance include lung disease, muscle pain, and electrolyte imbalances.

Other Data

1. In males, ischemic ST-segment displacement >0.1 mm of 80-msec duration during exercise but not found at rest means a five times greater risk of coronary heart disease.

2. Exertional hypotension may indicate left coronary artery disease, myocardial ischemia, or left ventricular dysfunction.

3. The exercise stress test may also be performed with radionuclide (thallium) or radiopharmaceutical (sestamibi) perfusion studies. See Heart scan—Diagnostic.

4. Shaw Olson, Kip et al (2006) found that the addition of functional capacity estimation via the Duke Activity Status Index in symptomatic females before exercise testing improved detection of clients most likely to benefit from the pharmacologic stress test (see Stress test, Pharmacologic—Diagnostic), combined with activities to manage their specific risks for coronary heart disease.

5. See also Stress test, Pharmacologic—Diagnostic.

Stress Test, Pharmacologic—Diagnostic

Norm. Negative.

Usage. Coronary artery disease; detection of ischemia and assessment of myocardial viability; evaluation of left ventricular function; preoperative cardiac risk stratification; and valvular competence.

Description. Pharmacologic stress testing is used to evaluate individuals with suspected or proven coronary artery disease who are unable to perform satisfactory levels of exercise to reach 85% of their maximal heart rate. A pharmacologic agent is used to elevate heart rate and blood pressure, and cardiac response is examined through an imaging technique. The *dobutamine echocardiographic stress test* induces pharmacologic stress by the infusion of dobutamine, a synthetic amine that increases myocardial contractility. Dobutamine directly stimulates cardiac alpha$_1$- and beta$_1$-adrenergic receptors, thereby increasing oxygen demand. When this occurs in the presence of an impaired oxygen supply, echocardiography can directly visualize myocardial wall motion abnormalities in individuals with fixed coronary artery stenosis. The *adenosine pharmacologic stress test* is a potent vasodilator that mimics the effect of exercise on the heart. Use of adenosine is preferred over dobutamine because adenosine's short duration of action and the fact that reversal agents are not needed.

Professional Considerations
Consent form IS required.

Risks of Dobutamine Infusion
Cardiac ischemia, including myocardial infarction and dysrhythmias, dizziness, flushing, hypertension, hypotension, and palpitations.

Contraindications for Adenosine
Active bronchospasm, asthma history, atrioventricular block (high-degree). Drugs include methylxanthines such as theophylline, aminophylline, caffeine or Cafergot, and oral dipyridamole.

Contraindications for Dobutamine
Tachyarrhythmias (atrial, ventricular). Drugs include beta blockers.

Preparation
1. Have emergency equipment readily available.
2. Establish intravenous access.
3. See Client and Family Teaching.
4. Just before beginning the procedure, take a "time out" to verify the correct client, procedure, and site.

Procedure
1. The stress test is performed by specially trained (that is, ACLS-certified) nurses and echocardiographers. The American Association of Cardiovascular and Pulmonary Rehabilitation has recommended direct physician supervision of all initial stress tests and tests for individuals considered at high risk for complications.
2. Attach electrocardiogram leads and a blood pressure cuff.
3. Obtain a baseline 12-lead ECG and blood pressure cuff.
4. The individual is placed in the best position to obtain echocardiographic images (usually left lateral decubitus), and baseline images are obtained.
5. Dobutamine is diluted according to institutional policy and procedure and administered by means of an infusion pump at an initial rate of 5 mg/kg/minute.
6. The infusion rate is increased every 3 minutes to 10, 20, and a maximum of 40 mg/kg/minute unless end points develop.
7. Heart rate and ECG rhythm strip are monitored continuously, and blood pressure and 12-lead ECG are recorded at each stage of drug infusion.
8. Continuous echocardiography is also performed. Direct recordings of images are made at rest, at mid infusion, at peak infusion, and at 1-2 minutes after infusion.
9. The test is terminated when any of the following occurs:
   a. Signs of ischemia are present (ST-segment depression of <1-2 mm for a duration >0.06 second, or ST-segment elevation).
   b. Heart rate is >75%-85% of predicted maximum for age.
   c. There is development of new wall motion abnormality.

d. Hypertension >210-260 mm Hg systolic blood pressure or diastolic blood pressure >100 mm Hg occurs.

e. New dysrhythmias occur.

f. Chest pain with or without ECG changes occurs.

g. Symptomatic hypotension or blood pressure decrease more than 20 mm Hg occurs.

h. Heart rate decreases more than 20 beats per minute.

i. Prespecified dosage of dobutamine has been reached or target heart rate has been reached.

j. The client requests to terminate test.

Postprocedure Care

1. The client should be monitored until the heart rate, blood pressure, and electrocardiogram are at baseline values.

2. Remove the electrodes and the blood pressure cuff.

Client and Family Teaching

1. The entire procedure lasts approximately 60 minutes.

2. According to physician preference and instructions, gradually discontinue beta-blocker drugs before the test. Antianginal agents may also be discontinued 24-48 hours before testing to maximize test sensitivity.

3. Fast from food and fluids and refrain from smoking and caffeine usage for 4 hours before the test.

4. Clients may take all their medications as usual.

5. The administration of dobutamine is associated with mild side effects such as chest tightness, dyspnea, flushing, nausea, headache, paresthesias, chills, anxiety, or palpitations. Individuals are instructed to immediately report any side effects they experience to the technician. Side effects generally subside quickly after the dobutamine is discontinued.

6. Do not take caffeine-containing foods, herbs, or drinks for 24 hours before the test. These include coffee, colas and chocolate.

Factors That Affect Results

1. Chest wall deformities, emphysema, and severe obesity limit visualization of the heart with transthoracic probes.

Other Data

1. The half-life of dobutamine is 2 minutes.

2. Side effects may be treated with intravenous beta-adrenergic blockers.

3. Abnormalities of ventricular contraction detected by echocardiography precede ECG signs or symptoms of ischemia.

4. The adenosine or dipyridamole stress tests also induce pharmacologic cardiac stress that is examined through radionuclide (thallium, sestamibi) imaging. See also Heart scan—Diagnostic.

5. See also Stress/exercise test—Diagnostic.

Striational Autoantibody—Specimen

Norm. Negative, titer <60.

Positive. Autoimmune liver disorders, Lambert-Eaton myasthenic syndrome, myasthenia gravis, myopathic disorders, and small cell lung carcinoma. Recipients of D-penicillamine and bone marrow allografts may have positive titers.

Description. Striational autoantibodies are immunoglobulins that react to contractile elements of skeletal muscle. They are detected by enzyme-linked immunoassay or immunofluorescence microscopy. Striational autoantibodies are a valuable marker of myasthenia gravis in the adult and are associated with thymoma. Their prevalence increases with the age of onset of myasthenia gravis. They are rarely positive at ages <20 years.

Professional Considerations

Consent form NOT required.

Preparation

1. Tube: Red topped, red/gray topped, or gold topped.

2. Specimens MAY be drawn during hemodialysis.

Procedure

1. Draw a 7-mL blood sample.

Postprocedure Care

1. None.

Client and Family Teaching

1. Results are normally available in 1 week.

Factors That Affect Results
1. None found.

Other Data
1. Titer rarely positive in adolescence.

Stuart-Prower Factor

See Factor X—Blood.

Sucrose Hemolysis Test—Diagnostic

Norm. <5% hemolysis, or negative.

Usage. Screening for paroxysmal nocturnal hemoglobinuria (PNH).

Description. Paroxysmal nocturnal hemoglobinuria is an acquired anemia characterized by the production of abnormal hemopoietic cells, red blood cells with an abnormal sensitivity to complement, and erythrocyte hemolysis. Symptoms include leukopenia or thrombocytopenia as well as nocturnal hemoglobinuria, chronic anemia, and thrombosis. Symptom severity is related to the degree of red blood cell sensitivity to complement and varies from client to client. In this test, sucrose provides a medium of low ionic strength that promotes the binding of complement to red blood cells. Blood from clients with PNH demonstrates the results of excessive lysis.

Professional Considerations
Consent form NOT required.

Preparation
1. Tube: Blue topped.
2. Specimens should NOT be drawn during hemodialysis.

Procedure
1. Draw a 5-mL blood sample.
2. Mix the washed red blood cells with ABO-compatible normal serum and 10% isotonic sucrose.

3. Incubate the tube 30 minutes at room temperature.
4. Centrifuge the tube.
5. Read the percentage of hemolysis that results.

Postprocedure Care
1. None.

Client and Family Teaching
1. Results are normally available within 2 hours of the test.

Factors That Affect Results
1. Hemolysis or clotting of the specimen invalidates the results.
2. False-positive results occur with megaloblastic anemia, autoimmune hemolytic anemias, dyserythropoietic anemia, lymphoma, adenocarcinoma of the colon, eosinophilia, renal failure, or bronchogenic carcinoma.
3. False-negative results may occur in clients who have received recent blood transfusions or if the specimen has been collected in a lavender topped tube containing EDTA or a green topped tube containing heparin.

Other Data
1. Recent advances in the diagnosis of PNH include direct identification of affected cells by flow cytometry, detection of impaired synthesis of GPI anchor, and cytogenic analysis of the abnormal expression of the PIG-A gene.

SUDS

See Acquired Immune Deficiency Syndrome Evaluation Battery—Diagnostic.

Sugar Water Test Screen

See Sucrose Hemolysis Test—Diagnostic.

Supreme BG

See Glucose Monitoring Machines—Diagnostic.

Swan-Ganz Catheter Pulmonary Wedge Pressure

See Pulmonary Artery Catheterization—Diagnostic.

Sweat Gland Nerve Fiber Density Test (SGNFD)—Specimen

Norm. No standard norms exist. See Other Data below.

Usage. May be used in conjunction with epidermal nerve fiber density (ENFD) testing, or after an ENFD test is negative. Detects neuropathy of the small fiber autonomic nerves.

Description. Small diameter nerve fiber (SDNF) neuropathy is characterized by damage to the small nerve fibers located in the internal organs, skin, and nerves of the periphery of the body. When the unmyelinated and thin-myelinated small autonomic nerve fibers are damaged, the symptoms that result can include irregularities in body temperature and sweating, orthostatic hypotension, tachycardia, bowel and bladder problems including constipation, diarrhea, difficulty urinating, sexual hypo- or hypersensitivity, and cutaneous symptoms including hair loss, skin dryness, and brittle nails (Gibbons, Illigens, Wang, 2009). Routine evaluation for neuropathy includes electromyelogram (EMG) testing; however, this type of testing only measures large nerves. When an EMG test is negative, a deep tissue biopsy can be used to count the number of small fiber nerves to measure the density of autonomic nerves, which are small-fiber nerve tissue. This test may be used in conjunction with the epidermal nerve fiber density test, which measures small nerve fiber density of sensory nerve fibers, which can also be affected in small fiber neuropathy.

Professional Considerations

Consent form NOT required.

Preparation

1. Obtain test kit. Place cool pack in freezer for return shipping.
2. Obtain 2% lidocaine, 1mL syringe, test kit vials containing Zamboni's fixative and dry sterile dressing, sterile scissors, and chemocautery solution.

Procedure

1. Cleanse the biopsy site with an alcohol swab.
2. Inject approximately 0.5 mL of 2% lidocaine with epinephrine in a 1-cm circle or "V" pattern around the site.
3. Obtain biopsy of the thigh, calf, or foot using a 3mm punch to a depth of 4 mm. Specific locations recommended are those where an established norm is known:
   a. Thigh: at the pubis level, 20 cm distal to the iliac spine
   b. Calf: lateral side, 10 cm above the lateral malleolus
   c. Foot: dorsum, above the extensor digitorum brevis muscle.
4. Remove the sample without damaging the epithelium by pushing down on the epithelium next to the sample, then attaching forceps to the dermal side and lifting the sample, then cutting the base to detach the specimen.
5. Split sample into two vials and label with location of the biopsy site.
6. Leave in fixative overnight. Pour off fixative, then rinse with buffer solution × 2. Fill vial with cryoprotectant, than place inside a cool pack and mail to the testing lab.

Postprocedure Care

1. Apply an aluminum-based chemocautery to the site. Apply pressure dressing to site.
2. Remove pressure, apply triple-antibiotic, then apply a dry sterile dressing.

Factors That Affect Results

1. Because sweat glands are located deep in dermal tissue, the full length of the punch biopsy needle should be inserted when obtaining the sample.

Other Data

1. There is no "gold standard" technique for measuring sweat gland nerve fiber density. Measurement and standardization of results is complex due to the complex structure of sweat glands, as well as the variable size and number of sweat glands. For this reason, some payers consider this procedure to be investigational.

2. Conditions causing small fiber autonomic neuropathy include autoimmune autonomic ganglionopathy, diabetes, human immunodeficiency virus-1, Guillain-Barré syndrome, anhidrosis, hyperhidrosis, familial amyloidosis, and Parkinson's disease.

3. See also Epidermal nerve fiber density test—Specimen.

Sweat Test

See **Chloride, Sweat**—Specimen.

Synovial Fluid Analysis

See **Body Fluid Analysis**—Specimen.

Synovial Fluid Mucin Test

See **Mucin Clot Test**—Specimen.

Syphilis

See **Microhemagglutination** *Treponema pallidum* (MHA-TP) **Test**—Serum.

TAG 72

See **CA 72-4**—Blood.

Tape Test

See **Parasite Screen**—Stool.

T- and B-Lymphocyte Subset Assay (Lymphocyte [T & B] Assay, Lymphocyte Subset Typing, Lymphocyte Marker Studies)—Blood

Norm.

T-cells	60%-80% of total lymphocyte count
B-cells	5%-15% of total lymphocyte count

T-Cell and B-Cell Lymphocyte Subset Percentages and Counts

| Age (years) | CD3+ | | CD19+ | |
	% (median)	Count × 10⁹/l	% (median)	Count × 10⁹/l
18-39	57-82 (70)	0.66-2.40	6-26 (13)	0.09-0.57
40-69	57-83 (71)	0.57-2.21	6-27 (14)	0.08-0.50
70-79	47-82 (65)	0.60-2.82	3-31 (11)	0.06-0.79

Age (years)	CD3+		CD19+	
	% (median)	Count × 10^9/l	% (median)	Count × 10^9/l
80-89	47-88 (67)	0.51-2.62	2-26 (8)	0.04-0.57
≥90	40-91 (67)	0.44-2.43	3-24 (8)	0.03-0.58

Age (years)	CD3+CD4+		CD3+CD8+	
	% (median)	Count × 10^9/l	% (Median)	Count × 10^9/l
18-39	28-57 (43)	0.34-1.70	16-38 (24)	0.22-0.88
40-69	30-60 (46)	0.34-1.54	12-47 (26)	0.15-0.98
70-79	18-53 (35)	0.28-1.77	11-65 (25)	0.17-1.75
80-89	21-60 (40)	0.31-1.48	8-70 (25)	0.11-1.73
≥90	16-63 (39)	0.26-1.44	9-57 (24)	0.10-1.34

Adapted from McNerlan SE, Alexander HD, Rea IM: Age-related reference intervals for lymphocyte subsets in whole blood of healthy individuals, *Scand J Clin Lab Invest* 59(2):89-92, 1999.

Usage. Acquired immune deficiency syndrome, autoimmune diseases, common variable immunodeficiency (CVID), DiGeorge syndrome, Graves' disease, Hodgkin's disease, humoral immune deficiency, leukemia, lymphoma, multiple myeloma, systemic lupus erythematosus, Waldenström's macroglobulinemia, and X-linked agammaglobulinemia.

Description. Quantification of T and B cells as a percentage of total peripheral blood lymphocytes to determine immune deficiency states. Lymphocyte stem cells are produced in the bone marrow and released into the peripheral circulation. The tissue that traps the lymphocyte stem cells determines whether they mature into a T or B lymphocyte. T lymphocytes mature in the thymus gland or the precortical areas of lymph nodes and are responsible for cell-mediated immunity. B lymphocytes mature in the tonsils, spleen, germinating centers of the lymph nodes, and nodules of the intestinal tract and are responsible for antibody-mediated immunity. This test is performed by use of flow cytometry and monoclonal antibody technology.

Professional Considerations
Consent form NOT required.

Preparation
1. Tube: Two EDTA-anticoagulated, lavender topped tubes.

2. Do NOT draw specimens during hemodialysis.

Procedure
1. Draw two 7-mL blood samples.

Postprocedure Care
1. Keep the specimens at room temperature and process them within 3 hours.

Client and Family Teaching
1. Explain the rationale for the test and explain the results, which should be available the same day.

Factors That Affect Results
1. Drugs that may increase lymphocytes include steroids and immunosuppressives.
2. Refrigerating or freezing blood decreases lymphocyte counts.
3. Some lymphocyte subset counts vary with age. See Norms.

Other Data
1. Fresh tissue, bone marrow, and suspensions of lymph node or spleen can also be used for analysis.
2. This test is also useful for monitoring clients on chemotherapy or immunosuppressive agents.
3. CD4 is commonly used to monitor progression of and response to treatment of HIV infection.
4. See also Acquired immune deficiency syndrome evaluation battery—Diagnostic when applicable.

T$_3$ or T$_4$ Thyroid Test

See Thyroid Test: Thyroxine—Blood or Thyroid Test: Triiodothyronine—Blood.

T₃ Resin Uptake Test

See Thyroid Hormone Binding Ratio—Blood.

TA90 Immune Complex Assay (TA90 IC)—Serum

Norm. Negative or ≤1.

Usage. Identifies subclinical metastasis of early-stage malignant melanoma; helps predict the risk of recurrence of melanoma; helps guide decisions about treatment after surgery. Significant predictor of survival for stage II and stage III clients.

Description. Detects the presence of an immune complex of a 90-kDa tumor-associated antigen and its antibody, which are found in the sera of clients with malignant melanoma. When found in the sera of clients who have had removal of a malignant melanoma, this test has a sensitivity of 70% and specificity of 85% for predicting recurrence of the disease.

Professional Considerations
Consent form NOT required.

Preparation
1. Tube: Red topped, red/gray topped, or gold topped.

Procedure
1. Draw a 2-mL blood sample.

Postprocedure Care
1. Write the collection time and date on the laboratory requisition.

Client and Family Teaching
1. Results are normally available within 2 days.

Factors That Affect Results
1. Reject specimens received more than 1 hour after collection.

Other Data
1. None.

Tartrate-Resistant Acid Phosphatase (TRAP) Stain—Specimen

Norm. Negative.

Positive. Leukocytes are not inhibited by L-tartrate: hairy cell leukemia, lipid storage disease (Gaucher cells), lymphoma, mononucleosis, and prolymphocytic leukemia. Also stains positive in the presence of mast cells and normal osteoclasts.

Description. Tartrate-resistant acid phosphatase (TRAP) is an enzyme produced by osteoclasts and contained in hairy cells. The presence of tartrate resistance to acid phosphatase is diagnostic for hairy cell leukemia (leukemic reticuloendotheliosis), a chronic form of leukemia characterized by distinctive cells called "hairy cells," which have many fine, cytoplasmic projections. Thus this test is used to help diagnose hairy cell leukemia and assess response to treatment and is a marker for the rate of bone resorption. Newer research has found that TRAP is produced by some osteoclasts causing bone dysplasia. This test may be performed on bone marrow or blood. If bone marrow is

positive for hairy cells, other confirmatory morphologic testing is needed because TRAP-positive specimens may be caused by conditions other than hairy cell leukemia.

Professional Considerations
Consent form NOT required.

Preparation
1. Obtain four glass microslides for smears and fixative (glutaraldehyde-acetone).
2. Blood specimens MAY be drawn during hemodialysis.

Procedure
1. Draw a 2-mL blood sample in a heparinized syringe.
2. Place two drops of blood on each of the four slides.
3. Bone marrow specimen is obtained via bone marrow aspiration.

Postprocedure Care
1. Spray fixative on the slides immediately.
2. See Bone marrow aspiration analysis—Specimen.

Client and Family Teaching

1. Results are normally available in 1-2 days.
2. See Bone marrow aspiration analysis—Specimen.

Factors That Affect Results

1. Rare false-negative results occur.
2. Results should be interpreted with caution in jaundiced clients because hyperbilirubinemia skews the accuracy of the results.
3. Abnormal erythrocyte or platelet levels will affect results.

Other Data

1. Serum levels of acid phosphatase isoenzyme 5 may also be elevated in hairy cell leukemia.

Tau Test (hTau Antigen)—CSF

Norm. <200 pg/mL^{-1}

Note: Tapiola (2001) used a cutoff of <380 pg/mL and found that the combination of the Tau test and the Beta-amyloid protein 40/42—CSF test had a specificity of 95% to differentiate Alzheimer's disease from control subjects and 85% to differentiate Alzheimer's disease from those with other dementias.

Usage. Biologic marker for Alzheimer's disease; helps differentiate causes of cognitive impairment; evaluation of disease progression; evaluation of response to treatment for Alzheimer's disease. This test is not used alone but is compared to the Ab42 test in determining consistency with a diagnosis of Alzheimer's disease. Increased levels of Tau with corresponding decreased levels of Ab42 in cerebral spinal fluid would be consistent with Alzheimer's disease. Kapaki (2005) found the Tau/Beta-amyloid protein 42 ratio reliable in differentiating early-stage Alzheimer's disease from alcohol-related cognitive disorder.

Description. While there are no definitive tests to diagnose Alzheimer's disease, there are some tests that may be used to assist in the complex diagnosis. Alzheimer's disease, the most common form of dementia, is characterized by the presence of senile plaques and neurofibrillary tangles containing abnormal masses of cytoplasmic proteins. The neurofibrillary tangles of Alzheimer's disease contain mainly the Tau protein in an (abnormal) hyperphosphorylated state. Elevated levels of the abnormal Tau proteins can be detected in the cerebrospinal fluid in more than 90% of clients with Alzheimer's disease, even before the dementia symptoms appear. Levels also correlate with elevated apolipoprotein E concentration (see Apolipoprotein E-4 genotyping—Plasma), a known risk factor for Alzheimer's disease. This test is sometimes performed in conjunction with beta-amyloid protein 40/42 (see Beta-amyloid protein—CSF), which is often decreased when the Tau test is elevated. There are six isoforms of the Tau protein, which can be detected by monoclonal antibodies. The AT8 monoclonal antibody is highly specific for the most common abnormal isoform of the Tau protein found in Alzheimer's disease and can detect its presence even before the neurofibrillary tangles appear. This test is an enzyme-linked immunosorbent assay using monoclonal antibodies for the detection of Tau proteins in cerebrospinal fluid (CSF).

Professional Considerations

Consent form IS required for the procedure used to obtain the specimen. Informed consent is recommended for genetic testing.

Risks

See Lumbar puncture—Diagnostic.

Contraindications

See Lumbar puncture—Diagnostic.

Preparation

1. See Lumbar puncture—Diagnostic.
2. Obtain a sterile container for CSF.

Procedure

1. Collect a 1-mL sample of CSF during the lumbar puncture procedure.

Postprocedure Care

1. See Lumbar puncture—Diagnostic.

Client and Family Teaching

1. See Lumbar puncture—Diagnostic.
2. Refer to section in this book on "Informed Consent for Genetic Testing".

Factors That Affect Results

1. Levels increase as the number of neurofibrillary tangles increase.

2. The use of this test in the diagnosis of Alzheimer's disease must also be correlated to both physical and neurologic testing of the client being evaluated for a diagnosis of dementia.

3. An abnormal result with one of these markers (Tau or beta-amyloid protein 40/42) without a corresponding change in the other would help to rule out Alzheimer's disease.

Other Data

1. The trade name of the monoclonal antibody test is INNOTEST hTAU Antigen, manufactured by Innogenetics® N.V.

2. Tau antigen testing can be performed on nasal secretions to detect CSF leakage.

3. The Genetic Information Nondiscrimination Act of 2008 prohibits health plans from using genetic family history or genetic test results from influencing eligibility or premiums for health insurance. It also prohibits employers from using this information to influence decisions about hiring, terminating employment, or employment pay, promotions, or privileges.

TB Test

See Mantoux Skin Test—Diagnostic.

TBPA PALB

See Transthyretin—Serum or Vitreous Fluid.

TBUT

See Schirmer Tearing Eye Test—Diagnostic.

Tear Break-Up Time

See Schirmer Tearing Eye Test—Diagnostic.

TEE

See Transesophageal Ultrasonography—Diagnostic.

Teichoic Acid Antibody—Blood

Norm. Titer ≤1:2 or less than a fourfold rise in titer between acute and convalescent samples.

Increased. Endocarditis, infections caused by *Staphylococcus aureus*, osteomyelitis, and subacute bacterial endocarditis.

Description. Teichoic acid is a macromolecule present on the cell wall of gram-positive bacteria. Antibodies to teichoic acid can be seen in some infections, such as prolonged exposure to *Staphylococcus* endocarditis. Monitoring teichoic acid antibody levels may be helpful in assessing response

to therapy in clients with gram-positive infections. Although the sensitivity of all methods for measuring teichoic acid is low, the enzyme-linked immunosorbent assay (ELISA) method is the most sensitive.

Professional Considerations

Consent form NOT required.

Preparation

1. Tube: Red topped, red/gray topped, or gold topped.

2. Specimens MAY be drawn during hemodialysis.

Procedure

1. Draw a 5-mL sample as soon as possible after symptoms appear or diagnosis is suspected, and label the tube as the acute sample.
2. Repeat the test in 14 days, and label the tube as the convalescent sample.
3. Serial testing may also be performed.

Postprocedure Care

1. See Client and Family Teaching.

Client and Family Teaching

1. The client must return in 2 weeks for convalescent sample testing.

Factors That Affect Results

1. Technical variability.

Other Data

1. Patients with invasive *S. aureus* infections with a low teichoic acid antibody level are more likely to have fatal outcomes.

Telomerase Enzyme Marker—Blood, Sputum, or Urine

Norm. Negative for the presence of active telomerase enzyme.

Usage. Early marker for detection of cancers.

Description. Approximately 80%-90% of cancer cells have an active ribonucleoprotein telomerase enzyme preventing their telomeres (chromosome ends) from wearing out, and such prevention allows them to divide indefinitely. This is in contrast to noncancerous cells in which telomerase is repressed, causing the telomeres to shorten with each division. The detection of the active telomerase enzyme in a person's blood, sputum, or urine can serve as an early marker for the presence of cancer. It is believed that if drugs can be developed that will selectively inactivate telomerase this may stop the growth or even destroy cancer cells.

Professional Considerations

Consent form NOT required.

Preparation

1. Tube: Gold topped. For urine study (used in evaluating bladder cancer), obtain a clean-catch container.

Procedure

1. Draw a 2- to 3-mL blood sample, or obtain a urine clean-catch specimen if urine sample is to be studied.

Postprocedure Care

1. None

Client and Family Teaching

1. For urine collection, teach clean-catch technique.

Factors That Affect Results

1. None found.

Other Data

1. None.

Temazepam

See **Benzodiazepines**—Plasma and Urine.

Tensilon Test—Diagnostic

Positive. Unequivocal improvement in a single weakened muscle. Frequency of positive test in persons with myesthenia gravis is lower in patients with muscle specific kinase (MuSK) antibodies.

Negative. Equivocal or no improvement in a weakened muscle. False-negative tests are fairly common, and repeated tests are helpful.

Usage. Diagnosis of myasthenia gravis.

Description. Myasthenia gravis is an autoimmune neuromuscular disease characterized by fatigue of the limb, facial, bulbar, and ocular muscles with repetitive activity and by improvement with rest. Respiratory muscle fatigue can also occur. It is caused by circulating antibodies directed toward the skeletal muscle acetylcholine receptor.

The factors that trigger the autoimmune response are unknown. In the Tensilon (edrophonium chloride) test, a short-acting anticholinesterase is administered intravenously, and muscle response is observed. The test is most useful if improvement in ptosis or the strength of an extraocular muscle is demonstrated because of the objective nature of this response. After intravenous administration of Tensilon, muscle strength will improve quickly in clients with myasthenia gravis.

Professional Considerations
Consent form NOT required.

Preparation
1. Assess for use of medications that affect muscle function, allergies, and respiratory disease.
2. Establish intravenous access with a butterfly needle or an infusion of 5% dextrose in water or 0.9% saline.
3. Obtain baseline vital signs.
4. Have emergency respiratory support equipment and atropine available for use in the event of complications.

Procedure
1. Determine the muscle to observe for response.
2. An initial test dose is administered because some people may be sensitive to Tensilon and may experience bradycardia or bronchospasm. These individuals should not receive additional Tensilon.
3. Administer an initial dose of Tensilon intravenously as follows:
   a. Adults: 2 mg.
   b. Children weighing >75 pounds: 2 mg.
   c. Children weighing <75 pounds: 1 mg.
   d. Infants: 0.5 mg.
4. Muscle strength may improve within 45 seconds. If no improvement is noted, additional Tensilon should be infused as follows:
   a. Adults: up to 8 mg over 30 seconds.
   b. Children weighing >75 pounds: up to 8 mg at a rate of 1 mg/30-45 seconds.
   c. Children weighing <75 pounds: up to 5 mg at a rate of 1 mg/30-45 seconds.
   d. Infants: Do not administer further Tensilon.
5. Flush the IV access line between doses to ensure that the medication has infused.
6. Be prepared for possible respiratory distress because Tensilon may stimulate a cholinergic crisis that causes extreme muscle weakness. If this occurs, up to 1 mg of intravenous atropine should be administered promptly.
7. Atropine may be administered during the test to clients with respiratory diseases, such as asthma, to minimize the side effects of Tensilon.
8. Once an unequivocal response is noted, the test is complete, and Tensilon administration should be stopped.

Postprocedure Care
1. Monitor vital signs every 5 minutes × 4.

Client and Family Teaching
1. Instruct the client about the procedure and the potential side effects of Tensilon.

Factors That Affect Results
1. Prednisone delays the effect of Tensilon.
2. Quinidine and anticholinergics inhibit the action of Tensilon.
3. Skeletal muscle relaxants may mask the effect of Tensilon.

Other Data
1. The side effects of Tensilon include abdominal cramps, bradycardia, diaphoresis, diarrhea, hypotension, incontinence, pupillary constriction, respiratory distress, and salivation.

Terminal Deoxynucleotidyltransferase (TdT)—Blood or Bone Marrow

Norm.

	Blood	Bone marrow
Adult	0-4 TdT U/10 cells or 0-0.67 pU/cell	0-5.7 TdT U/10 cells or 0-0.95 pU/cell
Child	0-3.5 TdT U/10 cells or 0-0.58 pU/cell	2.9-8.9 TdT U/10 cells or 0.48-1.49 pU/cell

Usage. Acute lymphoblastic leukemia, blast crisis, blastic plasmacytoid dendritic cell (BPDC) neoplasm, granulocytic sarcoma, Hodgkin's disease, lymphoma, and myelogenous leukemia.

Description. Terminal deoxynucleotidyl-transferase (TdT) is an intracellular protein that is a biochemical marker that aids in the diagnosis and classification of acute leukemias. It acts as a catalyst in the polymerization of deoxynucleotide triphosphates in the absence of a template. Approximately 1%-5% of normal mononuclear cells express TdT in normal peripheral blood and bone marrow.

Professional Considerations
Consent form NOT required for blood sample. Consent form IS required for bone marrow aspiration. See Bone marrow aspiration analysis—Specimen for procedural risks and contraindications.

Preparation
1. Contact the laboratory to determine if the test must be prescheduled.
2. Tube: Lavender topped for blood sample. Container of formalin for bone marrow specimen.

3. Blood specimens should NOT be drawn during hemodialysis.
4. See Bone marrow aspiration analysis—Specimen for bone marrow specimen.

Procedure
1. Draw a 10-mL blood sample.
2. For bone marrow sample, see Bone marrow aspiration analysis—Specimen.

Postprocedure Care
1. For bone marrow sample, see Bone marrow aspiration analysis—Specimen.

Client and Family Teaching
1. Results are normally available in 1-2 days.
2. See Bone marrow aspiration analysis—Specimen.

Factors That Affect Results
1. Heparin in the blood tube may decrease the results.
2. Insufficient bone marrow may produce indeterminate results.

Other Data
1. Some children with acute lymphoblastic leukemia have low TdT activity.
2. TdT-positive leukemics that relapse can show a change in phenotype and can then be TdT-negative.

Testicles Ultrasonography

See Scrotum and Testicular Ultrasonography—Diagnostic.

Testosterone, Free (Bioavailable) and Total—Blood
Norm.

Adult and Pubertal Male Testosterone Levels
Chemilucent Immunoassay

	Value	SI Units
Free Testosterone		
Male Adults		
≥18 years	44-244 pg/mL	
Male Children		
10-17 years	0.6-159 pg/mL	
% Free Testosterone	1.6%-2.9%	
Total Testosterone		
Male Adults		
20-39 years	400-1080 ng/dL	13.88-37.48 nmol/L
40-59 years	350-890 ng/dL	12.15-30.88 nmol/L
60 years and older	350-720 ng/dL	12.15-24.98 nmol/L
Male Children		
14-15 years	100-320 ng/dL	3.47-11.10 nmol/L
16-19 years	200-970 ng/dL	6.94-33.66 nmol/L

Prepubertal Male Testosterone Levels
High-Performance Liquid Chromatography And Tandem Mass Spectrometry

	Value	SI Units
Free Testosterone		
1-6 years	0.1-0.6 pg/mL	
7-9 years	0.1-0.8 pg/mL	
10-11 years	0.1-5.2 pg/mL	
12-13 years	0.4-79.6 pg/mL	
14-15 years	2.7-112.3 pg/mL	
16-17 years	31.5-141.6 pg/mL	
Bioavailable Testosterone		
1-6 years	0.2-1.3 ng/dL	0.007 -0.045 nmol/L
7-9 years	0.2-2.3 ng/dL	0.007-0.079 nmol/L
10-11 years	0.2-14.8 ng/dL	0.007-0.513 nmol/L
12-13 years	0.3-232.8 ng/dL	0.010-8.082 nmol/L
14-15 years	7.9-274.5 ng/dL	0.274-9.525 nmol/L
16-17 years	24.1-416.5 ng/dL	0.836-14.452 nmol/L
Total Testosterone		
Premature (26-28 weeks)	59-125 ng/dL	2.047-4.337 nmol/L
Premature (31-35 weeks)	37-198 ng/dL	1.284-6.871 nmol/L
Newborn	75-400 ng/dL	2.602-13.877 nmol/L
1 week	20-50 ng/dL	0.694-1.735 nmol/L
Second month	60-400 ng/dL	2.082-13.877 nmol/L
Seventh month until puberty	3-10 ng/dL	0.104-0.347 nmol/L
7-9 years	0-8 ng/dL	0-0.277 nmol/L
10-11 years	1-48 ng/dL	0.035-1.666 nmol/L
12-13 years	5-619 ng/dL	0.173-21.480 nmol/L
Sex Hormone Binding Globulin		
Male Adults		
≥18 years		11-80 nmol/L
Male Children		
1-30 days		13-85 nmol/L
1 month-1 year		70-250 nmol/L
1-3 years		50-180 nmol/L
4-6 years		45-175 nmol/L
7-9 years		28-190 nmol/L
10-12 years		23-160 nmol/L
13-15 years		13-140 nmol/L
16-17 years		10-60 nmol/L

Female Testosterone Levels
High-Performance Liquid Chromatography And Tandem Mass Spectrometry

	Value	SI Units
Free Testosterone		
Female Adults		
Premenopausal	0.8-9.2 pg/mL	
Postmenopausal	0.6-6.7 pg/mL	
Female Children		
1-6 years	0.1-0.6 pg/mL	
7-9 years	0.1-1.6 pg/mL	
10-11 years	0.1-2.9 pg/mL	

	Value	SI Units
12-13 years	0.6-5.6 pg/mL	
14-15 years	1.0-6.2 pg/mL	
16-17 years	1.0-8.3 pg/mL	

Bioavailable Testosterone

Female Adults

	Value	SI Units
Premenopausal	1.9-22.8 ng/dL	0.066-0.791 nmol/L
Postmenopausal	1.6-19.1 ng/dL	0.055-0.662 nmol/L

Female Children

	Value	SI Units
1-6 years	0.2-1.3 ng/dL	0.007-0.045 nmol/L
7-9 years	0.2-4.2 ng/dL	0.007-0.146 nmol/L
10-11 years	0.4-19.3 ng/dL	0.014-0.670 nmol/L
12-13 years	1.1-15.6 ng/dL	0.038-0.541 nmol/L
14-15 years	2.5-18.8 ng/dL	0.087-0.652 nmol/L
16-17 years	2.7-23.8 ng/dL	0.094-0.826 nmol/L

Total Testosterone

Female Adults

	Value	SI Units
Premenopausal	10-54 ng/dL	0.347-1.873 nmol/L
Postmenopausal	7-40 ng/dL	0.243-1.388 nmol/L

Female Children

	Value	SI Units
Premature (26-28 weeks)	5-16 ng/dL	0.173-0.555 nmol/L
Premature (31-35 weeks)	5-22 ng/dL	0.173-0.763 nmol/L
Newborn	20-64 ng/dL	0.694-2.220 nmol/L
1 month until puberty	<10 ng/dL	<0.347 nmol/L
7-9 years	1-12 ng/dL	0.035-0.416 nmol/L
10-11 years	2-35 ng/dL	0.069-1.214 nmol/L
12-13 years	5-53 ng/dL	0.173-1.839 nmol/L
14-15 years	8-41 ng/dL	0.278-1.423 nmol/L
16-17 years	8-53 ng/dL	0.278-1.839 nmol/L

Sex Hormone Binding Globulin

Female Adults

	Value	SI Units
≥18 years		30-135 nmol/L

Female Children

	Value	SI Units
1-30 days		14-60 nmol/L
1 month-1 year		60-215 nmol/L
1-3 years		60-190 nmol/L
4-6 years		55-170 nmol/L
7-9 years		35-170 nmol/L
10-12 years		17-155 nmol/L
13-15 years		11-120 nmol/L
16-17 years		19-145 nmol/L

Increased Total Testosterone. Adrenal hyperplasia, adrenal tumor, arrhenoblastoma, central nervous system lesions, eating disorders (male), hirsutism (idiopathic), hyperthyroidism, ovarian tumor (virilizing), pollutants (polychlorobiphenyls, hexachlorobenzene), testicular feminization, testicular tumor, virilizing luteoma, and virilization. In women, idiopathic hirsutism, cystic ache, polycystic ovary syndrome, adrogenic alopecia, abnormal menstruation, anovulation, adrenogenital syndrome with virilization, ovarian tumor, smokers, and Stein-Leventhal syndrome with virilization. Drugs include anticonvulsants, atrial natriuretic hormone (long-acting), barbiturates, cimetidine, clomiphene, estrogens, gonadotropin (males), kaliuretic hormone, oral contraceptives, and vessel dilator hormone.

Increased Free Testosterone. Acne (severe, in females), androgen resistance, hirsutism, pollutants (polychlorobiphenyls, hexachlorobenzene), polycystic ovary syndrome, tumor (virilizing). See also Increased total testosterone.

Decreased Total Testosterone. Alcohol consumption >24 g/week, anemia, body mass index increased, cirrhosis, cryptorchidism, COPD (moderate to severe), Down syndrome, end-stage renal disease, epilepsy, erectile dysfunction, gynecomastia, hemochromatosis, human immunodeficiency virus, hypogonadism (male), hypopituitarism, hysterectomy, impotence, infertility, inflammatory arthritis, insulin resistance in non-diabetic older men, Klinefelter's syndrome, male climacteric, obesity, orchiectomy, osteoporosis, sellar mass or status post sellar radiation, and Type 2 diabetes mellitus. Drugs include androgens, cyproterone, dexamethasone, diethylstilbestrol, digitalis, digoxin (males), estrogens (males), ethyl alcohol (ethanol), glucose, glucosteroids, gonadotropin-releasing hormone analogs, halothane, ketoconazole, metoprolol, metyrapone, opioids, phenothiazines, spironolactone, and tetracycline.

Decreased Free Testosterone. Body mass index increased, epilepsy, hypogonadism, P-450$_{c17}$ enzyme deficiency. See also decreased total Testosterone.

Description. Testosterone is the dominant androgen found in the adrenal glands, brain, ovary, pituitary, skin, kidney, and testes. It circulates both freely and bound to plasma proteins (sex hormone–binding globulin [SHBG]). Testosterone promotes the growth and development of the male sexual organs and increases body mass and hair replacement. This test measures total testosterone levels in clients with normal SHBG levels. Free testosterone is that portion of circulating testosterone that is not bound to the sex hormone–binding globulin (SHBG) plasma protein. Free testosterone is a better indicator of clinical status than total testosterone level. The free testosterone test is used to differentiate true abnormal testosterone levels from those caused by abnormally low or high amounts of circulating SHBG. Some conditions that increase SHBG are hyperthyroidism and low estrogen-production states (pregnancy; taking oral contraceptives or anticonvulsant drugs). Some conditions that decrease SHBG include excess androgen states, hypothyroidism, and obesity. Free testosterone may be measured directly, or calculated after total testosterone and SHBG levels are known.

Professional Considerations
Consent form NOT required.

Preparation
1. Tube: Green topped (plasma) or red topped, red/gray topped, or gold topped (serum).
2. Specimens MAY be drawn during hemodialysis.

Procedure
1. Because of the diurnal pattern of testosterone secretion, several morning specimens or pooled specimens should be tested.
2. Draw a 1.5-mL blood sample.

Postprocedure Care
1. None.

Client and Family Teaching
1. Discuss the test results and the implications thereof with the physician.
2. Results may not be available for several days.

Factors That Affect Results
1. In adult men, serum testosterone levels peak in the early morning and after exercise and decrease after glucose loading and immobilization. Because of this diurnal rhythm of circulating testosterone levels, the blood is generally drawn in the morning.
2. Results are invalidated if the client has undergone a radioactive scan within the previous 7 days.
3. During pregnancy, free testosterone values are lower because estradiol occupies space on the sex hormone–binding globulin sites.
4. The immunoassay method of measurement is accurate for males but not for females and children. High-performance liquid chromatography and tandem mass spectrometry are recommended for measuring testosterone levels in females and in children.

Other Data
1. Breast cancer risk in women is not associated with any androgens (Danforth et al, 2010).

TFI

See Pulse Volume Recorder Testing of Peripheral Vasculature—Diagnostic.

TG

See Thyroid Function Tests—Blood.

Thallium—Serum or 24-Hour Urine

Norm.

		SI Units
Serum	<10 ng/mL	<49 nmol/L
Urine		
Adult	<2 µg/L or <10 µg/24 hours	<9.8 µmol/L
Panic level	>2 µg/L	>9.8 µmol/L

Panic Level Symptoms and Treatment

Symptoms. Abdominal pain, alopecia, ataxia, constipation, coma, delirium, diaphoresis, hypertension, intractable insomnia, optic neuritis, pulmonary edema, rash, tachycardia, and vomiting.

Treatment. NOTE: Treatment choice(s) depend(s) on client's history and condition and episode history.

1. Prussian blue (ferric ferrocyanide) binds to thallium and prevents absorption in the gastrointestinal tract. The dose is 125 mg/kg in 50 mL of 15% mannitol twice daily by nasogastric tube. Continue this until excretion of thallium is <0.5 mg/day.
2. Neither chelating agents nor hemodialysis seems beneficial.
3. Hemoperfusion may be helpful.

Increased. Metal poisoning.

Description. Thallium is an extremely toxic heavy metal used in manufacturing and found in chlorinated chemicals, cosmetics, dyes, fireworks, jewelry, medications, pesticides, photoelectric cells, rat poison, and semiconductors. Thallium accumulates in the bone, kidney, liver, and muscle tissue. Thallium poisoning may cause blindness, liver damage, paralysis, paresthesia, peripheral neuropathy, and renal damage. This test helps identify clients who have acquired abnormal body amounts of thallium through ingestion or inhalation or through skin absorption.

Professional Considerations
Consent form NOT required.

Preparation
1. *Serum:*
   a. Tube: Metal-free green topped.
   b. Specimens MAY be drawn during hemodialysis.
2. *Urine:*
   a. Obtain a 3-L, metal-free urine collection container.
   b. Provide a plastic, metal-free urinal or bedpan for specimen collection.

Procedure
1. *Serum:* Draw a 5-mL blood sample in a metal-free, green topped tube.
2. *Urine:*
   a. Collect all the urine voided in a 24-hour period in a plastic, metal-free bedpan or urinal.
   b. The urine is mixed with 0.4% sodium bismuth in 20% nitric acid and 10% sodium iodine. If thallium is present, a red precipitate forms.

Postprocedure Care

1. Observe the client for symptoms of thallium poisoning.

Client and Family Teaching

1. For urine collection, urinate before defecating and avoid contaminating the specimen with stool or toilet tissue. If any urine is accidentally discarded, discard the entire specimen and restart the collection the next day.
2. Blood and urine thallium levels tend to decrease rapidly after exposure.

Factors That Affect Results

1. Urine or blood allowed to come into contact with metal will falsely elevate results.

Other Data

1. Poisoning occurs 1-10 days after exposure. A lethal dose is 1 g or 8-12 mg/kg.
2. The urine of a client with thallium poisoning will also show proteinuria, increased red cells, casts, eosinophils, lymphocytes, or polymorphonuclear leukocytes.

Thallium-Dipyridamole Stress Test and Scan

See **Heart Scan**—Diagnostic.

Thallium Exercise Scintigraphy

See **Heart Scan**—Diagnostic.

Thallium Imaging

See **Heart Scan**—Diagnostic.

Theophylline (Aminophylline)—Blood

Norm. NOTE: Measurement should be a peak specimen, after steady state has been reached.

	Peak	SI Units
Therapeutic	10-20 µg/mL	55-111 µmol/L
Toxic level	>20 µg/mL	>109 µmol/L
Panic level	>30 µg/mL	>165 µmol/L

Panic Level Symptoms and Treatment

75% of persons with levels >25 µg/mL have toxic symptoms.

Signs and Symptoms. Dysrhythmias, gastrointestinal bleeding, headache, hyperglycemia, hypokalemia, hypotension, nausea, peripheral vasodilation, restlessness, serum myoglobin increased, seizures, syncope, tachycardia, ventricular dysrhythmias and vomiting.

Treatment

NOTE: Treatment choice(s) depend(s) on client's history and condition and episode history.

1. Maintain a patent airway.
2. Withhold theophylline.
3. Perform gastric lavage if it can be done within 6 hours of ingestion.
4. Give activated charcoal only if client has ingested a life-threatening amount of theophylline.
5. Provide hydration.
6. Give diazepam for convulsions.
7. Provide continuous ECG monitoring for dysrhythmias.
8. Monitor theophylline levels every 2 hours.
9. Monitor and treat electrolyte imbalance.
10. Monitor for hypoglycemia.
11. Administer charcoal hemoperfusion for severe overdose or implement molecular adsorbent recirculating system (MARS) for 8 hours. MARS consists of a closed circuit containing an albumin-rich solution that permits

diffusion of protein-bound and water-soluble substances from the patient's circulation.

12. 40% of theophylline may be removed by hemodialysis. A higher clearance rate can be achieved with hemoperfusion but is associated with more complications. Peritoneal dialysis will NOT remove theophylline.

13. There might be a positive effect of oral administration of N-acetylcysteine in severe theophylline intoxication (Kisters et al, 2007).

14. Monitor for acute pancreatitis after severe overdoses.

Increased. Congestive heart failure, chronic obstructive pulmonary disease, liver dysfunction, and overdose. Drugs that may cause increased levels include allopurinol, cimetidine, ciprofloxacin, clindamycin, erythromycin, lincomycin, oral contraceptives, and probenecid.

Decreased. Smoking. Drugs that may cause decreased levels include barbiturates, carbamazepine, furosemide, isoniazid, nortriptyline, phenytoin, and rifampin. Herbal or natural remedies include *Andrographis paniculata* extract (rat study) and St. John's wort (*Hypericum perforatum*).

Description. Theophylline is a methylxanthine drug that decreases breakdown of intracellular cyclic adenosine monophosphate (cAMP), which in turn stimulates dilation of the smooth muscles of the bronchial airways and relaxation of the pulmonary blood vessels. However, this therapeutic effect does not occur until levels are at or near the top of the therapeutic range. At lower levels, theophylline exhibits antiinflammatory properties, enabling the sparing of steroid medication. It is for the latter reason that there has been a return to use of intravenous theophylline for acute exacerbation of obstructive pulmonary disease. Theophylline is 60% plasma protein bound, with a half-life of 6-10 hours in adults and 2-5 hours in children (half-life is reduced 40% in cigarette smokers); 90% of theophylline is metabolized in the liver. Steady-state levels occur in 15-20 hours in adults and in 5-40 hours in children.

Professional Considerations
Consent form NOT required.

Preparation
1. Tube: Red topped, red/gray topped, or gold topped.
2. The client should not ingest substances that contain xanthene for 12 hours before the test. The substances to avoid include chocolate, cocoa, coffee, cola, and tea.
3. Do NOT draw specimens during hemodialysis.

Procedure
1. Draw a 3-mL PEAK blood sample. Obtain serial measurements at the same time each day.

Postprocedure Care
1. Refrigerate the specimen. Do not freeze it.

Client and Family Teaching
1. Explain the significance of therapeutic drug levels and the periodic monitoring thereof.
2. If activated charcoal was given for elevated levels, the client should drink 4-6 glasses of water each day for 2 days to prevent constipation. The activated charcoal will cause stools to be black for a few days.
3. For intentional overdose, refer client and family for crisis intervention.
4. Referrals to appropriate rehabilitation centers and therapeutic community programs should be offered to all addicted clients who may be interested.

Factors That Affect Results
1. Peak levels with oral dosing occur 1-3 hours after uncoated or liquid preparations and 4-7 hours after enteric-coated or extended-release preparations.
2. Ingestion of xanthines within 12 hours before the test may elevate levels.

Other Data
1. A minor metabolite of theophylline is caffeine.

Thiamine

See **Vitamin B₁**—Blood or Urine.

Thiocyanate—Blood or Urine

Norm.

		SI Units
Serum		
Nonsmokers	1-4 µg/mL	0.02-0.07 mmol/L
Smokers	3-12 µg/mL	0.05-0.21 mmol/L
Pediatric	≤0.1 µg/mL	≤0.02 mmol/L
Nitroprusside therapy	6-29 µg/mL	0.10-0.51 mmol/L
Panic level	>35 µg/mL	>0.63 mmol/L
Urine		
Nonsmokers	1-4 mg/24 hours	
Smokers	7-17 mg/24 hours	
Panic levels	>0.2 mg/dL	>0.03 mmol/L

Poisoning Symptoms and Treatment

Symptoms. Agitation, confusion, focal brain damage, hyperreflexia, hypotension, metabolic acidosis, myocardial damage, psychotic behavior, thrombophlebitis, and thyroid enlargement.

Treatment

NOTE: Treatment choice(s) depend(s) on client's history and condition and episode history.

1. Perform gastric lavage.
2. Administer intravenous fluids at 3 L/day (if normal renal function is present) to maintain adequate output.
3. Monitor amyl nitrate inhalation.
4. Give sodium nitrite and sodium thiosulfate infusions.
5. Both hemodialysis and peritoneal dialysis WILL remove thiocyanate.

Increased. Iodine deficiency, poisoning from nitroprusside; smoking (including pregnant mothers).

Description. Thiocyanate is a major metabolite of the drug nitroprusside and is the important gauge of nitroprusside-induced toxicity during prolonged administration or with unusually high rates of infusion (see also Cyanide—Blood, which has a more important role in early toxicity of nitroprusside). Both sodium thiocyanate and potassium thiocyanate depress the metabolic activities of all cells but mostly those of the brain and heart. Half-life is 7 days. Formerly this drug was used to treat hypertension by producing peripheral vasodilation. More recently this measure has been studied for detection of smoking deceivers in smoking-cessation programs.

Professional Considerations

Consent form NOT required.

Preparation

1. Tube: Red topped, red/gray topped, or gold topped.
2. Obtain a sterile plastic container for urine sample.
3. Do NOT draw specimens during hemodialysis.

Procedure

1. Blood: Draw a 2-mL blood sample.
2. Urine: Obtain a 20-mL fresh urine sample in a sterile plastic cup.

Postprocedure Care

1. Tighten the top of the plastic urine container.

Client and Family Teaching

1. The treatment for poisoning will take at least 1 week.
2. Death is possible from thiocyanate poisoning.

Factors That Affect Results

1. Eating cabbage or smoking cigarettes can falsely increase blood and urine results.
2. Concurrent use of salicylates makes results unreliable.

Other Data

1. It takes 1 week to reduce thiocyanate levels by 50% if normal kidney function is present.
2. Some clients show a temporary improvement for several days, only to relapse and die as long as 2 weeks later.

Thiopurine S-Methyltransferase (TPMT, Tpmp RBC) Genotyping, Phenotyping and Activity—Blood

Norm.

Genotyping Results

Normal	Homozygous normal
Deficient	Heterozygous with 1 variant nonfunctional alleles
Absent	Homozygous with 2 variant nonfunctional alleles

Phenotyping Results

	Result	Implication
High	Greater than 65 U/mL	Leads to higher than expected drug inactivation. May need higher than usual/standard dosage of thiopurine.
Normal	25-65 U/mL	No thiopurine dose adjustment needed.
Abnormal	Less than 25 U/mL	Thiopurine dosage reduction; or select a different drug class for treatment. Close monitoring is needed if thiopurines are used.

TPMT Activity

Normal	Greater than 12 nmol/hr/mL RBC
Heterozygote or low metabolizer	4-12 nmol/hr/mL RBC
Homozygote deficient range	Less than 4 nmol/hr/mL RBC

Usage. Used prior to initiating 6-mercaptopurine or azathioprine therapy in clients with leukemia, inflammatory bowel disease, rheumatic disease, or solid organ transplant to help guide selection of appropriate drug therapy.

Description. Thiopurine S-methyltransferase (TPMT) is an enzyme contained in red blood cells that helps metabolize immunosuppressive thiopurine drugs. 89% of the population displays normal levels of TPMT, while 0.3% have little or no TPMT, and the remaining 11% have intermediate activity. Clients who have low or no TPMT are at high risk for intolerance of thiopurine therapy, and may develop life-threatening bone marrow toxicity (Nguyen, Mendes, Ma, 2011).

TPMT levels are controlled by the TPMT gene. Varying alleles of this gene lead to reductions in the amount of TPMT present in the body. The TPMT Genotyping and Phenotyping tests identify different genetic aspects: The genotyping test identifies the TPMT*1, *2, *3A, *3B, and/or *3C alleles causing sub-normal TPMT enzyme levels,

but does not quantify TPMT levels. The phenotyping test reveals the red blood cells' TPMT enzyme activity and provides quantitative results.

Professional Considerations

Informed consent is recommended for genetic testing.

Preparation

1. Tube: Lavender topped, pink topped, or green topped.

Procedure

1. Genotyping test: Collect a 6-mL blood sample for each test that is ordered.
2. Phenotyping test: Collect two 3-mL blood samples.

Postprocedure Care

1. Refrigerate sample until testing. Ship with cold pack to testing laboratory.

Client and Family Teaching

1. Do not take drugs that affect the results during the 48 hours prior to testing. (See Factors That Affect Results.)

2. If abnormal results are found, then there may be a dose reduction or a different type of drug may be therapy selected.
3. Refer to Appendix B, "Informed Consent for Genetic Testing".

Factors That Affect Results

1. Testing should be done before initiating thiopurine therapy, because the therapy itself will cause falsely low phenotyping results.
2. Other drugs that will cause falsely low phenotyping results include benzoic acid inhibitors, furosemide, mefenamic acid, naproxen, ibuprofen and ketoprofen NSAIDS, mesalamine, olsalazine, sulfasalazine aminosalicylates, and thiazide diuretics.
3. Red blood cell aging can falsely decrease the result. Testing should be performed within 2 weeks of sample collection.
4. Recent blood transfusion can falsely elevate the result of the phenotype test.

The genotype test should be considered for use in this situation.
5. Freezing of the specimen invalidates results.
6. The TPMP genotype test does not detect rare alleles.

Other Data

1. The phenotyping method is preferred (by the American College of Gastroenterology treatment guidelines) over genotyping because of the quantification provided with the results.
2. The Genetic Information Nondiscrimination Act of 2008 prohibits health plans from using genetic family history or genetic test results from influencing eligibility or premiums for health insurance. It also prohibits employers from using this information to influence decisions about hiring, terminating employment, or employment pay, promotions, or privileges.

Thioridazine

See **Phenothiazines**.

Thoracentesis—Diagnostic

Norm.

Amount	<20 mL	Cells	Few lymphocytes, few red blood cells
Color	Clear		
Specific gravity	<1.016	Lactate dehydrogenase	Equal to serum level
pH	Equal to serum level		
Protein	<3 g/dL	Glucose	Equal to serum level
Fibrinogen	None	Amylase	Equal to serum level

Usage.

Therapeutic: Relieves dyspnea because of pleural effusion or pneumothorax.
Diagnostic: Evaluates underlying cause of pleural effusion. Abnormal accumulation of fluid in the pleural space may be classified as either transudate or exudate.

	Transudate	Exudate
Color	Clear	Cloudy, turbid
Specific gravity	<1.016	>1.016
pH	Equal to serum level	<7.3
Protein	<3 g/dL	>3 g/dL
Fibrinogen	None or may be present	Present
Cells	Few lymphocytes	Many; may be a few red blood cells or purulent

	Transudate	Exudate
Lactate	Equal to serum level	May be >lactate dehydrogenase, serum
Glucose	Equal to serum level	May be <serum
Amylase	Equal to serum level	May be >serum

Description. Thoracentesis is the removal of fluid or air from the pleural space by transthoracic aspiration. It is performed to determine the nature or cause of an effusion, to relieve dyspnea caused by an effusion, or to obtain fluid for testing.

Professional Considerations
Consent form IS required.

Preparation
1. The procedure may be preceded by ultrasonography or chest radiography.
2. Identify the upper border of the effusion by the loss of fremitus and the presence of flat percussion. The thoracentesis will be performed in the interspace below this level and 5-10 cm lateral to the spine.
3. Obtain sterile gloves, injectable lidocaine, a thoracentesis tray, collection bottles with heparin, sterile 4- × 4-inch gauze pads, tape, a container of ice, and povidone-iodine solution.
4. Obtain baseline vital signs.
5. List any recent antibiotic therapy on the laboratory requisition.
6. Just before beginning the procedure, take a "time out" to verify the correct client, procedure, and site.

Procedure
1. The client is positioned sitting upright, often in the orthopneic position, with arms and head supported by a table at the bedside. Clients who cannot sit up are placed in the lateral decubitus position, lying on the side of the effusion, near the edge of the bed. This procedure can be performed on those who are ventilator dependent. Ultrasound is often used to confirm insertion site.
2. The skin is cleansed with povidone-iodine solution.
3. The underlying tissue at the previously identified effusion site is anesthetized.
4. A 20-gauge or larger needle is placed immediately above the superior aspect of the lower rib and advanced until the parietal membrane is penetrated and no more than 1 L of fluid is aspirated.

5. At least 50 mL of fluid is needed for diagnostic studies. Place syringe on ice for transport to the laboratory.

Postprocedure Care
1. Apply a pressure dressing and assess the puncture site for bleeding and crepitus every 5 minutes × 6.
2. Assess vital signs every 30 minutes × 4.
3. A follow-up chest radiograph should be taken within several hours of the procedure, or immediately if respiratory distress is exhibited.

Client and Family Teaching
1. Describe the procedure and the usual sensations the client may expect related to the test.
2. Do not cough, breathe deeply, or move during the procedure.

Factors That Affect Results
1. Complications that affect results include air embolism, hemothorax, pneumothorax, pulmonary edema, and subcutaneous seroma.
2. Transudate in the pleural space may be caused by ascites, cirrhosis (hepatic), congestive heart failure, hypertension (pulmonary, systemic), nephritis, and nephrosis.
3. Exudate in the pleural space may be caused by blocked lymphatic drainage, empyema (usually *Enterobacter* or gram-positive cocci), esophageal rupture, infarction (pulmonary), infection, neoplasm, pancreatitis, rheumatoid arthritis, systemic lupus erythematosus, thoracic duct disruption, accidental injury, and tuberculosis.
4. Allowing fluid to stand for a prolonged period before processing may cause deterioration and artifacts.

Other Data
1. If the thoracentesis is performed below the tenth intercostal space, care should be taken to avoid laceration of the spleen or liver or penetration of the diaphragm (ipsilateral shoulder pain is a sign of diaphragmatic penetration).

2. Malignant cells cannot be recovered from all fluids for clients with malignancies.
3. Increased amylase levels in the effusion are associated with pancreatitis, lung cancer, and esophageal perforation.
4. The most common pathogens found in pleural effusions are *Mycobacterium tuberculosis, Staphylococcus aureus, Streptococcus pneumoniae,* and *Haemophilus influenzae.*
5. Oral Uracil-Tegafur (UFT) at 400 mg/day induces pleural effusion following lung cancer surgery.

Throat Culture for *Candida albicans*—Culture

Norm. Negative, no growth.

Usage. Immunosuppressive diseases, stomatitis, and thrush.

Description. *Candida albicans* is an opportunistic fungus that occurs in the aged, debilitated, newborns, and clients with acquired immune deficiency syndrome (AIDS) or cancer who are immunosuppressed. Steroid use is also a causative factor. This fungus occurs mostly on the buccal mucosa, tongue, palate, and mucous membranes. It appears as patches or plaques that are white to gray in color.

Professional Considerations
Consent form NOT required.

Preparation
1. Obtain a sterile cotton swab, a sterile container, and a tongue blade.

Procedure
1. Swab suspicious lesions and place the swab in a sterile container.

Postprocedure Care
1. List the specific site of the specimen on the laboratory requisition.
2. Deliver the swab to the laboratory immediately or refrigerate the sample immediately.

Client and Family Teaching
1. The turnaround time for results is normally 3-7 days.

Factors That Affect Results
1. Dry swab or insufficient specimen volume.

Other Data
1. A Gram stain or potassium hydroxide (KOH) preparation may be requested to obtain a more rapid diagnosis.
2. Other *Candida* species (*C. tropicalis, C. glabrata, C. krusei*) are being reported in individuals after lengthy imidazole or triazole antifungal therapy. These species are less susceptible to treatment.

Throat Culture for *Corynebacterium diphtheriae*—Culture

Norm. Negative.

Positive. Diphtheria.

Description. *Corynebacterium* is an anaerobic, gram-positive, non–acid-fast, motile bacteria that does not produce endospores. *C. diphtheriae* liberates a cytotoxin that causes diphtheria, an acute infection of the oropharynx, larynx, nose, and other mucous membranes characterized by a patchy gray pseudomembrane over a lesion surrounded by reddened, inflamed tissue. The mode of transmission is usually direct contact with the discharges from lesions of an infected client. Culture of the throat is taken for incubation and study of the appearance and growth patterns of bacteria as well as the microscopic appearance and staining properties to identify the presence or absence of *Corynebacterium.*

Professional Considerations
Consent form NOT required.

Preparation
1. See Client and Family Teaching.
2. Obtain a tongue blade, sterile swab, and Culturette.
3. Call the laboratory so that it can have on hand the special culture medium for *C. diphtheriae.*

Procedure

1. With the client's head tilted back and mouth opened, depress the tongue with the tongue blade. Have the client say "ah" to elevate the uvula and expose the infective lesions.
2. Shine a light into the oropharynx to locate the characteristic gray lesions. Remove the patchy gray pseudomembrane by rubbing it firmly with a sterile swab.
3. Press a sterile Culturette swab firmly against the lesion for a few seconds. For asymptomatic clients, culture the tonsillar fossae, the posterior pharynx, and the retrouvular areas.
4. Remove the swab, taking care to avoid touching any area except the infected site.

Postprocedure Care

1. Return the swab to the Culturette tube and crush the ampule of the medium.
2. Transport the specimen to the laboratory immediately. The specimen should be refrigerated if it is not tested immediately.

Client and Family Teaching

1. Antiseptic gargles or mouthwashes before the procedure may prevent bacterial growth. Avoid using these products for 8 hours before the test.
2. Erythromycin is used to treat this disease.

3. If started on empiric therapy, you should continue taking the prescribed drug(s) unless and until the test results are found to be negative.
4. Results are normally available within 4 days.

Factors That Affect Results

1. Obtain cultures before starting the client on antibiotics.

Other Data

1. Diphtheria is communicable for up to 4 weeks from the appearance of the bacilli in the lesions.
2. A positive throat culture may also indicate a carrier state.
3. Cultures of the nose and the pseudomembrane are also helpful in making a positive diagnosis.
4. Toxic strains of this disease have recently been found in Russia, and nontoxigenic strains have been isolated with increasing frequency in the United Kingdom, France, and Australia.
5. Treatment includes beta-lactam and aminoglycoside antibiotics though 20% of strains are rifampin resistant.
6. Low protection rate against diphtheria correlates with female gender and latest vaccination within 3 years of life.

Throat Culture for Group A Beta-Hemolytic Streptococci—Culture

Norm. Negative, no growth.

Usage. Glomerulonephritis, pharyngitis, scarlet fever, strep throat, and tonsillitis.

Description. Group A beta-hemolytic streptococci are bacteria usually introduced into the respiratory tract whose incubation period is 3-5 days. The onset of streptococcal sore throat is sudden, with frank chills, headache, malaise, fever, throat soreness, and exudative gray-white patches on the tonsils or pharynx.

Professional Considerations

Consent form NOT required.

Preparation

1. Obtain a sterile cotton swab or Culturette, and a tongue blade.
2. Obtain the specimen before initiating antibiotic therapy.

Procedure

1. Depress the tongue and take a swab of the throat and pharynx (both tonsils). Avoid swabbing the tongue, saliva, buccal mucosa, or the lips.
2. Place the swab in a sterile container, or return the swab to the Culturette tube and crush the distal end to release the ampule of medium.

Postprocedure Care

1. Send the specimen to the laboratory within 2 hours or refrigerate the specimen.

Client and Family Teaching

1. It is important to obtain the specimen before beginning antibiotics. Strep throat remains contagious until 24 hours after antibiotic therapy is started.

2. If there is no improvement within 2 days, return to the health professional for further examination.
3. Place a cool mist humidifier in the bedroom to relieve any tight, dry feeling in the throat. A sore throat may be relieved with salt-water gargle (1 cup of warm water + 1 teaspoon of salt).
4. For a schoolchild with positive culture, wait 24 hours after antibiotics have been started before letting the child return to school.
5. Call the physician if the client develops a rash or coughs up green, yellow, or bloody sputum.

Factors That Affect Results

1. Technical proficiency is required to avoid false-positive and false-negative results.
2. Previous antibiotic therapy may cause false-negative results. Up to 10% of clients who deny the use of antibiotics have been shown to have taken unprescribed antibiotics before contact with the health professional.
3. The use of antibacterial gargles may cause false-negative results.

Other Data

1. For a faster diagnosis, the swab can be incubated for 2 hours and then examined for fluorescent organisms; a rapid strep test for direct antigen detection can obtain results in 7-20 minutes (the highest sensitivity with high colony counts); however, results should be confirmed with a throat culture.
2. Left untreated, symptoms usually subside within 3-5 days. Treatment will not shorten this time frame, but will reduce the risk of future rheumatic fever. Penicillin is the treatment of choice, but erythromycin and clindamycin are also effective.

Throat Culture for *Neisseria gonorrhoeae*—Culture

Norm. Negative; no *Neisseria gonorrhoeae* isolated.

Usage. Gonococcal infection of pharynx, gonorrhea, and pharyngitis.

Description. *N. gonorrhoeae* is a pyogenic, gram-negative, oxidase-positive cocci that is an obligate parasite of humans. It is the causative organism of the sexually transmitted infection gonorrhea. *N. gonorrhoeae* inhabits the mucous membranes of the genital tract and may also be found in the oral mucosa of clients who engage in oral sex (gonococcal pharyngitis). Left untreated, gonorrhea leads to skin lesions, arthritis, meningitis, and reproductive problems.

Professional Considerations

Consent form NOT required.

Preparation

1. Obtain a Thayer-Martin culture medium, sterile cotton swabs, and a tongue blade.

Procedure

1. Depress the tongue and swab from the tonsillar regions and the posterior pharynx.
2. Place the specimen immediately onto the Thayer-Martin medium and incubate it in a carbon dioxide environment.

Postprocedure Care

1. Transport the specimen to the laboratory within 2 hours.

Client and Family Teaching

1. Gonorrhea infection is treatable with antibiotics.
2. Evaluate the client's knowledge of safe sex practices and review appropriate measures.
3. If the results are positive, provide the client with the appropriate information on sexually transmitted diseases.
   a. Notify all sexual partners from the previous 90 days to be tested for gonorrhea infection.
   b. Do not have sexual relations until the physician confirms that the infection is gone.

Factors That Affect Results

1. Refrigerating the specimen invalidates the culture.

Other Data

1. Preliminary reports are available within 24 hours and the final report within 48 hours.
2. For a faster diagnosis, the swab can be incubated for 2 hours and then examined for fluorescent organisms.

3. Penicillin is the treatment of choice (plus probenecid), but erythromycin and clindamycin are also effective.
4. For positive results, the client should also be serologically tested for syphilis. Consider also testing for AIDS.

5. Positive results must usually be reported to the local health department.

Throat Culture, Routine

See **Culture**—Routine.

Throat Culture, Swab

See **Culture**—Routine.

Thrombin Time—Serum

Norm. Within 2 seconds of 9-second to 13-second control value; or within 5 seconds of 15-second to 20-second control value; or <1.5 times control value.

Increased. Acute leukemia, afibrinogenemia, amyloidosis, cirrhosis, disseminated intravascular coagulation (DIC), dysfibrinogenemia, epistaxis, factor deficiency, fibrinopenia, lymphoma, obstetric complications, polycythemia vera, shock, and stress. Drugs include asparaginase, fibrin degradation products, heparin, streptokinase, tissue plasminogen activator (TPA), uremia, and urokinase.

Decreased. Thrombocytosis.

Description. Thrombin is an enzyme that functions in the release of fibrin from fibrinogen in the final stage of the clotting cascade. This test measures the clotting time of a sample of plasma to which thrombin has been added. Thrombin time is longer than normal when abnormalities in the conversion of fibrinogen into fibrin are present.

Professional Considerations
Consent form NOT required.

Preparation
1. Tube: 2.7-mL blue topped or 4.5-mL blue topped tube and a control tube, and a waste tube or syringe.

Procedure
1. Withdraw 2 mL of blood into a syringe or vacuum tube. Remove the syringe or tube,

leaving the needle in place. (From a heparinized line, discard an amount equal to the volume of the tubing prime.) Attach a second syringe, and draw a blood sample volume of 2.4 mL for a 2.7-mL tube and 4.0 mL for a 4.5-mL tube.
2. Gently tilt the tube five or six times to mix the sample.

Postprocedure Care
1. Send the sample to the laboratory within 2 hours.
2. Refrigerate the sample. The plasma should be frozen if it is not tested promptly.

Client and Family Teaching
1. Results can be available within an hour.

Factors That Affect Results
1. Hemolyzed specimens invalidate the results.
2. Failure to discard the first 1-2 mL of blood may result in specimen contamination with tissue thromboplastin.
3. Heparin therapy within 2 days before the test increases the results. Collecting a sample from a heparinized line without discarding the first blood withdrawn can falsely prolong results.
4. A recent blood or plasma transfusion will invalidate the results.

Other Data
1. The test is used as a rapid screening device to detect profound fibrinogen deficiency.

2. This test is not reliable to monitor heparin therapy in clients with DIC.

3. This test will NOT differentiate primary fibrinolysis from DIC.

Thromboplastin Time, Activated Partial

See Activated Partial Thromboplastin Time and Partial Thromboplastin Time—Plasma.

Thymidylate Synthase (TS)—Specimen

Norm. Negative. NOTE: No definite norms have been established for this test.

Gastric cancer patients that were cisplatin responders had TS levels <40 ng/mg protein.

Immunoreactivity Grades

Grade 1	Negative to weakly positive
Grade 2	Moderately positive
Grade 3	Positive
Grade 4	Strongly positive

Usage. Evaluation of colorectal, gastric, cervical, and other epithelial cancers.

Description. Thymidylate synthase is an enzyme that acts as a catalyst in the thiamine DNA conversion. Cells that are producing DNA need larger amounts of thymidylate synthase to fuel the DNA production. In the cell cycle more thymidylate synthase (20% more) is produced during S and G2 phase because this is the phase when the most rapid cell proliferation takes place. In some cancers, such as those of the gastrointestinal tract (such as gastric and rectal), thymidylate synthase is being studied as a possible tumor marker. Normal gastrointestinal tract cells are rapid proliferators, and tumors in these tissues can be very rapid in growth, elevating thymidylate synthase expression. Research is also being done to examine chemotherapeutics to block thymidylate synthase and therefore to promote a slowdown or to deny altogether tumor cell reproduction in some cancers. Immunohistochemical staining is used on a sample of tissue, and thymidylate synthase reactivity is observed and graded. This test involves staining specimens and identifying the amount of immunoreactivity in the specimen.

Professional Considerations

Consent form NOT required for this test but IS required for the procedure used to obtain the specimen.

Preparation

1. See Biopsy, Site-specific—Specimen.

Procedure

1. See Biopsy, Site-specific—Specimen.

Postprocedure Care

1. See Biopsy, Site-specific—Specimen.

Client and Family Teaching

1. See Biopsy, Site-specific—Specimen.

Factors That Affect Results

1. None found.

Other Data

1. Low reactivity is associated with better colorectal cancer and bladder cancer 5-year survival rates than is high reactivity.

Thyrocalcitonin

See Calcitonin—Serum.

Thyroglobulin

See Thyroid Function Tests—Blood.

Thyroid Antimicrosomal Antibody

See Thyroid Peroxidase Antibody—Blood.

Thyroid Antithyroglobulin Antibody—Serum

Norm. Negative, or titer <1:100 or <2.0 IU/mL.

Positive or Increased. Anemia (autoimmune hemolytic, pernicious), goiter (nontoxic nodular), granulomatous thyroiditis, Graves' disease, Hashimoto's (chronic) thyroiditis, hyperthyroidism, hypothyroidism, myxedema, rheumatoid arthritis, Sjögren's syndrome, systemic lupus erythematosus, thyroid cancer, and thyrotoxicosis. Drugs include lithium.

Description. Thyroid antiglobulin antibody is an autoantibody directed against the antigen thyroglobulin, a thyroid glycoprotein that functions in the synthesis of triiodothyronine (T_3) and thyroxine (T_4). This antibody may be present in inflammation of the thyroid gland or may be the cause of hypothyroidism secondary to thyroid tissue destruction. The test is also helpful in identifying thyroid autoimmunity in clients who have other autoimmune diseases.

Professional Considerations
Consent form NOT required.

Preparation
1. Tube: Red topped, red/gray topped, or gold topped.

Procedure
1. Draw a 7-mL blood sample.

Postprocedure Care
1. None.

Client and Family Teaching
1. Results are normally available within a few days.

Factors That Affect Results
1. Antibody may be present in a small number of clients with no disease symptoms.

Other Data
1. The thyroid antimicrosomal antibody test should also be performed to eliminate other causes of thyroiditis.

Thyroid Echogram

See Thyroid Ultrasonography—Diagnostic.

Thyroid Function Tests—Blood

Norm.

Free Thyroxine Index		SI Units
		Mean
Puberty through adulthood	4.2-13.0	8.0
Cord blood	6.0-13.2	9.8
First 72 hours	9.9-17.5	13.9
7 days	7.5-15.1	11.2
4-52 weeks	5.0-13.0	8.4
1-3 years	5.4-12.5	8.1
3-10 years	5.7-12.8	8.2

		SI Units
Thyroxine (T$_4$) Radioimmunoassay		
Adults	4.5-12.0 µg/dL	58.5-155 nmol/L
Pregnant >14 weeks	9.1-14.0 µg/dL	117-181 nmol/L
Elderly (>60 years)		
Female	5.5-10.5 µg/dL	71-135 nmol/L
Male	5.0-10.0 µg/dL	65-129 nmol/L
Children		
Cord blood	7.4-13.0 µg/dL	95-168 nmol/L
First 72 hours	11.8-22.6 µg/dL	152-292 nmol/L
7-14 days	9.8-16.6 µg/dL	126-214 nmol/L
4-16 weeks	7.2-14.4 µg/dL	93-186 nmol/L
4-12 months	7.8-16.5 µg/dL	101-213 nmol/L
12 months-5 years	7.3-15.0 µg/dL	94-194 nmol/L
5-10 years	6.4-13.3 µg/dL	83-172 nmol/L
10-15 years	5.6-11.7 µg/dL	72-151 nmol/L
Triiodothyronine (T$_3$) Radioimmunoassay		
Adults	80-230 ng/dL	1.2-3.5 nmol/L
Children		
Cord blood	15-75 ng/dL	0.23-1.16 nmol/L
First 72 hours	32-216 ng/dL	0.49-3.33 nmol/L
7-14 days	Average 250 ng/dL	Average 3.85 nmol/L
2-4 weeks	160-240 ng/dL	2.46-3.70 nmol/L
4-16 weeks	117-209 ng/dL	1.80-3.22 nmol/L
16-52 weeks	110-280 ng/dL	1.70-4.31 nmol/L
1-5 years	105-269 ng/dL	1.62-4.14 nmol/L
5-10 years	94-241 ng/dL	1.45-3.71 nmol/L
10-15 years	83-213 ng/dL	1.28-3.28 nmol/L
Thyroid-Stimulating Hormone (TSH)		
Adults	0.4-4.7 µU/mL	0.4-4.7 mU/L
>60 years		
Female	2.0-16.8 µU/mL	2.0-16.8 mU/L
Male	2.0-7.3 µU/mL	2.0-7.3 mU/L
0.5-16 years	0.35-5.5 µU/mL	0.35-5.5 mU/L
Newborn (1-3 days)	3.0-20.0 µU/mL	3.0-20.0 mU/L
Premature Infant	0.5-29.0 µU/mL	0.5-29.0 mU/L
Thyroglobulin (Tg)	Undetectable (NOTE: Tg is only measured after total thyroid ablation to detect recurrent thyroid cancer.)	

Usage. Work-up of suspected thyroid disorder and differentiation of primary thyroid disease from secondary causes and from abnormalities in thyroid-binding globulin levels.

Description. Thyroid function testing involves performing several measurements on one sample of blood. These tests have largely been replaced by the third-generation thyroid-stimulating hormone assay. Tests included are as follows: Thyroid Test: Free Thyroxine Index—Serum; Thyroid-Stimulating Hormone, Sensitive Assay—Blood; Thyroid Test: Thyroxine—Blood; and Thyroid Test: Triiodothyronine—Blood. See individual test listings for further description. Many clients are found to have subclinical thyroid disease as described below, which may or may not be treated. Subclinical hypothyroidism is more common than subclinical hyperthyroidism.

Subclinical Thyroid Disease Findings

	Imaging findings	Sensitive tsh	Thyroxine	Triiodothyronine
Subclinical hyperthyroidism	Asymptomatic abnormalities	Suppressed	Normal	Normal
Subclinical hypothyroidism	Asymptomatic abnormalities	Mildly elevated	Normal	

Conditions Causing Changes in Thyroid Function Tests

	Low Free T_3 or Free T_4	Normal Free T_3 or Free T_4	High Free T_3 or Free T_4
High TSH	Endogenous Causes	Endogenous Causes	Endogenous Causes
	Amyloid goiter	Pendred's syndrome	Anti-TPO antibodies
	Iodine organification defect	Heterophile antibody	Familial dysalbuminemic hyperthyroxinemia
	Iodine transport abnormalities	Subclinical autoimmune hypothyroidism	Pituitary tumor that secretes TSH
	Riedel's thyroiditis	State of recovering from non-thyroid illness	Psychiatric illness(acute)
	Thyroglobulin synthetic defect	TSH receptor defects	Thyroid hormone resistance
	Thyroid dysgenesis	TSH-resistance	
	Thyroiditis (chronic autoimmune)		
	Thyroiditis (transient, hypothyroid phase)		
	TSH-receptor defects		
	TSH-resistance		
	TTF2 mutations		
	Exogenous Causes	Exogenous Causes	Exogenous Causes
	Amiodarone therapy	Amiodarone therapy	Amiodarone therapy
	Lithium therapy	Cholestyramine therapy	Intermittent T_4 therapy
	Interferon therapy	Intermittent T_4 therapy	
	Interleukin therapy	Sertraline therapy	
	After radioiodine treatment		
	After neck radiation therapy		
	Iodine deficiency		
	Iodine-excess goiter		
	Post thyroidectomy		
Normal TSH	Eating disorders (sick euthyroid syndrome)		Same as above
Low TSH	Endogenous Causes	Endogenous Causes	Endogenous Causes
	Congenital deficiency Hypothyroidism (secondary)	Hyperthyroidism (subclinical)	Activating germline TSH-receptor mutation
	Nonthyroidal illness	Nonthyroidal illness	Graves' disease
	TSH suppression secondary to recent treatment for hyperthyroidism		Hydatidiform mole
			Hyperthyroidism (primary)

Continued

High TSH	Low Free T$_3$ or Free T$_4$ Endogenous Causes	Normal Free T$_3$ or Free T$_4$ Endogenous Causes	High Free T$_3$ or Free T$_4$ Endogenous Causes
	Eating disorders (sick euthyroid syndrome)		Iodine excess* Multinodular goiter Pregnancy: thyrotoxicosis with hyperemesis gravidarum or familial gestational hyperthyroidism Presence of ectopic thyroid tissue* Thyroiditis (lymphocytic)* Thyroiditis (postpartum)* Thyroiditis (postviral)* Thyroiditis (transient)* Toxic nodule
		Exogenous Causes	**Exogenous Causes**
	Thyroxine ingestion Dobutamine therapy Dopamine therapy Steroid therapy		Amiodarone therapy* Thyroxine ingestion*

Modified from Dayan CM: Interpretation of thyroid function tests, *Lancet* 57(9256):619-624, 2001 (review).
*Accompanied by low radioiodine uptake.

Professional Considerations
Consent form NOT required.

Preparation
1. Tube: Red topped, red/gray topped, or gold topped.

Procedure
1. Completely fill the tube with venous blood.

Postprocedure Care
1. None.

Client and Family Teaching
1. Results are normally available within a few days.

Factors That Affect Results
1. Results are invalidated if the client has undergone a radionuclide scan within 7 days before the test.
2. Abnormal thyroid test findings often found in critically ill clients should be repeated after the critical nature of the condition is resolved.
3. The production, circulation, and disposal of thyroid hormone are altered throughout the stages of pregnancy.
4. An herb or botanical that may interfere with success of thyroid replacement therapy is kelp, which contains iodine.

Other Data
1. Many illnesses affect thyroid test values, but are not indicative of thyroid disease. For this reason, routine thyroid testing of hospitalized clients is not recommended.
2. An herbal or natural remedy that interferes with thyroid medication is kelp.
3. Abnormal thyroid function test (hyper and hypothyroidism) present in 18% of patients with atrial flutter and fibrillation.
4. Need for invasive mechanical ventilation and an increase in hospital mortality occur in respiratory failure patients with low T$_3$ and T$_4$.

Thyroid Hormone Binding Ratio—Blood

Norm.

		SI Units
T_3 Uptake		
Adults >60 Years	24%-39%	24-39 Arb units*
Female	22%-32%	22-32 Arb units
Male	24%-32%	24-32 Arb units
Neonates	25%-37%	25-37 Arb units
Thyroid Hormone Binding Ratio		
Adults ≤50 Years	0.85-1.14	0.85-1.14 Arb units
Adults >50 Years		
Female	0.80-1.04	0.80-1.04 Arb units
Male	0.87-1.11	0.87-1.11 Arb units
Children		
Cord blood	0.75-1.05	0.75-1.05 Arb units
First 72 hours	0.90-1.40	0.90-1.40 Arb units
7-14 days	0.82-1.15	0.82-1.15 Arb units
4-16 weeks	0.75-1.05	0.75-1.05 Arb units
1-15 years	0.88-1.12	0.88-1.12 Arb units

		Mean
Free Thyroxine Index		
Puberty Through Adulthood	4.2-13.0	8.0
Infants and Children		
Cord blood	6.0-13.2	9.8
First 72 hours	9.9-17.5	13.9
7 days	7.5-15.1	11.2
4-52 weeks	5.0-13.0	8.4
1-3 years	5.4-12.5	8.1
3-10 years	5.7-12.8	8.2

*Arb means arbitrary.

Increased T3 Uptake and THBR. Decreased TBG (from genetic deficiency or other causes), hyperandrogenic state, hyperthyroidism, hypoproteinemia, liver disease (severe), malnutrition, metastasis, nephrosis, nephrotic syndrome, protein loss, and thyrotoxicosis factitia. Drugs include adrenocorticotropic hormone, androgens, barbiturates, corticosteroids, glucocorticoids, furosemide, penicillin (large doses), phenylbutazone, phenytoins, salicylates (high doses), thyroid extract, and thyroxine.

Decreased T3 Uptake and THBR. Cretinism, endocrine-secreting tumors, hepatitis (acute), hypothyroidism, increased TBG (from congenital excess or other causes), and pregnancy. Drugs include chlorpromazine, estrogens, heroin, lithium carbonate, methadone, oral contraceptives, perphenazine (long-term use), and propylthiouracil.

Description. This test measures the amount of unbound thyroid hormone binding sites on thyroxine-binding globulin (TBG), a major protein carrier of thyroid hormones. The measurement is obtained by determination of the amount of radiolabeled T_3 bound by a T_3-binding resin (T_3 uptake) after all TBG-binding sites in a client's blood sample are saturated. The number of sites available is dependent on the amount of thyroxine (T_4) present because it is present in greater quantities than triiodothyronine (T_3) and has a greater affinity for TBG than T_3. The greater the number of TBG-binding sites available, the lower the T_3 uptake by the resin. The greater the amount of T_4 present, the smaller the proportion of unbound TBG-binding sites and the greater the T_3 uptake by the resin. T_3 uptake is used to calculate the thyroid hormone binding ratio (THBR) as follows:

$$THBR = \frac{(\% \ T_3 \ uptake)}{(Mean \ \% \ T_3 \ uptake \ of \ reference \ serum)}$$

THBR compared to T_4 level is useful in determining whether thyroid hormone changes are attributable to thyroid disease or to abnormalities in TBG. If the values show parallel changes, a problem in thyroid function is indicated. However, if the results show opposite changes, an abnormality in the amount of TBG is more likely. Use of these results in a further calculation provides an indirect measurement of free T_4 in the bloodstream by multiplication of the T_3 uptake by the client's T_4 level to obtain the free thyroxine index (FTI).

Professional Considerations
Consent form NOT required.

Preparation
1. Tube: Red topped, red/gray topped, or gold topped.

Procedure
1. Draw a 7-mL blood sample.

Postprocedure Care
1. Refrigerate specimens until tested. Freeze specimens at −20 degrees C if the test is not performed within 1 week after collection.

Client and Family Teaching
1. Results are normally available within 72 hours.

Factors That Affect Results
1. THBR results may be falsely increased in acidosis (severe) and atrial fibrillation.
2. Drugs that cause falsely elevated results include dicumarol, heparin, phenytoin, and salicylates.
3. Because thyroid hormone is bound to proteins, protein levels should be considered when interpreting the results.

Other Data
1. "THBR" replaces nomenclature of "T_3 uptake."
2. See also Thyroid test: Thyroxine—Blood; Thyroid test: Triiodothyronine—Blood.

Thyroid Peroxidase (TPO, Antimicrosomal Antibody, Antithyroid Microsomal Antibody) Antibody—Blood

Norm. 0.0-2.0 IU/mL.

Usage. Lends evidence for thyroid disease in clients with concomitant illnesses, which can affect other thyroid tests. Helps predict the progression of chronic thyroiditis and complications during pregnancy (preeclampsia, caesarean delivery, postpardum thyroiditis, abnormal neonatal thyroid function).

Increased. Graves' disease, hypothyroidism (idiopathic), thyroiditis (Hashimoto's, postpartum). Others include anemia (pernicious), lupus erythematosus, rheumatoid arthritis, and Sjögren's syndrome.

Decreased. Not applicable.

Description. Thyroid peroxidase (TPO) is now known to be the thyroid microsomal antigen. TPO is a membrane-bound enzyme essential for the synthesis of thyroid hormones thyroxine (T_4) and triiodothyronine (T_3). Thyroid peroxidase autoantibodies are autoimmune antibodies that inhibit the synthesis of the thyroid hormones and can also cause cytotoxic cell changes. TPO antibodies are present in 90% of clients with autoimmune diseases of the thyroid. This test has replaced the *thyroid antimicrosomal antibody test* because it is a more sensitive indicator of thyroid cells' antimicrosomal component.

Professional Considerations
Consent form NOT required.

Preparation
1. Tube: Red topped.

Procedure
1. Draw a 5-mL blood sample.

Postprocedure Care
1. None.

Client and Family Teaching
1. None.

Factors That Affect Results
1. Reject hemolyzed or anticoagulated specimens.

Other Data

1. TPO antibodies may be present in up to 10% of all clients and up to 30% of healthy elderly clients.
2. One study found that women with TPO antibodies present during pregnancy had almost three times the risk for postpartum depression as compared with the average pregnancy. Another study determined that supplementation with thyroxin during pregnancy had no impact on the incidence of postpartum depression.

Thyroid Profile

See Thyroid Function Tests—Blood.

Thyroid Test: Free Thyroxine Index (FT$_4$I, T$_7$)—Serum

Norm.

		Mean
Puberty Through Adulthood	4.2-13.0	8.0
Infants and Children		
Cord blood	6.0-13.2	9.8
First 72 hours	9.9-17.5	13.9
7 days	7.5-15.1	11.2
4-52 weeks	5.0-13.0	8.4
1-3 years	5.4-12.5	8.1
3-10 years	5.7-12.8	8.2
T-Uptake	32.0%-48.4%	

Increased. Dehydration, dysalbuminemia, hyperthyroidism, hyperthyroxinemia, and psychiatric illness (acute). Drugs include amiodarone, furosemide, propranolol, radiographic dyes, and thyroxine.

Decreased. Anorexia nervosa, heparin, hypothyroidism, and illness (severe). Drugs include carbamazepine and diphenylhydantoin.

Description. Thyroxine (T$_4$) is a hormone produced in the thyroid gland from iodide and thyroglobulin in a multistep process. Less than 0.05% of thyroxine circulates freely and is thus biologically active. Biologically active T$_4$ stimulates the basal metabolic rate, including use of carbohydrates and lipids, protein synthesis, bone calcium release, and vitamin metabolism. In infants, T$_4$ plays an important role in central nervous system growth and development. Circulating T$_4$ levels affect the release of thyroid-stimulating hormone (TSH) and hypothalamic thyroid-releasing hormone (TRH) through a negative-feedback mechanism. Because of the tiny quantity of free T$_4$ normally present, direct measurement is difficult and expensive. An alternative—the free thyroxine index (FT$_4$I)—is derived from a calculation and provides an indirect measurement of free T$_4$ levels, based on total T$_4$ levels and thyroid uptake (T-uptake) expressed as the percentage of hormone unbound to the thyroid-binding protein. T-uptake measures the binding sites that are saturated with thyroxine, and then is used in a calculation with the total serum T$_4$ level to determine the amount of thyroxine circulating freely in the blood. This is done in clients with conditions that can alter the number of thyroxine-binding sites, which leads to misleading free T$_4$ values alone. The calculation is as follows:

$$FT_4I = (\text{T-uptake \%})/(T_4 \times \text{Mean TU\%})$$

This calculation takes into account both the quantity of total T$_4$ and the availability of thyroxin-binding globulin binding sites.

Professional Considerations

Consent form NOT required.

Preparation

1. Tube: Red topped, red/gray topped, or gold topped.

T

Procedure

1. Draw a 5-mL blood sample.

Postprocedure Care

1. None.

Client and Family Teaching

1. Results are normally available in 72 hours.

Factors That Affect Results

1. Results are invalidated if the client has undergone a radionuclide scan within 7 days before the test. Schedule any needed scans after the thyroid profile tests.
2. During pregnancy, both T_4 and THBR are elevated, but the FT_4I is normal.

3. The value may be normal in hypothyroid clients receiving phenytoin or salicylate therapy.
4. The National Cholesterol Education Program found that ingestion of 56 mg of soy isoflavones per day resulted in a small, but insignificant increase in the free thyroxine index in postmenopausal women.

Other Data

1. See also Thyroid test: Thyroxine—Blood; Thyroid test: Thyroid hormone binding ratio—Blood.
2. Older methods calculated the FT_4I by multiplying total T_4 and T_3 uptake.
3. An herbal or natural remedy that interferes with thyroid medication is kelp.

Thyroid Scan—Diagnostic

Norm. Homogeneous uptake of radioactive tracer and normal size, shape, and position of the thyroid gland.

Usage. Differentiation of hyperfunctioning nodule and of thyroid tissue hyperplasia; help in diagnosis of thyroid cancer; evaluation of thyroid in client with history of irradiated head and neck; monitoring of the thyroid gland during therapy; used for clients with differentiated thyroid carcinoma to screen for recurrence or persistence.

Description. A thyroid scan is a nuclear medicine scan of the thyroid after injection of a radioactive tracer (^{123}I, ^{125}I, ^{131}I, or ^{99m}Tc) for the purpose of detecting areas of increased or decreased tracer uptake by the thyroid gland and surrounding area tissue. Hyperfunctioning thyroid nodules, which are usually nonmalignant, cause areas of increased uptake, labeled as "hot nodules." "Cold nodules" are nodules that do not take up the tracer (that is, tissue is not functioning as normal thyroid tissue) and are more likely to be malignant. For detection of metastatic thyroid cancer, whole-body scanning with ^{131}I in conjunction with levothyroxine withdrawal or stimulation with recombinant human TSH is done.

Professional Considerations

Consent form NOT required.

Risks

Allergic reaction to tracer (itching, hives, rash, tight feeling in the throat, shortness of breath, anaphylaxis).

Contraindications

Previous allergy to iodine, shellfish, or radioactive tracer; pregnancy (because of the radioactive iodine crossing the blood-placental barrier); breast-feeding.

Preparation

1. See Client and Family Teaching.
2. Have emergency equipment readily available.
3. Jewelry and metal objects near the head or neck area should be removed before scanning.

Procedure

1. Oral radioactive tracer is administered 6 hours before scanning. Intravenous radioactive tracer is administered ½ hour before scanning.
2. The client is positioned supine, with a pillow, rolled towel, or sponge beneath the shoulder blades, and the neck hyperextended.
3. The thyroid gland is scanned with a gamma camera that moves over one or more sections of the thyroid gland.
4. Scan takes ½ hour.

Postprocedure Care

1. Resume previous diet 2 hours after oral radioactive tracer administration.

2. Observe the client carefully for up to 60 minutes after the study for a possible (anaphylactic) reaction to the radionuclide.
3. Rubber gloves should be worn by health care providers when discarding urine for 24 hours after the procedure. Wash the gloved hands with soap and water before removing the gloves. Wash the ungloved hands after the gloves are removed. An incontinent client requires special handling of any soiled linen or disposable pads. These should be placed in special storage for a few weeks before cleaning or discarding. Consult with your radiation safety officer for details.

Client and Family Teaching
1. Drugs that may be discontinued up to 21 days before the scan include anticoagulants, antihistamines, corticosteroids, cough syrup, iodides, phenothiazines, radiopaque dyes (28-42 days), salicylates, thyroxine (10 days), triiodothyronine (3 days), vitamins, and antithyroid medications such as propylthiouracil or methimazole (Tapazole) (3 days).
2. Foods that should not be ingested for 14-21 days before the test include shellfish and salt or salt substitutes containing iodine.
3. Fast from food and fluids for 4 hours before and 1 hour after the test if radioactive tracer will be administered orally.
4. There is no discomfort with this test.

5. Describe the procedure and expected sensations.
6. Meticulously wash your hands with soap and water after each void for 24 hours. The toilet should be flushed 2-3 times after each voiding.

Factors That Affect Results
1. If a radioactive iodine tracer is used, uptake may be increased in clients on a diet with subnormal iodine levels or those on phenothiazine therapy.
2. Ingestion of drugs listed under Client and Family Teaching within 2-3 weeks before the test may cause decreased tracer uptake.
3. Gastroenteritis may interfere with the absorption of orally administered radioactive tracer.
4. Receipt by the client of intrathecal or intravenous contrast material within 21 days before the scan invalidates the results.

Other Data
1. Health care professionals working in a nuclear medicine area must follow federal standards set by the Nuclear Regulatory Commission. These standards include precautions for handling the radioactive material and monitoring of potential radiation exposure.
2. Technetium half-life is 6 hours. Iodine-131 half-life is 8 days. Iodine-123 half-life is 13.3 hours.

Thyroid-Stimulating Hormone
See Thyroid-Stimulating Hormone, Sensitive Assay—Blood.

Thyroid-Stimulating Hormone, Filter Paper—Blood
Norm.

Newborn		SI Units
At birth, peak occurs up to	30 µU/mL	30 mU/L
3 days old	<20 µU/L	<20 mU/L
10 days old	<10 µU/mL	<10 mU/L

Usage. Newborn screening for congenital hypothyroidism. May also be used to follow children known to have congenital hypothyroidism. Must be interpreted in light of T₄ levels.

Description. See also Thyroid-stimulating hormone, Sensitive assay—Blood. Thyroid screening is recommended for all newborns from birth to up to 4 weeks. With congenital hypothyroidism, TSH levels will be elevated.

Test kits using filter paper are considered specific enough to use for screening purposes. Early detection of congenital hypothyroidism enables treatment and prevents complications, which include mental retardation and subnormal growth patterns.

Professional Considerations
Consent form NOT required.

Preparation
1. Obtain alcohol wipe, lancet, and TSH filter paper card.
2. Prewarming the heel is not necessary.

Procedure
1. Cleanse the lateral curvature of the infant's heel with alcohol and allow it to dry.
2. Puncture the lateral heel curvature with a lancet.

3. Saturate a spot on the TSH filter paper card with heelstick blood.
4. Allow the blood spot to dry before sending the sample to the lab.

Postprocedure Care
1. Apply pressure to the puncture site until the bleeding stops. Let the site air-dry.

Client and Family Teaching
1. Results are normally available immediately.

Factors That Affect Results
1. The test must be repeated if the blood amount is not enough to completely saturate a spot on the card.
2. Touching the filter paper or exposure to extremes of heat and light can cause errors in the results.

Other Data
1. None.

Thyroid-Stimulating Hormone, Sensitive Assay (Sensitive TSH Assay, Sensitive Thyrotropin Assay)—Blood

Norm.

	SI Units
Adults	0.4-4.2 mU/L
Adults >80 years	0.4-10 mU/L
Children	0.35-4.94 mIU/L
First trimester:11-13 weeks	0.13-3.71 mIU/L
Cord blood	2-40 mU/L
Newborn by day 3	<20 mU/L
Newborn by day 7	0.4-15 mU/L
Infant 8 days-1 month	0.4-10 mU/L
1 month and older	0.3-5 mU/L
Diagnostic Values	
Borderline hyperthyroidism	0.1-0.29 mU/L
Primary hyperthyroidism	<0.1 mU/L
Borderline hypothyroidism	5.1-7.0 mU/L
Probable hypothyroidism	>7.0 mU/L
Desired level when receiving thyroxine therapy	0.5-3.5 mU/L

Increased. Acute sleep loss, Addison's disease (primary), anti-TSH antibodies, eclampsia, euthyroid goiter (with enzyme defect), fasting state, goiter (iodine-deficiency type), hyperpituitarism, hypertension, hypothermia, hypothyroidism (primary), longevity (with associated decreased T_3 and T_4), metabolic syndrome, pituitary adenoma (that secretes thyrotropin), postoperatively (subtotal thyroidectomy), preeclampsia, pregnancy breech presentation, psychiatric illness (acute), status after therapy with radioactive iodine, and thyroiditis. Drugs include amiodarone, benserazide, clomiphene, iopanoic acid, ipodate, lithium, methimazole, metoclopramide, morphine, propylthiouracil, radiographic dye, sorafenib, SSKI, and thyroid-releasing hormone. Foods include ingestion of seaweed. Exposures include organophosphate pesticides.

Decreased. Hashimoto's thyroiditis, hyperthyroidism, hypothyroidism (secondary, tertiary) (sometimes), low bone mineral density in males, and organic brain syndrome. Drugs include ASA, heparin, ketoconazole, T_3, and TSH. Drugs that decrease TSH function include dopamine, glucocorticoids, and octreotide.

Description. The serum TSH assay is an ultrasensitive indicator that has largely replaced all the other tests used to screen for and diagnose hypothyroidism and monitor treatment. Third-generation TSH-sensitive assay is considered to be the most appropriate initial test when thyroid disorder is suspected. If the assay is normal, further testing is not indicated. If the assay is abnormal, a T_4 assay should be prescribed. Clients are considered to have subclinical hypothyroidism if the sensitive thyrotropin level is elevated but the free thyroxine level is normal. Subclinical hyperthyroidism is diagnosed when serum thyrotropin level is low in association with normal free thyroxine and triiodothyronine levels. There is a two-step assay that uses monoclonal antibodies directed against TSH.

Professional Considerations
Consent form NOT required.

Preparation
1. Tube: Red topped, red/gray topped, or gold topped.
2. MAY be drawn during hemodialysis.

Procedure
1. Draw a 4-mL blood sample.

Postprocedure Care
1. None.

Client and Family Teaching
1. Results are normally available within 24 hours.

2. Samples may be stored up to 4 days refrigerated, or at room temperature.

Factors That Affect Results
1. Levels are elevated temporarily when the client is recovering from illness, but they return to normal after recovery.
2. Previous treatment with corticosteroid therapy may result in lower TSH levels while thyroid hormone levels are normal. Therefore thyroid hormones should also be measured in clients who have had previous corticosteroid therapy for chronic conditions such as rheumatoid arthritis.
3. Because TSH levels are often low in early pregnancy, further testing for abnormal results should include free thyroid hormones and thyroid-releasing hormone measurements.
4. The National Cholesterol Education Program found that ingestion of 90 mg of soy isoflavones per day resulted in a small, but insignificant increase in the TSH level in postmenopausal women.
5. Conditions in which the results of this test should not be evaluated in isolation include recent treatment for thyrotoxicosis, disease of the pituitary gland including TSH-secreting tumor, nonthyroidal illness, and resistance to thyroid hormone (Dayan, 2001).
6. Maternal serum concentrations of T_3, T_4, and TSH are lower in Blacks than Caucasians.

Other Data
1. Sensitive TSH measurement has been found to be accurate for detection of neonatal thyroid disease.
2. Clients more than 60 years of age with sensitive TSH ≤0.1 mIU/L are at risk for atrial fibrillation.
3. Girls with initial levels >7.5 are at greater risk for sustained abnormal TSH levels.

Thyroid Test: Thyroxine (T₄)—Blood
Norm.

		SI Units
Radioimmunoassay		
Adults	5-12 µg/dL	65-155 nmol/L
Pregnant >14 weeks	9.1-14.0 µg/dL	117-181 nmol/L

Continued

		SI Units
Elderly >60 years		
Female	5.5-10.5 µg/dL	71-135 nmol/L
Male	5.0-10.0 µg/dL	65-129 nmol/L
Children		
Cord blood	7.4-13.0 µg/dL	95-168 nmol/L
First 72 hours	11.8-22.6 µg/dL	152-292 nmol/L
7-14 days	9.8-16.6 µg/dL	126-214 nmol/L
4-16 weeks	7.2-14.4 µg/dL	93-186 nmol/L
4-12 months	7.8-16.5 µg/dL	101-213 nmol/L
12 months-5 years	7.3-15.0 µg/dL	94-194 nmol/L
5-10 years	6.4-13.3 µg/dL	83-172 nmol/L
10-15 years	5.6-11.7 µg/dL	72-151 nmol/L
Whole Blood Newborn Screening (Filter Paper Method)		
Infants		
First 5 days	>7.5 µg/dL	>97 nmol/L
6 days	>6.5 µg/dL	>84 nmol/L
Panic Levels		
Thyroid storm possible	>20 µg/dL	>257 nmol/L
Myxedema possible	<2.0 µg/dL	<26 nmol/L

Panic Level Symptoms and Treatment

Thyroid Storm Symptoms. Hyperthermia, diaphoresis, vomiting, dehydration, and shock.

Thyroid Storm Treatment

NOTE: Treatment choice(s) depend(s) on client's history and condition and episode history.

1. Provide supportive treatment for shock.
2. Administer fluid and electrolyte replacement for dehydration.
3. Administer antithyroid drugs (propylthiouracil and Lugol's solution).

Myxedema Symptoms. Hypothermia, hypotension, bradycardia, hypoventilation, CO_2 narcosis, lethargy, and coma.

Myxedema Treatment

1. Support airway and blood pressure.
2. Perform neurologic checks every hour.
3. Administer thyroid hormone (levothyroxine) intravenously.

Increased. Acute intermittent porphyria, cirrhosis (primary biliary), congenital excess of thyroxine-binding globulin, excess dietary iodine intake, familial dysalbuminemic hyperthyroxinemia, goiter (toxic multinodular, uninodular), Graves' disease, hyperemesis gravidarum, hyperthyroidism, liver disease (early stage), lymphoma, newborn infants, obesity, pregnancy, psychiatric disorder (acute), subacute thyroiditis (first stage), and thyrotoxicosis. Drugs include amiodarone (within the previous 4 months), amphetamines, Betadine, clofibrate, dextrothyroxine, dinoprost tromethamine, estrogens (within the previous 4 weeks), Floraquin, furosemide, 5-fluorouracil, halothane, heparin, heroin, iodinated radiographic contrast dyes, iodinated vaginal suppositories (within the previous 4 weeks), iodothiouracil (within the previous several weeks), iopanoic acid, ipodate, levarterenol, levodopa, methadone, Metrical, oral contraceptives, perphenazine (long-term use, occasional increase), phenylbutazone (first few days of therapy), progesterone, beta-blockers, thyroid extract (within the previous 6 weeks), thyroid-releasing hormone, thyrotropin, thyroxine (within the previous 4 weeks), and Vioform (clioquinol). Exposures include organophosphate pesticides.

Decreased. Acromegaly, cirrhosis, cretinism, eclampsia, exercise (strenuous), genetic deficiency of thyroxine-binding globulin, goiter (some), Hashimoto's thyroiditis (chronic thyroiditis), hypoproteinemia, hypothyroidism (primary, secondary), iodide deficiency (severe), liver disease (chronic), longevity (with associated decreased T_3 and increased TSH), malnutrition, myxedema, nephrosis, nephrotic syndrome, pancreatic malabsorption, panhypopituitarism, postoperatively (caused by stress), preeclampsia, radioactive iodine therapy, Sheehan's syndrome, Simmonds' disease, subacute thyroiditis (third stage), thyroidectomy, thyroid gland agenesis, and tumor (pituitary). Drugs include adrenal corticoids (within the previous 2 weeks), adrenocorticotropic hormone (within the previous 2 weeks), amiodarone (rare), androgens (within the previous 3 weeks), anabolic steroids, antithyroid drugs, asparaginase, barbiturates, carbamazepine, chlorpromazine, corticotropin, cortisone (long-term use), danazol, diphenylhydantoin, ethionamide, fenclofenac, furosemide (high doses), gold salts (within the previous several weeks), iodides, isoniazid (long-term use), isotretinoin, lithium carbonate, L-triiodothyronine (within the previous 4 weeks), methimazole (within the previous 7 days), oxyphenbutazone, penicillin, phenobarbital, phenytoin (within the previous 10 days), prednisone, propranolol, propylthiouracil (within the previous 7 days), reserpine, rifampicin, salicylates, somatotropin, SSKI (early in therapy), sorafenib, sulfonamides, and thiocyanate (within the previous 3 weeks).

Description. Thyroxine (T_4) is a hormone produced in the thyroid gland from iodide and thyroglobulin in a multistep process. Production occurs in response to the effects of pituitary thyroid-stimulating hormone (TSH) on the thyroid gland. T_4 is the major hormone synthesized by the gland and the hormone from which triiodothyronine (T_3) is derived. When released from the thyroid gland, almost all (99.96%) of T_4 is bound to protein (thyroxine-binding globulin, thyroxine-binding prealbumin, and albumin). The remainder of T_4 (0.04%) is called "free thyroxine" and is the only portion of this hormone that is biologically active. Biologically active T_4 stimulates the basal metabolic rate, including use of carbohydrates and lipids, protein synthesis, bone calcium release, and vitamin metabolism. In infants, T_4 plays an important role in central nervous system growth and development. Circulating T_4 levels affect the release of TSH and hypothalamic thyroid-releasing hormone (TRH) through a negative-feedback mechanism. This test measures total T_4 (protein-bound and free).

Professional Considerations
Consent form NOT required.

Preparation
1. Tube: Red topped; for whole-blood newborn screening, obtain an alcohol wipe, a lancet, and filter paper for T_4 testing.
2. The most accurate picture of T_4 levels is obtained when the client has been free of thyroid medications for 1 month.
3. Newborn screening for hypothyroidism should be performed at least 72 hours after birth and after the newborn has been taking feedings containing protein for at least 24 hours.

Procedure
1. Draw a 4-mL blood sample.
2. Do NOT draw specimens during hemodialysis.
3. Whole-blood newborn screening:
   a. Prewarming the heel is not necessary.
   b. Cleanse the lateral curvature of the heel with an alcohol wipe, and allow the area to dry.
   c. Puncture the lateral curvature of the heel with a lancet until free flow of blood is obtained.
   d. Completely saturate all test circles on the filter paper with heelstick blood. The circles should be completely filled.
   e. Place the filter paper in a light-protected container for delivery to the laboratory.
   f. Cord blood may also be used.

Postprocedure Care
1. Let the heelstick site air-dry.
2. Indicate pregnancy status on the laboratory requisition.

Client and Family Teaching
1. Results are normally available within 72 hours.

Factors That Affect Results
1. Results are invalidated if the client has undergone a radionuclide scan within 14 days before the test.
2. Results are invalidated in hemolyzed or lipemic specimens.
3. With the double-antibody testing method, results may be increased in the presence of anti-thyroxine antibodies.
4. With the single-antibody testing method, results may be decreased in the presence of anti-thyroxine antibodies.
5. Cord blood levels are lower in premature infants than in full-term infants.

T

6. The following iodine contrast media may increase test results:
   a. *Cholecystography*: Telepaque within the previous 6 weeks; Oragrafin.
7. Maternal serum concentrations of T_3, T_4, and TSH are lower in Blacks than Caucasians.

Other Data

1. Test results are usually evaluated in conjunction with free T_4 and TSH levels.
2. An herbal or natural remedy that interferes with thyroid medication is kelp.

Thyroid Test: Thyroxine by Ria

See Thyroid Test: Thyroxine—Blood.

Thyroid Test: Thyroxine Free (FT₄)—Serum

Norm. Norms vary among newer test kits and should be compared with those from the manufacturer.

Radioimmunoassay		SI Units
Adults	0.58-1.64 ng/dL	7.48-18.06 pmol/L
Pregnancy		
Trimester 1		0.1–2.5 mIU/L
Trimester 2		0.2–3.0 mIU/L
Trimester 3		0.3–3.0 mIU/L
Premature Infants		
25-30 weeks	0.5-3.3 ng/dL	6.4-42.5 pmol/L
31-36 weeks	1.3-4.7 ng/dL	16.7-60.5 pmol/L
Full-Term Infants		
0-1 month	0.8-2.2 ng/dL	10.32-28.38 pmol/L
1-6 months	0.8-1.8 ng/dL	10.32-23.22 pmol/L
≥6-12 months	0.8-1.6 ng/dL	10.32-20.64 pmol/L
1-12 years	0.9-1.4 ng/dL	11.61-18.06 pmol/L
≥12 years	1.3-2.8 ng/dL	16.77-36.12 pmol/L

Increased. Dehydration, hyperthyroidism and psychiatric illness (acute). Drugs include amiodarone, heparin, propranolol, radiographic dyes, and thyroxine. Exposures include organophosphate pesticides.

Decreased. Anorexia nervosa, hypothyroidism, illness (severe), post-dialysis, pregnancy, and thyroid cancer. Drugs include carbamazepine, phenylbutazone (after the first few days of therapy), heparin, rifampicin, and thiocyanate.

Description. Thyroxine (T_4) is a hormone produced in the thyroid gland from iodide and thyroglobulin in a multistep process. Less than 0.05% of thyroxine circulates freely and is thus biologically active. Biologically active T_4 stimulates the basal metabolic rate, including use of carbohydrates and lipids, protein synthesis, bone calcium release, and vitamin metabolism. In infants, T_4 plays an important role in central nervous system growth and development. Circulating T_4 levels affect the release of thyroid-stimulating hormone (TSH) and hypothalamic thyroid-releasing hormone (TRH) through a negative-feedback mechanism. Because of the tiny quantity of free T_4 normally present, direct measurement is difficult and expensive. Equilibrium dialysis is the common standard used for measuring free T_4. Radioimmunoassay is often used but is subject to the influence of the serum albumin and lipid levels. Newer testing kits are being developed to improve the accuracy and ease of direct measurement of free T_4.

Professional Considerations

Consent form NOT required.

Preparation

1. Tube: Red topped, red/gray topped, or gold topped.
2. Do NOT draw specimens during hemodialysis.

Procedure

1. Draw a 4-mL blood sample.

Postprocedure Care

1. The serum should be separated within 48 hours after collection.

Client and Family Teaching

1. Results are normally available within 72 hours.

Factors That Affect Results

1. RIA results are invalidated if the client has undergone a radionuclide scan within 14 days before the test.
2. Values may be normal in hypothyroid clients receiving phenytoin or salicylate therapy.

3. Because thyroxine is affected by protein binding, findings may be altered (lower) in pregnancy when hemodilution occurs.

Other Data

1. van Wassenaer et al (2002) found that, "in untreated infants, low FT_4 values during the first 4 weeks after birth in infants born at <30 weeks' gestation are associated with worse neurodevelopmental outcome at 2 and 5 years. In T_4-treated infants, high FT_4 is not associated with worse outcome."
2. An herbal or natural remedy that interferes with thyroid medication is kelp.
3. In hyperthyroidism a free thyroxine level >19 pmol/L increases risk of venous thrombosis.
4. Critically ill children in PICU have a 30 times increased mortality with decreased T_3 and T_4 levels.
5. See also Thyroid test: Thyroxine—Blood; Thyroid test: Thyroid hormone binding Ratio—Blood.

Thyroid Test: Triiodothyronine (T₃)—Blood

Norm.

		SI Units
Adults	80-230 ng/dL	1.2-3.5 nmol/L
Children 1 month-18 years	1.5 – 6.0 pg/mL	
Cord blood	14-86 ng/dL	0.22-1.32 nmol/L
First 72 hours	32-216 ng/dL	0.49-3.33 nmol/L
7-14 days	Avg. 250 ng/dL	Avg. 3.85 nmol/L
2-4 weeks	160-240 ng/dL	2.46-3.70 nmol/L
4-16 weeks	117-209 ng/dL	1.80-3.22 nmol/L
16-52 weeks	110-280 ng/dL	1.70-4.31 nmol/L
1-5 years	105-269 ng/dL	1.62-4.14 nmol/L
5-10 years	94-241 ng/dL	1.45-3.71 nmol/L
10-15 years	83-213 ng/dL	1.28-3.28 nmol/L

Increased. Congenital excess of thyroxine-binding globulin, familial dysalbuminemic hyperthyroxinemia, fasting state, Graves' disease, high altitudes, hyperthyroidism, pregnancy, psychiatric illness (acute), and T_3 thyrotoxicosis. Drugs include amiodarone (rarely), antithyroid medications, dextrothyroxine, dinoprost tromethamine, estrogens, heroin, lithium, L-triiodothyronine, methadone, oral contraceptives, rifampicin, terbutaline, and thyroxine.

Decreased. Anorexia nervosa, eclampsia, elderly, genetic deficiency of thyroxine-binding globulin, goiter (caused by iodine deficiency), hepatic cirrhosis, iodine deficiency (severe), longevity (with associated decreased T_4 and increased TSH), myxedema, obesity, post-dialysis, postoperatively (caused by stress), preeclampsia, radioactive iodine therapy, renal failure, starvation, and thyroidectomy. Drugs include amiodarone, androgens, antithyroid drugs, asparaginase, cimetidine, dexamethasone, fenclofenac, fenoprofen, iodinated radiographic contrast dyes, iopanoic acid, ipodate, isotretinoin, lithium compounds, phenytoin, propranolol, propylthiouracil, radiographic dyes, salicylates, sorafenib, and valproic acid.

Description. Triiodothyronine (T_3) is a hormone produced primarily in peripheral tissues from conversion of thyroxine (T_4) but also is produced in small amounts by the thyroid gland; 99.96% of T_3 is bound to protein (thyroxine-binding globulin, thyroxine-binding prealbumin, and albumin); and the remainder is the biologically active form. About four times as much T_3 as T_4 circulates freely, partly because of its lower affinity for serum proteins. Additionally, T_3 has a shorter half-life than T_4. Biologically active T_3 stimulates the basal metabolic rate, including use of carbohydrates and lipids, protein synthesis, bone calcium release, and vitamin metabolism. In infants, T_3 plays an important role in central nervous system growth and development. Circulating T_3 levels affect the release of thyroid-stimulating hormone (TSH) and hypothalamic thyroid-releasing hormone (TRH) through a negative-feedback mechanism. T_3 levels are used to confirm a diagnosis of hyperthyroidism when T_4 levels are borderline high and to help diagnose T_3 thyrotoxicosis. This test is a radioimmunoassay measurement of total T_3 levels.

Professional Considerations
Consent form NOT required.

Preparation
1. Tube: Red topped, red/gray topped, or gold topped.

2. List the dose and administration time of any thyroid drugs on the laboratory requisition
3. Do NOT draw specimens during hemodialysis.

Procedure
1. Draw a 4-mL blood sample. Cord blood may be used.

Postprocedure Care
1. Indicate pregnancy status on the laboratory requisition.

Client and Family Teaching
1. Results are normally available within 72 hours.

Factors That Affect Results
1. Results are invalidated if the client has undergone a radionuclide scan within 14 days before the test.
2. Results are invalidated in hemolyzed or lipemic specimens.
3. With the double-antibody testing method, results may be increased in the presence of anti-thyroxine antibodies.
4. With the single-antibody testing method, results may be decreased in the presence of anti-thyroxine antibodies.
5. Maternal serum concentrations of T_3, T_4, and TSH are lower in Blacks than Caucasians.

Other Data
1. Critically ill children in PICU have a 30 times increased mortality with decreased T_3 and T_4 levels.

Thyroid Test: Triiodothyronine by Ria

See Thyroid Test: Triiodothyronine—Blood.

Thyroid Ultrasonography (Thyroid Echogram, Thyroid Ultrasonogram)—Diagnostic

Norm. Proper size, shape, and position of the thyroid gland. Negative for cyst or tumor. Thyroid tissue demonstrates an even mixture of medium-level echoes. Suspicious for malignancy: hypoechogenicity, poorly defined irregular margins, and microcalcifications.

Usage. Differentiation between cyst and tumor not distinguishable by other studies;

guidance for aspiration of thyroid cyst or suspected thyroid tumor; monitoring of thyroid nodules during pregnancy; ongoing monitoring of size and density of thyroid during radioactive therapy; provides information about vascular flow and velocity when used with color-flow Doppler.

Description. High-frequency B-mode sonography and color-power Doppler are used to evaluate the thyroid gland size, shape, and positions. Ultrasound creates an oscilloscopic picture from the echoes of high-frequency sound waves passing over the neck area (acoustic imaging). The time required for the ultrasonic beam to be reflected back to the transducer from differing densities of tissue is converted by a computer to an electrical impulse displayed on an oscilloscopic screen to create a three-dimensional picture of the thyroid gland. The differing tissue densities of cysts and tumors enable the ultrasonogram to be helpful in determining which is present. Cysts are clearly demarcated by smooth borders and do not demonstrate internal echoes. Adenoma appearances vary but usually demonstrate halo. Multinodular goiter may also demonstrate a halo. In thyroiditis, the gland appears enlarged, with a greater than normal amount of low-level echoes. Ultrasound is a cost-effective procedure for screening for thyroid cancer because thyroid tissue has a high echogenicity. Thyroid cancer is usually poorly defined, with low-level echoes and without a halo. Advantages of this test are that it is safe for use during pregnancy because it does not use radiation, it can visualize the entire area of the anterior neck, it can detect smaller nodules (2 mm) than a nuclear scan, it can differentiate cysts from solid nodules (which a nuclear scan cannot), and it can improve the sensitivity of fine-needle aspiration biopsy.

Professional Considerations
Consent form NOT required.

Preparation
1. Remove any metallic objects or jewelry from the head and neck area.
2. Obtain ultrasonic gel.

Procedure
1. The client is positioned supine, with a towel roll, pillow, or sponge beneath the shoulder blades, and the neck hyperextended, with the head turned away from the side of the thyroid gland being scanned. This permits better transducer access to the area because the mandible is moved out of the scanning area.
2. The neck area is covered with ultrasonic gel, and a lubricated transducer is passed slowly and firmly over the thyroid gland and neck at specific intervals. Each lobe of the thyroid gland is examined separately and completely, beginning with transverse scanning followed by longitudinal scanning. Finally the isthmus is scanned transversely.
3. Photographs are taken of the oscilloscopic display.
4. The procedure takes less than 20 minutes.

Postprocedure Care
1. Remove ultrasonic gel from the skin.
2. If thyroid cyst aspiration is performed under ultrasonogram guidance, see separate test listing: Needle aspiration—Diagnostic.

Client and Family Teaching
1. The procedure is painless.

Factors That Affect Results
1. Thyroid volume is larger in males than in females, and varies with body surface area.

Other Data
1. Ultrasound alone should not be relied on for diagnosis of malignant thyroid nodules. Aspiration biopsy cytologic examination is necessary to confirm or add to the diagnosis.
2. The incidence of thyroid cancer among familiar adenomatous polyposis patients is high.
3. Abnormalities of thyroid function common in microdeletion of chromosome 22q11.

Thyroxine
See Thyroid Test: Thyroxine—Blood.

Tilt Table Test (Head-Up Tilt Table Test)—Diagnostic

Norm. Negative or absence of hypotension or bradycardia with position changes.

Usage. Evaluation of recurrent idiopathic syncope once cardiac causes have been ruled out. Vasovagal syncope (also known as vasodepressor, neurodepressor, dysautonomia, or neurogenic syncope) is a sudden, short-term loss of consciousness caused by malfunction in the regulatory mechanisms between the nervous and cardiac systems.

Description. The head-upright table, by sudden assumption of an upright position, can produce passive orthostatic stress, which induces syncope in individuals affected by vasovagal (neurally mediated) syncope. Administration of an intravenous isoproterenol (Isuprel) infusion increases sensitivity of the tilt table test for those susceptible to vasovagal syncope by producing the elevation of circulating catecholamines associated with this type of event.

Professional Considerations
Consent form IS required.

Risks
Dizziness, dysrhythmias, hypotension, tachycardia.
Contraindications
Gradual loss of more than 500 mL of blood, hypertension, hypotension.

Preparation
1. See Client and Family Teaching.
2. Start an IV at KO (keep-open) rate for administration of isoproterenol or emergency medication.

Procedure
1. The test can be run while the client is medicated or unmedicated.
2. Baseline monitoring of heart rate (HR), rhythm (ECG), blood pressure (BP), with the client in a supine resting state every 5 minutes for 15-30 minutes.
3. The table is then tilted up to 90 degrees for usually 5-7 minutes (up to 30 minutes). NOTE: Duration of the tilt has been found to be a more important variable than tilt angle. Duration of the tilt should be determined based on the suspected cause of the orthostatic intolerance: approximately 5 minutes to document orthostatic hypotension, approximately 10 minutes to identify orthostatic tachycardia, or neurally mediated syncope.
4. BP and HR are monitored and documented every minute for 25-45 minutes by automatic cuff or arterial line and ECG.
5. The test is terminated, and the client is returned to the supine position when presyncopal hypotension and bradycardia or full syncope develop.
6. Isoproterenol provocation may be added if no symptoms are produced during the unmedicated test.
   a. Return the client to the supine position for 5 to 10 minutes for the recovery period.
   b. Isoproterenol may then be added as a single-stage protocol (1 μg/minute for 5 minutes) or as a multi-stage protocol (repeated 3 times with progressively increasing doses of 1, 2, and 3 μg/minute).
   c. The table is tilted 60-80 degrees after each stage, and the test proceeds as previously described.

Postprocedure Care
1. Monitor vital signs for 15 minutes.
2. Full return to consciousness and baseline BP and HR is usually rapid when the client is placed in the supine position.
3. Normal intake and activity can be resumed immediately after the test.
4. Occasionally temporary residual pallor, weakness, headache, and bradycardia (rarely) last up to 30 minutes.

Client and Family Teaching
1. Any medication known to cause orthostatic hypotension or bradycardia should be stopped at least 3 days before the test. Your physician will tell you which drugs to stop.
2. Fast from food and fluids for 4-8 hours before the test.
3. Describe the procedure and the usual sensations the client can expect related to the tilt table test (see under Procedure). With the medicated test, mild stomach

cramping, salty taste in the mouth, and minor vision changes are not unusual. Increased heart rate and light-headedness are common.
4. An IV line will be inserted before the test.
5. The goal of the test is to reproduce syncope or near-syncope in a carefully controlled environment in which the client will not fall.
6. Usual testing time takes 1-2 hours.
7. Normal diet and activity may be resumed after the test is complete.
8. If you develop chest pain after the procedure, call 911. Do not drive yourself to the hospital.
9. Call the doctor if you experience shortness of breath, a fainting spell, a severe headache or dizziness, or pain in your back.

Factors That Affect Results
1. The positive effect of the isoproterenol-tilt table declines with age.
2. The syncopal homozygotes 825TT GNB3 gene significantly lowers the chance of syncope during tilt testing whereas those with a Gly389 allele have a higher chance of fainting.

Other Data
1. Abrupt infusion of 5 g of isoproterenol may cause intolerable changes in HR and BP.
2. This test is up to 75% effective in reproducing vasovagal syncope.
3. 67% elderly have a positive response to tilt table test with 30% having a severe response including second degree AV-block, severe bradycardia or hypotension and cardiac arrest.

Tissue Pathology

See **Histopathology**—Specimen.

Tissue Polypeptide Antigen (TPA)—Serum or Plasma

Norm. 78-5,000 pg/mL.

Usage. Indicates the presence of malignancy when cancers such as non-small cell lung cancer (Buccheri, Torchio, Ferrigno, 2003), bladder, and gynecologic cancers are present. Helps monitor response to treatment for bladder and lung cancer in males.

Description. Tissue polypeptide antigen (TPA) is a complex of polypeptide fragments that circulates in the blood and is elevated when there is higher-than-normal cell proliferation, as occurs in conditions where tumors are present. This enzyme-linked immunoassay of blood has a sensitivity for detecting early stage cancer of 31% to 64% and thus is not often used in clinical practice. Instead, chest CT and bronchoscopy provide higher sensitivity.

Professional Considerations
Consent form NOT required.

Preparation
1. Tube: Red topped or lavender topped.

Procedure
1. Collect a 3-mL sample.

Postprocedure Care
1. Store sample refrigerated until testing.
2. After using centrifuge, sample is stable for 5 days when refrigerated, or 1 month when frozen.

Client and Family Teaching
1. Not applicable.

Factors That Affect Results
1. High levels may be present in the absence of malignancy, in clients with cirrhosis or chronic liver damage and portal hypertension.

Other Data
1. None.

Tissue Typing

See **Human Leukocyte Antigen Typing**—Blood.

T-Lymphocytes—Blood

Norm.

	SI Units
500-2400/mm³ or 500-2400/μL	500-2400 × 10⁶ cells/L
45%-85% of total lymphocytes	0.45-0.85 fraction of total lymphocytes
75%-80% of circulating lymphocytes	0.75-0.80 fraction of total circulating lymphocytes

Increased. Autoimmune disease, delayed hypersensitivity reactions, and Graves' disease. Herbal or natural remedies include *Astragalus mongholicus, Acanthopanax senticosus,* and *Panax ginseng.*

Decreased. Agammaglobulinemia (sex-linked, Swiss-type), AIDS, antibody to human T-cell lymphotropic virus, ataxia telangiectasia, chronic mucocutaneous candidiasis, Hodgkin's disease, immunosuppression, lepromatous leprosy, leukemia (chronic lymphocytic), lymphoma, Nezelof syndrome, systemic lupus erythematosus, thymic hypoplasia, transplant rejection, and Wiskott-Aldrich syndrome. Drugs include immunosuppressives and steroids.

Description. T-lymphocytes are white blood cells with a long life span that are produced by and receive an antigenic imprint in the thymus gland. T-lymphocytes are responsible for a cell-mediated type of immunity and control of the immune system response. Subsets of T-lymphocytes secrete lymphokines such as interferon, chemotaxin, and macrophage migration–inhibition factor that function in cell-mediated immune response to varying antigens. Three of the T-lymphocyte subsets are "helper T cells" (OKT-4 cells), which help B cells produce certain antibodies; "suppressor T cells" (OKT-8 cells), which prevent unnecessary formation of antibodies; and "cytotoxic killer T cells," which have the ability to cause lysis of specific targeted cells such as those containing viral antigens. Overall, T-lymphocytes function in both good and bad ways. The T-cell characteristics that are beneficial by helping provide resistance to tumor and immunoresistance to bacterial and viral antigens can also harm the body via delayed hypersensitivity reactions, autoimmune responses, and rejection of transplanted tissue. This test is used to type and classify lymphocytic leukemias and lymphomas as well as define immunedeficient states such as AIDS. Identification of T-lymphocytes is accomplished by the "rosette technique," in which sheep erythrocytes gather around T cells to form a rosette pattern.

Professional Considerations

Consent form NOT required.

Preparation

1. Tube: Heparinized green topped tube.
2. Do NOT draw specimens during hemodialysis.

Procedure

1. Draw a 5-mL blood sample.

Postprocedure Care

1. Send specimens to the laboratory for processing within 2 hours.

Client and Family Teaching

1. Results are normally available within 24 hours.

Factors That Affect Results

1. Prolonged refrigeration decreases levels of helper T cells (OKT-4 cells).

Other Data

1. See also Acquired immune deficiency syndrome evaluation battery—Diagnostic; T- and B-lymphocyte subset assay—Blood.

Tobramycin—Serum

Norm. Negative.

Tobramycin Therapy		SI Units
Trough		
Therapeutic	0.5-2 μg/mL	1-4 μmol/L
Serious infection	0.5-1 μg/mL	1-2 μmol/L

Tobramycin Therapy		SI Units
Life-threatening infection	1-2 µg/mL	2-4 µmol/L
Peak		
Therapeutic	4-10 µg/mL	8-12 µmol/L
Serious infection	6-8 µg/mL	12-17 µmol/L
Life-threatening infection	8-10 µg/mL	17-21 µmol/L

Panic Level Symptoms and Treatment
Both sustained high peak and trough levels can be toxic.
Symptoms. Ototoxicity, nephrotoxicity, neuromuscular toxicity.
Treatment
NOTE: Treatment choice(s) depend(s) on client's history and condition and episode history.
1. Hydrate to keep urine output ≥3 mL/ kg/hour.
2. Hemodialysis and peritoneal dialysis remove tobramycin. High-permeability dialysis is likely to remove tobramycin.
3. The use of activated charcoal has not been shown to increase elimination of tobramycin.

Usage. Monitoring for therapeutic and safe levels during tobramycin therapy.

Description. Tobramycin is an aminoglycoside antibiotic used to treat infections caused by certain gram-negative bacilli that are resistant to gentamicin. It causes misreading of the genetic code to prevent protein synthesis by the bacterial ribosome. Tobramycin is minimally metabolized, with most of it being excreted in the urine, with a half-life of 2 hours and peak levels reached within 30 minutes (IV doses) or 30-60 minutes (IM doses). Nephrotoxicity (probably reversible) and ototoxicity (probably irreversible) are possible at levels only slightly above the therapeutic peak and trough levels. Therefore it is very important to monitor tobramycin levels during its usage. Clients with any degree of preexisting renal failure are at higher risk for toxicity because of impaired ability to clear the drug from the body.

Professional Considerations
Consent form NOT required.

Preparation
1. Tube: Red topped, red/gray topped, or gold topped.

2. Do NOT draw specimens during hemodialysis.

Procedure
1. Draw trough levels just before the dose. Draw peak levels 30 minutes after the last intravenous dose or 30 minutes to 3 hours after the last intramuscular dose.
2. Draw a 4-mL blood sample. Label the specimen as "trough" or "peak."

Postprocedure Care
1. Record the collection time on the laboratory requisition.

Client and Family Teaching
1. The information is needed to make sure the safe and effective dose of tobramycin is being given.
2. Drink 2-3 liters of water each day when taking tobramycin.
3. Results are normally available within 4 hours.

Factors That Affect Results
1. In clients with normal renal function, 24-36 hours are required before steady-state levels are reached.
2. Hyperlipidemia may cause falsely elevated results.
3. Cross-reactivity may occur from clients co-treated with gentamicin or netilmicin.
4. For aerosolized tobramycin delivery, use of a holding chamber results in greater delivery of the medication than use of a T-piece.
5. Peak tobramycin levels drawn from central venous access devices (CVADs) flushed with 3 mL flush volume are falsely elevated compared to peripheral venipuncture samples. Use of a 10-20 mL flush in the CVAD, however, provided 87% accurate information for clinical decision making.

Other Data
1. Renal function (creatinine, beta$_2$-microglobulin, muramidase, albumin)

and hearing should be monitored throughout therapy with tobramycin.

2. A once-daily dosing regimen has been shown to be safe and effective for mother and fetus during pregnancy.

3. An every-6-hour dosing regimen with a larger daily dosage administered has been shown in one study to provide better pulmonary function and longer time of wellness in clients with cystic fibrosis than an every-8-hour dosing regimen.

4. Usual methods of continuous ambulatory peritoneal dialysis (CAPD) result in relatively low drug clearance during any specific dialysate exchange, but cumulative drug removal may necessitate dosage supplementation with increased flow rates. Tobramycin added to the peritoneal dialysate is absorbed into the bloodstream.

5. Aminoglycosides are inactivated when used concomitantly with antipseudomonal penicillins in the treatment of gram-negative infections in the client with renal failure.

6. Nebulized tobramycin at 300 mg over 30 minutes every 12 hours reveals low systematic absorption and no renal effects.

Tolbutamide Tolerance Test (TTT)—Diagnostic

Norm.

Response to Tolbutamide Administration

	Serum Glucose Level			Serum Insulin Level
	30 Minutes, G_{30}	90-120 Minutes, G_{90-120}	180 Minutes, G_{180}	
Normal	50% below baseline	80%-100% of baseline	Baseline	Remains ≤150 µIU/mL
Abnormal		40%-64% of baseline		Rapid serum insulin increase above baseline at 10, 20, and 30 minutes. >150 µIU/mL at 60 minutes
Fasting hypoglycemia		<55 mg/dL (lean persons) <62 mg/dL (obese persons)		

Usage. Helps diagnose insulinoma; also used in the differential diagnosis of types of hypoglycemia.

Description. There are primarily three types of hypoglycemia: one type that involves an insulin-secreting tumor of the pancreas known as "insulinoma;" one that that is the result of hyperactive islet cells; and a third type that is a result of liver disease. Insulinomas secrete disproportionately high levels of insulin in response to blood glucose levels, causing frequent hypoglycemic episodes. Insulinoma can be diagnosed through this indirect test that administers intravenous tolbutamide, a sulfonylurea that stimulates the pancreas to produce insulin. When administered to a person with insulinoma, there is an exaggerated response, causing abnormally rapid and high insulin levels and abnormally prolonged hypoglycemic response.

Professional Considerations
Consent form IS required.

Risks
Acute hypoglycemic reaction.
Contraindications
In pediatric or pregnant clients or in clients with baseline glucose levels less than 60 mg/dL.

Preparation
1. Tubes: Red topped, red/gray topped, or gold topped. Also obtain ice for the blood sample for insulin measurement.

2. Obtain baseline blood samples for glucose and insulin levels. Evaluate results before beginning tolbutamide infusion.
3. Because of the risk of acute hypoglycemia during this test, have oral glucose/rapid-acting carbohydrate and/or 50% dextrose in water available for emergency treatment.
4. Establish patent intravenous access.
5. Just before beginning the procedure, take a "time out" to verify the correct client, procedure, and site.

Procedure

1. Draw a 3-mL baseline blood sample immediately before tolbutamide injection for glucose in a red topped tube.
2. Draw a 7-mL blood sample for insulin immediately before tolbutamide injection in a red topped, red/gray topped, or gold topped tube. Place tube immediately on ice.
3. Administer tolbutamide 1 g (or 25-40 mg/kg) IV push over 2-3 minutes.
4. Client should rest comfortably over the next 2 hours while being monitored closely for signs of acute hypoglycemia.

5. Draw serial glucose and insulin samples at 0, 2, 10, 20, 30, 60, 90, 120, 150, and 180 minutes after the tolbutamide infusion is completed.

Postprocedure Care

1. Client should eat a meal containing rapid-acting carbohydrates.

Client and Family Teaching

1. Eat a high-carbohydrate meal for each of the 3 days before this test. Then fast after midnight the night before the test or for at least 8 hours, if the test is not done in the early morning.
2. This test can take up to 3 hours.

Factors That Affect Results

1. Concurrent use of beta-adrenergic blockers will diminish response to the test.
2. Response to tolbutamide may be altered in clients taking MAO inhibitors, sulfonylureas (oxyphenbutazone, phenylbutazone), probenecid, and salicylates.

Other Data

1. The treatment for insulinoma is surgical removal; the other types of hypoglycemia can often be managed medically.

Tonometry Test for Glaucoma—Screen

Norm. 10-22 mm Hg; mean 16 mm Hg with standard deviation of 3 mm Hg.
Warning: 22-28 mm Hg. More testing required.
Normal values of 21 mm Hg or less can occur in a condition known as normal or low-tension glaucoma.
Major concern: >38 mm Hg.
Panic levels: There is lack of definitive intraocular pressure cutoff level for glaucoma.

Usage. Screening (not diagnostic) for glaucoma. Ongoing monitoring for clients with glaucoma.

Description. In glaucoma, the intraocular pressure increases either because of blocked drainage or because of excessive production of aqueous humor. Applanation tonometry testing involves measurement of intraocular pressure using a tonometer, an instrument that is lightly pressed directly against the anesthetized eye. The tonometry test can be conducted in any of three ways. In contact tonometry, in which the instrument touches the eye, the Schiøtz method, the Goldmann applanation method (commonly known as the "blue light" test), or a handheld method with a small penlike tonometer may be used. Contact tonometers make an indentation in the eye with a specific amount of weight and record the amount of resistance to the indentation, which is then converted to an intraocular pressure. In noncontact (indentation) tonometry, pneumotonometry or "air" tonometry may be used. Noncontact tonometry measures eye pressure indirectly. Noncontact tonometry has been found to improve compliance with testing in children, and there has been improvement in the accuracy of the handheld units. However, noncontact tonometry results in the same client may be higher than the results from applanation tonometry. Pneumotonometry is the gentlest method and preferred for clients after LASIK surgery. The new dynamic contour tonometer is the most accurate. Overall, tonometry is superior to *digital tension*, which tends to underestimate pressure, for obtaining intraocular pressure in young children. The Goldmann applanation method is considered the criterion standard for this procedure.

Professional Considerations
Consent form NOT required.

Risks
Corneal abrasion or infection.

Contraindications
Corneal infection or ulcer, unless absolutely necessary. It is also contraindicated in clients who may be unable to hold very still during the test (that is, those with persistent coughing or sneezing).

Preparation
1. Remove contact lenses and loosen any jewelry or clothing (e.g., tie, tight collar, necklace) around the neck area.
2. For all methods except the noncontact methods, anesthetic eye drops are instilled bilaterally.
3. Schiøtz method: Obtain sterile tonofilms for the contact tonometer.

Procedure
1. Schiøtz method:
   a. The client is positioned supine.
   b. One eye is tested at a time. After the tonometer is zeroed, the eyelids are held open as the tonometer is placed against the eyeball. The tonometer is pressed against the eye with a specific amount of weight, and the tonometer scale reflects a number that is converted to millimeters of mercury (mm Hg) for an intraocular pressure (IOP) reading.
2. Goldmann applanation method:
   a. A fluorescein-stained paper is touched against the surface of the eye and removed.
   b. The slit-lamp is advanced until the tonometer touches the eye surface.
   c. A digital measurement of the pressure required to flatten a small portion of the eye surface is recorded.
3. Handheld tonometer method:
   a. A small, penlike handheld tonometer is lightly pressed against the surface of the eye and a digital measurement of the eye pressure is taken.
4. Noncontact "air puff" method (indentation tonometry):

a. The client's head is positioned on a chin rest and the equipment is aligned to the eye. As a calibrated puff of air is expelled from the equipment against the eye surface, this causes an indentation in the eye surface and a photoelectric cell measures the amount of corneal deformity indicated by changing reflections back to the light source from the corneas.
5. Noncontact pneumotonometry method:
   a. A handheld pneumotonometer connected to a long tube is placed against the cornea. A stream of air flows through the tube and is directed into the sensing tip, where ocular pressure, standard deviation, and ocular pulse pressure are measured and displayed on a screen.

Postprocedure Care
1. Eyeglasses may be worn in place of contact lenses.
2. See Client and Family Teaching.

Client and Family Teaching
1. Provide a thorough explanation of the procedure, emphasizing that the client must cooperate by keeping the eyes open during testing.
2. Contact lenses must be removed. Bring eyeglasses to wear, if needed, after the test.
3. Avoid rubbing the eyes or replacing contact lenses until the local anesthetic has worn off (about 2 hours). Rubbing the eyes before this time can cause corneal abrasion, which is painful and takes several days to heal.

Factors That Affect Results
1. Diurnal variation exists, with levels higher in the evening than in the morning.
2. It may be necessary to adjust the weight placed against the eyeball to obtain a consistent pressure reading.
3. Clients who have undergone laser eye surgery may test normal, yet still have increased intraocular pressure, because laser eye surgery results in thinner corneas.
4. Thick corneas lead to overestimates; while thin corneas lead to underestimated findings.

Other Data
1. IOP evaluation in the detection of glaucoma has approximately 50% specificity.

2. Pneumotonometry is another specialized method of measuring IOP and is used in cases of irregular corneas or after keratoplasty when the applanation tonometer cannot be used.

3. For abnormal findings, the client should have a full ophthalmologic examination, including cup-to-disk ratio and field studies.

TORCH

See **Toxoplasmosis, Other, Rubella, Cytomegalovirus, Herpes Virus Serology**—Blood.

Total Body Scan

See **Bone Scan**—Diagnostic.

Total Iron-Binding Capacity (TIBC)

See **Iron and Total Iron-Binding Capacity/Transferrin**—Serum.

Toxicology, Drug Screen—Blood or Urine

Norm. Negative.

Overdose Symptoms and Treatment
(See individual test listings.)
Treatment of Overdose
(See individual test listings.)

Usage. Monitor toxic, overdose, or newly comatose situations; screen for drug abuse; determine causes for agranulocytosis, impotence, and pruritus; screen for substance use in on-the-job injuries.

Description. Toxicology drug screening is normally done with a urine test via immunoassay for several drugs. Positive results are confirmed by gas chromatography and additional blood testing may be requested. Common drugs included in this test are acetaminophen, alcohol, amphetamines, barbiturates, benzodiazepines, cannabinoids, cocaine metabolite, hypnotics, methadone, methaqualone, narcotics, opiates, organic bases, phencyclidine, phenothiazines, phenytoins, salicylates, and tricyclic antidepressants. Drugs NOT detected by this rapid test method include clonidine, calcium-channel blockers, beta-adrenergic blockers, and albuterol. (See also Toxicology, volatiles group by GLC—Blood or Urine, and many are also in individual test listings.)

Professional Considerations
Consent form NOT required unless results may be used for legal purposes.

Preparation
1. *Blood:* Tube: red topped, red/gray topped, or gold topped or lavender topped.
2. *Urine:* Obtain a clean container with a tight-fitting lid.

Procedure
1. If the specimen may be used as legal evidence, have the specimen collection witnessed.
2. *Blood*: Draw a 2-mL blood sample in a red topped, red/gray topped, or gold topped tube, or draw a 5-mL blood sample in a lavender topped tube.
3. *Urine*: Obtain a 50-mL random urine specimen in a clean container. Tightly cap the container.

Postprocedure Care
1. Specify suspected drug(s) on the requisition.
2. If the specimen may be used for legal purposes, write the client's name, date, exact time of collection, and specimen source on the laboratory requisition. Sign and have the witness sign the laboratory requisition. Transport the specimen to the laboratory immediately in a sealed plastic bag marked as legal evidence. All clients handling the specimen should sign and

mark the time of receipt on the laboratory requisition.

3. Assess for possible signs of drug withdrawal.

Client and Family Teaching

1. Results are normally not available for days.
2. If activated charcoal was given for elevated levels, the client should drink 4-6 glasses of water each day for 2 days to prevent constipation. The activated charcoal will also cause stools to be black for a few days.
3. For intentional overdose, refer the client and family for crisis intervention and offer resource information for counseling.
4. Referrals to appropriate rehabilitation centers and therapeutic community programs should be offered to all addicted clients who may be interested.
5. Ethanol-based hand sanitizer if ingested can cause acute ethanol poisoning in children.

Factors That Affect Results

1. Failure to maintain a clear chain of custody may invalidate results for legal purposes.
2. Failure to tightly cap the specimen container may cause falsely decreased results for volatiles.
3. False positive results possible:
   Amphetamines/Methamphetamines: Brompheniramine, Bupropion, Chlorpromazine, Phenylpropanolamine, Promethazine, Ranitidine, Trazodone.
   Barbiturates: Ibuprofen, Naproxen.
   Benzodiazepines: Sertraline.
   Cannabinoids: Ibuprofen, Naproxen.
   Methadone: Chlorpromazine, Clomipramine, Diphenhydramine, Doxylamine, Quetiapine, Thioridazine, Verapamil.

Opiates: Quinolones (ciprofloxacin, clinafloxacin, enoxacin, gatifloxacin, levofloxacin, lomefloxacin, moxifloxacin, norfloxacin, ofloxacin, pefloxacin, sparfloxacin).

Phencyclidine: Dextromethorphan, Ibuprofen, Venlafaxine.

Other Data

1. The test provides only qualitative detection of drugs. Any drug identified in a screening should be confirmed by a test specific to that drug.
2. The blood drug screening is usually performed with urine drug screening.
3. Barbiturates co-ingested with other substances have the highest incidence of mortality out of all cases of sedative-hypnotic overdose.
4. The AdultaCheck 4 Test Strip can be used to identify if a urine specimen has been tampered with or adulterated.
5. The Advanced Quality One Step Multi-Drug Screen test (barbiturates, benzodiazepines, cocaine, MDMA) is reliable for abuse screening in postmortem urine.
6. Morphine is secreted by neutrophils during sepsis.
7. Infants with hypoxic ischemic encephalopathy have elevated serum morphine levels during infusion rate >10 microg/kg/hour.
8. Morphine in low concentrations depresses seizure activity but in higher concentrations enhances seizures (mice research).
9. Ceftriaxone antibiotic decreases efficacy of morphine (rat research).
10. See also individual listings of specific drugs or classes of drugs for therapeutic ranges and panic levels.

Toxicology, Volatiles Group by Gas Liquid Chromatography (GLC)—Blood or Urine

Norm. Negative for acetone, ethyl alcohol (ethanol), ethylene glycol, isopropanol, and methyl alcohol (methanol).

Positive. Ingestion of substances.

		SI Units
Blood Panic Levels		
Acetone	>20 mg/dL	>3.44 mmol/L
Ethyl alcohol (ethanol)	>100 mg/dL	>21.7 mmol/L

		SI Units
Ethylene glycol	>20 mg/dL	>3.2 mmol/L
Lethal level	>30 mg/dL	>4.8 mmol/L
Isopropanol	>400 mg/L	>6.64 mmol/L
Methanol	>200 mg/L	>6.24 mmol/L
Urine Panic Levels		
Acetone	>27 mg/dL	>4.65 mmol/L
Ethyl alcohol (ethanol)	>100 mg/dL	>21.7 mmol/L
Ethylene glycol	Presence of oxalate crystals in urine	Presence of oxalate crystals in urine
Isopropanol (isopropyl alcohol)	>500 μg/mL; >150 mg/dL	>8.32 mmol/L
Methanol	>50 mg/L	>1.56 mmol/L

Overdose Symptoms and Treatment

NOTE: Treatment choice(s) depend(s) on client's history and condition and episode history.

Acetone Panic Level Symptoms. Coma, hypotension, respiratory depression.

Acetone Panic Level Treatment

1. Support airway, breathing, and circulation.
2. Perform hourly neurologic checks.
3. Measure blood glucose; monitor serum and urine acetone levels; and provide arterial pH monitoring.
4. Hemodialysis WILL remove acetone. Hemoperfusion will NOT remove acetone.

Ethyl Alcohol (Ethanol) Poisoning Symptoms

<50 mg/dL	Muscular incoordination
50-100 mg/dL	Worsening incoordination of movement
100-150 mg/dL	Mood and behavior changes
150-200 mg/dL	Delayed reactions
200-300 mg/dL	Ataxia, double vision, nausea, vomiting
300-400 mg/dL	Amnesia, dysarthria, hypothermia
400-700 mg/dL	Respiratory failure, coma, death possible

Ethyl Alcohol Poisoning Treatment

1. Support oxygenation and breathing.
2. Consider NG aspiration and rapid lavage if within 4 hours of ingestion. Do NOT use gastric lavage.
3. Hemodialysis WILL remove ethanol but is seldom necessary unless levels rise

>300 mg/dL. During hemodialysis, levels drop an average of 62 mg %/hour.

Isopropanol Panic Level Symptoms. Coma, confusion, dizziness, headache, hypotension, nausea, oliguria initially; followed by diuresis, respiratory depression, stupor, uncoordinated movement, vomiting. Death is possible. Levels >150 mg/dL produce coma and hypotension and levels >400 mg/dL are incompatible with life.

Isopropanol Panic Level Treatment

1. Implement aspiration precautions and support airway.
2. Administer vasopressors for hypotension.
3. Hemodialysis is usually indicated when levels exceed 400 mg/dL. Peritoneal dialysis is minimally effective in removing isopropanol. Hemodialysis will not remove isopropanol but will remove its acetone metabolite.
4. Monitor electrolytes and treat imbalance.
5. Monitor for hepatic or renal damage.
6. Monitor closely for central nervous system depression. Administer thiamine and D_5W if client is obtunded.

Methanol Poisoning Symptoms. Half-life is 5 minutes with peak absorption 30-60 minutes. Indications for treatment include plasma concentration 0.20mg/dL or 200 mg/L, osmolar gap >10 mOsm/kg, arterial pH <7.3, serum bicarbonate >20 meq/L. At 8-36 hours after ingestion: headache, weakness, blurred vision, abdominal and back pain, nausea and vomiting, dizziness, hallucinations and confusion, high anion gap metabolic acidosis, possible blindness, respiratory depression, and coma; death is possible. Lethal dose of pure methanol is 1-2 mL/kg. Permanent blindness and death reported between 0.1mL/kg (6-10 mL in adults).

Methanol Poisoning Treatment (within 2 hours of ingestion)

1. Support airway, breathing, and circulation.
2. Consider NG aspiration and rapid lavage if within 4 hours of ingestion.
3. Administer ethyl alcohol (ethanol) IV or PO to block breakdown of methanol into its toxic metabolites. Adjust infusion rate to maintain blood ethanol level of 100-150 mg/dL (may need higher doses in alcoholics). Remeasure ethanol levels frequently. Continue this treatment until methanol level is <20 mg/dL.
4. As an alternative to ethanol, fomepizole has been found to be effective as an antidote to methanol, and can eliminate the need for dialysis, but not in clients with renal problems or levels above 50 mg/dL. Administer IV loading dose of 15 mg/kg followed by maintenance dose of 10 mg/kg every 12 hours × 4, followed by 15 mg/kg every 12 hours to reach therapeutic fomepizole level >8.6 mg/mL. Continue until methanol concentrations are undetectable. Dosing frequency must be increased if dialysis is also used.
5. Dialyze to eliminate methanol and its toxic formic acid metabolites. Use forced diuresis if dialysis is not available. Indications for hemodialysis include methanol level >50 mg/dL, or pH <7.20, or renal failure, or presence of visual symptoms.
6. Correct acidemia with $NaHCO_3$ if pH is <7.20.
7. Keep environment dark to reduce stress on vision.
8. Consider using folic acid (leucovorin) in clients with folic acid deficiency. Give leucovorin 50 mg IV every 4 hours for several days. Folic acid potentiates metabolism of formic acid into carbon dioxide and water.

Usage. Evaluation for poisoning; monitoring response to treatment for poisoning. This test is frequently routine for clients who are newly unconscious with unknown cause.

Description. The toxicologic volatiles' screen tests for the presence of acetone, ethyl alcohol (ethanol), ethylene glycol, isopropanol, and methanol in a blood sample.

Acetone level helps identify isopropyl alcohol (isopropanol, rubbing alcohol) ingestion or toxicity because, when ingested, isopropanol is converted to acetone.

Isopropanol is a portion of rubbing alcohol (70% isopropanol), perfumes, aftershaves, and antifreeze that is metabolized to acetone, carbon dioxide, and water in the blood and urine. This alcohol is readily absorbed by the gastrointestinal tract, having a half-life of 30-180 minutes, and produces central nervous system depression. Isopropanol is often ingested in desperation by alcoholics.

Ethyl alcohol, also known as grain alcohol (ethanol), is a substance, often abused, that depresses the central nervous system and may lead to coma progressing to death at levels above the panic level listed above.

Ethylene glycol is the main compound contained in antifreeze—also found in other automotive products—that, when ingested and metabolized, causes toxicity to humans. Ethylene glycol may be ingested as an inexpensive substitute for alcohol. Methanol and isopropanol may be ingested by alcoholics accustomed to taking ethyl alcohol (ethanol) when ethyl alcohol is unavailable. After ingestion, oxalic acid is excreted by the kidneys, causing oxalate crystals in the urine, acidosis, tetany, and renal failure. Stages of clinical presentation include neurologic symptoms (vomit, euphoria, CNS depression), cardiopulmonary (hyperventilation, ARDS, heart failure), then renal symptoms (oliguria, flank pain, renal failure). The minimum lethal dose is approximately 100 mL, but any amount ingested may produce toxic symptoms. Half-life is 3 hours without treatment, 2.5 hours with dialysis, and 17 hours with concomitant orally administered ethyl alcohol.

Methyl alcohol—clear, colorless with a faint alcoholic odor, also known as wood alcohol (methanol)—is an alcohol produced in the distillation process and is sometimes found in improperly prepared alcohols, such as moonshine. It is also an ingredient in antifreeze, some varnishes, paints, paint thinners, windshield washer fluid, and camp stove fluid. Poisoning has led to Parkinsonism and polyneuropathy (days-weeks post ingestion).

Both blood and urine levels of these substances are important. Although blood levels reflect the most recently ingested substance(s), urine levels may reflect substances ingested over a longer period. This test is frequently routine for clients who are newly unconscious with unknown cause.

Professional Considerations
Consent form NOT required unless results may be used as legal evidence.

Preparation
1. Tube: Gray topped (contains glycolytic inhibitor) for the blood sample.
2. Obtain a clean container with a tight-fitting lid, and a container of ice for the urine sample.
3. Do NOT draw specimens during hemodialysis.

Procedure
1. Specimen collection should be witnessed if it may be used as legal evidence.
2. *Blood sample*: Do NOT use alcohol for venipuncture. Instead, cleanse the site with a povidone-iodine wipe and allow the area to dry. Draw a 5-mL blood sample. Tightly cap the tube.
3. *Urine sample*: Obtain a 50-mL random urine specimen in a clean container. Tightly cap the container. Transport it on ice.

Postprocedure Care
1. Place the urine specimen on ice.
2. Write the client's name, the date, the contents of the tube, and the exact time of specimen collection, along with your signature and the signature of the witness, on the tube label and laboratory requisition if the specimen may be used as legal evidence. Transport the specimen on ice to the laboratory in a sealed plastic bag labeled as legal evidence.
3. Store the blood or urine sample at 4 degrees C.
4. Monitor for panic level symptoms.

Client and Family Teaching
1. Results may be available within hours.
2. For intentional overdose, refer client and family for crisis intervention.
3. Referrals to appropriate rehabilitation centers and therapeutic community programs should be offered to all addicted clients who may be interested.

Factors That Affect Results
1. Failure to tightly cap the specimen container may cause falsely low results.
2. Failure to maintain a clear chain of custody may invalidate the results for legal purposes.

Other Data
1. Because of the low molecular weight of these volatiles, an osmolar gap results (see Osmolality, Calculated test—Blood).
2. Ethylene glycol can also be detected in gastric secretions.
3. The highest known ethylene glycol concentration in which a person survived is 1889 mg/dL.
4. See also Ethylene glycol—Serum and urine.

Toxoplasmosis, Other, Rubella, Cytomegalovirus, Herpesvirus Serology (TORCH)—Blood

Norm. Negative for all diseases.

Usage. Maternal and infant screening.

Description. This serologic test is performed to detect the congenitally acquired diseases of toxoplasmosis, rubella, cytomegalic inclusion disease, herpes, and others such as syphilis and varicella infections in infants who manifest symptoms of viral or other infections during the first year of life. The test may also be performed on the mother during pregnancy to screen for diseases that are likely to cause birth defects. The literature discounts the value of routine TORCH screening and discusses the value of various methods of testing (Abdel-Fattah et al, 2005). TORCH screening IS recommended in HIV-infected pregnant women who have not had previous TORCH screening. IgM enzyme-linked immunosorbent assay (ELISA) is recommended to detect recent toxoplasmosis or rubella, and culture is required to confirm herpes or cytomegalovirus infection.

Professional Considerations
Consent form NOT required.

Preparation
1. Tube: Red topped, red/gray topped, or gold topped.

Procedure
1. Draw a 3-mL blood sample.

Postprocedure Care
1. Any individual positive test or higher-than-normal titer should be repeated in 7-10 days to observe for changing titer.

Client and Family Teaching
1. Return in 7-10 days for repeat testing if the results are positive.

Factors That Affect Results
1. See individual test listings.

Other Data
1. For positive tests, genetic counseling may be indicated.
2. See individual test listings for full descriptions.
3. TORCH test sera should be held in the laboratory for 1 year in the event repeat testing is necessary.

Toxoplasmosis Serology—Serum

Norm.

Immunofluorescence	
Adults	IgM titer <1:64
	IgG titer <1:1024
Neonates	IgM undetectable
Indirect Hemagglutination	
No previous infection	Titer <1:4
Probable past infection	Titers >1:4 and <1:256
Suggestive of recent infection	Titer >1:256

Increased. Current or past infection with *Toxoplasma gondii*.

Decreased. Not applicable.

Description. Toxoplasmosis is a systemic, parasitic disease caused by the protozoon *T. Gondii* and associated with surface antigen 2 gene (SAG2). Estimated acute infections are 18.5% with *T. Gondii* antibodies found in 15.33 (India) to 59.5% (Poland) of population. It is transmitted to humans by ingestion of the undercooked meat of infected animals, unpasteurized milk or often by the ingestion of oocysts acquired from handling cat litter containing contaminated cat feces. High risk occupations include forestry and animal workers. It may also be transmitted to a fetus through the placenta of an infected mother. After ingestion, this parasite travels to various body tissues and is found grouped together in oocysts. Acquired toxoplasmosis often causes no symptoms in clients with intact immune systems. In immunosuppression, it may cause hyperpyrexia, lymphadenopathy, lymphocytosis, and, in some cases, encephalitis, pneumonitis, myocarditis, myositis, and possibly death. Fetal congenital toxoplasmosis can cause severe birth defects, including blindness, hydrocephalus, and mental retardation, and may lead to fetal or postnatal death. Serologic testing for *T. gondii* antibody titer is recommended for all pregnant females. If antibody titer is low positive, indicating past infection, there is no risk to the fetus. However, the fetus is at risk for birth defects if the disease is acquired during pregnancy. Thus if antibody titer is initially high (indicative of current active infection) or initially negative, the test should be repeated at each prenatal checkup throughout the first 5 months of pregnancy and just before delivery. Toxoplasmosis occurs in advanced AIDS.

Professional Considerations
Consent form NOT required.

Preparation
1. Assess whether the woman has handled cat feces during pregnancy.
2. Assess whether the client has eaten any raw or undercooked meat.
3. Tube: Red topped, red/gray topped, or gold topped.

Procedure
1. Draw a 3-mL blood sample as soon as pregnancy is known or as soon as possible after symptoms appear. Label the specimen as the acute sample. Repeat the test in 7-14 days to detect rising antibody titer

and label the tube as the convalescent sample. For pregnancy, repeat the test as described under Description.

Postprocedure Care

1. None.

Client and Family Teaching

1. Cat owners who are pregnant or who have AIDS must feed the cat commercially prepared or well-cooked food and prevent the cat from roaming and scavenging. Avoid handling the cat litter if possible. Cat litter should be handled (preferably by another household member) with gloved hands and discarded every day, with daily disinfection of the litter container by rinsing with boiling water. If you must handle the cat litter or litter box, avoid touching anything else afterward until you have performed meticulous handwashing. Also avoid handling other cats and avoid gardening (where you may come into contact with contaminated cat feces).
2. Thoroughly cook any meat to be ingested.
3. Avoid unpasteurized milk.

4. Treatment includes parasite treatment and use of antioxidant vitamins.

Factors That Affect Results

1. None found.

Other Data

1. Except for placental-fetal transfer or cord-blood/bone marrow transplant, toxoplasmosis is not communicable between clients. Patients from northern Africa have higher, Asians a lower, probability of being immune.
2. Fatal acute disseminated breakthrough toxoplasmosis after haploidentical stem cell transplant has occurred (Garcia de la Fuente et al, 2010). After allogenic stem cell transplant all patients are at risk for toxoplasmosis and need to be monitored.
3. When toxoplasmosis is acquired early in pregnancy, abortion may be recommended.
4. Pyrimethamine, sulphonamides, and bumped kinase inhibitors are used to treat toxoplasmosis. Co-trimoxazole is treatment for toxoplasmotic lymphadenitis.

Toxoplasmosis Skin Test—Diagnostic

Norm. Negative.

Positive. Current or past infection with *Toxoplasma gondii*.

Description. Toxoplasmosis is a systemic, parasitic disease caused by the protozoon *T. gondii*. It is transmitted to humans by ingestion of the undercooked meat of infected animals or often by the ingestion of oocysts acquired from handling cat litter containing contaminated cat feces. It may also be transmitted to a fetus through the placenta of an infected mother. After ingestion, this parasite travels to various body tissues and is found grouped together in oocysts. Acquired toxoplasmosis often causes no symptoms in clients with intact immune systems. In immunosuppression, it may cause hyperpyrexia, lymphadenopathy, lymphocytosis, and, in some cases encephalitis, pneumonitis, myocarditis, myositis, and possibly death. Fetal congenital toxoplasmosis can cause severe birth defects, including blindness, hydrocephalus, and mental retardation, and may lead to fetal or postnatal death.

Professional Considerations

Consent form NOT required.

Preparation

1. Assess whether a pregnant woman has handled cat feces during her pregnancy.
2. Assess whether the client has eaten any raw or undercooked meat.
3. Obtain an alcohol wipe, a 4-mL syringe, an intradermal needle, *Toxoplasma* antigen, and a control.

Procedure

1. Cleanse the forearm injection site with an alcohol wipe, and allow the area to dry.
2. Inject *Toxoplasma* antigen intradermally and record the site of injection. Inject the control in the other arm, and record the site of injection.
3. Read the skin test in 24-48 hours. A positive test is indicated by redness and induration >10 mm in diameter.

Postprocedure Care

1. See Toxoplasmosis serology—Serum for pregnancy precautions and precautions for persons with AIDS.

Client and Family Teaching

1. After the injection, return in 24-48 hours for a skin test reading.

Factors That Affect Results

1. None found.

Other Data

1. Many clients may be infected with *T. gondii* but are free of symptoms. Therefore any pregnant woman should be tested for the presence of antibodies to *T. gondii*. See Toxoplasmosis serology—Serum.

TPA

See Tissue Polypeptide Antigen (TPA)—Serum or Plasma.

Tracer

See Glucose Monitoring Machines—Diagnostic.

Transcranial Cerebral Oximetry

See Transcranial Near-Infrared Spectroscopy—Diagnostic.

Transcranial Doppler Ultrasonography

See Doppler Ultrasonographic Flow Studies—Diagnostic.

Transcranial Near-Infrared Spectroscopy (NIRS, Cerebral Near-Infrared Spectroscopy, NIRS Phlebotomy, Transcranial Cerebral Oximetry)—Diagnostic

Norm. Norms not well established. Some studies indicate that a decrease in cerebral oxygen saturation (COS) of more than 25% indicates potentially correctable impending cerebral ischemia and the need for intervention.

Usage. Used in conjunction with transcranial Doppler to monitor cerebral oxygen metabolism during cardiac and neurologic surgical procedures in anesthetized clients; used in conjunction with EEG to assess cerebral activity in clients thought to be in a coma. COS values primarily represent the venous oxygenation of the brain (75% weight), and to a lesser extent the arterial oxygenation (25%). Also used to evaluate sleep apnea and epilepsy, and in phlebotomy to facilitate venipuncture. Other uses include helping to diagnose sinusitis, detecting dental decay, evaluating coronary arteries (use of indocyanine green or methylene blue), evaluating medication administration in ICUs to avoid medication errors, and detecting status epilepticus after pediatric cardiac surgery.

Description. Transcranial near-infrared spectroscopy (NIRS) is a bedside neuro-monitoring technique for detection of cerebral hypoxia by identifying changes in COS. The technique involves measuring changes in the absorption of light at a variety of wave lengths in the spectral range of 690 to 1100nm as it is transmitted through the skull, bone, brain, and cerebrospinal fluid. COS values change as the proportion of oxygen supply to oxygen consumption changes. Cerebral oxygen metabolism can be affected by any of five variables: mean arterial pressure, hemoglobin level, peripheral oxygen saturation, partial pressure of carbon dioxide, and core temperature. Use of NIRS during surgery can alert the physicians to possible inadequate anesthetic in which the waking brain uses more oxygen, or to cerebral seizures. Both conditions cause the COS to drop.

Professional Considerations

Consent form NOT required.

Preparation

1. Obtain near-infrared light emitter and receiver.
2. Verify that other monitoring systems are in place to co-assess the underlying variables that can affect COS: arterial monitoring, peripheral oxygen saturation, carbon dioxide monitoring, core temperature, cerebral seizures.

Procedure

1. For synchronous, bilateral monitoring, place sensors as high as possible on the forehead. Sensors should be shielded from ambient light.
2. Monitoring is carried out using a light emitter and sensors positioned near the forehead. Light emitted is reflected back to the receiver, which produces a graphical tracing of COS.

Postprocedure Care

1. Remove sensors.

Client and Family Teaching

1. This technique is used to help determine how well the brain is using oxygen.

Factors That Affect Results

1. Endovascular procedures in which arterial vasospasm occurs cause unreliable results.

2. Although decreased COS indicates impending ischemia, a stable COS does not necessarily signify intact cerebral processes.
3. Placement of sensors affects results. Readings are only indicative of the status of cerebral oxygenation in the region of the brain located near the sensors. Positioning sensors laterally instead of high on the forehead omits data from the sagittal sinus. Results are erroneous if sensors are placed near areas of damaged brain tissue or implants such as metal plates.
4. Areas of localized pooling of blood within the cranium will affect results. If pooled blood is unoxygenated, the results are not useful. Superficial or deep hematomas can cause false-negative results.
5. Factors that interfere with the validity of the results include the presence of strong ambient light in the room, use of electrocautery, recent injection of dyes in the client's bloodstream, mechanical motion, abnormal hemoglobin levels, and abnormal bilirubin levels.

Other Data

1. Interpretation of NIRS changes requires complex knowledge of physiologic mechanisms and consideration of all variables affecting the COS.

Transesophageal Echocardiogram

See Transesophageal Ultrasonography—Diagnostic.

Transesophageal Ultrasonography (Transesophageal Echocardiogram, TEE)—Diagnostic

Norm. Negative or normal structure or function and absence of a pathologic condition.

Usage. Transesophageal echocardiogram (TEE) is especially indicated for examination of prosthetic heart valves; detection of mitral valve regurgitation, pulmonary vein stenosis, aortic dissection (site and extent), congenital heart disease of the adult, cardiac tumors and masses, embolic or thrombotic disorders (particularly of the left atrium), vegetative endocarditis; and intraoperative guide to left ventricular function. Used for clients with conditions making standard transthoracic echocardiograms unreliable, such as obesity, chest deformities, chronic lung disease, or intubation; provides guidance for pericardiocentesis in cardiac tamponade; helps evaluate for transvenous pacemaker malposition; newer use in ruling out the presence of atrial thrombus before cardioversion as an alternative to anticoagulation.

Description. Ultrasound uses high-frequency sound waves to induce vibrations that echo or reflect from the solid structures within the body. These echoes create images from which chamber and valve size, function, and pericardial effusion can be determined. A specially adapted flexible gastroscope is fitted with a high-frequency transducer to send, receive, and translate the reflected vibrations. This tube, when swallowed or advanced into the esophagus, is positioned behind the heart and related structures. It can be rotated anteriorly, laterally, or posteriorly to allow an unimpeded route for sound-wave reflection off the heart chambers, walls, and valves. Abnormalities that are missed by standard diagnostic techniques can be displayed. Only the upper aortic view is limited by the interference of the left mainstem bronchus. The newest echocardiographic equipment includes three-dimensional capabilities, which can provide many views of the heart structures. A micro-TEE exists for use in small infants.

Professional Considerations
Consent form IS required.

Risks
Air embolism (post saline contrast); vasovagal bradycardia and drug-induced tachycardia are likely dysrhythmias; esophageal, oropharyngeal and gastric perforation/trauma; bleeding; transient hypoxemia; transient global amnesia; oversedation. Those with active infections who undergo TEE are at higher risk for methemoglobinemia.

Contraindications
Esophageal obstructions, stenosis, fistula, dysphagia or varices (> grade 2); history of radiation therapy to the esophagus or surrounding area (mediastinum); acute penetrating chest injuries. Neonates and young children are not candidates because of the unavailability of specially sized TEE scopes. Sedatives are contraindicated in clients with central nervous system depression. Also contraindicated in clients who cannot tolerate lying flat.

Preparation
1. See Client and Family Teaching.
2. Obtain a chest radiograph, ECG, and laboratory work, including CBC, electrolytes, PT, and PTT.

3. Start an IV infusion at KVO (keep-vein-open) rate for administration of conscious sedation (not necessary in routine adult cases) or emergency medications.
4. Remove dentures and glasses. Have the client void before the procedure.
5. A drying agent is typically given to reduce secretions (that is, glycopyrrolate 0.1-0.2 mg IV). Some clients require a small IV dose of an antianxiety agent (such as midazolam or diazepam). Prophylactic antibiotics are usually given if the client has a prosthetic valve.
6. Just before beginning the procedure, take a "time out" to verify the correct client, procedure, and site.

Procedure
1. The client is monitored continuously: heart rate and rhythm by cardiac monitor, blood pressure by noninvasive monitor, and O_2 by pulse oximetry.
2. Position the client in the left lateral decubitus position.
3. Topical anesthesia per physician preference is used to numb the throat and suppress the gag reflex. This may be repeated several times during the procedure.
4. The client should be awake enough to follow commands but drowsy. This procedure may also be performed on a fully anesthetized or intubated client.
5. The client is asked to open the mouth and flex the neck forward in a chin-to-chest position.
6. The lidocaine-lubricated probe is inserted, and the client is asked to swallow.
7. Over the next 5-20 minutes the probe is gently withdrawn, and cardiac images are viewed or recorded at different levels.
8. The nurse remains with the client to monitor respiratory status, vital signs, and cardiac rhythm and to assess the need for further sedation or suctioning.

Postprocedure Care
1. Continue assessment of respiratory status. If deep sedation was used, follow institutional protocol for post sedation monitoring. Typical monitoring includes continuous ECG monitoring and pulse oximetry with continual assessments (every 5-15 minutes) of airway, vital signs, and neurologic status until client reaches level 3, 2, or 1 on the Ramsay Sedation Scale.

2. Once the gag reflex has returned, the client can resume fluid intake. Full diet is not recommended until 3 hours after procedure.

Client and Family Teaching

1. Ask if the healthcare personnel is certified in perioperative TEE.
2. Fast for 6-8 hours before the test. Medications may be taken with a small amount of water as directed by the physician. You will have to remove your dentures/partials (can cause airway obstruction) and eyeglasses, but you should keep your hearing aid on so that you can hear the physician's instructions.
3. You may be given a sedative for the procedure. You should arrange for someone to drive you home because you may be drowsy after the procedure and will not be permitted to drive.
4. Do not eat or drink for 4-6 hours before the procedure. Take any prescription medications with a small sip of water.
5. This procedure lets the physician look at your heart and its major blood vessels from the back, without the lungs blocking the view. A flexible tube about the thickness of a pen is inserted into the mouth and moved down into the esophagus. The tip of the tube produces sound waves that bounce off the heart and are changed into pictures on a video screen.
6. Breathe through the nose and swallow during introduction of the probe, and breathe through the mouth for the remainder of the procedure, which takes about 30 minutes.
7. Your tongue and throat may feel swollen after the topical anesthetic; your mouth and lips will feel sticky and dry if a drying agent is used. Do not eat or drink after the procedure until the numbness is gone.
8. The doctor must review the videotape of the procedure before discussing the test results.
9. Discharge instructions: Promptly report persistent sore throat, dysphagia, stiff neck, and epigastric, substernal, or abdominal pain that worsens with breathing or movement.

Factors That Affect Results

1. See the description of the test.

Other Data

1. None.

Transfer Factor

See **Diffusing Capacity for Carbon Monoxide**—Diagnostic.

Transfer Function Index

See **Pulse Volume Recorder Testing of Peripheral Vasculature**—Diagnostic.

Transferrin, Carbohydrate-Deficient (CDT)—Serum

Norm. Quantitative: <6 units %; qualitative: not detected.

Quantitative Test	% of Transferrin
Pentasialo-	13%-23%
Tetrasialo-	38%-49%
Trisialo-	17%-31%
Disialo-	2%-15%
Monosialo-	0%-5%

Usage. Used sometimes with MCV and GGTP to detect recent heavy alcohol consumption; monitor for relapse after alcohol rehabilitation; helps diagnose carbohydrate-deficient glycoprotein syndromes. Also used to detect carbohydrate-deficient glycoprotein syndromes; rare autosomal recessive genetic traits in which levels of transferrin, haptoglobin, thyroxine-binding globulin, antithrombin II, and protein C are reduced (causing multisystemic symptoms such as skeletal problems and muscular weakness, ataxia, peripheral neuropathy, psychomotor or mental retardation, lipodystrophy); and problems with sight or vision.

Increased. Alcohol abuse, body builders, chemical use (nitro-based lacquer, plant protecting chemicals spread on farms), heavy intake protein, iron-depletion treatment.

Decreased. Carbohydrate-deficient glyco-protein syndrome. Drugs include iron compounds.

Description. Carbohydrate-deficient trans-ferrin (CDT) is transferrin with less than the normal amount of sugar chains. CDT is a sensitive and specific biologic marker for alcohol abuse in persons with normal iron states. The mechanism by which CDT increases in response to alcohol consumption is not yet well understood. Heavily influenced by mean alcohol consumption within 30 days before testing, CDT is elevated in clients who have had high alcohol consumption (>50-60 g/day) during this time. Many studies have found moderate sensitivity and specificity (80%-90%), but newer tests using lecithin-affinity chromatography have sensitivities and specificities close to 100%. CDT is equal in sensitivity but more specific than gamma-glutamyltranspeptidase for detection of long-term heavy alcohol consumption.

Professional Considerations
Consent form NOT required.

Preparation
1. *Qualitative* test: Tube: red topped. Also obtain dry ice.
2. *Quantitative* test (used for infants): Obtain alcohol wipe, capillary tube, lancet, and filter paper.

Procedure
1. *Quantitative* test: Obtain a 5-mL blood sample. Place tube on dry ice.
2. *Qualitative* test:
   a. Cleanse the lateral curvature of the infant's heel with alcohol and allow it to dry.
   b. Puncture the lateral heel curvature with a lancet.
   c. Collect blood in a capillary tube and completely saturate two spots on the filter paper card with heelstick blood.
   d. Allow the blood spot to dry before sending the sample to the lab.

Postprocedure Care
1. Apply pressure to the puncture site until the bleeding stops. Let the site air-dry.
2. Test is usually performed at a reference laboratory.

Client and Family Teaching
1. 5-14 days may be required for testing.
2. Offer resources for alcoholism treatment or genetic counseling if appropriate.

Factors That Affect Results
1. The test must be repeated if the blood amount is not enough to completely saturate both spots on the filter paper card.
2. Touching the filter paper or exposure to extremes of heat and light can cause errors in the results.
3. When the test is used to monitor for relapse after treatment, results should be compared to initial baseline specimen values.
4. Unexplained false-positive and false-negative results have been found in several studies. Iron overload accounts for some false-negative results. Therefore a negative result does not exclude the possibility of alcohol consumption. False-positive results may occur with pregnancy, liver abnormalities, metabolic syndrome, obesity, smoking, and chronic hemodialysis.
5. Concomitant liver disease reduces the specificity of this test.

Other Data
1. Only FDA approved test for identification of heavy alcohol use.

Transferrin—Serum

Norm.

		SI Units
Transferrin saturation	10%-55%	10%-55%
Adult	200-400 mg/dL	2-4.0 g/L
Maternal (term)	305 mg/dL	3.0 g/L
Fetal	190 mg/dL	1.9 g/L
Newborn	130-275 mg/dL	1.3-2.8 g/L

Increased. Iron-deficiency states with normal protein levels and pregnancy. Drugs include oral contraceptives.

Decreased. Congenital absence of transferrin (autosomal recessive hereditary atransferrinemia or hypotransferrinemia), hemolytic states, hepatic disease (acquired), inflammation (chronic), iron overload, low iron states combined with protein malnutrition, neoplasm, proteinuria (severe) and other protein-losing states, and renal disease.

Description. Transferrin is a beta globulin and glycoprotein with a short (7-day) half-life. Formed in the liver, transferrin transports dietary iron from the intestinal mucosa to iron-storage sites and hemoglobin-synthesis sites in the body (bone, muscle, erythrocytes, lymphocytes). Transferrin enables iron storage by binding to transferrin receptors at the iron-storage sites. Transferrin is capable of binding more than its own weight in iron. That is, 1 g of transferrin can carry 1.43 g of iron. Normally, iron saturation of transferrin (transferrin saturation) is between 20% and 45%. Because of its short half-life, values will decrease more quickly in protein malnutrition states than albumin will. Thus transferrin is sometimes used to evaluate nutritional status. Transferrin also has growth-stimulating properties that are separate from its iron-transport properties.

Professional Considerations

Consent form NOT required.

Preparation

1. See Client and Family Teaching.
2. Tube: Red topped, red/gray topped, or gold topped.

Procedure

1. Draw the specimen during the morning hours if it is to be used to evaluate transferrin saturation because a diurnal pattern with a morning peak exists.
2. Draw a 4-mL blood sample.

Postprocedure Care

1. None.

Client and Family Teaching

1. Fast from food and fluids (except water) for 12 hours before the test.
2. Results are normally available within 24 hours.

Factors That Affect Results

1. None found.

Other Data

1. Transferrin is also called "siderophilin" and "iron-binding protein."
2. See also Iron and total iron-binding capacity/transferrin—Serum; Soluble transferrin receptor assay—Serum.

Transferrin, Soluble Receptor

See Soluble Transferrin Receptor Assay—Serum.

Transferrin Saturation

See Iron and Total Iron-Binding Capacity/Transferrin—Serum; Transferrin—Serum.

Transfusion Reaction Work-Up—Diagnostic

Norm. Not applicable.
Transfusion Reaction Symptoms and Treatment

NOTE: Treatment choice(s) depend(s) on client's history and condition and episode history.

Mild Febrile Reaction

Symptoms	Treatment
Slight, nonsustained temperature increase <1 degree C Urticaria, rash, or hives Headache Malaise Mild chills	Slow the transfusion rate. Verify that the information on the client's blood band, hospital bracelet, blood bag, and blood transfusion requisition all correspond properly and notify the physician. *If all information matches properly, possible courses of action available to the physician include:* Continue the transfusion while monitoring the recipient closely for further development of hemolytic or nonhemolytic reaction. Add a microaggregate filter to filter the blood if not already being used. Administer antipyretic and antihistamine and continue the transfusion while monitoring the client closely for further development of hemolytic or nonhemolytic reaction. Stop the transfusion, and return the blood to the blood bank. Stop the transfusion, and complete the transfusion reaction blood work and urine tests as described below.

Hemolytic Reaction

Symptoms	Treatment
Early signs Sustained rise in temperature >1 degree C Nausea or vomiting Monitor vital signs every 5-15 minutes Pronounced chills and shivering Palpitations Pain in the chest or low back Apprehension Infusion-site tenderness and warmth *Progressive signs* Shock Oliguria Hemoglobinuria Bleeding tendencies (disseminated intravascular coagulation) Acute renal failure Anaphylaxis	Stop the transfusion immediately, and leave a normal saline infusion at a keep-open rate. Notify the physician immediately. Completely fill a red topped tube and a lavender topped tube with a blood sample. Obtain a 50-mL random, fresh urine sample in a clean container. Document pretransfusion and posttransfusion vital signs on the blood bank requisition. Return the blood bank requisition, laboratory requisition for the transfusion reaction work-up, the bag of blood, the urine specimen, and the red topped and lavender topped tubes to the blood bank promptly. If DIC is suspected, additional testing should include fibrinogen level, fibrin split products, platelet count, PT/PTT, and thrombin time. Prepare for the administration of RH immune globulin if the reaction was caused by transfusion of RH-incompatible blood

Acute Nonimmune Febrile Reaction

Symptoms	Treatment
Sustained rise in temperature >1 degree C	*In addition to following the procedures described above for a hemolytic reaction:*
Hematemesis	Draw blood for aerobic and anaerobic culture and Gram stain.
Diarrhea	
Hypotension	
Tachycardia	
Shock	
Sepsis	

Anaphylactic Reaction

Symptoms	Treatment
Tachycardia	*In addition to following the procedures described above for a hemolytic reaction:*
Dyspnea, wheezing (bronchospasm and upper airway edema)	Have an emergency cart readily available.
Apprehension	Maintain a patent airway and blood pressure.
Flushing	Administer epinephrine intravenously as follows:
Urticaria, hives	Bolus with epinephrine 0.2-0.5 mg of 1:1000 dilution mixed in 10 mL of 0.9% saline over 5-10 minutes.
Angioedema	
Shock	Follow the bolus with a continuous infusion of epinephrine at 1-4 mg/minute.
Circulatory collapse	
Bowel spasm, with diarrhea	Other drugs used to treat anaphylaxis may include aminophylline, atropine (for bradycardia), cimetidine, diphenhydramine, and hydrocortisone.
	Use IgA-deficient blood or plasma-deficient blood for future transfusions.

Transfusion-Related Acute Lung Injury (Trali)

Symptoms	Treatment
Increased capillary permeability	*In addition to following the procedures described above for a hemolytic reaction:*
Pulmonary edema	Have an emergency cart readily available.
Dyspnea	Maintain a patent airway and blood pressure.
Hypoxia	Prepare for blood gas measurement.
	Provide supportive care and usual transfer to intensive care setting.

Usage. Helps determine the cause of transfusion reaction.

Description. An acute transfusion reaction work-up is indicated whenever an unexpected reaction to transfusion of blood products is noted. Symptoms are most likely to occur within the first 15-30 minutes of transfusion and may be stimulated by as little as 10 mL of incompatible blood. Recombinant erythropoietin should be considered as an alternative to transfusion for anemic clients with nonmyeloid cancers.

Mild febrile reactions and urticaria may occur in clients who have been immunized to blood protein constituents through past receipt of donor blood or past pregnancies. A microaggregate filter used with transfusion can minimize the transfusion of such blood constituents.

Hemolytic transfusion reaction: With correctly administered blood, a hemolytic transfusion reaction may be attributable to recipient antibodies reacting to donor antigens not identified during type-and-crossmatch or type-and-screen procedures. Reactions are more likely to occur in clients who have had recent transfusions of blood because new antibodies to past donor blood may have developed since the last type-and-crossmatch procedure was performed. In blood administered incorrectly (that is, to the wrong recipient), a transfusion reaction is most likely caused by ABO incompatibility or antigen-antibody reactions. An incompatible or contaminated transfusion may cause fatal hemolytic reactions and disseminated intravascular coagulation. Thus it is important to observe recipients closely for early signs of reaction, so that the transfusion may be promptly stopped and complications minimized.

Acute nonimmune febrile reactions may be caused by bacterial contamination of the donor blood. This type of reaction may cause fever and erythrocyte hemolysis and may progress to shock and sepsis.

Anaphylactic transfusion reactions may occur in clients with subnormal immunoglobulin A (IgA) who have a history of recurrent infections. The receipt of IgA in donor blood stimulates an antibody response to IgA that causes anaphylaxis.

Delayed transfusion reactions include delayed hemolytic reactions, graft-versus-host disease, purpura, hemosiderosis, and transfusion-related acute lung injury (TRALI). Delayed hemolytic reactions usually are caused by recipient anti-Rh antibodies, anti-Duffy antibodies, and anti-Kidd antibodies that were not detected during type-and-crossmatch procedures. TRALI is thought to occur when a client with a preexisting systemic inflammatory condition experiences an antigen-antibody attack either from or against the contents of the blood product. A transfusion of blood containing these antigens causes delayed hemolysis and continued anemia. Graft-versus-host disease is usually fatal and occurs in immunosuppressed clients whose immune systems are unable to provide resistance against donor lymphocytes. Purpura with thrombocytopenia may develop about 7 days after transfusion in clients deficient in and who have developed antibodies to platelet antigen PLA-1. Hemosiderosis (iron overload) may occur in clients receiving multiple transfusions over a short period of time.

Laboratory procedures for an acute transfusion reaction work-up include direct Coombs' testing; repeated type and crossmatch on original recipient and donor samples; type and crossmatch on post-reaction recipient sample with donor sample; hemoglobin and hematocrit level; serum haptoglobin; urea nitrogen, plasma or serum; recipient and donor blood culture and Gram stain; and urine measurement of bilirubin, hemoglobin, urobilinogen, and hemosiderin.

Professional Considerations
Consent form NOT required.

Preparation
1. Assess the client during the transfusion for signs of a transfusion reaction listed previously.

Procedure
1. Follow procedures described under Transfusion Reaction Symptoms and Treatment.

Postprocedure Care
1. Continue monitoring vital signs every 5-15 minutes until they are stable.

Client and Family Teaching
1. Complete results may take several days.
2. See Other Data and provide information appropriate to the type of reaction that occurred.

Factors That Affect Results
1. See individual test listings.

Other Data
1. For delayed transfusion reactions, the following should be performed if future transfusions are needed:
   a. Delayed hemolytic reactions: The client should be advised to carry the information in writing that any blood transfusions received must be negative for Rh (c and E), Duffy, and Kidd antigens.
   b. Graft-versus-host disease: If the client survives this complication, future

donor blood should be irradiated before transfusion.

c. Purpura: The client should be advised to carry the information in writing that any blood transfusions received must be PLA-1 negative.

d. Hemosiderosis: Hemosiderosis may be fatal. The risk for developing this complication may be minimized in clients who need multiple transfusions by performing lead chelation therapy.

2. Card or slide hemagglutination or dipstick methods are available for use in ABO blood grouping at the bedside just before transfusion.

Transrectal Ultrasonography

See **Prostate Ultrasonography**—Diagnostic.

Transthyretin (TTR, Prealbumin-Thyroxine binding, Tbpa Palb, Tryptophan-Rich Prealbumin)—Serum or Vitreous Fluid

Norm.

		SI Units
Adult	10-40 mg/dL	100-400 mg/L
Male	(mean) 21.5 mg/dL	(mean) 215 mg/L
Female	(mean) 18.2 mg/dL	(mean) 182 mg/L
Maternal	17-18.6 mg/dL	170-186 mg/L
Children		
Cord blood	(mean) 13 mg/dL	(mean) 130 mg/L
Newborn	10.4-11.4 mg/dL	104-114 mg/L
12 months	(mean) 10 mg/dL	(mean) 100 mg/L
24-36 months	16-28.1 mg/dL	160-281 mg/L
Vitreous fluid (eye)	4-24 mg/L	

Increased. Adrenal hyperfunction, cardiac amyloidosis (V122L mutation), cardiomyopathy, Hodgkin's disease, shigellosis. Drugs include corticosteroids (high dose) and NSAIDs (high dose). Vitreous fluid increased found in retinal dysfunctions.

Decreased. Abdominal peritoneal dialysis, allele of V30M familial amyloidotic polyneuropathy found in Portuguese and Japanese patients, chronic illness (with concomitant subnormal nutritional status), cirrhosis, cystic fibrosis, diabetes mellitus, disseminated malignant disease, epithelial ovarian carcinoma, familial amyloidotic polyneuropathy (FAP), hereditary amyloidosis, protein and calorie malnutrition (<300 mg/L), and senile systemic amyloidosis (SSA). Drugs include amiodarone, estrogens, and oral contraceptives (containing estrogen).

Description. Transthyretin (TTR) is a transport protein synthesized in the liver that carries and helps maintain normal levels of thyroxine and retinol-binding protein in the body. Transthyretin migrates ahead of albumin on protein electrophoresis, and because of that, has been called "prealbumin". Transthyretin is otherwise unrelated to albumin. The half-life of 2-4 days makes it a much more sensitive marker for nutritional status and for liver dysfunction than albumin, which has a half-life of 22 days. Because transthyretin reflects changes in nutritional status more quickly than albumin, it is frequently used to evaluate nutritional needs in postoperative and critically ill clients. Transthyretin mutations have been associated with many familial amyloidosis diseases, autosomal dominant disorders in which amyloid deposits accumulate in peripheral nerves, resulting in neuropathy.

Professional Considerations

Informed consent is recommended if the purpose is for genetic testing for familial amyloidosis. Refer to Appendix B, "Informed Consent for Genetic Testing".

Preparation

1. Tube: Red topped, red/gray topped, or gold topped.
2. Do NOT draw specimens during hemodialysis.

Procedure

1. Draw a 4-mL blood sample without hemolysis.

Postprocedure Care

1. None.

Client and Family Teaching

1. Results are normally available within 24 hours.

Factors That Affect Results

1. Hemolyzed or lipemic specimens interfere with the nephelometric testing method.

Other Data

1. Swedish V30M haplotype carriers display later age at onset of symptoms.
2. Pre-albumin concentrations <20 mg/dL associated with increased risk of death, even with normal albumin levels, in maintenance hemodialysis patients.

Tranylcypromine

See **Amphetamines**—Blood.

TRAP

See **Tartrate-Resistant Acid Phosphatase Stain**—Specimen.

Trazodone

See **Tricyclic Antidepressants**—Plasma or Serum.

Triazolam

See **Benzodiazepines**—Plasma and Urine.

Trichinosis Serology—Serum

Norm. None detected, negative, or titer <1:16. Possible current or past infection: titer >1:5.

Positive. A fourfold rise in titer is diagnostic for trichinosis. May also see increased leptin and macrophage migration inhibitory factor.

Description. Trichinosis is a parasitic disease caused by the larvae of *Trichinella spiralis*, a roundworm acquired in humans by ingestion of raw or poorly cooked pork or other animals it inhabits (cats, dogs, horses, swine, and some wild animals such as bears, boars, and walruses). The ingested worm larvae mature and reproduce in the intestinal tract and then migrate through the lymphatic system and bloodstream to other sites in the body. Those reaching muscle tissue become encapsulated as cysts, causing inflammation and necrosis. The symptoms of trichinosis are progressive. Soon after ingestion, fever, diarrhea, facial edema, eosinophilia, and muscle edema occur. These symptoms are followed by muscle soreness and may progress to neurotoxicity and myocarditis. Clients with chronic trichinosis may experience myalgia, eye burning, headache, and easy fatigability. This test detects the presence of *T. spiralis* antibodies by mixing of serial dilutions of the client's serum with *T. spiralis* antigen and observation for antigen-antibody reactions. Titers may be negative soon after symptoms appear but begin rising about 21 days after infection. Levels peak about 60 days after infection and then slowly return to higher-than-baseline levels until about 2 years later.

Professional Considerations
Consent form NOT required.

Preparation
1. Tube: Red topped, red/gray topped, or gold topped.
2. Assess for history of recent ingestion of raw pork or poorly cooked pork or other susceptible animals.
3. The test may need to be prescheduled with the laboratory.
4. Specimens MAY be drawn during hemodialysis.

Procedure
1. Draw a 5-mL blood sample. Repeat the test every 3-5 days to detect rising titer.

Postprocedure Care
1. None.

Client and Family Teaching
1. Thoroughly cook pork or meat from other susceptible animals.
2. Serial testing is necessary to confirm *T. spiralis* infection.

Factors That Affect Results
1. Titers may be negative in the presence of infection if drawn during the first 3 weeks after exposure.

Other Data
1. Other tests used to diagnose trichinosis include skin testing, muscle biopsy, or examination of cerebrospinal fluid for *T. spiralis*.
2. Trichinosis has been treated with albendazole (20-30mg/kg/day × 5-7 days), mebendazole or thiabendazole (intestinal phase), mebendazole (muscular stage), and corticosteroids.

Trichinosis Skin Test—Diagnostic

Norm. Negative.

Positive. Current or past infection with *T. spiralis*.

Description. Trichinosis is a parasitic disease caused by the larvae of *Trichinella spiralis*, a roundworm acquired in humans by ingestion of raw or poorly cooked pork or other animals it inhabits (cats, dogs, swine, and some wild animals such as walruses, and bears). The ingested worm larvae mature and reproduce in the intestinal tract and then migrate through the lymphatic system and bloodstream to other sites in the body. Those reaching muscle tissue become encapsulated as cysts, causing inflammation and necrosis. The symptoms of trichinosis are progressive. Soon after ingestion, hyperpyrexia, gastrointestinal upset, eosinophilia, and muscle edema occur. These symptoms are followed by muscle soreness and may progress to neurotoxicity and myocarditis. This test is based on an immediate hypersensitivity reaction. The presence of *T. spiralis* antibodies is indicated when intradermal injection of the killed larvae of *T. spiralis* produces signs of an antigen-antibody reaction.

Professional Considerations
Consent form NOT required.

Preparation
1. Obtain an alcohol wipe, a 4-mL syringe with an intradermal needle, *T. spiralis* antigen, and a control.
2. Assess for history of recent ingestion of raw pork or poorly cooked pork or other susceptible animals.

Procedure
1. Cleanse the forearm site for injection with an alcohol wipe and allow the area to dry.
2. Inject *T. spiralis* antigen intradermally. Inject the control into the site in the opposite forearm. Record the sites of injection.
3. 20 minutes later, observe the injection site for a blanched wheal with surrounding erythema, a symptom of a positive reaction.

Postprocedure Care
1. None.

Client and Family Teaching
1. Thoroughly cook pork or meat from other susceptible animals.

2. In positive tests, the wheal and redness should disappear within a few hours.

Factors That Affect Results

1. Positive results may also indicate past trichinosis infection.

Other Data

1. Injected corticosteroids may help mediate an excessive reaction to the skin test.
2. See also Trichinosis serology—Serum.

Trichomonas Preparation—Specimen

Norm. Negative. No *Trichomonas* identified.

Positive. Trichomoniasis.

Description. Trichomoniasis is a sexually transmitted protozoan infection of the genitourinary tract. This infection causes considerable foamy, yellow drainage as well as petechiae and vaginal burning and itching in females; in males a persistent, white urethral discharge may exist or frequently no symptoms may be present. The causative organism, *Trichomonas vaginalis*, is transmitted by direct contact with the vaginal and urethral fluids of infected individuals. Diagnosis of trichomoniasis is made by direct microscopic examination of a wet mount of the secretions of infected individuals.

Professional Considerations

Consent form NOT required.

Preparation

1. Obtain a speculum, a pipette, a sterile tube to which 1 mL of sterile nonbacteriostatic 0.9% saline has been added, and a sterile swab approved for microbiologic use.
2. See Client and Family Teaching.
3. The client should disrobe below the waist for the collection of a vaginal, cervical, or urethral swab.

Procedure

1. *Female: vaginal, cervical, or urethral specimen:*
   a. Place the client in the dorsal lithotomy position and drape her for comfort and privacy.
   b. Collect the vaginal specimen by pipette aspiration from the vaginal pool or by swabbing the circumference of the vagina with a sterile swab. Express the secretions into the sterile tube of saline and cover the tube.
   c. For the cervical swab, place the speculum over the cervical os and gently express secretions onto the sterile swab. Alternatively, aspirate endocervical secretions through a pipette. Transfer the secretions to the sterile tube of saline and cover the tube.
2. *Male or female: urethral specimen:*
   a. Insert the cotton-tipped end of a sterile swab into the urethral meatus. Rotate the swab and hold it in place for 10 seconds to allow absorption of secretions. Transfer the secretions to the sterile tube of saline and cover the tube.
3. *Male: prostatic specimens:* Provide privacy for the client.
   a. Instruct the client to stimulate ejaculation by masturbation. The semen should be collected into a clean container. If the client is uncomfortable with masturbation or unable to collect the specimen, it may be collected into a plastic condom at home and brought in within 1 hour. The client should be instructed to empty the condom into a clean container and cover it tightly to prevent the specimen from drying out.
4. *Urine collection for examination of sediment:*
   a. Instruct the client to cleanse the area surrounding the urethral meatus with four soapy sponges and then to rinse and dry the area.
   b. While holding the labia open or the foreskin back, the client should void about 20 mL of urine into a clean container and then stop the stream and cap the container.

Postprocedure Care

1. Write the specimen source and the collection time on the laboratory requisition.
2. Send the specimen to the laboratory immediately.
3. Do not refrigerate the specimen.

Client and Family Teaching

1. For vaginal or cervical specimens, avoid douching for 72 hours.

2. If results are positive, notify any sexual contacts to be tested. Do not have sexual relations until your physician confirms that follow-up testing is negative.
3. Assess the client's knowledge of safe sex and teach safe sex practices.

Factors That Affect Results
1. Results are invalidated if the specimen dries before microscopic examination.

2. The test is less sensitive for asymptomatic females. Wet mounts are negative in 30%-50% of females positive for *Trichomonas*. Unfortunately, negative microscopy results give false reassurance.

Other Data
1. Trichomoniasis may be treated with metronidazole.
2. Consider testing for *Chlamydia* and *Neisseria gonorrhoeae* with positive results.

Tricyclic Antidepressants—Plasma or Serum

Norm. Negative.

Tricyclic Antidepressant	Therapeutic Trough Levels	SI Units
Amitriptyline	100-250 ng/mL	360-900 nmol/L
Panic level	>400 ng/mL	>1275 nmol/L
Amoxapine	20-100 ng/mL	64-319 nmol/L
Panic level	>500 ng/mL	>1594 nmol/L
Desipramine	150-300 ng/mL	563-1126 nmol/L
Panic level	>400 ng/mL	>1500 nmol/L
Doxepin	50-200 ng/mL	180-720 nmol/L
Panic level	>400 ng/mL	>1440 nmol/L
Imipramine	75-250 ng/mL	279-890 nmol/L
Panic level	>400 ng/mL	>1440 nmol/L
Maprotiline	150-400 ng/mL	541-1442 nmol/L
Panic level	>1000 ng/mL	>3605 nmol/L
Nortriptyline	50-150 ng/mL	190-570 nmol/L
Panic level	>200 ng/mL	>760 nmol/L
Protriptyline	50-150 ng/mL	190-570 nmol/L
Panic level	>400 ng/mL	>1520 nmol/L
Trazodone	300-2500 ng/mL	1000-6000 nmol/L
Panic level	>4000 ng/mL	>9600 nmol/L

Overdose Symptoms and Treatment

Symptoms. Confusion, agitation, hallucinations, lethargy, seizures, coma, dysrhythmias (atrial flutter in children, Brugada pattern, tachycardia, torsades de pointes, absent R wave), hyperthermia, flushing, and dilation of the pupils; death may occur. Sodium-channel blockade manifesting as early prolonged QRS interval, rightward axis of 40 msec, presence of an R wave in aV_R lead and an S wave in leads I and aV_L. Life-threatening cardiac toxicity or seizures are seen if concentrations are >1000 ng/mL.

Treatment

NOTE: Treatment choice(s) depend(s) on client's history and condition and episode history.
1. Give bicarbonate 1-2 mmol/kg IV for delayed cardiac conduction or ventricular dysrhythmias, hypotension, reduced level of consciousness, or convulsion. Adjust the dose according to arterial pH and correction of symptoms. Alternatively, hypertonic saline may be used for hypotension. Use of 150 mEq intravenous sodium bicarbonate treats Brugada pattern in amitriptyline overdose.
2. Administer IV fluids for hypotension. Follow with vasopressor, if needed.
3. Monitor cardiac pattern for QRS elongation, dysrhythmias, and conduction abnormalities for 72 hours (adults) or 96 hours (children).
4. Hemodialysis and peritoneal dialysis will NOT remove amitriptyline, desipramine, doxepin, imipramine, maprotiline, nortriptyline, or protriptyline. They are unlikely to remove amoxapine and trazodone.

5. Hemoperfusion will remove amitriptyline.
6. Severe amitriptyline and tianeptine poisoning can be treated with naloxone and amitriptyline toxicity can be treated with intravenous fat emulsion or plasma exchange.
7. Provide supportive intervention for lethargy, confusion, hallucinations, urinary retention, hypertension, hyperpyrexia, respiratory depression, and declining level of consciousness.
8. Pharmacobezoars can be removed by endoscopic gastroscopy.

Usage. Monitoring for therapeutic or toxic levels during tricyclic antidepressant therapy or for toxic levels in attempted suicide.

Description. "Tricyclic antidepressants" is a term describing a group of drugs with similar cyclic chemical structures, frequently used to treat depression on a long-term basis. These drugs act by blocking norepinephrine and serotonin reuptake in the central nervous system and have anticholinergic properties. They are metabolized in the liver, with a variable half-life and peak levels occurring 4-8 hours after an oral dose. One common side effect is weight gain. Because certain drugs of this group are metabolized to others in the group, the levels of all of these drugs should be measured and considered when one is evaluating clinical symptoms. Therapeutic blood monitoring is important, both because the drugs have a narrow window of therapeutic effectiveness and because levels have been shown to correlate poorly with clinical effectiveness. Thus toxicity is a risk when doses are increased to improve clinical symptoms.

Professional Considerations
Consent form NOT required.

Preparation
1. Draw specimen 1 week after drug therapy starts in order to ensure that the drug has reached steady state.
2. Tube: Red topped, red/gray topped, or gold topped (for serum); green topped (for plasma).
3. Samples for amitriptyline, desipramine, doxepin, imipramine, nortriptyline, or protriptyline levels MAY be drawn during hemodialysis. Do NOT draw samples for amoxapine, maprotiline, or trazodone during hemodialysis.
4. Write the name of the drug ingested (if known) on the laboratory requisition.

Procedure
1. Draw TROUGH blood 10-12 hours after the previous dose. Obtain serial measurements at the same time each day.
2. Draw a 7-mL blood sample into a syringe and then eject the blood into the tube. For a plasma specimen, gently roll the tube several times to mix the blood with the anticoagulant.

Postprocedure Care
1. Send the specimen to the lab promptly. Serum should be separated within 2 hours, and the sample should be frozen or refrigerated if not tested promptly.
2. If concurrent MAO inhibitors have been ingested, monitor the client for hyperpyrexia and provide convulsion precautions.

Client and Family Teaching
1. 7-21 days is needed for a steady state.
2. For overdose, intensive care may be required.
3. For an intentional overdose, refer the client and family for crisis intervention and offer counseling resources.
4. Referrals to appropriate rehabilitation centers and therapeutic community programs should be offered to all addicted clients who may be interested.
5. Cardiac deaths have occurred up to 6 days after an overdose.

Factors That Affect Results
1. Drugs that may cause increased levels include barbiturates, bupropion, cimetidine, corticosteroids, methylphenidate, neuroleptics, oral contraceptives, selective serotonin reuptake inhibitors (SSRIs) (citalopram, desmethylcitalopram, didesmethylcitalopram, fluoxetine, milnacipran, norfluoxetine, paroxetine, sertraline, venlafaxine), and valproic acid.
2. Drugs that may cause decreased levels include barbiturates, chloral hydrate, glutethimide, nicotine (cigarette smoking), and phenobarbital.
3. Levels for African-Americans may be up to 50% higher than those for Caucasian clients taking the same-dosage regimen.

4. Toxicity occurs more readily and at lower levels with advancing age as a result of slowed metabolism and also with concomitant phenothiazine use.

Other Data

1. Tricyclic antidepressants cause serum glucose level to increase and glucose tolerance to decrease. Monitor diabetic clients for hyperglycemia when using these drugs.
2. Neurotoxicity and cardiotoxicity are less likely to occur with trazodone than with other drugs of this group.

3. Amitriptyline or maprotiline provokes torsades de pointes, prolonged QT interval, absent R wave on ECG.
4. Maprotiline has selective antiproliferative effects against Burkitt's lymphoma.
5. Children are more sensitive than adults to toxic effects.
6. When tricyclic antidepressants are taken concurrently with the herb *Pausinystalia yohimbe*, the risk for hypertension is increased.

Trifluoperazine

See **Phenothiazines**.

Triglycerides—Blood

Norm.

Serum Values		SI Units
Adult Females		
20-29 years	10-100 mg/dL	0.11-1.13 mmol/L
30-39 years	10-110 mg/dL	0.11-1.24 mmol/L
40-49 years	10-122 mg/dL	0.11-1.38 mmol/L
50-59 years	10-134 mg/dL	0.11-1.51 mmol/L
>59 years	10-147 mg/dL	0.11-1.66 mmol/L

Serum Values		SI Units
Adult Males		
20-29 years	10-157 mg/dL	0.11-1.77 mmol/L
30-39 years	10-182 mg/dL	0.11-2.05 mmol/L
40-49 years	10-193 mg/dL	0.11-2.18 mmol/L
50-59 years	10-197 mg/dL	0.11-2.22 mmol/L
>59 years	10-199 mg/dL	0.11-2.24 mmol/L
Children		
Female: 1-19 years	10-121 mg/dL	0.11-1.36 mmol/L
Male: 1-19 years	10-103 mg/dL	0.11-1.16 mmol/L

NOTE: Plasma values are lower by about 3%.

Classification of Triglyceride Levels		
Borderline high	200-400 mg/dL	2.3-4.5 mmol/L
High	400-1000 mg/dL	4.5-11.3 mmol/L
Very high	>1000 mg/dL	>11.3 mmol/L

Increased. Alcoholism, aortic aneurysm, aortitis, arteriosclerosis, cancers (colon, respiratory, kidney, melanoma for men and respiratory, cervical and non-melanoma skin cancers for women), coronary artery disease, depression, diabetes mellitus, diet (recent high-carbohydrate, prolonged high-fat), familial hypertriglyceridemia, fat embolism, gene variation of lipoprotein lipase (LPL) or adipose triglyceride lipase (ATGL) genes, glycogen storage diseases, gout, hepatic cholesterol ester storage disease, hypercholesterolemia, hyperlipoprotein-emia, hypothyroidism, insulin resistance, metabolic syndrome (>150 mg/dL), mothers of large for gestational age newborns, myocardial infarction (for up to 1 year), myxedema, nephrotic syndrome, obesity, pancreatitis, pregnancy, renal insufficiency (chronic), starvation (early), stress, Tangier disease, and von Gierke's disease. Tobacco use. Drugs include cholestyramine, cortico-steroids, estrogens, ethyl alcohol (ethanol), miconazole (intravenous), oral contracep-tives, and spironolactone.

Decreased. Abetalipoproteinemia, acan-thocytosis, aerobic exercise, chronic obstruc-tive pulmonary disease, cirrhosis (portal), hemorrhagic stroke, hyperalimentation, hyperthyroidism, malabsorption, and mal-nutrition. Drugs include ascorbic acid, asparaginase, biotin, clofibrate, dextrothy-roxine, docosahexaenoic or eicosapentae-noic acid, endurance exercise (women), fenofibrate, gemfibrozil, heparin, lovastatin, metformin, niacin, olmesartan (40 mg/day), phenformin, pravastatin, and sulfonylureas. Herbal or natural remedies include *Cordy-ceps sinensis*, fish or seal oil diet of omega-3 fatty acids, garlic (aged extract taken over time), hazelnuts, olive oil enriched with n-3 PUFA, soy, and vinegar ingestion 15mL/day.

Description. Also known as "fat," triglycer-ide is a compound consisting of fatty acid or glycerol ester that constitutes a major part (up to 70%) of very-low-density lipopro-teins (VLDLs) and a small part (<10%) of low-density lipoproteins (LDLs) in fasting serum samples. Dietary triglycerides are carried as part of chylomicrons through the lymphatic system and bloodstream to adipose tissue, where they are released for storage. Triglycerides are also synthesized in the liver from fatty acids and from protein and glucose above the body's current needs and then stored in adipose tissue. They may be later retrieved and formed into glucose through gluconeogenesis when needed by the body. Triglyceride levels are taken into consideration with total choles-terol, high-density lipoprotein cholesterol, and chylomicron levels when categorizing a client's serum into lipoprotein phenotypes that represent genetic lipoprotein abnor-malities. Treatments differ for the different phenotypes.

Professional Considerations
Consent form NOT required.

Preparation
1. Tube: Red topped, red/gray topped, or gold topped; or lavender topped.
2. A fasting specimen is preferred.
3. See Client and Family Teaching.

Procedure
1. Draw a 4-mL blood sample.

Postprocedure Care
1. None.

Client and Family Teaching
1. Avoid variations in diet and weight for 21 days; avoid alcohol and refined carbohy-drates for 3 days.
2. Fast 12 hours before the test. Water is permitted.

Factors That Affect Results
1. Drugs that may cause falsely elevated results include cholestyramine, estrogens, furosemide, miconazole, and oral contraceptives.
2. Triglyceride levels for African-American clients have been demonstrated to be lower than those for Caucasian clients.

Other Data
1. The following national guidelines, avail-able at http://www.guideline.gov, provide a good summary of triglycerides in context with other lipids and treatment recommendations: National Cholesterol Education Program: Third report of the National Cholesterol Education Program (NCEP) expert panel on detection, evalu-ation, and treatment of high blood cho-lesterol in adults (Adult Treatment Panel III) and Implications of recent clinical trials for the National Cholesterol Educa-tion Program Adult Treatment Panel III Guidelines, National Heart, Lung, and Blood Institute, September 1993 (updated 2004).
2. Metabolic syndrome consists of a group of findings occurring together: general obesity, central obesity, elevated triglycer-ides, low levels of high-density lipopro-tein cholesterol, hyperglycemia, and hypertension. This condition is becoming more prevalent and is associated with an increased risk of developing cardiovascu-lar disease and type 2 diabetes.

3. Low-density lipoproteins become morphologically smaller and more dense in the presence of hypertriglyceridemia. This change is associated with an increased risk of atherogenesis.
4. Triglycerides <1.70 mml/L might be associated with increased cancer risk which is attenuated in presence of use of statins (Yang X et al, 2011).
5. High triglycerides and TSH and low free T_4 associated with insulin resistance.

Triiodothyronine

See Thyroid Test: Triiodothyronine—Blood.

Troponin I—Plasma and Troponin T (cTnI or cTnT)—Serum

Norm.

		SI Units
Troponin I		
Negative	<0.05 ng/mL	<0.05 µg/L
Indeterminate or suspicious for injury to myocardium	00.06-0.49 ng/mL	0.06-0.49 µg/L
Positive for myocardial injury	greater than or equal to 0.50 ng/mL	greater than or equal 0.50 to µg/L
Troponin T	<0.1 ng/L	<0.1 µg/L

Ranges vary according to the specific method and technology used.

Usage. Confirmation of acute myocardial infarction (including cocaine associated), including extent; indicator of reperfusion after treatment with thrombolytic therapy.

Increased Troponin I. Acute myocardial infarction, angina, coronary syndromes, electrical countershock, myocarditis, and pregnancy-induced hypertension. Transient increase with rapid atrial pacing.

Increased Troponin T. Acute myocardial infarction, angina, heart failure, idiopathic inflammatory myopathies, muscle damage, pregnancy-induced hypertension, and renal failure. A hypothesis exists in the literature that increases may possibly be a marker for ruptured plaques and severe coronary artery disease.

Description. Cardiac troponin I is a subunit of the actin-myosin complex contractile protein of the myofibril manufactured only in the myocardium. Troponin T and cardiac-specific troponin I are two isoforms that leak into the bloodstream during myocardial necrosis. Because of the low-to-undetectable values in the serum of healthy people and the quick elevation (detectable within 1 hour after myocardial cell injury), these ultrasensitive markers have been praised for their usefulness in the early diagnosis of acute myocardial infarction (MI), especially in the detection of silent MIs and microinfarctions and in the case of chest pain not accompanied by typical electrocardiogram changes. Both tests show similar accuracy in identifying acute myocardial injury and results are influenced by kidney function. Some studies have found an even correlation between the degree of elevation of troponins I and T and the severity and extent of coronary lesions, angina, and ECG changes, and thus these values may be useful in predicting outcome for cardiac conditions. Some research has found that troponin levels are predictive of later intracoronary thrombus and obstruction in the distal microvasculature. A Troponin T level of >0.8microg/L is associated with major cardiac adverse events after cardiac operations. Troponin T has been found to be an independent predictor of outcome for chronic hemodialysis clients. Newer ultrasensitive tests for measurement of both types of troponin are available.

Professional Considerations
Consent form NOT required.

Preparation
1. Tube for Troponin I: Pink topped, green topped, or blue topped.
2. Tube for Troponin T: Red topped or serum gel tube.

Procedure
1. Draw a 5-mL blood sample.

Postprocedure Care
1. None.

Client and Family Teaching
1. Results are normally available within 4 hours.

Factors That Affect Results
1. It is not yet known definitively whether troponins can also be found in myocardial ischemia or strain, but levels have been found to be elevated in the absence of myocardial necrosis when other diseases, such as septic shock, renal failure, pulmonary embolism, and arterial hypertension, are present.

Other Data
1. Cardiac troponin-T and I elevation after nonemergent PCI indicates long-term mortality.
2. The troponin I assay costs less than the troponin T assay.
3. The American College of Emergency Physicians recommends that the cause of acute myocardial infarction should not be ruled out for chest pain unless a repeat CK-MB taken 6-10 hours after the onset of symptoms and a repeat troponins I and T taken 8-12 hours after the onset of symptoms are both negative.
4. The release of a new peptide, protein fragment Caspase-3 p17, has been discovered in heart failure patients.
5. A high sensitivity troponin test is undergoing study. This test detects clients with myocardial injury at much lower levels of troponin.

Trus

See **Prostate Ultrasonography**—Diagnostic.

Trypanosomiasis Serologic Test (Chagas' Disease Serologic Test)—Blood

Norm. Negative titer.

Positive. American trypanosomiasis (Chagas' disease).

Description. American trypanosomiasis, also known as "Chagas' disease," is endemic in Latin America; its cause is thought to be either autoimmune or parasitic. Symptoms may include central nervous system (CNS) changes, CNS lesions in immunocompromised clients, and meningoencephalitis in children. The course of the disease may run months to years and is frequently fatal. Serologic testing is useful after the acute stage of the disease, when blood films are not very sensitive. Serologic tests have good sensitivity but lack specificity for detection of Chagas' disease. Newer molecular assays based on the polymerase chain reaction hold promise for more specific testing.

Professional Considerations
Consent form NOT required.

Preparation
1. Tube: Red topped, red/gray topped, or gold topped.
2. Obtain a container of ice.
3. Specimens MAY be drawn during hemodialysis.

Procedure
1. Draw a 5-mL blood sample. Place the tube on ice.

Postprocedure Care
1. Write the name of the suspected parasite and the place and date of recent travel on the laboratory requisition.

Client and Family Teaching
1. Results may not be available for several days because testing is performed by the

Centers for Disease Control and Prevention (Atlanta) or sent to a parasitology laboratory.

Factors That Affect Results
1. Reject specimens that are not frozen.

Other Data
1. Transmission of American trypanosomiasis is possible by transfusion of contaminated blood to immunocompromised clients.
2. Drugs used for treatment of Chagas' disease include nitrofurans and nitroimidazoles and eflornithine (African). For clients with immunosuppression, the nitroimidazole benznidazole has been used.
3. Staging of Chagas' disease is done via examination of cerebrospinal fluid, after serologic diagnosis has been confirmed.
4. Monitor for digitalis toxicity in chronic heart failure patients with Chagas.
5. See also African trypanosomiasis— Blood; Parasite screen—Blood.

Trypsin—Plasma or Serum

Norm.

Behringwerke Antibody Method

Young adult 18-36 years	185-272 µg/L
Middle adult 37-66 years	185-272 µg/L
Older adult >66 years	147-1438 µg/L

Immunoreactive (Cationic) Trypsin by RIA Method

Adults	16.7-32.3 µg/L

RIA Double-Antibody (Geokas') Method

Adults	22.2-44.4 µg/L
Children	
Cord	21.4-25.2 µg/L
<6 months	25.9-36.7 µg/L
6-12 months	30.2-44.0 µg/L
1-3 years	28.0-31.6 µg/L
3-5 years	25.1-31.5 µg/L
5-7 years	32.1-39.3 µg/L
7-10 years	32.7-37.1 µg/L

Sorin Antibody Method

Adults	5.0-85.0 µg/L
Children	11.1-51.3 µg/L

Increased. Beta-thalassemia, chronic renal failure, cystic fibrosis (initial years), hepatic disease, malnutrition (acute), pancreatic viral infection, pancreatitis (acute), peptic ulcer disease, and recent endoscopic retrograde cholangiopancreatography. Drugs include bombesin, cerulein, cholecystokinin, and secretin.

Decreased. Beta-thalassemia, cystic fibrosis (advanced), diabetes mellitus, malnutrition (chronic), pancreatic cancer, and pancreatitis (chronic).

Description. Trypsin is a proteolytic enzyme produced in the pancreas in the precursor form of inactive trypsinogen. Trypsinogen is converted to trypsin in the duodenum by enterokinase. Trypsin exists in several forms in the bloodstream. One form includes a trypsinogen that is bound to alpha-antitrypsin, another to alpha-macroglobulin, and a third as free trypsin. During the initial years of cystic fibrosis, serum trypsin levels are elevated as a result of pancreatic cell destruction and liberation of trypsin into the bloodstream. Over time, pancreatic insufficiency leads to abnormally low trypsin levels. Because of the possibility of overlap with normal values as pancreatic function declines, the value of this test is limited when one is diagnosing cystic fibrosis. Elevations reflect either pancreatic damage or impairment of organs involved in its clearance. Trypsin is thought to play a role in activating the complement cascade.

Professional Considerations
Consent form NOT required.

Preparation
1. Tube: Red topped, red/gray topped, or gold topped (serum sample); or green topped (plasma sample).
2. Specimens MAY be drawn during hemodialysis.
3. See Client and Family Teaching.

Procedure
1. Draw a 7-mL blood sample.

Postprocedure Care
1. Transport the specimen to the laboratory and refrigerate it at 4 degrees C or freeze it at −20 degrees C until testing.

Client and Family Teaching

1. Fast from food for 8 hours before the test.

Factors That Affect Results

1. Levels are elevated in nonfasting samples.
2. Trypsin levels demonstrate a diurnal variation, with the highest levels occurring during the late evening.
3. Because of the problem of wide variability in trypsin norms, values should be compared to the norms of the laboratory performing the test.
4. Values are not affected by hemodialysis.

Other Data

1. Sensitivity is 90%; false-negative rate is approximately 7%.
2. For elevated immunoreactive trypsin levels, refer clients for confirmatory sweat testing.

Trypsin—Stool

Norm. Positive.

Gelatin	2+ to 4+ digestion
≤1 year	Positive at dilutions >1:80
>1 year	Positive at dilutions >1:40
Cystic fibrosis	Negative at dilutions >1:10

Negative. Cystic fibrosis (advanced), trypsin insufficiency and malabsorption in children; pancreatic insufficiency (chronic).

Description. Trypsin is a proteolytic enzyme produced in the pancreas in the precursor form of inactive trypsinogen. Trypsinogen is converted to trypsin in the duodenum by enterokinase. Trypsin is present in the stool of young children but amounts lessen in older children and adults as a result of intestinal bacterial destruction of trypsin. In clients with pancreatic insufficiency, stool trypsin tests are negative. One performs this test by observing the digestive activity of serial dilutions of stool or duodenal fluid on the gelatin of unexposed radiographic film after incubation. A negative result necessitates test repetition on at least two more stool samples.

Professional Considerations

Consent form NOT required.

Preparation

1. Obtain a tongue blade and a clean container.
2. See Client and Family Teaching.

Procedure

1. Obtain a dime-sized sample of stool and place it in a covered, dry, clean container.

Postprocedure Care

1. Send the specimen to the laboratory promptly. The specimen must be tested within 2 hours.

Client and Family Teaching

1. Defecate in a bedpan. For infants the stool sample may be taken from a diaper.
2. Avoid laxatives or barium procedures the week before the specimen collection.

Factors That Affect Results

1. The stool from constipated samples may produce false-negative results because of the extended time allowed for intestinal bacteria to destroy trypsin.
2. False-positive results may be caused by the presence of bacterial proteases in the sample.

Other Data

1. See also Trypsin—Plasma or serum.

Trypsinogen-2—Urine

Norm. Negative or <50 ng/mL.

Positive (≥50 ng/mL). Possible pancreatitis.

Description. Trypsinogen is a pancreatic proteinase with two main isoenzymes, 1 and 2. The pancreas secretes these in high concentrations in pancreatic fluid, with much smaller concentrations appearing in the serum. Trypsinogens, being small in size, are usually readily filtered through the glomeruli. The kidney has a much higher reabsorption of trypsinogen-1, thus leaving trypsinogen-2 concentration higher in the urine. In people with acute pancreatitis, the trypsinogen-2 level in the urine will dramatically increase. This test can be used as a rapid screening of clients with possible acute pancreatitis, thus avoiding a costly acute abdominal work-up.

Professional Considerations
Consent form NOT required.

Preparation
1. See Client and Family Teaching.
2. Obtain a clean container for urine sample.

Procedure
1. Obtain a 5- to 10-mL clean-catch or catheter urine sample.

Postprocedure Care
1. Send the specimen to the laboratory within 1 hour.

Client and Family Teaching
1. Instruct client on proper technique for clean-catch specimen.

2. Test is a quick 3-minute dipstick test, and results will be immediately available.
3. Clients with positive results will likely be referred for further testing.

Factors That Affect Results
1. Extremely high concentrations of trypsinogen-2 in the urine might result in a false-negative reading.
2. Trypsinogen-2 is present in the epithelium cells of the bile ducts and peribiliary glands. Inflammation in these structures may cause a positive result that is attributable not to pancreatitis but to cholangitis.

Other Data
1. Dipstick kits for point-of-care testing are available.

Tryptophan—Plasma

Norm.

		SI Units
Adults	0.51-1.49 mg/dL	25-73 μmol/L
Infants (first day of life)		
Premature	0.32-0.92 mg/dL	15-45 μmol/L
Full-term	0.51-1.49 mg/dL	25-73 μmol/L

Increased. Allergic rhinitis, hemodialysis patients, non-responders to subcutaneous immunotherapy, sepsis, and tryptophanuria.

Decreased. Blue diaper syndrome (tryptophan malabsorption syndrome), carcinoid syndrome, depression, Hartnup disease, hypothermia, kwashiorkor, lung cancer, postoperative abdominal surgery (first 48 hours), postoperative delirium in elderly, and tobacco smokers. Drugs include alclofenac, aspirin, glucose, and indomethacin.

Description. Tryptophan is an essential amino acid that functions as a precursor for serotonin and niacin. Some tryptophan also occurs naturally in the body. Tryptophan metabolism involves action by the enzyme tryptophan pyrrolase. Tryptophanuria is an inherited, X-linked trait in which an enzyme (tryptophan pyrrolase) is deficient. The resulting accumulation of nonmetabolized tryptophan results in elevated serum levels as well as tryptophan excretion in the urine

after renal reabsorption sites for tryptophan become saturated. Symptoms of tryptophanuria include dwarfism, photosensitivity, and ataxia. In blue diaper syndrome, an autosomal recessive trait, intestinal absorption of tryptophan is impaired. Dietary tryptophan is broken down into indoles and excreted in the stool, where the indoles are hydrolyzed to the blue-tinged pigment indigo blue. Other symptoms of blue diaper syndrome include hypercalcemia, growth defects, nephrocalcinosis, and frequent infections. This test helps diagnosis of these two genetic traits.

Professional Considerations
Consent form NOT required.

Preparation
1. Tube: Heparinized, green topped tube.
2. Obtain a container of ice-water.
3. Specimens MAY be drawn during hemodialysis.
4. See Client and Family Teaching.

Procedure

1. Draw a 7-mL blood sample. Place the tube immediately in a container of ice-water.

Postprocedure Care

1. Send specimens to the laboratory promptly. Plasma should be separated and frozen within 60 minutes of collection.

Client and Family Teaching

1. Fast for 8 hours before the test.

Factors That Affect Results

1. A delay in sample separation and freezing over 1 hour invalidates the results.

Other Data

1. Dietary supplementation of tryptophan is associated with an eosinophilia-myalgia syndrome, which includes myalgia, arthralgia, fatigue, rash, hair loss, edema, impaired motion of the joints, muscle cramping, and paresthesias as well as several laboratory value abnormalities.
2. Tryptophan levels have been found to be higher, and serotonin levels have been found to be lower, in the plasma of violent offenders.

Tryptophan-Rich Prealbumin

See **Transthyretin**—Serum or Vitreous Fluid.

T-Scan

See **Mammography**—Diagnostic.

TSH Assay

See **Thyroid-Stimulating Hormone, Sensitive Assay**—Blood.

T-SPOT®.TB

See **RD1-Interferon Tests for Tuberculosis**—Blood.

TST

See **Mantoux Skin Test**—Diagnostic.

TTR

See **Transthyretin**—Serum or Vitreous Fluid.

T-Tube Cholangiography, Postoperative—Diagnostic

Norm. Even filling of the biliary ductal system. Absence of strictures, obstruction, calculi, abnormal pathways, or delays in emptying.

Usage. Evaluation of biliary ducts for calculi, leakage, stricture, biliopancreatic reflux, and instrumentation injuries after gallbladder surgery or liver transplantation.

Description. T-tube cholangiography is the instillation of radiographic contrast medium through a T-tube (percutaneously inserted, T-shaped, bile duct drainage tube), followed by fluoroscopic examination of the biliary ducts. Use of intraoperative cholangiography minimizes the number of biliary calculi remaining after surgery, but up to 3% of surgeries miss some calculi, and bile duct damage, resulting in strictures, can result. Because of this possibility, T-tube cholangiography is usually performed 7-10 days after exploratory gallbladder or duct surgery or cholecystectomy for the purpose of evaluating duct patency and identifying any remaining stones or further ductal obstruction. Biliary duct obstruction or anastomotic leakage is also possible after liver transplantation; thus a T-tube is also placed after this type of surgery. If retained stones are identified, the T-tube is left in place because this is the route of choice for removal of the remaining stones. A total 4-6 weeks are required for the sinus tract surrounding the T-tube to be well healed before percutaneous removal of remaining stones.

Professional Considerations
Consent form IS required.

Risks
Allergic reaction to dye (itching, hives, rash, tight feeling in the throat, shortness of breath, anaphylaxis, death); renal toxicity from contrast medium.

Contraindications
Previous allergy to iodine, shellfish, or radiographic dye; pregnancy (because of the radioactive iodine crossing the blood-placental barrier); renal insufficiency.

Preparation
1. A cleansing enema may be prescribed.
2. Have emergency equipment readily available.
3. The T-tube may be clamped for 24 hours before the procedure.
4. See Client and Family Teaching.
5. Just before beginning the procedure, take a "time out" to verify the correct client, procedure, and site.

Procedure
1. The client is positioned supine.
2. Local anesthetic may be injected around the T-tube site if the site is inflamed and painful.
3. After the T-tube is cleansed with 70% alcohol, radiographic contrast medium is instilled through the tube via a large-caliber catheter.
4. Fluoroscopic radiographs are taken in a variety of positions to track dye progress

through the biliary duct system. Upright films are taken to detect inadvertent injection of air through the T-tube.
5. The procedure is concluded with films of contrast medium emptying into the duodenum. Delays in emptying prolong the procedure, which normally takes less than $\frac{1}{2}$ hour.
6. If findings are normal, the T-tube is removed, and a dry, sterile dressing is applied to the site.

Postprocedure Care
1. If the T-tube has been removed, assess the site for redness, edema, pain, or drainage every hour × 4 and then every 4 hours until 24 hours after removal. A T-tube left in place should be reconnected to drainage.
2. Assess for allergic reaction to the dye (listed above) for 24 hours.
3. Resume previous diet.

Client and Family Teaching
1. Fast from food and fluids for 6 hours before the procedure.

Factors That Affect Results
1. Inadvertent injection of air may cause bubbles that look like biliary calculi. One may differentiate these by observing for movement when the client is positioned upright. Calculi move down with gravity, whereas air bubbles rise.

Other Data
1. This procedure uses a low-dilution or high-dilution iodine contrast medium. A low-dilution medium requires longer x-ray exposure than a high-dilution medium.
2. The preoperative administration of morphine sulfate 0.05 mg/kg intravenously may result in spasm of the ampulla of Vater and duodenum, resulting in improved quality of cholangiography. Post-operative morphine in well positioned t-tubes improved output by 85%-93% (Saad et al, 2009).
3. Routine antibiotic prophylaxis after the procedure has not been found to be necessary for most clients.
4. See also Magnetic resonance cholangiopancreatography—Diagnostic.

Tuberculin Skin Test

See **Mantoux Skin Test**—Diagnostic.

Tuberculosis Test

See **Mantoux Skin Test**—Diagnostic; **RD1-Interferon Tests for Tuberculosis**—Blood.

Tularemia Agglutinins—Serum

Norm. <1:40. Current or past tularemia infection: >1:80.

Positive. A fourfold rise in titer is considered diagnostic of *Francisella tularensis* infection.

Negative. Normal finding. May also occur the first few days after infection.

Description. Tularemia is a highly contagious, serious infectious disease caused by the organism *F. tularensis*, which inhabits wild animals such as rabbits, muskrats, and beavers; some domestic animals, such as cats; and also ticks and deerflies. The pneumonic aerosolized form of the disease is considered a biologic weapon and can cause respiratory collapse and death. The mode of transmission is through direct contact of human skin or mucous membranes with the blood, tissue, or lesions of infected animals; ingestion of poorly cooked, infected animal meat; or through the bite of infected ticks. Airborne transmission is also possible from contaminated dust. Tularemia infection causes ulceration, lymph node edema, headache, pharyngeal inflammation, or pneumonia in humans 2-10 days after exposure. After infection, antibody levels begin rising in the conventional tube agglutination test within 7-21 days, peak in 60-90 days, and then decline over several months to higher-than-normal levels. After recovery, lifetime immunity exists. Titers at peak antibody levels are as high as 1:640. This test is a febrile agglutinin test in which the sample is heated and observed for clumping and unclumping. A sample that clumps upon warming and unclumps upon cooling is considered a positive test. A positive reaction is followed by serial dilutions of serum and retesting. The results are expressed as the highest titer showing agglutination. Agglutination at a titer greater than 1:80 indicates the presence of *F. tularensis* antibodies. A newer method, called the micro agglutination test, detects serum agglutinins of the immunoglobulin M type up to 9 days earlier and at levels 8-64 times higher than the conventional test. Therefore the newer test offers earlier and more specific results.

Professional Considerations

Consent form NOT required.

Preparation

1. Tube: Red topped, red/gray topped, or gold topped. Cool the tube in the refrigerator or on ice before specimen collection.
2. This test should be performed before skin testing for tularemia.

Procedure

1. Draw a 5-mL blood sample without hemolysis. Draw the first sample about 1 week after suspected exposure, and repeat the test every 3-5 days to observe for rising titers.

Postprocedure Care

1. Send sample to the laboratory immediately.

Client and Family Teaching

1. If routinely handling wild animals (such as skinning rabbits), wear gloves and goggles during contact, and thoroughly cook any wild animal meat to be ingested.
2. Serial testing is required to interpret the results.

Factors That Affect Results

1. Hemolysis of the specimen invalidates the results.
2. False-positive results may occur in the presence of *Brucella abortus* or *Proteus vulgaris* (OX-19) with the Weil-Felix agglutination test.
3. False-negative results may occur when the specimen is drawn early in the infective process.

4. False-positive results may occur if skin testing for tularemia has been performed within the previous 7 days.

Other Data

1. Avoid contact with open lesions of clients suspected of having tularemia.

2. If present, lesions should be cultured for *F. tularensis.*
3. Streptomycin, tetracyclines, gentamicin, fluoroquinolones, and chloramphenicol are used to treat tularemia.
4. See also Febrile agglutinins—Serum.

Tularemia Skin Test—Diagnostic

Norm. Negative. No redness, induration, or wheal.

Positive. Current or past infection with *Francisella tularensis.*

Negative. Normal finding. May also occur the first few days after infection.

Description. See Tularemia agglutinins—Serum for a description of the infectious disease of tularemia. The Foshay skin test for tularemia is based on a delayed hypersensitivity reaction. Results will be positive for clients with current infection of at least 7 days or for up to 5 years after recovery.

Professional Considerations
Consent form NOT required.

Preparation

1. Obtain a 4-mL syringe with an intradermal needle and purified *F. tularensis* antigen.

Procedure

1. Cleanse the forearm site for injection with an alcohol wipe and allow the area to dry.
2. Inject *F. tularensis* antigen, derived from culture, intradermally.

3. Record the site of injection.
4. Inspect the injection site in 48 hours. Reaction is positive if redness and induration of >5 mm diameter are present at the site.

Postprocedure Care

1. Let the site air-dry.

Client and Family Teaching

1. If routinely handling wild animals (such as skinning rabbits), wear gloves and goggles during contact, and thoroughly cook any wild animal meat to be ingested.
2. Return in 48 hours to have the injection site viewed and the skin test interpreted.

Factors That Affect Results

1. False-negative results may occur during the first week after infection as a result of insufficient antibody formation. If tularemia is suspected, the test should be repeated in 1 week.

Other Data

1. If serum testing for tularemia agglutinins is to be done, it should be performed before this test.

Tumor-Associated Glycoprotein 72

See CA 72-4—Blood.

Tuning Fork Test, of Weber, Rinne, and Schwabach Tests—Diagnostic

Norm. *Weber's test:* The tone is heard equally well in both ears.
Rinne's test: The tone is heard twice as long by air conduction (AC) as by bone conduction (BC).
Schwabach's test: The tone is heard for the same length of time by both the client and the examiner.

Usage. Assists in the differential diagnosis of conduction and perceptive or sensorineural hearing loss, hearing disorders, and tinnitus.

Description. The Weber, Rinne, and Schwabach tests are three simple tuning-fork hearing tests.

Weber's test helps determine whether hearing loss is the result of conductive or sensorineural causes. In clients with normal hearing, a vibrating tuning fork positioned midline on the skull is heard equally well by both ears. However, in conductive hearing loss, the tone seems loudest in the affected ear; in sensorineural hearing loss, the tone seems loudest in the unaffected ear.

Rinne's test also helps differentiate conductive from sensorineural hearing loss by comparing the duration of tone perception by bone conduction to the duration of tone perception by air conduction. In a client with normal hearing, a vibrating tuning fork that can no longer be heard by bone conduction can still be heard by air conduction for twice as long. Conductive hearing loss may be secondary to blocked pathways of sound conduction in the middle or external ear; thus bone conduction will be longer than air conduction (BC > AC). Perceptive or sensorineural loss may be secondary to inner ear disease or vestibulocochlear (eighth cranial nerve) disorders; thus air conduction will be longer than bone conduction (AC > BC) but not as high as the 2:1 ratio expected in normal clients.

Schwabach's test helps evaluate bone conduction by comparing the length of time the client hears a tuning fork placed against his or her mastoid process with the length of time it is heard by a client with normal hearing.

Professional Considerations
Consent form NOT required.

Preparation
1. Obtain a low-frequency tuning fork of 256-512 Hz.
2. The test should take place in a quiet room, free of noise and visual distractions.

Procedure
1. *Weber's test:*
   a. The examiner sets the tuning fork into light vibration by pinching the prongs between the thumb and index finger or by tapping it on his or her own knuckles.
   b. The tuning fork is placed on the skull at the midpoint or on the maxillary incisors.
   c. The client is asked to state whether the sound can be heard better in one ear

than the other and, if so, to state which ear hears the tone more loudly.
2. *Rinne's test:*
   a. The examiner sets the tuning fork into light vibration by pinching the prongs between the thumb and index finger or by tapping it on his or her own knuckles.
   b. The ear not being tested should be masked from detecting sound by bone conduction by providing a sound stimulus into it during step c.
   c. The vibrating fork is held by its stem on the mastoid process of the ear until vibration is no longer heard by the client.
   d. The fork is then held close to the external auditory meatus (within 2.5 cm of the pinna). If the client still hears the vibrations, this is called a positive Rinne's test. If the fork is not heard by air conduction, the test is repeated, but air conduction is first tested until the sound is no longer heard, and then the stem of the fork is placed on the mastoid process of the ear. If the sound is still heard, this is called a negative Rinne's test.
3. *Schwabach's test:*
   a. The examiner sets the tuning fork into light vibration by pinching the prongs between the thumb and index finger or by tapping it on his or her own knuckles.
   b. The ear not being tested should be masked from detecting sound by bone conduction by providing a sound stimulus into it during step c.
   c. The vibrating fork is held by its stem on the mastoid process of the client, who is instructed to indicate whether the tone is heard. Each time he or she hears the tone, the tuning fork is quickly transferred to the mastoid process of the examiner, who listens for the tone. This process continues back and forth between the client and the examiner until the tone is no longer heard by one of them, and the results are recorded. The process is then repeated in the other ear.

Postprocedure Care
1. None.

Client and Family Teaching

1. Testing is noninvasive and can take up to 15 minutes.
2. Thorough audiologic testing is indicated if results are abnormal.

Factors That Affect Results

1. The examiner should strike the tuning fork with equal intensity for each repetition of the tests.

2. For the Schwabach test, the examiner must have normal hearing for the results to be meaningful.

Other Data

1. Not to be used as a general screening test.

Tuttle Test

See **Esophageal Acidity Test**—Diagnostic.

Type-and-Crossmatch—Blood

Norm. Recipient blood type is determined to be either type A, B, O, or AB, and either Rh positive or Rh negative. Antibodies present in the recipient sample and donor blood are identified. Recipient and donor samples are mixed and observed for antigen-antibody reactions.

Usage. Determination of compatibility of recipient and donor blood before blood-product transfusion. A two specimen requirement prior to blood transfusion decreases human error.

Description. The type-and-crossmatch technique includes a series of procedures designed to identify donor blood that may be potentially safe to transfuse into a particular recipient with the lowest possible risk of causing a hemolytic reaction. The ABO group and Rh type of the recipient's blood sample are first determined. Donor blood of the same ABO blood group and Rh type is then chosen for further testing before transfusion. Many facilities use an electronic crossmatch system to detect ABO incompatibility and verify the correct ABO/RhD type of the donor blood. General antibody screening (indirect Coombs' testing) is then performed on both recipient and donor blood. If antibody screening is positive, more specific antibody identification is performed to determine the specific nature of irregular antibodies, which may cause a transfusion reaction. One identifies the exact antibody by combining the recipient or donor serum with a panel of red blood cell samples, each containing a known antigen, and observing for antigen-antibody reactions. Finally, recipient and donor blood samples are combined (crossmatched) and observed for antigen-antibody reactions that may cause a transfusion reaction. Newer techniques substitute a computerized crossmatch procedure. If no such reaction occurs, the donor blood is considered to be compatible for transfusion into the recipient. Absence of antigen-antibody reaction during crossmatching decreases but does not completely eliminate the possibility of a hemolytic transfusion reaction.

Professional Considerations
Consent form NOT required.

Preparation

1. Tube: Red topped, red/gray topped, or gold topped AND lavender topped. Also obtain a 30-mL syringe; a blood band (if required); two labels, stamped with the client's addressograph plate; and blood.
2. Note the client's age, medications, past transfusions of blood products, and number of pregnancies on the laboratory requisition.
3. Consult institutional protocol for any additional requirements.
4. Do NOT draw specimens during hemodialysis.

Procedure

1. The entire procedure should be performed by the person who performs the venipuncture.
2. Ask the client to state his or her full name and social security number. Verify that

this information matches the client's wrist identification band and addressograph stamp on the blood bank requisition and labels.

3. Some institutions use bar-coded or numeric-coded blood bands as an extra precaution to validate the proper recipient:

   a. Write the client's name, social security number, hospital number, and the date on the blood band, and place the band on the client's wrist, cutting off the distal end of the number stickers.

   b. Write the blood band number on both addressograph labels, and place a label on each tube. Alternatively, place addressograph labels on each tube, and place a number sticker from the blood band on each tube.

   c. Place a blood band number sticker on the blood bank requisition.

4. Do NOT draw specimens from an extremity into which blood or dextran is infusing. Draw a 25-mL blood sample, without hemolysis, in a 30-mL syringe. Completely fill the red topped tube and the lavender topped tube with the sample.

5. The caregiver performing this procedure should initial the following after drawing the blood: the blood band (if used), the label on each tube, and the blood bank requisition.

6. Staple the remaining blood band number stickers (if used) to the requisition.

Postprocedure Care

1. Send both tubes with the requisition and blood band number stickers (if used) to the blood bank.

2. Testing must be performed within 48 hours of specimen collection.

Client and Family Teaching

1. Screening for antibodies may take longer, up to several hours, if initial screening is positive.

2. Type-and-crossmatches are good for only 72 hours because of the possibility of the recipient developing irregular antibodies in response to a recent blood transfusion.

3. A type-and-crossmatch takes approximately 1 hour to complete.

Factors That Affect Results

1. Hemolysis of the specimen invalidates the results.

2. Drugs causing a false-positive Rh test include levodopa, methyldopa, and methyldopate hydrochloride.

Other Data

1. A type-and-screen involves only the ABO group and Rh-type determinations and the general antibody screening. It is sometimes prescribed instead of a type-and-crossmatch if there is only a small possibility of the client needing blood or if the blood must be transfused in an emergency. Donor blood should not be transfused if the general antibody screen is positive.

2. Identification of cold-reacting antibodies reactive at 30 degrees C may require the use of a blood warmer during transfusion.

3. See also ABO group and Rh type—Blood; Antibody identification, Red cell—Blood; Coombs' test, Indirect—Serum; Transfusion reaction work-up—Diagnostic.

Typhus Titer

See **Weil-Felix Agglutinins—Blood.**

Tzanck Smear—Specimen

Norm. Absence of multinucleated giant cells.

Usage. Helps diagnose viral infections in which blistering vesicles are present such as Chikungunya, clear cell acanthoma, cutaneous leishmaniasis, Dorfman-Chanarin syndrome, herpes simplex, pemphigus, and varicella zoster.

Description. The Tzanck smear is a rapid and sensitive inexpensive staining technique that can confirm the presence of herpes simplex virus or varicella zoster virus by examination of the morphology of cells present in fluid from the vesicles. Both viruses contain multinucleated giant cells, which can be seen under a microscope with this staining technique. The Tzanck smear cannot differentiate the type of virus present; thus viral culture should also be performed.

Professional Considerations
Consent form NOT required.

Preparation
1. Obtain scalpel blade, matches, and 3-4 glass slides.

Procedure
1. Using a scalpel, carefully and gently rupture the surface of the vesicle. Using the curved edge of the scalpel blade, scrape the soft (mushy) epidermis from the base of the vesicle and smear it onto a glass slide.
2. Light a match and hold it under the slide for about 10 seconds to "fix" the specimen. Repeat on 2-3 additional vesicles.
3. Add Giemsa, PAP, or Wright's stain to the slide. Wait 1 minute, and then rinse under water.
4. Add immersion oil and a coverslip and examine under microscope.

Postprocedure Care
1. Gently blot vesicle with sterile gauze. Leave site open to air.

Client and Family Teaching
1. The test may cause mild discomfort, but it will be brief.
2. It is important to prevent transferring the virus to others when vesicles are present. Keep your hands away from the vesicles, use careful handwashing, and avoid skin-to-skin contact with other people when vesicles are present or are moist or draining.

Factors That Affect Results
1. Several samples may be needed to locate the multinucleated giant cells.

Other Data
1. Tzanck smear staining can also identify noninfectious pustular eruptions by the presence of eosinophils and neutrophils.

UBT
See **Urea Breath Test**—Diagnostic.

UDS
See **Toxicology, Drug Screen**—Blood or Urine.

UFP
See **Pap Smear, Ultrafast and Fine-Needle Aspiration**—Diagnostic.

UGI
See **Upper Gastrointestinal Series**—Diagnostic.

UGP
See **Urinary Chorionic Gonadotropin Peptide**—Urine.

Ulcerative Lesions, Culture
See **Body Fluid, Routine**—Culture; Culture, Routine.

Ultra—Diagnostic

See Glucose Monitoring Machines—Diagnostic.

Ultrafast Computed Tomography

See Computed Tomography of the Body—Diagnostic.

Ultrasonography, Abdomen

See Abdominal Aorta Ultrasonography—Diagnostic; Gallbladder and Biliary System Ultrasonography—Diagnostic; Liver Ultrasonography—Diagnostic; Obstetric Ultrasonography—Diagnostic; Pancreas Ultrasonography—Diagnostic; Spleen Ultrasonography—Diagnostic.

Ultrasonography, Abdominal Aorta

See Abdominal Aorta Ultrasonography—Diagnostic.

Ultrasonography, Bone

See Breast Ultrasonography—Diagnostic.

Ultrasonography, Brain

See Brain Ultrasonography—Diagnostic.

Ultrasonography, Breast

See Breast Ultrasonography—Diagnostic.

Ultrasonography, Carotid Artery

See Doppler Ultrasonographic Flow Studies—Diagnostic.

Ultrasonography, Color Duplex

See Color Duplex Ultrasonography—Diagnostic.

Ultrasonography, Compression

See Compression Ultrasound—Diagnostic.

Ultrasonography, Coronary

See Coronary Intravascular Ultrasonography—Diagnostic.

Ultrasonography, Endoscopic

See Endoscopic Ultrasonography—Diagnostic; Transesophageal Ultrasonography—Diagnostic.

Ultrasonography, Eye and Orbit

See Eye and Orbit Ultrasonography—Diagnostic.

Ultrasonography, Gallbladder

See Gallbladder and Biliary System Ultrasonography—Diagnostic.

Ultrasonography, Gynecologic

See Gynecologic Ultrasonography—Diagnostic.

Ultrasonography, Heart

See Echocardiography—Diagnostic.

Ultrasonography, Kidney

See Kidney Ultrasonography—Diagnostic.

Ultrasonography, Liver

See Liver Ultrasonography—Diagnostic.

Ultrasonography, Obstetric

See Obstetric Ultrasonography—Diagnostic.

Ultrasonography, Pancreas

See Pancreas Ultrasonography—Diagnostic.

Ultrasonography, Pelvic

See Gynecologic Ultrasonography—Diagnostic.

Ultrasonography, Prostate

See Prostate Ultrasonography—Diagnostic.

Ultrasonography, Scrotum

See Scrotum and Testicular Ultrasonography—Diagnostic.

Ultrasonography, Spleen

See **Spleen Ultrasonography**—Diagnostic.

Ultrasonography, Thyroid

See **Thyroid Ultrasonography**—Diagnostic.

Ultrasonography, Transcranial

See **Doppler Ultrasonographic Flow Studies**—Diagnostic.

Ultrasonography, Transesophageal

See **Transesophageal Ultrasonography**—Diagnostic.

Ultrasonography, Transrectal

See **Prostate Ultrasonography**—Diagnostic.

Ultrasonography, Transvaginal

See **Gynecologic Ultrasonography**—Diagnostic; **Obstetric Ultrasonography**—Diagnostic; **Urinary Bladder Ultrasonography**—Diagnostic.

Ultrasonography, Urinary Bladder

See **Urinary Bladder Ultrasonography**—Diagnostic.

Upper GI Endoscopy

See **Esophagogastroduodenoscopy**—Diagnostic.

Upper Gastrointestinal (UGI) Series—Diagnostic

Norm. Mucosa is smooth and regular and free of lesions, polyps, narrowing, or filling defects. Barium fills smoothly and does not leak into the abdominal cavity. The passage of barium progresses at a normal rate, and there is no reflux into the esophagus (indicating hiatal hernia or incompetent cardiac sphincter). Gastric folds measure approximately 5 mm in the antrum and body of the stomach and are slightly wider near the fundus than near the esophagus.

Usage. Investigation of abnormal gastrointestinal symptoms; evaluation for leaks after gastric bypass surgery; evaluate resolving mural hematomas in children; evaluate "candy cane" Roux syndrome post gastric bypass; evaluate risk of obstruction prior to capsule endoscopy; allows fluoroscopic visualization of the esophagus, stomach, and duodenum; helps evaluate organ size, lumen size, outline, and position of the examined areas; and detection of obstructions, polypoidal lesions, strictures, scarring, stenosis (e.g., pyloric), superior mesenteric artery syndrome, varices, ulcers, tumors (e.g., Brunner's gland adenoma), hiatal hernia, or inflammation of the upper gastrointestinal tract.

Description. Upper gastrointestinal (UGI) series involves examining the upper gastrointestinal tract under fluoroscopy after the client drinks barium sulfate. Barium sulfate is a chalky substance of "milkshake" consistency that has radiopaque properties. Films of specific portions of the tract are taken as the barium passes through and outlines the structures. Barium-swallow studies of the esophagus with or without a small bowel series may be performed with this test. (See Barium swallow—Diagnostic; Small bowel series—Diagnostic.)

Professional Considerations
Consent form NOT required.

Risks
Aspiration of contrast material, bowel obstruction, constipation. Human error when central venous line mistaken for gastrostomy tube during barium sulfate injection includes symptoms of fever, vomiting, and rigors.

Contraindications
Suspected ileus, obstruction, or gastrointestinal perforation.

Precautions
During pregnancy, risks of cumulative radiation exposure to the fetus from this and other previous or future imaging studies must be weighed against the benefits of the procedure. Although formal limits for client exposure are relative to this risk:benefit comparison, the United States Nuclear Regulatory Commission requires that the cumulative dose equivalent to an embryo/fetus from occupational exposure not exceed 0.5 rem (5 mSv). Radiation dosage to the fetus is proportional to the distance of the anatomy studied from the abdomen and decreases as pregnancy progresses. For pregnant clients, consult the radiologist/radiology department to obtain estimated fetal radiation exposure from this procedure.

Preparation
1. Notify the physician before preparation if the client is pregnant.
2. When it is possible, medications that affect the motility of the gastrointestinal tract should be withheld for 24 hours before the study.
3. If this test is to be followed by a small bowel series for a bowel cleansing routine, see also Small bowel series—Diagnostic.
4. The client should disrobe and put on a gown. All jewelry and metal objects should be removed.
5. Obtain 8 ounces of barium sulfate solution.
6. See Client and Family Teaching.

Procedure
1. The client is positioned supine on the fluoroscopic tilt table and strapped into place. The hydraulic table is then moved into a vertical position.
2. Baseline fluoroscopic radiographs are taken of the area to be studied.
3. The client is then given 8 ounces of barium sulfate solution and is instructed to drink portions of it at specified intervals as the table is tilted to various angles.
4. Initial films are taken of the esophagus as the barium travels downward.
5. Stomach films are taken as barium mixed with air enters the stomach. The lower esophagus is examined for reflux of the barium from the stomach or for free-flowing barium between the stomach and the esophagus, both conditions indicating hiatal hernia.
6. As the client finishes ingesting the barium, the filled stomach and the emptying of the barium into the duodenum are radiographed from several angles. Gastric folds are examined for thickening, indicated by a rugal pattern that is not obliterated by filling of the stomach with barium sulfate.
7. The test takes less than 1 hour.

Postprocedure Care
1. Resume previous diet.
2. See Client and Family Teaching.

Client and Family Teaching
1. Fast from food and fluids, and do not chew gum or smoke overnight before the study.
2. A laxative or suppository may be prescribed to be taken the night before the study.
3. If this test is to be followed by a small bowel series, bring something to read, if desired, because the procedure time may increase to 4-6 hours.
4. After swallowing a chalky barium solution, you will be asked to move to

several positions and at times to hold your breath while the radiographs are taken.

5. Drink 6-8 glasses of water or other fluids each day for 2 days after the test to help pass the barium through the gastrointestinal system.

6. Observe stools for passage of barium for 1-3 days. This will make the stools look chalky white.

7. Call the physician if unable to defecate. A mild laxative may be prescribed prophylactically, or cathartics or enemas may be prescribed as needed if pending impaction is suspected.

Factors That Affect Results

1. The client must be able to cooperate in swallowing the barium sulfate.

Other Data

1. *Helicobacter pylori* infection should be suspected if isolated thickened gastric folds are found.

2. Routine use of this procedure for morbid obesity as part of presurgery evaluation is controversial.

Urea

See **Urea Nitrogen**—Plasma or Serum.

Urea Breath Test (UBT, ^{13}C-UBT, ^{14}C-UBT)—Diagnostic

Norm. Negative for *Helicobacter pylori*.

Usage. Diagnosis of gastric *H. pylori* colonization. This test is useful in children and adults and is a sensitive indicator of *H. pylori* eradication 4-6 weeks after treatment with antibiotics. Considered the test of choice to confirm *H. pylori* infection.

Description. *H. pylori* infection is an underlying cause found in most cases of gastritis and duodenal ulcer/peptic ulcer. In addition, *H. pylori* is a carcinogen that causes gastric cancer and is also associated with stroke, coronary artery disease, and vitamin B$_{12}$ deficiency. *H. pylori* infection is thought to be acquired in childhood, with the highest rates of seroconversion occurring in those ages 4-5 years. This organism is the most common type of bacterial pathogen, in that it is colonized in more than half of adults >40 years. The source of infection is thought to be direct person-to-person transmission, but isolates have inconsistently been found in water, food, or animals.

The urea breath test detects exhaled labeled carbon dioxide absorbed into the bloodstream from the stomach when the urease enzyme produced by *H. pylori* degrades ingested radiolabeled urea. The labeled carbon dioxide (CO_2), known as ^{13}C or ^{14}C, is present in exhalations within 10-30 minutes. After the radiolabeled urea is ingested, a test meal is given to delay emptying from the stomach so as to allow the urease enzyme to act. The addition of citric acid to the test meal improves the sensitivity and specificity of the urea breath test. The difference between the ^{13}C and ^{14}C tests is that the ^{14}C is radioactive, is inexpensive, and can be interpreted using a liquid scintillation counter, widely available in radiology settings. The ^{13}C test is not radioactive and may be performed in any setting, but is much more expensive, and the mass spectrometer equipment needed for interpretation is not widely available.

Professional Considerations

Consent form NOT required for the ^{13}C test. Consent form IS required for the ^{14}C test.

Risks

There is a very small amount of radiation with the ^{14}C test.

Contraindications

The ^{14}C test is contraindicated during pregnancy.

Preparation

1. Obtain 200 mL of test drink for client ingestion.

2. Remove dentures, if present, to avoid trapping of the mixture under them.

3. See Client and Family Teaching.

4. Just before beginning the procedure, take a "time out" to verify the correct client, procedure, and site.

Procedure

1. *^{14}C test:*
   a. The client must rinse his/her mouth before drinking the mixture.
   b. A baseline breath is taken by having the client blow into a solution that contains an acid/base indicator.
   c. The client drinks a mixture or ingests a pill of radiolabeled ^{14}C-urea. A standard meal may be given.
   d. Breath samples are measured at frequent intervals (e.g., 6, 12, 20, and 30 minutes) after ingestion.
   e. Alternatively, the client will blow into a balloon 10 minutes after urea ingestion and the balloon contents are transferred to a trapping solution for analysis.

2. *^{13}C test:*
   a. The client drinks a mixture of radiolabeled ^{13}C-urea or ^{14}C-urea. A standard meal may be given.
   b. Breath samples are taken by being blown into a bag or balloon.
   c. In the ^{13}C test, breath samples are measured at 0 and at 30 minutes after ingestion of the urea mixture.

Postprocedure Care

1. The client may resume eating and drinking and all medications.

Client and Family Teaching

1. Do not take antibiotics (except vancomycin, nalidixic acid, trimethoprim, amphotericin B) or bismuth mixtures (e.g., Pepto-Bismol) within 1 month before the test.
2. Do not take omeprazole, lansoprazole, or pantoprazole within 14 days before the test.
3. Do not take cimetidine, famotidine, nizatidine, or ranitidine within 24 hours before the test.

4. Do NOT eat or drink for at least 6 hours before the test.
5. The test takes about 30 minutes.
6. *^{13}C test only:* There is no radioactivity exposure from this test.
7. *^{14}C test only:* The radioactivity received from this test is much less than that received from a regular chest radiograph and less than what you normally receive from a natural day of radiation.

Factors That Affect Results

1. A fatty meal profoundly affects results by increasing values at 30-, 40-, 50-, 60-, 90-, and 120-minute intervals.
2. Taking antibiotics or Pepto-Bismol for 1 month or Prilosec or Carafate for 1 week before the test can cause false-negative results.
3. Taking drugs that inhibit bacterial growth, such as antibiotics, within 1 month before the test can cause false-negative results.
4. Antacids and proton pump inhibitors (PPI) can produce false-negative results.
5. Substituting orange juice for citric acid reduces diagnostic accuracy (specificity) of this test. Citric acid has 100% specificity, but orange juice has only 88% specificity.
6. False positive results occur in up to 12% of children <6 years of age.

Other Data

1. *H. pylori* infection is treated with a 7-day cycle of tetracycline, metronidazole, and bismuth subsalicylate.
2. See also *Campylobacter*-like organism test—Specimen; *Helicobacter pylori*, Quick office serology, Serum and titer—Blood.

Urea Nitrogen (BUN, Blood Urea Nitrogen)—Plasma or Serum

Norm. Note reference interval provided with test results. Plasma and serum levels are about 12% higher.

	Blood Urea Nitrogen	SI Units
Young adult <40 years	5-18 mg/dL	1.8-6.5 mmol/L
Adult	5-20 mg/dL	1.8-7.1 mmol/L
Elderly >60 years	8-21 mg/dL	2.9-7.5 mmol/L
Mild azotemia	20-50 mg/dL	7.1-17.7 mmol/L

Continued

	Blood Urea Nitrogen	SI Units
Children		
Cord blood	21-40 mg/dL	7.5-14.3 mmol/L
Premature infant, first 7 days	3-25 mg/dL	1.1-7.9 mmol/L
Full-term newborn	4-18 mg/dL	1.4-6.4 mmol/L
Infant	5-18 mg/dL	1.8-6.4 mmol/L
Child	5-18 mg/dL	1.8-6.4 mmol/L
Panic Level	>100 mg/dL	>35.7 mmol/L

Panic Level Symptoms and Treatment

Symptoms. Acidemia, agitation, coma, confusion, fatigue, nausea, stupor, and vomiting.

Treatment

NOTE: Treatment choice(s) depend(s) on client's history and condition and episode history.
1. Correct the cause.
2. Administer sodium bicarbonate IV for severe acidemia.
3. Prescribe a low-protein diet.
4. Hemodialysis and peritoneal dialysis WILL remove urea nitrogen.
5. Avoid or reduce drug usage of long-acting barbiturates, narcotics, sulfonamides, anticoagulants, and antibiotics such as vancomycin, kanamycin, and polymyxins.

Increased. Acute necrotizing pancreatitis (continued elevation associated with mortality), Addison's disease, allergic purpura, amyloidosis, analgesic abuse, blood transfusions, cachexia, cardiac failure, congenital hypoplastic kidneys, dehydration, diabetes mellitus, diabetic ketoacidosis, diet (high-protein), eating disorders (dehydration), Fanconi syndrome, fluid therapy (excessive), gastrointestinal bleeding, glomerulonephritis, Goodpasture's syndrome, gout, heavy-metal poisoning, hemoglobinurias, infection, intestinal obstruction, multiple myeloma, myocardial infarction (acute), nephritis, nephropathy (hypercalcemic, hypokalemic), nephrosclerosis, pancreatitis, peritonitis, pneumonia, polyarteritis nodosa, polycystic disease, postoperative state, protein intake (excessive), pyelonephritis, renal artery stenosis or thrombosis, renal cortical necrosis, renal hypoperfusion states, renal malignancy, renal tuberculosis, renal vein thrombosis, scleroderma, sepsis, shock, sickle cell anemia, starvation, stress, subacute bacterial endocarditis, suppuration, systemic lupus erythematosus, thyrotoxicosis, tumor necrosis, uremia, and urinary tract obstruction. Drugs include acetohexamide, acetone, alkaline antacids, aminophenol, ammonium salts, amphotericin B, anabolic steroids, androgens, antimony compounds, arginine, arsenicals, ascorbic acid, asparaginase, bacitracin, calcium salts, capreomycin, captopril, carmustine, carbutamide, cephaloridine, chloral hydrate, chloramphenicol, chlorobutanol, chlorothiazide sodium, chlorthalidone, clonidine, colistimethate sodium, dextran, dextrose infusions, disopyramide phosphate, doxapram, ethacrynic acid, fluorides, fluphenazine, fosinopril, furosemide, guanethidine sulfate, gentamicin sulfate, guanochlor, guanethidine analogs, hydroxyurea, indomethacin, kanamycin, Lipomul (maize oil, corn oil emulsion), lithium carbonate, marijuana, meclofenamate sodium, mephenesin, mercurial diuretics, mercury compounds, methicillin, methoxyflurane, methsuximide, methyldopa, methylprednisolone sodium succinate, methysergide, metolazone, metoprolol tartrate, minoxidil, mithramycin, morphine, nalidixic acid, naproxen sodium, neomycin, nitrofurantoin, paramethasone, pargyline, polymyxin B, propranolol, salicylates, spectinomycin, streptodornase, streptokinase, sulfonylureas, tetracycline, thiazide diuretics, tolmetin sodium, triamterene, and vancomycin.

Decreased. Acromegaly, alcohol abuse, amyloidosis, celiac disease, cirrhosis, diet (inadequate protein), eating disorders (laxatives), fluid intake (excessive), hemodialysis, hepatitis, infancy, liver destruction, malnutrition, nephrosis, plasma volume expansion, and pregnancy (late). Drugs include chloramphenicol, streptomycin, and thymol. Herb or natural remedy is *Cordyceps sinensis*.

Description. Commonly referred to as BUN (blood urea nitrogen), this measurement is actually performed on plasma or serum. Plasma or serum levels of urea nitrogen are about 12% higher than BUN levels, resulting from the relatively higher percentage of protein contained in erythrocytes. Urea nitrogen is the nitrogen portion of urea, a substance formed in the liver through an enzymatic protein-breakdown process. Urea is normally freely filtered through the renal glomeruli, with a small amount reabsorbed in the tubules and the remainder excreted in the urine. Elevated urea nitrogen in the bloodstream is called "azotemia." However, the value is nonspecific as to cause and thus may be a result of prerenal, renal, or postrenal causes. Prerenal causes may be grouped under factors that result in inadequate renal circulation or conditions resulting in abnormally high levels of blood protein. Renal causes are those of impaired renal filtration and excretion of urea nitrogen. Postrenal causes are lower urinary tract obstructive conditions that result in diffusion of urea nitrogen in dormant urine back into the bloodstream through the tubules. "Uremia" is a term used to describe symptoms occurring at very high elevations of urea in the bloodstream and may occur at urea nitrogen levels of about 200 mg/dL (>70 mmol/L). Also of significance are low urea nitrogen levels in severe hepatic disease. A damaged liver that is unable to synthesize urea from protein results in a buildup of blood ammonia (NH_3), causing hepatic encephalopathy.

Professional Considerations

Consent form NOT required.

Preparation

1. Tube: Red topped, red/gray topped, or gold topped.
2. Do NOT draw specimens during hemodialysis.

Procedure

1. Draw a 4-mL blood sample without hemolysis.

Postprocedure Care

1. Separate plasma or serum and refrigerate until testing.

Client and Family Teaching

1. This test result alone is of little diagnostic value but must be compared to itself over time or used with other test results.

Factors That Affect Results

1. Falsely elevated results may occur in hemolyzed specimens.
2. Values are somewhat affected by hemodilution.
3. In contrast to creatinine level, dietary protein intake does influence the urea nitrogen level.

Other Data

1. Both creatinine levels and urea nitrogen levels should be considered when evaluating renal function.
2. See also Blood urea nitrogen/creatinine ratio—Blood.

Uric Acid—Serum

Norm. Norms vary based upon instrumentation.

		SI Units
Adult females	2.4-6.0 mg/dL	143-357 µmol/L
Adult males	3.4-7.0 mg/dL	202-416 µmol/L
Children	2.5-5.5 mg/dL	119-327 µmol/L
Oxidative stress begins	>6.38 mg/dL	>380 µmol/L
Panic level	>12 mg/dL	>714 µmol/L

Panic Level Symptoms and Treatment
Symptoms. Painful swelling of great toe, hypertension, arthritis.
Treatment
NOTE: Treatment choice(s) depend(s) on client's history and condition and episode history.

Acute phase: allopurinol, colchicine, indomethacin, or phenylbutazone, orally; corticotropin (ACTH) intramuscularly; also analgesics for severe pain.

Chronic phase: allopurinol, probenecid, or sulfinpyrazone, orally.

Increased. Alcoholism, anemia (hemolytic, pernicious, sickle cell), arterial disease legs (women), arteriosclerosis, arthritis, atrial fibrillation, berylliosis (chronic), Blackfoot Indians, body size (larger than average), calcinosis universalis and circumscripta, chronic kidney disease (CKD), cirrhosis, congestive heart failure, coronary artery ectasia, coronary bypass graft (CABG—predicts mortality), dehydration, dementia, diabetes mellitus, diet (high-protein, excess nucleoproteins), Down syndrome, eclampsia, exercise, fasting, Filipinos, glomerulonephritis (chronic), Graves' disease, gout, heart transplant (predicts mortality), hemolysis (prolonged), hepatic disease, hypertension or hypertensive vascular damage, hyperuricemia, hypoparathyroidism, hypothyroidism, infections (acute), insulin resistance, intestinal obstruction, ketoacidosis, ketosis, lead poisoning, Lesch-Nyhan syndrome, leukemia, lipoproteinemia (type III), lymphoma, maple syrup urine disease, metabolic syndrome, mononucleosis (infectious), multiple myeloma, multiple sclerosis, neoplasm (disseminated), nephritis, nephropathy, New Zealand Maoris, Pima Indians (Akimel O'odham), pneumonia (resolving), polycystic kidneys, polycythemia vera, pregnancy (low–birth-weight, onset of labor, twin pregnancy), psoriasis, pulmonary hypertension, renal failure, rheumatoid arthritis, sarcoidosis, silent brain infarction, starvation, stress, toxemia of pregnancy, transplant rejection (cardiac), uremia, urinary obstruction, and von Gierke's disease. Drugs include acetazolamide, asparaginase, busulfan, chlorothiazide sodium, chlorthalidone, corticosteroids, cyclophosphamide, dactinomycin, daunorubicin hydrochloride, dextran, diazoxide, diltiazem, diuretics (except spironolactone, mercurials, and ticrynafen), epinephrine, ethacrynic acid, ethambutol, ethyl alcohol (ethanol), fructose, furosemide, gentamicin sulfate, glucose, hydralazine, hydrocortisone, hydroxyurea, ibufenac, levodopa, mecamylamine, mechlorethamine hydrochloride, 6-mercaptopurine, methicillin, methotrexate, methyldopa, metoprolol tartrate, niacin, nicotinic acid (large doses), nitrogen mustards, norepinephrine, phenothiazines, pitavastatin, probenecid, propranolol, propylthiouracil, pyrazinamide, quinethazone, rifampin, salicylates (low doses), theophylline, thiazide diuretics, 6-thioguanine, triamterene, and vincristine. Foods include sugar sweetened soda and orange juice.

Decreased. Acromegaly, amyotrophic lateral sclerosis (ALS), bronchogenic carcinoma, celiac disease, Dalmatian dog mutation, Fanconi syndrome, Hodgkin's disease, myeloma, pernicious anemia, post hemodialysis, transsexual (male to female), Wilson's disease, xanthinuria, and yellow atrophy of liver. Drugs include acetohexamide, ACTH, allopurinol, anticoagulants, atorvastatin, azathioprine, azlocillin, bacitracin, benziodarone, chlorine, chlorpromazine hydrochloride, chlorprothixene, chlorthalidone, cinchophen, corticosteroids, corticotropin, cortisone, coumarins, dicumarol, ethacrynic acid, glyceryl guaiacolate, lithium carbonate, mannitol, marijuana, oxyphenbutazone, phenothiazines, phenylbutazone, piperazine, potassium oxalate, probenecid, radiographic dyes, rosuvastatin, salicylates (long-term, large doses), saline infusions, sodium oxalate, sulfinpyrazone, thyroid hormone and triamterene. Herbal or natural remedies include products containing aristolochic acids (*Akebia* spp., *Aristolochia* spp., *Asarum* spp., birthwort, *Bragantia* spp., *Clematis* spp., *Cocculus* spp., *Diploclisia* spp., Dutchman's pipe, *Fang chi*, *Fang ji*, *Guang fang ji*, *Kan-Mokutsu*, *Menispermum* spp., *Mokutsu*, *Mu tong*, *Sinomenium* spp., and *Stephania* spp.).

Description. Uric acid (lithic acid) is formed as the purines adenine and guanine are continuously metabolized during the formation and degradation of ribonucleic acid (RNA) and deoxyribonucleic acid (DNA) and from metabolism of dietary purines. After synthesis in the liver triggered by the action of xanthine oxidase, part of the uric acid is excreted in the urine. Elevated amounts of serum uric acid (uricemia) become deposited in joints and soft tissues and cause gout, an inflammatory reaction to the urate crystal deposition. Conditions of both fast cell turnover and slowed renal excretion of uric acid may cause uricemia. Elevated amounts of urinary uric acid precipitate into urate stones in the kidneys.

Professional Considerations
Consent form NOT required.

Preparation

1. Tube: Red topped, red/gray topped, or gold topped.
2. See Client and Family Teaching.

Procedure

1. Draw a 4-mL blood sample.

Postprocedure Care

1. None.

Client and Family Teaching

1. Fast for 8 hours before sampling.
2. Foods high in purines that can contribute to gout include caffeine-containing beverages, legumes, mushrooms, organ meats, spinach, gravies, and baker's and brewer's yeast.
3. Switching from a normal diet to a low-purine diet may potentially decrease urine uric acid levels by half.

Factors That Affect Results

1. Drugs that may cause falsely elevated results include aminophylline, caffeine, and vitamin C.
2. African men have slightly lower uric acid norms, about 0.1 mg/dL lower than Caucasian men.

Other Data

1. Mortality for women with ischemic heart disease increases fivefold if their uric acid level is ≥7 mg/dL (416 μmol/L).
2. Predictor of 24-month mortality in persons seen in emergency departments with acute dyspnea with unknown cause (Reichlin et al, 2009).
3. High uric acid treated with rasburicase or allopurinol.

Uric Acid—Urine

Norm.

		SI Units
Adult female	250-750 mg/24 hours	1.5-4.5 mmol/day
Adult male	250-800 mg/24 hours	1.5-4.8 mmol/day

Usage. Determines whether renal calculi may be the result of hyperuricosuria. Excretion increased in some children with an ethnic background of sleep apnea (e.g., Greeks) and in perinatal asphyxia.

Description. Uric acid (lithic acid) is formed as the purines adenine and guanine are continuously metabolized during the formation and degradation of ribonucleic acid (RNA) and deoxyribonucleic acid (DNA) and from metabolism of dietary purines. After synthesis in the liver triggered by the action of xanthine oxidase, part of the uric acid is excreted in the urine. Elevated amounts of serum uric acid (uricemia) become deposited in joints and soft tissues and cause gout, an inflammatory reaction to the urate crystal deposition. Conditions of both fast cell turnover and slowed renal excretion of uric acid may cause uricemia. Elevated amounts of urinary uric acid precipitate into urate stones in the kidneys.

Professional Considerations

Consent form NOT required.

Preparation

1. Obtain a 3-L container to which 10 mL of 12.5 M sodium hydroxide solution has been added.
2. Write the beginning time of collection on the laboratory requisition.

Procedure

1. Discard the first morning-voided urine.
2. Save all the urine voided for the next 24 hours in a 3-L container to which 10 mL of 12.5 M sodium hydroxide solution has been added. For specimens collected from an indwelling urinary catheter, empty the urine into the collection container hourly. Document the quantity of urinary output during the collection period. Do not refrigerate the specimen.

Postprocedure Care

1. Write the ending time on the laboratory requisition.
2. Compare the quantity of urine with the urinary output record for the collection. If the specimen contains less than what was recorded as output, some urine may have been discarded, thus invalidating the test.

Client and Family Teaching

1. Save all the urine voided during the collection period, urinate before defecating, and avoid contaminating the specimen with stool or toilet tissue. If any urine is accidentally discarded, discard the entire specimen and restart the collection the next day.
2. Foods high in purines that can contribute to gout include caffeine-containing beverages, legumes, mushrooms, organ meats, spinach, gravies, and baker's and brewer's yeast.
3. Switching from a normal diet to a low-purine diet may potentially decrease urine uric acid levels by half.

Factors That Affect Results

1. Drugs that increase the rate of uric acid excretion include ascorbic acid, cytotoxics, probenecid, radiographic dyes, salicylates (long-term, large doses), and sulfinpyrazone.
2. Drugs that slow uric acid excretion include diuretics and insulin.
3. Trauma has been shown to increase the rate of urinary uric acid excretion.

Other Data

1. Herbal or natural remedies that can cause Fanconi syndrome and increased uric acid in the urine include products containing aristolochic acids (*Akebia* spp., *Aristolochia* spp., *Asarum* spp., birthwort, *Bragantia* spp., *Clematis* spp., *Cocculus* spp., *Diploclisia* spp., Dutchman's pipe, *Fang chi, Fang ji, Guang fang ji, Kan-Mokutsu, Menispermum* spp., *Mokutsu, Mu tong, Sinomenium* spp., and *Stephania* spp.).

Urinalysis (UA)—Urine

Norm.

Albumin	Negative
Appearance	Clear to faintly hazy
Bilirubin	Negative
Color	Yellow
Glucose or reducing substances	Negative
Ketones	Negative
Leukocyte esterase	Negative
Nitrite	Negative
Occult blood	Negative
Odor	Faint (not fruity, musty, fishy, or fetid)
pH	4.5-8.0
Protein	Negative
Specific gravity	1.003-1.030
Urobilinogen	Negative or 0.1-1 Ehrlich U/dL
Cells	
Erythrocytes	<3 cells/high power field (HPF)
Leukocytes	≤4 cells/HPF
Urinary Tract Epithelium	≤10 cells/HPF
Casts	Moderate clear protein casts
Crystals	Small amount
Bacteria or fungi	None or <1000/mL
Parasites	None

Increased or Decreased. For specific causes of increased or decreased values of constituents, see individual test listings as follows: Albumin—Serum, Urine, and 24-Hour Urine; Bilirubin—Urine; Glucose, Qualitative, Semiquantitative—Urine; Ketone, Semiquantitative—Urine; Nitrite, Bacteria screen—Urine; Occult blood—Urine; pH—Urine; Protein—Urine; Urinalysis—Urine; Urobilinogen—Urine.

Changes in Urine Color. A variety of substances may alter urine color as follows:

Color	Possible Cause
Black	Ferrous sulfate, homogentisic acid, indicans, indigo carmine dye used in renal function tests and cystoscopy, levodopa, melanin, methemoglobin, phenols, urobilinogen; herbal or natural remedies include cascara sagrada (*Rhamnus purshiana*)
Blue	Amitriptyline, some diuretics, methylene blue, nitrofurans, *Pseudomonas*
Brown	Acid hematin, Addison's disease, bile pigment, furazolidone, levodopa, metronidazole, myoglobin, nitrofurantoin, porphyrinuria, renal disease, some sulfonamides
Dark yellow	Bilirubin, chlorpromazine, food (carrots), nitrofurantoin, phenacetin, to amber quinacrine, riboflavin, urobilinogen; herbal or natural remedies include cascara sagrada (*Rhamnus purshiana*)
Green	Bacterial infection, biliverdin, some diuretics, vitamins
Light	Diuresis caused by alcohol ingestion or diuretics, diabetes insipidus, glycosuria
Orange	Bile pigment, chlorzoxazone, dehydration, fever, fluorescein sodium, jaundice, some oral anticoagulants, phenazopyridine, phenothiazines, pyridium, rifampin, sulfasalazine
Red	Deferoxamine mesylate, foods (beets, rhubarb, senna), hemoglobin, malaria, myoglobin, porphobilinogen, phenolphthalein, phenolsulfonphthalein, porphyrins, renal injury, rifampin, sulfobromophthalein

Automated Microscopy. >2 white blood cells (WBC)/HPF indicates urinary tract inflammation causing pyuria.

Description. A frequently performed screening test that gives a general indication of the client's overall state of health as well as the health of the urinary tract. The dipstick reagent strip method is commonly used to measure pH, ketones, leukocyte esterase, protein, sugars, and other reducing substances. Additional reagent strips are available to measure bilirubin and urobilinogen levels. The sample is also centrifuged, with the sediment then examined microscopically for determination of the presence and type of cells, casts, crystals, and organisms such as bacteria or fungi. Urine color should correlate with specific gravity. That is, dilute urine with low specific gravity should be almost colorless, and concentrated urine with high specific gravity should be dark yellow. Glucose content should also correlate positively with specific gravity. pH should correlate inversely with ketone (acetone) level. A sweet or fruity urine odor indicates the presence of ketones in the sample. A fish or fetid odor indicates urinary tract infection. An odor of maple syrup may indicate maple syrup urine disease. A musty urine odor may be caused by recent ingestion of asparagus.

An increase in epithelial cells may signal an inflammatory process in the kidneys. Erythrocytes present in the urine signal damage to the renal glomeruli. Elevated leukocyte levels indicate inflammation or infection in the urinary tract and indicate the need for urine culture. Both erythrocytes and leukocytes, if present, will appear trapped in casts and can be observed microscopically. Crystals may form at room temperature in voided urine before being tested or may be caused by a variety of drugs. More detailed descriptions of other aspects of urine analysis may be found under individual test listings described above under Increased or Decreased.

Professional Considerations

Consent form NOT required.

Preparation

1. Obtain a soapy sponge and a clean specimen container.
2. If bilirubin or urobilinogen results are of specific interest, the specimen container should be wrapped in foil to protect it from light.

Procedure

1. A first morning void is preferred.
2. *Female*: Instruct the client to wash the area surrounding the urethral meatus with soap and water. Then, while holding

the labia open, position the specimen container beneath the urethral meatus and void into the container, filling it about half full (about 50 mL). Also see Client and Family Teaching.

3. *Male*: Instruct the client to retract the foreskin if present. Then wash the distal end of the penis surrounding the urethral meatus with soap and water. The client should then void into the specimen container, filling it about half full (about 50 mL).

Postprocedure Care

1. Write the collection method, date, and time on the laboratory requisition.
2. Send the specimen to the laboratory promptly and refrigerate it until testing. The best results are obtained if testing is performed within 2 hours.

Client and Family Teaching

1. Urinate before defecating and avoid contaminating the specimen with vaginal or perineal secretions or stool.
2. Menstruating females should insert a tampon into the vagina before cleansing and voiding.

Factors That Affect Results

1. First morning-voided specimens provide the most accurate reflection of the presence of bacteria and formed elements such as casts and crystals.
2. A delay in testing after collection may cause falsely decreased glucose, ketone, bilirubin, and urobilinogen values. Delayed testing with specimens left at room temperature may cause falsely elevated bacteria levels because of bacterial overgrowth. Delays also inhibit microscopic clarity because of the dissolution of urates and phosphates.
3. Increased accuracy of results can be obtained by waiting 5 minutes before reading the dipstick.
4. Drugs that interfere with results of the leukocyte esterase test include vitamin C and phenazopyridine.
5. For detailed listings of factors that affect results, see individual test listings described under Increased or Decreased.

Other Data

1. Abnormal results should be confirmed by more specific, or quantitative, follow-up testing.

Urinalysis, Fractional—Urine

Norm. Sugars: negative. Acetone: negative. Calculated albumin excretion rate (nephorimetric [combined nephelometric, calorimetric] method).

		SI Units
Adult		
At rest	2-80 mg/24 hours	0.03-0.08 g/day
Ambulatory	<150 mg/24 hours	<0.15 g/day
Child <10 years	<100 mg/24 hours	<0.10 g/day

Usage. Monitoring for clients with diabetes mellitus (infrequently used). Assessment of urinary albumin excretion rate.

Description. A fractional urine involves testing as many as four timed urine collections within a 24-hour period for the presence of sugars, acetone, or albumin, all of which are abnormal. Glucose results reflect serum glucose levels because levels above the renal threshold for glomerular glucose reabsorption into the bloodstream are excreted in the urine. Acetone levels are an indication of the state of fatty acid metabolism in diabetic clients. The detection of microalbuminuria in an aliquot of a fractional specimen can be predictive of diabetic nephropathy at an early and potentially reversible stage. This test used to be performed more frequently for diabetic clients. However, as studies demonstrated that renal thresholds for glucose reabsorption vary from client to client, this test is no longer considered the most accurate reflection of insulin needs. Routine daily blood glucose monitoring has replaced fractional urine analysis for ongoing diabetes monitoring. Fractional urine testing is more often used to measure the excretion rate of albumin.

Professional Considerations

Consent form NOT required.

Preparation

1. Obtain four clean 1-L specimen containers to which toluene preservative has been added (for glucose measurement) or without preservative (for albumin measurement), reagent strips, or Clinitest and Acetest tablets.
2. Number the containers sequentially.

Procedure

1. Specimens for albumin measurement should be refrigerated.
2. *First collection period*:
   a. The first morning void, 1 hour before breakfast, is discarded.
   b. The client should drink 8 ounces of water.
   c. One-half hour later, the client should void and test the specimen for sugar and acetone, then transfer the specimen to container 1, and record the results as well as the beginning time of the collection period.
   d. The client should eat breakfast.
   e. All additional urine voided until 1 hour before the midday meal should be added to container 1, and the ending time of the collection period should be recorded.
3. *Second collection period:*
   a. The client should drink 8 ounces of water 1 hour before the midday meal.
   b. One-half hour later, the client should void and test the specimen for sugar and acetone, then transfer the specimen to container 2, and record the results as well as the beginning time of the collection period.
   c. The client should eat the midday meal and an afternoon snack.
   d. All additional urine voided until 1 hour before the evening meal should be added to container 2, and the ending time of the collection period should be recorded.
4. *Third collection period:*
   a. The client should drink 8 ounces of water 1 hour before the evening meal.
   b. One-half hour later, the client should void and test the specimen for sugar and acetone, then transfer the specimen to container 3, and record the results as well as the beginning time of the collection period.

c. The client should eat the evening meal.
   d. All additional urine voided until 1 hour before the bedtime snack should be added to container 3, and the ending time of the collection period should be recorded.
5. *Fourth collection period:*
   a. The client should drink 8 ounces of water 1 hour before the bedtime snack.
   b. One-half hour later, the client should void and test the specimen for sugar and acetone, then transfer the specimen to container 4, and record the results as well as the beginning time of the collection period.
   c. The client should eat a bedtime snack.
   d. All additional urine voided until 1 hour before breakfast the next day should be added to container 4.
   e. The client should include the void at 1 hour before breakfast in container 4, and record the time ended.

Postprocedure Care

1. Send all four containers to the laboratory.

Client and Family Teaching

1. Collect specimens according to the procedure described above.
2. All testing should be performed on freshly voided urine with reagent strips (Keto-Diastix, Multistix) or Clinitest and Acetest tablets according to manufacturer's directions. Compare the results with the color chart on the container.

Factors That Affect Results

1. Expired reagent strips, Clinitest tablets, or Acetest tablets, or those that have had prolonged exposure to air or moisture should not be used because the results will be invalid.
2. Many drugs and factors affect the accuracy of the test media used. For detailed information, see the specific test listing for the method used as follows: Acetone—Urine; Albumin—Serum, Urine, and 24-Hour Urine; Glucose, Qualitative, Semiquantitative—Urine.

Other Data

1. None.

Urinary Bladder Ultrasonography (Urinary Bladder Echogram, Urinary Bladder Ultrasonogram)—Diagnostic

Norm. Negative for tumor, cyst, overdistention, or residual urine. Proper size, shape, and position of the urinary bladder.

Usage. Assessment for residual urine in bladder, female stress incontinence, or for volume or overdistention of bladder; search for radiolucent stones; evaluation of large diverticulae; confirmation of suspicious filling defects seen on other imaging studies; guidance for suprapubic placement of needles and catheter in the bladder; detection of inguinal bladder hernia; evaluation of the size, shape, and position of the urinary bladder; diagnose bladder schistosomiasis; helps diagnose, localize, monitor, and stage bladder tumors and evaluate hemorrhagic cystitis after bone marrow transplantation as well as detect urinary bladder involvement in Crohn's disease; differentiation of superficial from deep infiltrative bladder tumors (transurethral ultrasonography); and measurement of urinary bladder volumes (transrectal ultrasonography or transvaginal ultrasonography).

Description. Evaluation of the urinary bladder size, shape, and position by the creation of an oscilloscopic picture from the echoes of high-frequency sound waves passing over the bladder area (acoustic imaging) by the transabdominal or transurethral route. The time required for the ultrasonic beam to be reflected back to the transducer from differing densities of tissue is converted by a computer to an electrical impulse displayed on an oscilloscopic screen to create a three-dimensional picture of the urinary bladder. Additionally, transvaginal or transrectal endosonography can provide an advantage in evaluating the neck of the bladder, the bladder base, and the urethra in females. Because ultrasonography cannot confirm diagnosis of lesions found, when these lesions are found they should be followed by urinary bladder biopsy via cystoscopy.

Professional Considerations

Consent form NOT required for transabdominal method. Consent form IS required for transrectal, transurethral, and transvaginal methods.

Preparation

1. The client should disrobe below the waist or wear a gown.
2. Obtain ultrasonic gel or paste.
3. For transrectal ultrasonography, an enema may be prescribed.
4. See Client and Family Teaching. NOTE: Verify with the physician whether preprocedure water should be ingested. Some research shows that middle urethral stones are more reliably identified when the ultrasound is done before the client ingests water.

Procedure

1. *Transabdominal ultrasonography:*
   a. The client is positioned supine.
   b. Ultrasonic gel or paste is applied to the skin overlying the bladder.
   c. A lubricated transducer is placed firmly against the skin over the bladder area and moved slowly back and forth at intervals 1-2 cm apart. The oscilloscope displays a three-dimensional image of the full bladder.
   d. The client is instructed to void, and the procedure is repeated to check for the presence of residual urine.
   e. Photographs are taken of the oscilloscopic display.
   f. The procedure takes less than 30 minutes.
2. *Transvaginal ultrasonography:*
   a. After uroflowmetry studies are completed, 0.9% saline solution is instilled through a urethral catheter to fill the bladder.
   b. A transducer probe is inserted into an ultrasonic gel–filled condom. The condom is covered with a sterile lubricant.
   c. The probe is inserted into the vagina by the client or the examiner and moved to touch the vesicourethral area.
   d. The bladder and urethra are identified by sonography. Pictures are taken of the oscilloscopic display, with the client at rest or during micturition.
3. *Transrectal ultrasonography:*
   a. The client is positioned supine, and short transabdominal ultrasonography

is performed to evaluate for kidney distention.

b. The rectum is examined digitally for obstruction.

c. The client is assisted to a knee-elbow, lateral decubitus, or sitting position.

d. The probe is covered with an air-free, sterile, transparent cover or condom. The condom is then coated with a sterile lubricant, and the probe is slowly inserted into the rectum.

e. After the probe is inserted into the rectum, the condom is inflated with 20-60 mL of deaerated water.

f. The probe is angled anteriorly, and ultrasonography of the bladder is performed.

g. Photographs of the oscilloscopic display are taken.

4. *Transurethral ultrasonography:*

a. The bladder is filled with sterile 0.9% saline solution.

b. The probe is covered with an air-free, sterile, transparent cover and inserted into the bladder through a cystoscope.

c. The probe is rotated within the bladder as transverse sectional scans are taken.

d. Oscilloscopic images may be recorded on videotape or photographs.

Postprocedure Care

1. Remove the gel from the skin.

2. Sterilize the endosonography probes by soaking in glutaraldehyde solution for 10 minutes.

Client and Family Teaching

1. This test should be performed before intestinal barium tests or else after the barium is cleared from the system.

2. Drink three to four 8-ounce glasses of fluid within 2 hours before the test (where not contraindicated because the purpose of the test is to evaluate the bladder when full), and refrain from voiding.

3. The transabdominal procedure is painless and carries no risks.

Factors That Affect Results

1. Dehydration interferes with adequate contrast between organs and body fluids.

2. Lower intestinal barium contrast medium obscures results by preventing proper transmission and deflection of the high-frequency sound waves.

3. The more lower-abdominal fat present, the greater is the attenuation (reduction in sound-wave amplitude and intensity), which interferes with the clarity of the transabdominal picture.

Other Data

1. Computed tomography is preferred to ultrasonography for staging and measuring urinary bladder tumors.

Urinary Chorionic Gonadotropin Peptide (UGP, Urinary Gonadotropin Fragment, UGF)—Urine

Norm. Negative or <0.2 ng/mL or <5 fmol/mg creatinine.

Increased. Down syndrome, gynecologic cancers (cervical, endometrial, ovarian, and vulvovaginal), pregnancy, recurrence of gynecologic cancer, transitional cell carcinoma of the bladder.

Decreased. Survival rate from gynecologic cancer is increased; nonpregnant.

Description. Urinary chorionic gonadotropin (CG) peptide (UGP) is a beta-subunit core fragment that is found in pregnancy and is also known to originate from cancer tissue itself. It is elevated in gynecologic cancers, especially when the disease is advanced. UGP is secreted into the circulation, is rapidly cleared, and is generally not detected in the serum. The urine test uses immunohistochemical staining to identify the CG-beta expression at the level of messenger RNA.

Professional Considerations

Consent form NOT required.

Preparation

1. Obtain a soapy sponge and a clean specimen container.

Procedure

1. Wash the area around the meatus with a soapy sponge.

2. Hold the labia open, and position the specimen container beneath the urethral meatus.
3. Void into the container at least 10 mL of urine. A first morning specimen is preferred.

Postprocedure Care

1. Write the collection date and time and the suspected diagnosis on the laboratory requisition.
2. Send the specimen to the laboratory within 2 hours.
3. Freeze the specimen.

Client and Family Teaching

1. This test shows sensitivity as a survival and prognostic indicator for cancers of the cervix, ovary, and vulvovaginal area.

Factors That Affect Results

1. The sensitivity of the test is increased when results are corrected for urinary concentration.
2. False positive results post high orchiectomy.

Other Data

1. Use of UGP alone or together with serum CA 125 levels as a test for ovarian cancer—performed as a single diagnostic test, or in conjunction with an annual Pap smear test, or in women with benign pelvic masses—should be carefully evaluated.
2. False-positive results have been detected in 2% of healthy postmenopausal women.
3. A history of gynecologic malignancy does not falsely increase UGP levels.

Urine, Anaerobic Culture, Suprapubic Puncture

See **Body Fluid, Routine**—Culture.

Urine, Culture and Sensitivity (C & S)

See **Body Fluid, Routine**—Culture.

Urine, Fungus

See **Body Fluid, Fungus**—Culture.

Urine, Mycobacteria

See **Body Fluid, Mycobacteria**—Culture.

Urine Culture, Routine, Catheterized

See **Body Fluid, Routine**—Culture.

Urine Culture, Routine, Clean-Catch

See **Body Fluid, Routine**—Culture.

Urine Culture, Routine, Suprapubic Puncture

See **Body Fluid, Routine**—Culture.

Urine Culture, Routine

See **Body Fluid, Routine**—Culture.

Urine Culture and Nucleic Acid Amplification Tests for *Neisseria gonorrhoeae*—Urine

Norm. Negative. No *Neisseria gonorrhoeae* isolated.

Positive. Gonorrhea.

Description. Gonorrhea is a sexually transmitted disease caused by the organism *N. gonorrhoeae*. *N. gonorrhoeae* is a gonococcus transmitted from client to client by direct contact with exudates from the mucous membranes of infected clients. This disease causes purulent urethral discharge within 7 days of infection. Other symptoms may include rectal pruritus, cervicitis, endometritis, epididymitis, salpingitis, pelvic peritonitis, or vulvovaginitis. A culture is performed on the sediment of centrifuged urine. Although cultures are considered the criterion standard for diagnosis of cervical infections because of their specificity, it can take 48 hours or longer for growth to occur. Newer nucleic acid amplification tests (NAATs) and antigen/antibody detection methods are becoming available that can detect the organisms in a urine specimen.

Professional Considerations

Consent form NOT required.

Preparation

1. Obtain four soapy sponges and a sterile specimen container.

Procedure

1. Instruct the client to void and discard the urine.
2. Cleanse the penis or vulva × 4 with the soapy sponges, moving distally to proximally or front to back, discarding each sponge after one use.
3. Collect the first 10 mL of the first morning-voided urine in a sterile container; OR collect the entire first morning void in a sterile container; OR at least 2 hours after the previous void, collect the first 10 mL of urine voided in a sterile container.

Postprocedure Care

1. Write the collection date and time, any recent antibiotic therapy, and the suspected diagnosis on the laboratory requisition.
2. Send the specimen to the laboratory within 1 hour. Do not refrigerate it.

Client and Family Teaching

1. At least 2 days are required for results.
2. Gonorrhea is a reportable disease in the United States.
3. The follow-up culture should be performed 7-10 days after treatment.
4. Gonorrhea infection is treatable with antibiotics.
5. If results are positive, provide the client with the appropriate information on sexually transmitted diseases.
   a. Notify all sexual partners from the previous 90 days to be tested for gonorrhea infection.
   b. Do not have sexual relations until your physician confirms that the infection is gone.
6. Do not use feminine hygiene sprays or douche during treatment.
7. Wear underpants and pantyhose that have a cotton lining in the crotch.
8. Take showers instead of tub baths until the infection is gone.

Factors That Affect Results

1. False-negative results may occur for some strains of *N. gonorrhoeae* when Thayer-Martin or Martin-Lewis growth medium is used (because of vancomycin content of the medium).
2. Specimen contamination with other genital flora may result in overgrowth of normal flora.

Other Data

1. Gonorrhea is treated with aqueous procaine penicillin G (remember that a penicillin-resistant strain has been reported), ampicillin, spectinomycin, tetracycline, or ciprofloxacin (remember that ciprofloxacin-resistant gonococci have been reported).
2. The client should also be tested for syphilis.
3. Dipstick methods are available for purposes of screening for *N. gonorrhoeae*.

Urine Cytology
See **Cytologic Study of Urine**—Diagnostic.

Urine Drug Screen
See **Toxicology, Drug Screen**—Blood or Urine.

Urobilinogen—Urine
Norm.

Urine Specimen Type		SI Units
24-hour specimen	0.5-4.0 mg or 0.5-4.0 Ehrlich units	0.9-7.2 μmol
2-hour specimen		
Female	0.1-1.1 mg or 0.1-1.1 Ehrlich units	0.2-1.9 μmol
Male	0.3-2.1 mg or 0.3-2.1 Ehrlich units	0.5-3.6 μmol

Random Specimen (Dipstick Method)	Ehrlich Units/dL	Color
Normal or negative	0.1-1	Yellow to yellow-green
Positive	0.2-4	Yellow-orange
	0.8-12	Orange-brown

Increased. Anemia (hemolytic, pernicious), bananas eaten within 48 hours before the test, cholangitis, cirrhosis, congestive heart failure causing hepatic dysfunction, Dubin-Johnson syndrome, hemolytic processes, hepatic parenchymal damage, hepatitis (early), idiopathic pulmonary hemosiderosis, infectious mononucleosis, jaundice (hemolytic), lead poisoning, malaria, polycythemia vera, portal hypertension, pulmonary infarction, sickle cell disease, thalassemia major, and tissue hemorrhage. Drugs include sodium bicarbonate.

Decreased. Carcinoma of the head of the pancreas, cholelithiasis, complete common bile duct obstruction, diarrhea (severe), inflammation (severe), and renal insufficiency. Drugs include antibiotics that suppress the normal flora of the intestine such as chloramphenicol, cholestatics, and vitamin C.

Description. Urobilinogen is a reduction product formed by the action of bacteria on conjugated bilirubin in the gastrointestinal tract. The majority of urobilinogen is excreted in the stool. A small portion is reabsorbed by the enterohepatic pathway and re-excreted in bile. The remainder is excreted in the urine. A random dipstick check for urine bilinogen is normally negative because of its rapid oxidation to urobilin. An increase in urine urobilinogen indicates that some type of hemolytic process or hepatic dysfunction is occurring in the body. Urine urobilinogen levels are usually the highest in early to mid-afternoon. Thus when reagent strips test positive, a 2-hour urine collection between 1 and 3 PM is indicated.

Professional Considerations
Consent form NOT required.

Preparation
1. *Dipstick method:*
   a. A dipstick method should not be used for clients taking the drug phenazopyridine.
   b. Obtain a container of Bili-Labstix, Multistix, Urobilistix, or other reagent strip for urine urobilinogen testing, and a clean container.
2. *2-hour specimen:*
   a. Obtain a light-protected, 1- to 2-L urine collection container without

preservatives, a cup for drinking, and a pitcher of water (500 mL).

3. *24-hour specimen:*
   a. Obtain a light-protected, 3-L urine collection container without preservative.
   b. Instruct the client to save all the urine voided for the next 24 hours, to urinate before defecating, and to avoid contaminating urine with stool or toilet tissue.
   c. Write the beginning time of collection on the container and the laboratory requisition.
   d. Plan collection so that the test ends during laboratory open hours.
4. See Client and Family Teaching.

Procedure

1. *Dipstick method:*
   a. Obtain a 20-mL random urine sample in a clean plastic container.
   b. Immediately dip the reagent strip into the specimen and slide the strip along the edge of the container to remove excess urine.
   c. Hold the strip horizontally next to the color chart on the container, and time the reading according to the manufacturer's directions (most are 45-60 seconds).
   d. When the timing is completed, compare the color of the reagent pad for the urobilinogen measurement to the color chart, and record the measurement as follows:
2. *2-hour specimen:*
   a. Collect the specimen during early to mid-afternoon.
   b. Instruct the client to void and to discard the urine.
   c. Instruct the client to drink all 500 mL of water in the pitcher over the next 10 minutes.
   d. Save all the urine voided over the next 2 hours in a refrigerated, light-protected, urine collection container. The urine must be transferred into the container immediately after each void.
3. *24-hour specimen:*
   a. Discard the first morning-void urine.
   b. Save all the urine voided in a refrigerated, light-protected, 3-L container without preservatives. For specimens collected from an indwelling urinary catheter, keep the foil-covered drainage bag on ice, and empty the urine into the light-protected collection container hourly. Document the quantity of urinary output during the collection period.

Postprocedure Care

1. *2-hour collection:*
   a. Send the specimen to the laboratory immediately for prompt measurement.
2. *24-hour collection:*
   a. Write the ending time of collection on the laboratory requisition.
   b. Compare the urine quantity in the container with the urinary output record for the test. If the container has less urine than what was recorded as output, some of the urine may have been discarded, thus invalidating the test. The test must be restarted.
   c. Send valid specimens to the laboratory immediately for prompt measurement.

Client and Family Teaching

1. Avoid eating bananas for 2 days before the test.
2. Collect specimens according to the appropriate procedure, as described above.

Factors That Affect Results

1. Drugs that may cause falsely increased results include acetazolamide, aminosalicylic acid, antipyrine, aspirin, chlorpromazine, 5-hydroxyindoleacetic acid, phenazopyridine, phenothiazines, sulfobromophthalein (Bromsulphalein), and sulfonamides. Herbal or natural remedies include cascara sagrada (*Rhamnus purshiana*).
2. Urine alkalinization increases the excretion rate of urine urobilinogen. Urine acidification decreases the excretion rate of urine urobilinogen.
3. Dipstick methods can detect only abnormally high levels, not abnormally low levels.
4. The level may be normal in clients with incomplete common bile duct obstruction.
5. False-positive or falsely increased results may occur in porphyria.

Other Data

1. None.

Uroflowmetry—Diagnostic

Norm. Normal uroflow curve, with normal peak and normal voiding time for quantity voided.

		Rate (q[max])	
	Volume	Female	Male
Postvoid residual amount			
Normal		≤50 mL	≤50 mL
Equivocal		100-200 mL	100-200 mL
Abnormal		>200 mL	>200 mL
Adults			
Young <45 years	≥150 mL	18 mL/second	21 mL/second
Middle 46-65 years	≥150 mL	15 mL/second	15 mL/second
Older >65 years	>150 mL	10-15 mL/second	10-15 mL/second
	1100-2000 mL/24 hr		
Children			
Younger <8 years	≥100 mL	10 mL/second	10 mL/second
Older 8-13 years	≥100 mL	15 mL/second	12 mL/second

Usage. Part of diagnostic evaluation for voiding abnormalities (e.g., evaluating cystourethrocele or erectile dysfunction, identifying postvoiding residual volumes, determining voiding speed as an indicator of obstruction, post prostate cryoablation, recurrent stricture post urethral reconstructive surgery).

Description. Uroflowmetry, a non-invasive test, involves measuring the voiding duration, amount, and rate of urine voided into a funnel with a urine flowmeter that records the above information in a graphic format aiding in identifying voiding abnormalities. The Q[max] is the maximum number of milliliters of urine per second. A Q[max] of less than 12 mL/second is associated with a higher risk for urinary retention. This simple, noninvasive test is usually performed with other tests such as cystometry and voiding cystourethrography.

Professional Considerations
Consent form NOT required.

Preparation
1. Provide a private environment for voiding.

Procedure
1. Several types of urine flowmeters are available. The exact procedure depends on the type of flowmeter used and should be followed according to the manufacturer's instructions and institutional protocol.

2. In general, the flowmeter is activated just before the void, as described above. The client voids while standing to avoid straining pressure effects on urine volume. The volume voided and the rate, pattern, and duration of voiding are analyzed and displayed graphically by the urine flowmeter. A uroflow curve displays the changes in the urine flow rate throughout the void. NOTE: In persons not accustomed to sitting while voiding it is best to perform the test in either the standing or squatting position.

3. Serial recordings of each void over 2-3 days may be performed to provide the most accurate evaluation of the client's urine flow patterns. This helps correct for aberrancies such as hesitancy as a result of nervousness, or single voided specimens of extremely small or large volume.

4. The client's position during each void and the amount and route of fluid intake throughout testing should be recorded.

Postprocedure Care
1. None.

Client and Family Teaching
1. Do not void for several hours before the test. Drink several glasses of water at least 1 hour before the test so that your bladder is full and you are feeling like you have to urinate.

2. When the urge to void is felt, assume a standing voiding position and perform a

normal void, completely emptying the bladder urine into the funnel of the flowmeter. The void should be performed without straining and while the rest of the body is held as motionless as possible. Urinate before defecating, and do not allow stool or toilet tissue to enter the funnel.

Factors That Affect Results

1. The quantity of urine voided affects the flow rate. Optimal amounts for evaluation of bladder function are between 150 and 400 mL. Quantities greater than 400 mL cause deterioration of bladder detrusor muscle function.
2. Recent urethral instrumentation may cause decreased flow rates
3. Sildenafil improves Q[max] and Q[avg] in patients suffering from erectile dysfunction.

Other Data

1. None.

Urography, Excretory

See Intravenous Pyelography—Diagnostic.

UroVysion™ Fish Test

See Fluorescence In Situ Hybridization Test—Urine.

Uterosalpingography

See Hysterosalpingography—Diagnostic.

Uterotubal Insufflation

See Rubin's Test—Diagnostic.

Vaginal Aspirate for Motile/Nonmotile Sperm

See Sims-Huhner Test—Diagnostic.

Vaginal Culture

See Genitals, *Neisseria gonorrhoeae*—Culture.

Vaginal Cytology

See Hormonal Evaluation, Cytologic—Specimen.

Valproic Acid—Blood

Norm. Negative.

Valproic Acid Therapy	Trough	SI Units
Therapeutic level	50-100 µg/mL	350-690 µmol/L
Toxic level	>100 µg/mL	>690 µmol/L
Panic level	>200 µg/mL	>1380 µmol/L

Panic Levels Symptoms and Treatment

Symptoms. Burning feet paresthesia, numbness, tingling, weakness, mental changes.

Treatment

NOTE: Treatment choice(s) depend(s) on client's history and condition and episode history.

1. Administer naloxone.
2. Hemodialysis and peritoneal dialysis will NOT remove valproic acid. High-permeability dialysis WILL remove valproic acid.
3. The use of activated charcoal did NOT enhance valproic acid elimination in animal studies.

Usage. Monitoring for therapeutic levels during valproic acid therapy.

Description. Valproic acid is an anticonvulsant effective against myoclonus and grand mal, petit mal, and complex partial seizures, and also used for long-term control of manic episodes in bipolar disorders. It is being used experimentally for panic disorders and migraine treatment. Newer research has found that it has a role in resistance to cancer activity by suppressing tumor growth. After oral or rectal administration, it is metabolized by the liver and excreted in the urine, with a half-life of 6-8 hours and elimination half-life of 15-20 hours.

Professional Considerations

Consent form NOT required.

Preparation

1. Tube: Red topped, red/gray topped, or gold topped (for serum level); or green topped (for plasma level).
2. Specimens MAY be drawn during hemodialysis.

Procedure

1. Draw a 44-mL blood sample. Draw the trough level immediately before dose administration. Draw the peak level 1-3 hours after dose administration.

Postprocedure Care

1. Specimens must be kept in a tightly capped tube until testing to prevent evaporation of valproic acid from the sample.

Client and Family Teaching

1. Long-term use of this drug may result in hepatotoxicity.
2. Overdose of this drug can cause neurotoxicity.
3. For an intentional overdose, refer the client and family for crisis intervention and offer resource information for counseling.

Factors That Affect Results

1. Absorption is slowed by the presence of food in the gastrointestinal tract; thus peak levels occur later for doses given on a full stomach than for doses given on an empty stomach.
2. Valproic acid reaches steady-state levels in about 96 hours.
3. Drugs that decrease valproic acid half-life include carbamazepine, carbapenem, ertapenem, fluoxetine, imipenem, phenobarbital, phenytoin, and primidone.
4. Hepatic failure or use of the drugs riluzole (in autism patients) or topiramate (in epilepsy patients) may cause elevated results.
5. Concurrent administration of methsuximide decreases valproic acid levels.

Other Data

1. Periodic liver function tests should be performed throughout valproic acid therapy.
2. Valproic acid increases serum levels of phenobarbital.
3. A case has been reported of fatal acute pancreatitis caused by valproic acid.
4. Levels >80 μg/mL require close monitoring for thrombocytopenia in females.

Vancomycin—Serum

Norm. Negative.

		SI Units
Trough		
Therapeutic	5-10 μg/mL	3-7 μmol/L
Potential nephrotoxicity	>10 μg/mL	>7 μmol/L

		SI Units
Panic level	>15 µg/mL	>10 µmol/L
Toxic level	>20 µg/mL	>13 µmol/L
Peak		
Therapeutic	30-40 µg/mL	20-27 µmol/L
Ototoxicity	>40 µg/mL	>27 µmol/L
Panic level	>60 µg/mL	>41 µmol/L
Toxic level	>80 µg/mL	>53 µmol/L

Panic Levels Symptoms and Treatment

Symptoms. Hypotension, leukopenia, or neutropenia (agranulocytosis, granulocytopenia); exfoliative dermatitis, lacrimation, thrombocytopenia, dermatitis, tubular necrosis, deafness, colitis; ototoxicity (prolonged levels >30 mg/mL).

Treatment

NOTE: Treatment choice(s) depend(s) on client's history and condition and episode history.

1. Administer ipecac (within 30 minutes of oral vancomycin ingestion) or perform gastric lavage (within 60 minutes).
2. Provide supportive therapy for hypotension.
3. The use of activated charcoal orally has NOT been shown to enhance the elimination of vancomycin (see American Academy of Clinical Toxicology, 1999).
4. Hemodialysis, hemofiltration, and peritoneal dialysis will NOT remove vancomycin. Charcoal hemoperfusion will NOT remove vancomycin. High permeability dialysis WILL remove vancomycin.

Usage. Monitoring for therapeutic (and safe) levels during vancomycin therapy.

Description. Vancomycin is an aminoglycoside antibiotic that inhibits cell wall synthesis of gram-positive bacteria. It is frequently used in the treatment of infections caused by methicillin-resistant *Staphylococcus aureus* (MRSA) and in treatment for pseudomembranous colitis. Vancomycin is metabolized in the liver, with 80% excreted through the kidneys and a small amount in bile. Oral doses are primarily excreted in the feces. Vancomycin half-life is very dependent on renal glomerular function. Rapid infusions of this drug have been associated with histamine release causing "red-man syndrome," in which the skin becomes flushed, erythematous, and pruritic. The predictability of therapeutic effect is better at trough levels than at peak levels; thus peak levels are not routinely recommended unless the client has renal failure or in other situations where the volume distribution is increased (see Factors That Affect Results).

Professional Considerations
Consent form NOT required.

Preparation
1. Tube: Red topped or green topped.
2. Specimens MAY be drawn during hemodialysis.

Procedure
1. Draw the trough level just before administering the dose. Peak levels are not routinely recommended, but if measured should be drawn 30 minutes after intravenous administration.
2. Draw a 3-mL blood sample.

Postprocedure Care
1. Send the sample to the laboratory promptly. Serum should be separated and frozen within 4 hours.

Client and Family Teaching
1. Overdoses can cause renal failure and hearing loss.
2. Slowing the rate of drug infusion can decrease feelings of the skin being flushed, red, and itchy.

Factors That Affect Results
1. Minimum inhibitory concentration (MIC) of vancomycin varies for different organisms and will affect the therapeutic trough level needed. MIC should be included in sensitivity testing results. In general, an average peak vancomycin level that is two to four times higher than the MIC is considered adequate for control of the organism. Minimum inhibitory concentration is the lowest concentration that results in a negative test.

2. Clients with impaired glomerular renal function will have elevated levels if dosages are not adjusted accordingly.
3. Clients receiving extracorporeal membrane oxygenation, clients treated with indomethacin, and neonates with patent ductus arteriosus are likely to have an increased volume distribution of vancomycin as compared to those clients without these situations. Close monitoring of both trough and peak levels is indicated.
4. Falsely elevated plasma concentrations (Wright et al, 2010) can occur from samples obtained from central line ports (port-a-caths).

Other Data

1. Renal function and hearing should be assessed before and throughout vancomycin therapy. Clients who demonstrated increased nephrotoxicity in one study were those also receiving another aminoglycoside concurrently, those who received vancomycin for more than 3 weeks, and those who had trough levels >10 mg/L.
2. Vancomycin administered intravenously over 2 hours, as compared to 1 hour, has been shown to reduce the occurrence of red-man syndrome.

Vanillylmandelic Acid (VMA)—Urine

Norm.

	24-Hour Aliquot		SI Units
	μg/mg of Creatinine	μg/g of Body Weight	mmol/mol of Creatinine
Adults	≤7	≤150	4.0
Children			
Birth-35 months	≤28	≤180	15.4
3-5 years	<13	<150	7.4
6-17 years	<10	<150	2.91

Norms	24-Hour Quantity	SI Units
Adults	<7.0 mg/24 hours	<35 μmol/day
Children		
≤12 months	≤1.8 mg/24 hours	≤9 μmol/day
13 months-4 years	≤3 mg/24 hours	≤15 μmol/day
4-15 years	≤4 mg/24 hours	≤20 μmol/day

Increased. Anxiety (severe), exercise (intense), ganglioblastoma, ganglioneuroma, hypertension (essential), neuroblastoma, and pheochromocytoma. Drugs include aspirin, aminosalicylic acid, epinephrine, glyceryl guaiacolate, levodopa, lithium carbonate, mephenesin, methocarbamol, nalidixic acid, norepinephrine, oxytetracycline, penicillin, phenazopyridine, phenolsulfonphthalein, salicylates, sulfobromophthalein (Bromsulphalein), and sulfonamides. Herbal or natural remedies include *Coffea*.

Decreased. Familial dysautonomia (Riley-Day syndrome). Drugs include chlorpromazine, clofibrate, clonidine, guanethidine analogs, imipramine, levodopa, methyldopa, monoamine oxidase (MAO) inhibitors, reserpine, and salicylates.

Description. Vanillylmandelic acid (VMA) occurs as an end product of epinephrine and norepinephrine metabolism and is freely excreted in the urine. This test aids in the diagnosis and monitoring for clients with catecholamine-secreting tumors.

Professional Considerations
Consent form NOT required.

Preparation

1. Withhold drugs that may cause increased or decreased results (listed above) for 72 hours before the test. Diuretics, antihypertensives, and sympathomimetics (including nonprescriptive cold and

allergy medications) must be withheld for 5-14 days.
2. Obtain a clean, 3-L container.
3. Write the starting time of collection on the laboratory requisition and container.
4. See Client and Family Teaching.

Procedure

1. Discard first morning urine specimen.
2. Save all the urine voided for a 24-hour period in a refrigerated, clean, 3-L plastic container. For specimens collected from indwelling urinary catheters, keep the drainage bag on ice and empty urine into the collection container hourly. Document the quantity of urine output throughout the collection period.

Postprocedure Care

1. Compare the urine quantity in the container with the record of urine output during the collection period. If the container contains less urine than what was documented as output, some may have been discarded, invalidating the test.

Client and Family Teaching

1. Avoid the following foods for 72 hours before the test: avocados, bananas, beer, cheese (aged), Chianti wines, chocolate, citrus fruits, cocoa, fava beans, grains, tea, vanilla, walnuts, and wine. Also avoid the herb coffee (*Coffea*) for 72 hours before the test.

2. Save all the urine voided for 24 hours, urinate before defecating, and avoid contaminating urine with stool or toilet tissue. If any urine is accidentally discarded, discard the entire specimen and restart the collection the next day.
3. Avoid stress, strenuous exercise, and smoking of tobacco before and throughout the urine collection period.

Factors That Affect Results

1. Drugs that cause decreased results in normal clients may not suppress levels to below normal in clients with catecholamine-secreting tumors.
2. Drugs that cause unpredictable changes in the results include amphetamines, appetite suppressants, bromocriptine, buspirone, caffeine, chlorpromazine, clonidine, disulfiram, diuretics (sodium-depleting), glucagon, guanethidine, histamine, hydrazine derivatives, imipramine, melatonin, morphine, nitroglycerin, nose drops, propafenone (Rythmol), radiographic agents, *Rauwolfia* alkaloids (reserpine), tricyclic antidepressants, and vasodilators.

Other Data

1. Consistency in results has been demonstrated between random, 6-hour, 12-hour, and 24-hour specimens.

Varicella-Zoster Virus Serology—Serum

Norm. Less than a fourfold increase in titer between acute and convalescent samples.

Enzyme-Linked Immunosorbent Assay

IGG Index Value (IV)		IGM Immune Status Ratio (ISR)	
≤0.89	Negative	≤0.89	Negative
0.9-1.09	Equivocal	0.90-1.09	Equivocal
	Repeat testing in 2 weeks		Repeat testing in 2 weeks
≥1.10	Positive	≥1.10	Positive
	Suggests current or past exposure		Suggests current or recent infection
	May indicate immunity if no symptoms are present		

Increased. Chickenpox and herpes zoster (shingles).

Description. Varicella-zoster virus, also known as human herpesvirus 3, is the causative agent of chickenpox and shingles, which are time-limited viral infections that produce skin lesions or vesicles. The mode of transmission is either directly from client to client (by airborne spread of infected respiratory secretions or vesicle fluid) or indirectly (through contact with contaminated secretions on inanimate objects). The virus multiplies in the respiratory tract and then spreads through the bloodstream to the skin and internal organs. After causing chickenpox in childhood, the latent virus may reemerge to cause shingles in the elderly. In this test, complement fixation, indirect immunofluorescence, or agglutination methods are used to detect the antibody to the varicella-zoster virus.

Professional Considerations
Consent form NOT required.

Preparation
1. Tube: Red topped, red/gray topped, or gold topped.

Procedure
1. Draw a 4-mL blood sample as soon as possible after symptoms appear. Label the tube as the "acute sample." Repeat the test in 10-14 days and label the tube as the "convalescent sample."

Postprocedure Care
1. Transport sample to the laboratory and refrigerate.

Client and Family Teaching
1. Return for convalescent sampling in 10-14 days.

Factors That Affect Results
1. Low levels of IgM antibodies may persist for up to 12 months after infection or immunization.
2. Reduction in serum PSA in males following varicella-zoster infection.

Other Data
1. Chickenpox and shingles are contagious for up to 6 days after lesions or vesicles appear. Immunocompromised clients may be contagious for longer periods of time.
2. For clients exposed to varicella-zoster, varicella-zoster immune globulin from zoster-convalescent clients or human immune globulin given within 4 days may limit or prevent symptoms.
3. The incidence of varicella in children younger than age 4 years is increasing. Because maternal antibody protection lasts only about 5 months after birth, the varicella vaccine is recommended to be given between the ages of 5 and 12 months. Humoral immunity remains low in children with biliary atresia.
4. Seroprevalence rate exceed 90% population in South Korea and 75% in the United States (primary vaccine only).

Vascular Endothelial Growth Factor (VEGF, Vascular Permeability Factor, VPF)—Specimen

Norm. CSF: None detected. Blood: Consult norms provided with report. Levels may be measured serially to gauge the progression of tumor growth or the effectiveness of anti-VEGF drug therapy. Tissue bone marrow: None detected.

Increased. Increased levels of vascular endothelial growth factor have been associated with many forms of cancers (e.g., NSCLC) and are a useful predictor of prognosis in Kawasaki disease. CSF levels are increased in brain tumors, levels found to be present in 89% of astrocytomas versus 27% of nonastrocytomas. Drugs include statins.

Decreased. Not applicable.

Description. Vascular endothelial growth factor (VEGF) is a glycoprotein substance secreted by some cancers such as renal cell carcinomas. When secreted, VEGF acts directly on endothelial cells to induce development of tiny blood vessels (angiogenesis), which helps provide the blood flow and nourishment necessary to enable continued growth of the tumor. In addition to stimulating angiogenesis, VEGF enhances the permeability of blood vessels associated with the tumor, causing edema, and thus is also known by the term vascular permeability factor (VPF). Because of its role in stimulating angiogenesis near tumors, VEGF is also thought to be an important factor in allowing metastasis to occur. However, the introduction of VEGF is thought to stimulate the growth of new blood vessels, a process called angiogenesis. VEGF is present in normal tissues such as the lungs, which are dependent on good blood flow.

Professional Considerations

Consent form NOT required for this test, but IS required if the test specimen is obtained via biopsy or lumbar puncture.

Preparation

1. Tube: Lavender topped.

Procedure

1. For blood test, obtain a 7-mL blood sample.
2. For biopsy, see Biopsy, Site-specific—Specimen.
3. For CSF specimen, see Lumbar puncture—Diagnostic.
4. For bone marrow specimen, see Bone marrow aspiration analysis—Specimen.

Postprocedure Care

1. See appropriate invasive procedure information for Postprocedure Care.
2. Transport specimen to the pathology laboratory. Serum samples must clot for 2-6 hours before testing.

Client and Family Teaching

1. Educate the client/family on purpose of test, procedure for obtaining sample, and turnaround time for results (2-4 days). Tell them that their physician will discuss findings and implications with them.

Factors That Affect Results

1. Failure to allow the blood specimen to clot will yield falsely elevated results because the neutrophils, which contain the most VEGF, will spill their contents into lysed whole blood.
2. Platelet count and VEGF levels are normally positively correlated. Thus VEGF levels must be corrected when platelets are elevated.

Other Data

1. Vascular endothelial growth factor has been shown to improve outcomes for some clients suffering from vascular disease by promoting the growth of new blood vessels.
2. Some recombinant antibodies that inhibit VEGF are being studied as possible anticancer drugs. Recently, bevacizumab has been approved as an anti-VEGF therapy for metastatic colorectal carcinoma.

Vasoactive Intestinal Polypeptide (VIP)—Blood

Norm. Adults and children: <61 pg/mL (<61 ng/L, SI units).

Increased. Achlorhydria (WDHA) syndrome, bronchogenic carcinoma, ectopic islet cell tumor, ganglioneuroblastoma, gastric adenocarcinoma, hypokalemia, islet cell hyperplasia, islet cell tumor, laxative abuse, medullary thyroid carcinoma, pancreatic cholera syndrome, pheochromocytoma, retroperitoneal histiocytoma, tachycardia, Verner-Morrison syndrome, vipoma, and watery diarrhea.

Decreased. Asthma exacerbation.

Description. Vasoactive intestinal polypeptide (VIP) is a gastrointestinal hormone produced by neuroendocrine cells in the small and large intestines, pancreas, brain, and peripheral nervous system. Its actions include stimulating watery pancreatic secretions with a high pH, stimulating glycogenolysis, inhibiting stomach secretions, stimulating the release of insulin and glucagon, causing peripheral vasodilation, exhibiting a positive inotropic and chronotropic effect on the cardiovascular system, slowing gastric motility, stimulating intestinal chloride secretion, and inhibiting intestinal sodium absorption. Clients with vipoma neoplasms have symptoms of watery diarrhea that is high in potassium and bicarbonate. VIP is also found abundantly in the human lung and is thought to cause bronchodilation.

Professional Considerations

Consent form NOT required.

Preparation

1. When possible, medications should be withheld for 1-2 days.
2. Observe clients with watery diarrhea closely for symptoms of dehydration during the 12-hour preparation fast.
3. Preschedule this test with the laboratory, and verify collection instructions with the laboratory performing the test.

4. Obtain a chilled plastic syringe to which 1.2 mg of EDTA has been added.
5. See Client and Family Teaching.

Procedure

1. Draw a 5-mL blood sample.

Postprocedure Care

1. Transport the specimen to the laboratory immediately.
2. The specimen must be separated and transferred to a special VIP container and then frozen.

Client and Family Teaching

1. Fast from food and fluids for 12 hours before the test.

Factors That Affect Results

1. Results are invalidated if the client has undergone a radioactive scan within 1 week before the test.

Other Data

1. None.

VDRL

See **Venereal Disease Research Laboratory Test—Serum.**

Vectorcardiogram—Diagnostic

Norm. Requires interpretation by an expert. P, QRS, and T loops are evaluated for direction, magnitude, and inscription.

Usage. Identification and classification of myocardial infarction; evaluation of risk for myocardial infarction progression to complete heart block; aids in diagnosis of ventricular preexcitation and localization of ventricular bypass tracts.

Description. A vectorcardiogram (VCG) is a spatial representation of the sequence of changes in the heart's electrical activity measured three-dimensionally along the x-(horizontal, transverse, left-to-right) axis, y-(vertical, head-to-foot) axis, and z-(sagittal, anteroposterior) axis. A vector represents the heart's electrical potential with respect to specific direction and magnitude. The vectorcardiograph simultaneously records two lead axes at a time to represent the frontal plane vector (x, y), the horizontal plane vector (x, z), and the sagittal plane vector (y, z) and provides a screen display or graphic recording of P, QRS, and T vector loops that move in the same direction as the heart's electrical activity. The literature demonstrates controversy regarding the ability of VCG to better detect and classify myocardial infarction than ECG, though it is advantageous to patients with AMI treated with thrombolytic therapy (Gill et al, 2002). This expensive procedure is infrequently performed in clinical settings but is used as a teaching tool.

Professional Considerations

Consent form NOT required.

Preparation

1. Obtain a vectorcardiogram machine, electrodes, and conductive gel.

Procedure

1. The client is positioned supine.
2. Conductive electrodes are applied according to institutional protocol (usually to the anterior and posterior upper torso, left lower extremity, and the forehead or nape of the neck).
3. The machine is activated, and the vectorcardiogram is completed in about 10 minutes.

Postprocedure Care

1. Remove the electrodes. Cleanse the skin of conductive gel.

Client and Family Teaching

1. It is important to relax, breathe normally, and lie very still throughout the recording.

Factors That Affect Results

1. The client's sex, age, medications, and clinical picture must be considered when one is interpreting the results.

2. One study recommends that respiratory status be identical for serial vectorcardiograms to diminish the effects of respiration and ventilation on the results (Leanderson et al, 2003).

Other Data

1. The vectorcardiogram is most useful when evaluated in combination with an electrocardiogram.

Venereal Disease Research Laboratory Test (VDRL)—Serum

Norm. Negative. Nonreactive.

Treponema pallidum titer <1:2.

NOTE: Titers are indicated when samples are weakly positive or positive.

Positive. Treponemal disease: bejel, pinta, syphilis, yaws.

Description. Syphilis is a complex sexually transmitted disease characterized by a wide range of symptoms that imitate other diseases. It is caused by the organism *Treponema pallidum*. The Venereal Disease Research Laboratory test (VDRL) is a screening test for the presence of reagin, the antibody specific for the treponemal spirochete. In this test, the sample is heat inactivated and then mixed with an antigen (cardiolipin phospholipid derived from beef heart in complex with lecithin and coated on particles of cholesterol) to reagin. The mixture is then examined microscopically to detect flocculation of the cholesterol particles, indicating a positive test. The VDRL test is less sensitive than the rapid plasma reagin (RPR) test for primary syphilis. The test becomes reactive during primary-stage syphilis (about 14 days after a chancre is visible) and is reactive in virtually all cases of secondary-stage syphilis. Results will revert to negative with treatment or by the tertiary stage. Many biologic false-positive results are possible; thus specificity is low. Positive results should be confirmed with the fluorescent treponemal antibody-absorbed double-stain test (see Fluorescent treponemal antibody-absorbed double-stain test—Serum).

Professional Considerations

Consent form NOT required.

Preparation

1. Tube: Red topped, red/gray topped, or gold topped.

Procedure

1. Draw a 4-mL blood sample.

Postprocedure Care

1. None.

Client and Family Teaching

1. Syphilis is a sexually transmitted disease; information regarding sexual partners is necessary for control of the disease.
2. If testing positive for syphilis and diagnosis is confirmed:
   a. Notify all sexual contacts from the previous 90 days (if early stage) to be tested for syphilis.
   b. Syphilis can be cured with antibiotics. These may worsen the symptoms for the first 24 hours.
   c. Do not have sex for 2 months and until after repeat testing has confirmed that the syphilis is cured. Use condoms after that for 2 years. Return for repeat testing every 3-4 months for the next 2 years to make sure the disease is cured.
   d. Do not become pregnant for 2 years because syphilis can be transmitted to the fetus.
   e. If left untreated, syphilis can damage many body organs, including the brain, over several years.

Factors That Affect Results

1. Refrigeration destroys *Treponema* spirochetes in 72 hours.
2. Conditions that may cause false-positive results include active immunization in children, antinuclear antibodies, blood loss (with multiple transfusions), brucellosis, chancroid, chickenpox, cirrhosis, the common cold, diabetes mellitus, fever (relapsing), first week of life, hepatitis (infectious), hypergammaglobulinemia, leprosy, leptospirosis (Weil's disease), Lyme disease, lymphogranuloma venereum, lymphoma, infection (chronic), malaria, measles, mononucleosis (infectious), mycoplasmal pneumonia, nonsyphilitic treponemal diseases (bejel, pinta, yaws), periarteritis nodosa, pneumococcal pneumonia, pneumonia, pregnancy, rat-bite fever, rheumatic fever, rheumatic heart disease, rheumatoid

arthritis, scarlet fever, scleroderma, senescence, subacute bacterial endocarditis, systemic lupus erythematosus, tuberculosis (advanced pulmonary), treponematosis, trypanosomiasis, tuberculosis, typhus fever, and vaccinia.

Other Data

1. The greatest risk for transmission of syphilis occurs in freshly drawn blood products that must be administered immediately (platelets) or those not refrigerated for 72 hours before infusion.
2. Syphilis is treated with penicillin.
3. A newer test, the *Treponema pallidum* enzyme-linked immunosorbent assay (ELISA), is being studied for possible replacement of this test for large-scale screening for syphilis.

Venereal Disease Research Laboratory Test (VDRL), Test, Cerebrospinal Fluid—Specimen

Norm. Nonreactive. *Treponema pallidum* titer <1:2. NOTE: Titers are indicated when samples are weakly positive or positive.

Usage. The only test approved for cerebrospinal fluid testing for neurosyphilis.

Description. Syphilis is a complex, sexually transmitted disease characterized by a wide range of symptoms that imitate other diseases. It is caused by the organism *Treponema pallidum*. The Venereal Disease Research Laboratory test (VDRL) is a screening test for the presence of reagin, the antibody specific for the treponemal spirochete. In this test, the sample is heat inactivated and then mixed with an antigen (cardiolipin phospholipid derived from beef heart in complex with lecithin and coated on particles of cholesterol) to reagin. The mixture is then examined microscopically to detect flocculation of the cholesterol particles, indicating a positive test. Unlike serum results, cerebrospinal fluid (CSF) results may remain positive long after treatment; thus this test is not useful for monitoring response to therapy.

Professional Considerations

Consent form NOT required for the test but IS required for the procedure used to obtain the specimen. For procedural risks and contraindications, see Lumbar puncture—Diagnostic.

Preparation

1. See Lumbar puncture—Diagnostic.

Procedure

1. Obtain at least a 1-mL sample of CSF in a sterile, capped vial by lumbar puncture, or from the ventricles of the brain during special procedures (see Lumbar puncture—Diagnostic).

Postprocedure Care

1. Transport specimen to the laboratory and refrigerate until tested.
2. See Lumbar puncture—Diagnostic.

Client and Family Teaching

1. Syphilis is a sexually transmitted disease; information regarding sexual partners is necessary for control of the disease.
2. See also Venereal disease research laboratory test—Serum for additional teaching related to syphilis.

Factors That Affect Results

1. False-negative results may occur in clients with tabes dorsalis.

Other Data

1. Serial testing is recommended for clients with AIDS who are suspected of having syphilis but have a negative VDRL test.

Venezuelan Equine Encephalitis Virus Serology—Serum

Norm. A less than fourfold rise in titer between acute and convalescent samples.

Usage. Confirmation of diagnosis of Venezuelan equine encephalitis.

Description. Venezuelan equine encephalitis is caused by a group A arbovirus (arthropod-borne virus) that results in fever and mild flulike symptoms (most commonly) but may progress to severe encephalitis symptoms of disorientation, convulsions, paralysis, coma, and death in children. The virus was relatively inactive between 1973 and 1991, but then reemerged primarily in South America, Central America, and Mexico. Mode of transmission to humans from horses is through the bite of an infected mosquito. Identification of the virus is performed through viral neutralization, complement fixation, hemagglutinin inhibition, fluorescent antibody, and agar gel precipitation. There is no vaccine for Venezuelan equine encephalitis, but there is some literature suggesting antiviral therapy with VEEV-specific human or "humanized" monoclonal antibodies may help protect those exposed from developing the symptoms (Phillpotts et al, 2003). Mouse-model research shows treatment with carbocyclic cytosine (Carbodine) is effective (Julander et al, 2008).

Professional Considerations
Consent form NOT required.

Preparation
1. Tube: Red topped, red/gray topped, or gold topped.

Procedure
1. Draw a 7-mL blood sample as soon as possible after symptoms appear and label it as the "acute sample." Repeat the test in 10 days and label the sample as the "convalescent sample."

Postprocedure Care
1. None.

Client and Family Teaching
1. The mode of transmission is a mosquito bite.
2. Hypertension can be a result of this viral infection.
3. Return in 10 days for a follow-up test.

Factors That Affect Results
1. None found.

Other Data
1. Testing may also be performed on cerebrospinal fluid.
2. Venezuelan equine encephalitis is not transmitted client to client.
3. There is no specific treatment for this illness.

Venlafaxine

See **Selective Serotonin Reuptake Inhibitors**—Blood.

Venography (Phlebography)—Diagnostic

Norm. Negative. Normal finding. Absence of thrombosis. No obstructions to flow or filling defects identified.

Positive. Abnormal finding. An intraluminal filling defect in the deep venous contrast column indicates deep venous thrombosis (DVT). An abrupt cutoff of a deep vein with the development of collateral circulation may also indicate the presence of DVT.

Usage. Detection of site and presence of venous thrombosis of the lower extremities; radiographic guidance for insertion of peripherally inserted central catheter (PICC); used with magnetic resonance imaging for the detection and evaluation of arteriovenous malformations and vascular venous lesions.

Description. Venography is an invasive, radiographic, or nuclear medicine procedure whereby radiopaque dye or a radionuclide is injected intravenously and the lower extremities are radiographed for the DVT. Although considered to be the criterion standard for detection of deep venous thromboses, venography is similar in accuracy to newer ultrasonographic techniques for symptomatic clients. In asymptomatic clients, however, it remains superior in accuracy but higher in risk compared to ultrasonography for the detection of DVT. For initial detection of proximal DVT, venography has largely been replaced by the use of compression ultrasonography (CUS) and color duplex ultrasonography. Venography is more often reserved for detection of calf

DVT, and for further testing for repeat symptoms during the first 6 months after an acute DVT.

Professional Considerations

Consent form IS required.

Risks

Allergic reaction to dye (itching, hives, rash, tight feeling in the throat, shortness of breath, anaphylaxis), bacteremia, cellulitis (onset 2-12 hours; peak 12-24 hours), congestive heart failure, embolism, renal toxicity from contrast medium, thrombophlebitis, vasospasm, venipuncture-site infection, venous thrombosis.

Contraindications

Severe congestive heart failure; severe pulmonary hypertension; previous allergy to radiographic dye, iodine, or shellfish; pregnancy (because of the radioactive iodine crossing the blood-placental barrier); renal insufficiency.

Preparation

1. This test is normally performed in a radiology department.
2. Have emergency equipment readily available.
3. Obtain radiographic dye, heparin and saline flush solution, and a tourniquet.
4. Just before beginning the procedure, take a "time out" to verify the correct client, procedure, and site.

Procedure

1. The client is positioned supine or semi-upright on the fluoroscopic table, with the weight placed on the nonexamined extremity.

2. A tourniquet may be placed on the extremity to control the speed of blood flow.
3. After intravenous access is established in a foot vein, radiographic dye is injected, and several rapid, sequential radiographs are taken of the extremity as the dye flows in the bloodstream. Alternatively, one may conduct a nuclear medicine study whereby a radionuclide is injected, followed by scintigraphic scanning of the extremity.
4. The intravenous access site is flushed with heparin/saline solution, and the access is removed.

Postprocedure Care

1. Assess injection site for symptoms of dye infiltration (redness, edema, warmth, tenderness).
2. Assess vital signs; peripheral pulses; and color, motion, temperature, and sensation of lower extremities every 15 minutes × 4, then every 30 minutes × 4, then hourly × 4, and then every 4 hours until 24 hours after the procedure.

Client and Family Teaching

1. A feeling of warmth around the neck and face is normally felt after the injection.
2. Procedure time is 1-1½ hours.

Factors That Affect Results

1. Only 25% of symptomatic clients have a thrombus.

Other Data

1. Limitations of this procedure include poor visualization when a client has previously had a DVT in the affected extremity, intralimb contrast material dilution, and difficulties obtaining pedal venous access secondary to client characteristics.

Ventilation/Perfusion Lung Scan

See Lung Scan, Perfusion and Ventilation—Diagnostic.

Ventriculography—Diagnostic

Norm. Normal cardiac ventricular structure; lack of disease process.

Usage. Noninvasive test to detect changes in heart function, assess for cardiac damage, and evaluate heart-wall motion and pumping function. Conditions include atrial septal defect, cardiomyopathy, heart failure, Lyme disease (secondary), mitral stenosis, and superior vena cava obstruction. May be used before coronary angiography to detect those clients with severe coronary artery disease who are at risk for angiographic procedural complications.

Description. Ventriculography is a noninvasive nuclear medicine test that allows for the heart chambers and major blood vessels to be outlined. A small dose of a radioactive isotope is injected in the client's veins. The isotope attaches itself to red blood cells that then pass through the heart. Special scanners or cameras can track the radioactive isotopes as they flow through the heart. The image is often synchronized with an electrocardiogram. Frequently the test is given in two stages: one at rest, one with exercise.

Professional Considerations
Consent form MAY be required.

Risks
Small exposure to radiation from the radioactive isotopes. With exercise testing, potential for cardiac ischemia, myocardial infarction, dysrhythmias, blood pressure changes.

Contraindications
Clients unable to lie motionless for the scan, previous allergy to radioisotope.

Precautions
During pregnancy, risks of cumulative radiation exposure to the fetus from this and other previous or future imaging studies must be weighed against the benefits of the procedure. Although formal limits for client exposure are relative to this risk:benefit comparison, the United States Nuclear Regulatory Commission requires that the cumulative dose equivalent to an embryo/fetus from occupational exposure not exceed 0.5 rem (5 mSv). Radiation dosage to the fetus is proportional to the distance of the anatomy studied from the abdomen and decreases as pregnancy progresses. For pregnant clients, consult the radiologist/radiology department to obtain estimated fetal radiation exposure from this procedure.

Preparation
1. Have emergency equipment available.
2. Obtain baseline ECG.
3. Review for history of allergic type of responses to radiographic dyes.

Procedure
1. Insert an intravenous access device.
2. Inject the isotope.
3. A scanner will be placed over the chest area.
4. Imaging takes place; depending on the type of test, the client may have a resting image, a resting and then an exercise image, or an exercise and then a resting image.

Postprocedure Care
1. Assess for any chest pain or discomfort.
2. For scans that involved exercise, monitor the client until vital signs return to baseline values.
3. Ensure proper disposal of any radioactive waste.

Client and Family Teaching
1. Do not ingest caffeine or any stimulants for 3-6 hours before the test.
2. Because this test may take some time, bring items to occupy yourself while waiting.
3. Wear comfortable clothing.
4. In women who are breast-feeding, formula should be substituted for breast milk for 1 or more days after the procedure.

Factors That Affect Results
1. Client's ability to remain motionless for the scan.
2. Drugs that alter cardiac contractility.
3. Recent MI (within 24 hours).
4. Recent previous exposure to radioactive tracers may interfere with the quality of the scan.
5. The decrement of the R-wave amplitude changes can indicate clients with three-vessel disease at risk of angiographic complications.
6. Standard volumes of contrast material are often associated with ventricular ectopy, which makes the readings uninterpretable. Reducing the volume of contrast material from 15 mL/second for 3 seconds to 15 mL/second for 1 second has been shown to reduce ectopy without affecting results.

Other Data
1. Abnormal findings in the scan may indicate the need for more extensive studies.
2. Health care professionals working in a nuclear medicine area must follow federal standards set by the Nuclear Regulatory

Commission. These standards include precautions for handling the radioactive material and monitoring potential radiation exposure.

Vestibular Evoked Myogenic Potential

See **Audiometry Test**—Diagnostic.

Video-Assisted Mediastinoscopy

See **Mediastinoscopy**—Diagnostic.

Viral Culture—Specimen

Norm. Negative. No virus isolated.

Usage. This procedure isolates the following viruses: enteroviruses; herpes simplex virus; influenza A and B; parainfluenza types 1, 2, 3; adenovirus; varicella-zoster virus; cytomegalovirus; and respiratory syncytial virus.

Positive. Acquired immune deficiency syndrome, adenovirus, chickenpox, conjunctivitis, cytomegalovirus, enteroviruses, herpes simplex, herpes zoster, keratitis, mumps virus, parainfluenza, pneumonia (viral), respiratory syncytial virus, rhinovirus, and varicella-zoster virus.

Description. Viruses are the tiniest known infectious agents and are composed of a single type of deoxyribonucleic acid (DNA) or ribonucleic acid (RNA) surrounded by an envelope of protein (proteinaceous coat). Viruses are parasites in that they reproduce with the aid of the enzymes of their living host. Thus they will not grow on artificial (nonliving) media. Viruses must be inoculated onto special viral culture media consisting of growing cells. The availability of viral culture methodology allows the rapid diagnosis and treatment of viral illnesses, as well as pattern tracking for outbreaks of viral illnesses.

Professional Considerations
Consent form NOT required.

Preparation
1. Blood cultures MAY be drawn during hemodialysis.
2. Clarify specific instructions with the laboratory performing the test.

3. Obtain the proper supplies, as listed below, depending on the site to be cultured.
   Blood: Chilled, heparinized green topped tube.
   Biopsy: Biopsy tray and sterile container.
   Conjunctivae: Virocult or Culturette swab, or sterile spatula and viral transport medium.
   Cerebrospinal fluid: Sterile vial with cap.
   Lesion: Virocult or Culturette swab, and 4-mL syringe with intradermal needle.
   Pharynx: Virocult or Culturette swab.
   Rectal swab: Virocult or Culturette swab.
   Stool: Clean, dry container.
   Urine: Sterile specimen container.
4. Obtain ice for packing around specimens to be cultured for Influenzavirus or cytomegalovirus.

Procedure
1. *Blood*: Draw a 5-mL blood sample as soon as possible after symptoms appear. Label the tube as the acute specimen. Repeat the test in 14-28 days, and label the sample as the convalescent specimen.
2. *Biopsy*: Using a sterile technique, collect an individual tissue sample into a cold, sterile container. Label it with the collection site and date.
3. *Conjunctivae*: Gently pull the lower eyelid down. Firmly swab the lower conjunctival border back and forth several times with a sterile swab. Place the swab in a chilled viral transport medium. Alternately, gently but firmly scrape the conjunctiva with a sterile spatula and smear the sample onto a chilled viral transport medium.

4. *Cerebrospinal fluid*: Obtain a 5-mL sample of cerebrospinal fluid by lumbar puncture into a chilled, sterile vial.
5. *Lesion*: Aspirate fluid from the vesicle with an intradermal needle and a 4-mL syringe. Eject the fluid into 1-2 mL of chilled viral transport medium. Firmly swab the base of the opened lesion and place the swab into a chilled viral transport medium.
6. *Pharynx*: With the client's head tilted back and the mouth open, have the client say "ah" to elevate the uvula. Firmly swab any visible lesions as well as the posterior surface of the nasopharyngeal area. Place the swab into a chilled viral transport medium.
7. *Rectal swab*: Insert a sterile swab into the rectum about 2-4 inches. Leave the swab in place for 10 seconds to allow absorption of fluid. Firmly rub the swab several times around the circumference of the rectum. Remove the swab and place it in a chilled viral transport medium.
8. *Stool*: Place a marble-sized stool sample in a clean, dry container.
9. *Urine*: Obtain a midstream, clean-catch urine specimen in a sterile container. See Urine culture from a clean-catch specimen instructions in the test Body fluid, Routine—Culture.

Postprocedure Care
1. Keep the specimen cold (not frozen) and transport it to the laboratory immediately. Specimens for Influenzavirus or cytomegalovirus culture should be transported in an ice bath.
2. Write the client's name, age, specimen source, recent antibiotic therapy, symptoms, and suspected diagnosis on the laboratory requisition.

Client and Family Teaching
1. The convalescent blood sample is needed 14-28 days after the first blood sample.
2. Results may take up to 4 weeks, but prophylactic antibiotics are normally started immediately.

Factors That Affect Results
1. Failure to keep the specimen cold after collection invalidates the results.

Other Data
1. None.

Viscosity—Blood

Norm. Serum: 1.4-1.8 cP (relative to water). Whole blood, <1 month: 3.6-6.5 cP. Whole blood, >1 month: 3.6-6.0 cP.

Increased. Arthritis (rheumatoid), cardiovascular risk, dysproteinemias, hyperfibrinogenemia, hyperviscosity syndrome, multiple myeloma (IgA), polycythemia, sickle cell anemia, systemic lupus erythematosus, and Waldenström's macroglobulinemia. May also be increased in neonates who experienced intrauterine hypoxia, delayed umbilical cord clamping, twin-to-twin transfusion, and maternal-fetal transfusion, as well as those neonates with mothers who have diabetes.

Decreased. Drugs include aspirin and dipyridamole. Herb or natural remedies are *Cordyceps sinensis* or Naoxinqing tablets.

Description. "Serum viscosity" is a term describing a physical property of fluid related to the resistance to flow generated by friction. Low-viscosity fluids flow freely, whereas high-viscosity fluids flow more slowly. In hyperviscosity syndrome, of which most cases occur in clients with Waldenström's macroglobulinemia, death can occur as a result of the impact of high serum viscosity. Sequelae include retinal hemorrhage, bleeding, pulmonary hypertension, congestive heart failure, and neurologic deficits. Increased viscosity is thought to contribute to the development of heart disease, thrombosis, arteriosclerosis, and several other conditions.

In this test, the viscosity of serum is compared to that of water at room temperature. Serum is normally more viscous than water.

Professional Considerations
Consent form NOT required.

Preparation
1. Tubes: Two red topped, red/gray topped, or gold topped. For evaluation of polycythemia vera and neonatal hyperviscosity syndrome, whole-blood viscosity should

be measured. Draw the specimen in a heparinized, green topped tube.

Procedure

1. Completely fill two tubes with blood.

Postprocedure Care

1. None.

Client and Family Teaching

1. Clinical symptoms do not correlate well with test results.

Factors That Affect Results

1. Increased levels found in persons exposed to carbon monoxide.

Other Data

1. Increased viscosity may cause dilation of the retinal veins, causing fundus changes in clients.

Visual Acuity Tests—Diagnostic

Norm.

	Distance Vision
Snellen Chart	
Adults	20/20 (near vision, 14/14)
Children	
Infants	3/60 or better
1-4 years	20/40 or better
4-7 years	20/30 or better
>7 years	20/20
Allen Cards	
3 years	15/30
4 years	20/30
Infant testing for optokinetic nystagmus	Present at 2 months of age
Strabismus	Absent
Stereopsis	Present
Color vision	Present bilaterally
Peripheral vision	Intact bilaterally

Usage. Part of routine ophthalmologic examination; community health screening for vision testing.

Description. Visual acuity testing involves testing a client's ability to read a standard Snellen chart of symbols (usually letters) at a specified distance to test distance vision, and a Jaeger card to test near vision. A Snellen chart consists of numbered rows of letters that progressively decrease in size from top to bottom. A Jaeger card contains text in progressively decreasing size. For young children and infants, substitute testing in place of the Snellen chart is performed as described below. Children are tested for distance vision, nystagmus, strabismus, stereopsis, color vision, and peripheral vision. The tests may be performed with and without current corrective lenses. For unsatisfactory tests, they will be repeated with new combinations of corrective lenses, until the best possible vision correction is obtained.

Professional Considerations

Consent form NOT required.

Preparation

1. Obtain charts, a handheld eye-occluder wand, an eye patch for children, and glasses for testing for stereopsis.

Procedure

1. The client is positioned sitting 20 feet away from the Snellen chart.
2. Each eye is tested separately as follows:
   a. The eye not being tested is occluded.
   b. The client is instructed to read the line closest to the bottom of the chart that he or she can read and then to attempt to read one line lower.
   c. The fractionated visual acuity is recorded as follows: The distance in feet the client is positioned away from the chart is the numerator (that is, 20), and the number of the lowest line read correctly is the denominator. If the client can read one symbol of a line farther down, the results are recorded as:

   20/Number of the lowest line read perfectly + Number of symbols read correctly on the line below

   For example, "20/100 + 1" means the client, at a distance of 20 feet, read the line at which a normal eye could read at 100 feet, plus 1 symbol on the line below. A passing score for a line requires that the client read the entire line with no more than one error.

V

3. *Near-vision testing:*
   a. The client is instructed to read a Jaeger card at normal reading distance. The numerator score is the distance at which the card was read, and the denominator score is the line number of the smallest-sized letters read correctly.

4. *Testing in young children:*
   a. For young children, the "E" chart is substituted for the Snellen chart. The child must indicate which direction the letter E is pointing. Pictures of familiar objects may be placed above, below, left, and right of the chart for the child to use in identification of direction. The test is performed for each eye separately.
   b. Other substitutes for young children are Allen cards, which contain pictures of objects familiar to children. The numerator score is the distance at which three of the objects can be recognized by the child, and the denominator is 30. The eyes are tested separately.
   c. *Strabismus testing:* A light is shined into the child's eyes from 16 inches away, and the bilateral reflection of the light in the eyes is observed. Strabismus causes an off-center reflection in one eye. A second test involves occluding one eye at a time, as the child gazes at an object 1 foot away, and observing for inward or outward movement of the uncovered eye, which indicates strabismus.
   d. *Stereopsis testing:* Wearing stereoscopic glasses, the child is shown a stereo picture and asked if the object is on the page or in front of the page. With intact stereopsis, the child should be able to see a three-dimensional object that appears to be in front of the page. Without stereopsis, the object appears flat on the page.
   e. *Color-vision testing:* The child is asked to identify objects made of specifically patterned colored dots fused into gray dots.
   f. *Peripheral-vision testing:* As the child gazes ahead, he or she is asked to indicate on which side of the visual field an object is appearing.

5. *Testing of infants:*
   a. Infants can be tested for optokinetic nystagmus by passing a bright object back and forth in front of the eyes and observing whether nystagmus occurs.
   b. The infant is also assessed for the ability to follow a lighted object moved in front of the visual field.
   c. Mirror fixation distance increases with age in infants and correlates with acuity card (Bowman et al, 2010).
   d. *Peripheral-vision testing:* As the child is distracted, a bright object is moved into the peripheral visual field, and the child's response to the object is noted.

6. This test is usually followed by visual field testing. Testing time for both procedures can take up to 60 minutes.

Postprocedure Care

1. None.

Client and Family Teaching

1. Young children may cooperate best if testing is practiced at home before this test.
2. Eye exercises may be prescribed for very young children with strabismus. Simple exercises that can be performed at home involve using small pictures pasted on Popsicle sticks to strengthen the muscle. The child holds the stick at arm's length in front of the visual field. While focusing on the picture, he or she slowly and steadily moves the stick in toward the eyes and attempts to maintain single vision. When double vision occurs, the child restarts the exercise.

Factors That Affect Results

1. The client must be able to follow directions.

Other Data

1. Client questionnaires are also used to assess the client's subjective functional impact of visual impairments. Three that are often used include the Activities of Daily Vision Scale, the National Eye Institute Visual Function Questionnaire, and the Visual Function Index.
2. See Visual field testing—Diagnostic.

Visual Evoked Potential—Diagnostic

Norm. P-100 is of normal latency. Latency is equivalent bilaterally (test results require expert interpretation).

Usage. Diagnosis or monitoring of demyelinating diseases, epilepsy (measure of cortical lateral interactions), glaucoma, maculopathy, migraine headaches, nitrous oxide toxicity (chronic), papilledema, Parkinson's disease, pressure on the optic pathway as a result of tumors or granulomas, pseudotumor cerebri, retinal diseases of the optic nerve, toxic optic neuropathies, and vitamin B deficiency. Also used intraoperatively during eye surgery to provide early warning of potential optic nerve damage.

Description. Visual evoked potential (VEP) is a low-amplitude, electrical waveform representation of the brain's response to a visual stimulus. Because the amplitude is too low to be noted on a traditional electroencephalogram (EEG), sophisticated computer signal-averaging techniques are used to average out the effect of other brain activity during testing. The test involves placing repetitive, patterned stimuli such as a striped, checkerboard, or dotted pattern in the visual field while VEP waveforms are recorded and the amount of time taken for the VEP to occur is measured. Variations of the technique include varying the pattern size, intensity, and visual field size as well as alternating the pattern itself in an effort to selectively stimulate portions of the visual field. Results are analyzed according to an algorithm and are related to the "P-100" wave. The P-100 wave occurs at about 100 milliseconds after each stimulus in normal clients. Of significance is the amount of time required for the VEP to occur after stimulation (latency) and a comparison of latency measurements of both eyes. Factors that affect latency include head size, electrode location, visual field position of the stimulus, and integrity of the visual nerve pathways.

Professional Considerations
Consent form NOT required.

Preparation
1. See Client and Family Teaching.
2. Obtain EEG electrodes, a machine and cap, and electroconductive gel.

3. Remove jewelry and metal objects from the client's head.

Procedure
1. The client is positioned sitting with his or her eyes located about 1 meter away from the screen. One eye is patched.
2. Scalp electrodes are placed in occipital, parietal, and midline locations.
3. The client is instructed to focus the eyes on the screen.
4. The chosen pattern(s) is (are) displayed in a rapid, flashing sequence as the client gazes at the screen, and a recording of VEPs is made. A computer signal average of the brain's electrical activity at a specifically chosen time after each stimulus is displayed.
5. The other eye is patched, and the test is repeated on the opposite eye.

Postprocedure Care
1. Remove the electrodes and cleanse the scalp of electroconductive gel.

Client and Family Teaching
1. The client must gaze continuously at a lighted screen of flashing patterns.
2. Hair should be shampooed the night before the examination and should be free of hair spray or other hair fixatives.
3. The test may take more than 1 hour.

Factors That Affect Results
1. Results must be compared with the norms of the laboratory performing the test, as different patterns and variations of the test will be performed, depending on the client's history and the purpose of the test.
2. Cataracts or a miotic pupil may increase the latency of the response.
3. Female P-100 latency has been shown to be shorter than that of male latency.
4. After 50 years of age, latency increases by about 2 milliseconds every 10 years.
5. The client must be able to concentrate on the test. Breaking the gaze on the screen hinders the usefulness of the results.

Other Data
1. An acute migraine attack produces prolonged peak latency.
2. Multifocal pattern electroretinography can help differentiate VEP delays caused by macular degeneration from delays resulting from optic nerve disease.

Visual Field Testing—Diagnostic

Usage. Confirmatory testing in conjunction with visual field loss for glaucoma in clients with elevated intraocular pressures obtained on tonometry testing; monitoring glaucoma progression in response to treatment; measuring impact of ptosis on visual field; evaluating optic nerve and brain visual pathways function.

Description. Visual field testing identifies whether the client's scope of vision is normal or impaired. It involves a variety of techniques designed to pinpoint specific areas of the visual field that are impaired and helps pinpoint whether there are abnormalities in the visual pathway from the brain, or whether there are mechanical problems such as lid droop, which impairs the visual field.

Professional Considerations

Consent form NOT required.

Preparation

1. This test requires the client to be able to sit completely still and erect, and to follow commands such as to press a button or move a hand when visual cues are given.
2. One eye is covered while testing is performed on the alternate eye. Then the eye covering and procedure is reversed to test the other eye.

Procedure

1. A series of confrontational, perimeter and light intensity maneuvers performed with the client seated and staring straight ahead to detect gaps or limitations in the field of vision. These tests are normally carried out with computerized equipment.
   a. Static perimetry testing involves having the client respond when visualizing fixed light sources displayed in the peripheral field of vision.
   b. Kinetic perimetry testing involves a moving light source and produces a map of the intensity of the visual perception.
   c. Frequency doubling analysis is more specific to identifying field loss caused by glaucoma and involves using shimmering light in specific sections of the both the peripheral and central visual fields.

Postprocedure Care

1. None.

Client and Family Teaching

1. It is important to sit up erect and be very still during this testing.

Factors That Affect Results

1. Test results include the number of fixation errors (how many times the client's eyes left the visual field), the number of false negatives (quantity of lights shone when client did not press the button), number of data points tested, reliability index for the client response, comparison of client results to a standard group of clients, and a map of the client's visual fields with any altered patterns identified.

Other Data

1. See also Amsler grid test—Screen.

Vitamin A (Retinol)—Serum

Norm.

	Vitamin A (Retinol)	SI Units
Normal Values		
Newborn to 1 month	0.18-0.50 mg/L	
2 months to 12 years	0.20-0.50 mg/L	
13-17 years	0.26-0.70 mg/L	
≥18 years	0.30-1.20 mg/L	

Continued

	Vitamin A (Retinol)	SI Units
Deficiency		
Borderline deficiency in clients	11-20 μg/dL	0.38-0.70 μmol/L older than 1 month
Deficiency in clients older than 1 month	<10 μg/dL	<0.35 μmol/L

Normal Value	Retinol Palmitate
All ages	<0.10 mg/L

Toxic Level Symptoms and Treatment

NOTE: The dose estimated to be toxic is 25,000 IU/kg.

Symptoms of Acute Toxicity. Long bone tenderness, neurologic changes similar to increased intracranial pressure.

Symptoms of Chronic Toxicity. Alopecia, anemia, ataxia, benign intracranial hypertension, brittle nails, cheilitis, conjunctivitis, diplopia, edema, erythema, exanthema, hepatic cirrhosis, hepatosplenomegaly, hyperostosis, neuritis (peripheral), papilledema, petechiae, premature closure of epiphyses, skin desquamation.

Treatment of Toxicity

NOTE: Treatment choice(s) depend(s) on client's history and condition and episode history.
1. Treatment is primarily supportive:
2. Maintain observation, particularly neurologic status.
3. Hydrate if dehydrated or hypercalcemic.
4. Discontinue vitamin A supplements.

Symptoms of Deficiency. Changes in vision, including night blindness, Bitot's spots; reduced growth; dry skin; and weak dental enamel.

Treatment of Deficiency. High-dose vitamin A replacement. Consult medication guidelines reference.

Increased. Excessive supplementary or dietary intake, intrahepatic cholestasis.

Decreased. Asthma (children), autoimmune hepatitis, biliary atresia, Brazilian children (5.8%), breast cancer (predicts poorer prognosis), celiac disease, congenital diaphragmatic hernia, cystic fibrosis of the pancreas, hearing impairment, infectious hepatitis, intestinal worms, intrauterine growth retardation, Iranian pregnant women, iron deficiency, jaundice (obstructive), low prealbumin level, malabsorption, nephritis (chronic), night blindness, obesity, oligozoospermia, otitis media, post Roux-en-Y gastric bypass, protein-calorie malnutrition, sepsis, smokers, tuberculosis (severe), and Vietnamese preschool children.

Description. Vitamin A is a fat-soluble vitamin obtained from animal-based foods and the carotenes of dietary plants and stored in the liver. It is absorbed from the intestines in the presence of bile and lipase, transported to the liver in the form of chylomicrons, and stored in the liver as retinyl ester. Vitamin A is necessary for mucous membrane epithelial-cell integrity, proper growth, and proper night vision. Vitamin A deficiency is more common in children from lower socioeconomic groups.

Professional Considerations

Consent form NOT required.

Preparation
1. Tube: Green topped and a paper bag.
2. See Client and Family Teaching.

Procedure
1. Draw a 4-mL blood sample without hemolysis. Place the tube in the paper bag to protect it from light.

Postprocedure Care
1. None.

Client and Family Teaching
1. Fast from food and fluids (except for water) overnight before the test.
2. Do not drink alcohol for 24 hours before sampling.
3. Tobacco smoke exposure of infants significantly decreases serum antioxidant vitamins A, C, and E levels.

Factors That Affect Results
1. Hemolysis invalidates the results.
2. Using plastic tubing or prolonged exposure of the specimen to light causes falsely low results.

3. Vitamin A levels may be low in the third trimester for about 30% of pregnant clients.
4. Levels less than 10 μg/dL (μmol/L, SI units) are common from birth to 30 days of age.

Other Data
1. None.

V

Vitamin B₁ (Thiamine)—Blood or Urine

Norm. *Whole blood* (preferred specimen): 1.6-4.0 μg/dL.
Plasma: 0.2-2.0 μg/dL.
Serum: 5.3-7.9 μg/dL.
Urine: 100-200 μg/24 hours.

Increased. Excessive supplemental intake. Drugs include spironolactone.

Decreased. Alcoholism (chronic), beriberi, chronic fatigue syndrome, chronic renal failure clients receiving dialysis, diarrhea (chronic), hyperthyroidism, lactic acidosis, pregnancy, postcoronary bypass graft (CABG) surgery, and Wernicke-Korsakoff syndrome (cerebral beriberi). Drugs include diuretics (long-term use).

Description. Vitamin B₁ is a water-soluble vitamin of particular salt compounds. It is found widely in foods, especially organ meats, yeast, and whole grains. Vitamin B₁ is absorbed in the duodenum in the presence of folic acid and excreted in the urine. About 80% of Vitamin B₁ found in whole blood is contained within the red blood cells. This vitamin acts as an enzyme in alpha-ketoacid decarboxylation, connects the glycolytic cycle to the Krebs cycle, and activates the guanylate cyclase-cyclic guanosine monophosphate system. Deficiency of B₁ causes three types of beriberi. "Wet" beriberi is characterized by congestive heart failure. "Dry" beriberi is characterized by peripheral neuritis, muscle paralysis and atrophy, myelin sheath degeneration, weakness, and confusion. "Cerebral" beriberi (Wernicke-Korsakoff syndrome) occurs in chronic alcoholics and is characterized by encephalopathy, ataxia, ocular disturbances, and ocular neuropathy.

Professional Considerations
Consent form NOT required.

Preparation
1. Tube: Green topped, lavender topped, or pink topped (for serum level), and a paper bag.

2. For urine level, obtain a clean, brown, 3-L container. Write the beginning time of collection on the laboratory requisition.
3. Do NOT draw specimens during hemodialysis.
4. See Client and Family Teaching.

Procedure
1. *Serum level:*
   a. Draw a 4-mL blood sample for whole blood measurement or a 7-mL blood sample for plasma or serum measurement. Place the sample immediately in a paper bag to protect it from light.
2. *24-hour urine collection:*
   a. Discard the first morning void.
   b. Save all the urine voided in a 24-hour period in a refrigerated, clean, light-protected, 3-L container without preservatives. For catheterized specimens, keep the drainage bag on ice and empty the urine into the collection container hourly. Document the quantity of urine output during the collection period.

Postprocedure Care
1. Send the serum specimen to the laboratory immediately.
2. For urine collections, write the ending time and total 24-hour urine output quantity on the laboratory requisition. Send the specimen to the laboratory and refrigerate it.

Client and Family Teaching
1. Fast overnight before blood draw.
2. For the urine test, save all the urine voided, void before defecating, and avoid contaminating the specimen with stool or toilet tissue. Empty each void into the refrigerated, light-protected collection container. If any urine is accidentally discarded, discard the entire specimen and restart the collection the next day.

Factors That Affect Results
1. Prolonged exposure of the specimen to light invalidates the results.

2. Clients who consume a diet high in freshwater fish or tea made from tea leaves may have low levels because these foods contain thiamine antagonists.
3. Hemodialysis will reduce vitamin B$_1$ levels.

4. An increase in the percent of carbohydrates in the diet has been shown to reduce vitamin B$_1$ levels.

Other Data

1. None.

Vitamin B$_6$ (Pyridoxine, Pyridoxal, and Pyridoxamine)—Plasma

Norm. Norms are method-dependent.

Radioenzymatic Assay	SI Units
5-30 ng/mL	20-121 nmol/L

Increased. Pyridoxine megavitaminosis caused by excessive dietary supplementation.

Decreased. Alcoholism (chronic), anemia (sideroblastic), common variable immunodeficiency (CVID), diabetes (gestational), inadequate dietary intake, lactation, malabsorption, malnutrition, pregnancy, retinal vein occlusion, small bowel inflammatory disease and smokers. Drugs include cycloserine, disulfiram, hydralazine, isoniazid, levodopa, oral contraceptives, penicillamine, and pyrazinoic acid.

Description. Vitamin B$_6$ is a term that collectively refers to three water-soluble vitamins: pyridoxine, pyridoxal, and pyridoxamine. After absorption, pyridoxine is converted to the active forms of pyridoxal and pyridoxamine phosphates. These vitamins are found in many foods, including meats, egg yolks, fish, fowl, whole grains (such as wheat germ, rye meal, soybean meal, barley, soybeans, brown rice), and vegetables. Recommended Dietary Allowance for Americans is 3-4.9 mg/day. The B vitamins are important in the function of the central nervous system and heme synthesis, and they function as coenzymes in amino acid metabolism and glycogenolysis. Because vitamin B$_6$ is partially destroyed by heat, overheating of infant formula makes infants particularly prone to vitamin B$_6$ deficiency. A sign of vitamin B$_6$ deficiency includes peripheral neuropathy, and a sign of toxicity is severe sensorimotor neuropathy.

Professional Considerations
Consent form NOT required.

Preparation

1. Tube: Lavender topped or pink topped and a paper bag.

Procedure

1. Draw a 5-mL blood sample. Place the sample immediately in a paper bag to protect it from light.
2. Write the collection time on the laboratory requisition.

Postprocedure Care

1. Send the specimen to the laboratory within 30 minutes.
2. The plasma must be quickly separated and frozen.

Client and Family Teaching

1. Symptoms of B$_6$ deficiency may include colic, enhanced startle reflex, convulsions, and irritability.

Factors That Affect Results

1. Prolonged exposure of the specimen to light invalidates the results.
2. Reject specimens received more than 30 minutes after collection.
3. Plasma levels of vitamin B$_6$ tend to decrease with age, but no age-related norms have been established.

Other Data

1. Concurrent testing recommended for evaluation of vitamin B$_6$ status includes plasma pyridoxal 5'-phosphate (PLP) and urinary 4-pyridoxic acid.
2. Vitamin B$_6$ may be measured indirectly by tryptophan loading and measurement of subsequent xanthurenic acid in the urine.
3. Low levels are associated with increased risk for vascular disease in some studies.
4. Low levels are associated with elevated plasma homocysteine levels.

Vitamin B₆ (4-Pyridoxic Acid)—Urine

Norm. 0.5-1.3 mg/dL (2.7-7.1 µmol/day, SI units).

Increased. Pyridoxine megavitaminosis caused by excessive dietary supplementation; renal insufficiency.

Decreased. Anemia, asthma, carpal tunnel syndrome, chronic alcoholism, gestational diabetes, industrial exposure to hydrazine compounds, lactation, malnutrition, pellagra, peripheral neuritis, peritoneal dialysis, and vitamin B₆ deficiency. Drugs include amiodarone, anticonvulsants, cyclosporin A, disulfiram, ethyl alcohol (ethanol), hydralazine, isoniazid, oral contraceptives, penicillamine, pyrazinoic acid, and tricyclic antidepressants.

Description. Urinary 4-pyridoxic acid is a major metabolite of vitamin B₆ and can be used to evaluate vitamin B₆ deficiency. As a coenzyme, vitamin B₆ aids in the synthesis and breakdown of amino acids, aids in the synthesis of unsaturated fatty acids from essential fatty acids, is essential for conversion of tryptophan to niacin, and is involved in formation of the precursor to porphyrin compound. Urinary testing of 4-pyridoxic acid is not widely used and is of limited value. Plasma values are preferred.

Professional Considerations

Consent form NOT required.

Preparation

1. Obtain a clean 3-L container that is free of preservative. For pediatric/infant collections, also obtain tape and a pediatric urine collection device/bag.
2. Write the beginning time of the 24-hour collection on the laboratory requisition.

Procedure

1. Early morning is the preferred time to begin a 24-hour collection.
2. Discard the first morning urine specimen.
3. Save all the urine voided for 24 hours in a refrigerated, clean, 3-L container that is free of preservatives. Document the quantity of urine output during the specimen collection period. Include the urine voided at the end of the 24-hour period. For catheterized clients, keep the drainage bag on ice and empty the urine into the refrigerated collection container hourly.
4. Pediatric/infant specimen collection:
   a. The child is placed in a supine position with the knees flexed and the hips externally rotated and abducted.
   b. Cleanse, rinse, and thoroughly dry the perineal area.
   c. To prevent the child from removing the collection device/bag, a diaper may be placed over the genital area.
   d. *Females:* Tape the pediatric collection device/bag to the perineum. Starting at the area between the anus and vagina, apply the device/bag in an anterior direction.
   e. *Males:* Place the pediatric collection device/bag over the penis and scrotum and tape it to the perineal area.
   f. Empty the collection bag into the refrigerated collection container after each void.

Postprocedure Care

1. Compare the urine quantity in the specimen container with the urinary output record for the test. If the specimen contains less urine than what was recorded as output, some of the sample may have been discarded, thus invalidating the test.
2. Document the urine quantity and ending time on the laboratory requisition.
3. Isoniazid (INH) is a pyridoxal antagonist. Observe if the client is using the drug.

Client and Family Teaching

1. Save all the urine voided in a 24-hour period, urinate before defecating to avoid loss of urine, and avoid contamination of the specimen with stool, toilet tissue, or prostatic or vaginal secretions. If any urine is accidentally discarded, discard the entire specimen and restart the collection the next day.
2. Inform the client of the possible need for a vitamin B₆ supplement during pregnancy and lactation or with the use of oral contraceptives.

Factors That Affect Results

1. None.

Other Data

1. Recommended daily requirements of vitamin B$_6$ are complicated by differences in protein intake and the use of alcohol and oral contraceptives.
2. Daily allowances for vitamin B$_6$ generally are 1.6-2.0 mg.
3. Foods rich in vitamin B$_6$ include yeast, wheat germ, pork, glandular meats, whole grain cereal, legumes, potatoes, bananas, and oatmeal.

Vitamin B$_9$

See Folic Acid—Serum.

Vitamin B$_{12}$ (Cyanocobalamin, CBL, Extrinsic Factor)—Serum

Norm.

		SI Units
Low	<100 pg/mL	<74 pmol/L
Indeterminate	100-200 pg/mL	74-147 pmol/L
Normal	200-1100 pg/mL	147-810 pmol/L
High	>1100 pg/mL	>810 pmol/L

Increased. Chronic obstructive pulmonary disease, colorectal cancer, congestive heart failure, diabetes, hepatic cellular damage, leukemia (chronic granulocytic), liver disease (chronic decompensated), obesity, polycythemia vera, renal failure (chronic) and Still's disease (adult onset).

Decreased. Anemia (pernicious), atrophic gastritis, bacterial overgrowth syndromes, Brazilian adults, congenital deficiency of transcobalamin II, Crohn's disease, depression, fish tapeworm infestation, gastrectomy or gastric bypass (with removal of parietal cells), hepatitis (alcoholic), ileal disease or resection, inflammatory bowel disease, intestinal tapeworm, intrinsic factor deficiency (pernicious anemia), neural tube defects (NTD), polycystic ovary syndrome (PCOS), protein-bound cobalamin malabsorption, malnutrition, pancreatic insufficiency, sickle cell anemia, and (strict) veganism. Drugs include p-aminosalicylic acid, antibacterials (neomycin), anti-diabetics, anti-epileptics, anti-gout agents (colchicine), omeprazole, and proton pump inhibitors (PPI).

Description. Vitamin B$_{12}$ (cyanocobalamin) is a water-soluble vitamin obtained from dietary animal sources that is necessary for proper deoxyribonucleic acid (DNA) synthesis. It can be absorbed from the gastrointestinal tract only when intrinsic factor glycoprotein secreted from the stomach's parietal cells is present. Although the body stores up to a 12-month supply of this vitamin in the liver, kidneys, and heart, rapid growth states or conditions causing rapid turnover of cells increase the body's need for vitamin B$_{12}$. Symptoms of vitamin B$_{12}$ deficiency include anemia; a smooth, red, painful tongue (glossitis); and neurologic abnormalities of extremity paresthesias.

Professional Considerations

Consent form NOT required.

Preparation

1. Hold blood transfusion or B$_{12}$ administration until blood is drawn, when possible.
2. Ascertain baseline hematocrit.
3. Tube: Red topped, red/gray topped, or gold topped, and a paper bag.
4. See Client and Family Teaching.

Procedure

1. Draw a 4-mL blood sample. Place the tube immediately in a paper bag to protect it from light.

Postprocedure Care

1. Send the specimen to the laboratory immediately. Samples must be quickly spun, with serum separated, frozen, and protected from light.

Client and Family Teaching
1. Fast overnight before the test.

Factors That Affect Results
1. Hemolysis or prolonged exposure of the specimen to light invalidates the results.
2. Administration of radiographic dyes within 7 days before the test invalidates the results.
3. Falsely normal results may occur in myeloproliferative disorders such as chronic myelogenous leukemia and polycythemia vera, and in hepatic disease, congenital transcobalamin II deficiency, and overgrowth of intestinal bacteria.

4. Falsely decreased results may occur during pregnancy and in clients with folic acid deficiency, multiple myeloma, or congenital deficiency of serum haptocorrins.
5. Drugs that may cause falsely decreased results include oral contraceptives.

Other Data
1. B_{12} is involved in the suppression of viral replication during anti-hepatitis C treatment.
2. See also Vitamin B_{12}, Unsaturated binding capacity—Serum.

Vitamin B_{12}, Unsaturated Binding Capacity (UBC)—Serum

Norm. 870-2000 pg/mL (640-1473 pmol/L, SI units).

Increased. Hepatoma, leukemia (chronic myelogenous), myeloproliferative state, polycythemia vera, pregnancy, and reactive leukocytosis. Drugs include oral contraceptives.

Decreased. Hypoproteinemia.

Description. Vitamin B_{12} (cyanocobalamin) is a water-soluble vitamin obtained from dietary animal sources that is necessary for proper deoxyribonucleic acid (DNA) synthesis. It is absorbed from the gastrointestinal tract only when bound by intrinsic factor glycoprotein secreted from the stomach's parietal cells. After absorption, it is transported in the bloodstream by transcobalamin-binding proteins, primarily transcobalamin I. In this test, intrinsic factor is added to a mixture of the client's serum and radiolabeled vitamin B_{12}. The mixture is incubated, and then the fraction of bound, radiolabeled vitamin B_{12} is measured by a scintillation counter after removal of the unbound vitamin. The results are an indication of the level of transcobalamin-binding proteins, which are known to be elevated in certain conditions (listed above).

Professional Considerations
Consent form NOT required.

Preparation
1. Preschedule this test with the laboratory.
2. Tube: Red topped, red/gray topped, gold topped, or lavender topped (depending on laboratory requirements).

Procedure
1. Draw a 7-mL blood sample.

Postprocedure Care
1. Send the specimen to the laboratory immediately or else refrigerate it.

Client and Family Teaching
1. Results are normally available within 48 hours.

Factors That Affect Results
1. Clotting of the specimen may cause elevated results.
2. Falsely elevated results may occur if intrinsic factor that is not highly purified is used.

Other Data
1. See also Vitamin B_{12}—Serum.

Vitamin C (Ascorbic Acid)—Plasma or Serum
Norm.

		SI Units
Normal level	0.6-2 mg/dL	34-114 μmol/L
Possible (or risk for) deficiency	<0.2-0.4 mg/dL	1-22.7 μmol/L
Deficiency	<0.2 mg/dL	<11 μmol/L

Increased. Preterm delivery. Drugs that include ascorbic acid.

Decreased. Alcoholism, hyperthyroidism, malabsorption, peritoneal dialysis, pregnancy, renal failure, scurvy, and in smokers.

Description. Vitamin C is a water-soluble vitamin found in citrus fruits and leafy (raw) vegetables and tomatoes. It is absorbed from the diet through the small intestine and stored in the adrenal glands, kidney, spleen, liver, and leukocytes. Excess amounts of the vitamin are excreted in the urine. Vitamin C is important in cellular structure, collagen synthesis, capillary integrity, wound healing, intestinal iron absorption, and resistance to infection.

Professional Considerations
Consent form NOT required.

Preparation
1. Clarify the type of tube needed with the testing laboratory because requirements vary.
2. Tube: CHILLED green topped, red topped, red/gray topped, gold topped, lavender topped, or black topped.
3. Obtain a container of ice.
4. See Client and Family Teaching.

Procedure
1. Draw a 10-mL blood sample according to specific laboratory requirements. Use a chilled tube.
2. Place the specimen immediately on ice.

Postprocedure Care
1. Send the specimen to the laboratory immediately. Serum or plasma must be promptly separated and frozen.

Client and Family Teaching
1. Fast overnight before the test.
2. Results are normally available within 24 hours.

Factors That Affect Results
1. Chronic tobacco smoking decreases levels.

Other Data
1. For clients ingesting inadequate vitamin C, scurvy can develop in about 90 days.
2. Signs of vitamin C deficiency include petechiae, corkscrew hairs, and perifollicular petechiae.
3. Supplements of Vitamin C, Vitamin E, and glutathione may be used in preventive measures in malaria.

Vitamin D (Cholecalciferol)—Plasma or Serum

Norm. Norms vary according to the test method used.

	Radioimmunoassay	SI Units
Serum vitamin D_3 (1,25-dihydroxy-)	15-75 pg/mL	39-195 nmol/L
Plasma vitamin D_3 (25-hydroxy-)		
Summer	15-80 ng/mL	37-200 nmol/L
Winter	14-42 ng/mL	35-105 nmol/L

Increased. Hyperparathyroidism, hypervitaminosis D, and sarcoidosis.

Decreased. Alzheimer's, atherosclerosis, congestive heart failure, diabetic retinopathy, hemodialysis (long-term), hepatic failure, hyperparathyroidism (primary), hypocalcemia post parathyroidectomy, inflammatory bowel disease, malabsorption, multiple sclerosis, osteomalacia, Parkinson's disease, post-kidney transplant, pseudohypoparathyroidism, renal failure, renal osteodystrophy, and rickets. Drugs include anticonvulsants and isoniazid.

Description. Vitamin D is a fat-soluble vitamin found as a dietary supplement in milk and is synthesized in the skin from the body's cholesterol stores in conjunction with exposure to sunlight, and is important in maintaining bone health. Vitamin D is a pro-hormone and becomes biologically active through hepatic hydroxylation to 25-hydroxyvitamin D and then to 1,25-dihydroxyvitamin D through renal hydroxylation. It works in conjunction with calcitonin and parathyroid hormone and is necessary for proper dietary calcium absorption from the intestinal tract, for regulation of skeletal calcium resorption, and for release of parathyroid hormone. The 2011 Endocrine Society Clinical Practice Guidelines recommend no routine screening of individuals for Vitamin D deficiency; however this test is recommended as the initial evaluation in individuals with suspected deficiency.

A meta-analysis (Tice, 2011) found that vitamin D supplementation reduces the risk of subsequent bone fracture only when combined with calcium supplementation, and the combination therapy did not increase cardiovascular events. The Institute of Medicine's recommendations for Vitamin D supplementation are geared toward the goal of bone health and recommend 600 IU per day for clients age 70 and under, and 800 IU per day for those over age 70.

Professional Considerations
Consent form NOT required.

Preparation
1. Tube: Lavender topped or pink.
2. See Client and Family Teaching.

Procedure
1. Draw a 4-mL blood sample.

Postprocedure Care
1. None.

Client and Family Teaching
1. Fast overnight before the test.
2. Results are normally available within 24 hours.

Factors That Affect Results
1. Insufficient dietary phosphorus intake causes decreased 1,25-dihydroxyvitamin D.
2. Clients who have no exposure to sunlight may have decreased levels.

Other Data
1. Concurrent measurement of parathyroid hormone is recommended.
2. Hypervitaminosis D may be nephrotoxic.
3. 25-hydroxyvitamin D is being studied for correlation of its levels to the risk for cardiovascular disease. Findings to date are inconsistent and inconclusive.
4. For treatment in clients without severe renal failure, Cholecalciferol (D3) is preferred over Ergocalciferol (D_2) because it is more potent and has a longer duration of action.

Vitamin E (Alpha-Tocopherol)—Serum

Norm.

	Vitamin E (Alpha-tocopherol)
Adults	≤6.0 mg/L or ≤25.94 µmol/L SI units
Children	
Newborn to 60 days	1.0-3.5 mg/L
2-5 months	2.0-6.0 mg/L
6-23 months	3.5-8.0 mg/L
2-12 years	5.5-9.0 mg/L
>12 years	≤6.0 mg/L
	Vitamin E (Gamma-tocopherol)
All ages	<6.0 mg/L or 5.25 µmol/L SI units

Increased. Atherosclerosis, excessive intake of supplemental vitamin E. Drugs include atorvastatin and other statins.

Decreased. Alzheimer's, brown-bowel syndrome, certain neurologic degenerative diseases, chronic alcoholism, chronic fatigue syndrome, human immunodeficiency virus (HIV), malabsorption caused by intestinal bile deficiency (biliary atresia, cystic fibrosis), non-alcoholic steatohepatitis (NASH), and smokers.

Description. Vitamin E is a fat-soluble vitamin found widely in foods such as green vegetables, grains, eggs, oils, liver, chicken, and fish. This vitamin prevents oxidation of vitamin A, deoxyribonucleic acid (DNA), and cell-membrane phospholipids by free radicals. It is necessary for proper reproductive function, muscle growth and development, and hemolytic resistance of red blood cell membranes. Deficiency of vitamin E causes hemolytic anemia and neurologic abnormalities.

Professional Considerations
Consent form NOT required.

Preparation
1. Tube: Green topped, and a paper bag.
2. Client should fast overnight before the test.

Procedure
1. Draw a 4-mL blood sample. Label the tube, and place it promptly in a paper bag to protect it from light.

Postprocedure Care
1. Send the specimen to the laboratory.
2. Serum must be separated within 2 hours of collection.

Client and Family Teaching
1. Fast overnight before the test. Do not drink alcohol for 24 hours before the test.
2. Results are normally available within 72 hours.

Factors That Affect Results
1. Hemolysis or prolonged exposure of the specimen to light invalidates the results.

Other Data
1. The specimen is stable at room temperature or refrigerated for 30 days, or frozen for up to 1 year.

VLDL
See Low-Density Lipoprotein Cholesterol—Blood.

Voiding Cystourethrography
See Cystourethrography, Voiding—Diagnostic.

Volatile Screen
See Toxicology, Volatiles Group by GLC—Blood or Urine.

von Willebrand Factor Activity (Ristocetin Cofactor)—Blood

Norm. Aggregation occurs after addition of ristocetin to the sample.

Adults	44%-195%
Children	
<7 years	44%-195%
7-9 years	51%-172%
10-11 years	61%-195%
12-13 years	47%-183%
14-15 years	50%-215%
16-17 years	47%-206%

Usage. Helps differentiate between hemophilia A (classical hemophilia) and von Willebrand's disease.

Description. Von Willebrand's disease is an autosomal dominantly transmitted factor VIII defect. It is a coagulation disorder that results in varying degrees of bleeding abnormalities. Coagulation factor VIII has three properties, namely, procoagulant activity (low or absent in hemophilia A), antigenic activity, and von Willebrand factor activity. The von Willebrand factor activity of factor VIII enhances the formation of platelet plugs. In this test, the von Willebrand factor activity of factor VIII is measured by use of a modified platelet aggregation test. In normal clients or those with hemophilia A, the antibiotic ristocetin induces platelet aggregation on a test sample. In clients with von Willebrand's disease, however, addition of ristocetin to the client's serum does not result in platelet aggregation. The lower the percentage of platelet aggregation, the lower the amount of von Willebrand factor.

Professional Considerations

Consent form NOT required.

Preparation

1. Preschedule this test with the laboratory.
2. Tube: Two 2.7-mL or 4.5-mL blue topped tubes and a control tube.

Procedure

1. The blood draw is best performed by a laboratory technician.
2. Completely fill a 4.5-mL tube with blood.
3. Gently roll the tube several times to mix the blood with the anticoagulant.
4. Serum should be immediately separated into a plastic vial and frozen before it is sent to the laboratory.

Postprocedure Care

1. Send the specimen to the laboratory immediately. Specimen should be immediately centrifuged. Plasma should be frozen if not tested immediately.

Client and Family Teaching

1. If ordered by your physician, avoid warfarin for 14 days before this test and avoid heparin for 2 days before this test.
2. Results are normally available within 72 hours.

Factors That Affect Results

1. Hemolysis or clotting of the specimen invalidates the results.
2. Contamination of the specimen with tissue thromboplastins invalidates the results. This is the reason for the double-draw technique.
3. Results are invalidated if the specimen is received by the laboratory more than 2 hours after collection.
4. Levels may increase 200%-300% during pregnancy.
5. An acute-phase reactant, von Willebrand factor increases may occur during stress, infection, inflammatory conditions, postoperatively, or after extreme physical exercise.
6. ABO blood type O clients may have up to 30% lower levels of von Willebrand factor than clients with other blood types.

Other Data

1. To establish a diagnosis of von Willebrand's disease, plasma factor VIII levels and von Willebrand factor antigen measurements are used in conjunction with this test.
2. See also von Willebrand factor antigen—Blood; Factor VIII—Blood.

von Willebrand Factor Antigen (vWF Ag, Factor VIII R:Ag, Factor VIII–Related Antigen)—Blood

Norm.

	Percent of Control Sample Activity
Adults	51-185
Children	
<7 years	51-185
7-9 years	62-176
10-11 years	61-201
12-13 years	61-186
14-15 years	57-204
16-17 years	51-211
von Willebrand's disease, all ages	<40

Usage. Differentiation between hemophilia A (classical hemophilia) and von Willebrand's disease when bleeding time tests are inconclusive.

Description. von Willebrand's disease is an autosomal dominantly transmitted factor VIII defect. It is a coagulation disorder that results in varying degrees of bleeding abnormalities. Coagulation factor VIII has three properties, namely, procoagulant activity (circulating von Willebrand factor is newly recognized as initiating platelet adhesion), antigenic activity, and von Willebrand factor activity. In this test, factor VIII antigenic activity is determined by measurement of von Willebrand factor antigen (vWF Ag). In hemophilia A and in carriers of hemophilia A, vWF Ag activity is normal, but in von Willebrand's disease, vWF Ag is characteristically low (that is, <40% of control sample activity).

Professional Considerations

Consent form NOT required.

Preparation

1. Preschedule this test with the laboratory.
2. Tube: 2.7-mL or 4.5-mL blue topped tube.

Procedure

1. Collect a 4.5-mL blood sample.
2. Gently roll the tube several times to mix the blood with the anticoagulant.

Postprocedure Care

1. Send the specimen to the laboratory immediately. Specimen should be promptly separated and frozen until testing.

Client and Family Teaching

1. If ordered by your physician, avoid warfarin for 14 days before this test and avoid heparin for 2 days before this test.
2. Results are normally available within 72 hours.

Factors That Affect Results

1. Hemolysis invalidates the results.
2. Contamination of the specimen with tissue thromboplastins invalidates the results. This is the reason for the double-draw technique.

3. Results are invalidated if the specimen is received by the laboratory more than 2 hours after collection.
4. Levels may increase 200%-300% during pregnancy.
5. An acute-phase reactant, von Willebrand factor increases may occur during stress, infection, inflammatory conditions, post-operatively, or after extreme physical exercise.
6. ABO blood type O clients may have up to 30% lower levels of von Willebrand factor than clients with other blood types.

Other Data

1. To establish a diagnosis of von Willebrand's disease, plasma factor VIII levels and von Willebrand factor assay are used in conjunction with this test.
2. See also von Willebrand factor activity—Blood; Factor VIII—Blood.

VPF

See Vascular Endothelial Growth Factor—Specimen.

V/Q Scan

See Lung Scan, Perfusion and Ventilation—Diagnostic.

Vulva Smear

See Pap Smear—Diagnostic.

Washing Cytology

See Bronchial Washing—Specimen.

Water Deprivation Test for Vasopressin Deficiency

See Concentration Test—Urine.

Water Loading Test—Diagnostic

Norm. ≥500-mL urine output over 4 hours after water ingestion.
Urine osmolality < serum osmolality or <180 mOsm/kg by 5 hours after water ingestion.

Usage. Diagnosis of syndrome of inappropriate antidiuretic hormone secretion (SIADHS).

Description. The water loading test involves administering a large quantity of water and then comparing the osmolality of timed urine and serum collections. In a normal client, increased fluid intake increases urine output and decreases urine osmolality. In clients with SIADHS, however, excess secretion of antidiuretic hormone causes a lower-than-normal urine output in response to the water loading and a urine osmolality that does not decrease below serum osmolality.

Professional Considerations
Consent form NOT required.

Risks
Fluid overload, congestive heart failure. Complications of nasogastric tube insertion include bleeding, dysrhythmias, esophageal perforation, laryngospasm, and decreased mean pO_2.

Contraindications and Precautions
Perform with extreme caution in clients with a history of congestive heart failure.

Preparation
1. The baseline serum sodium level should be at least 125 mEq/L before this test is started.
2. Withhold diuretics for 12 hours before the test.
3. Tube: Six red topped, red/gray topped, or gold topped.
4. Also obtain six clean plastic specimen containers.
5. Insert a nasogastric tube if the client will be unable to drink 1 L of water over a short period of time.

Procedure
1. Draw a 4-mL blood sample for the baseline serum osmolality. Obtain a 20-mL random urine sample in a clean plastic container for baseline urine osmolality.
2. Have the client drink 1 L of water, or 20 mL/kg of body weight, over 15-20 minutes, or instill it through a nasogastric tube.
3. Document the quantity of urine output, starting with the time of water ingestion and ending 5 hours later.
4. Obtain samples for serum and urine osmolality as in step 1 every hour for 5 hours. Label each tube sequentially, and write the collection time on the label.

Postprocedure Care
1. Refrigerate the serum samples if they are not tested within 4 hours.
2. Refrigerate all urine samples until they are tested.

Client and Family Teaching
1. The client will be asked to drink or have instilled at least 1 L of water within 20 minutes.

Factors That Affect Results
1. Diuretics administered within 12 hours before the test invalidate the results.

Other Data
1. Terlipressin increases water excretion in nonazotemic cirrhotic patients without hyponatremia.

Weber Test
See Tuning Fork Test, of Weber, Rinne, and Schwabach Tests—Diagnostic.

Weil-Felix Agglutinins—Blood

Norm. A less than fourfold rise in titer between acute and convalescent samples; or titer <1:160.

Usage. Helps in the diagnosis of rickettsial infections.

Description. A test performed for the purpose of detecting and differentiating rickettsial antibodies in the serum. Rickettsial organisms cause Rocky Mountain spotted fever, Q fever, Brill-Zinsser disease, epidemic typhus, murine typhus, scrub typhus, and rickettsialpox. Three *Proteus* antigens are known to cross-react in specific relationships with rickettsial antibodies. The test is performed by mixture of serial dilutions of test serum with suspensions of *Proteus* strains OX-2, OX-19, and OX-K and observation for agglutination. A single titer >1:320 or a fourfold rise in titer between acute and convalescent samples is considered diagnostic.

Professional Considerations
Consent form NOT required.

Preparation
1. Tube: Red topped, red/gray topped, or gold topped.
2. Specimens MAY be drawn during hemodialysis.

Procedure
1. Draw a 10-mL blood sample and label it as the "acute sample." Repeat the test every 3-5 days. Draw a final sample in 10-14 days, and label it as the "convalescent sample."

Postprocedure Care
1. None.

Client and Family Teaching
1. Return for serial sampling as prescribed and then in 10-14 days for final follow-up testing.

Factors That Affect Results
1. Hemolysis invalidates the results.
2. Immunosuppressed clients may be infected but have low or negative titers.
3. Antibiotic therapy causes low initial titers.

Other Data
1. Because the test is based on a known cross-reaction, caution must be used in interpreting the results. Although differentiation between Rocky Mountain spotted fever and typhus fever is not possible with this test, interpretation of results can rule out certain rickettsial infections.
2. See also Febrile agglutinins—Serum.

Westergren Sedimentation Rate
See **Sedimentation Rate, Erythrocyte**—Blood.

Western Blot
See **Acquired Immune Deficiency Syndrome Evaluation Battery**—Diagnostic.

Western Equine Encephalitis Virus Serology—Serum

Norm. Negative. A less than fourfold rise in titer between acute and convalescent samples; HI (hemagglutination inhibition) antibody titer <1:10; no IgM antibody detected; IFA IgG <1:16 and IgM <1:16.

Positive. Aseptic meningitis and meningoencephalitis.

Description. Western equine encephalitis is caused by a group A arbovirus (arthropod-borne virus), specifically, togavirus, which results in inflammation of parts of the brain, meninges, and spinal cord in horses and humans. Occurrence is primarily in the Western Hemisphere and in summer to early fall. Mode of transmission to humans is from small birds and mammals through the bite of an infected mosquito. Symptoms are short in duration and may range from mild to fatal (10%) encephalitis symptoms (stiff neck, lethargy, sore throat, vomiting, stupor, coma, paralysis in children). Identification of the virus is performed through viral neutralization, complement fixation, hemagglutinin inhibition, fluorescent antibody, and agar gel precipitation. A positive IgG or IgM result indicates current or recent infection.

Professional Considerations
Consent form NOT required.

Preparation
1. Tube: Red topped, red/gray topped, or gold topped.

Procedure
1. Draw a 7-mL blood sample as soon as possible after symptoms appear, and label it as the "acute sample." Repeat the test in 14 days, and label it as the "convalescent sample."

Postprocedure Care
1. None.

Client and Family Teaching

1. The mode of transmission is by a mosquito bite. Wear insect-repellant spray or lotion on skin when outdoors.
2. Return in 2 weeks for follow-up testing.

Factors That Affect Results

1. Cross-reactions may occur with eastern equine encephalitis virus, another group A togavirus.

2. Disease cannot be excluded if sample is drawn within 2 weeks of symptom onset.

Other Data

1. Testing may also be performed on cerebrospinal fluid.
2. Western equine encephalitis is not transmitted client to client.

WFDC2

See Human Epididymis Protein 4—Blood.

White Blood Cell Count Differential

See Differential Leukocyte Count—Peripheral Blood.

White Blood Count

See Differential Leukocyte Count—Peripheral Blood.

Whole-Body Scan

See Bone Scan—Diagnostic.

Wintrobe Sedimentation Rate

See Sedimentation Rate, Erythrocyte—Blood.

Wound, Fungus

See Biopsy, Site-Specific—Specimen; Body Fluid, Fungus—Culture.

Wound, Mycobacteria

See Biopsy, Site-Specific—Specimen; Body Fluid, *Mycobacteria*—Culture.

Wound Culture

See Culture, Routine—Specimen.

Xeromammogram

See **Mammography**—Diagnostic.

X-Ray

See **Radiography, various types of radiography.**

Xylose

See D-**Xylose Absorption Test**—Diagnostic.

Xylose Tolerance Test

See D-**Xylose Absorption Test**—Diagnostic.

Xpert *C. difficile* Assay

See *C. difficile* **Amplified probe**—Stool.

Yersinia enterocolitica Antibody—Blood

Norm. <1:160. A fourfold increase between acute and convalescent specimens (such as convalescent titer 1:1280) is diagnostic for yersiniosis.

Increased. Gastroenterocolitis or endocarditis caused by *Yersinia* (yersiniosis) and terminal ileitis.

Decreased. Titers decrease to normal levels 2-6 months after recovery from *Yersinia* infections.

Description. *Yersinia enterocolitica* is a bacterium found in animal carriers and bodies of water that is transmitted to humans by the fecal-oral route or by ingestion of food or water contaminated with the organism. *Y. enterocolitica* causes gastroenterocolitis accompanied by diarrhea, anorexia, fever, vomiting, headache, arthritis, and abscesses and may progress to septicemia. Incidence is more common in children and teens than in adults. In this test, an indirect Coombs' test is performed to identify the presence of the antibody to *Y. enterocolitica*.

Professional Considerations

Consent form NOT required.

Preparation

1. Tube: Red topped, red/gray topped, or gold topped.

Procedure

1. Draw a 5-mL blood sample as soon as possible after symptoms appear. Label the sample as the acute specimen.
2. Repeat the test in 2-3 weeks and label as the convalescent specimen.

Postprocedure Care

1. None.

Client and Family Teaching

1. Return in 2-3 weeks for a convalescent blood sample.
2. Because *Yersinia* infection is transmitted from stool to other persons, avoid contaminating your hands with stool and wash your hands vigorously for 15 seconds with antibacterial soap after each defecation. Cleanse the toilet seat with disinfectant after each defecation until the physician confirms that you are no longer contagious.
3. *Yersinia* infection may be treated with amphotericin B.

Factors That Affect Results

1. Results may not be elevated in clients who are infected with *Yersinia* but who are immunosuppressed or receiving antifungal therapy.

Other Data
1. Diagnosis should be confirmed by blood culture.
2. Standard precautions are adequate for preventing transmission of *Yersinia* infection to others. Use strict Standard Precautions when handling feces of infected clients because fecal shedding of *Yersinia* occurs throughout the period of active symptoms.
3. Reactive arthritis may be triggered by *Yersinia*.
4. Higher antibody levels are detected in patients with gastrointestinal symptoms rather than reactive arthritis.

Zeta Sedimentation Rate
See Sedimentation Rate, Erythrocyte—Blood.

Zeta Sedimentation Ratio
See Sedimentation Rate, Erythrocyte—Blood.

Zinc—Blood

Norm.

		SI Units
All ages	60-150 µg/dL	9.2-149 µmol/L
Zinc deficiency	<60 µg/dL	<9.2 µmol/L

Toxic Level Symptoms and Treatment
NOTE: Treatment choice(s) depend(s) on client's history and condition and episode history.

Symptoms of Zinc Toxicity. Cough, chest discomfort, tachycardia, hypertension, gastrointestinal irritation, nausea, vomiting, diarrhea, and metallic taste in the mouth.

Treatment of Zinc Toxicity
1. Eliminate dietary zinc or reduce zinc additives to hyperalimentation.
2. Peritoneal dialysis WILL remove excess zinc.

Symptoms of Zinc Deficiency. May progress from decreased weight, low sperm count, and impaired wound healing to alopecia, hypogonadism, ataxia, tremors, and impaired resistance to infection.

Treatment of Zinc Deficiency
1. Replace zinc through diet, medication, or hyperalimentation.

Increased. Anemia, arteriosclerosis, coronary heart disease, dietary intake of acidic food or beverages from galvanized containers, industrial exposure to zinc (welding), and primary osteosarcoma of bone. Drugs include cisplatin, corticosteroids, denture adhesive (overuse), estrogens, interferon, oral contraceptives (containing estrogen), phenytoin, and thiazides.

Decreased. Acrodermatitis enteropathica, alcoholism, alopecia, Alzheimer's, anemia (hemolytic), bariatric surgery (post), burning mouth syndrome, burns (severe), celiac sprue, chronic kidney disease (CKD), cirrhosis (43% prevalence), critical illness, depression, diabetes (type 2), diarrhea, Ethiopian pregnant women, gallbladder disease, hepatic metastasis, hyperactivity, hypoalbuminemia, hypogonadal dwarfism, hypothyroidism (transient), infection (acute), leukemia, liver disease, lymphoma, malabsorption, mood disorders, myocardial infarction, neural tube defects (NTD), New Zealand children, organ failure, orofacial cleft, pancreatitis, Parkinson's disease, poor dietary intake, pregnancy (third trimester), receiving parenteral nutrition, renal failure (chronic), seizures (febrile in children), stress (acute), stroke, thalassemia major, typhoid fever, tuberculosis (pulmonary), viral warts, and Wilson's disease. Drugs include antimetabolites, chlorthalidone, cisplatin, diuretics, estrogens, histidine, and penicillamine.

Description. Zinc is a nutritional trace metal important for cellular growth and metabolism. Both zinc toxicity and serious zinc deficiency are possible (see symptoms listed above). Zinc levels are usually measured as part of a heavy-metal screen for suspected zinc toxicity. Routine levels are measured for clients receiving parenteral nutrition and to monitor progress during replacement for zinc deficiency.

Professional Considerations
Consent form NOT required.

Preparation
1. Obtain a stainless-steel needle and a metal-free, navy blue topped BD Vacutainer tube from the laboratory.
2. Do NOT draw specimens during hemodialysis.

Procedure
1. Draw a 7-mL blood sample without hemolysis directly into the tube through a stainless-steel needle.

Postprocedure Care
1. Send the specimen to the laboratory promptly for spinning and separation of the serum into a metal-free container.

Client and Family Teaching
1. Results are normally available within 72 hours.

Factors That Affect Results
1. Collecting the specimen in a regular, rubber topped tube other than that specified above invalidates the results.
2. Hemolysis invalidates results.
3. Fever, myocardial infarction, sepsis, and stress may cause abnormally low results.

Other Data
1. None.

ZSR

See **Sedimentation Rate, Erythrocyte**—Blood.

APPENDIX A
REPORTABLE DISEASES

Reportable Disease (in Many Areas)	Report Immediately? (Inform Health Dept.)	Quarantine Required?	Sexually Transmitted?
AIDS	No	No	**Yes**
Anthrax	**Yes**	No	No
Botulism (all types)	**Yes**	No	No
Brucellosis	No	No	No
California serogroup virus disease	No	No	No
Chancroid	No	No	**Yes**
Chlamydia infections	No	No	No
Cholera	**Yes**	**Yes**	No
Coccidioidomycosis	No	No	No
Cryptosporidiosis	No	No	No
Cyclosporiasis	No	No	No
Diphtheria	**Yes**	No	No
Eastern equine encephalitis virus disease	No	No	No
Ehrlichiosis	No	No	No
Giardiasis (acute)	No	No	No
Gonococcal infection	No	No	**Yes**
Haemophilus influenzae (invasive)	No	No	No
Hansen's disease (leprosy)	No	No	No
Hantavirus pulmonary syndrome	**Yes**	No	No
Hemolytic uremic syndrome, post diarrheal	No	No	No
Hepatitis (A, B, C)	No	No	**Yes**
HIV infection	No	No	**Yes**
Influenza-associated pediatric mortality	No	No	No
Legionellosis	No	No	No
Listeriosis	No	No	No
Lyme disease	No	No	No
Malaria	No	No	No
Measles (rubeola)	No	No	No
Meningococcal infections	No	No	No
Mumps	No	No	No
Novel influenza A virus infection (e.g., avian and swine)	**Yes**	Possible	No
Pertussis (whooping cough)	No	No	No
Plague	**Yes**	**Yes**	No
Poliomyelitis, paralytic	**Yes**	No	No
Poliovirus infection, nonparalytic	**Yes**	No	No
Powassan virus disease	No	No	No
Psittacosis	No	No	No
Q fever	No	No	No
Rabies (human or animal) or bite from animal that may be rabid	**Yes**	No	No
Rocky Mountain spotted fever (spotted fever rickettsiosis)	No	No	No
Rubella (German measles)	**Yes**	No	No

Continued

Reportable Disease (in Many Areas)	Report Immediately? (Inform Health Dept.)	Quarantine Required?	Sexually Transmitted?
Rubella, congenital syndrome	No	No	No
Salmonellosis	No	No	No
Severe acute respiratory syndrome-associated Coronavirus (SARS-CoV) disease	**Yes**	**Yes**	No
Shiga toxin producing *Escherichia coli*	No	No	No
Shigellosis	No	No	No
Smallpox	**Yes**	**Yes**	No
St. Louis encephalitis virus disease	No	No	No
Streptococcal disease, invasive group A	No	No	No
Streptococcal pneumonia	No	No	No
Streptococcal toxic shock syndrome	No	No	No
Syphilis (all types and stages)	No	No	**Yes**
Tetanus	No	No	No
Toxic shock syndrome (other than streptococcal)	No	No	No
Toxoplasmosis	No	No	No
Trichinellosis (Trichinosis)	No	No	No
Tuberculosis	No	No	No
Tularemia	No	No	No
Typhoid fever (*Salmonella typhi*)	No	No	No
Vancomycin intermediate resistant *Staphylococcus aureus* (VISA)	No	No	No
Vancomycin-resistant *Staphylococcus aureus* (VRSA)	No	No	No
Varicella morbidity	No	No	No
Vibriosis	No	No	No
Viral hemorrhagic fevers (New World Arena, Crimean-Congo, Dengue, Ebola, Lassa, Marburg viruses)	Yes	Yes	No
West Nile virus disease	**Yes**	**Yes**	No
Western equine encephalitis virus disease	No	No	No
Yellow fever	**Yes**	No	**Yes**

Centers for Disease Control and Prevention: Nationally Notifiable Infectious Diseases, 2010. Available at http://www.cdc.gov/mmwr/PDF/wk/mm5953.pdf.

APPENDIX B
INFORMED CONSENT FOR GENETIC TESTING

To perform genetic testing for inherited syndromes, germline genetic analysis begins with an affected individual.

Prior to genetic testing, genetic counseling is recommended, and informed consent should be obtained and according to practice parameters published by The American Society of Clinical Oncology (ASCO) these include the following:

1. Information on the specific test being performed
2. Implications of positive and negative results
3. Possibility that the test may not be informative
4. Options for risk estimation without genetic testing
5. Risk of passing a mutation to children
6. Technical accuracy of the test
7. Fees involved in counseling and testing
8. Risks of psychological distress
9. Risks of insurer or employment discrimination
10. Confidentiality issues
11. Options and limitations of medical surveillance and screening following testing

Reference: American Society of Clinical Oncology Policy Statement: Update: Genetic testing for cancer susceptibility, *J Clin Oncol*, 21(12):1-10, 2003.

REFERENCES

Abdel-Fattah SA, Bhat A, Illanes S et al: TORCH test for fetal medicine indications: Only CMV is necessary in the United States, *Prenatal Diagn* 25(11):1028-1031, 2005.

Abraham J: OVA1 test for preoperative assessment of ovarian cancer, *Community Oncology* 7(6):249-250, 2010.

Alexander M, Baker L, Clark C et al: Management of ventricular arrhythmias in diverse populations in California, *Am Heart J* 144(3):431-439, 2002.

Al-Fozan HM, Tulandi T: Fertility preservation in children and young adults undergoing treatment for malignancy, *Saudi Med J* 25(2):141-144, 2004.

Allison JE, Potter MB: New screening guidelines for colorectal cancer: A practical guide for the primary care physician, *Prim Care* 36(3):575-602, 2009.

American College of Obstetricians and Gynecologists Committee on Genetics: ACOG committee opinion No. 469: Carrier screening for Fragile X syndrome, *Obstet Gynecol* 116(4):1008-10, 2010.

American College of Obstetricians and Gynecologists Committee on Gynecologic Practice: ACOG committee opinion No. 483: Primary and preventive care: Periodic assessments, *Obstet Gynecol* 117:1008–15, 2011.

American Diabetes Association: Standards of medical care in diabetes—2011, *Diabetes Care* 34(Suppl 1):S11-61, 2011.

American Thoracic Society: Guidelines for methacholine and exercise challenge testing—1999, *Am J Respir Crit Care Med* 161(1):309-29, 2000.

Anastasi E: HE4: A new potential early biomarker for the recurrence of ovarian cancer, *Tumour Biol* 31(2):113-9, 2010a.

Anastasi E: Ovarian tumor marker HE4 is differently expressed during the phases of the menstrual cycle in healthy young women, *Tumour Biol* 31(5):411-5, 2010b.

Anderson SD, Brannan JD: Bronchial provocation testing: The future, *Curr Opin Allergy Clin Immunol* 11(1):46-52, 2011.

Asali MG: [Numerical aberrations of chromosomes 11 and 17 detected by fish—fluorescence in situ hybridization combined with cytology in exfoliated cells from voided urine in patients with urothelial carcinoma of the bladder], *Harefuah* 146(12):914-9,1000, 2007.

Bayer-Carter JL, Green PS, Montine TJ: Diet intervention and cerebrospinal fluid biomarkers in amnestic mild cognitive impairment, *Arch Neurol* 68(6):743-752, 2011.

Bennett IC, Muller J, Cockburn L et al: Outcomes of multimodality breast screening for woman at increased risk for familial breast cancer, *World J Surg* 34(5):979-986, 2011.

Berman DS: SPECT/PET myocardial perfusion imaging versus coronary CT angiography in patients with known or suspected CAD, *Q J Nucl Med Mol Imaging* 54(2):177-200, 2010.

Bilavsky E, Yarden-Bilavsky H, Ashkenazi S et al: C-reactive protein as a marker of serious bacterial infections in hospitalized febrile infants, *Acta Paediatrica* 98(11):1776-80, 2009.

Bowman R, McCulloch DL, Law E et al: The 'mirror test' for estimating visual acuity in infants, *Br J Ophthalmol* 94(7):882-5, 2010.

Brown L, Ferlo Todd J, DoLov HM: Breast implant adverse events during mammography: Reports to the Food and Drug Administration, *J Women's Health* 13(4):371-378, 2004.

Buccheri G, Torchio P, Ferrigno D: Clinical equivalence of two cytokeratin markers in non–small cell lung cancer: A study of tissue polypeptide antigen and cytokeratin 19 fragments, *Chest* 124:622-632, 2003.

Burns JL, Englund J, Prince AS: Infectious complications in special hosts. In Long SS, Pickering LK, Prober CG, editors: *Principles and practice of pediatric infectious diseases*, ed 3, 2009, New York: Churchill Livingstone.

Chan WS, Ray JG, Murray S et al: Suspected pulmonary embolism in pregnancy: Clinical presentation, results of lung scanning, and subsequent maternal and pediatric outcomes, *Arch Intern Med* 162(10):1170-1175, 2002.

Chyka PA, Erdman AR, Christianson G et al: Salicylate poisoning: An evidence-based consensus guideline for out-of-hospital management, *Clin Tox* 45:95-131, 2007.

Cooper LT, Baughman KL, Feldman AM et al: The role of endomyocardial biopsy in the management of cardiovascular disease: A scientific statement from the American Heart Association, the American College of Cardiology, and the European Society of Cardiology endorsed by the Heart Failure Society of America and the Heart Failure Association of the European Society of Cardiology, *J Am Coll Cardiol* 50:1914-1931, 2007.

Crowther MA, Douketis JD, Schnurr T et al: Oral vitamin K lowers the international normalized ratio more rapidly than subcutaneous vitamin K in the treatment of warfarin-associated coagulopathy: A randomized, controlled trial, *Ann Intern Med* 137(4):I39 (comment), 2002.

Cummings DE, Weigle DS, Frayo RS et al: Plasma ghrelin levels after diet-induced weight loss or gastric bypass surgery, *N Engl J Med* 346(21):1623-1630, 2002.

Cushman A, Patterson C, Yarnell J et al: Fibrinolytic activation markers predict myocardial infarction in the elderly: The cardiovascular health study, *Arterioscler Thromb Vasc Biol* 19(3):493-498, 1999.

Danforth KN, Eliassen AH, Tworoger SS et al: The association of plasma androgen levels with breast, ovarian and endometrial cancer risk factors among postmenopausal women, *Int J Cancer* 1;126(1):199-207, 2010.

Dayan CM: Interpretation of thyroid function tests. *Lancet* 357(9256):619-624, 2001 (review).

Deruisseau KC, Roberts LM, Kushnick MR: Iron status of young males and females performing weight-training exercise, *Med Sci Sports Exerc* 36(2):241-248, 2004.

Devigili G, Tugnoli V, Penza P et al: The diagnostic criteria for small fibre neuropathy: From symptoms to neuropathology, *Brain* 131(Pt 7):1912-19, 2008.

Ellfolk M, Malm H: Risks associated with in utero and lactation exposure to selective serotonin reuptake inhibitors (SSRIs), *Reprod Toxicol* 30(2):249-60, 2010.

Evans RW, Armon C, Frohman EM, Goodin DS: Assessment: Prevention of post-lumbar puncture headaches—report of the therapeutics and technology assessment subcommittee of the American Academy of Neurology, *Neurology* 55(7):909-914, 2000.

Fragile X Clinical and Research Consortium: Practice guidelines for Fragile X-associated disorders: fragile X-associated tremor/ataxia syndrome (FXTAS), Retrieved August 31, 2012, from http://www.fxcrc.org/index.php/document-library/81.

Friedrich MG, Hellstem A, Hautmann SH et al: Clinical use of urinary markers for the detection and prognosis of bladder carcinoma: A comparison of immunology with monoclonal antibodies against Lewis S and 486p3/12 with the BTA STAT and NMP22 tests, *J Urol* 168(2):470-474, 2002.

Froom P, Barak M: Falsely elevated prothrombin international normalized ratio values, *Am J Clin Pathol* 134(1):86-9, 2010.

Fujikawa T, Shiraha H, Yamamoto K: Significance of des-gamma-carboxy prothrombin production in hepatocellular carcinoma, *Acta.Med Okayama* 63(6):299-304, 2009.

Ganau S, Sentís M, Tortajada L: Use of serum progesterone concentration for timing breast MRI examinations and avoiding false-negative findings, *AJR Am J Roentgenol* 195(1), 2010.

Gansevoort RT, Matsushita K, van der Velde M et al: The chronic kidney disease prognosis consortium. Lower estimated GFR and higher albuminuria are associated with adverse kidney outcomes. A collaborative meta-analysis of general and high-risk population cohorts, *Kidney Int* 80(1):93-104, 2011.

Garcia de la Fuente I, Ansari M, Rougemont AL et al: Acute disseminated fatal toxoplasmosis after haploidentical stem cell transplantation despite atovaquone prophylaxis in a young man, *Pediatr Infect Dis J* 29(11):1059-60, 2010.

Gibbons CH, Illigens BM, Wang N et al: Quantification of sweat gland innervation: A clinical-pathologic correlation, *Neurology* 72:1479-86, 2009.

Gill S, Haastrup B, Haghfelt T et al: Continuous vectorcardiography is superior to standard electrocardiography in the prediction of long-term outcome after thrombolysis in patients with acute myocardial infarction, *Coron Artery Dis* 13(3):169-175, 2002.

Giuliano AE, Hawes D, Ballman KV et al: Association of occult metastases in sentinel lymph nodes and bone marrow with survival among women with early-stage invasive breast cancer, *JAMA* 306(4):385-93, 2011.

Gobal F, Deshmukh A, Shah S et al: Triad of metabolic syndrome, chronic kidney disease, and coronary heart disease with a focus on microalbuminuria death by overeating, *J Am Coll Cardiol* 57(23):2303-2308, 2011.

Goel A, Jain V, Gupta I, Varma N: Serial serum ferritin estimation in pregnant women at risk of preterm labor, *Acta Obstet Gynecol Scand* 82(2):129-132, 2003.

Goldenberg I, Moss AJ, Bradley J et al: Long-QT syndrome after age 40, *Circulation* 117(17):2192-2201, 2008.

Goldenberg SD: Two-step glutamate dehydrogenase antigen real-time polymerase chain reaction assay for detection of toxigenic *Clostridium difficile*, *J Hosp Infect* 74(1): 48-54, 2010.

Green DM, Ropper AH, Kronmal RA et al: Serum potassium level and dietary potassium intake as risk factors for stroke, *Neurology* 59(3):314-320, 2002 (comment).

Grundy SM, Cleeman JI, Merz CN: Implications of recent clinical trials for the national cholesterol education program adult treatment panel III guidelines, *J Am Coll Cardiol* 44(3): 720-732, 2004 (review).

Guller U, Turek J, Eubanks S et al: Detecting pheochromocytoma: Defining the most sensitive test, *Ann Surg* 243(1):102-107, 2006.

Hagerman PJ, Hagerman RJ: The Fragile X premutation: A maturing perspective, *Am J Hum Genet* 74(5):805-16, 2004.

Hatoum IJ, Cook NR, Nelson JJ et al: Lipoprotein-associated phospholipase A2 activity improves risk discrimination of incident coronary heart disease among women, *Am Heart J* 161(3):516-22, 2011.

He WJ, Hu Y, Zhang XP et al: Activated protein C ratio, plasma tissue factor activity and activated factor VII in Chinese patients with coronary heart disease, *Eur J Med Res* 13(2):47-51, 2008.

Helbig JH, Uldum SA, Bernander S et al: Clinical utility of urinary antigen detection for diagnosis of community-acquired, travel-associated, and nosocomial legionnaire's disease, *J Clin Microbiol* 41(2):830-840, 2003.

Henry MJ, Major CA, Reinsch S: Accuracy of self-monitoring of blood glucose: Impact on diabetes management decisions during pregnancy, *Diabetes Educ* 27(4):521-529, 2001.

Houben ML, Bont L, Wilbrink B et al: Clinical prediction rule for RSV bronchiolitis in healthy newborns: Prognostic birth cohort study, *Pediatrics* 127(1), 2011.

Huang ES, Liu JY, Moffet HH et al: Glycemic control, complications, and death in older diabetic patients: The diabetes and aging study, *Diabetes Care* 34(6):1329-36, 2011.

Innis SM, Palaty J, Vaghri Z, Lockitch G: Increased levels of mercury associated with high fish intakes among children from Vancouver, Canada, *J Pediatr* 148(6):759-763, 2006.

Ishibashi Y, Yamauchi M, Musha H et al: Impact of contrast-induced nephropathy and cardiovascular events by serum cystatin C in renal insufficiency patients undergoing cardiac catheterization, *Angiology* 61(8):724-30, 2010.

Itoh T, Itoh H, Kikuchi T: Five cases of MRSA-infected patients with cerebrovascular disorder and in a bedridden condition, for whom bu-zhong-yi-qi-tang (hochu-eddi-to) was useful. *Am J Chin Med* 28(3-4):401-408, 2000.

Izawa J, Kedar D, Wong F, Pettaway CA: Sentinel lymph node biopsy in penile cancer: Evolution and insights, *Can J Urol* 12(Suppl 1):24-29, 2005.

Julander JG, Bowen RA, Rao JR et al: Treatment of Venezuelan equine encephalitis virus infection with (-)-carbodine, *Antiviral Res* 80(3):309-15, 2008.

Kalman L, Wilson JA, Buller A et al: Development of genomic DNA reference materials for genetic testing of disorders common in people of Ashkenazi Jewish descent. *J Mol Diagn* 11(6):530-6, 2009.

Kapaki E, Liappas I, Paraskevas G et al: The diagnostic value of tau protein, beta-amyloid (1-42) and their ratio for the discrimination of alcohol-related cognitive disorders from Alzheimer's disease in early stages. *Int J Geriatr Psychiatry* 20(8):722-729, 2005.

Kato K, Sato N, Yamamoto T et al: Valuable markers for contrast-induced nephropathy in patients undergoing cardiac catheterization, *Circulation* 72(9):1499-1505, 2008.

Kisters K, Cziborra M, Funke C et al: Positive effect of N-acetylcysteine in theophylline intoxication, *Clin Nephrol* 68(4):266, 2007.

Kiuru MJ, Pihlajamaki HK, Hietanen HJ, Ahovuo JA: MR imaging, bone scintigraphy, and radiography in bone stress injuries of the pelvis and lower extremeties, *Acta Radiol* 43(2):207-212, 2002.

Kong W, Wei J, Abidi P et al: Berberine is a novel cholesterol-lowering drug working through a unique mechanism distinct from statins, *Nat Med* 10(12):1344-1351, 2004.

Lauria G, Devigli G: Skin biopsy as a diagnostic tool in peripheral neuropathy, *Nat Clin Pract Neurol* 3:546-57, 2007.

Leanderson S, Laguna P, Sornmo L: Estimation of the respiratory frequency using spatial information in VCGs, *Med Engin Physics* 25(6):501-507, 2003.

Lee JM, Wu E-L, Tarini B et al: Diagnosis of diabetes using hemoglobin A1c: Should recommendations in adults be extrapolated to adolescents? *J Pediatr* 158(6):947-952, 2011.

Lemire M, Mergler D, Fillion M et al: Elevated blood selenium levels in the Brazilian Amazon, *Sci Total Environ* 336(1):101-111, 2006.

Lidstone V, James S, Stross P: INR: Intervals of measurement can safely extend up to 14 weeks, *Clin Lab Hematol* 22(5): 291-293, 2000.

Linder A, Akesson P, Brink M et al: Heparin-binding protein: A diagnostic marker of acute bacterial meningitis, *Crit Care Med* 39(4):812-7, 2011.

Lindor NM: Familial colorectal cancer type X: The other half of hereditary nonpolyposis colon cancer syndrome, *Surg Oncol Clin N Am* 18(4): 637-45, 2009.

Lokeshwar VB, Schroeder GL, Selzer MG et al: Bladder tumor markers for monitoring recurrence and screening comparison of hyaluronic acid-hyaluronidase and BTA-STAT tests, *Cancer* 95(1):61-72, 2002.

Lowe GD, Sweetnam PM, Yarnell JW et al: C-reactive protein, fibrin, D-dimer, and risk of ischemic heart disease: The Caerphilly and Speedwell studies, *Arterioscler Thromb Vasc Biol* 24(10):1957-1962, 2004.

Machiko T, Katsutaro N, Chika O: A study of psychoneuroendocrinological effects of music therapy (Japanese), *Psychiatr Neurol Japan* 105(4):468-472, 2003.

Madsen TE, Pearson RR, Muhlestein JB et al: Risk of nephropathy is not increased by the administration of larger volume of contrast during coronary angiography. *Crit Pathw Cardiol* 8(4): 167-71, 2009.

Malyszko J, Bachorzewska-Gajawska H, Poniatowski B et al: Urinary and serum biomarkers after cardiac catheterization in diabetic patients with stable angina and without severe chronic kidney disease, *Renal Failure* 31(10):910-919, 2009.

Matheson EM, Mainous AG, Everett CJ et al: Tea and coffee consumption and MRSA nasal carriage, *Ann Fam Med* 9(4):299-304, 2011.

Matsuura H, Hakomori S: The oncofetal domain of fibronectin defined by monocolonal antibody FDC-6: its presence in fibronectins from fetal and tumor tissues and its absence in those normal adult tissues and plasma, *Proc Natl Acad Sci USA* 82(19):6517-6521, 1985.

McArthur JC, Stocks EA, Hauer P et al: Epidermal nerve fiber density normative reference range and diagnostic efficiency, *Arch Neurol* 55:1513-1520, 1998.

McNerlan SE, Alexander HD, Rea IM: Age-related reference intervals for lymphocyte subsets in whole blood of healthy individuals, *Scand J Clin Lab Invest* 59(2):89-92, 1999.

Michiels JJ, Kasbergen H, Oudega R et al: Exclusion and diagnosis of deep vein thrombosis in outpatients by sequential noninvasive tools, *Int Angiol* 21(1):9-19, 2002.

Miglioretti DL, Rutter CM, Geller BM et al: Effect of breast augmentation on the accuracy of mammography and cancer characteristics, *JAMA* 29(4):442-450, 2004.

Miller MA, Hyland M, Ofner-Agostini M et al: Morbidity, mortality, and healthcare burden of nosocomial *Clostridium difficile*–associated diarrhea in Canadian hospitals, *Infect Control Hosp Epidemiol* 23(3):137-140, 2002.

Moss AJ, Shimizu W, Wilde AA et al: Clinical aspects of type-1 long-QT syndrome by location, coding type, and biophysical function of mutations involving the KCNQ1 gene, *Circulation* 115(19):2481-2489, 2007.

Murano T, Tateishi U, Iinuma T et al: Evaluation of the risk of radiation exposure from new 18FDG PET/CT plans versus conventional X-ray plans in patients with pediatric cancers, *Ann Nucl Med* 24(4):261-7, 2010.

Naoe M: Use of the CellSearch circulating tumor cell test for monitoring urothelial cancer: Two case reports of metastatic urothelial cancer, *South Med J* 101(4): 439-41, 2008.

Ned RM, Melillo S, Marrone M: Fecal DNA testing for colorectal cancer screening: The ColoSure™ test, *PLoS Curr* 3:RRN1220, 2011.

Nemmar A, Melghit K, Al-Salam S et al: Acute respiratory and systemic toxicity of pulmonary exposure to rutile Fe-doped TiO(2) nanorods, *Toxicology* 279(1-3):167-75, 2011.

Nguyen CM, Mendes M, Ma JD: Thiopurine methyltransferase (TPMT) genotyping to predict myelosuppression risk, *PLoS Curr* 3: RRN1236, 2011.

Noah Z, Budeck C, Patwari PP, Weese-Mayer DE: Congenital central hypoventilation syndrome, rapid onset obesity with hypothalamic dysfunction, hypoventilation, and autonomic dysregulation, and diaphragm pacing. In Kliegman RM, Stanton BF, Schor NC, St. Geme III JW, Behrman RE, eds: *Nelson Textbook of Pediatrics*, Philadelphia: Elsevier-Saunders, 1520-1522, 2011.

Nozaki Y, Nagare Y, Hino S et al: Therapeutic strategy and significance of serum rheumatoid factor in patients with rheumatoid arthritis during infliximab treatment, *Nihon Rinsho Meneki Gakkai Kaishi* 33(3):135-41, 2010.

Ozcakir HT, Goker EN, Terek MC et al: Relationship of follicle number, serum estradiol level, and other factors to clinical pregnancy rate in gonadotropin-induced intrauterine insemination cycles, *Arch Gynecol Obstet* 266(1):18-20, 2002.

Palomino JC: Newer diagnostics for tuberculosis and multi-drug resistant tuberculosis, *Curr Opin Pulmon Med* 12(3):172-178, 2006.

Park EY, Shim JY, Kim DS et al: Elevated serum soluble E-selectin levels in Korean children with measles, *Pediatr Int* 50(4):519-22, 2008.

Paynter NP, Mazer NA, Pradhan AD et al: Cardiovascular risk prediction in diabetic men and Women Using Hemoglobin A1c vs Diabetes as a High-Risk Equivalent, *Arch Intern Med* 171(19): 1712-8, 2011.

Peralta CA, Shlipak MG, Judd S et al: Detection of chronic kidney disease with creatinine, cystatin c, and urine albumin-to-creatinine ratio and association with progression to end-stage renal disease and mortality, *JAMA* 305(15):1545-1552, 2011.

Phillpotts RJ, Jones LD, Lukaszewski RA et al: Antibody and interleukin-12 treatment in murine models of encephalitogenic flavivirus (St. Louis encephalitis, tick-borne encephalitis) and alphavirus (Venezuelan equine encephalitis infection), *J Interferon Cytokine Res* 23(1):47-50, 2003.

Picano E: [Risk-benefit balance in cardiovascular imaging: The radiation issue]. *[Article in Italian] G Ital Cardiol (Rome)* 9(12):808-14, 2008.

Pratap T, Sloand JA, Narins CR: Potential pitfalls of renal angiography: A case of atypical fibromuscular dysplasia, *Angiology* 59(6):753-6, 2008.

Prosen G, Klemen P, Strnad M et al: Combination of lung ultrasound (a comet-tail sign) and N-terminal pro-brain natriuretic peptide in differentiating acute heart failure from chronic obstructive pulmonary disease and asthma as cause of acute dyspnea in prehospital emergency setting, *Crit Care* 15(2):R114, 2011.

Reichlin T, Potocki M, Breidthardt T et al: Diagnostic and prognostic value of uric acid in patients with acute dyspnea, *Am J Med* 122(11): 1054.e7-1054.e14, 2009.

Rhodes AR: Prognostic usefulness of sentinel lymph node biopsy for patients who have clinically node negative, localized, primary invasive cutaneous melanoma: A Bayesian analysis using informative published reports, *Arch Dermatol* 147(4):408-15, 2011.

Rosati E, Chitano G, Dipaola L et al: Indications and limitations for a neonatal pulse oximetry screening of critical congenital heart disease, *J Perinatal Med* 33(5):455-457, 2005.

Saad WE, Wilson IJ, Davies MG et al: Intravenous morphine for augmentation of postoperative T-tube cholangiograms in liver transplant recipients with choledocho-choledochal anastomoses, *J Vasc Interv Radiol* 20(10):1320-8, 2009.

Salani R, Backes FJ, Fung MFK et al: Posttreatment surveillance and diagnosis of recurrence in women with gynecologic malignancies: Society of Gynecologic Oncologists recommendations, *Am J Obstet Gynecol* 204(6):466-478, 2011.

Samuels J, Ng CS, Nates J et al: Small increases in serum creatinine are associated with prolonged ICU stay and increased hospital mortality in critically ill patients with cancer, *Support Care Cancer* 19(10):1527-32, 2011.

Schneider J, Bitterlich N, Schultz G: Improved sensitivity in the diagnosis of gastro-intestinal tumors by fuzzy logic-based tumor marker profiles including the tumor M2-PK, *Anticancer Res* 25(3A):1507-1515, 2005.

Schneir AB, Ly BT, Clark RF: A case of withdrawal from the GHB precursors gamma-butyrolactone and 1,4-butanediol, *J Emerg Med* 21(1):31-33, 2001.

Seliger SL, DeFilippi C: Role of Cystatin C as a Marker of Renal Function and Cardiovascular Risk, *Medscape Nephrology*, October 27, 2006.

Sevinc A, Sari R, Fadillioglu E: The utility of lactate dehydrogenase isoenzyme pattern in the diagnostic evaluation of malignant and nonmalignant ascites, *J Natl Med Assoc* 97(1):79-84, 2005.

Sexton K, Adgate JL, Fredrickson AL et al: Using biologic markers in blood to assess exposure to multiple environmental chemicals for inner-city children 3-6 years of age, *Environ Health Perspect* 114(3):453-459, 2006.

Shaw LJ, Olson MB, Kip K et al: The value of estimated functional capacity in estimating outcome: Results from the NHBLI-sponsored Women's Ischemia Sydrome (WISE) study, *J Am Cardio* 47(Suppl 3):S36-S43, 2006.

Shire N: Effects of race, ethnicity, gender, culture, literacy, and social marketing on public health, *J Gender Specif Med* 5(2):48-54, 2002.

Shteinshnaider M, Almoznino-Sarafian D, Tzur I et al: Shortened erythrocyte sedimentation rate evaluation is applicable to hospitalised patients, *Eur J Intern Med* 21(3):226-9, 2010.

Silver LD, Farley TA: Sodium and potassium intake. Mortality effects and policy implications, *Arch Intern Med* 171:1191-1192, 2011.

Smith A, Patterson C, Yarnell J et al: Which hemostatic markers add to the predictive value of conventional risk factors for coronary heart disease and ischemic stroke? The Caerphilly Study, *Circulation* 112(20):3080-3087, 2005.

Smith NL, Barzilay JI, Shaffer D: Fasting and 2-hr postchallenge serum glucose measures and risk of incident cardiovascular events in the elderly: the Cardiovascular Health Study, *Arch Intern Med* 162(2):209-216, 2002.

Smyth CM, Stead RH: Survey of flexible fiberoptic bronchoscopy in the United Kingdom, *Eur Respir J* 20(3):789, 2002.

Stolbach AI, Hoffman RS, Nelson LS: Mechanical ventilation was associated with acidemia in a case series of salicylate-poisoned patients, *Acad Emerg Med* 15(9):866-9, 2008.

Tapiola T, Soininen H, Pirttila T: CSF tau and Abeta42 levels in patients with Down's syndrome, *Neurology* 56(7):979-980, 2001.

Tice JA: Vitamin D for the prevention of osteoporotic fractures: a technology assessment, California Technology Assessment Forum, February 16, 2011. Available at http://www.ctaf.org/content/assessment/detail/1250/. Accessed August 4, 2011.

Ueland FR, Desimone CP, Seamon LG et al: Effectiveness of a multivariate index assay in the preoperative assessment of ovarian tumors, *Obstet Gynecol* 117(6):1289-1297, 2011.

Ueland FR: Replacing CA-125 with OVA1 correctly identifies over 70% of malignancies missed by ACOG criteria, *Community Oncology* 7(6):250-251, 2010.

Umar A, Boland CR, Terdiman JP et al: Revised Bethesda Guidelines for hereditary nonpolyposis colorectal cancer (Lynch syndrome) and microsatellite instability, *J Natl Cancer Inst* 96(4): 261-8, 2004.

Van Crevel JA, de Gans J: Lumbar puncture and the risk of herniation: When should we first perform CT? *J Neurol* 249(2):129-137, 2002 (review).

Van Wassenaer AG, Briet JM, van Baar et al: Free thyroxine levels during the first weeks of life and neurodevelopmental outcome until the age of 5 years in very preterm infants, *Pediatrics* 110(3): 534-539, 2002.

Vashi AR, Oesterling JE: Percent free prostate-specific antigen: Entering a new era in the detection of prostate cancer, *Mayo Clin Proc* 72: 337-344, 1997.

Wakugawa Y, Kiyohara Y, Tanizaki Y et al: C-Reactive protein and risk of first-ever ischemic and hemorrhagic stroke in a general Japanese population: The Hisayama study, *Stroke* 37(1): 27-32, 2006.

Ware Miller R, Smith A, Desimone CP et al: Performance of the American College of Obstetricians and Gynecologists' ovarian tumor referral guidelines with a multivariate index assay, *Obstet Gynecol* 117(6):1298-1306, 2011.

Wilhelm SM, Kale-Pradhan PB: Estimating creatinine clearance: A meta-analysis, *Pharmacotherapy* 31(7):658-664, 2011.

Wilmot GR, Warren ST: A new mutational basis for disease. In Wells RD, Warren ST, editors: *Genetic instabilities and hereditary diseases*, San Diego, 1998, Academic Press.

Wong KS, Wong AY, Tse LH, Tang LC: Use of fetal-pelvic index in the prediction of vaginal birth following previous cesarean section, *J Obstet Gynaecol* 29(2):104-108, 2003.

Wright DF, Al-Sallami HS, Jackson PM et al: Falsely elevated vancomycin plasma concentrations sampled from central venous implantable catheters (portacaths), *Br J Clin Pharmacol* 70(5):769-72, 2010.

Xi Z: Human epididymis protein 4 is a biomarker for transitional cell carcinoma in the urinary system, *J Clin Lab Anal* 23(6):357-6, 2009.

Yang Q, Liu T, Kuklina EV et al: Sodium and potassium intake and mortality among US adults. Prospective data from the Third National Health and Nutrition Examination Survey, *Arch Intern Med* 171:1183-1191, 2011.

Yang X, Ma RC, So WY et al: Low triglyceride and nonuse of statins is associated with cancer in type 2 diabetes mellitus: The Hong Kong Diabetes Registry, *Cancer* 117(4):862-71, 2011.

Zhang MH, Zhang H, Zhao JH et al: Relationship between red cell volume distribution width and cardiac function in acute coronary syndrome patients, *Zhonghua Yi Xue Za Zhi* 13;90(26):1833-1835, 2010.

INDEX

Page numbers followed by "t" indicate tables.